BASIC to ADVANCED
Clinical
Echocardiography

A Self-Assessment Tool for the Cardiac Sonographer

BASIC to ADVANCED
Clinical
Echocardiography

A Self-Assessment Tool for the Cardiac Sonographer

Bonita Anderson, DMU (Cardiac), MAppSc (Medical Ultrasound), ACS, FASE, FASA
Clinical Fellow, School of Clinical Science
Faculty of Health, Queensland University of Technology
Brisbane, Australia
Advanced Cardiac Scientist, Cardiac Sciences Unit
The Prince Charles Hospital
Brisbane, Australia

Margaret M. Park, BS, ACS, RDCS, RVT, FSDMS, FASE
Lead Imaging Specialist
C5 Imaging Research
Heart, Vascular and Thoracic Institute
Cleveland Clinic
Cleveland, Ohio

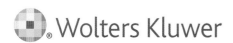 Wolters Kluwer

Philadelphia • Baltimore • New York • London
Buenos Aires • Hong Kong • Sydney • Tokyo

Executive Editor: Sharon Zinner
Development Editor: Eric McDermott
Editorial Coordinator: Chester Anthony Gonzalez
Editorial Assistant: Nicole Dunn
Marketing Manager: Phyllis Hitner
Production Project Manager: Bridgett Dougherty
Design Coordinator: Elaine Kasmer
Manufacturing Coordinator: Beth Welsh
Prepress Vendor: TNQ Technologies

9 8 7 6 5 4 3 2 1

Printed in China

Library of Congress Cataloging-in-Publication Data

ISBN-13: 978-1-975136-25-3

Cataloging in Publication data available on request from publisher.

shop.lww.com

CONTRIBUTORS

Bonita Anderson, DMU (Cardiac), MAppSc (Medical Ultrasound), ACS
Advanced Cardiac Scientist
Cardiac Sciences Unit
The Prince Charles Hospital
Brisbane, Australia
Clinical Fellow
Faculty of Health
Queensland University of Technology
Brisbane, Australia

Alicia Armour, MA, BS, RDCS
Clinical Operations Supervisor, Diagnostics
Duke Triangle Heart Associates
Duke University Health System
Durham, North Carolina

Lisa A. Bienvenu, BS, ACS, RDCS
Technical Director, Echocardiography Laboratory
John Ochsner Heart and Vascular Institute
Ochsner Medical Center
New Orleans, Louisiana

Laura T. Boone, BS, RDCS, RVT, RDMS, RT(R)
Program Director Cardiovascular Technology
Health Care Division
Piedmont Technical College
Greenwood, South Carolina

Heidi S. Borchers, BS, RDCS (AE, PE)
Pediatric Cardiac Sonographer
Heart Center
Seattle Children's Hospital
Seattle, Washington

Daniel P. Bourque, MS, RCS
Lead Sonographer/Technical Director
Orlando Regional Medical Center
Orlando, Florida

Paul F. Braum, BS, RDCS, RCS, RVT, RVS, ACS
Technical Director/Manager Northeast Georgia
    Medical Center
Echo/Vascular Laboratory
Gainesville, Georgia
Associate Professor/Program Director of
    Cardiovascular Technology
School of Health Sciences
Piedmont College
Demorest, Georgia

Merri L. Bremer, EdD, RN, ACS, RDCS
Assistant Professor
Mayo Clinic College of Medicine and Science
Mayo Clinic
Rochester, Minnesota

Colleen D. Cailes, AS, RDCS, RCS
Pediatric Cardiac Sonographer
Pediatric Cardiology
Island Health
Victoria, British Columbia, Canada

Jayne Cleve, BS, RDCS
Cardiac Sonographer III
Cardiac Diagnostic Unit
Duke University Hospital
Durham, North Carolina

Keith A. Collins, MS, RDCS
Lead Cardiac Sonographer-New Technology
Department of Cardiology-Adult Echo Lab
Northwestern Medicine
Chicago, Illinois

Ashlee Davis, BS, ACS, RDCS
Cardiac Sonographer, III
Cardiac Diagnostic Unit
Duke University Health System
Durham, North Carolina

Amy Dillenbeck, MS, ACS, RDCS
Coordinator of Education and Training
Cardiovascular Imaging Lab
Heart, Vascular and Thoracic Institute
Cleveland Clinic
Cleveland, Ohio

Bryan Doldt, BS, RDCS
Associate Professor, Diagnostic Medical Sonography
School of Medical Imaging and Therapeutics
MCPHS University
Boston, Massachusetts

Kellie D'Orsa, BSc, DMU (Cardiac), GCHELT
Director Cardiac Skills Australia
Adjunct tutor, School of Medicine, Deakin University
    Geelong
Victoria, Australia

Erik Echegaray, BS, ACS, RDCS (AE, PE, FE)
Lead Congenital Cardiac Sonographer
Non-invasive Cardiovascular Lab
UC San Diego Health
Cardiovascular Institute
La Jolla, California

Natalie F. A. Edwards, M Cardiac Ultrasound, B Ex Sci, ACS
Senior Cardiac Scientist
Echocardiography Laboratory, Cardiac Sciences Unit
The Prince Charles Hospital
Brisbane, Queensland, Australia

Tony Forshaw, BExSci, M Cardiac Ultrasound
Adjunct Senior Lecturer
School of Clinical Sciences
Queensland University of Technology
Brisbane, Queensland, Australia

Robert W. Gill, BE, MS, PhD
Conjoint Associate Professor
School of Women's and Children's Health
University of New South Wales
Randwick, New South Wales, Australia

Theresa A. Green, RDCS
Echocardiography Advanced Coordinator
Department of Cardiology
Piedmont Heart Institute
Atlanta, Georgia

Joy Guthrie, PhD, ACS, RDMS, RDCS, RVT
Associate Clinical Professor- UCSF Fresno,
    Echocardiography
Technical Director-Community Regional Medical
    Center -Pediatric/Fetal Echo Lab
Program Director-CRMC DMS and Advanced Cardiac
    Sonography Programs
Fresno, California

Karen Helfinstine, MAEd, ACS, RCS, RDCS
Instructor in Health Care Administration
Operations Administrator
Mayo Clinic
Rochester, Minnesota

Jeffrey C. Hill, BS, ACS
Associate Professor, Diagnostic Medical Sonography
School of Medical Imaging and Therapeutics
MCPHS University
Worcester, Massachusetts

Kenneth Horton, ACS, RCS
Echo Research Coordinator
Intermountain Heart Institute
Intermountain Medical Center
Murray, Utah

Lanqi Hua, BS, ACS, RDCS
Technical Director
Cardiac Ultrasound Laboratory
Massachusetts General Hospital
Boston, Massachusetts

Bonnie J. Kane, BS, RDCS
Senior Cardiovascular Research and Clinical
    Sonographer
Northwestern University Feinberg School of Medicine
Chicago, Illinois

Amy Kanta, RDCS
Imaging Specialist
C5 Imaging Research
Heart, Vascular and Thoracic Institute
Cleveland Clinic
Cleveland, Ohio

Peg Knoll, RDCS, RCS
Retired
Manager, University of California Health
Cardiovascular Services, Cardiology Faculty Practice,
    Diagnostic Testing & Cardiac Rehabilitation

Christopher J. Kramer, BA, ACS, RDCS
Echocardiography Education Program Director
Advanced Clinical and Research Sonographer
Cardiovascular Ultrasound Imaging and Hemodynamic
    Laboratory
Advocate Aurora Health Care
Milwaukee, Wisconsin

Eric Kruse, BS, ACS, RDCS, RVT
Technical Imaging Coordinator
Heart and Vascular Imaging Center
University of Chicago Medicne
Chicago, Illinois

**Kate A. Marriott, BSc App (HMS), M Cardiac
Ultrasound**
Lecturer in Cardiac Ultrasound
School of Clinical Sciences, Faculty of Health
Queensland University of Technology (QUT)
Brisbane, Australia
Senior Sonographer
Hearts 1st
Greenslopes Private Hospital
Brisbane, Australia

Jane E. Marshall, BS, RDCS
Technical Director, Emeritus
Cardiac Ultrasound Laboratory
Massachusetts General Hospital
Boston, Massachusetts

Rick Meece, ACS, RDCS, RCIS
Cardiac Imaging Specialist
Perioperative and Structural Heart Division
Saint Thomas West Hospital
Nashville, Tennessee

Jennifer Mercandetti, BS, ACS, RDCS (AE/PE)
Lead Sonographer
Echocardiography
University of Colorado Hopsital
Aurora, Colorado

Sally J. Miller, BS, RDCS, RT(R)
Assistant Professor of Medicine, Mayo Clinic College
    of Medicine and Science
Department of Cardiovascular Medicine, Division of
    Cardiovascular Ultrasound
Mayo Clinic
Rochester, Minnesota

Raymond R. Musarra, ACS, RCS, RDCS
Manager Adult Echocardiography
Advanced Cardiac Sonographer
Harrington Heart & Vascular Institute
University Hospitals Cleveland Medical Center
Cleveland, Ohio

Stephanie Nay, MBA, RCCS
Cardiology Administration-Molecular Imaging
Department of Cardiology
Intermountain Healthcare
Murray, Utah

Joan J. Olson, BS, RDCS, RVT
Lead Cardiac Sonographer
Echocardiography Lab
Nebraska Medicine
Omaha, Nebraska

Maryellen H. Orsinelli, RN, RDCS
Lead Cardiac Sonographer
The Ross Heart Hospital
The Ohio State Wexner Medical Center
Columbus, Ohio

Richard A. Palma, BS, ACS, RCS, RDCS
Director of the Duke Cardiac Ultrasound Program
Duke School of Medicine
Duke Heart Center
Durham, North Carolina

Margaret M. Park, BS, ACS, RDCS, RVT
C5 Imaging Research
Heart, Vascular and Thoracic Institute
Cleveland Clinic
Cleveland, Ohio

Sarah H. Park, RDCS
Cardiac Sonographer III
Harrington Heart & Vascular Institute
University Hospitals Ahuja Medical Center
Hudson, Ohio

Bharatbhushan Patel, RDCS, RDMS, RVS
Senior Cardiac Sonographer
Cardiology Department
Carepoint health, Hoboken University Medical
    center
Hoboken, New Jersey

Andy Pellett, PhD, RDCS
Professor
Department of Cardiopulmonary Science
School of Allied Health Professions
Louisiana State University Health Sciences Center
New Orleans, Louisiana

Jason B. Pereira, MS, RCS
Technologist II and Research Cardiac Echo
    Sonographer
Department of Heart and Vascular (Echocardiography)
Yale-New Haven Hospital
New Haven, Connecticut

Rebecca Perry, PhD, DMU (Cardiac), BSc
Senior Lecturer
School of Health Sciences
University of South Australia
Adelaide, South Australia

Evelina Petrovets, BASc, RDCS
Adult Cardiac Sonographer
Heart, Vascular and Thoracic Institute
Cleveland Clinic
Cleveland, Ohio

Michael Rampoldi, ACS, RDCS, RVT
Manager, Non-Invasive Cardiology
Baylor Scott & White Heart and Vascular Hospital –
    Dallas
Baylor Scott & White Heart and Vascular Hospital –
    Fort Worth
Dallas, Texas

Jennifer L. Schaaf, BS, ACS, RDCS
Assistant Manager, Cardiovascular Imaging Services
Technical Director, Echocardiography Laboratory
The Christ Hospital Health Network
Cincinnati, Ohio

Elaine A. Shea, ACS, RCCS, RCIS
Manager, Cardiovascular Services/Interventional
    Radiology/EEG
Sutter Hospital/Alta Bates Summit Medical Center
Berkeley/Oakland, California

Neha Soni-Patel, BS, RDCS (AE/PE), RCCS
Education Coordinator and Trainer
Pediatric Non-Invasive Lab
Cleveland Clinic Children's
Cleveland, Ohio

G. Monet Strachan, ACS, RDCS (AE, PE)
Manager & Technical Director
Non-invasive Cardiovascular Lab
UC San Diego Health
Cardiovascular Institute
La Jolla, California

Matt Umland, BS, ACS, RDCS
Echocardiography Quality Director
Advanced Clinical and Research Sonographer
Cardiovascular Ultrasound Imaging and Hemodynamic
    Laboratory
Advocate Aurora Health Care
Milwaukee, Wisconsin

Thomas Van Houten, MPH, ACS, RDCS
Principal Cardiac Sonographer
Non-invasive Cardiovascular Lab
UC San Diego Health
Cardiovascular Institute
La Jolla, California

Ashwin Venkateshvaran, PhD, RCS, RDCS
Sonographer Scientist
Department of Cardiology
Karolinska University Hospital
Stockholm, Sweden

Anthony Wald, BTech, PDM, GDCT
PoCUS Educator
MonashHeart, Monash Health
Melbourne, Australia

Steven Walling, BS, RCS, RDCS
Director and Clinical Coordinator
Hoffman Heart School of Cardiovascular Technology
Trinity Health of New England Corporation, Inc.
Hartford, Connecticut

Melissa A. Wasserman, RDCS (AE/PE), RCCS
Satellite Operations Sonographer Lead
Department of Cardiology
The Children's Hospital of Philadelphia
Philadelphia, Pennsylvania

Cathy West, DMU (Cardiac), EACVI CHD, MSc
Principal Echocardiographer
Echocardiography Laboratory
Royal Brompton Hospital
London, United Kingdom

Gillian Whalley, PhD, DMU (Cardiac), BAppSci, MHSc (Hons)
Professor
Department of Medicine
University of Otago
Dunedin, New Zealand

Alison White, BSc, MSc, DMU (Cardiac)
Senior Lecturer
School of Environment and Science
Griffith University
Brisbane, Queensland, Australia

Ashley Woolf, BS, RDCS
Supervisor of Echocardiography
Heart and Vascular Institute
Cleveland Clinic Akron General
Cleveland, Ohio

Leah Wright, BSc, DMU (Cardiac), PhD
Senior Echocardiographer
Baker Heart and Diabetes Institute
Melbourne, Australia

Megan Yamat, RDCS, RCS, ACS
Technical Imaging Coordinator
Lead Advanced Cardiac Sonographer
University of Chicago Medicine
Chicago, Illinois

Karen G. Zimmerman, BS, ACS, RDCS (AE/PE), RVT
Facilitator Clinical Quality Imaging
Cardiology
Henry Ford Health System
Detroit, Michigan

We are delighted to introduce *Basic to Advanced Clinical Echocardiography: A Self-Assessment Tool for the Cardiac Sonographer by Bonita Anderson and Margaret M. Park*. This 38-chapter book presents the essentials of echocardiography in a precise question and answer format, following along the lines of the "Socratic method" of information sharing and teaching. Written by leading sonographers and educators, this unique book of more than 1200 self-assessment questions has been designed to test your level of expertise and applicability of knowledge in chapters ranging from cardiac anatomy and physiology, the fundamentals of ultrasound, the use of echocardiography in the interventional suite and managing an echo laboratory. Each question is supported by a detailed answer outline and suggested readings to further enhance comprehension, critical thinking and skill development. Using a star-rating similar to a Sudoku puzzle, the questions are identified as beginner, intermediate, or advanced, therefore making it easy to select the appropriate level for review. As we all know, a picture is worth a thousand words. Consequently, this text contains more than 950 figures and over 400 online real-time videos. Many chapters also include highlighted Key Points and Teaching Points. All mathematical formulas are shown in a step by step format for the reader to easily follow. An appendix of all equations and formulas used throughout the book, listing the chapter and question in which they were used, is included for easy reference.

It is with our deepest appreciation that we sincerely thank our contributing authors for their exceptional contributions. All are friends and/or colleagues who are deeply dedicated to the practice of Echocardiography. We feel very fortunate to have captured their passion, experience, and knowledge to share with our readers. We could not have completed this project without their support.

We owe our sincerest gratitude and appreciation to Craig Asher for his devotion and time in the review of each chapter for suggestions, corrections, and medical accuracy. We are also incredibly grateful to Andy Pellet who volunteered to meticulously review each question and answer for content and grammatical perfection, a task in which he has done commendably well.

We wholeheartedly thank Allan Klein for his perseverance and encouragement for us to write this book fashioned after *Clinical Echocardiography Review: A Self-Assessment Tool, 2nd Edition, edited by Allan L. Klein MD, and Craig R. Asher, MD, 2017* and wish to acknowledge the contributors of *Clinical Echocardiography Review: A Self-Assessment Tool, 2nd Edition* for their insight and inspiration to our contributing authors.

The completion of this book was laborious and at times unrelentless, but we are proud of the final product. We hope that you will find it comprehensive and valuable to enriching your knowledge and advancing your career and skills in Echocardiography.

Last but not least, we wish to acknowledge Wolters Kluwer for their assistance and guidance in the preparation of this text and our families for their patience and support. ■

Margaret M. Park and Bonita Anderson

CONTENTS

Cardiac Anatomy and Embryology

Contributors: Laura T. Boone, BS, RDCS, RVT, RDMS, RT(R) and Alison White, BSc, MSc, DMU (Cardiac)

✪ Question 1

In which body cavity is the heart located?
- **A.** Abdominal
- **B.** Pelvic
- **C.** Pleural
- **D.** Thoracic

✪✪ Question 2

Which section of the mediastinum is the heart located within?
- **A.** Anterior mediastinum
- **B.** Middle mediastinum
- **C.** Posterior mediastinum
- **D.** Superior mediastinum

✪ Question 3

The left ventricular apex points:
- **A.** Inferiorly toward the left hip.
- **B.** Inferiorly toward the right hip.
- **C.** Superiorly toward the left hip.
- **D.** Superiorly toward the right hip.

✪ Question 4

The membrane that lines the pericardial cavity and encases the heart is called the:
- **A.** Endocardium.
- **B.** Myocardium.
- **C.** Pericardium.
- **D.** Pleura.

✪✪ Question 5

Two of the main functions of the pericardium are to:
- **A.** Allow the heart to move freely within the mediastinum and provide a highly permeable covering for the heart.
- **B.** Allow the heart to move freely within the mediastinum and provide a protective covering for the heart.
- **C.** Secure the heart within the mediastinum and provide a protective covering for the heart.
- **D.** Secure the heart within the pleural cavity and provide a protective covering for the heart.

✪ Question 6

The outer connective tissue layer of the pericardium is called the:
- **A.** Epicardial pericardium.
- **B.** Fibrous pericardium.
- **C.** Serous pericardium.
- **D.** Visceral pericardium.

✪✪ Question 7

Which layer of the serous pericardium is in contact with the myocardium?
- **A.** Endocardial
- **B.** Fibrous
- **C.** Parietal
- **D.** Visceral

✪✪✪ Question 8

The fibrous pericardium limits distention of the heart and prevents overfilling of the cardiac chambers. The resultant effect on the cardiac chambers in cardiac tamponade is that:

A. The chambers can become compressed, which aids cardiac output.

B. The chambers can become compressed, which can compromise cardiac output.

C. The chambers can expand easily, which aids cardiac output.

D. The degree of chamber expansion or compression is unaffected

✪ Question 9

What is the correct order of the heart layers from innermost to outermost?

A. Endocardium, myocardium, epicardium

B. Endocardium, epicardium, myocardium

C. Epicardium, myocardium, endocardium

D. Endocardium, mesocardium, epicardium

✪ Question 10

Which ventricular wall layer is the thickest?

A. Endocardium

B. Epicardium

C. Mesocardium

D. Myocardium

✪ Question 11

The atrial muscle fibers are isolated electrically from the ventricular muscle fibers by:

A. The adipose tissue in the epicardium.

B. The chordae tendineae.

C. The coronary arteries.

D. The fibrous skeleton of the heart.

✪✪ Question 12

The cardiac or fibrous skeleton of the heart has several functions including assisting with the normal function of the cardiac valves. The cardiac skeleton also prevents:

A. The flow of blood through the semilunar valves.

B. The overstretching of the chordae tendineae.

C. The overstretching of the valve openings.

D. The flow of blood through the coronary arteries.

✪✪✪ Question 13

The cardiac skeleton can be described as:

A. An inflexible structure that does not distribute the forces of contraction.

B. A flexible structure that assists the distribution of the forces of contraction.

C. A flexible structure that inhibits the distribution of the forces of contraction.

D. An inflexible structure that has no relationship to the forces of contraction.

✪✪✪ Question 14

The fibrous band that separates the orifices of the inferior vena cava (IVC) and coronary sinus in the right atrium (RA) is the:

A. Eustachian ridge.

B. Koch's triangle.

C. Moderator band.

D. Tendon of Todaro.

✪✪ Question 15

The wall of the left ventricle (LV) is thicker than the wall of the right ventricle (RV) because the LV:

A. Accommodates a greater volume of blood than the RV.

B. Pumps blood at a higher pressure.

C. Pumps blood more quickly than the RV.

D. Pumps blood through a smaller valve orifice area.

✪✪ Question 16

When comparing the internal structural surfaces of the left and right atria, which of the following statements is most correct?

A. Both the left and right atria have a smooth zone located within the posterior region of the atrial wall.

B. Both the left and right atria have a rough zone located within the posterior region of the atrial wall.

C. Both the left and right atria have a smooth zone located within the anterior region of the atrial wall.

D. Neither the left nor the right atria have a smooth zone within the posterior region of the atrial wall.

✪✪✪ Question 17

Which of the following statements correctly describes the entry location of the great veins into the right atrium (RA) in relation to the crista terminalis (CT)?

  A. The superior vena cava (SVC) enters the RA slightly above the superior bend of the CT while the inferior vena cava (IVC) enters slightly below the inferior bend of the CT.
  B. The SVC enters the RA slightly below the superior bend of the CT while the IVC enters slightly above the inferior bend of the CT.
  C. The SVC enters the RA slightly below the superior bend of the CT while the IVC enters slightly below the inferior bend of the CT.
  D. The SVC enters the RA slightly below the inferior bend of the CT while the IVC enters slightly below the superior bend of the CT.

✪ Question 18

In adults, the partition that divides the superior left and right chambers into separate chambers is called the:

  A. Atrioventricular septum.
  B. Fossa ovalis.
  C. Interatrial septum.
  D. Interventricular septum.

✪✪ Question 19

Which of the following statements regarding the atrial appendages is false?

  A. The appendages are the remnants of the primitive common atrium.
  B. The appendages serve no physiological function in the developed heart.
  C. The inner surface of the appendages is consistently irregular and rough.
  D. The appendages are located on the outer side of the heart.

✪✪ Question 20

The chamber that forms most of the anterior and inferior surfaces of the heart is the:

  A. Left atrium.
  B. Left ventricle.
  C. Right atrium.
  D. Right ventricle.

✪ Question 21

The outflow portion of the right ventricle (RV) is also referred to as the:

  A. Apical segment.
  B. Basal segment.
  C. Infundibulum.
  D. Sinus portion.

✪✪✪ Question 22

When comparing the anatomic features of the right ventricle (RV) and the left ventricle (LV), which of the following statements is false?

  A. The right ventricular apex is more coarsely trabeculated than the left ventricular apex.
  B. The chordal attachments to the interventricular septum (IVS) are present in the RV and absent in the LV.
  C. The inlet and outlet components of the RV are separated by a muscular arch while the inlet and outlet components of the LV are in continuity.
  D. The middle myofiber layer is absent in the LV and present in the RV.
  E. The RV has multiple papillary muscles while the LV has only two.

✪ Question 23

The coronary sulcus forms an external boundary between which chambers of the heart?

  A. The atria and the ventricles
  B. The left and right atria
  C. The left and right ventricles
  D. The ventricles and the great vessels

✪✪ Question 24

When comparing the anatomic features of the aortic valve (AV) and the pulmonary valve (PV), which of the following statements is false?

  A. Both the AV and PV have fibrous tissue nodes (nodules of Arantius) in the center of their cusps.
  B. The AV is in fibrous continuity with the left atrioventricular valve and is supported by the interventricular septum (IVS) while the PV is not in continuity with the right atrioventricular valve and is not supported by the IVS.
  C. The PV is situated anterior and leftward relative to the AV.
  D. The names of the AV cusps are right coronary, left coronary, and noncoronary while the PV cusps are anterior, posterior, and right.

✪✪ Question 25

The components of the semilunar valves include:
   A. The annulus, the root of the great veins, the commissures, and the interleaflet triangles.
   B. The annulus, the leaflets, the papillary muscles, and the interleaflet triangles.
   C. The annulus, the cusps, the commissures, and the interleaflet triangles.
   D. The annulus, the cusps, the chordae tendineae, and the interleaflet triangles.

✪✪ Question 26

When comparing the anatomic features of the mitral valve (MV) and the tricuspid valve (TV), which of the following statements is false?
   A. Both the MV and TV have septal chordal attachments.
   B. The MV has a high septal attachment and the TV has a low septal attachment.
   C. At the mid-leaflet level, the MV orifice is elliptical in shape while the TV orifice is triangular.
   D. The anterior leaflet of each valve is a mid-cavitary structure that divides its ventricle into inflow and outflow regions.

✪ Question 27

The role of the papillary muscles is to:
   A. Assist in the conduction of the electrical potential to the atrioventricular (AV) valves.
   B. Contract during ventricular systole resulting in tightening of the chordae tendineae to assist with the complete closure and correct positioning of AV valves.
   C. Relax during ventricular systole and support the chordae tendineae to ensure correct AV valve position.
   D. Block the conduction of the electrical potential to the AV valves.

✪✪ Question 28

The atrioventricular (AV) node is located within:
   A. The floor of the right atrium (RA) near the interatrial septum (IAS).
   B. The inner wall of the left atrium near the IAS.
   C. The roof of the RA near the entrance of the superior vena cava.
   D. The interventricular septum.

✪✪ Question 29

In which direction does the primitive heart tube fold to form the normal bulboventricular loop?
   A. Anteriorly and leftward
   B. Anteriorly and rightward
   C. Posteriorly and leftward
   D. Posteriorly and rightward

✪✪ Question 30

Which portion of the interatrial septum (IAS) acts as a flap at the level of the foramen ovale?
   A. Membranous
   B. Outlet
   C. Primum
   D. Secundum

✪ Question 31

What is the last portion of the interventricular septum (IVS) to form?
   A. Inlet
   B. Membranous
   C. Muscular
   D. Outlet

✪ Question 32

The septum that originates from conotruncal ridges is the _____ septum.
   A. Aorticopulmonary
   B. Interatrial
   C. Membranous
   D. Ventricular

✪✪ Question 33

What is essential for normal development of the primum atrial septum, inlet ventricular septum, and atrioventricular orifices?
   A. Aorticopulmonary septum
   B. Conotruncal ridges
   C. Endocardial cushions
   D. Truncus arteriosus

✪ Question 34

Which of the six pairs of aortic arches forms the aortic arch?
   A. First
   B. Third
   C. Fourth
   D. Sixth

✪ Question 35

Which segment of the primitive heart tube develops into the aorta and the pulmonary artery?
   A. Bulbus cordis
   B. Primitive ventricle
   C. Sinus venous
   D. Truncus arteriosus

✪ Question 36

Which segment of the primitive heart tube develops into the definitive right ventricle (RV)?
   A. Bulbus cordis
   B. Conus cordis
   C. Primitive ventricle
   D. Sinus venous

✪✪ Question 37

What is the position of the bulbus cordis after the completion of normal cardiac looping?
   A. Anterior, inferior, and to the right
   B. Anterior, superior, and to the left
   C. Posterior, inferior, and to the right
   D. Posterior, superior, and to the left

✪✪ Question 38

What structure directs blood flow from the inferior vena cava (IVC) toward the foramen ovale during normal fetal circulation?
   A. Chiari network
   B. Eustachian valve
   C. Thebesian valve
   D. Tricuspid valve

✪✪✪ Question 39

Which of the following receives the least amount of blood in normal fetal circulation?
   A. Descending thoracic aorta
   B. Ductus arteriosus
   C. Foramen ovale
   D. Pulmonary veins

✪✪ Question 40

Which hemodynamic event occurs postdelivery resulting in the close of the foramen ovale?
   A. Foramen ovale flow increases.
   B. Left atrial pressure increases.
   C. Pulmonary artery blood flow decreases.
   D. Pulmonary vascular resistance increases.

✪✪ Question 41

Which of the following statements regarding the ductus arteriosus is false?
   A. The ductus arteriosus is formed from the left distal sixth aortic arch.
   B. In the fetal circulation, the ductus arteriosus directs blood away from the fetal lungs.
   C. The blood in the ductus arteriosus has a low oxygen content.
   D. Closure of the ductus arteriosus by contraction of its muscular wall occurs almost immediately after birth.

✪ Question 42

What is the remnant of the ductus arteriosus called?
   A. Ligamentum ductus
   B. Ligamentum arteriosum
   C. Ligamentum teres
   D. Ligamentum venosum

ANSWERS

1. **Answer: D.** The body consists of internal cavities that are sealed to the outside environment and these internal cavities house the organs (**Figure 1-1**). The thoracic cavity is a large cavity positioned toward the anterior surface of the body. It extends from the clavicles to the diaphragm and is surrounded by the ribs, the muscles of the chest wall, and the thoracic vertebrae of the spinal column. The heart is located in the middle of the thoracic cavity, with two-thirds of the heart located to the left of the midline.

2. **Answer: B.** The mediastinum is the middle (or central) cavity of the thorax. The mediastinum is the cavity that lies between the two pleural cavities and is bordered by the sternum anteriorly, the vertebral column posteriorly, the first rib superiorly, and the diaphragm inferiorly. The mediastinum consists of two regions, the superior and inferior regions, which are divided horizontally at the level of the fourth vertebrae and the manubriosternal joint (**Figure 1-2**). The inferior mediastinum can be further subdivided

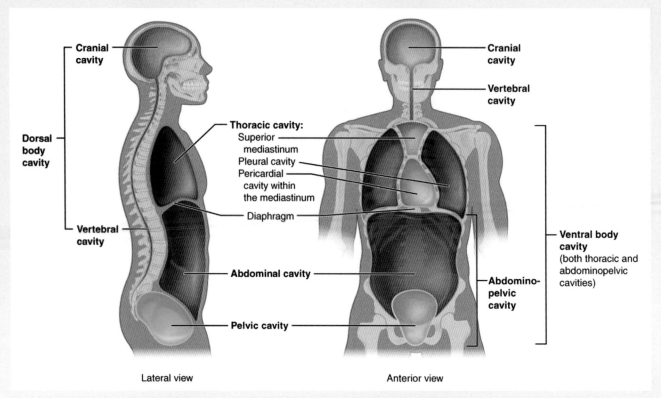

Figure 1-1 Body cavities. (From An Introduction to the human body (1.15 Dorsal and Ventral Body Cavities). In: Young KA, Wise JA, DeSaix P, et al, eds. *Anatomy and Physiology*. https://creativecommons.org/licenses/by/4.0/. Copyright © May 2, 2019 OpenStax.)

into the anterior, middle, and posterior compartments. The heart and pericardium are housed within the middle mediastinum. The compartments of the mediastinum have no real features that separate

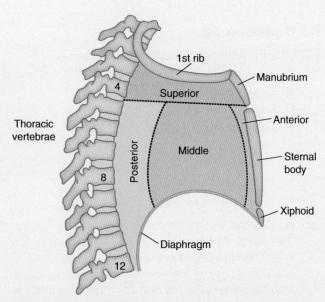

Figure 1-2 Mediastinum, shown schematically. Viewed from a right lateral perspective, the mediastinum has four divisions. The heart is located in the middle mediastinum. (Reprinted with permission from Maleszewski JJ, Edwards WD. Cardiac anatomy and examination of cardiac specimens. In: Allen HD, Shaddy RE, Penny DJ, et al, eds. *Moss and Adams' Heart Disease in Infants, Children, and Adolescents. Including the Fetus and Young Adult*. 9th ed. Philadelphia, PA: Wolters Kluwer; 2016:chap 6.)

them anatomically. However, the clinical importance of this nomenclature becomes apparent when describing the presence and position of abnormal pathologies such as infiltration of tumors or localized regions of inflammation.

3. **Answer: A.** The apex of the heart is normally conical in shape, positioned inferiorly and is made primarily of the tip of the left ventricle. Following embryological development, the apex of the heart is oriented anteriorly, inferiorly, and pointing toward the left hip. This orientation means that the heart is rotated slightly, resulting in the right side of the heart sitting more anteriorly, toward the surface of the body, than is the left side of the heart.

4. **Answer: C.** The pericardium is a tough and dense fibroserous sac, which covers the external surface of the heart and the origins of the great vessels.

5. **Answer: C.** The pericardium is bound inferiorly to the diaphragm by the central tendon of the diaphragm and helps to secure the heart anteriorly within the mediastinum via sternopericardial ligaments and adherence to the pleura.

   The pericardium also provides a barrier to infection by separating the heart from other structures in the mediastinum, including the lungs and pleural spaces.

6. **Answer: B.** The pericardium is not just a simple container in which the heart is housed. The pericardium is a complex triple-layered membranous structure that lines the pericardial cavity and covers the heart. The fibrous pericardium is a tough fibrous outer sac that

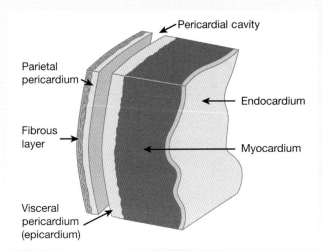

Figure 1-3 This image represents the structure of the wall of the ventricle and demonstrates the pericardium schematically. The diagram shows the outermost layer (fibrous pericardium) lined by the double-walled sac of the serous pericardium. The two layers of the serous pericardium are separated by the pericardial cavity. (Reproduced with permission by Echotext Pty Ltd, from Anderson B. *A Sonographer's Guide to the Assessment of Heart Disease*. 1st ed. Australia: Echotext Pty Ltd; 2014:343.)

has an open end and the inside of this outer sac is a second, double-walled closed sac. The fibrous pericardium has no direct contact with the surface of the heart and is made of a dense, highly tensile layer of irregular connective tissue that is relatively noncompliant.

7. **Answer: D.** The serous pericardium is the inner, closed, double-layered sac that sits inside the outer sac, that is, the fibrous pericardium. The serous pericardium consists of an inner and outer surface (**Figure 1-3**). The parietal layer is the outer surface that adheres to the fibrous pericardium. The inner surface of the serous pericardium is called the visceral layer. The visceral layer adheres directly to the heart and is also known as the epicardial layer of the heart wall. It is often considered to be part of the wall of the heart. The visceral layer is a moist serous membrane made primarily of simple squamous epithelial cells that produce an oily serous fluid substance (pericardial fluid), and these cells are connected to a thin layer of connective tissue (a basement membrane). The pericardial cavity is a small slit or gap that separates the parietal layer and visceral layer and normally contains a small volume of lubricating pericardial fluid.

8. **Answer: B.** The highly tensile noncompliant connective tissue of the fibrous pericardium resists rapid expansion and helps to prevent the cardiac chambers from overfilling. In a patient with cardiac tamponade, this function becomes detrimental to the maintenance of normal cardiac output. Due to the relatively inflexible nature of the pericardium, as the pressure builds within the pericardial cavity in tamponade, the increased pressure compresses the heart and limits the extent of ventricular filling (venous return is decreased), which will in turn decrease cardiac output.

9. **Answer: A.** The heart wall comprises three distinct layers (see **Figure 1-3**). The innermost layer, the endocardium, consists of a single layer of simple endothelial cells attached to a thin connective tissue basement membrane and is in direct contact with the blood contained within the cardiac chambers. The middle layer of the wall of the heart is the myocardium and consists of striated muscle tissue surrounded by connective tissue that binds the muscle cells together. The outermost layer of the heart wall is the epicardium or visceral layer of the serous pericardium. The epicardium is a thin layer of mesothelial cells overlying a layer of fibroelastic tissue and adipose tissue.

10. **Answer: D.** The myocardium is the thickest of the three layers of the ventricular wall, constituting almost 90% of the width of the wall. This is due to the large number of muscle cells that are present in the myocardial layer.

11. **Answer: D.** The fibrous skeleton of the heart, also known as the cardiac skeleton, is located between the atria and the ventricles. Although the name is suggestive of a bony structure, it is composed of interconnecting arrangements of dense connective tissue (**Figure 1-4**). Traditionally the cardiac skeleton was viewed as a defined structure consisting of four distinct and complete interconnecting rings (one for each valve) anchoring the valves to the mass of the ventricular muscle. However, a more anatomically correct description of the cardiac skeleton reveals that only three of the valves (aortic, mitral, and tricuspid valves) do have fibrous rings, while the pulmonary valve is not connected to a fibrous ring but is instead supported by the muscle of the right ventricle outflow tract. The components that collectively join to make the fibrous skeleton include the aortic-mitral continuity (or mitral curtain), the fibrous trigones (thickened areas of tissue between the aortic and atrioventricular valves), the membranous portion of the interventricular septum, the interleaflet triangles of the aortic valve, the subvalvar collar of the septal leaflet of the mitral valve, the tendon of Todaro, and potentially the conus ligament (the ligament situated between the right coronary cusp of the aortic valve and the septal pulmonary valve cusp) (**Figure 1-4**). The connective tissue of the cardiac skeleton is electrically inert, meaning that it cannot conduct electrical impulses. Thus, an important function of the cardiac skeleton is to prevent direct electrical connection of the atria to the ventricles.

12. **Answer: C.** The dense and highly tensile nature of the collagen fibers in the connective tissue of the cardiac skeleton aids valvular function by providing support for the base of the valve cusps/leaflets. Also, the relatively noncompliant property of the collagen fibers in the connective tissue of the cardiac skeleton helps to prevent overstretching of the valve opening as blood flows through the valves.

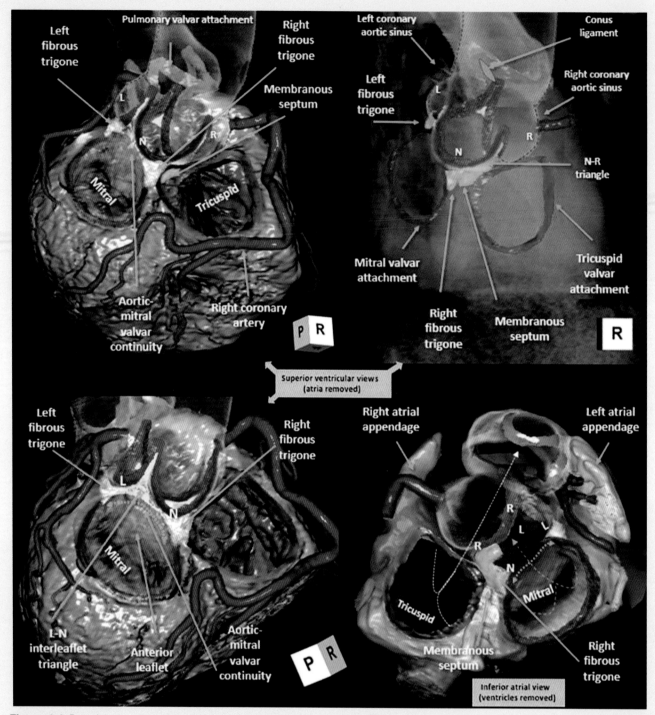

Figure 1-4 Essential components of the fibrous skeleton. Color-coded computed tomographic (CT) images show basal views of the heart after removal of the atria (superior ventricular views) and removal of the ventricles (inferior atrial view). Essential components of the fibrous skeleton include the fibrous aortic-mitral continuity, right and left fibrous trigones, membranous septum, interleaflet triangles, parts of the mitral and tricuspid annuli, tendon of Todaro, and conus ligament. L, left coronary sinus; N, noncoronary sinus; R, right coronary sinus. (From Saremi F, Sánchez-Quintana D, Mori S, et al. Fibrous skeleton of the heart: anatomic overview and evaluation of pathologic conditions with CT and MR imaging. *Radiographics*. 2017;37(5):1330-1351, with permission.)

13. **Answer: B.** Historically, the fibrous cardiac skeleton was thought to operate as a rigid structure whose primary function was to serve as an anchor for the ventricular muscle fibers. Current evidence shows that the fibroelastic sheets of connective tissue that wrap and separate the muscle layers in the chambers of the heart are continuous with the denser bundles of connective tissue that make up the fibrous skeleton. The stretchy elastic fibers that are present throughout the muscle of the heart are in continuity with the stiff central band of the cardiac skeleton. This continuity and arrangement of fibers enables the distribution of kinetic energy created during contraction (thus distributing the force of contraction) and facilitates the heart returning to its initial shape during relaxation.

14. **Answer: A.** The Eustachian ridge (option A) runs across the inferior border of the RA and separates the orifice of the IVC from the coronary sinus. Koch's triangle (option B) is located in the lower medial portion of the right atrium, overlying the atrioventricular node and the proximal His bundle. The moderator band (option C) is located in the right ventricle and is a muscular bridge that connects the distal septum and the right ventricular free wall at the anterior papillary muscle. The tendon of Todaro (option D) is a band of collagen that lies deep in the subendocardium of the atria and forms part of the central portion of the fibrous skeleton of the heart. It is not visible from the inner surface of the atria but can be located by identifying the Eustachian ridge, beneath which it is located.

15. **Answer: B.** Normally, the left and right ventricles simultaneously pump and eject an equal volume of blood with each contraction. However, there are major differences when comparing the function of the left and right ventricles regarding output requirements and workload. The LV is required to pump blood over a greater distance at a higher pressure into the high-resistance systemic circulation. This is in comparison to the RV, whose workload as a pump is less because it is required to pump blood into a lower pressure, lower resistance pulmonary circulation over a shorter distance. Thus, to achieve the same volume and same rate of blood flow with each contraction, the left ventricular workload must be greater than the right ventricular workload.

16. **Answer: A.** Both atria have a smooth zone, with the right atrium (RA) also having a rough zone due to the presence of pectinate muscles. The smooth zone of the RA is separated from the rough zone by a large C-shaped muscular ridge called the crista terminalis. The smooth zone is located in the posterior portion of the atrium where the inferior vena cava enters the RA (**Figure 1-5A**). The rough zone is located in the anterior portion of the atrium superior to the crista terminalis.

    In contrast to the right atrial internal surface, the internal surface of the left atrium (LA) is relatively smooth throughout and does not have two distinct zones (**Figure 1-5B**). Thus, both the posterior and anterior portions of the LA are smooth in appearance. This is due to the absence of pectinate muscles within the body of the LA. In the LA, the pectinate muscles are usually confined to the left atrial appendage.

TEACHING POINT

Pectinate muscles are horizontal ridges of muscles seen in the left atrial appendage and in the rough zone of the RA. These muscles are described as having an appearance like the teeth on a comb. The protrusions of the ridges of pectinate muscle cause the surface to be irregular and rough in appearance.

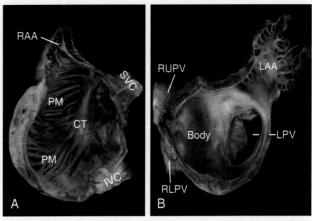

Figure 1-5 The internal right atrial surface (A, viewed from a left lateral perspective) has a rough zone containing the pectinate muscles (PM) that is separated from the smooth zone by the crista terminalis (CT). The left atrial wall (B, viewed from an anterior perspective) contains neither a crista terminalis or pectinate muscles; pectinate muscles are isolated to the left atrial appendage (LAA). IVC, inferior vena cava; LPV, left pulmonary vein; RAA, right atrial appendage; RLPV, right lower pulmonary vein; RUPV, right upper pulmonary vein; SVC, superior vena cava. (Reprinted with permission from Maleszewski JJ, Edwards WD. Cardiac anatomy and examination of cardiac specimens. In: Allen HD, Shaddy RE, Penny DJ, et al, eds. *Moss and Adams' Heart Disease in Infants, Children, and Adolescents. Including the Fetus and Young Adult.* 9th ed. Philadelphia, PA: Wolters Kluwer; 2016:chap 6.)

17. **Answer: C.** The CT is a distinct ridge of smooth fibrous muscle that extends along the posterolateral aspect of the right atrial wall (see **Figure 1-5A**). The CT originates from the atrial septal wall, passes anteriorly to where the SVC enters the RA, then creates the characteristic "C" shape as it descends posteriorly and laterally, and then turns anteriorly to hug the right side of the entry point of the IVC. The orifices of the SVC and IVC can be described in relation to the position of the CT; that is, the SVC opens into the RA slightly below the superior bend of the muscle ridge, while the IVC opens into the RA slightly below the inferior bend of the muscle ridge.

TEACHING POINT

The importance of understanding the location of the CT is that if this fibromuscular band is larger than normal, it can be mistaken for a mass or a tumor within the RA on the echocardiogram.

18. **Answer: C.** The superior chambers of the heart are the atria. The thin membrane of tissue that longitudinally divides the left and right atria into separate chambers is the interatrial septum (IAS). The IAS is normally 1 to 2 mm in thickness. It is mainly composed of fibrous connective tissue (septum secundum portion) with some myocardial muscle fibers (mainly in the septum primum).

    The atrioventricular (AV) septum (option A) is the portion of the interventricular septum that lies between the right atrium and the left ventricle. The AV node is located along the right atrial aspect of the AV septum. The fossa ovalis (option B) is an oval-shaped indent in the IAS visualized from the right atrial side and is the thinnest part of the septum. The interventricular septum (option D) divides the left and right ventricles into separate chambers.

TEACHING POINT

By understanding the normal features of the IAS, the cardiac sonographer can quickly identify alterations to the thickness of the septum that may be due to either physiological or pathological causes ranging from inflammation or deposition of adipose tissue to the presence of a mass or tumor.

19. **Answer: B.** The appendages are flap-like structures that are extensions of each atrium located on the outer side of the heart and are the remnants of the embryological primitive common atrium. The inner surface of the appendages is irregular and rough due to a high concentration of pectinate muscles (see **Figure 1-5**). The physiological function of appendages includes the accommodation of an additional blood volume during atrial diastole; and in atrial systole, the appendages deflate as the pectinate muscles in the wall of the appendage contract, forcing the blood forward through the atrioventricular valves.

20. **Answer: D.** The right ventricle (RV) wraps around the left ventricle to form most of the anterior and inferior surfaces of the heart. The RV is a complex structure that has been described as cone-shaped when viewed anteriorly or crescent-shaped when viewed from a cross-section through the chamber.

21. **Answer: C.** The outflow portion of the RV is a smooth-walled muscular conduit that leads to the pulmonary valve. The outflow portion of the RV is also called the conus (meaning cone-shaped) or infundibulum (meaning funnel-like). There are several approaches used to describe the complex internal anatomy of the RV as listed in **Table 1-1**.

TEACHING POINTS

In the embryological development of the heart, the RV can be divided into two main segments or portions, the sinus portion (superior end) and the conus portion (subpulmonary channel). These two portions of the RV are separated internally by the moderator band, which spans from the interventricular septum to the anterior wall of the RV at the base of the anterior papillary muscle. The sinus portion is a rough-walled compartment due to the presence of a series of irregular muscle folds called the trabeculae carneae.

In the developed heart, the RV can be divided into three segments: inflow or inlet, apical, and outflow or outlet. The inlet portion of the RV begins at the base of the ventricle and continues until the insertions of the papillary muscles. It supports the tricuspid valve annulus. The apical portion of the RV contains numerous irregular muscular ridges or trabeculations (trabeculae carneae). The right ventricular wall is thinnest at the apex. The outflow segment is almost tubular in shape, is smooth-walled, and supports the cusps of the pulmonary valve (hence the terminology of subpulmonary channel). The posterior aspect of the outflow segment consists of a pronounced muscle ridge called the crista supraventricularis or supraventricular crest. The supraventricular crest demarcates the inlet from the outlet portions of the RV and it separates the tricuspid and pulmonary valves. The muscular structure of the supraventricular crest consists of three sections or bands, which are the parietal band, infundibular septum, and septal band. These three muscle bands can act as individual structures or can combine.

22. **Answer: D. Table 1-2** summarizes the anatomic features that differentiate the RV from the LV. Transmurally through the ventricular wall, the myocardium is composed of a complex helical arrangement of myofibrils in three layers: (1) superficial (subepicardial), (2) middle, and (3) deep (subendocardial) layers. The middle layer is only present in the LV.

23. **Answer: A.** The coronary sulcus is a deep groove that denotes the boundary between the atria and the ventricles and is also known as the atrioventricular (AV) groove. The AV groove defines the base of the ventricles externally.

Table 1-1. Methods to Describe the Internal Anatomy of the Right Ventricle

Method	Anatomical Sections
Embryologically	Sinus (superior end), conus (subpulmonary channel)
Direction of blood flow (physiologically)	Inlet (inflow), apical, outlet (outflow), or infundibulum
In relation to the left ventricle and thorax	Anterior, lateral, and inferior
Imaging descriptors (echocardiography, magnetic resonance imaging [MRI])	Basal, middle, and apical

Table 1-2. Distinguishing Anatomic Features of the Left and Right Ventricles

	Right Ventricle (RV)	Left Ventricle (LV)
Geometry	Complex shape From the side appears triangular; in cross-section appears crescent-shaped	Ellipsoid Ventricular septum convex into the right ventricular cavity
Ventricular components	Inlet and outlet components separated by a muscular arch	Continuity between the inlet and outlet components
Trabeculations	Heavily trabeculated at the apex; moderator band	Fine trabeculations at the apex
Atrioventricular valves	Trileaflet configuration of the tricuspid valve with septal papillary attachments Apical displacement of the septal tricuspid leaflet relative to anterior mitral leaflet	Bileaflet mitral valve with no attachments to the ventricular septum
Papillary muscles	Multiple (>3) papillary muscles	Two prominent papillary muscles
Tendinous chords	Multiple attachments of chords from the septal leaflet to the interventricular septum	No chordal attachments to the interventricular septum
Wall thickness	3-5 mm base to middle (RV mass one-sixth of LV mass)	12-15 mm at base Gradual thinning from base to apex
Myofiber architecture	Two layers only: 1. Superficial (subepicardial) 2. Deep (subendocardial)	Three layers: 1. Superficial (subepicardial) 2. Middle 3. Deep (subendocardial)

(Reproduced with permission by Echotext Pty Ltd, from Anderson B. *A Sonographer's Guide to the Assessment of Heart Disease.* 1st ed. Australia: Echotext Pty Ltd; 2014:24.)

TEACHING POINT

There are three major grooves or sulci on the external surface of the heart. The significance of the external sulci is that the coronary blood vessels course along these external grooves and the sulci also demarcate the external boundary between two chambers in the heart. The coronary sulcus, or AV groove, denotes the boundary between the atria and the ventricles. The interventricular groove is the superficial (external) landmark that defines the position of the interventricular septum internally. This groove is subdivided into diaphragmatic (posterior) and anterior components based on its course along the surface of the heart. The anterior groove travels parallel to the obtuse margin of the ventricle spanning the distance between the AV groove and the acute margin (just right of the cardiac apex). This groove then continues posteriorly as the diaphragmatic (posterior) groove near the midpoint of the ventricle and it terminates at the diaphragmatic AV groove near the point of entry of the coronary sinus to the right atrium.

24. **Answer: D.** Table 1-3 summarizes the anatomic features of these two valves. The nomenclature of the AV cusps is related to the origin of the coronary arteries, while the nomenclature of the PV cusps is related to their relative position to the AV. The pulmonary valve is situated anterior and leftward relative to the AV. Therefore, the names of the cusps of the PV are anterior, left (or left posterior), and right (or right posterior) (**Figure 1-6**).

TEACHING POINT

The structural anatomy of aortic and pulmonary valves is very similar, with the two valves sharing many components. The minor differences in anatomy between the aortic and pulmonary valves are due to the differences in pressure and function of their respective locations in the heart. For example, the aortic valve cusps are slightly thicker than the pulmonary valve cusps due to the higher pressure that they must withstand on the left side of the heart in comparison to the right side.

25. **Answer: C.** The anatomy of both semilunar valves consists of four principal components, which are the annulus, the cusps of the valve, the commissures, and the interleaflet triangles. The annulus of the semilunar valves is a crown-shaped region at the base of the valve that lacks a well-defined fibrous structure and marks the junction or hinge point between the valve and the fibroelastic walls of the associated great artery. The cusps of the valves are the thin pieces of tissue that are flap-like and open and close during the cardiac cycle. The commissures define the region where the cusps touch each other (zone of apposition) and insert into the annulus. Lastly, the interleaflet triangles are triangular-shaped regions of tissue that lie underneath the top of the crown-like annulus and are extensions of the fibrous tissue of the outflow tract.

Table 1-3. The Comparative Anatomy of the Aortic and Pulmonary Valves

	Aortic Valve (AV)	Pulmonary Valve (PV)
Names of cusps	Right coronary, left coronary, noncoronary	Anterior, left, right
Continuity with AV valve	In fibrous continuity with the MV and is supported by the IVS	Not in continuity with the TV and is not supported by the IVS
Position in the chest	Lies to the left of the sternum opposite the third left intercostal space	Lies behind the medial end of the third costal cartilage and anterior to the AV
Fibrous tissue node (nodules of Arantius)	Present in the center of the aortic side of the cusps	Present in the center of the pulmonary arterial side of the cusps and are slightly smaller in size than the AV

IVS, interventricular septum; MV, mitral valve; TV, tricuspid valve.

TEACHING POINT

The semilunar valves are located between the ventricles and the great arteries at the exit point of the ventricles. The name "semilunar" stems from the crescent moon–shaped pieces of tissue that compose the cusps of the valve. The semilunar valve located between the right ventricle and the pulmonary trunk is called the pulmonary valve, while the semilunar valve located between the left ventricle and the aorta is called the aortic valve. The pulmonary valve connects the infundibulum of the right ventricular outflow tract and the main trunk of the pulmonary artery.

26. **Answer: A.** **Table 1-4** summarizes the anatomic features of the mitral and tricuspid valves. Each valve is similar in structure consisting of five components: the annulus, leaflets, and commissures form the

valvular apparatus, and the chordae tendineae (tendinous cords) and papillary muscles form the subvalvular apparatus (**Figure 1-7**). Only the tricuspid valve has septal chordal attachments; this is a reliable distinguishing feature of the tricuspid valve.

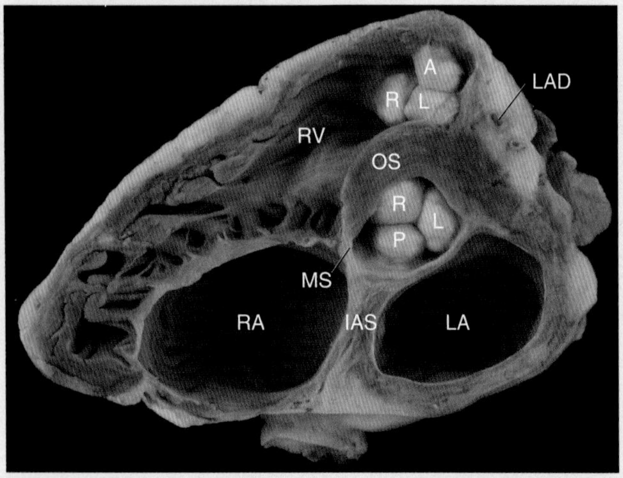

TEACHING POINTS

The tricuspid valve has three leaflets, commissures, and papillary muscles, whereas the mitral valve has only two of each. The tricuspid valve can also be differentiated from the mitral valve by the lower septal insertion of the anterior tricuspid leaflet compared to the anterior mitral leaflet and the insertion of numerous chords directly onto the interventricular septum. Once the atrioventricular valves have been identified, then the ventricles can be identified; the tricuspid valve virtually always connects to a morphologic right ventricle, whereas the mitral valve connects to a morphologic left ventricle.

Figure 1-6 Short-axis view at the level of the aortic valve. The aortic valve (center) has three cusps: right coronary (R), left coronary (L), and the noncoronary or posterior (P). The pulmonary valve is anterior to the aortic valve and also has three cusps: anterior (A), right (R), and left (L). IAS, interatrial septum; LA, left atrium; LAD, left anterior descending coronary artery; MS, membranous septum; OS, outlet (infundibular) septum; RA, right atrium; RV, right ventricle. (Reprinted with permission from Maleszewski JJ, Edwards WD. Cardiac anatomy and examination of cardiac specimens. In: Allen HD, Shaddy RE, Penny DJ, et al, eds. *Moss and Adams' Heart Disease in Infants, Children, and Adolescents. Including the Fetus and Young Adult.* 9th ed. Philadelphia, PA: Wolters Kluwer; 2016:chap 6.)

27. **Answer: B.** When the ventricles contract during ventricular systole, the papillary muscles contract, which increases the tension on the chordae, which in turn pulls the AV leaflets toward each other resulting in complete closure of the valve. This prevents the backflow of blood into the atria during systole. The tension on the chordae also prevents inversion of the leaflets into the atria. During ventricular diastole the papillary muscles relax and the tension on the chordae decreases. This chordal slackening allows the leaflets to open when the pressure in the atria exceeds the pressure in the ventricles. Therefore, the role of the papillary muscles is to contract during ventricular systole resulting in tightening of the chordae tendineae to assist with the complete closure and correct positioning of the AV valve.

28. **Answer: A.** The AV node is located in the floor of the RA near the IAS. The sinoatrial (SA) node is located in the roof of the RA near the entrance of the superior vena cava. The internodal pathways are located within the walls of the right atrium and extend from the SA node to the AV node. The right and left bundle branches are located within the interventricular septum.

Table 1-4. The Comparative Anatomy of the Mitral and Tricuspid Valves

	Mitral Valve (MV)	Tricuspid Valve (TV)
Names of leaflets	Anterior, posterior	Septal (medial, conal), anterior (anterosuperior, infundibular or superior), posterior (inferior, marginal)
Orifice	Elliptical orifice (mid-leaflet level)	Triangular orifice (mid-leaflet level)
Size of leaflets	The surface area of the anterior leaflet is greater than the posterior leaflet	Anterior is the largest; septal is usually the smallest
Septal attachments	High septal attachment	Low septal attachment
Chordal attachments	No septal chordal attachments	Septal chordal attachments
Papillary muscles	Usually two; posterior (posteromedial) and lateral (anterolateral)	Number is variable; usually a minimum of three; septal, anterior, and inferior (posterior)
Relationship to the semilunar valves	In direct fibrous continuity with the AV (aortomitral fibrosa)	No direct continuity with the PV (infundibulum separates TV from PV)
Position in the chest	Lies to the left of the sternum opposite the fourth costal cartilage	Lies toward the right of the sternum opposite the fourth intercostal space

AV, aortic valve; PV, pulmonary valve.

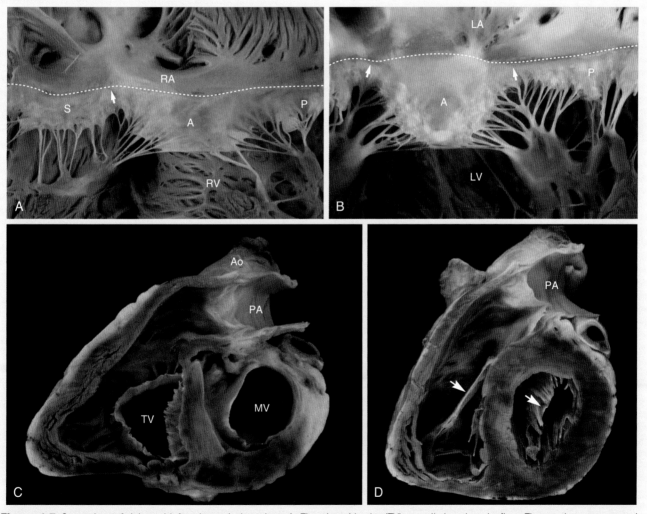

Figure 1-7 Comparison of right and left atrioventricular valves. A, The tricuspid valve (TV) normally has three leaflets. The membranous septum is located along its annulus (*dashed line*), at the anteroseptal commissure (*arrow*). B, The mitral valve (MV) has two leaflets, with papillary muscles beneath each commissure. C and D, In short-axis views, the tricuspid orifice is shaped like a reversed D at the annular level (C) and like a triangle at the mid-leaflet level (D). In contrast, the mitral orifice is elliptical at both levels. As shown in D, the anterior leaflet (*arrow*) of each valve is a mid-cavitary structure that divides its ventricle into inflow and outflow regions. Ao, aorta; PA, pulmonary artery. (From Maleszewski JJ, Edwards WD. Cardiac anatomy and examination of cardiac specimens. In: Allen HD, Shaddy RE, Penny DJ, Feltes TF, Cetta F, eds. *Moss and Adams' Heart Disease in Infants, Children, and Adolescents. Including the Fetus and Young Adult.* 9th ed. Wolters Kluwer; 2016:chap 6.)

TEACHING POINT

Electrical conduction through the heart commences at the SA node. Thus, the SA node is known as the pacemaker of the heart. Once the SA node initiates electrical activity, the electrical signal then spreads across the atria via the internodal pathways (which are directly connected to the atrial contractile muscle cells) to the next cluster of autorhythmic cells at the AV node. The AV node slows the speed of electrical conduction allowing time for the ventricles to fill following atrial contraction. From the AV node the electrical signal travels through the bundle of His, to the left and right bundle branches, and to the subendocardial (Purkinje) fibers.

29. **Answer: B.** The embryologic heart begins as a pair of tubes on either side of the embryo that fuse into a single heart tube. As development continues, a series of alternating constrictions and dilatations occur forming distinct segments (from superior to inferior): truncus arteriosus (TA), conus cordis (CC), bulbus cordis (BC), primitive ventricle (PV), common atria (CA) (**Figure 1-8**, left). As the superior and inferior ends of the heart tube are anchored in position, the heart continues to grow, the heart tube folds over itself anteriorly and rightward to form the normal dextral bulboventricular loop (**Figure 1-8**, right). This leaves the apex of the heart pointing toward the left of the embryo.

TEACHING POINT

In abnormal looping, the primitive heart tube folds anteriorly and leftward within the embryo. A complete inversion of the cardiac loop results in the apex pointing toward the right of the embryo and is referred to as dextrocardia. Abnormal looping can be referred to as levo-looping and can cause congenitally corrected transposition of the great arteries, which is when the left and right ventricles switch places.

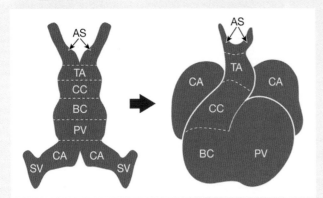

Figure 1-8 This image represents the transformation of the primitive heart tube into the bulboventricular cardiac loop. AS, aortic sac; BC, bulbus cordis; CA, common atria; CC, conus cordis; PV, primitive ventricle; SV, sinus venosus; TA, truncus arteriosus. (Reproduced with permission by Echotext Pty Ltd, from Anderson B. *A Sonographer's Guide to the Assessment of Heart Disease.* 1st ed. Australia: Echotext Pty Ltd; 2014:464.)

30. **Answer: C.** There are four stages in the formation of the IAS (**Figure 1-9**). Stage 1: the primum septum grows inferiorly toward the endocardial cushions from the roof of the common atrium. Stage 2: the primum septum continues its growth toward the endocardial cushions. Before it fuses with the endocardial cushions, perforations appear in the middle to upper septum to form the foramen secundum. Stage 3: the secundum septum begins to form and grow inferiorly from the roof of the atria and to the right of the primum septum. This secundum septum does not block flow from crossing the foramen secundum. Stage 4: the initial primum septum disappears and the remaining primum septum acts as a flap or valve at the level of the foramen secundum that is now called the foramen ovale.

31. **Answer: B.** There are four stages in the development of the IVS (**Figure 1-10**). Stage 1: the trabecular or muscular septum begins forming from the apex toward the base of the heart, stopping short of the atrioventricular canal, allowing blood to flow between the bulbus cordis and primitive ventricle toward the truncus arteriosus. Stage 2: trabeculations from the inlet region grow perpendicular to the trabecular IVS, forming the inlet IVS. Stage 3: the conotruncal (or aorticopulmonary) septum grows in a spiral direction, dividing the truncus arteriosus into the aorta and pulmonary artery. This conotruncal septum also divides the conus cordis into right and left ventricular outflow tracts also known as the outlet IVS. Stage 4: the outlet septum fuses with the endocardial cushions, inlet septum, and trabecular septum to form the membranous IVS that completes the IVS development.

32. **Answer: A.** At the end of the fifth week, two swellings of tissue appear on the sides of the truncus arteriosus and are referred to as conotruncal ridges. The aorticopulmonary septum develops from the conotruncal ridges. The aorticopulmonary septum is also known as the conotruncal septum.

33. **Answer: C.** The endocardial cushions are pairs of thickened tissue located on each side of the common atrioventricular canal; this includes the superior and inferior endocardial cushions and two lateral endocardial cushions. The endocardial cushions swell as cells migrate from the primitive endocardium and subsequently convert to mesenchymal tissue. The growth or swelling of the endocardial cushions occurs predominantly in the superior and inferior cushions (**Figure 1-11**). As these cushions grow toward each other, they protrude into the common atrioventricular (AV) canal. As the tissue continues to grow, the superior and inferior endocardial cushions eventually fuse to form a septum dividing the canal into two

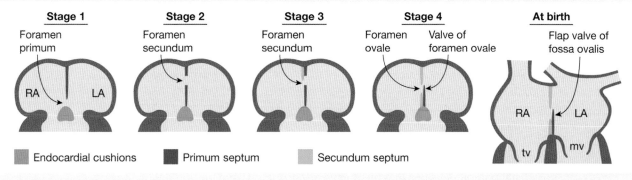

Figure 1-9 Formation of the interatrial septum. LA, left atrium; mv, mitral valve; RA, right atrium; tv, tricuspid valve. (Reproduced with permission by Echotext Pty Ltd, from Anderson B. *A Sonographer's Guide to the Assessment of Heart Disease.* 1st ed. Australia: Echotext Pty Ltd; 2014:432.)

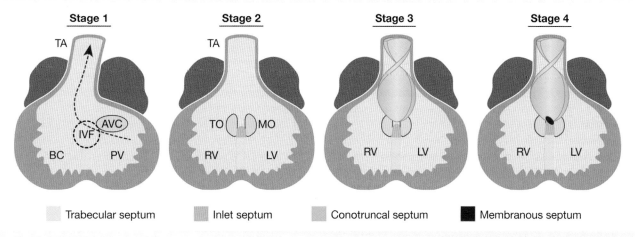

Figure 1-10 Formation of the interventricular septum. AVC, atrioventricular canal; BC, bulbis cordis; IVF, interventricular foramen; LV, left ventricle; MO, mitral orifice; PV, primitive ventricle; RV, right ventricle; TA, truncus arteriosus; TO, tricuspid orifice. (Reproduced with permission by Echotext Pty Ltd, from Anderson B. *A Sonographer's Guide to the Assessment of Heart Disease.* 1st ed. Australia: Echotext Pty Ltd; 2014:440.)

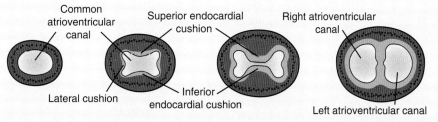

Figure 1-11 Formation of the septum in the atrioventricular canal. (Reprinted with permission from Sadler TW. The cardiovascular system. In: *Langman's Medical Embryology.* 14th ed. Philadelphia, PA: Wolters Kluwer; 2018:chap 13.)

channels, the right AV canal and the left AV canal. These separate channels eventually become the orifices of the mitral and tricuspid valves.

KEY POINTS

The endocardial cushions are essential for normal development of the primum atrial septum, inlet ventricular septum, and AV orifices. An endocardial cushion defect, also known as an atrioventricular canal defect, will occur if the endocardial cushions fail to develop. The endocardial cushion defect is characterized by a primum atrial septal defect, an inlet ventricular septal defect, and a common AV valve.

34. Answer: C. There are three stages in the formation of the aorta. Stage 1: the aortic sac is adjacent to the truncus arteriosus and there are six pairs of aortic arches that branch off the aortic sac. Stage 2: as the embryo develops, the aortic arch system is greatly modified and gradually loses its original symmetry. Stage 3: ultimately, the aortic arch is formed by segments of the aortic sac, the fourth left aortic arch and the left dorsal aorta. The fate and evolution of the aortic arches and other related structures are summarized in **Table 1-5** and illustrated in **Figure 1-12**.

Table 1-5. Important Derivatives of the Aortic Arches

Origin	Left	Right
Aortic sac	Proximal segment of aortic arch	Right brachiocephalic artery
Third arches	Left common carotid artery Proximal portion of left internal carotid arteries	Right common carotid artery Proximal portion of right internal carotid arteries
Fourth arches	Definitive aortic arch	Proximal right subclavian artery
Sixth arches	Proximal portion develops into left pulmonary artery Distal portion develops into the ductus arteriosus	Proximal portion develops into right pulmonary artery Distal portion degenerates
Seventh intersegmental arteries	Left subclavian artery	Distal part of right subclavian artery (in conjunction with right dorsal aorta)
Dorsal aortas	Distal aortic arch and descending aorta Distal portion of left internal carotid artery	Right subclavian artery Distal portion of right internal carotid artery

35. **Answer: D.** The aorticopulmonary septum divides the truncus arteriosus into the aorta and pulmonary artery.

36. **Answer: A.** The bulbus cordis forms the definitive RV. The conus cordis (option B) is divided by the truncus arteriosus into the right and left ventricular outflow tracts. The primitive ventricle (option C) forms the definitive left ventricle. The sinus venosus (option D) develops into the superior vena cava, inferior vena cava, and coronary sinus. **Table 1-6** summarizes the major derivatives of the primary heart tube segments.

37. **Answer: A.** Following normal cardiac looping, the bulbus cordis is located anterior, inferior, and to the right. The bulbus cordis eventually forms the right ventricle. **Table 1-7** summarizes the major derivatives of the primary heart tube segments and their positions following normal cardiac looping.

38. **Answer: B.** The Eustachian valve is the valve of the IVC and sits at the entrance to the right atrium (RA). In fetal circulation, the Eustachian valve serves to direct flow through the foramen ovale into the left atrium. This ensures that oxygenated blood from the maternal placenta is directed toward the fetal brain and also prevents "flooding" of the underdeveloped lungs.

The Chiari network (option A) is a fenestrated variant of the Eustachian valve. The thebesian valve (option C) is located at the entrance of the coronary sinus. It protects the coronary sinus from regurgitation when the RA contracts. The tricuspid valve (option D) is the right atrioventricular valve between the RA and right ventricle.

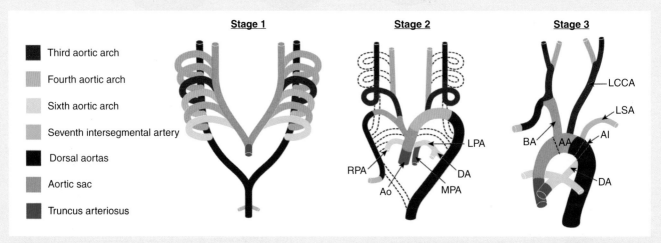

Figure 1-12 Formation of the aorta and fate of the embryological aortic arches. AA, aortic arch; AI, aortic isthmus; Ao, aorta; BA, brachiocephalic artery; DA, ductus arteriosus; LCCA, left common carotid artery; LPA, left pulmonary artery; LSA, left subclavian artery; MPA, main pulmonary artery; RPA, right pulmonary artery. (Reproduced with permission by Echotext Pty Ltd, from Anderson B. *A Sonographer's Guide to the Assessment of Heart Disease.* 1st ed. Australia: Echotext Pty Ltd; 2014:456.)

Table 1-6. Major Derivatives of the Primitive Heart Tube

Origin	Derivative
Truncus arteriosus	Aortic and pulmonary artery trunks
Conus cordis	Right and left ventricular outflow tracts
Bulbus cordis	Right ventricle
Primitive ventricle	Left ventricle
Common atria	Right and left atria
Sinus venosus	SVC, IVC, coronary sinus

IVC, inferior vena cava, SVC, superior vena cava.

39. **Answer: D. Figure 1-13** shows the normal fetal circulation. Inferior vena caval flow is directed across the foramen ovale by the Eustachian valve. The flow through the foramen ovale is circulated through the left side of the heart and ejected into the aorta and circulates through the systemic system. Superior vena caval flow enters the right atrium and is directed through the tricuspid valve into the right ventricle (RV). The flow from the RV is ejected into the pulmonary artery. The pulmonary arteries are extremely resistant to flow in the fetus and therefore most pulmonary artery flow is redirected through the ductus arteriosus, which is a connection between the pulmonary artery and aorta at the level of the aortic isthmus. Very little blood flow reaches the lungs and therefore very little blood reaches the pulmonary veins. Therefore, in fetal circulation, the left atrium receives most of its blood from the right side of the heart through the foramen ovale.

40. **Answer: B.** After birth, the lungs inflate with air and pulmonary vascular resistance decreases. This causes blood flow to increase through the pulmonary arteries and through to the pulmonary bed. The right atrial pressure decreases, and the left atrial pressure increases resulting in the closure of the foramen ovale. In the majority of individuals,

the septum primum flap fuses to the septum secundum, resulting in the permanent closure of the foramen ovale.

41. **Answer: C.** The ductus arteriosus is formed from the left distal sixth aortic arch. In the fetal circulation, the resistance in the pulmonary vessels is high and therefore most of the blood entering the pulmonary trunk is directed to the ductus arteriosus and away from the fluid-filled and underdeveloped fetal lungs. The oxygen content of blood entering the ductus arteriosus is quite high since oxygenated blood from the placenta enters the inferior vena cava, mixes with a small amount of deoxygenated blood from the right atrium, travels to the right ventricle and the pulmonary trunk, and is then directed to the ductus arteriosus (see **Figure 1-13**). Closure of the ductus arteriosus occurs almost immediately after birth due to the release of bradykinin from the lungs during initial inflation, which constricts the muscular wall of the ductus arteriosus.

42. **Answer: B.** The obliterated ductus arteriosus forms the ligamentum arteriosum. Other postnatal changes to the fetal adaptations necessary for normal fetal circulation are summarized in **Table 1-8**. In normal circumstances, these adaptations all close and become remnants.

Table 1-7. Major Derivatives of the Primitive Heart Tube and Positions After Normal Cardiac Looping

Origin	Derivative	Position After Looping
Truncus arteriosus	Aortic and pulmonary artery trunks	Slightly rightward
Conus cordis	Right and left ventricular outflow tracts	Rightward and anterior
Bulbus cordis	Right ventricle	Anterior, inferior, and to the right
Primitive ventricle	Left ventricle	Leftward
Common atria	Right and left atrium	Posterior and superior
Sinus venosus	SVC, IVC, coronary sinus	Posterior

IVC, inferior vena cava, SVC, superior vena cava.

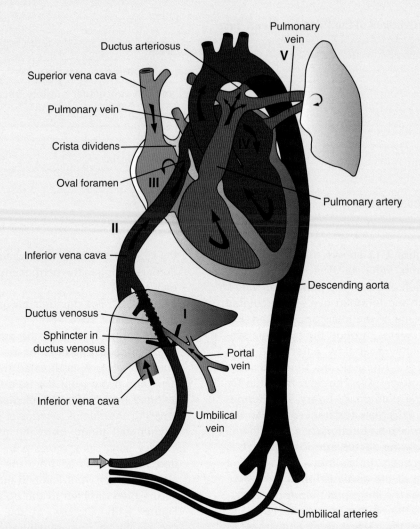

Figure 1-13 Fetal circulation before birth. *Arrows*, direction of blood flow. Note where oxygenated blood mixes with deoxygenated blood in: the liver (I), the inferior vena cava (II), the right atrium (III), the left atrium (IV), and at the entrance of the ductus arteriosus into the descending aorta (V). Shades of red and pink indicate oxygenated blood; blue indicates deoxygenated blood. (Reprinted with permission from Sadler TW. The cardiovascular system. In: *Langman's Medical Embryology*. 14th ed. Philadelphia, PA: Wolters Kluwer; 2018:chap 13.)

Table 1-8. Adaptations and Remnants of Fetal Circulation

Adaptation	Adaptation Function	Remnant
Ductus venosus	Bypass the liver	Ligamentum venosum
Foramen ovale	Bypass high resistant pulmonary circulation	Fossa ovalis
Ductus arteriosus	Bypass high resistant pulmonary circulation	Ligamentum arteriosum
Umbilical vein	Brings oxygenated blood from the placenta to the fetus	Ligamentum teres

SUGGESTED READINGS

Anderson B. Introduction to congenital heart disease. In: *A Sonographer's Guide to the Assessment of Heart Disease*. Echotext Pty Ltd; 2014:chap 15.

Drake RL, Vogl W, Mitchell AW. *Gray's Anatomy for Students*. 4th ed. Philadelphia, PA: Elsevier Inc; 2020.

Fuster V, Harrington RA, Narula J, Eapen ZJ, McGraw-Hill Companies. Functional anatomy of the heart. In: *Hurst's the Heart*. 14th ed. New York: McGraw-Hill Education; 2017:chap 14.

Gosling JA, Harris PF, Humpherson JR, Whitmore I, Willan PL. Thorax. In: *Human Anatomy, Color Atlas and Textbook E-Book*. Elsevier Health Sciences; 2016:chap 2.

Maleszewski JJ, Edwards WD. Cardiac anatomy and examination of cardiac specimens. In: Allen HD, Shaddy RE, Penny DJ, Feltes TF, Cetta F, eds. *Moss and Adams' Heart Disease in Infants, Children, and Adolescents. Including the Fetus and Young Adult.* 9th ed. Wolters Kluwer; 2016:chap 6.

McKinley MP, O'Loughlin VD, Bidle TS. Cardiovascular system: the heart. In: *Anatomy & Physiology: An Integrative Approach.* New York, NY: McGraw-Hill; 2013:chap 19.

Moore K, Persaud T, Torchia M. Cardiovascular system. In: *The Developing Human: Clinically Oriented Embryology.* 10th ed. Elsevier; 2015:chap 13.

Sadler TW. The cardiovascular system. In: *Langman's Human Embryology.* 14th ed. Wolters Kluwer; 2019:chap 13.

Saremi F. Anatomy of the heart for a dissector. In: *Revisiting Cardiac Anatomy: A Computed-Tomography-Based Atlas and Reference.* John Wiley & Sons; 2011:chap 1.

Saremi F, Sánchez-Quintana D, Mori S, et al. Fibrous skeleton of the heart: anatomic overview and evaluation of pathologic conditions with CT and MR imaging. *Radiographics.* 2017;37(5):1330-1351.

Schoenwolf G, Bleyl S, Brauer P, Francis-West P. Development of the heart. In: *Larsen's Human Embryology.* 5th ed. Churchill Livingstone; 2014:chap 12.

Tortora GJ, Peoples G, Derrickson B, et al. The cardiovascular system: the heart. In: *Principles of Anatomy and Physiology.* First Asia-Pacific ed. Milton, QLD: Wiley; 2016.

CHAPTER 2

Cardiac Physiology

Contributors: Andy Pellett, PhD, RDCS and Matt Umland, BS, ACS, RDCS

✪ Question 1

Cardiac muscle contraction is initiated by the binding of which ion to a regulatory contractile protein in the cell?
  A. Calcium
  B. Magnesium
  C. Potassium
  D. Sodium

✪✪ Question 2

In **Figure 2-1**, showing the left ventricular, aortic, and left atrial pressure traces, the letter "B" corresponds to which phase of the cardiac cycle?

  A. Diastasis
  B. Ejection
  C. Rapid filling
  D. Isovolumetric contraction

✪✪ Question 3

In **Figure 2-2**, showing left ventricular, aortic, and left atrial pressure traces, the letter "D" corresponds to which valvular event?
  A. Mitral valve closure
  B. Mitral valve opening
  C. Aortic valve closure
  D. Aortic valve opening

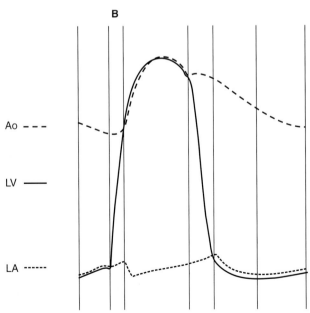

Figure 2-1 Ao, aortic pressure trace; LA, left atrial pressure trace; LV, left ventricular pressure trace.

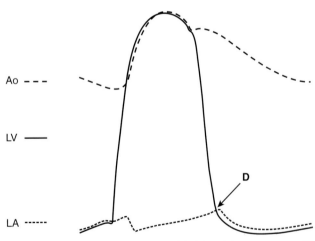

Figure 2-2 Ao, aortic pressure trace; LA, left atrial pressure trace; LV, left ventricular pressure trace.

✪ Question 4

On the spectral Doppler trace, the left ventricular inflow E-wave occurs immediately after which event of the electrocardiogram (ECG)?

A. P wave
B. P-R interval
C. QRS complex
D. T wave

✪✪ Question 5

Which of the following events will cause an increase in venous return to the right side of the heart?

A. Forced expiration against a closed glottis
B. Deep inspiration
C. Moving from a supine to a standing position
D. Rolling from a supine to a prone position

✪✪✪ Question 6

▶ According to the law of Laplace, if the patient's blood pressure is normal, the left ventricle seen in **Video 2-1** likely has an increased:

A. Contractility.
B. Coronary blood flow.
C. Stroke volume.
D. Wall stress.

✪✪ Question 7

Parasympathetic stimulation will primarily cause which of the following variables to decrease?

A. Heart rate
B. Stroke volume
C. Systemic vascular resistance
D. Venous return

✪✪ Question 8

The Frank-Starling mechanism states that an increase in end-diastolic volume will cause an increase in:

A. Heart rate.
B. Mean arterial pressure.
C. Stroke volume.
D. Ventricular contractility.

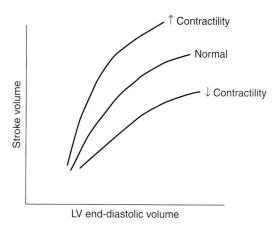

Figure 2-3

✪ Question 9

The normal range of left atrial pressure is:

A. 2 to 6 mm Hg.
B. 4 to 12 mm Hg.
C. 10 to 20 mm Hg.
D. 15 to 30 mm Hg.

✪✪ Question 10

Short-term control of mean arterial pressure is primarily affected by:

A. Arterial baroreceptors.
B. Arterial chemoreceptors.
C. Cardiopulmonary baroreceptors.
D. The kidneys.

✪✪ Question 11

Administration of a drug that dilates systemic arterioles will cause an immediate:

A. Increase in blood pressure.
B. Decrease in stroke volume.
C. Decrease in systemic vascular resistance.
D. Increase in venous return.

✪ Question 12

Atrial contraction occurs immediately after which electrocardiographic event?

A. P wave
B. QRS complex
C. T wave
D. U wave

✪ Question 13

The arrow in **Figure 2-4** points to which phase of the cardiac cycle?

    A. Atrial contraction
    B. Diastasis
    C. Isovolumetric relaxation
    D. Rapid filling

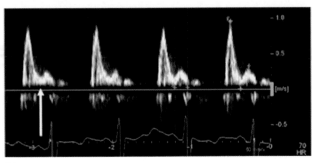
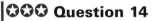

Figure 2-4

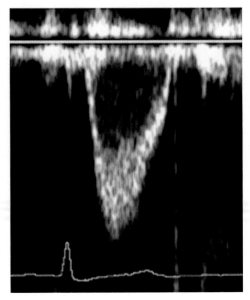

Figure 2-5

✪✪✪ Question 14

The speed of electrical conduction is slowest through the:

    A. Atrial muscle.
    B. Atrioventricular node.
    C. Bundle of His.
    D. Purkinje fibers.

✪✪✪ Question 15

A patient in cardiac tamponade may exhibit tachycardia. This increased heart rate is likely due to:

    A. A direct effect of a decrease in venous return.
    B. A direct effect of an increase in venous return.
    C. Reflex activation of the parasympathetic nervous system.
    D. Reflex activation of the sympathetic nervous system.

✪ Question 16

The left ventricular outflow tract (LVOT) velocity waveform in **Figure 2-5** is associated with which phase of the cardiac cycle?

    A. Isovolumetric contraction
    B. Isovolumetric relaxation
    C. Rapid filling
    D. Ventricular ejection

✪✪ Question 17

What is the relationship between the mean arterial pressure (MAP), heart rate (HR), stroke volume (SV), and systemic vascular resistance (SVR)?

    A. $MAP = HR + SV + SVR$
    B. $MAP = (HR \times SV) - SVR$
    C. $MAP = HR \times SV \times SVR$
    D. $MAP = (HR - SV) + SVR$

✪✪✪ Question 18

A premature ventricular complex typically causes:

    A. A decrease in ventricular contractility.
    B. A decrease in peak aortic velocity.
    C. An increase in left ventricular end-diastolic volume.
    D. An increase in the peak velocity of tricuspid regurgitation.

✪✪ Question 19

What is the greatest determinant of resistance to blood flow?

    A. Blood flow velocity
    B. Blood vessel length
    C. Blood vessel radius
    D. Blood viscosity

✪✪ Question 20

Which of the following conditions involves an increase in left ventricular afterload?

- A. Systemic hypotension
- B. Aortic stenosis
- C. Mitral regurgitation
- D. Mitral stenosis

✪ Question 21

Which of the following represents the normal pressures in the pulmonary artery?

- A. 20/15 mm Hg with a mean of 18 mm Hg
- B. 25/10 mm Hg with a mean of 15 mm Hg
- C. 30/10 mm Hg with a mean of 25 mm Hg
- D. 45/20 mm Hg with a mean of 15 mm Hg

✪ Question 22

Cardiac output is increased by:

- A. Exercise.
- B. Carotid sinus massage.
- C. Hypothyroidism.
- D. Hemorrhage.

✪ Question 23

Regarding ventricular depolarization, which occurs first?

- A. Depolarization of the apex of the left ventricle
- B. Depolarization of the base of the left ventricular free wall
- C. Depolarization of the base of the right ventricular free wall
- D. Depolarization of the interventricular septum

✪✪ Question 24

The rapid initial depolarization of a ventricular myocyte during an action potential (phase 0) is caused by a sudden:

- A. Increase in permeability of the membrane to chloride ions.
- B. Decrease in the rate at which sodium ion is pumped out of the cell.
- C. Increase in permeability of the membrane to sodium ions.
- D. Decrease in permeability of the membrane to potassium ions.

✪ Question 25

Phase 4 of the ventricular myocyte action potential correlates with which portion of the cardiac cycle?

- A. Diastole
- B. Systole
- C. Isovolumic contraction
- D. Isovolumic relaxation

✪ Question 26

The ability of a cardiac muscle cell to respond to a stimulus is known as:

- A. Automaticity.
- B. Excitability.
- C. Conductivity.
- D. Rhythmicity.

✪✪✪ Question 27

The renin-angiotensin-aldosterone system is most important in:

- A. Preventing hypotension when standing up rapidly.
- B. Maintenance of blood pressure during hemorrhage.
- C. Long-term control of blood pressure and volume.
- D. Increasing myocardial blood flow during exercise.

✪ Question 28

The initial event of diastole is:

- A. Aortic valve closure.
- B. Atrial contraction.
- C. Isovolumetric relaxation.
- D. Mitral valve opening.

✪ Question 29

What is the intrinsic rate of depolarization of the atrioventricular junction?

- A. 20 to 40 beats per minute (bpm)
- B. 40 to 60 bpm
- C. 60 to 80 bpm
- D. 80 to 100 bpm

✪✪ Question 30

Cardiac reserve is defined as the:

- A. Cardiac output divided by the body surface area.
- B. Difference between myocardial contractility at rest compared to stress.
- C. Difference between resting and maximal cardiac output.
- D. End-systolic volume following ventricular ejection.

✪✪ Question 31

Which portion of the systemic circulation has the highest vascular resistance?

   A. Arteries
   B. Arterioles
   C. Capillaries
   D. Veins

✪ Question 32

Which heart sound is associated with atrial contraction?

   A. S_1 (first heart sound)
   B. S_2 (second heart sound)
   C. S_3 (third heart sound)
   D. S_4 (fourth heart sound)

✪ Question 33

Which term is utilized to describe the amount of stretch of the left ventricular myocardium at end-diastole?

   A. Afterload
   B. Cardiac output
   C. Preload
   D. Stroke volume

✪ Question 34

The bundle of His receives an electrical impulse from the:

   A. AV node.
   B. Purkinje fibers.
   C. Right and left bundle branches.
   D. SA node.

✪✪ Question 35

Left ventricular ejection fraction is decreased by a sudden:

   A. Decrease in heart rate.
   B. Decrease in systemic vascular resistance.
   C. Increase in afterload.
   D. Increase in preload.

ANSWERS

1. **Answer: A.** Both sodium and calcium enter the cardiac muscle cell during the myocardial action potential. Calcium entry triggers the release of more calcium from the sarcoplasmic reticulum, whereupon the released calcium binds to the regulatory protein troponin C. Binding of calcium to troponin C causes the protein tropomyosin to shift, allowing myosin to bind to actin, beginning the process by which these contractile filaments slide past one another, shortening the muscle.

2. **Answer: D.** Isovolumetric contraction, which is the period of time during which the ventricles contract and all four valves are closed, extends from mitral valve closure (MVc) to aortic valve opening (AVo) for the left side of the heart (**Figure 2-6**). The mitral valve closes when left ventricular (LV) pressure rises above left atrial (LA) pressure at the onset of systole, and the aortic valve opens when LV pressure surpasses aortic (Ao) pressure. During isovolumetric contraction, although the ventricles are contracting, there is no change in the ventricular volume, hence, the term isovolumetric meaning same (iso) volume.

3. **Answer: B.** The mitral valve opens when the LV pressure falls below the LA pressure, after which rapid filling of the LV occurs.

4. **Answer: D.** The T wave of the ECG represents ventricular repolarization, which leads to ventricular relaxation, during which the LV pressure decreases.

When the LV pressure falls below the LA pressure, the mitral valve opens, and rapid filling occurs. The flow of blood into the LV is associated with the transmitral E-wave velocity that is measured across the mitral valve.

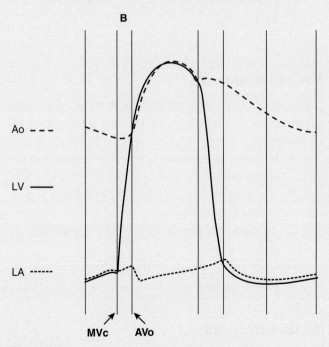

Figure 2-6

5. **Answer: B.** Deep inspiration causes a decrease in intrathoracic pressure, including right atrial (RA) pressure, which represents the downstream pressure for venous return. Thus, blood is "sucked" into the RA. At the same time, inferior movement of the diaphragm compresses abdominal veins, pushing blood toward the heart. Forced expiration (answer A) will have the opposite effect, causing an immediate decrease in venous return. Moving from a supine to a standing position (answer C) allows gravity to pull blood away from the heart, thereby decreasing venous return. Turning over from a supine to a prone position (answer D) should have no significant effect on the return of blood to the RA.

6. **Answer: D.** The law of Laplace states that ventricular wall stress (σ) is equal to ventricular transmural pressure (P) multiplied by the radius (r) divided by two times wall thickness (h):

$$\sigma = \left(P \times r \right) \div \left(2 \times h \right)$$

The ventricle in **Video 2-1** is dilated, leading to an increase in wall stress, which can be derived from the Laplace equation, given the increased radius, normal blood pressure, and lack of significant wall thickening. Answers A and C are incorrect since poor systolic function is associated with decreased contractility and stroke volume. While an increase in wall stress may lead to an increase in coronary blood flow, the law of Laplace makes no inferences about blood flow, and the poor ventricular systolic function may be associated with chronic ischemia, making answer B an incorrect choice.

KEY POINT

The law of Laplace describes the relationship between the tension or wall stress, intracavity pressure, radius, and the thickness of a thinned-walled sphere. This law explains why a dilated ventricle requires more tension to generate the same pressure as a normal ventricle.

7. **Answer: A.** Parasympathetic (vagal) nerves primarily innervate the sinoatrial (SA) and atrioventricular (AV) nodes, the atria, and some arterioles. In the heart, parasympathetic (vagal) stimulation causes local release of acetylcholine, which results in slowing of SA node impulse formation and slowed conduction with lengthening of the refractory period in the AV node, thus, causing a decrease in heart rate.

Answer B is incorrect since strong parasympathetic stimulation may decrease heart rate sufficiently to allow more time for filling of the ventricles and cause an increase (not a decrease) in stroke volume. Parasympathetic stimulation also relaxes arteriolar smooth muscle in some vascular beds, but not enough to affect systemic vascular resistance; therefore, answer C is incorrect. Parasympathetic nerves do not innervate veins and thus do not directly affect venous return; therefore, answer D is incorrect.

8. **Answer: C.** **Figure 2-3** shows the Frank-Starling mechanism in the heart, which expresses the length-tension relationship of cardiac muscle fibers and, in the ventricle, relates end-diastolic volume (EDV) to stroke volume (SV). When cardiac muscle is stretched, as it would be with an increased EDV, more myosin heads are able to bind to actin, causing a more forceful contraction and the ejection of more blood; thus, the stroke volume increases. Also shown in **Figure 2-3** is how changing contractility affects the Frank-Starling curve. Changes in EDV involve movement to the left or right along the "Normal" curve in **Figure 2-3**, whereas alterations in contractility shift the curve up and to the left (increased contractility), or down and to the right (decreased contractility), and are independent of EDV. Ventricular contractility is specifically related to an increase in calcium ion concentration in the cardiac muscle cell, which is not a cause of the myocardial length-tension relationship; therefore, answer D is incorrect.

KEY POINT

An increase in venous return to the heart increases the EDV, which stretches the muscle fibers, thereby increasing preload. This increase in EDV, with no change in the end-systolic volume, will result in an increase in stroke volume. The overall result of increased preload, within a physiological limit, is an increase in the force of ventricular contraction. Decreasing preload has the opposite effects. A decrease in venous return results in a decrease in preload (EDV), which leads to a decrease in SV and a decrease in the force of ventricular contraction.

9. **Answer: B.** The normal range of left atrial pressure is 4 to 12 mm Hg. Left atrial pressure is a variable with which sonographers and cardiologists should be familiar, as it is a measure of filling pressure for the left side of the heart, and therefore may influence patient symptoms and prognosis.

10. **Answer: A.** Arterial baroreceptors are high-pressure stretch receptors located in the carotid sinus and aortic arch. These receptors rapidly convey the status of blood pressure in the form of action potential frequency, traveling via cranial nerves, to the medulla. Arterial chemoreceptors (answer B) are located in the carotid sinus and aortic arch but are involved with control of the rate and depth of breathing. Cardiopulmonary baroreceptors (answer C) are low-pressure receptors located in the heart and lungs that are more involved in regulating blood volume. The kidneys (answer D) are involved

in long-term (not short-term) control of blood pressure through mechanisms that take hours to days to exert their effects.

11. **Answer: C.** The degree of contraction of smooth muscle in arterioles determines systemic vascular resistance (SVR), which in turn directly affects MAP. SVR decreases when the systemic arterioles dilate. Answers A and B are incorrect since systemic arteriolar dilation will cause blood pressure to decrease, which may immediately increase stroke volume, as the heart spends less energy overcoming pressure and more energy on ejecting blood. Answer D is incorrect as arteriolar vasodilation will not increase venous return, as blood will tend to pool rather than return to the heart.

12. **Answer: A. Figure 2-7** shows the main waveforms of the ECG. The P wave represents atrial depolarization, which immediately precedes atrial contraction. The QRS complex (answer B) represents ventricular depolarization, which is followed by ventricular contraction. The T wave (answer C) represents the repolarization of the ventricles; the end of the T wave coincides with the end of ventricular systole. The U wave (answer D) is a small deflection that is sometimes seen immediately following the T wave; the U wave is thought to represent delayed repolarization of Purkinje fibers.

TEACHING POINT

Depolarization is an electrical event that results in myocardial contraction. Repolarization is also an electrical event and results in myocardial relaxation.

13. **Answer: B.** The arrow is pointing to the period of time between the mitral inflow E and A waves, during which little blood is flowing between the LA and LV. This period is known as diastasis. During diastasis, the LV and LA pressures are almost equal. Pressure equalization occurs due to the simultaneous decrease in the LAP as the atrium empties and the rise in the LV pressure as the ventricle fills. A small amount of blood continues to flow across the mitral valve during diastasis due to inertia. The duration of diastasis is determined by the heart rate; with slower heart rates

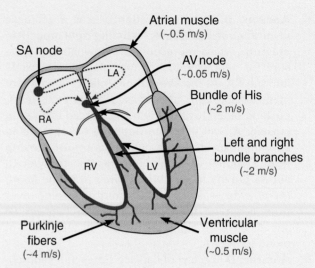

Figure 2-8 Conduction velocities of different regions within the conduction system of the heart. Note that Purkinje fibers have the highest conduction velocity and the atrioventricular (AV) node has the lowest conduction velocity. LA, left atrium; LV, left ventricle; RA, right atrium; RV, right ventricle; SA, sinoatrial. (Reprinted with permission from Klabunde RE. *Cardiovascular Physiology Concepts.* 2nd ed. Philadelphia, PA: Wolters Kluwer Health/Lippincott Williams & Wilkins; 2012:22.)

diastasis is longer, while at faster heart rates diastasis is shortened or it may be totally absent.

14. **Answer: B. Figure 2-8** illustrates the conduction system within the heart and the conduction velocities through the different regions. Cells in the atrioventricular (AV) node have a slow response action potential, which is associated with a relatively slow influx of positive ions, and therefore slow spread of the action potential. The slow conduction velocity is beneficial in that it allows complete atrial depolarization prior to ventricular depolarization, ensuring that subsequent contraction of the atria and ventricles will occur sequentially, rather than simultaneously.

15. **Answer: D.** Cardiac tamponade occurs when there is an increase in the intrapericardial pressure due to accumulation of an effusion, blood, clots, pus, gas, or combinations of these within the pericardium. This ultimately leads to compression of the heart, impeded diastolic filling of both ventricles, systemic and pulmonary congestion, and a decreased stroke volume, blood pressure, and cardiac output. The decreased blood pressure will decrease stretch of the arterial baroreceptors, leading to reduced action potential frequency in the afferent nerves traveling to the medulla. This leads to activation of the sympathetic nervous system, in an attempt to maintain blood pressure. One of the consequences of sympathetic stimulation is an increase in heart rate. Venous return will be reduced in tamponade, but this will not have a direct effect on heart rate.

16. **Answer: D.** Forward flow in the LVOT, occurring after the QRS complex, is associated with ventricular contraction and blood flowing across the aortic valve, which is the ventricular ejection phase of the cardiac cycle.

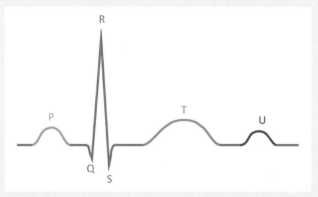

Figure 2-7

17. **Answer: C.** MAP is determined by the cardiac output (CO), SVR, and central venous pressure (CVP) as expressed below:

$$MAP = (CO \times SVR) + CVP \qquad (1)$$

Because CVP is usually at or near 0 mm Hg, this relationship is often simplified to:

$$MAP \approx (CO \times SVR) \qquad (2)$$

Cardiac output is derived from the heart rate (HR) and stroke volume (SV) as:

$$CO = (HR \times SV) \qquad (3)$$

Therefore, by combining Equations 2 and 3, the MAP is:

$$MAP \approx (HR \times SV \times SVR) \qquad (4)$$

This is an important relationship to keep in mind when attempting to figure out how blood pressure will be affected by various physiologic and pathologic conditions.

TEACHING POINT

More commonly, the MAP is estimated from the systolic blood pressure (SBP) and diastolic blood pressure (DBP) as:

$$MAP = DBP + 1/3(SBP - DBP)$$
or
$$MAP = SBP + [(2 \times DBP) \div 3]$$

18. **Answer: B.** A premature ventricular complex (PVC) shortens the normal filling time of the ventricles. Thus, the end-diastolic volume will decrease and, according to the Frank-Starling mechanism, the force of contraction of both ventricles will be reduced. This will result in a decrease in both peak aortic and tricuspid regurgitant velocities. Contractility is affected primarily by the sympathetic nervous system and is not directly affected by the amount of blood filling the ventricles (see answer outline for Question 8). It is important not to confuse the events of the PVC with those of the ensuing beat, which normally occurs after a compensatory pause, thereby increasing filling of the ventricles and the subsequent force of contraction.

19. **Answer: C.** Poiseuille equation expresses the relationship between volumetric flow rate (Q) determined by pressure difference (ΔP) and the resistance (R):

$$Q = \Delta P \div R \qquad (1)$$

Resistance to flow is determined by the viscosity of blood (η), the radius of the vessel lumen (r), and the length of the vessel (L) and is expressed by the following equation:

$$R = [8 \times L \times \eta] \div [\pi \times r^4] \qquad (2)$$

Therefore, since resistance is inversely proportional to the radius of a vessel raised to the fourth power, small changes in radius produce large changes in resistance. Blood flow viscosity and blood vessel length are also proportional to resistance but exert lesser effects than does radius.

20. **Answer: B.** Afterload may be described as the "load" or "pressure" that the heart must eject against. The most accurate clinical definition of afterload for the LV is the end-systolic wall stress (σ). As previously described, the wall stress can be determined by the law of Laplace. That is, wall stress is determined by the pressure, radius, and wall thickness (see the answer outline for Question 6); however, other variables may be substituted. For example, any variable that represents the work that the ventricle must pump against during systole, such as the MAP or SVR, can be used as a representation of afterload. Thus, systemic hypotension (answer A), which involves a decrease in MAP, causes a decrease in afterload. In a patient with aortic stenosis (answer B), the narrowed aortic orifice offers significantly increased resistance against which the LV must pump. The LV must develop higher systolic pressures, which in turn increases end-systolic wall stress. Mitral regurgitation (answer C) actually decreases afterload, as the LV can now pump blood both forward into the aorta and backward into the LA, effectively decreasing the resistance against which the LV must pump. Mitral stenosis (answer D) does not increase LV or aortic pressures or LV cavity size, and therefore does not increase afterload.

21. **Answer: B.** The normal pulmonary artery systolic and diastolic pressures are about 25 and 10 mm Hg, respectively with a normal mean pulmonary artery pressure of about 15 mm Hg. Pulmonary hypertension is defined as a mean pulmonary artery pressure ≥25 mm Hg. Echocardiography labs most commonly detect pulmonary hypertension using pulmonary artery systolic pressure (PASP). Although a threshold value of PASP for pulmonary hypertension has not been defined, a value of 35 to 40 mm Hg is consistent with American Society of Echocardiography guidelines.

22. **Answer: A.** Exercise is associated with activation of the sympathetic nervous system and thus increased heart rate, contractility, and venous return, all of which contribute to an increase in cardiac output. Carotid sinus massage (answer B) stimulates arterial baroreceptors, which leads to an activation of

the parasympathetic nervous system and a decrease in heart rate and cardiac output. Hypothyroidism (answer C) is associated with decreased total body metabolism and a decrease in cardiac output. Hemorrhage (answer D) decreases venous return and therefore decreases cardiac output.

23. **Answer: D.** Depolarization of the interventricular septum creates the "Q" wave of the electrocardiogram. The left and right ventricular free walls then depolarize, spreading from the apex to the base.

24. **Answer: C.** The action potential curve shows the electrical changes in the myocardial cell during the depolarization-repolarization cycle (**Figure 2-9**). Depolarization (phase 0) is the process of decreasing the potential difference across a cell membrane and during an action potential, reversing the polarity of that charge difference. Thus, the inside of the cell membrane becomes positive relative to the outside. This is caused by a rapid influx of sodium ions due to the opening of voltage-sensitive sodium channels.

25. **Answer: A.** In the ventricular myocyte, phase 4 occurs when the cell is at rest, in diastole. During this period potassium ions (K^+) are leaking out of the cell and sodium ions (Na^+) are leaking in (see **Figure 2-9**). To help to maintain a constant membrane electrical potential, an energy (ATP)-dependent pump system (Na^+/K^+-adenosine triphosphatase [ATPase]) is pumping these ions in the opposite directions; that is, Na^+ is pumped out and K^+ is pumped into the cell.

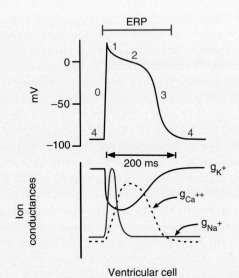

Figure 2-9 Changes in ion conductance associated with a ventricular myocyte action potential. Phase 0 (depolarization) primarily is due to the rapid increase in sodium conductance (gNa^+) accompanied by a fall in potassium conductance (gK^+); the initial repolarization of phase 1 is due to opening of special potassium channels; phase 2 (plateau) primarily is due to an increase in slow inward calcium conductance (gCa^{++}) through calcium channels; phase 3 (repolarization) results from an increase in gK^+ and a decrease in gCa^{++}. Phase 4 is a true resting potential that primarily reflects a high gK^+. ERP, effective refractory period. (Reprinted with permission from Klabunde RE. *Cardiovascular Physiology Concepts.* 2nd ed. Philadelphia, PA: Wolters Kluwer Health/Lippincott Williams & Wilkins; 2012:17.)

26. **Answer: B.** Ventricular muscle cells generate action potentials in response to an initial depolarization caused by the spread of electrical activity from adjacent depolarized cells. This ability to respond to the stimulus of depolarization by generating action potentials is known as excitability. Conductivity (answer C) permits a rapid spread of electrical activity following excitability. Automaticity (answer A) is the ability to generate an action potential in the absence of an external stimulus. Rhythmicity (answer D) refers to the repetitive manner in which spontaneous depolarization and repolarization occurs; that is, this is the rhythmic contraction of the heart.

27. **Answer: C.** Renin is an enzyme produced by cells in the afferent arterioles in the kidneys. Renin converts the plasma protein angiotensinogen to angiotensin I, which is then converted to angiotensin II by angiotensin-converting enzyme. Angiotensin II stimulates the release of aldosterone from the adrenal cortex. Aldosterone increases reabsorption of sodium and water by the kidneys. This process takes hours to days and thus is important in long-term control of blood pressure and volume. Blood pressure maintenance during hemorrhage (answer B) and movement from a supine to a standing position (answer A) involve the arterial baroreceptor reflex and activation of the sympathetic nervous system, which are rapid responses. Increasing myocardial blood flow during exercise (answer D) is caused by an increase in myocardial oxygen consumption and associated production of local vasodilators, which decreases coronary arterial resistance.

28. **Answer: A.** The events of the cardiac cycle are illustrated in **Figure 2-10**. Diastole begins when the LV stops contracting and starts relaxing. This immediately causes LV pressure to decrease below aortic pressure, which causes the aortic valve to close. Isovolumetric relaxation, which can be described as the initial "phase" of diastole, then ensues, followed by mitral valve opening and early rapid LV filling. Diastasis (also known as reduced filling) is the "middle" stage of diastole. Atrial contraction occurs in late diastole, right before systole begins.

29. **Answer: B.** The AV junction's normal intrinsic rate without stimulation is 40 to 60 times/min. This property, known as automaticity, is important because loss of this automatic depolarization by the SA node should still result in pacing of the ventricles by the slower pacemaking ability of the AV junction.

30. **Answer: C.** Cardiac reserve is the difference between resting and maximal cardiac output. The cardiac output divided by the body surface area (answer A) is the cardiac index. The difference between myocardial contractility at rest compared to stress (answer B) is the contractile reserve. The end-systolic volume following ventricular ejection (answer D) is simply the volume of blood remaining in the LV at the end of ventricular contraction, or systole.

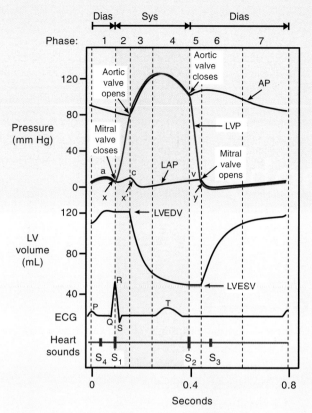

Figure 2-10 The seven phases of the cardiac cycle are (1) atrial systole; (2) isovolumetric contraction; (3) rapid ejection; (4) reduced ejection; (5) isovolumetric relaxation; (6) early rapid filling; and (7) diastasis. Sys, systole; Dias, diastole; AP, aortic pressure; LVP, left ventricular pressure; LAP, left atrial pressure; a, a wave; c, c wave; v, v wave; x, x descent; x', x' descent; y, y descent; LV, left ventricle; ECG, electrocardiogram; LVEDV, left ventricular end-diastolic volume; LVESV, left ventricular end-systolic volume, S1-S4, four heart sounds. (Reprinted with permission from Klabunde RE. *Cardiovascular Physiology Concepts.* 2nd ed. Philadelphia, PA: Wolters Kluwer Health/Lippincott Williams & Wilkins; 2012:63.)

31. **Answer: B.** Arterioles have muscular walls (usually only one to two layers of smooth muscle) and relatively small luminal diameters and are the primary site of vascular resistance as well as physiologic control of resistance. Arteries and veins also have smooth muscle in their walls, but their larger lumens create less resistance. Individual capillaries have very small luminal diameters, but their overall resistance is low because there are so many vessels arranged in parallel.

32. **Answer: D.** The fourth heart sound (S4), also known as the "atrial gallop," occurs just before S1 when the atria contract to force blood into the ventricles (see **Figure 2-10**). This heart sound is associated with a stiff, noncompliant ventricle and is always considered pathological. The first heart sound (S1) is associated with closure of the mitral and tricuspid valves, and the second heart sound (S2) is associated with closure of the aortic and pulmonic valves. The third heart sound (S3) is associated with rapid filling of the ventricles, which may be normal in younger individuals or pathological.

33. **Answer: C.** Preload is the amount of ventricular stretch at end-diastole. Clinical measures of LV preload include LV end-diastolic volume, LV end-diastolic pressure, and LA pressure. Afterload (answer A) is the pressure against which the heart must work to eject blood during systole. Cardiac output (answer B) is the volume of blood being pumped by the heart per minute. Stroke volume (answer D) is the volume of blood being pumped by the heart per beat.

34. **Answer: A.** The bundle of His receives impulses from the AV node and transmits to the bundle branches, followed by the Purkinje fibers, which spread electrical activity along the ventricular endocardium.

35. **Answer: C.** Ejection fraction is equal to stroke volume divided by end-diastolic volume. As previously described, afterload is the pressure against which the heart must work to eject blood during systole. With a sudden increase in afterload, the heart will eject less blood with each contraction, as more energy must be expended generating pressure and less energy is available to eject blood. As this stroke volume decreases, the end-systolic and end-diastolic volumes will increase, thus reducing the ejection fraction. Answer A is incorrect since a decrease in heart rate will allow more time for the left ventricle to fill, thus increasing preload, stroke volume, and ejection fraction. Answer B is incorrect as a decrease in systemic vascular resistance will increase stroke volume and ejection fraction. Answer D is incorrect since an increase in preload (end-diastolic volume) will increase stroke volume and ejection fraction.

SUGGESTED READINGS

Klabunde RE. *Cardiovascular Physiology Concepts.* 2nd ed. Philadelphia, PA: Lippincott Williams & Wilkins; 2012.

Pappano AJ, Wier WG. *Cardiovascular Physiology.* 10th ed. Philadelphia, PA: Mosby; 2012.

Mohrman DE, Heller LJ. *Cardiovascular Physiology.* 9th ed. New York, NY: McGraw-Hill Education; 2018.

CHAPTER 3

Electrocardiography

Contributors: Elaine A. Shea, ACS, RCCS, RCIS and Peg Knoll, RDCS, RCS

✪ Question 1

The standard 12-lead electrocardiogram (ECG) comprises how many electrodes?

A. 2
B. 3
C. 10
D. 12

✪ Question 2

The chest leads are also called:

A. Augmented leads.
B. Bipolar leads.
C. Limb leads.
D. Precordial leads.

✪ Question 3

Electrical impulses originating in the sinoatrial (SA) node produce the:

A. P wave.
B. QRS complex.
C. T wave.
D. U wave.

✪✪ Question 4

A Q wave that is greater than 0.04 seconds wide and one-third the height of the QRS complex is defined as:

A. Normal.
B. Isoelectric.
C. Pathologic.
D. Physiologic.

✪ Question 5

A wave of depolarization traveling away from a positive electrode will produce a:

A. Biphasic waveform.
B. Isoelectric waveform.
C. Negative waveform.
D. Positive waveform.

✪ Question 6

What is the normal duration for the PR interval?

A. <0.08 seconds
B. 0.08 to 0.10 seconds
C. 0.12 to 0.20 seconds
D. 0.20 to 0.26 seconds

✪ Question 7

What is the normal duration for the QRS interval?

A. <0.12 seconds
B. >0.12 seconds
C. 0.12 to 0.20 seconds
D. 0.20 to 0.26 seconds

✪ Question 8

The QRS complex represents:

A. Atrial depolarization.
B. Ventricular depolarization.
C. Atrial repolarization.
D. Ventricular repolarization.

✪ Question 9

The T wave represents:
- **A.** Atrial depolarization.
- **B.** Ventricular depolarization.
- **C.** Atrial repolarization.
- **D.** Ventricular repolarization.

✪✪ Question 10

Leads II, III, and aVF represent:
- **A.** Anterior leads.
- **B.** Inferior leads.
- **C.** Lateral leads.
- **D.** Posterior leads.

✪✪ Question 11

Leads I, aVL, V5, and V6 represent:
- **A.** Anterior leads.
- **B.** Inferior leads.
- **C.** Lateral leads.
- **D.** Posterior leads.

✪✪ Question 12

Leads V1, V2, V3, and V4 represent:
- **A.** Anterior leads.
- **B.** Inferior leads.
- **C.** Lateral leads.
- **D.** Posterior leads.

✪✪ Question 13

A short PR interval combined with a delta wave is defined as:
- **A.** Brugada syndrome.
- **B.** Lown-Ganong-Levine syndrome.
- **C.** Wellen syndrome.
- **D.** Wolff-Parkinson-White syndrome.

✪ Question 14

What is the heart rate range for normal sinus rhythm?
- **A.** 40 to 60 beats per minute (bpm)
- **B.** 60 to 80 bpm
- **C.** 60 to 100 bpm
- **D.** 100 to 120 bpm

✪✪ Question 15

An acute coronary event due to a coronary blockage without ST elevations on the electrocardiogram (ECG) is called:
- **A.** NSTEMI.
- **B.** PCI.
- **C.** STEMI.
- **D.** Thrombolysis.

✪✪✪ Question 16

The 12-lead electrocardiogram (ECG) in **Figure 3-1** might exhibit which finding on the echocardiogram?
- **A.** Anteroseptal hypokinesis
- **B.** Inferior wall hypokinesis
- **C.** Lateral wall akinesis
- **D.** Posterior wall akinesis

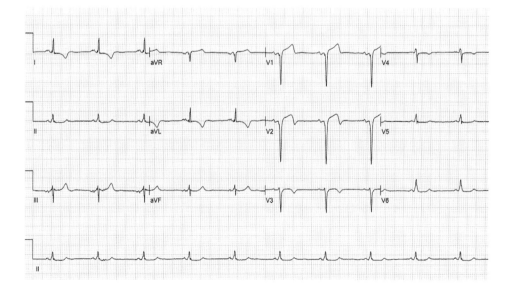

Figure 3-1

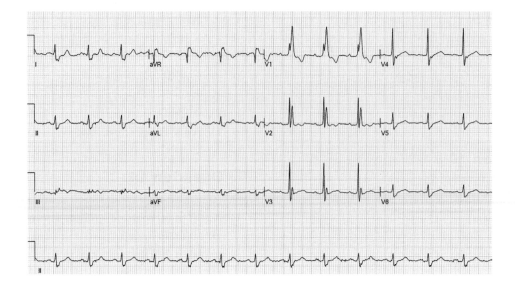

Figure 3-2

✪✪✪ Question 17

The 12-lead electrocardiogram (ECG) in **Figure 3-2** indicates what cardiac rhythm?

A. Sinus rhythm with left bundle branch block (LBBB)

B. Sinus rhythm with right bundle branch block (RBBB)

C. Sinus bradycardia with RBBB

D. Sinus bradycardia with LBBB

✪✪✪ Question 18

What is the rhythm on the 12-lead electrocardiogram (ECG) shown in **Figure 3-3**?

A. Atrial flutter

B. Atrial fibrillation

C. Sinus tachycardia

D. Sinus rhythm with premature atrial contractions

✪✪✪ Question 19

What is the paced rhythm on the 12-lead electrocardiogram (ECG) shown in **Figure 3-4**?

A. Ventricular paced with abnormal sensing

B. Atrial paced

C. Ventricular paced with normal sensing

D. Atrioventricular (AV) sequential pacing

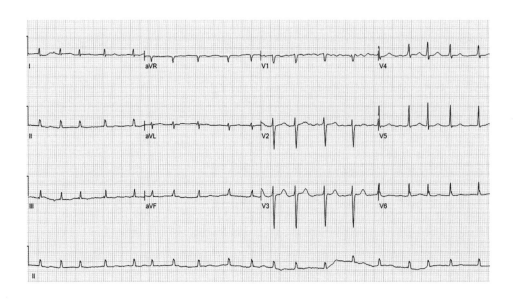

Figure 3-3

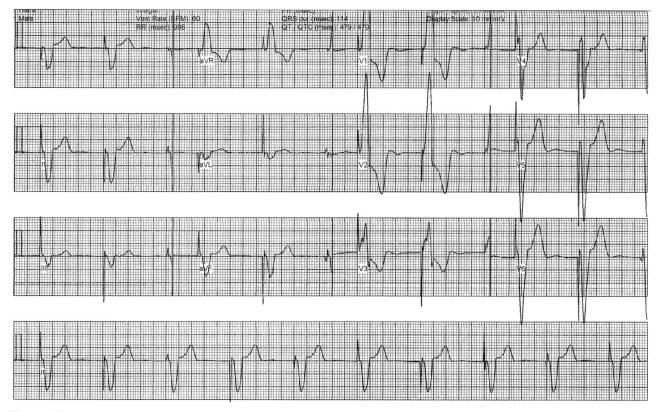

Figure 3-4

✪✪✪ Question 20

Which segments of the left ventricle will likely show regional wall motion abnormalities based on the 12-lead electrocardiogram (ECG) shown in **Figure 3-5**?
- **A.** Anterior wall
- **B.** Posterior wall
- **C.** Inferolateral wall
- **D.** Anterolateral wall

✪✪✪ Question 21

Which echocardiographic finding correlates with the 12-lead electrocardiogram (ECG) shown in **Figure 3-6**?
- **A.** Left atrial enlargement
- **B.** Left ventricular hypertrophy
- **C.** Right atrial enlargement
- **D.** Right ventricular hypertrophy

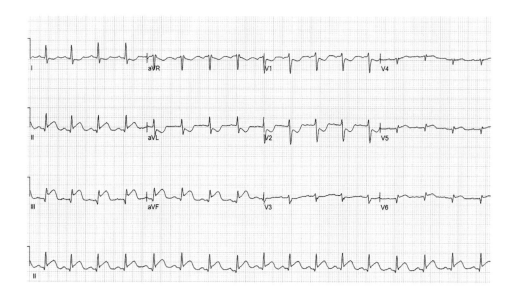

Figure 3-5

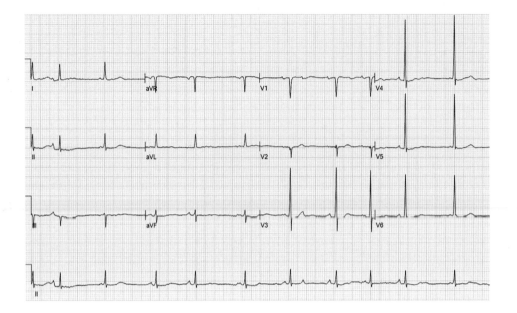

Figure 3-6

✪✪✪ Question 22

What is the rhythm shown on the 12-lead electrocardiogram (ECG) in **Figure 3-7**?

    A. Atrial fibrillation with premature atrial contractions (PACs)

    B. Atrial flutter with PACs

    C. Sinus tachycardia with premature ventricular contractions (PVCs)

    D. Sinus bradycardia with PVCs

✪✪✪ Question 23

What is the rhythm on the 12-lead electrocardiogram (ECG) shown in **Figure 3-8**?

    A. First-degree atrioventricular (AV) block

    B. Second-degree AV block Mobitz Type I

    C. Second-degree AV block Mobitz Type II

    D. Third-degree AV block

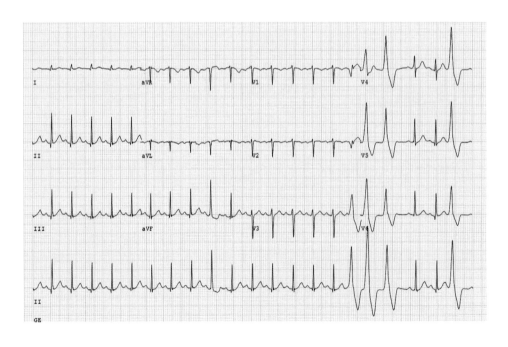

Figure 3-7

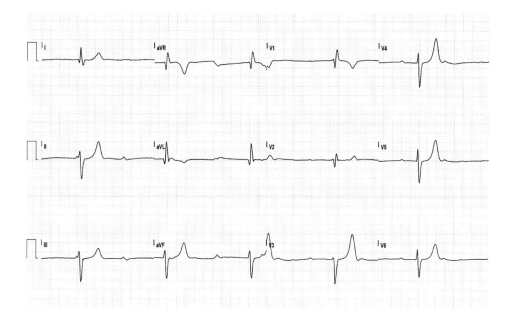

Figure 3-8

✪✪✪ Question 24

What echocardiographic finding is associated with the 12-lead electrocardiogram (ECG) shown in **Figure 3-9**?
- A. Left atrial enlargement
- B. Paradoxical septal motion
- C. Pulsus paradoxus
- D. Right ventricular volume overload

✪✪✪ Question 25

What is the rhythm on the 12-lead electrocardiogram (ECG) in **Figure 3-10**?

- A. Atrial fibrillation
- B. Atrial flutter
- C. Sinus tachycardia
- D. Sinus bradycardia

✪✪ Question 26

What is the rhythm on the 12-lead electrocardiogram (ECG) shown in **Figure 3-11**?
- A. Sinus tachycardia
- B. First-degree atrioventricular block
- C. Sinus bradycardia
- D. Ventricular tachycardia

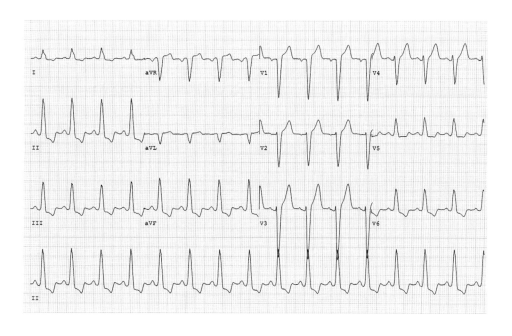

Figure 3-9

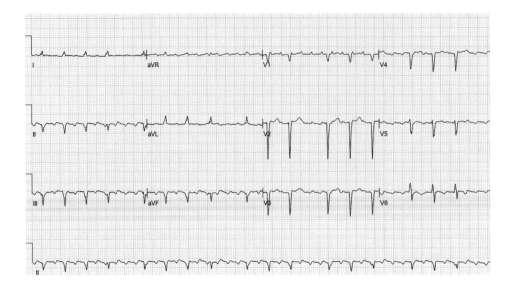

Figure 3-10

✪✪✪ Question 27

Which echocardiographic finding best correlates with the electrocardiographic rhythm shown in **Figure 3-12**?
- **A.** Pericardial effusion
- **B.** Mitral valve prolapse
- **C.** Left ventricular hypertrophy
- **D.** Right ventricular hypertrophy

✪✪✪ Question 28

What is the rhythm on the electrocardiogram (ECG) shown in **Figure 3-13**?
- **A.** Sinus arrest
- **B.** Junctional escape rhythm
- **C.** Complete heart block
- **D.** Wandering atrial pacemaker

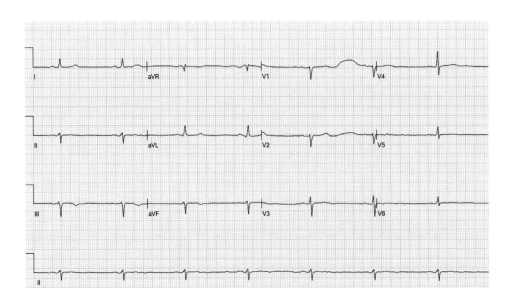

Figure 3-11

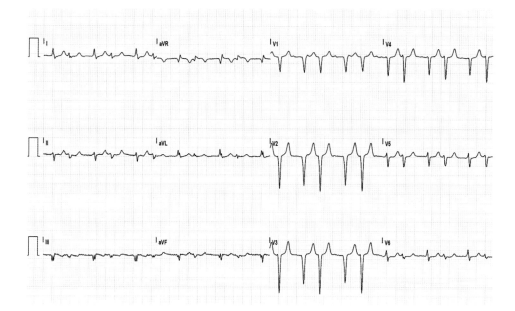

Figure 3-12

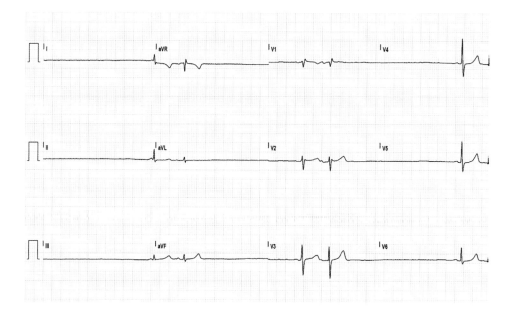

Figure 3-13

ANSWERS

1. **Answer: C.** There are 10 electrode positions for the 12-lead ECG. This includes six chest electrodes and four limb electrodes (**Figure 3-14**). Although it is called a 12-lead ECG, it uses only 10 electrodes.

2. **Answer: D.** Chest leads are also referred to as precordial leads. These precordial leads are unipolar leads that are composed of a single positive electrode and a reference point. The six precordial (chest or V leads) include V1, V2, V3, V4, V5, and V6.

   Augmented leads (answer A) are also unipolar leads that are composed of a single positive electrode and a reference point. There are three unipolar

limb leads: aVR (augmented vector right, positive electrode right shoulder), aVL (augmented vector left, positive electrode left shoulder), and aVF (augmented vector foot, positive electrode foot). These leads record a change in electrical potential in the frontal plane. A bipolar lead (answer B) refers to leads that are composed of two electrodes of opposite polarity. Limb leads (answer C) are bipolar leads. A 12-lead electrocardiogram consists of three bipolar limb leads (I, II, and III). Four electrodes are placed on the extremities: left and right wrist (or shoulders); left and right ankles (or legs). The lead

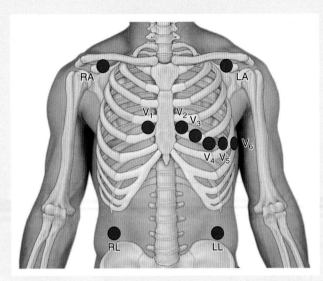

Figure 3-14 From https://www.wikilectures.eu/index.php?curid=8292.

connected to the right ankle is a neutral (ground) lead. It completes the electrical circuit and plays no role in the electrocardiogram.

3. **Answer: A.** The heart's electrical activity is represented on the electrocardiographic tracing by three basic waveforms: the P wave, the QRS complex, and the T wave; a U wave is also sometimes present (**Figure 3-15**). The P wave of the electrocardiogram (ECG) originates from the sinoatrial (SA) node and represents electrical depolarization of the atria, which initiates contraction of the atrial musculature.

The QRS complex (answer B) represents ventricular depolarization. The T wave (answer C) represents ventricular repolarization. The U wave (answer D) is thought to represent delayed repolarization of Purkinje fibers.

TEACHING POINT

The ECG graph paper consists of horizontal and vertical lines (**Figure 3-16**). The horizontal lines measure the duration (width) of the waveform. Each small square measured horizontally represents 0.04 seconds and 5 small squares represent 0.20 seconds. The vertical lines measure the amplitude or voltage (the height or depth of a waveform or complex) in millimeters (mm). Each small square represents 1 mm in height or depth and 5 small squares represent 5 mm.

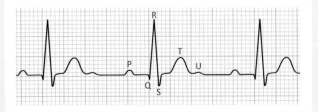

Figure 3-15

4. **Answer: C.** A Q wave is any negative deflection that precedes an R wave. Q waves may be normal or pathological. Normal small Q waves (<0.04 second in duration) typically occur in the lateral precordial (chest) leads and in one or more of the limb leads (except aVR). Q waves are considered pathological if >0.04 seconds wide (more than 1 small square on the ECG grid), >2 mm deep (2 small squares on the ECG grid), >25% of the depth of the QRS complex, and if seen in leads V1-3. Newer studies, however, suggest that Q waves with durations of over 0.03 seconds in leads I, II, aVL, aVF, or V4 to V6 may be abnormal. Pathological Q waves usually indicate current or prior myocardial infarction; however, pathological Q waves may also be seen with ventricular enlargement and altered ventricular conduction. The two most important conduction disturbances associated with pseudo-infarct Q waves are left bundle branch block (LBBB) and Wolff-Parkinson-White (WPW) preexcitation patterns.

Isoelectric refers to the baseline or isoelectric line on the ECG paper where there are no positive or negative charges of electricity to create deflections in the ECG trace.

5. **Answer: C.** The electrocardiogram (ECG) provides a view of the heart's electrical activity between two points or electrodes (a positive electrode and a negative electrode). The direction in which the electric current flows determines how the waveforms appear on the ECG tracing (**Figure 3-17**). A wave of depolarization traveling away from a positive electrode produces a negative waveform or deflection.

When a lead is perpendicular to the mean ventricular electrical axis, the vector changes throughout the course of ventricular depolarization producing a deflection (both positive and negative) and this is a biphasic waveform (answer A). Biphasic waveforms or deflections may be equally positive and negative, more negative than positive, or more positive than negative. Isoelectric (zero voltage) refers to the ECG baseline where there are no positive or negative changes; anything above the isoelectric line is "positive" waveform or deflection; below the line is "negative" waveform or deflection. A wave of depolarization traveling toward the positive electrode will produce a positive deflection or waveform (answer D).

6. **Answer: C.** The PR interval represents the time required for the depolarization wave to traverse the atria and the atrioventricular (AV) node; that is, the PR interval represents the time from the onset of atrial depolarization to the onset of ventricular depolarization. The PR interval is measured from the beginning of the P wave to the beginning of the QRS complex (**Figure 3-18**). The duration of the normal PR interval is 0.12 to 0.20 seconds (3-5 small squares on the electrocardiogram grid).

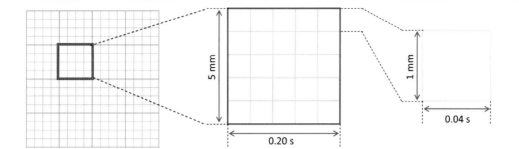

Figure 3-16

PR intervals <0.08 seconds (answer A) and between 0.08 and 0.10 seconds (answer B) are shortened PR intervals and indicate preexcitation. A PR interval between 0.20 and 0.26 seconds (answer D) is prolonged and is consistent with first-degree atrioventricular heart block.

7. **Answer: A.** The QRS interval is measured from the beginning of the QRS complex (as the first wave of the complex leaves baseline) to the end of the QRS complex (when the last wave of the complex begins to level out into the ST segment (**Figure 3-19**). The duration of the normal QRS interval is 0.06 to 0.1 seconds (less than 3 small squares on the ECG grid).

A QRS duration >0.12 seconds (answer A) is considered slightly prolonged while QRS durations of 0.12 to 0.20 seconds (answer C) and 0.20 to 0.26 seconds (answer D) are considered abnormal.

8. **Answer: B.** The QRS complex represents ventricular depolarization, which is followed by ventricular contraction.

Atrial depolarization (answer A) is reflected by the P wave and represents the spread of the electrical impulse throughout the left and right atria. Atrial repolarization (answer C) is not seen on the electrocardiogram because atrial repolarization occurs during ventricular depolarization and is hidden within the QRS complex. Ventricular repolarization (answer D) is reflected by the ST segment.

9. **Answer: D.** The T wave represents the repolarization of the ventricles; the end of the T wave coincides with the end of ventricular systole.

Atrial depolarization (answer A) is reflected by the P wave and represents the spread of the electrical impulse throughout the left and right atria. Ventricular depolarization (answer B) is reflected by the QRS complex and represents ventricular depolarization, which is followed by ventricular contraction. Atrial repolarization (answer C) is not seen on the electrocardiogram because atrial repolarization occurs during ventricular depolarization and is hidden within the QRS complex.

10. **Answer: B.** There are four main heart surfaces to consider when discussing the heart: anterior (front), posterior (back), inferior (bottom), and lateral (side). The electrocardiogram leads correspond to the surfaces of the heart. Leads II, III, and aVF are inferior leads and look at the electrical activity from the inferior surface of the heart.

Leads V3 and V4 are anterior leads (answer A) and these leads look at the electrical activity from the anterior wall of the right and left ventricles. Leads I, aVL, V5, and V6 are lateral leads (answer C) and these leads look at the electrical activity from the lateral wall of the left ventricle. Posterior leads (answer D) include V7-V9 leads and are recorded by moving V4-V6 electrodes to under the left scapula. This is done to detect posterior infarcts, which are

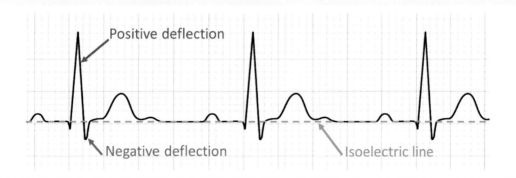

Figure 3-17

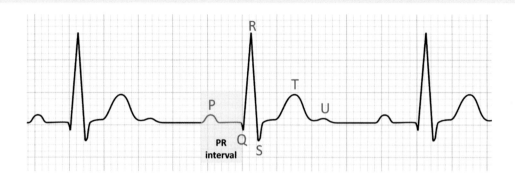

Figure 3-18

often associated with inferior or lateral wall acute myocardial infarctions.

11. **Answer: C.** Leads I, aVL, V5, and V6 are lateral leads and look at the electrical activity from the lateral wall of the left ventricle (LV).

Leads V3 and V4 are anterior leads (answer A) and these leads look at the electrical activity from the anterior wall of the right and left ventricles. Leads II, III, and aVF are inferior leads (answer B) and these leads look at the electrical activity from the inferior surface of the heart. Posterior leads (answer D) include V7-V9 leads and are recorded by moving V4-V6 electrodes to under the left scapula. This is done to detect posterior infarcts, which are often associated with inferior or lateral wall acute myocardial infarctions.

12. **Answer: A.** Leads V3 and V4 are anterior leads and these leads look at the electrical activity from the anterior wall of the right and left ventricles; leads V1 and V2 are anteroseptal leads and look at the electrical activity from the septal surface of the heart.

Leads II, III, and aVF are inferior leads (answer B) and these leads look at the electrical activity from the inferior surface of the heart. Leads I, aVL, V5, and V6 are lateral leads (answer C) and these leads look at the electrical activity from the lateral wall of the left ventricle. Posterior leads (answer D) include V7-V9 leads and are recorded by moving V4-V6

electrodes to under the left scapula. This is done to detect posterior infarcts, which are often associated with inferior or lateral wall acute myocardial infarctions.

KEY POINT

Based on changes in the various electrocardiographic leads, the location of myocardial infarction may be identified (**Table 3-1**).

13. **Answer: D.** Wolff-Parkinson-White (WPW) is a preexcitation syndrome that is characterized by a short PR interval (less than 0.12 seconds) and a broad QRS complex due to a delta wave (**Figure 3-20**).

Brugada syndrome (answer A) is a genetic disorder associated with an increased risk of ventricular tachyarrhythmias and sudden cardiac death. Typical electrocardiographic findings include a pseudo–right bundle branch block and persistent ST segment elevation in leads V1 to V2. Lown-Ganong-Levine (LGL) syndrome (answer B) is a preexcitation syndrome that is characterized by a short PR interval with a normal QRS complex. Wellen syndrome (answer C) or Wellen sign refers to the pattern of deeply inverted or biphasic T waves in V2 and V3, which is highly specific for a critical stenosis of the left anterior descending artery.

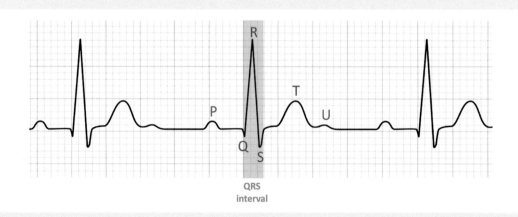

Figure 3-19

Table 3-1.

Leads	Myocardial Region
II, III, aVF	Inferior
V1-V2	Anteroseptal
V1-V4	Anterior
I, aVL, V5-V6	Lateral
I, aVL, V5-V6, II, III, aVF	Inferolateral
I, aVL, V1-V6	Anterolateral

14. Answer: C. The heart rate range for normal sinus rhythm is between 60 and 100 bpm. A heart rate less than 60 bpm is sinus bradycardia, while a heart rate over 100 bpm is sinus tachycardia.

TEACHING POINT

Sinus rhythm refers to a normal heart rhythm that originates in the sinoatrial node. The impulse follows the normal conduction pathway through the atria, the atrioventricular node, the bundle branches, and the ventricles, resulting in normal atrial and ventricular depolarization. Therefore, P waves are normal in size, shape, and direction, with one P wave preceding each QRS complex. The duration of the PR interval and the QRS complex is within normal limits.

15. Answer: A. Acute coronary syndromes (ACS) can be divided into three presentations: ST segment elevation myocardial infarction (STEMI), non-ST segment elevation myocardial infarction (NSTEMI), and unstable angina. NSTEMI and unstable angina are very similar, with NSTEMI having positive cardiac biomarkers. The distinction between STEMI and NSTEMI and unstable angina is important as the treatment strategies for each differ.

PCI (answer B) is the abbreviation for percutaneous coronary intervention, which refers to both non-stenting procedures and stent interventions for the treatment of coronary artery disease. Thrombolysis (answer D), also known as thrombolytic therapy, utilizes a thrombolytic agent to lyse coronary artery clots; this therapy was historically performed in patients with a STEMI. Most STEMI are now treated with primary PCI.

16. Answer: A. The 12-lead ECG shown in **Figure 3-1** shows ST segment elevation in leads V1 and V2. ST segment elevation is an indication of acute myocardial injury. As the ST segment elevation is isolated to V1 and V2, this indicates an acute anteroseptal myocardial infarction. Therefore, the echocardiogram would show evidence of anteroseptal hypokinesis. The anterior septum is best seen in the parasternal long-axis and apical long-axis views. This wall is usually supplied by the left anterior descending coronary artery.

Inferior wall hypokinesis (answer B) would be expected when there are acute changes demonstrated in leads II, III, and aVF representing the right coronary artery and/or posterior descending coronary artery. Lateral wall akinesis (answer C) would be expected when there are acute changes demonstrated in leads I, aVL, V5, and V6, which represent the left circumflex coronary artery. Posterior wall akinesis (answer D) would be expected when there is ST depression in leads V1-V4. Additional chest leads may be placed on the back of the patient in order to view the heart's posterior surface. In this case, ST elevation would be present in posterior leads V1-V4. The posterior wall is usually supplied by the left circumflex and sometimes the right coronary artery.

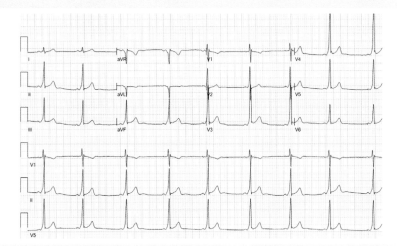

Figure 3-20 Example of WPW with a short PR interval and broad QRS complexes (160 ms) with a slurred upstroke (delta wave), seen best in leads II, III, aVF, and chest leads V3-V6. (From https://commons.wikimedia.org/wiki/File:Wolff-Parkinson-White_syndrome_12_lead_EKG.png. https://creativecommons.org/licenses/sa/3.0/deed.en. Under the terms of the GNU Free Documentation License, Version 1.2.)

The normal ST segment should be isoelectric. Abnormalities of the ST segment include elevation and depression. ST segment elevation or depression is abnormal if the displacement is greater than 1 mm (more than 1 small square) from baseline. ST segment elevation is an indicator of acute myocardial infarction, while ST segment depression is a marker of myocardial ischemia; the leads in which the elevation occurs indicate the location of myocardial injury or ischemia. The ST segment depression can represent a reciprocal change to ST segment elevation in the contralateral lead. Importantly, there are other causes for ST segment elevation and depression.

17. **Answer: B.** The ECG in **Figure 3-2** shows normal sinus rhythm with a right bundle branch block (RBBB). An RBBB occurs when the normal electrical activity in the His-Purkinje system to the right bundle branch is interrupted. As a result, the electrical conduction to the right ventricle (RV) is delayed, and this asynchronous activation of the two ventricles increases the QRS duration. The ECG hallmarks for RBBB include a wide QRS complex of 120 ms or more (greater than 3 small squares), an rSR′ "bunny ear" pattern in the anterior precordial leads (leads V1-V3), and slurred S waves in leads I, aVL, and frequently V5 and V6 (**Figure 3-21**). The heart rate can be calculated by counting the number of QRS complexes in 30 large squares (each representing 0.2 seconds) and then multiplying this number by 10 (the six-second method). In this example, the number of QRS complexes over 30 large squares is 9; therefore, the heart rate is approximately 90 bpm. As the heart rate is above 60 bpm, this is not sinus bradycardia.

The ECG criteria for left bundle branch block include a QRS >120 ms, supraventricular rhythm, and terminal waves, indicating that the left ventricle is depolarizing late.

TEACHING POINT

There are several methods for calculating the heart rate from the ECG. This includes:

1. The 1500 Method: Count the number of small squares (representing 0.04 seconds) between the QRS complexes and then divide this number into 1500. This method is ideal for faster heart rates.

2. The Six-Second Method: Count the number of QRS complexes over 30 large squares (each representing 0.2 seconds) and then multiply this number by 10. This method is ideal for slow or irregular rhythms.

3. The 300 Method: Count the number of large squares plus the fraction of a large square, if necessary, between two successive R waves and divide this number into 300.

4. The Square-Counting Method: Count the number of large squares between R waves and count using the following numbers: 300-150-100-75-60-50-etc. This is a simplification of the 1500 method. For example, one large square = 5 small squares, so 1500 ÷ 5 = 300, two large squares = 10 small squares, so 1500 ÷ 10 = 150, etc. (**Figure 3-22**). This method can only be used on regular rhythms.

18. **Answer: B.** Atrial fibrillation occurs when electrical impulses arise from multiple ectopic sites within the atria. These impulses depolarize at a rapid rate causing the atria to "quiver" instead of contracting

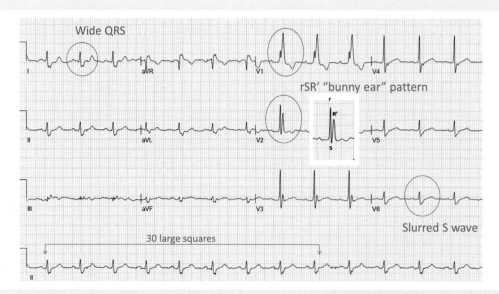

Figure 3-21 RBBB example showing a wide QRS with a slurred S wave is seen in lead I and V6. An rSR′ pattern is seen in lead V1 and V2 and T wave inversion in V1. There are 9 QRS complexes in 30 large squares; hence, the heart rate is approximately 90 bpm.

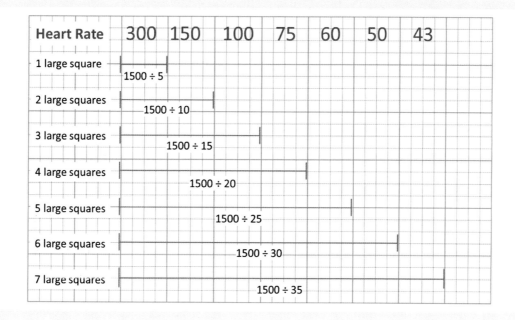

Figure 3-22

regularly, producing irregular, wavy deflections called fibrillatory waves (f waves). Because impulses arise from multiple sites and not from the sinoatrial node, there are no discernible P waves preceding the QRS complexes; furthermore, because the atrial impulses occur irregularly, the ventricular response will be irregular also (**Figure 3-23**). Using the six-second method, the heart rate in this example is about 120 bpm (12 QRS complexes over 30 large squares in the lead II rhythm strip at the bottom of the trace).

Atrial flutter (answer A) would display a regular or irregular ventricular rhythm with flutter waves before each QRS (presenting a sawtooth wave pattern); the atrial rate is between 25 and 400 bpm.

Sinus tachycardia (answer C) would show P waves prior to each QRS complex and a heart rate between 100 and 160 bpm. Sinus rhythm with premature atrial contractions (answer D) would show a normal ventricular rate with atrial beats originating from a single or multiple ectopic pacemaker sites in the atria; the premature P wave would have an abnormal appearance and be followed by a normal QRS and a pause.

19. **Answer: C.** Atrial and ventricular pacing can be seen on the ECG as a pacing stimulus (spike) followed by a P wave or QRS complex, respectively. When there is ventricular pacing, as shown in **Figure 3-4**, a single pacemaker spike followed by a wide, bizarre QRS complex is seen on the ECG. Ventricular

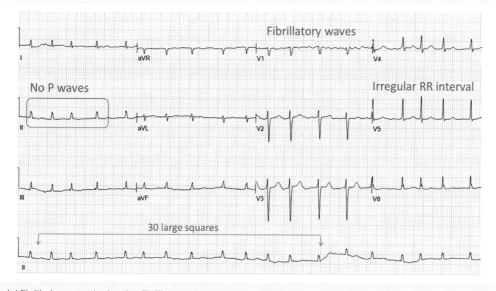

Figure 3-23 Atrial fibrillation example showing fibrillatory waves, no discernible P waves prior to QRS complexes, and irregular R-R intervals. There are 12 QRS complexes over 30 large squares; hence the heart rate is approximately 120 bpm.

paced with normal sensing is evident by a ventricular paced rhythm and continuous stimulation of the ventricles by the pacemaker, demonstrating 100% capture.

Answer A is incorrect as each pacemaker spike is followed by a QRS complex. Answer B is incorrect. With atrial pacing, there is a single pacemaker stimulus followed by a P wave, which is then followed by a QRS complex. The morphology of the P wave depends upon the location of the atrial lead; it may be normal, diminutive, biphasic, or negative. Answer D is incorrect. With atrioventricular (AV) sequential pacing (or dual chamber pacing) there are two pacemaker spikes: an atrial spike followed by a P wave and a ventricular spike followed by a wide QRS complex.

TEACHING POINT

The wide QRS complex associated with ventricular pacing occurs as the ventricles are depolarized sequentially (one after the other) rather than simultaneously. Because the pacemaker lead is usually in the right ventricular (RV) apex, the paced QRS complex has a left bundle branch block (LBBB) configuration since RV depolarization occurs before left ventricular depolarization.

20. **Answer: C.** ST segment elevation is seen in inferolateral leads (II, III, aVF, V5, and V6), indicating inferolateral ST segment elevation myocardial infarction (STEMI). There is also marked ST segment depression in leads V1, V2, and aVL. On echocardiographic examination, the regional motion of the inferolateral wall segments would be abnormal. These segments are best seen in the parasternal and apical long-axis views. These segments are usually supplied by the

right coronary artery and/or the left circumflex coronary artery.

Anterior wall regional wall motion abnormalities (answer A) are usually associated with ECG changes in leads V1-V4, which represent the segments of the heart supplied by the left anterior descending coronary artery. Posterior wall regional wall motion abnormalities (answer B) are usually associated with ST depression in leads V1-V4, which represent the segments of the heart supplied by the left circumflex coronary artery. As previously described, additional chest leads may be used to view the heart's posterior surface. Anterolateral wall regional wall motion abnormalities (answer D) are usually associated with ST elevation in leads I, AVL, V5, and V6, which represent the segments of the heart supplied by the proximal left anterior descending coronary artery.

21. **Answer: B.** Left ventricular hypertrophy (LVH) refers to an increase in the size of cardiac myocytes and usually occurs in response to a chronic pressure or volume load. On the echocardiographic examination, LVH appears as an increase in LV wall thickness. The ECG criterion for LVH based on the QRS voltages is a sum of the S wave in V1 and tallest R wave in V5 or V6 ≥ 35 mm. The sum of the S wave in V1 and the tallest R wave in V5 is 37 mm (**Figure 3-24**) which meets the voltage criteria for LVH.

With left atrial enlargement (answer A), the P waves are typically wide and notched but may be biphasic in some leads. Left atrial enlargement is classically associated with severe mitral stenosis and therefore the notched appearance of the P wave is often referred to as "P mitrale." With right atrial enlargement (answer C) the P wave is tall and

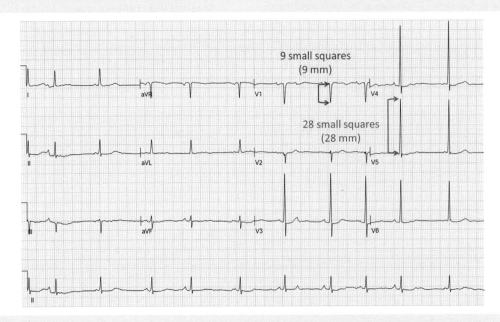

Figure 3-24 LVH by voltage criteria. The S wave in V1 is 9 small squares or 9 mm and the R wave in V5 is 28 small squares or 28 mm; the sum of these two waves is 37 mm.

peaked. As right atrial enlargement is commonly associated with chronic pulmonary diseases such as chronic obstructive pulmonary disease and asthma, these P waves are referred to as "P pulmonale." With right ventricular hypertrophy (answer D), the ECG shows a dominant R wave in V1 (>7 mm tall or R/S ratio >1) and a dominant S wave in V5 or V6 (>7 mm deep or R/S ratio <1).

22. **Answer: C.** The ECG in **Figure 3-7** shows sinus tachycardia with multiple multifocal premature ventricular contractions (PVCs). Recall that the heart rate is derived by counting the number of QRS complexes over 30 large squares and multiplying this number by 10. In this example, there are 13 QRS complexes in 30 large squares; hence, the heart rate is approximately 130 bpm. As there is a P wave preceding most of the beats and because the heart rate exceeds 100 bpm, this is sinus tachycardia. A premature ventricular contraction is a premature ventricular ectopic impulse that arises in the ventricles. PVCs are identified as premature beats with a wide QRS complex not preceded by a P wave, a T wave that is in the opposite direction to the preceding beat, and followed by a compensatory pause. PVCs may be unifocal or multifocal. Unifocal PVCs have the same appearance and originate from one ectopic ventricular focus. Multifocal PVCs display a different morphology to one another within the same lead; these PVCs may originate from different ectopic sites or may originate from a single site but are conducted along different ventricular pathways. Observe that the PVCs in V4 and in the lead II rhythm strip appear different from one another.

Atrial fibrillation with frequent PACs (answer A) would show an irregular ventricular rhythm with no P waves (there are no P waves because the atria are being irregularly depolarized by many ectopic pacemakers at once causing the atria to "quiver") and the PACs would appear as premature P waves of an abnormal appearance and followed by a normal QRS and a pause. Atrial flutter with frequent PACs (answer B) would show flutter waves before each QRS (presenting a sawtooth wave pattern, an atrial rate between 25 and 400 bpm, and a regular or irregular ventricular rhythm) and the PACs would appear as premature P waves of an abnormal appearance and followed by a normal QRS and a pause. Sinus bradycardia with frequent PVCs (answer D) would show a sinus rhythm with a heart rate <60 bpm and the PVCs would appear as described above.

23. **Answer: D.** AV block is defined as a delay or interruption in the conduction of an impulse from the atria to the ventricles. First-degree AV block (answer A) occurs when there is slowed conduction between the atria and the ventricles without missed beats; this is identified by prolongation of the PR interval >200 ms. With second-degree AV block, there is intermittent atrial conduction to the ventricle resulting in intermittent missed or dropped ventricular beats. Second-degree AV block is further classified into Mobitz type I (Wenckebach) and Mobitz type II AV block. In Mobitz type I AV block (answer B), there is progressive lengthening of the PR interval and then a dropped ventricular beat, followed by a conducted beat with a shorter PR interval and then a repetition of this cycle. In Mobitz type II AV block (answer C), the PR interval is constant and there is an occasional dropped ventricular beat. With third-degree block (answer D), also known as complete heart block or complete AV block, there is a complete absence of conduction between the atria and the ventricles with the atria and ventricles beating independently of each other. The atria are usually paced by the sinus node at the inherent rate of 60 to 100 bpm and the ventricles are paced from a ventricular focus at a much slower rate of 30 to 40 bpm.

The ECG in **Figure 3-8** is an example of third-degree AV block as evidenced by the complete dissociation between the P waves, wide QRS complexes, and a slow ventricular rate.

24. **Answer: B.** The ECG shown in **Figure 3-9** is an example of left bundle branch block (LBBB). A LBBB occurs when the normal electrical activity in the His-Purkinje system to the left bundle branch is interrupted. As a result, the electrical conduction to the left ventricle (LV) is delayed and this asynchronous activation of the two ventricles increases the QRS duration. The ECG hallmarks for LBBB includes a wide QRS complex of 120 ms or more (greater than 3 small squares), a dominant S wave in V1, ST segments and T waves in an opposite direction to the QRS complex, and a broad, often notched ("M" shaped) R wave in V6 (R wave is monophasic in this example).

The echocardiographic finding with LBBB is paradoxical septal motion. Paradoxical septal motion is defined as movement of the interventricular septum (IVS) away from the center of the LV during systole, which is the opposite of its normal movement, which is inward toward the LV throughout systole. Early and abrupt contraction of the interventricular septum occurs during the preejection period before the delayed commencement of contraction of the posterior wall of the LV.

With left atrial enlargement (answer A), the P waves are typically wide and notched but may be biphasic in some leads. Left atrial enlargement is classically associated with severe mitral stenosis and therefore the notched appearance of the P wave is often referred to as "P mitrale". Pulsus paradoxus (answer C) refers to an exaggerated fall in a patient's blood pressure (>10 mm Hg) during inspiration; there are no specific ECG findings associated with this condition. Right ventricular (RV) volume overload (answer D) refers to an increase in the volume/size of the right ventricle caused by valvular regurgitation and/or congenital heart disease. An RV strain pattern on the ECG may be seen with RV hypertrophy or dilatation; a characteristic feature of this includes T wave inversion in the right precordial (V1-4) and inferior (III, aVF) leads.

25. **Answer: B.** Atrial flutter is caused by a circular pathway (reentry) of electrical conduction within the atria at a characteristic rate of approximately 300 bpm. This produces V-shaped or sawtooth waveforms which are called flutter waves (F waves). There is typically 2:1 conduction across the atrioventricular (AV) node; as a result, the ventricular rate is usually one-half the flutter rate. However, AV conduction ratio can be variable as seen in this example. Atrial fibrillation (answer A) is excluded based on the sawtooth appearance of the regularly paced flutter waves. Sinus tachycardia (answer C) and sinus bradycardia (answer D) can be excluded due to the absence of P waves prior to each QRS complex.

26. **Answer: C.** The ECG in **Figure 3-11** shows sinus bradycardia. The heart rate estimated by the square-counting method (see **Figure 3-22**) is 43 bpm (**Figure 3-25**). Sinus bradycardia is sinus rhythm (rhythm originating at the sinoatrial node) with a heart rate less than 60 bpm. The patient's exercise capacity should be taken into consideration, as a highly trained athlete's heart rate will be lower. Sinus tachycardia (answer A) is excluded since the heart rate is below 100 bpm. First-degree atrioventricular block (answer C) is excluded since the PR interval is not prolonged. Ventricular tachycardia (answer D) is excluded since a P wave is observed prior to each QRS complex, the heart rate is <100 bpm, and the QRS complexes are of a normal width.

27. **Answer: A.** The electrocardiogram shown in **Figure 3-12** is an example of electrical alternans. Electrical alternans is recognized by an alternation of QRS complex amplitude or axis between beats. It is most often observed in the precordial (chest) leads where the QRS amplitude is greater. Observe that in **Figure 3-12**, there is an obvious alternation in amplitude of the QRS complexes in leads V2–V4. The most common cause of electrical alternans is a pericardial effusion where the alternating amplitude of the QRS complexes is the result of a "swinging" motion of the heart from beat to beat within the pericardial fluid; therefore, answer A is correct.

28. **Answer: A.** The ECG shown in **Figure 3-13** shows sinus arrest. Sinus arrest (a component of the sick sinus syndrome) occurs when the sinoatrial (SA) node fails to initiate an impulse to the atria. This is a conductivity disorder that is caused by SA node dysfunction secondary to damage to the SA node following an acute myocardial infarction, inflammatory, or infiltrative or fibrotic disease of the SA node, excessive vagal tone, sleep apnea, or drugs such as digitalis, beta-blockers, or calcium channel blockers.

Answer B is incorrect as a junctional escape rhythm will show a regular, slow heart rate (40-60 bpm). As the electrical activation occurs near or within the atrioventricular node, rather than from the SA node, the P waves are frequently hidden within the QRS complex; however, when visible, the P waves are often inverted. Answer C is incorrect as in complete degree block there is a complete absence of conduction between the atria and the ventricles with the two chambers beating independently of

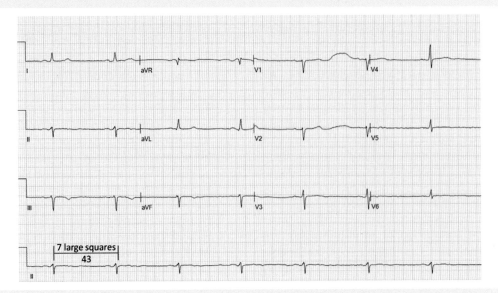

Figure 3-25 The heart rate is estimated via the square-counting method. There are 7 large squares between R waves; therefore, the heart is estimated at 43 bpm.

each other. The atria are usually paced by the sinus node at the inherent rate of 60 to 100 bpm and the ventricles are paced from a ventricular focus at a much slower rate of 30 to 40 bpm. Answer D is incorrect as a wandering atrial pacemaker is identified by the variation in P wave morphology (shape, size, and duration) across the rhythm strip. A wandering atrial pacemaker occurs when the atrial pacemaker site shifts back and forth between the SA node and ectopic atrial sites. As a result, the P wave morphology varies across the rhythm strip as the pacemaker "wanders" among the multiple sites.

SUGGESTED READINGS

Barbara JA. *ECGs Made Easy*. 5th ed. St. Louis, MO: Mosby/Elsevier Science; 2013.

Channer K, Morris F. ABC of clinical electrocardiography: myocardial ischaemia. *BMJ*. 2002;324(7344):1023-1026.

Edhouse J1, Brady WJ, Morris F. ABC of clinical electrocardiography: acute myocardial infarction-Part II. *BMJ*. 2002;324(7343):963-966.

Goodacre S, Irons R. ABC of clinical electrocardiography: atrial arrhythmias. *BMJ*. 2002;324(7337):594-597.

Huff J. *ECG Workout: Exercises in Arrhythmia Interpretation*. 7th ed. Philadelphia: Wolters Kluwer; 2016.

Meek S, Morris F. ABC of clinical electrocardiography. Introduction. I-Leads, rate, rhythm, and cardiac axis. *BMJ*. 2002;324(7334):415-418.

Morris F, Brady WJ. ABC of clinical electrocardiography: acute myocardial infarction-Part I. *BMJ*. 2002;324(7341):831-834.

CHAPTER 4

Basic Principles of Ultrasound Imaging

Contributor: Robert W. Gill, BE, MS, PhD

✪ Question 1

Ultrasound imaging uses sound waves with frequencies in which of the following ranges?
- **A.** 20 kHz to 200 kHz
- **B.** 200 kHz to 2 MHz
- **C.** 2 MHz to 20 MHz
- **D.** 20 MHz to 200 MHz

✪✪ Question 2

For frequencies typically used in echocardiography the ultrasound wavelength is approximately:
- **A.** 0.1 mm.
- **B.** 0.5 mm.
- **C.** 1.0 mm.
- **D.** 5.0 mm.

✪✪ Question 3

How does ultrasound affect the patient's tissues?
- **A.** The tissues are heated.
- **B.** Tissue pressure increases and decreases.
- **C.** Neither A nor B.
- **D.** Both A and B.

✪ Question 4

Why is the ultrasound pulse transmitted by an ultrasound machine so short?
- **A.** To minimize attenuation
- **B.** To minimize patient exposure
- **C.** To optimize axial resolution
- **D.** To reduce reverberation artifacts

✪✪ Question 5

The strength of the echo produced by a tissue interface separating two different tissues depends on:
- **A.** The difference in acoustic impedance of the two tissues.
- **B.** The incidence angle between the ultrasound beam and tissue interface.
- **C.** Neither A nor B.
- **D.** Both A and B.

✪✪ Question 6

What causes the speckle seen in soft-tissue ultrasound imaging?
- **A.** Reflection
- **B.** Refraction
- **C.** Reverberation
- **D.** Scattering

✪ Question 7

As it passes through the patient's tissues ultrasound is attenuated (grows weaker). Attenuation can be caused by:
- **A.** Absorption of ultrasound energy.
- **B.** Reflection of ultrasound energy.
- **C.** Neither A nor B.
- **D.** Both A and B.

✪ Question 8

Increasing the ultrasound frequency will improve image resolution. It will also:

A. Increase penetration.
B. Decrease penetration.
C. Increase temporal resolution.
D. Decrease temporal resolution.

✪ Question 9

The ultrasound machine calculates the depth at which each echo should be displayed using the:

A. Echo arrival time.
B. Pulse duration.
C. Echo amplitude.
D. Pulse frequency.

✪✪ Question 10

The elements in a phased array transducer transmit at slightly different times. What is the purpose of this?

A. It allows the heart to be imaged at different phases in the cardiac cycle.
B. It steers the ultrasound beam in different directions to build up a two-dimensional image.
C. It allows the machine to detect phase differences in the echoes from blood to calculate its speed of movement.
D. It enables the machine to quickly switch between transmitting and receiving.

✪ Question 11

Increasing the depth of the ultrasound image will:

A. Reduce the frame rate.
B. Increase tissue heating.
C. Improve the temporal resolution.
D. Improve spatial resolution.

✪ Question 12

Which one of the following will increase the frame rate (the number of images per second) and therefore improve temporal resolution?

A. Increasing image width
B. Decreasing image width
C. Increasing transmit power
D. Decreasing transmit power

✪ Question 13

The image shown in **Figure 4-1** lacks brightness throughout the image. Which of the following adjustments would correct for this?

A. Increase TGC slope
B. Reduce image width
C. Increase overall gain
D. Decrease dynamic range

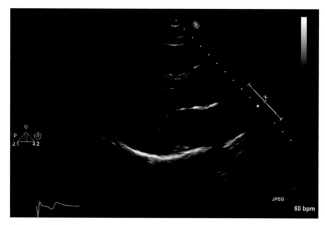

Figure 4-1

✪ Question 14

Image brightness varies with depth in the image shown in **Figure 4-2**. Which of the following controls could be used to correct for this?

A. TGC
B. Overall gain
C. Image width
D. Dynamic range

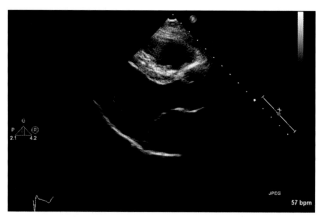

Figure 4-2

✪ Question 15

In **Figure 4-3A**, one of the following factors has been changed to improve resolution at the left ventricular apex, while in **Figure 4-3B**, it has been adjusted to improve resolution around the mitral valve. Which factor is that?

A. Gain
B. Focus
C. Frame rate
D. Dynamic range

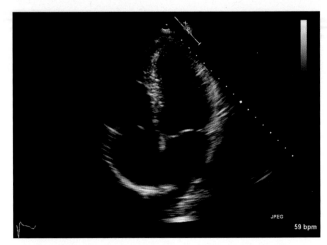

Figure 4-3A

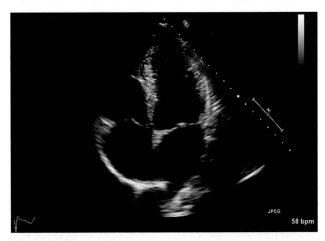

Figure 4-3B

✪ Question 16

After capturing the image shown in **Figure 4-4A**, another image was obtained by switching to the harmonic mode as shown in **Figure 4-4B**. The image in **Figure 4-4B** was created from reflections of ultrasound of:

A. Half the frequency of the transmitted waves.
B. Double the frequency of the transmitted waves.
C. Same frequency as the transmitted waves generated by resonating particles.
D. Half the frequency of the transmitted waves generated by nonlinear reflectors.

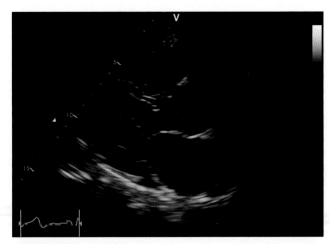

Figure 4-4A

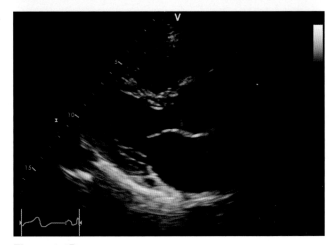

Figure 4-4B

✪✪✪ Question 17

Which of the following aspects of the image is **not** improved when the user switches from standard (fundamental or non-harmonic) imaging to harmonic mode imaging?

A. Speckle
B. Spatial resolution
C. Contrast resolution
D. Slice thickness artifact

✪ Question 18

What is meant by the term "spatial resolution"?

A. Ability to see weak echoes at the maximum image depth
B. Ability to see variations in soft tissue echo strength
C. Ability to see tissues clearly without blurring due to movement
D. Ability to see objects that are close together as separate entities

✪ Question 19

Figure 4-5 shows an M-mode trace. Which one of the following statements comparing M-mode with B-mode (greyscale) imaging is true?

A. The axial resolution of M-mode is better.
B. The lateral resolution of M-mode is better.
C. The temporal resolution of M-mode is better.
D. The patient exposure to ultrasound energy is lower.

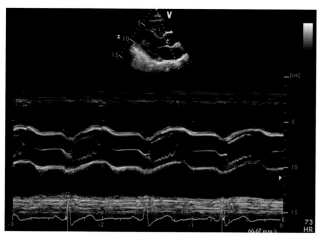

Figure 4-5

✪✪ Question 20

Which of the following is the main factor that determines the axial resolution of the image?

A. Focal depth
B. Transmit pulse amplitude
C. Transmit pulse duration
D. Transmit pulse repetition frequency (PRF)

✪ Question 21

Which of the following is the main factor that determines the lateral resolution of an image?

A. TGC setting
B. Beamwidth
C. Pulse duration
D. Pulse repetition frequency (PRF)

✪ Question 22

What does the term "contrast resolution" mean?

A. Ability to see small tissue structures
B. Ability to make accurate measurements
C. Ability to see low-level soft-tissue echoes adjacent to strong reflectors
D. Ability to see small variations in soft-tissue echo strength

✪✪ Question 23

How does a phased array transducer focus the ultrasound beam?

A. It adjusts the time at which each transducer element transmits
B. It adjusts the amount by which the received echo signal from each transducer element is delayed before the signals are combined
C. Both A and B
D. Neither A nor B

✪✪ Question 24

Why does the ultrasound transducer incorporate a "matching layer" in its design?

A. To ensure the transducer operates at the correct frequency
B. To accelerate the propagation speed and so increase the frame rate
C. To match the received echo frequency to the transmitted frequency
D. To correct for the acoustic impedance difference between the transducer and the tissues

✪ Question 25

What term is used to describe the material used to make the ultrasound transducer?

A. Photoelectric
B. Piezoelectric
C. Polymorphic
D. Pyroelectric

✪ Question 26

The ultrasound image is created and initially stored in the machine's image memory. The individual storage locations within the image memory are called:

A. Bits.
B. Bytes.
C. Pixels.
D. Photo cell.

✪✪✪ Question 27

Which of the following ultrasound exposure parameters must be known to calculate the rate at which the patient's tissues will be heated?

A. Energy
B. Power
C. Intensity
D. Pressure

✪✪ Question 28

Which of the following parameters relates directly to the likelihood of cavitation in the patient's tissues?

A. Pressure
B. Propagation speed
C. Acoustic impedance
D. Attenuation coefficient

✪ Question 29

Which of the following statements regarding the safety of ultrasound is correct?

A. It has been proven to be completely safe.
B. It cannot be proved to be completely safe.
C. It is not an ionizing radiation, so it cannot harm tissues.
D. Equipment manufacturers design machines, so they cannot exceed safe levels of exposure.

✪✪ Question 30

Which of the following operating modes is likely to cause the largest temperature rise in the patient's tissues?

A. M-mode
B. Color Doppler
C. Pulsed Doppler
D. B-mode (grayscale)

✪ Question 31

The parameters TI and MI are displayed on the screen. What does "TI" stand for?

A. Tissue index
B. Transmit index
C. Temporal index
D. Thermal index

✪ Question 32

What is the upper limit of the acceptable range of TI values?

A. 0.5
B. 1.0
C. 1.5
D. 2.0

✪ Question 33

What is the safe upper limit for the MI?

A. 0.9
B. 1.9
C. 9.0
D. 19

✪✪ Question 34

Which of the following changes will cause the heating of the patient's tissues to increase?

A. Increase frequency
B. Increase width
C. Increase gain
D. Increase dynamic range

✪✪ Question 35

The ALARA concept is an essential element in the safe use of ultrasound. What does the term "ALARA" mean?

A. Transmit power should be as low as possible.
B. Examination times should be as short as possible.
C. Ultrasound frequency should be as low as possible.
D. Neither A nor B nor C.

✪ Question 36

Which of the following statements in **not** true of the image shown in **Figure 4-6**?

A. It has higher temporal resolution than two-dimensional imaging.
B. It displays ultrasound reflections along a single scan line over time.
C. It allows simultaneous visualization of different anatomical structures.
D. It displays the power spectrum of velocities measured along a single scan line over time.

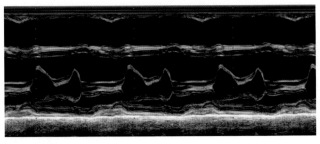

Figure 4-6

✪ Question 37

After capturing the image shown in **Figure 4-7A** (**Video 4-1A**), another image was obtained by increasing imaging frequency as shown in **Figure 4-7B** (**Video 4-1B**). The image in **Figure 4-7B** (**Video 4-1B**) has:

A. Greater imaging depth.
B. Better temporal resolution.
C. Better spatial resolution.
D. Less acoustic shadowing.

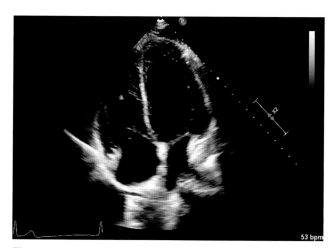

Figure 4-7A

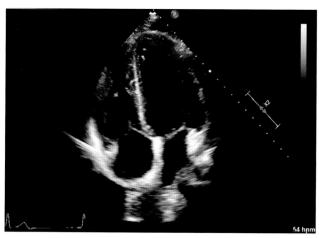

Figure 4-7B

✪✪✪ Question 38

How does the ultrasound machine scan the beam to create a two-dimensional (2D) image when a linear probe is being used?

- **A.** It uses a different group of transducer elements to form each beam.
- **B.** It uses phase differences to steer the beam in different directions.
- **C.** It uses time delays to steer the beam in different directions.
- **D.** It uses a lens to refract the beam in different directions.

✪ Question 39

What is meant by the term "refraction"?

- **A.** Ultrasound energy reflects repeatedly between two tissue interfaces.
- **B.** The beam intensity reduces due to beam divergence beyond the focal point.
- **C.** The direction in which the ultrasound is traveling changes due to differences in tissue density.
- **D.** The direction in which the ultrasound is traveling changes due to differences in propagation speed.

✪✪ Question 40

When is refraction clinically important?

- **A.** When it causes ring-down artifact
- **B.** When it causes multiple equally spaced echoes
- **C.** When it causes some structures to appear twice in the image
- **D.** When it causes structures to be displayed more superficially than their true position

✪✪ Question 41

Assuming that the propagation speed is 1540 m/s, the ultrasound wavelength when the machine is operating at 4.0 MHz is:

- **A.** 0.039 mm.
- **B.** 0.39 mm.
- **C.** 3.9 cm.
- **D.** 3.9 μm

✪ Question 42

Sometimes it is beneficial to zoom (magnify) the image so that a selected region of the heart fills the image. Two types of zoom function are available in most machines. Which is the preferred option?

- **A.** Preprocessing zoom because the frame rate will be higher
- **B.** Preprocessing zoom because image artifacts will be reduced
- **C.** Postprocessing zoom because the frame rate will be higher
- **D.** Postprocessing zoom because image artifacts will be reduced

✪ Question 43

The strength of the transmitted ultrasound wave is controlled by adjusting the:

A. Power control.
B. Overall gain control.
C. Compression control.
D. Time gain compensation controls.

✪ Question 44

Which machine control is used to adjust the dynamic range of echoes displayed on the screen?

A. Overall gain
B. Compression
C. Transmit power
D. Time gain compensation

ANSWERS

1. **Answer: C.** To maximize image resolution, ultrasound machines use the highest possible frequencies compatible with the required depth of penetration. Across the whole of diagnostic ultrasound frequencies in the range 2 to 20 MHz are used. In echocardiography, frequencies typically range from 2 to 8 MHz. Therefore, answer C is correct.

2. **Answer: B.** The wavelength (λ) is calculated by dividing the ultrasound propagation speed ($c = 1540$ m/s) by the frequency (f):

$$\lambda = c \div f \tag{1}$$

For frequencies in the range 2 to 8 MHz the wavelength will range from 0.77 mm at 2 MHz to 0.19 mm at 8 MHz (see Equations (2) and (3)). Therefore, answer B is correct. Wavelength is important since it is closely related to image resolution.

$$\begin{aligned}
\lambda &= c \div f \\
&= 1540 \div \left(2 \times 10^{6}\right) \\
&= 0.00077\,\text{m} \\
&= 0.77\,\text{mm} \tag{2}
\end{aligned}$$

$$\begin{aligned}
\lambda &= c \div f \\
&= 1540 \div \left(8 \times 10^{6}\right) \\
&= 0.0001925\,\text{m} \\
&= 0.19\,\text{mm} \tag{3}
\end{aligned}$$

3. **Answer: D.** Ultrasound is a traveling wave that increases and decreases the pressure at a rapid rate. A fraction of the ultrasound energy is absorbed by the tissues as it passes through them, causing the tissue temperature to rise. Therefore, answer D is correct. Importantly, if the ultrasound exposure is too high, this can have implications for patient safety.

4. **Answer: C.** Axial (or depth) resolution (AR) is directly related to the transmit pulse duration (T). It is calculated as:

$$AR = \left(c \times T\right) \div 2 \tag{1}$$

where c is the ultrasound propagation speed (1540 m/s). Best resolution will be achieved when the axial resolution is as small as possible.

For example, a transmit pulse with a duration of 0.5 µs will produce images with an axial resolution (AR) of 0.4 mm:

$$\begin{aligned}
AR &= \left(c \times T\right) \div 2 \\
&= \left(1540 \times 0.5 \times 10^{-6}\right) \div 2 \\
&= 0.000385\,\text{m} \\
&= 0.385\,\text{mm or } 0.4\,\text{mm} \tag{2}
\end{aligned}$$

Therefore, answer C is correct. Note that axial resolution is the same throughout the image, while lateral resolution varies with depth. Patient exposure is related to the ultrasound intensity, not the pulse duration. Attenuation is related to ultrasound frequency, not pulse duration. Pulse duration is not related to reverberation artifact.

5. **Answer: D.** When ultrasound is reflected at an interface between two tissues, the fraction of energy reflected is determined by the acoustic impedance difference between the two tissues. The amount of this reflected energy that reaches the probe depends on the incidence angle. As shown in **Figure 4-8**, at 90° incidence the echo will return directly to the probe. If the angle is less than 90° only a fraction of the echo energy will be detected and so it will be less strongly displayed in the image. Therefore, answer D is correct.

6. **Answer: D.** Ultrasound energy is scattered by small structures within the patient's tissues. Echoes from multiple scatterers arrive at the probe where they combine to determine the echo strength that will be displayed. Because of the wave nature of ultrasound and the random placement of the scatterers, the echo amplitude fluctuates randomly, causing the speckle appearance seen in ultrasound images. Therefore, answer D is correct. Reflection, refraction, and reverberation do not cause speckle.

7. **Answer: D.** In normal soft tissue, the main cause of attenuation is absorption of energy by the tissues. When strong reflectors are present (e.g., fibrous

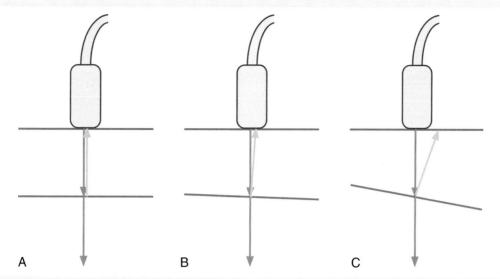

A   B   C

Figure 4-8 A, When the incidence angle is 90°, the echo returns directly to the probe and a strong echo will be seen. B, When the incidence angle is slightly less than 90°, the echo is slightly off-center and so the echo amplitude is reduced. C, When the incidence angle is significantly less than 90°, the echo does not reach the probe at all, so it will not be seen in the image.

tissues, calcification, prosthetic valves), these also reduce the ultrasound energy that passes through them to deeper tissues (i.e., they attenuate the ultrasound more than normal tissue) and cause shadowing in the image. Therefore, answer D is correct.

8. **Answer: B.** The rate of attenuation increases exponentially as frequency increases. Thus, at higher frequencies, ultrasound energy is more rapidly absorbed and so the penetration depth is reduced. Therefore, answer B is correct. Higher frequencies can therefore be used only when the depth is small, for example, in pediatric and transesophageal imaging. Temporal resolution refers to the ability to accurately display the position of moving structures at a particular instant in time. Adjusting the ultrasound frequency has no effect on temporal resolution.

9. **Answer: A.** Ultrasound travels at a known propagation speed ($c = 1540$ m/s) in tissue. Thus, there is a fixed relationship between the depth of the tissue causing an echo (d) and the time between the transmission of the ultrasound pulse and its return as an echo (t). The time can be calculated as:

$$t = (2 \times d) \div c \tag{1}$$

This equation can be rearranged to allow the machine to calculate depth from the echo arrival time:

$$d = (c \times t) \div 2 \tag{2}$$

Therefore, answer A is correct.

10. **Answer: B.** Phased array transducers steer the ultrasound beam by transmitting at slightly different times from each of the transducer elements. This allows the machine to steer the beam in a range of different directions to acquire echo information from a complete two-dimensional (2D) slice of the heart.

11. **Answer: A.** After each transmit pulse, the machine must wait until all echoes have been received before it transmits again. As the image depth increases the time taken for the deepest echoes to return increases and so the machine must wait longer before it can transmit again. Thus, the number of pulses that can be transmitted each second is inversely related to depth. This means that the frame rate (the number of images per second) is also inversely related to depth. Increasing the depth will therefore reduce the frame rate and worsen temporal resolution. Therefore, answer A is correct. Increasing the depth of the ultrasound image will have no direct effect on spatial resolution or tissue heating.

12. **Answer: B.** Decreasing the width of the image decreases the number of lines in the image. This reduces the number of transmit pulses required to make each image, and so increases the number of images the machine can produce per second (i.e., the frame rate). Therefore, answer B is correct. Changing the transmit power will have no impact on the frame rate.

13. **Answer: C.** When the image lacks intensity at all depths, the overall gain should be increased. Compare the original image where the 2D gain was set to 31% (**Figure 4-9A**) to the image when the overall gain was increased to 50% (**Figure 4-9B**). Observe that the myocardium and the mitral and aortic valves are much better seen by increasing the overall gain.

Adjusting the TGC (time gain compensation) control is not appropriate since it selectively alters gain

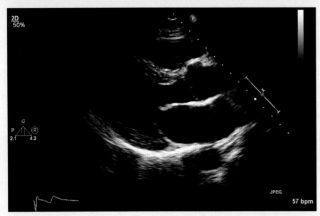

Figure 4-9A

Figure 4-9B

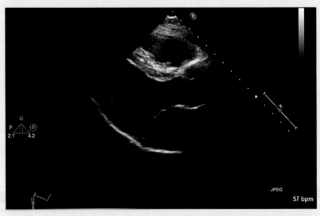

Figure 4-10A

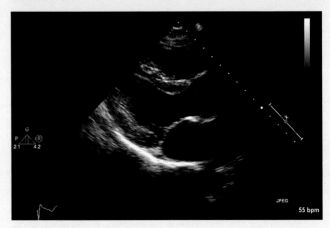

Figure 4-10B

at specific depths; therefore, answer A is incorrect. Reducing image width and dynamic range will not increase overall brightness (echo strength); therefore, answers B and D are incorrect.

14. **Answer: A.** The time gain compensation (TGC) control is used to correct or compensate for variation in echo strength with depth. In this image the brightness reduces as the depth increases, indicating that the TGC slope should be increased. Therefore, answer A is correct. Compare the original image (**Figure 4-10A**) to the image when the TGC slope was increased in the far field (**Figure 4-10B**). Observe that the myocardium of the interventricular septum and posterior left ventricular wall have a similar appearance.

   Answer B is not correct since adjusting the overall gain would make the superficial part of the image too bright. Adjusting the dynamic range and image width would not correct the lack of brightness in the deeper parts of the image; therefore, answers C and D are not correct.

KEY POINT

The TGC is adjusted to ensure structures of similar acoustic properties are displayed at similar echo amplitudes.

15. **Answer: B.** Adjusting the focus can improve the resolution around a region of interest. In the image shown the shift of focus is demonstrated on the right side of the screen where the focus, adjacent to the measurement lines, has been shifted downward from the apex in image A to the mitral valve level in image B. Therefore, answer B is correct.

16. **Answer: B.** Harmonic imaging (or more precisely, second harmonic imaging) uses ultrasound reflections that have twice the frequency of the transmitted waves. Therefore, answer B is correct. It is also possible to use higher harmonics such as third, fourth, and so on for image formation. Typically, only second harmonic imaging is available in commercial systems, because higher harmonic images are noisier and have not been shown to be useful.

17. **Answer: A.** Harmonic imaging reduces the effective beamwidth and slice thickness and so it improves lateral resolution and reduces slice thickness artifact. Contrast resolution is therefore improved. Harmonic imaging does not reduce soft tissue speckle; therefore, answer A is correct. Note that harmonic imaging also reduces penetration since the higher frequency content of the echoes used in harmonic imaging attenuates more rapidly.

18. **Answer: D.** The term refers to the ability of the machine to "resolve," that is, see as separate, two objects that are close together. It is common to differentiate between **axial resolution** (i.e., ability to resolve objects at slightly different depths) and **lateral resolution** (ability to resolve objects side by side at the same depth).

19. **Answer: C.** M-mode or motion mode traces are produced by pulsing repeatedly along a single stationary line of sight (beam position). The transmit pulse duration and beam focusing are the same as for B-mode (grayscale) imaging and so the axial and lateral resolution are the same. However, the rate at which the M-mode trace is updated is much higher than the frame rate of a B-mode image and so the temporal resolution is better. The exposure of the tissue along the beam will be higher than in B-mode imaging since the beam is stationary, whereas in B-mode the ultrasound energy is spread throughout the imaged region.

20. **Answer: C.** As stated earlier, **axial resolution** refers to the ability to resolve objects at slightly different depths. The transmit pulse duration determines how much the echo from a single reflector extends in depth and hence the axial (depth) resolution; therefore, answer C is correct. Beamwidth and focusing do not affect axial resolution. Neither does the pulse amplitude or the PRF.

21. **Answer: B.** Every echo in the image is smeared laterally by an amount equal to the beamwidth. Therefore, two reflectors at the same depth must be spaced by more than the beamwidth to be seen separately in the image, and so the lateral resolution is equal to the beamwidth. Beamwidth is not related to the pulse duration, PRF, or TGC setting.

22. **Answer: D.** The term "contrast resolution" refers to the user's ability to see subtle variations in echogenicity in soft tissue. The best contrast resolution will be obtained when (1) image artifacts are minimized and (2) settings such as frequency, gain, TGC, and dynamic range are optimized. As previously stated, contrast resolution is also improved with harmonic imaging (see the answer for Question 17).

23. **Answer: C.** The beamforming component of the machine is responsible for focusing the beam when the transducer is transmitting and receiving. Transmit focusing is achieved by delaying the transmit pulse by different amounts for each transducer element. Receive focusing is similarly achieved by delaying the echo signal from each element by a different amount. The beamformer also steers the beam in a range of different directions to build up a two-dimensional image. Therefore, answer C is correct.

24. **Answer: D.** The transducer has significantly different acoustic impedance from that of tissue. This would cause a fraction of the ultrasound energy to be reflected at the interface between the transducer and tissue, both when it is transmitting and receiving. The matching layer makes it seem as though the acoustic impedances are identical, so there is no reflection and ultrasound can pass through this interface without loss. Therefore, answer D is correct.

25. **Answer: B.** The term piezoelectric means that the material converts pressure into an electric signal (this is what the transducer does when receiving). It can also be used to describe the inverse effect where application of a varying electric signal to the material causes it to expand and contract, creating pressure variations (this is what the transducer does when transmitting).

26. **Answer: C.** The image memory consists of a large array of pixels. Each pixel stores a number that translates into the color and brightness that will be displayed at the corresponding point in the image. This is very similar to the way a digital camera stores its images.

27. **Answer: C.** The ultrasound intensity in the tissues, in combination with the tissue absorption coefficient, determines the rate of heating. Therefore, answer C is correct. Energy is a measure of the total amount of ultrasound deposited in the patient's body during the examination. It does not account for the time frame or the degree to which the energy is spread around within the body. Power is a measure of the energy deposited in the body per second, but it too does not take into account how the energy is spread around in the tissues. If the energy is concentrated in a relatively small amount of tissue (e.g., when the beam is stationary in M-mode or pulsed Doppler), the heating of that tissue will be greater than when the beam scans through a larger volume of tissue. Pressure is not directly related to heating.

28. **Answer: A.** Cavitation can occur when small gas bubbles are exposed to ultrasound. In some situations, it may lead to tissue damage and should be avoided. The likelihood of cavitation is related to (1) the peak rarefaction pressure (that is, the largest negative pressure caused by the ultrasound pulse), and (2) $1/\sqrt{f}$ where f is the ultrasound frequency. Therefore, answer A is correct.

29. **Answer: B.** It is not possible to **prove** that ultrasound is completely safe. There could (theoretically) be some subtle mechanism by which ultrasound harms patients that we have not yet thought of or detected. (Think of X-rays; they were initially thought to be completely harmless.) Therefore, answer B is correct.

30. **Answer: C.** Doppler uses a more intense transmit pulse than other modes to compensate for the weak scattering of ultrasound by blood. Pulsed Doppler has a greater heating effect on the exposed tissues than color Doppler because the beam is stationary in the tissues.

31. **Answer: D.** TI stands for thermal index. It indicates the likely maximum temperature rise in the patient's tissues (in degrees Celsius) with the current machine

settings. Variants of the TI are: TIs for soft tissue, TIb when tissue-bone interfaces are present in the focal region, and TIc for transcranial ultrasound.

32. **Answer: C.** As previously mentioned, TI refers to the thermal index. The value for this index is displayed on ultrasound machines as an on-screen guide to the user of the potential for tissue heating. A TI of 1.5 implies a temperature rise of approximately 1.5°C above physiological levels (37°C). A temperature rise of up to 1.5°C is considered safe even for extended periods of time. Therefore, answer C is correct. For a temperature rise of 1.5°C to 4.0°C, exposure for short periods of time is regarded as safe. A temperature of more than 4°C is considered unsafe for any period of time.

33. **Answer: B.** MI refers to the mechanical index. The value for this index is displayed on ultrasound machines as an on-screen guide to the user of the likelihood of inducing a nonthermal or mechanical effect. Most guidelines nominate 1.9 as the maximum safe value for MI. Lower values may be encountered in some practices performing fetal ultrasound examinations. The MI is especially noteworthy in echocardiographic examinations when ultrasound enhancing agents are used. In these studies, it is recommended that the MI be set low (0.15-0.3 for low-MI imaging) to avoid microbubble destruction.

34. **Answer: A.** As the frequency increases the rate at which ultrasound energy is absorbed in the tissues increases exponentially, and so the heating of the tissues increases. Therefore, answer A is correct. Increasing the image width will distribute the transmitted ultrasound energy more widely, reducing the heating effect at each point in the tissues. The gain and dynamic range controls alter the processing of the echo signals but have no effect on the transmitted ultrasound energy and its distribution in the tissues.

35. **Answer: D.** ALARA stands for As Low As Reasonably Achievable. This means that the exposure parameters and examination time should be kept reasonably low, but not so low that the clinical value of the examination is compromised. Another consequence of applying this principle is that ultrasound should not be used unless there is a medical indication. An exception is when it is being used for educational or research purposes.

KEY POINT

The likelihood of bioeffects occurring in diagnostic imaging is very low. However, because there is potential for bioeffects to occur, it is important that the sonographer operates the equipment as safely as possible by applying the "ALARA" principle.

36. **Answer: D.** M-mode imaging does not display the power spectrum of velocities measured along a single scan line over time, which can be obtained using the spectral Doppler mode. M-mode does indeed display ultrasound reflections along a single scan line over time. It has higher temporal resolution than 2D imaging because it is essentially one-dimensional. It uses a single scan line which allows formation of a much larger number of lines per second than the frame rate of a 2D image. M-mode does allow simultaneous visualization of different anatomical structures, as long as they can be connected by a straight line going through the transducer.

37. **Answer: C.** The image shown in **Figure 4-7B** (**Video 4-1B**) was obtained using higher frequency, which means that the wavelength was smaller. The smaller wavelength allows differentiation between two distinct objects located close to each other and so this image has better spatial resolution.

38. **Answer: A.** Each beam is formed using a different group of transducer elements. For example, the first beam may be formed using elements 1 to 128, the second beam may be formed using elements 2 to 129, the third beam may be formed using elements 3 to 130, and so on. This steps the beam along the face of the probe. The spacing from one beam to the next is equal to the spacing of the transducer elements, which is a fraction of a millimeter. The beams will all be parallel and so the image will be rectangular in shape. Note that time delays are used to achieve focusing of the beam. Also note that beam steering is used for compound imaging and in Doppler to achieve appropriate Doppler angles.

39. **Answer: D.** Refraction is the process where the beam alters direction as it passes through an interface separating tissues that have different propagation speeds (**Figure 4-11**). Note: the beam direction will **not** change if the incidence angle is 90°.

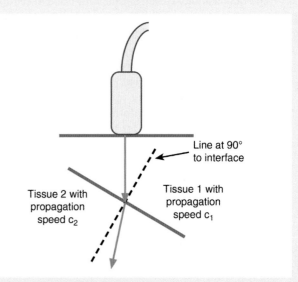

Figure 4-11 Refraction (or bending) of the ultrasound beam occurs when the ultrasound beam strikes an interface between tissues of different propagation speeds at an oblique angle. In this example, the propagation speed (c) is lower in the second tissue (i.e., $c_2 < c_1$).

40. **Answer: C.** Superficial structures such as muscles and cartilage can refract the ultrasound beam in such a way that deeper tissue structures are displayed twice at slightly different lateral positions. This is referred to as a refraction artifact.

41. **Answer: B.** As previously explained in the answer outline for Question 2, the wavelength can be calculated as:

$$\lambda = c \div f \tag{1}$$

where c is the propagation speed and f is the frequency.

Assuming a propagation speed of 1540 m/s and the frequency of 4×10^6 Hz (i.e., 4 MHz), the wavelength is calculated as:

$$\begin{aligned}
\lambda &= c \div f \\
&= 1540 \div \left(4 \times 10^6\right) \\
&= 0.000385\,m \\
&= 0.39\,mm
\end{aligned} \tag{2}$$

PRACTICAL TIP

Be careful to keep track of the units when performing this calculation. It can be helpful to write the propagation speed as $c = 1.54 \times 10^6$ mm/s rather than $c = 1540$ m/s so then:

$$\begin{aligned}
\lambda &= c \div f \\
&= \left(1.54 \times 10^6\right) \div \left(4 \times 10^6\right) \\
&= 0.39\,mm
\end{aligned}$$

42. **Answer: A.** When zooming the image while it is being acquired (preprocessing zoom), the machine will collect only the echo information required to image the reduced area in the heart. Each image will be acquired more quickly than a standard image and so the frame rate will be higher. Therefore, answer A is correct. Zooming after the image has been captured (postprocessing zoom) will have no effect on the frame rate since a full-sized image was obtained and then zoomed on the display. Both types of zoom have no effect on the level of image artifacts.

43. **Answer: A.** The strength of the transmitted ultrasound wave is controlled by adjusting the power control. Gain control determines to what extent the received signal is amplified, and the compression determines the dynamic range of received signals that are used to create the image. Time gain compensation has nothing to do with the strength of the transmitted power; it is part of the machine's processing and is designed to correct for beam attenuation as it travels through the body.

44. **Answer: B.** The dynamic range of echoes displayed on the screen is adjusted by the compression control. This control can be used to include or suppress weak echoes. Typically, the dynamic range is increased for high-quality images and decreased for difficult images.

Overall gain adjusts the amplification of received acoustic signals, the transmit power control adjusts the strength of the transmitted ultrasound wave, and the time gain compensation (TGC) adjusts the gains (amplification of signals) along the image depth to compensate for acoustic attenuation.

Acknowledgments: The authors thank and acknowledge Victor Mor-Avi, MD, Rajesh Jaganath, MD, Lynn Weinert, MD, and Jim D. Thomas, MD (Chapter 1, Physics: Fundamentals of Ultrasound Imaging and Instrumentation) in *Clinical Echocardiography Review: A Self-Assessment Tool*, 2nd ed., edited by Allan L. Klein, Craig R. Asher, 2017.

SUGGESTED READINGS

Anderson B. Basic principles of two-dimensional ultrasound imaging. In: *Echocardiography: The Normal Examination and Echocardiographic Measurements*. 3rd ed. Brisbane: Echotext Pty Ltd; 2017:chap 1.

Gill RW. *The Physics and Technology of Diagnostic Ultrasound: A Practitioner's Guide*. High Frequency Publishing; 2012.

Armstrong WF, Ryan T. Physics and instrumentation. In: *Feigenbaum's Echocardiography*. 8th ed. Philadelphia: Lippincott Williams and Wilkins; 2019:chap 2.

CHAPTER 5

Imaging Artifacts

Contributors: Ashwin Venkateshvaran, PhD, RCS, RDCS and Bonita Anderson, DMU (Cardiac), MAppSc (Medical Ultrasound), ACS

✪ Question 1

Which of the following basic assumptions related to the ultrasound beam and its interaction with tissue is false?

A. There is a constant rate of attenuation of 1 dB/cm/MHz.

B. All echoes arise from the center of a razor-thin ultrasound beam.

C. The distance to the reflecting object is inversely proportional to the round-trip travel time.

D. The ultrasound beam travels in a straight line and reflects just once.

E. The propagation speed in soft tissue is 1540 m/s.

✪ Question 2

Beam width artifacts demonstrate a direct relationship to which type of image resolution?

A. Axial

B. Lateral

C. Elevational

D. Temporal

✪ Question 3

Which of the following statements with respect to the echocardiographic appearance of beam width artifacts is false?

A. Reflectors producing the artifact lie behind or in front of the main beam plane.

B. A single reflector appears wider than it really is.

C. Strong reflectors at the edge of the beam appear within an echo-free space or cavity.

D. Two separate reflectors lying side by side appear as one reflector.

✪ Question 4

Which of the following statements regarding side lobe artifacts is true?

A. Side lobe artifacts are generated by a weakly reflective structure that is close to the main ultrasound beam.

B. A side lobe artifact will appear at the wrong location lateral to the true structure position.

C. Side lobe artifacts are created after echoes are returned from highly reflective structures located within the pathway of the main ultrasound beam.

D. Side lobe artifacts appear as diffraction or divergence reflections in the far field of the image.

✪ Question 5

Side lobe and beam width artifacts may have a similar ultrasound appearance. These artifacts can be differentiated based on the fact that:

A. Side lobe artifacts are usually wider than beam width artifacts.

B. Side lobe artifacts are usually brighter than beam width artifacts.

C. Side lobes are a lateral extension of a real structure while a beam width artifact is a replication of a real structure.

D. Side lobes are always curvilinear in appearance while beam width artifacts are strictly horizontal.

⭐ Question 6

Which of the following statements regarding refraction artifacts is false?
   A. Refraction of the ultrasound beam can result in misplacement of echoes.
   B. Refraction of the ultrasound beam can result in missing echoes.
   C. Refraction of the ultrasound beam can result in duplication of structures.
   D. Refraction of the ultrasound beam can result in distortion of structures.

⭐ Question 7

Acoustic shadowing and acoustic enhancement artifacts can be avoided by performing which of the following maneuvers?
   A. Switching to a high frequency transducer
   B. Altering overall gains
   C. Turning off harmonics
   D. Changing the probe position

⭐ Question 8

Which of the following artifacts does not result in the duplication of a structure?
   A. Mirror
   B. Refraction
   C. Reverberation
   D. Slice thickness

⭐ Question 9

The presence of a ring-down artifact should alert the sonographer to the presence of:
   A. Gas bubbles.
   B. Calcium.
   C. Metallic objects.
   D. Thrombus.

⭐ Question 10

As opposed to artifacts, true anatomical structures are characterized by:
   A. Poorly defined borders.
   B. The appearance being limited to a single view.
   C. Confinement to anatomical borders.
   D. A lack of attachment to adjacent structures.

⭐ Question 11

Which of the following statements regarding reverberation artifacts is true?
   A. Reverberation artifacts result from repeated reflections off the transducer or other strong reflectors.
   B. Reverberation artifacts appear as equally spaced lines perpendicular to the main axis of the beam.
   C. Reverberation artifacts increase in intensity as the distance from the transducer increases.
   D. Reverberation artifacts occur when the acoustic mismatch between two media through which ultrasound is passing is constant.

⭐ Question 12

A mirror-image artifact in 2D echocardiography is created when:
   A. A structure is located behind a strong reflector resulting in the display of a mirror-image copy of that structure in a shallower position.
   B. A structure in front of a highly reflective interface is detected and a mirror-image copy of that structure is displayed in a deeper position.
   C. A mirror-like interface is located parallel to the ultrasound beam.
   D. The assumption that all echoes arise from the center of a razor-thin ultrasound beam is violated.

⭐ Question 13

Which of the following artifacts can be minimized or eliminated by repositioning the focal zone?
   A. Attenuation shadow
   B. Beam width
   C. Grating lobe
   D. Mirror

⭐ Question 14

Which of the following statements regarding range ambiguity is true?
   A. Range ambiguity occurs when the propagation speed through a structure is lower than the assumed propagation speed.
   B. Range ambiguity occurs when the ultrasound machine is operating at a low pulse repetition frequency (PRF).
   C. Range ambiguity can be avoided by decreasing the image depth (field of view).
   D. Range ambiguity occurs when echoes from deep structures created by a first pulse arrive at the transducer after the second pulse has been transmitted.

✪✪ Question 15

In the corresponding apical four-chamber image of a prosthetic mitral valve (**Figure 5-1**), the artifact obscuring the left atrium is due to the interaction between the ultrasound beam and a structure with _____ attenuating properties.

    A. No
    B. Low
    C. Moderate
    D. High

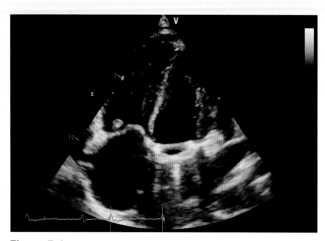

Figure 5-1

✪✪ Question 16

In the corresponding apical four-chamber image acquired from a patient with normal left ventricular systolic function and no regional wall motion abnormalities (**Figure 5-2**), the apical "mass" (arrow) is most likely a result of which of the following artifacts?

    A. Shadowing
    B. Refraction
    C. Near-field clutter
    D. Beam width

✪✪ Question 17

▶ The parasternal long-axis view reveals a "mass" posterior to the pericardium (**Video 5-1**). This is most likely:

    A. A left pleural effusion with a collapsed lung.
    B. A large pericardial effusion with hematoma.
    C. A pericardial tumor.
    D. The posterior left ventricular wall.

✪✪ Question 18

▶ In the corresponding zoomed views of the aortic valve acquired from the parasternal long- and short-axis views (**Videos 5-2A** and **5-2B**), the "mass" on the noncoronary cusp of the aortic valve in the parasternal short-axis view is likely due to which of the following artifacts?

    A. Slice thickness
    B. Refraction
    C. Range ambiguity
    D. Beam width

✪✪ Question 19

▶ In the corresponding subcostal short-axis view of the left ventricle (**Video 5-3**), which artifact is present?

    A. Mirror
    B. Reverberation
    C. Refraction
    D. Slice thickness

✪✪ Question 20

▶ Observe the corresponding videos of a St Jude mitral valve replacement (MVR) acquired from the apical four-chamber view (**Video 5-4A**) and a zoomed apical four-chamber view (**Video 5-4B**). Which of the following statements is true?

    A. Reverberation artifacts indicate that this MVR is functioning normally.
    B. Reverberation artifacts indicate dehiscence of the MVR at the medial annulus.
    C. Reverberation artifacts indicate dehiscence of the MVR at the lateral annulus.
    D. Reverberation artifacts indicate obstruction of the medial disk of the MVR.
    E. Reverberation artifacts indicate obstruction of the lateral disk of the MVR.

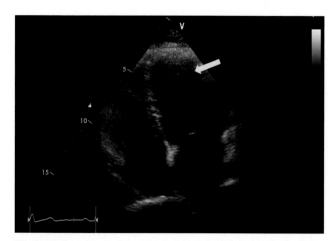

Figure 5-2

✪✪ Question 21

In the corresponding apical four-chamber view (**Figure 5-3**), the "structure" seen in the left atrium (arrow) is most probably attributable to which of the following artifacts?

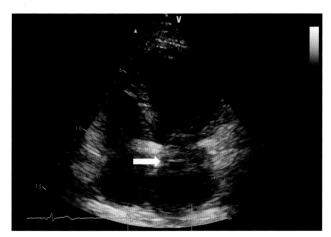

Figure 5-3

A. Reverberation
B. Beam width
C. Range ambiguity
D. Mirror

✪✪ Question 22

▶ In the corresponding apical two-chamber view (**Video 5-5**), the artifact seen within the left atrial (LA) cavity is a:

A. Range ambiguity.
B. Slice thickness
C. Grating lobe.
D. Propagation speed error.

✪✪ Question 23

▶ Which of the following statements is most accurate regarding the structure seen in the left atrium in **Video 5-6A** (parasternal long-axis view) and the structure seen in the right atrium in **Video 5-6B** (off-axis parasternal long-axis view of right ventricular inflow)?

A. The patient has undergone surgery for congenital heart disease.
B. The patient has undergone an interventional procedure.
C. There is a calcified atrial septal aneurysm.
D. There is a complex anomalous coronary artery.

✪✪ Question 24

▶ Observe the corresponding apical four-chamber view acquired from a patient with a Starr-Edwards

(ball-cage) mitral valve replacement (**Video 5-7**). Which of the following statements regarding the appearance of this valve is true?

A. The speed of sound in the silastic ball is faster than the speed of sound in tissue so that the shape of the ball appears distorted.
B. The speed of sound in the silastic ball is slower than the speed of sound in tissue so that the shape of the ball appears distorted.
C. Ball-cage valves cause a resolution-type artifact.
D. The propagation speed of ultrasound in tissue is assumed to be 13 μs to a depth of 1 mm.

✪✪ Question 25

▶ **Video 5-8** displays a 3D image showing a stitching artifact. Which of the following maneuvers is unlikely to resolve a stitching artifact?

A. Minimizing out-of-pane movement during ECG acquisition
B. Turning off electrocautery
C. Momentarily arresting respiration
D. Increasing the number of gated beats during acquisition

✪✪✪ Question 26

Which of the following best describes the artifacts depicted by the arrows in **Figure 5-4**?

A. Comet-tail
B. Ring-down
C. Reverberation
D. Refraction (lens-effect)
E. Any of the above (production is effectively the same)

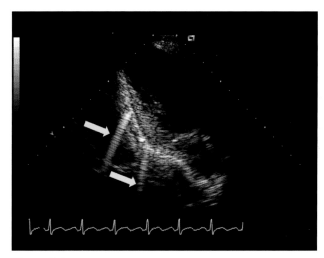

Figure 5-4

✪✪✪ Question 27

Regarding the artifacts in Question 26 (**Figure 5-4**), which fundamental assumptions are violated to produce these artifacts?

  A. There is a constant rate of attenuation of 1 dB/cm/MHz and a propagation speed of 1540 m/s.
  B. The ultrasound beam travels in a straight line and reflects just once.
  C. All echoes arise from the center of a razor-thin ultrasound beam and are reflected just once.
  D. The distance to the reflecting object is proportional to the round-trip travel time and attenuation is the same in all tissues imaged.
  E. The ultrasound beam travels in a straight line and all echoes detected are due to the most recently sent pulse.

✪✪✪ Question 28

▶ Observe the corresponding videos acquired from the apical four-chamber view (**Video 5-9A**) and a zoomed apical four-chamber view of the interatrial septum (**Video 5-9B**). The three prominent artifacts in the right and left atria as displayed in **Video 5-9B** are:

  A. Comet-tail, grating lobes, beam width.
  B. Slice thickness, comet-tail, beam width.
  C. Mirror, grating lobes, beam width.
  D. Refraction, grating lobes, comet-tail.

✪✪✪ Question 29

Figure 5-5 is a parasternal long-axis image acquired from a patient post cardiac surgery. The structure depicted by the arrow is:

  A. A normal anatomic structure.
  B. A reverberation artifact.

  C. A mirror artifact.
  D. A grating lobe artifact.
  E. A propagation speed artifact.

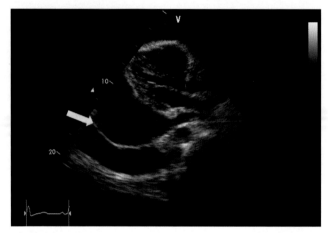

Figure 5-5

✪✪✪ Question 30

▶ In **Video 5-10**, there is an artifact in the right atrium, superior to the septal tricuspid valve leaflet. Which of the following statements regarding this artifact is false?

  A. This is a range ambiguity artifact.
  B. This artifact can be eliminated by increasing the image depth.
  C. This artifact can be eliminated by increasing the transducer frequency.
  D. This artifact is created when there is a high pulse repetition frequency.
  E. This artifact is caused by structures outside of the field of view.

ANSWERS

1. **Answer: C.** The round-trip time of a given echo is **directly** related to the depth of the reflecting object from the transducer. Therefore, answer C is a false statement. All other stated basic assumptions are true.

   Two-dimensional (2D) imaging artifacts may occur when the basic assumptions relating to the ultrasound beam and its interaction with tissue are violated. For example, it is assumed that there is a constant rate of attenuation through soft tissue of 1 dB/cm/MHz; however, the ultrasound beam encounters many different tissue types throughout the field of view, many of which have different attenuation rates. It is also assumed that the ultrasound beam travels in a straight line and reflects just once. However, bending of the ultrasound beam can occur and the ultrasound beam may be reflected more than once. The assumption that all echoes arise from the center of a razor-thin beam is frequently violated as echoes arise throughout the full width and thickness of the ultrasound beam as well as from secondary beams. While the propagation speed in soft tissue is

1540 m/s, the propagation speed varies depending upon the structure encountered. The round-trip time assumption may be compromised by numerous factors such as bouncing of the ultrasound beam between two interfaces.

2D imaging artifacts can be categorized based on the violation of these assumptions (**Table 5-1**). The four major 2D imaging artifact categories include attenuation artifacts, beam dimension artifacts, depth of origin artifacts, and beam path artifacts (**Table 5-2**).

KEY POINTS

The five key assumptions of ultrasound machines are (1) "there is a constant rate of attenuation of 1 dB/cm/MHz," (2) "all echoes arise from the center of a razor-thin beam," (3) "the propagation speed in soft tissue is 1540 m/s," (4) "the round-trip time of a given echo is directly related to the depth of the reflector from the transducer," and (5) "the ultrasound beam travels in a straight line and reflects just once." When one or more of these assumptions is violated, an artifact is created.

2. **Answer: B.** Lateral resolution refers to the ability of the ultrasound machine to detect echoes from two closely spaced reflectors positioned side by side across the lateral axis of the ultrasound beam and to then display these reflectors as being separate. Since beam width artifacts occur when echoes are generated from structures lying within the full width of the ultrasound beam, beam width artifacts are directly related to the **lateral resolution**. Therefore, answer B is correct.

Structures that lie side by side may not be clearly distinguishable (resolved) as separate objects by the transducer. As illustrated in **Figure 5-6**, an ultrasound beam focuses within a certain distance from the transducer; this is the focal zone. Beyond the focal zone, the ultrasound beam diverges. Hence, if two separate reflectors are encompassed within the ultrasound beam width beyond the focal zone, they will not be resolved (Depth B in **Figure 5-6**). However, when the same two reflectors are separated by a distance that is greater than the ultrasound beam width, they will be resolved and will appear as two separate points (Depth A in **Figure 5-6**).

Answer A is not correct as axial resolution refers to the ability to detect echoes from two closely spaced reflectors at different depths along the beam axis and to display reflectors as being separate. Answer C is not correct as elevational resolution refers to the ability to distinguish two planes lying in front of or behind the main image plane or across the elevation or slice thickness dimension of the ultrasound beam. Answer D is not correct as temporal resolution refers to the ability to accurately display the position of moving structures at an instant in time.

3. **Answer: A.** Reflectors producing a beam width artifact will always be imaged **adjacent** to the artifact, not behind or in front of the main beam plane. Therefore, answer A is a false statement. All other statements are true regarding the potential echocardiographic features of beam width artifacts. Recall that echoes are generated from reflectors lying within the full width of the ultrasound beam and echoes will continue to be generated if a reflector remains within the beam width. Therefore, beam width artifacts occur when (1) two separate reflectors lying side by side within the ultrasound beam appear as one (see **Figure 5-6**), (2) a narrow reflector within the ultrasound beam appears wider than it really is, and (3) a strong reflector

Table 5-1. Artifacts Occurring When Assumptions of Ultrasound Are Violated

Artifact	Violated Assumption(s) Producing Artifact
Attenuation artifacts (improper brightness): include acoustic enhancement, acoustic shadowing	Constant rate of attenuation of 1 dB/cm/MHz
Beam dimension artifacts (added structures): include beam width, slice thickness, slide lobe, or grating lobe	All echoes arise from the center of a razor-thin ultrasound beam
Depth of origin artifacts (wrong place or wrong size): include propagation speed or range ambiguity	Propagation speed in soft tissue is 1540 m/s Distance to the reflecting object is directly proportional to the round-trip travel time Ultrasound beam travels in a straight line and reflects just once
Beam path artifacts (duplication of structures or structures in the wrong place): include reverberation, mirror, refraction	Distance to the reflecting object is directly proportional to the round-trip travel time Ultrasound beam travels in a straight line and reflects just once

Table 5-2. 2D Imaging Artifacts

Artifact	Principal Assumption Violated	Mechanism of Formation	Overall Effect	Example
Acoustic enhancement	Attenuation of U/S beam = 1 dB/cm/MHz	Lower than expected attenuation of U/S beam	Improper brightness	Increased brightness posterior to PE
Acoustic shadow	Attenuation of U/S beam = 1 dB/cm/MHz	Higher than expected attenuation of U/S beam	Improper brightness Missing echoes	Absence of echoes distal to mitral annular calcification
Beam width	All echoes arise from central axis of U/S beam	Structures detected throughout full width of U/S beam	Wrong shape Wrong size Lateral extension	"Fuzziness" of atrial chamber walls
Side lobe and grating lobe	All echoes arise from central axis of U/S beam	Structures detected by secondary U/S beams	Replication	"Extra" echoes in RA arising from IVC
Mirror	U/S beam travels in a straight line and is reflected only once	U/S beam interrogates same structure twice	Duplication	"Two" mitral valves in the PLAX view
Range ambiguity	Round-trip time ∝ depth to reflector	Echo from pulse 1 is received after pulse 2 emitted	Improper depth	"Mass" within ventricular cavities in apical views
Refraction	U/S beam travels in a straight line and is reflected only once	Bending of U/S beam	Improper placement Duplication	Double LV in subcostal SAX
Reverberation	U/S beam travels in a straight line and is reflected only once	Bouncing of U/S beam between two interfaces	Improper placement Duplication	"Ladder" appearance within LA from mechanical MVR
Slice thickness	All echoes arise from central axis of U/S beam	Structures detected in front of or behind main imaging plane	Added echoes	Apparent mass within chamber cavity
Propagation speed	Round-trip time ∝ depth to reflector	Speed of sound ≠ 1540 m/s	Improper depth Wrong shape	Ball of Starr-Edwards MVR appears within LA cavity

IVC, inferior vena cava; LA, left atrium; MVR, mitral valve replacement; PE, pericardial effusion; PLAX, parasternal long axis; RA, right atrium; SAX, short axis; U/S, ultrasound.

Reproduced with permission by Echotext Pty Ltd, from Anderson B. Basic principles of two-dimensional ultrasound imaging. In: *Echocardiography: The Normal Examination and Echocardiographic Measurements*. 3rd ed. Australia: Echotext Pty Ltd; 2017:20, chap 1.

to the side of an echo-free cavity appears within this cavity. Beam width artifacts are most apparent within echo-free cavities.

KEY POINTS
Beam width artifacts may (1) result in the merger of two separate objects so they appear as one, (2) produce lateral smearing or extension of an object, or (3) generate a partial-volume effect where a strong reflector appears within an echo-free space. These artifacts can be minimized by placing the focal zone at the level of the structure of interest.

4. **Answer: B.** A side lobe artifact will appear as a structure in the wrong location and lateral to the true structure position. Recall that secondary weaker beams of ultrasound (side lobes) exist outside of the main beam. Side lobes have the capacity of sending and receiving ultrasound energy just like the main beam. Therefore, strong reflectors may produce echoes strong enough to return to the transducer and be recorded and displayed. Echoes received from these secondary beams are assumed to have originated from the main beam and will therefore be displayed at both sides of the strong reflector. In **Figure 5-7**, as the ultrasound beam sweeps left to right, the structure is interrogated by side lobe beams (light blue) as well as by the main beam (dark blue). On the final image display, echoes originating from the side lobe beams and the main beam are displayed with the weaker side lobe artifacts appearing lateral to the true structure. Most commonly, this artifact creates a linear "arc-like" artifact at both sides of the strong reflector.

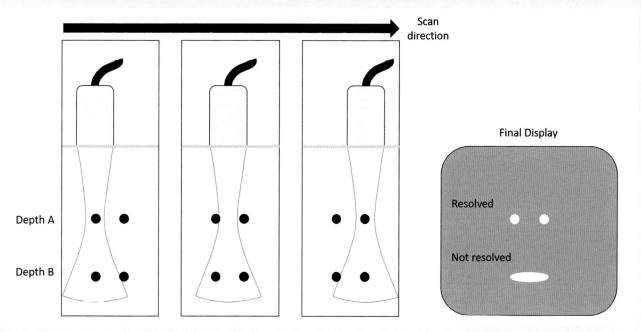

Figure 5-6

5. **Answer: A.** Side lobe artifacts can be differentiated from beam width artifacts as they are usually **wider** than beam width artifacts. Therefore, answer A is correct. The maximum width of a beam width artifact is limited by the actual beam width while side lobe artifacts are produced by secondary beams resulting in potentially "wider" artifacts.

   Answer B is not correct as side lobe artifacts are usually **less bright** than beam width artifacts as these artifacts are produced by weaker secondary beams while beam width artifacts are produced by the main beam. Answer C is not correct as side lobe artifacts are produced by the replication of the real structure while a beam width artifact is simply a lateral smearing of a real structure. Answer D is not correct as both side lobes and beam width artifacts may have a curvilinear appearance.

6. **Answer: D.** Distortion of structures occurs when propagation speed through a structure is not the assumed 1540 m/s; this is not a feature of refraction artifacts. Therefore, answer D is correct as this is a false statement.

   Refraction or bending of the ultrasound beam occurs when an ultrasound beam strikes an interface at an angle other than 90° and when the propagation speeds of the two media at either side of the interface are different. This can result in (1) improper positioning or misplacement of structures (**Figure 5-8A**), (2) missing echoes or shadowing at the edge of curved structures (**Figure 5-8B**), or (3) duplication of structures (**Figure 5-8C**). Therefore, answers A-C are true statements.

   In **Figure 5-8A**, the propagation speed through media 1 (C_1) is less than the propagation speed

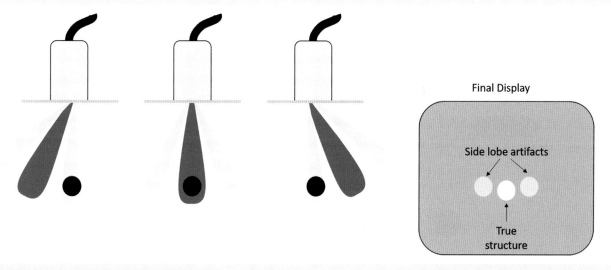

Figure 5-7

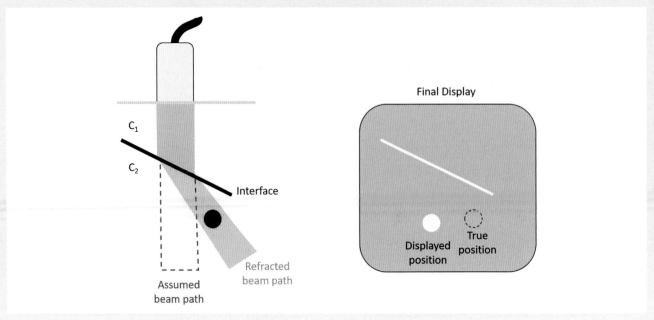

Figure 5-8A

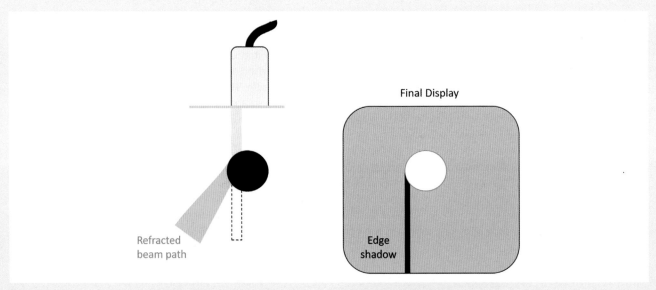

Figure 5-8B

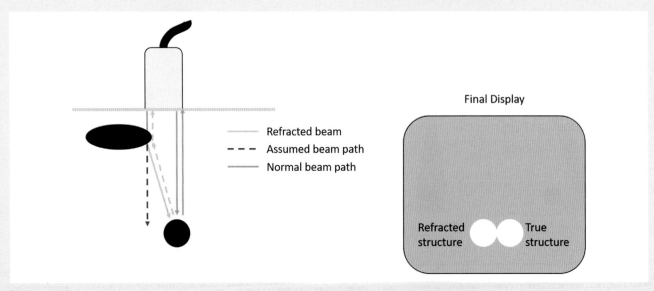

Figure 5-8C

through media 2 (C_2), resulting in bending of the beam away from the assumed (expected) path. This results in the misplacement of the structure on the final image display.

In **Figure 5-8B**, an edge shadowing is produced when the ultrasound beam strikes the edge of the circular structure. A combination of refraction and reflection occurs, causing the ultrasound beam to be deflected and broadened. This leads to a reduction on the beam intensity so that the echoes beyond the edge of the circular structure are reduced in amplitude. On the final image display, this results in a narrow shadow directly beneath the margins of the rounded structure.

In **Figure 5-8C**, duplication of a structure is produced when there is refraction of the ultrasound beam as it passes obliquely through a lens-shaped muscle. As a result, the single structure (black circle) is interrogated twice: once by the refracted beam and once by the "normal" beam. On the final image display, the single structure is displayed twice as either two separate structures (as shown) or as two overlapping structures.

KEY POINTS
Refraction of the ultrasound beam can result in the misplacement of echoes, missing echoes (edge shadow or refractive shadow), or the duplication of structures (also known as a lens artifact).

7. **Answer: D.** Acoustic shadowing and acoustic enhancement artifacts are 2D ultrasound artifacts that violate the assumption that the ultrasound beam is uniformly attenuated along the beam path. Shadowing occurs when there is excessive attenuation or weakening of the ultrasound beam through

a structure compared with the attenuation through adjacent structures. This results in an anechoic region distal to the "offending" structure. Conversely, enhancement occurs when there is a low level of attenuation through a structure compared with the attenuation through adjacent structures. This results in a hyperechoic region distal to the "offending" structure. Answer D is correct as both artifacts can be avoided by changing probe position to avoid the "offending" structures. For example, the loss of echo information within the left atrium secondary to a highly calcified mitral valve in the apical views may be addressed by switching to the parasternal view, thereby eliminating the "offending" reflector from the beam path.

Answer A is not correct as switching to a high frequency transducer will improve the spatial resolution but will not eliminate acoustic shadowing and acoustic enhancement artifacts.

Answer B is not correct as decreasing the overall gain simply reduces the amplitude of the echoes but will not eliminate acoustic shadowing and acoustic enhancement artifacts.

Answer C is not correct as turning off harmonics (or reverting to the fundamental transducer frequency) will not eliminate acoustic shadowing and acoustic enhancement artifacts.

8. **Answer: D.** Slice thickness artifacts occur when a structure is detected within the elevation plane of the ultrasound beam; that is, when the structure is detected in front of or behind the main beam. As illustrated in **Figure 5-9**, the slice thickness or elevation plane is shown from a side view of the transducer (left). When an echo-free structure within the main beam (middle) and a structure behind the

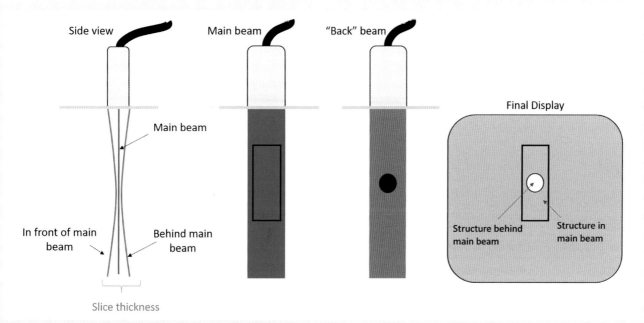

Figure 5-9

main beam (right) are detected, echoes are generated from both structures and then "collapsed" to produce a 2D image. As a result, the displayed image is composed of echoes that have originated from the main imaging plane as well as those that have arisen from structures in front of and behind the main imaging plane. Therefore, answer D is correct as slice thickness artifacts are **not duplications** or copies of real structures.

Answers A-C are not correct since these artifacts do result in the duplication of a real structure. Reverberation artifacts produce multiple reflections of the same structure when the ultrasound beam bounces between two or more strong reflectors that are positioned in close proximity. Mirror artifacts can produce duplication of structures when the ultrasound beam encounters a strongly reflecting interface that acts as a mirror. A refraction artifact can produce duplication of structures via the lens principle.

9. **Answer: A.** Ring-down artifacts are caused when fluid is trapped by air or gas bubbles. When the ultrasound beam encounters these gas bubbles, they continuously resonate or vibrate. These echoes are reflected to the transducer creating a bright continuous "streak" distal to the gas bubble; this is referred to as a ring-down artifact. Therefore, answer A is correct as the presence of ring-down artifacts should alert the sonographer to look for the potential source of gas bubbles.

Answer B is incorrect as the artifact associated with calcium is an acoustic shadow. Calcium usually attenuates the ultrasound; therefore, echoes beyond calcified structures are significantly reduced, creating an acoustic shadow.

Answer C is incorrect as the artifact associated with metallic objects is a comet-tail artifact. Comet-tail artifacts occur when there are highly reflective objects such as metallic needles and pacemaker wires. This results in a reverberation-type artifact

where there is ringing of the transducer to create a solid hyperechoic beam of ultrasound distal to the "offending" object.

Answer D is not correct as thrombus is not associated with ring-down artifacts.

10. **Answer: C.** True structures confine themselves strictly to anatomical borders and do not pass through cardiac or vascular walls. Therefore, answer C is correct. This is an important distinction between artifacts and anatomical structures. Unlike true structures, artifacts often cross anatomic borders, have poorly defined borders, demonstrate no clear attachment to adjacent structures, and are often visualized only in a single echocardiographic view. See **Table 5-3** for clues to the correct interpretation of common echocardiographic artifacts.

11. **Answer: A.** Reverberation artifacts occur when there are multiple reflections off the transducer or strong reflectors. In **Figure 5-10**, there is repeated "bouncing" of the ultrasound beam between two interfaces. Because the re-reflected echoes return to the transducer later, these echoes will be placed deeper than the true reflector. The distance between reverberation artifacts is equal to the distance (d) between the two interfaces. Echoes produced from multiple reflections appear progressively weaker since the ultrasound intensity of reverberation artifacts decreases.

Answer B is incorrect as reverberation artifacts appear as equally spaced reflections, **parallel** to the main beam.

Answer C is incorrect as reverberation artifacts become progressively **weaker** in intensity as the distance from the transducer increases.

Answer D is incorrect as reverberation artifacts occur when the acoustic mismatch between two media through which ultrasound passes is **large** resulting in some of the energy returning to the transducer and some of the energy being re-reflected from this interface.

Table 5-3. Clues to the Correct Interpretation of Common Echocardiographic Artifacts

	Favors Real Structure	Favors Artifact
Morphology	Distinct edges (unless thrombus)	Linear Lacks well-demarcated borders
Motion	Independent motion	Identical to other real structures (parallel or mirror) Appears to pass through other solid structures
Attachments	Attached to other structures	No clear attachments
Reproducibility	Consistently seen in multiple views	May not be reproduced in other imaging views
Color Doppler	Affected by real structure	Not affected by artifact
Others	Logical anatomic relationships	Logical physical explanation for its presence in that specific location

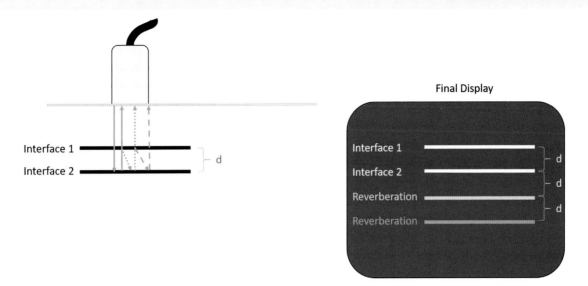

Figure 5-10 d, Depth.

12. Answer: B. A mirror artifact is produced when a structure in front of a highly reflective surface is detected resulting in the display of a mirror-image copy of that structure in a deeper position. Therefore, answer B is correct. As illustrated in **Figure 5-11**, the true structure is interrogated twice by the transducer: once as the ultrasound beam travels straight to the structure and then straight back to the transducer (solid lines), and a second time when the beam hits a mirror interface. When the beam hits the mirror interface, it is reflected off the "mirror" to the structure and then echoes from the structure, and return along the same path back to the transducer (dashed lines). On the final image display, the real structure is displayed on the transducer side of the mirror interface while the mirror artifact appears on the opposite side of the "mirror"

because the return time to the transducer is longer. The true reflector and the artifact appear at equal distances from the mirror.

Answer A is incorrect as mirror artifacts appear deeper in position as described above.

Answer C is not correct as the mirror interface is located perpendicular to the ultrasound beam.

Answer D is incorrect as the violated assumptions producing a mirror artifact are that the ultrasound beam has traveled in a straight line and is reflected only once.

13. Answer: B. As previously described, beam width artifacts occur when (1) two separate reflectors lying side by side within the ultrasound beam appear as one, (2) a narrow reflector within the ultrasound beam appears wider than it really is, or (3) a strong reflector to the side of an echo free cavity appears

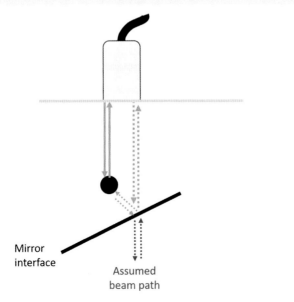

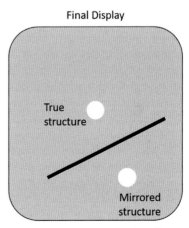

Figure 5-11

within this cavity. Moving the focus narrows the ultrasound beam and may therefore minimize or even eliminate a beam width artifact. Therefore, answer B is correct. Another maneuver that may minimize or eliminate beam width artifacts includes increasing the transducer frequency.

Answer A is not correct. Attenuation artifacts are created when the assumption that there is a constant rate of attenuation of 1 dB/cm/MHz is violated. Adjustment of the focus will not minimize or eliminate this artifact.

Answer C is not correct. Grating lobe artifacts are produced by secondary beams similar to side lobe artifacts. These artifacts may be avoided by changing the angle of insonation. Adjustment of the focus will not minimize or eliminate this artifact.

Answer D is not correct. Mirror artifacts are produced when a there is a large acoustic impedance mismatch between an interface and a specular reflector. The specular reflector acts like a mirror so that structures located in front of the "mirror" are interrogated and displayed twice. These artifacts may be avoided by changing the angle of insonation. Adjustment of the focus will not minimize or eliminate this artifact.

14. **Answer: D.** Range ambiguity occurs when echoes from deep structures created by a first pulse arrive at the transducer **after** the second pulse has been transmitted. It is assumed that all received echoes are produced by the most recently sent pulse and the depth placement of received echoes is based on the return time to the transducer. Range ambiguity artifacts may occur when a structure is detected outside the field of view by the first pulse. When the echoes generated from the first pulse arrive at the transducer after the second pulse has been emitted, the machine assumes that the returning echoes have originated from the second pulse and therefore incorrectly places the received echoes closer to the transducer than their actual location (**Figure 5-12**). These artifacts are especially apparent when the ultrasound beam passes through low-attenuating structures such as blood-filled cavities.

Answer A is not correct as propagation speed artifacts are not *mechanistically* the same as a range ambiguity artifact. Propagation speed artifacts occur when the propagation speed is slower or faster than the assumed propagation speed of 1540 m/s. This results in incorrect placement of echoes or the incorrect display of the size and shape of structures.

Answer B is not correct as range ambiguity occurs when the ultrasound machine is operating at a **high** PRF. At a high PRF, echoes from deep structures created by the first pulse arrive at the transducer after the second pulse has been transmitted.

Answer C is not correct as range ambiguity can be avoided by **increasing** the image depth or field of view, which effectively lowers the PRF. Therefore,

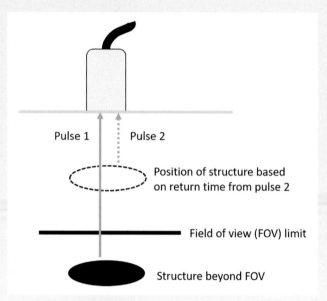

Pulse 1   Pulse 2

Position of structure based on return time from pulse 2

Field of view (FOV) limit

Structure beyond FOV

Figure 5-12

echoes from deep structures created by the first pulse arrive at the transducer before the second pulse has been transmitted.

KEY POINTS
Range ambiguity artifacts are commonly seen within the left ventricular cavity from the apical views especially when image quality is very good, and the image depth is shallow. Elimination of these artifacts can be achieved by increasing the image depth to lower the PRF.

15. **Answer: D.** The registered intensity of an echo signal is directly related to the attenuating properties of the tissue interface. When the ultrasound beam encounters structures with high attenuating properties such as a metallic prosthetic valve, shadowing occurs immediately distal to the structure along the path of the ultrasound beam. This results in hypoechoic or anechoic regions distal to the "offending" structure. In this example, shadowing created by the prosthetic mitral valve hinders the comprehensive assessment of the left atrium. Reverberation artifacts created by the metallic prosthetic valve are also seen within the left atrium.

16. **Answer: C.** High amplitude transducer oscillations sometimes obscure the near field, causing a near-field clutter artifact. These artifacts may give the false impression of an apical mass or thrombus. However, unlike a thrombus, this artifact is relatively unaffected by adjacent wall motion and often appears to cross anatomical borders (**Video 5-11**). Employing both higher frequencies and harmonic imaging may improve near-field resolution. Additionally, using contrast to opacify the apex or switching probe position to see if the mass persists in other views can also be performed to disprove the presence of a thrombus. Application of color Doppler with a reduced color

velocity scale to demonstrate blood flow through the apex may also be useful to disprove a suspected apical mass caused by near-field clutter.

17. ▶ **Answer: D.** This is a mirror image of the posterior wall of the left ventricle (LV). Mirror artifacts occur when the ultrasound beam encounters a strong reflective surface. The ultrasound beam bounces off this surface to another object closer to the transducer and back to the strong reflector surface, before it makes its way back to the transducer (see **Figure 5-11**). The ultrasound machine misinterprets the signal as originating at twice the distance from the transducer since the time taken by the pulse to return to the transducer is doubled. This generates a false image. In this example, the strong reflective surface is the pericardial-lung interface (yellow arrow) resulting in the mirrored appearance of the posterior wall (PW) (**Figure 5-13**). A mirror image of the mitral valve (MV) and cords are also appreciated on the real-time video clip. Mirror artifacts are generally easy to identify as they project a copy of structures located above the reflective surface. This artifact is best avoided by changing probe position to one that eliminates the highly reflective surface from the beam path.

In the same patient, a nice mirror artifact of the right atrial (RA) wall was seen from the apical four-chamber view (**Video 5-12**). Observe how the motion of this artifact mirrors the motion of the true RA wall.

18. **Answer: A.** In this example, the "mass" is only seen in the parasternal short-axis view. This is an example of a slice thickness artifact whereby the "belly" of the aortic valve has been detected behind the main beam and has been compressed onto the 2D image. Recall that the ultrasound machine assumes that all echoes are generated from the center of a razor-thin ultrasound beam. However, the ultrasound beam is three-dimensional such that echoes detected in front of or behind the main beam are assumed to have originated from the relatively thin central beam and the images will be superimposed accordingly (see **Figure 5-9**).

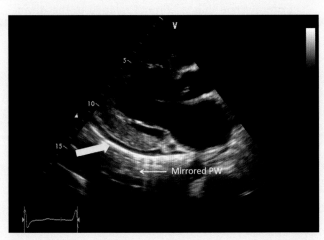

Figure 5-13

Answer B is not correct as refraction artifacts occur when there is bending of the ultrasound beam resulting is the improper placement or duplication of structures.

Answer C is unlikely. Range ambiguity artifacts may occur when a structure is detected outside the field of view in the setting of a high PRF. Given that this artifact is absent from the zoomed parasternal long-axis view, which would have a similar PRF as the zoomed parasternal short-axis view, a range ambiguity artifact is not likely.

Answer D is not correct. While both beam width and slice thickness artifacts are beam dimension artifacts, with a beam width artifact the "offending" structure creating the artifact will be seen in the imaging plane adjacent to the real structure.

KEY POINTS
Slice thickness artifacts arise when the assumption that all echoes arise from the center of a razor-thin beam is violated. The offending structure creating the slice thickness artifact is not seen in the same imaging plane as the artifact; it will be seen at 90° to this imaging plane.

19. **Answer: C.** This is an example of a refraction (lens) artifact, which can create the appearance of a double image, which in this case is the left ventricle. Refraction is produced when the transmitted ultrasound beam is deviated from its straight-line path (that is, there is bending of the ultrasound beam). This occurs when there is an oblique angle of incidence between two media of different propagation velocities (see **Figure 5-8C**). Refraction of the ultrasound beam causes displacement of structures laterally from their true location. Refraction artifacts violate the assumption that ultrasound travels in straight lines.

Answers A and B are not correct. Reverberation and mirror artifacts can produce duplication of structures; however, these artifacts are seen beyond the strong reflector/mirror interface (see **Figures 5-10** and **5-11**).

Answer D is not correct since slice thickness artifacts do not produce "double" images of a structure. Slice thickness artifacts occur when structures are detected in front of or behind the main imaging plane and are displayed as though they have originated from the central beam (see **Figure 5-9**).

KEY POINTS
Mirror and reverberation artifacts can be differentiated from refraction (lens) artifacts based on the position of the duplicated structure. Refraction artifacts typically appear at the same depth and to the side of the real structure while mirror and reverberation artifacts always appear deeper and behind the real structure.

20. ▶ **Answer: E.** There is obstruction of the lateral disk of the MVR. Observe that there is a fixed reverberation in the center of the left atrium that is

associated with the lateral disk. Compare this fixed reverberation artifact to the normal reverberation artifact associated with the medial disk. The absence of movement of the reverberation artifact should alert the sonographer to the possibility of thrombosis or pannus of the prosthetic valve. When imaged from the parasternal short-axis view (**Video 5-13**), the lateral disk appears fixed and immobile compared with the motion of the medial disk. The patient went to cardiac surgery as thrombolysis was unsuccessful. The appearance of the resected MVR shows that the lateral disk was completely thrombosed (**Figure 5-14**), thus, explaining the absence of disk motion on the 2D examination. This example illustrates how imaging artifacts may be useful to assist in a clinical diagnosis.

21. **Answer: B.** The aberrant presentation of a "structure" in the left atrium (LA) is most probably attributed to a beam width artifact. Observe the position of the focal zone close to the apex of the heart in this image with the LA positioned in the far field. Recall that beyond the focal zone, the ultrasound beam diverges (see **Figure 5-6**), leading to a poorer lateral resolution in the far field and the subsequent impaired ability of the ultrasound machine to distinguish structures that lie side by side as being separate structures. This loss of adequate spatial (lateral) definition can sometimes create the impression of a diffuse mass corresponding to the area of increasing beam divergence. Repositioning the focus to this level of the apparent "structure" or "mass" often resolves this issue.

22. **Answer: C.** Grating lobe artifacts occur in a similar manner to side lobe artifacts in that secondary grating lobe beams produce echoes strong enough to return to the transducer and be recorded and

displayed. Since it is assumed that all echoes received have originated from the central beam, grating lobe echoes appear lateral to the true structure. Compared with side lobes, grating lobes occur at more oblique angles (up to 90°) relative to the main beam and the strength of these beams is higher than side lobes (comparable to the main beam). These artifacts are most evident in echo-free cavities as in the example shown. Observe the arc-like "structure" within the LA that is characteristic of a grating lobe artifact; this artifact is produced by strong reflectors arising from the lateral LA wall.

Answer A is not correct. Range ambiguity occurs when the ultrasound machine is operating at a high PRF and a structure outside of the field of view is displayed within the echo-free cavity. This occurs because echoes from deep structures created by the first pulse arrive at the transducer after the second pulse has been transmitted. In this example, the PRF is unlikely to be high as the image depth is 20 cm.

Answer B is not correct. Slice thickness artifacts are produced from structures in front of or behind the main beam and these artifacts appear as added echoes within an echo-free cavity. However, the characteristic arc-like appearance of this artifact is most consistent with a grating lobe artifact.

Answer D is not correct. Propagation speed artifacts occur when the propagation speed through a structure is slower or faster than the assumed propagation speed of 1540 m/s. This results in incorrect placement of echoes or the incorrect display of the size and shape of structures. There is no intervening structure between the artifact and the transducer that could produce a propagation speed artifact.

23. **Answer: B.** The patient has undergone an interventional procedure. This patient has an Amplatzer atrial septal occluder device. **Videos 5-6A** and **5-6B** display a "figure-of-eight" artifact from the device (see still frame clips in **Figure 5-15A** and **B**). This artifact occurs in disk occluders that have a specific epitrochoidal mesh configuration and when imaged from a plane that is coronal relative to the device. The ultrasound physics resulting in the "figure-of-eight" appearance is quite complex (see Suggested Reading Bertrand PB, et al. *Echocardiography.* 2015;32(3):557-564).

KEY POINTS

The "figure-of-eight" artifact is a normal artifact that has been described with the Amplatzer closure device for left atrial appendage and atrial septal defect/patent foramen ovale closure. This artifact may be seen on 3D echocardiography, transesophageal echocardiography, and less frequently on transthoracic echocardiography. *Recognition of this normal imaging artifact is important for the correct interpretation of the images.*

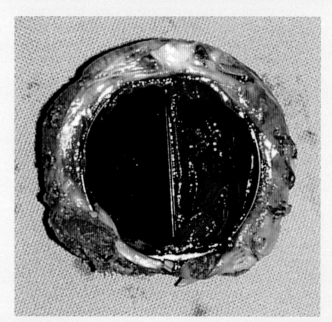

Figure 5-14

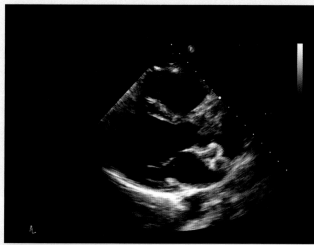

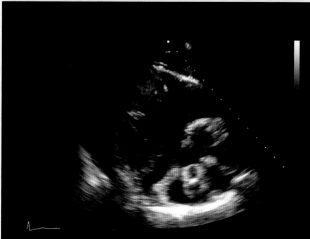

Figure 5-15

24. ▶ Answer: B. The speed of ultrasound in the silastic ball is slower than the speed of sound in tissue, resulting in the distorted appearance of the ball (or poppet). One of the basic assumptions of ultrasound is that the propagation speed of ultrasound in soft tissue is 1540 m/s (or 13 μs/cm). However, the propagation speed varies depending upon the structure encountered. For example, the propagation speed may speed up or slow down. The silastic ball of a Starr-Edwards valve slows the propagation speed. This has the effect of distorting the appearance of the ball from a round to a more oval shape as shown in **Video 5-7**. This type of artifact is referred to as a propagation speed artifact not a resolution-type artifact. Not all Starr-Edwards valves result in the distortion of the ball and this would relate to the composition of the ball. For example, if the propagation speed through the ball is not significantly different from the assumed propagation speed of 1540 m/s, then the ball will not appear distorted. **Video 5-14** is a nice example of a normal, rounded ball in a mitral Starr-Edwards valve.

25. Answer: D. 3D images are often produced over multiple consecutive cardiac cycles using ECG gating.

Multiple pyramidal data sets are then stitched together to create a single data set. Misalignment of one or more of the pyramidal data set leads to the presence of "fault lines" or "stitch" artifacts as seen in **Video 5-8**. These artifacts are created by patient or respiratory motion, transducer movement, or irregular cardiac rhythms. These artifacts can be minimized by avoiding the capture of transient arrhythmia, switching to single-beat acquisition mode, minimizing both out-of-plane and respiration-related movement and turning off electrocautery. Increasing the number of beats during acquisition does not resolve the occurrence of a stitch artifact and will likely worsen this artifact.

26. **Answer: A.** The artifacts depicted by the arrows are comet-tail artifacts. Comet-tail artifacts are produced when the ultrasound beam encounters highly reflective interfaces such as the pericardium or metallic objects. This interaction creates a continuous streak-like hyperechoic beam of ultrasound distal to the structure. Like the tail of a comet, these artifacts usually taper and fade over the image depth. In the image provided, the highly reflective pericardial interface generates a "comet-tail" of diminishing reverberations below the pericardium.

Answer B is not correct. While the ring-down artifact displays a similar continuous streak-like hyperechoic beam of ultrasound distal to the structure, these artifacts are produced when the ultrasound beam causes the liquid within gas bubbles to vibrate or resonate. Unlike comet-tail artifacts, these artifacts generally do not fade over the image depth as little energy is lost.

Answer C is not the best answer as "true" reverberation artifacts produce a more obvious "step ladder" effect of equally spaced reflectors of decreasing intensity over the image depth (see **Figure 5-10**).

Answer D is not correct as refraction artifacts are produced when there is bending of the ultrasound beam resulting is the improper placement or duplication of structures.

Answer E is not correct. As detailed above, while comet-tail, ring-down, and reverberation artifacts are similar, the physical basis and mechanism that produces each is different. The mechanism for creating a refraction is totally different from reverberation and reverberation-like artifacts.

KEY POINTS

Ring-down and comet-tail artifacts are reverberation-like artifacts that appear as continuous "streaking" of the ultrasound beam distal to a reflector. Ring-down artifacts are created by resonating gas bubbles. As little energy is lost, this artifact generally does not fade over the image depth. Comet-tail artifacts are created by highly reflective objects. The loss of energy in the creation of these artifacts results in fading of the artifact over the image depth.

27. Answer B. The artifacts displayed are comet-tail artifacts. These are reverberation-like artifacts and are produced when the assumptions that the ultrasound beam travels in a straight line and reflects just once are violated. These artifacts occur when energy is re-reflected from the "offending" structures resulting in the repeated reverberation of the ultrasound beam. Because re-reflected echoes return to the transducer later, these echoes will be placed deeper than the true reflector. Echoes become progressively weaker throughout the image depth due to a significant loss of energy.

28. ▶ Answer: A. **Video 5-9B** demonstrates how multiple artifacts may be seen within a given view. In this image, comet-tail, grating lobe, and beam width artifacts are evident (see **Figure 5-16** for labeled identifiers). The comet-tail artifact is generated from an implantable cardioverter defibrillator (ICD) lead within the right heart chambers. There are two prominent grating lobe artifacts present: (1) an arc-like structure within the right atrial (RA) cavity that is created from secondary beams that have been generated from echoes arising from the adjacent RA wall, and (2) a double interatrial septum that is created from secondary beams that have been generated from echoes arising from the interatrial septum. As previously described, beam width artifacts may result in smearing of a structure and this appears as fuzziness of the superior RA wall and more prominently of the superior LA wall.

Answer B is not correct as there is no obvious slice thickness artifact.

Answer C is not correct since the double interatrial septum is not a mirror artifact. This is because the duplicated structure appears adjacent to the real structure. Mirror artifacts are seen beyond the strong mirror interface (see **Figure 5-11**).

Answer D is not correct since the double interatrial septum is not due to refraction. Refraction artifacts can produce duplicated structures but only when the ultrasound beam passes obliquely through a lens-shaped object that has a different propagation speed from surrounding tissue (see **Figure 5-8C**). There is no intervening lens-like structure in this example that could cause refraction of the ultrasound beam. Therefore, the duplication of the interatrial septum in this example is most likely due to grating lobes.

29. ▶ Answer: A. The structure depicted by the arrow is the pericardium. There is a large pericardial effusion (PE) and a left pleural effusion (LPE) (see **Figure 5-17** with labels and **Video 5-15**).

Answers B and C are not correct. Reverberation and mirror artifacts are excluded since a large specular reflector must be present to create these artifacts and there is no evidence of a large specular reflector being present.

Answer D is not correct. A grating lobe artifact is produced when there is a strong reflector immediately adjacent to the "arc-like artifact" and there is no evidence of this.

Answer E is not correct. A propagation speed artifact occurs when the assumed propagation speed is not 1540 m/s. This results in the misplacement of structures or the distortion of the shape and size of structures.

30. ▶ Answer: C. This is a **range ambiguity** artifact which has the appearance of a "mass" within the right atrium. As previously described, these artifacts occur when a structure is detected **outside of the field of view** (FOV) and when the **pulse repetition frequency (PRF) is high**. As a result, echoes from deep structures outside the FOV are generated by the first pulse which arrives at the transducer after the second pulse has been transmitted. These structures are therefore incorrectly placed closer to the transducer than their actual location (see **Figure 5-12**). Lowering the PRF can eliminate these artifacts. Recall that PRF is the total number of pulses emitted per second and is measured in Hertz (Hz). PRF (Hz) is equal to 77,000 (cm/s)/depth of view

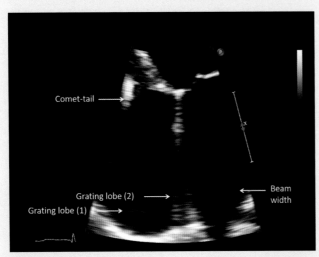

Figure 5-16

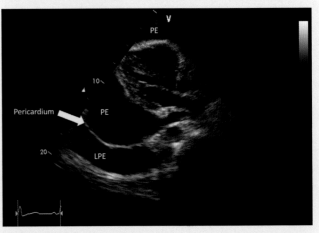

Figure 5-17

(cm). Hence, the PRF can be altered by changing the image depth. As there is an inverse relationship between the PRF and image depth, increasing the image depth (or FOV) decreases the PRF and avoids the artifact. Observe that after increasing the image depth to 18 cm in this patient, the artifact is no longer seen (**Video 5-16**). Therefore, answers A, B, D, and E are all true statements.

Answer C is correct as this is the false statement. As stated, range ambiguity artifacts are produced when there is a high PRF. Importantly, the PRF is not directly related to the transducer frequency. Hence, the PRF cannot be altered by changing the transducer frequency.

Acknowledgments: The authors thank and acknowledge the contributions from Juan-Carlos Brenes, MD, and Craig R. Asher, MD (Chapter 2, Cardiac Ultrasound Artifacts) in *Clinical Echocardiography Review: A Self-Assessment Tool*, Second Edition, edited by Allan L. Klein, Craig R. Asher, 2017.

SUGGESTED READINGS

Anderson B. *Echocardiography: The Normal Examination and Echocardiographic Measurements*. 3rd ed. Brisbane: Echotext Pty Ltd; 2017:chap 1.

Baad M, Lu ZF, Reiser I, Paushter D. Clinical Significance of US Artifacts. *Radiographics*. 2017;37(5):1408-1423.

Bertrand PB, Grieten L, Smeets CJ, et al. The figure-of-eight artifact in the echocardiographic assessment of percutaneous disc occluders: impact of imaging depth and device type. *Echocardiography*. 2015;32(3):557-564.

Bertrand PB, Levine RA, Isselbacher EM, Vandervoort PM. Fact or artifact in two-dimensional echocardiography: avoiding misdiagnosis and missed diagnosis. *J Am Soc Echocardiogr*. 2016;29(5):381-391.

Gill R. *The Physics and Technology of Diagnostic Ultrasound. A Practitioner's Guide*. Sydney: High Frequency Publishing; 2012.

Otto CM. *Textbook of Clinical Echocardiography*. 6th ed. Philadelphia, PA: Elsevier; 2018:chap 1.

CHAPTER 6

Two-Dimensional Examination

Contributors: Jayne Cleve, BS, RDCS and Steven Walling, BS, RCS, RDCS

✪✪ Question 1

Acoustic windows are best described as:
- **A.** The point on the body surface that allows ultrasound to be absorbed by the internal anatomy of interest.
- **B.** The point on the body surface that allows ultrasound to penetrate to the internal anatomy of interest.
- **C.** The point on the body surface that allows ultrasound to reflect off the internal anatomy of interest.
- **D.** The point on the body surface that allows ultrasound to refract off the internal anatomy of interest.

✪ Question 2

The four acoustic windows routinely used in a comprehensive transthoracic echocardiography (TTE) exam are:
- **A.** Left parasternal, left apical, subcostal, and suprasternal notch.
- **B.** Left parasternal, right parasternal, suprasternal notch, and left apical.
- **C.** Right parasternal, left apical, subcostal, and suprasternal notch.
- **D.** Right parasternal, right apical, subcostal, and suprasternal notch.

✪ Question 3

Alternative acoustic windows are often used when assessing the heart, when traditional acoustic windows are ineffective or unavailable. Which of the following are alternative acoustic windows?
- **A.** High left parasternal
- **B.** Right lateral

- **C.** Right parasternal
- **D.** Supraclavicular
- **E.** All of the above

✪ Question 4

Various terms are used to describe probe manipulations to acquire various echocardiographic views. Which of the following terms describes the movement of the probe from a fixed point on the chest wall to show a new structure?
- **A.** Angling
- **B.** Rotating
- **C.** Sliding
- **D.** Tilting

✪ Question 5

Which transthoracic echocardiographic view is used to image both the anterolateral and posteromedial papillary muscles?
- **A.** Parasternal long axis (PLAX)
- **B.** Parasternal short axis (PSAX)
- **C.** Subcostal 4 chamber
- **D.** Apical 4 chamber

✪✪ Question 6

Which two tricuspid valve leaflets are seen from the parasternal short-axis (PSAX) view at the level of the aorta?
- **A.** Septal and anterior
- **B.** Anterior and posterior
- **C.** Posterior and septal
- **D.** Any of the above combinations

✪✪ Question 7

Which of the following transthoracic echocardiographic views is used to image the infundibulum?
- A. Apical 4 chamber
- B. Parasternal long axis
- C. Parasternal short axis
- D. Right ventricular inflow tract (RVIT)

✪ Question 8

From which of the following transthoracic echocardiographic views can both the coronary sinus and the left atrial appendage (LAA) be imaged?
- A. Apical 2 chamber
- B. Apical 4 chamber
- C. Apical long axis
- D. Parasternal long axis

✪ Question 9

Which direction would the probe be tilted to see the coronary sinus from the apical 4-chamber view?
- A. Anteriorly
- B. Inferiorly
- C. Medially
- D. Posteriorly

✪ Question 10

Which is the best view to image an atrial septal defect?
- A. Apical 4 chamber
- B. Apical long axis
- C. Parasternal short axis at the level of mitral valve
- D. Subcostal 4 chamber

✪ Question 11

In which direction would the probe be tilted to see the pulmonary artery from the apical 4-chamber view?
- A. Anteriorly
- B. Laterally
- C. Medially
- D. Superiorly

✪ Question 12

What is the probe orientation (index marker direction) for acquiring the parasternal long-axis view (PLAX)?
- A. Toward the patient's left shoulder
- B. Toward the patient's left foot
- C. Toward the patient's right shoulder
- D. Toward the patient's right foot

✪ Question 13

What is the probe orientation (index marker direction) for acquiring the apical 4-chamber view?
- A. 9 o'clock
- B. 6 o'clock
- C. 3 o'clock
- D. 12 o'clock

✪✪ Question 14

In terms of anatomical nomenclature, the 4-chamber imaging plane of the heart is equivalent to which anatomic plane?
- A. Axial
- B. Coronal
- C. Sagittal
- D. Transverse

✪ Question 15

What is the probe orientation (index marker direction) for acquiring the subcostal 4-chamber view?
- A. Horizontal with indicator toward patient's left
- B. Horizontal with indicator toward patient's right
- C. Vertical with indicator toward patient's left
- D. Vertical with indicator toward patient's right

✪✪ Question 16

Which of the sector orientations below correctly describes the anatomic orientation for the subcostal 4-chamber view?
- A. Top is superior; bottom is inferior; right is left; left is right.
- B. Top is superior; bottom is inferior; right is right; left is left.
- C. Top is anterior; bottom is posterior; right is medial; left is lateral.
- D. Top is anterior; bottom is posterior; right is inferior; left is superior.

✪✪ Question 17

The structures numbered 1 to 3 in **Figure 6-1** are:
- A. 1 = noncoronary cusp of the aortic valve; 2 = posterior mitral valve leaflet; 3 = posterior left ventricular (LV) wall.
- B. 1 = noncoronary cusp of the aortic valve; 2 = anterior mitral valve leaflet; 3 = inferior LV wall.
- C. 1 = noncoronary cusp of the aortic valve; 2 = anterior mitral valve leaflet; 3 = posterior LV wall.

D. 1 = left-coronary cusp of the aortic valve; 2 = posterior mitral valve leaflet; 3 = posterior LV wall.

E. 1 = left-coronary cusp of the aortic valve; 2 = anterior mitral valve leaflet; 3 = lateral LV wall.

D. Posterior wall.

E. C or D.

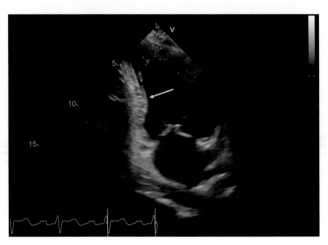

Figure 6-3

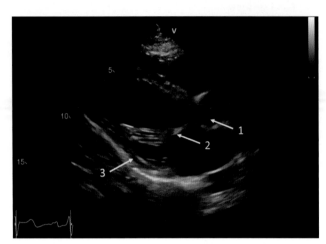

Figure 6-1

✪ Question 18

The echocardiographic view shown in **Figure 6-2** is:

A. An off-axis apical 4-chamber view.

B. A right ventricle (RV)-focused apical 4-chamber view.

C. The right ventricular inflow tract (RVIT) view.

D. The right ventricular outflow tract (RVOT) view.

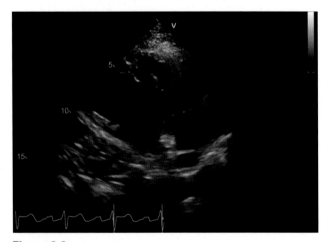

Figure 6-2

✪ Question 19

The left ventricular wall indicated by the arrow in **Figure 6-3** is the:

A. Anterior wall.

B. Inferior wall.

C. Inferolateral wall.

✪✪✪ Question 20

Which of the following adjustments of the ultrasound machine controls would improve the frame rate to maximize the temporal resolution?

A. Decreasing the depth of the image, decreasing the number of focal zones, and narrowing the sector width

B. Decreasing the depth of the image, increasing the number of focal zones, and narrowing the sector width

C. Increasing the number of focal zones, narrowing the sector width, and decreasing the overall gain

D. Narrowing the sector width, decreasing the overall gain, and decreasing the number of focal zones

E. Widening the sector width, increasing the image depth, and decreasing the number of focal zones.

✪✪ Question 21

In an obese patient, 2D images may be improved by:

A. Decreasing the transducer frequency, increasing the dynamic range, and increasing the gain.

B. Decreasing the transducer frequency, increasing the gain, and decreasing the dynamic range.

C. Decreasing the transducer frequency, decreasing the output power, and increasing the gain.

D. Increasing the transducer frequency, decreasing the output power, and increasing the dynamic range.

E. Increasing the transducer frequency, increasing the output power, and decreasing the dynamic range.

✪ Question 22

Which of the following statements regarding the measurement of the left ventricular outflow tract diameter (LVOTd) is true?

A. The LVOTd is measured inner-edge-to-leading-edge in mid-systole approximately 3 to 10 mm from the aortic valve plane.

B. The LVOTd is measured inner-edge-to-inner-edge in mid-systole at the aortic annulus.

C. The LVOTd is measured inner-edge-to-inner-edge in mid-systole at the aortic annulus or approximately 3 to 10 mm from the aortic valve plane.

D. The LVOTd is measured leading-edge-to-leading-edge in mid-systole at the aortic annulus.

E. The LVOTd is measured leading-edge-to-leading-edge in mid-systole approximately 3 to 10 mm from the aortic valve plane.

✪✪ Question 23

In the zoomed parasternal long-axis (PLAX) view of the aortic root (**Figure 6-4**), which structures are incorrectly measured?

A. Aortic root and sinotubular junction

B. Both left ventricular outflow tract (LVOT) diameter measurements

C. All measurements are inaccurate

D. All measurements are accurate

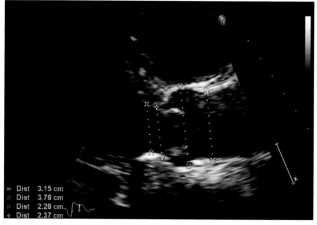

Figure 6-4 Mid-systolic frame of the aortic root acquired from a zoomed PLAX view. From left to right, the measurements are the LVOT diameter 5 mm from the annulus, LVOT diameter at the annulus, the aortic root, and the sinotubular junction.

✪✪ Question 24

Which of the following statements regarding diastolic linear measurements of the left ventricle (LV) is correct?

A. LV diastolic linear measurements are made in early diastole at a level just below the mitral valve leaflet tips, perpendicular to the long axis of the LV.

B. LV diastolic linear measurements are made at end-diastole at a level just below the mitral valve leaflet tips, parallel to the long axis of the LV.

C. LV diastolic linear measurements are made at end-diastole at a level of the papillary muscles, parallel to the long axis of the LV.

D. LV diastolic linear measurements are made at end-diastole at a level just below the mitral valve leaflet tips perpendicular to the long axis of the LV.

✪✪ Question 25

Which of the following sets of left ventricular (LV) measurements in **Figure 6-5** is most correct?

A. Set 1

B. Set 2

C. Set 3

D. Set 4

E. None of the above

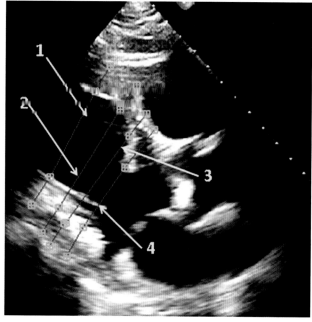

Figure 6-5

✪✪ Question 26

Which of the following methods is recommended by the American Society of Echocardiography guidelines for reporting of right atrial (RA) size?

A. Apical 4-chamber view, RA area
B. Apical 4-chamber view, RA volume indexed for body surface area
C. Apical 4-chamber view, RA volume indexed for body surface area and differentiated by gender
D. Biplane RA volume indexed for body surface area and differentiated by gender

✪ Question 27

Which of the following views is the recommended view for assessing right ventricular (RV) size?
A. Apical 4 chamber
B. Apical coronary sinus
C. Modified apical 4 chamber
D. Right ventricle–focused apical 4 chamber

✪✪ Question 28

Which of the following views is recommended for measuring right ventricular (RV) wall thickness?
A. Parasternal long axis
B. Parasternal short axis of basal RV
C. Apical 4 chamber
D. Subcostal 4 chamber

✪✪ Question 29

From the parasternal long-axis (PLAX) view, calipers placed from the anterior right ventricular (RV) wall to the interventricular septal-aortic junction at end-diastole is a measurement of the:
A. Distal RV outflow tract.
B. Proximal RV outflow tract.
C. Basal RV cavity.
D. Mid RV cavity.

✪✪ Question 30

Which of the inferior vena cava (IVC) end-expiratory measurements shown in **Figure 6-6** is correct?
A. Measurement 1
B. Measurement 2
C. Measurement 3
D. Measurement 4
E. Measurement 2 or 4

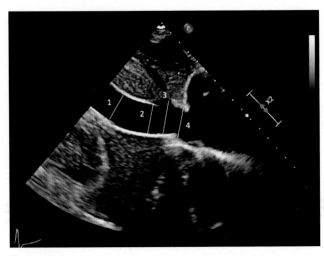

Figure 6-6

✪✪ Question 31

When tracing the left atrial (LA) border, which of the following is incorrect?
A. The LA appendage should be included.
B. The confluences of the pulmonary veins should be excluded.
C. The mitral annular plane should represent the atrioventricular interface.
D. The tip of the mitral leaflets should not represent the atrioventricular surface.

✪✪✪ Question 32

Which of the following statements regarding left ventricular (LV) volumes is incorrect?
A. LV volume measurements should be performed from the apical 4- and 2-chamber views.
B. Biplane method of disks summation is recommended for estimating LV volumes.
C. LV volumes should be reported indexed to BSA.
D. The Teichholz method can be used to estimate LV volumes in the presence of significant LV foreshortening.

✪✪✪ Question 33

Which of the following statements regarding mitral and tricuspid annular measurements is correct?
A. Mitral and tricuspid annular measurements are made at end-diastole at the insertion of the valve leaflets, using the inner-edge-to-inner-edge method.

B. Mitral and tricuspid annular measurements are made in mid-diastole at the leaflet tips, using the inner-edge-to-inner-edge method.

C. Mitral and tricuspid annular measurements are made in early diastole at the insertion of the valve leaflets, using the inner-edge-to-inner-edge method.

D. Mitral and tricuspid annular measurements are made in mid-systole at the leaflet tips, using the inner-edge-to-inner-edge method.

✪ Question 34

Which of the following methods is recommended for the calculation of left ventricular ejection fraction (LVEF)?

A. Area-length
B. Teichholz
C. Modified Quinones
D. Biplane method of disks (modified Simpson's)
E. Any of the above

✪✪ Question 35

Which of the following statements regarding left ventricular (LV) mass is incorrect?

A. LV mass should be reported indexed to the body surface area.
B. The normal values of LV mass by both the linear measurement and 2D methods are the same.
C. In a normally shaped LV, both M-mode and 2D echocardiography formulas may be used to calculate LV mass.
D. Three-dimensional (3D) echocardiography is the only echocardiographic method that directly measures myocardial volume.

✪✪✪ Question 36

A patient presents to the echo lab with an akinetic left ventricular (LV) apex. The remaining LV segments are normal. Using a 16-segment model, which is the regional wall motion score index?

A. 0.75
B. 1.5
C. 1.75
D. 24

✪✪✪ Question 37

Which of the following statements regarding right ventricular fractional area change (RV FAC) is incorrect?

A. An RV FAC <35% indicates systolic dysfunction.
B. RV FAC is a measurement that includes the RV end-diastolic and end-systolic areas of the entire RV.
C. RV FAC change provides an estimate of regional RV systolic function.
D. While tracing the RV area for the RV FAC calculation, care must be taken to include the trabeculae in the RV cavity.

✪✪ Question 38

Observe the left atrial volume (LAV) measurements shown in **Figure 6-7**. Based on these measurements, which of the following statements is correct regarding the left atrium (LA) or LAV?

A. The LA is mildly dilated.
B. The LA is moderately dilated.
C. The LA is severely dilated.
D. LAV is underestimated.
E. LAV is overestimated.

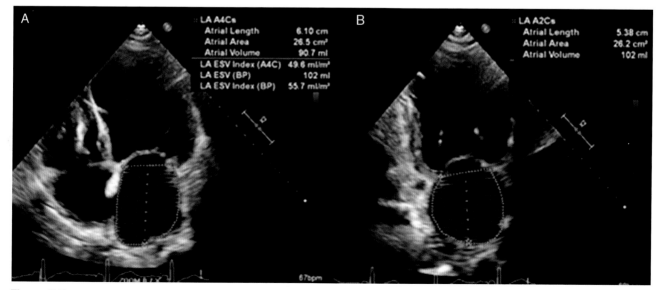

Figure 6-7

✪✪✪ Question 39

A 55-year-old man presents to the echocardiography laboratory for the evaluation of a cardiac murmur. He has a body surface area (BSA) of 2.0 m² and his ascending aorta was measured at 3.9 cm. Which of the following is correct with regard to his ascending aortic size?

- **A.** The ascending aorta is normal in size.
- **B.** The ascending aorta is dilated.
- **C.** The ascending aorta should not be measured for a cardiac murmur indication.
- **D.** Not enough information is provided.

✪✪✪ Question 40

Which of the following statements is true with regard to the LVOT diameter (LVOTd), aortic stenosis (AS) severity, and the continuity equation?

- **A.** Overestimation of the LVOTd will overestimate the LVOT stroke volume and therefore overestimate the AS severity.
- **B.** Underestimation of the LVOTd will overestimate the LVOT stroke volume and therefore underestimate the AS severity.
- **C.** Underestimation of the LVOTd will underestimate the LVOT stroke volume and therefore overestimate the AS severity.
- **D.** Overestimation of the LVOTd will underestimate the LVOT stroke volume and therefore underestimate the AS severity.

ANSWERS

1. **Answer: B.** Acoustic windows are the areas that allow ultrasound to penetrate to the region of interest. Ultrasound beams travel at different propagation speeds, depending on the material encountered. When the ultrasound beam traveling within soft tissue encounters air or bone, there is almost total reflection of ultrasound due to the abrupt change in acoustic impedance. For this reason, ultrasound imaging of the heart through the chest wall requires access to several acoustic windows where the heart does not lie directly beneath bony and air-filled structures.

2. **Answer: A.** The four acoustic windows routinely used in a TTE exam are the left parasternal, left apical, subcostal, and suprasternal notch windows (**Figure 6-8**). The left parasternal and left apical windows are often simplified to just the parasternal and apical windows. These windows allow for assessment of cardiac function, structure, hemodynamics, and pathology.

TEACHING POINT

For optimal parasternal and apical views, the patient is positioned in the left lateral decubitus position. This shifts the heart slightly leftward, out from under the sternum, and drops the left lung away from the mid-line of the chest; thus, creating a better acoustic window to image the heart. Using patient breathing to bring the heart into view is also valuable in improving acoustic windows. For the parasternal views, asking the patient to breathe all the way out often improves these views. For the apical views, asking the patient to take a small breath in often improves images. For the subcostal views, asking the patient to inspire and hold their breath fills the lungs and pushes the heart closer to the probe; an added advantage is that this stabilizes the images.

3. **Answer: E.** Often, there can be challenges while imaging the heart from the standard acoustic windows. Knowledge of other acoustic windows may help to enhance the examination. Rolling the patient on his or her right side (right lateral decubitus) will help when acquiring images from the right side, such as with the right parasternal window. The right parasternal window is especially useful when assessing the ascending aorta and for the continuous-wave (CW) Doppler interrogation of the pressure gradient across the aortic valve. The right lateral window, which can be performed with the patient in the supine position, is beneficial for imaging the inferior vena cava (IVC) when the subcostal views are unavailable. The high left parasternal and supraclavicular windows are both helpful for the CW Doppler interrogation for aortic stenosis and can be performed with the patient supine. Imaging from the right side of the sternum may also be useful in the assessment of certain congenital heart anomalies.

4. **Answer: A.** Angling the probe from a fixed position on the chest wall enables the sonographer to change the focus of the image. For example, from the parasternal short-axis (PSAX) view at the level of the great vessels, by angling the probe medially the image can be optimized for the tricuspid valve (**Figure 6-9**, left), and by angling the probe laterally the image can be optimized for the pulmonary valve and main pulmonary artery (**Figure 6-9**, right).

   Rotating (answer B) refers to "twisting" of the probe from a fixed position of the chest wall. For example, by rotating the probe 90° clockwise from the parasternal long-axis (PLAX) view, the PSAX view is achieved.

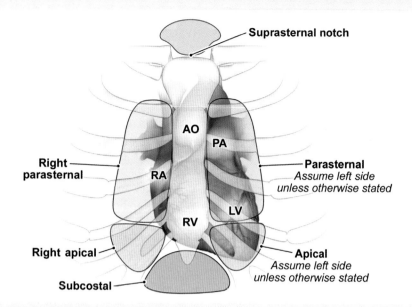

Figure 6-8 Echocardiographic acoustic windows. The windows used routinely in a TTE exam include the parasternal, apical, subcostal, and suprasternal notch windows. (From Mitchell C, Rahko PS, Blauwet LA, et al. Guidelines for performing a comprehensive transthoracic echocardiographic examination in adults: recommendations from the American Society of Echocardiography. *J Am Soc Echocardiogr.* 2019;32(1):1-64, with permission from Elsevier.)

Sliding (answer C) refers to the movement of the probe over the chest wall. For example, sliding the probe inferiorly refers to movement of the probe down toward the patient's feet.

Tilting (answer D) refers to the movement of the probe from a fixed position on the chest wall to a different imaging plane. For example, anterior tilting from the apical 4 chamber view, where the probe face is pointed/tilted upward toward the patient's

front, brings in the apical 5 chamber view while posterior tilting from the apical 4 chamber view, where the probe face is pointed/tilted down toward the patient's back, brings in the coronary sinus.

5. **Answer: B.** The PSAX view can be found by rotating the transducer clockwise approximately 90° from the PLAX view with the index marker pointed toward the patient's left shoulder. By tilting the probe superiorly and inferiorly, the heart can be imaged at

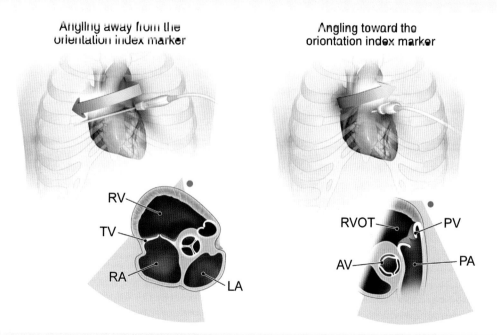

Figure 6-9 Probe angling from the PSAX view at the level of the great vessels. (From Mitchell C, Rahko PS, Blauwet LA, et al. Guidelines for performing a comprehensive transthoracic echocardiographic examination in adults: recommendations from the American Society of Echocardiography. *J Am Soc Echocardiogr.* 2019;32(1):1-64, with permission from Elsevier.)

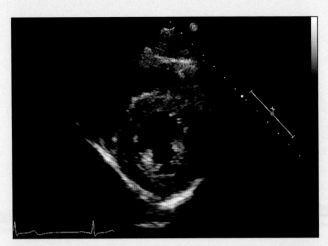

Figure 6-10 In this patient, the anterolateral papillary muscle located at the 3-o'clock position and the posteromedial papillary muscle is located at the 8-o'clock position.

several anatomic levels. This includes the level of the great vessels, the mitral valve, and the papillary muscle level. From the papillary muscle level, the anterolateral papillary muscle is situated between the 3- and 5-o'clock positions and the posteromedial papillary muscle is typically found between the 7- and 9-o'clock positions (**Figure 6-10**).

At this level, this PSAX view is useful in visualizing the left and right ventricles, assessing ventricular dimensions and systolic function, and for the detection of intraventricular lesions and pericardial fluid.

6. **Answer: D.** The tricuspid valve consists of three leaflets, which are the anterior, septal, and posterior leaflets. There is some degree of ambiguity when imaging the tricuspid valve leaflets from the various two-dimensional (2D) echocardiographic views. This uncertainty is based upon variability in the level at which the imaging plane transects the leaflets. In a recent study using multiplanar reconstruction (MPR) of three-dimensional (3D) data sets, it was found that from the 2D PSAX view, the tricuspid leaflet combination may include septal and anterior, anterior and posterior, or posterior and septal (**Figure 6-11**).

7. **Answer: C.** The infundibulum is a cone-shaped or pouch-like muscular structure that extends from the crista supraventricularis to the pulmonary valve; this structure is distinct from the rest of the right ventricle in origin and anatomy. The infundibulum, along with the pulmonary valve, encompasses the right ventricular outflow tract (RVOT). The infundibulum can be seen from the parasternal short-axis (PSAX) view at the level of the great vessels as well as from a parasternal long-axis view of the RVOT, an apical 4-chamber view with anterior tilt beyond the apical 5-chamber view, and from the subcostal views. From the PSAX view, the infundibulum and RVOT are located at the top of the image, anterior to the aortic valve (**Figure 6-12**).

8. **Answer: A.** To obtain the true apical 2-chamber view, it is useful to use the coronary sinus and the LAA as anatomic landmarks (**Figure 6-13**). The coronary sinus receives blood from the coronary veins and empties into the right atrium; it is located inferior to the left atrium (LA). In the apical 2-chamber view, it appears as an echolucent circular structure to the left of the LA in the image. The LAA is a finger-like extension originating from the main body of the LA. In the apical 2-chamber view, this normally echolucent structure is seen on the right side of the image. The apical 2-chamber is useful for assessing the inferior and anterior walls of the left ventricle, the LA, and the mitral valve.

9. **Answer: D.** The coronary sinus lies in the posterior left atrioventricular groove. From the apical 4-chamber, keeping the same degree of transducer rotation, tilting the probe posteriorly (aiming the face of the probe toward the patient's back) will bring the coronary sinus into view (**Figure 6-14**). From this view, the coronary sinus appears as a tube-like structure between the left ventricle and the left atrium.

10. **Answer: D.** The subcostal 4 chamber is the best view for evaluating the interatrial septum (IAS) for any defects. This is because "drop-out" of the IAS, which may occur in the parasternal and apical views, does not occur from the subcostal view as the IAS lies perpendicular to the interrogating ultrasound beam. This view is also helpful for interrogating the IAS by color and spectral Doppler. From this view, any blood flow across a defect in the IAS would be parallel to the ultrasound beam and would therefore be readily assessed by color and spectral Doppler.

Answer A is not correct as "drop-out" of the IAS is frequently seen in the apical 4-chamber view. This "drop-out" artifact occurs as a result of poor backscatter of echoes from the relatively thin and smooth IAS, which lies almost parallel to the ultrasound beam.

Answers B and C are not correct since the IAS is not seen from the apical long-axis view or parasternal short-axis view at the level of the mitral valve.

11. **Answer: A.** Tilting the probe in an anterior direction from the apical 4-chamber view will, in some patients, bring the pulmonary artery into view (**Figure 6-15**). The pulmonary artery is the most anterior vessel arising from the heart.

12. **Answer: C.** All ultrasound probes have a probe orientation marker or an orientation index marker. This marker may be in the form of a groove, external ribbing, or a button. Importantly, this marker indicates the edge of the imaging plane. In echocardiography, this edge is always displayed to the right of the 2D sector and this is also reflected on the 2D image display by the positioning of the machine "logo" at the top right of the 2D sector. To

Aorta and single leaflet

PSAX view

Anterior or septal leaflet

Posterior or anterior leaflet

A — Anterior leaflet — Aorta

A / P S / Septum

Aorta and two leaflets

B — Anterior leaflet — Aorta — Posterior leaflet

A / P S / Septum

LVOT/septum and two leaflets

C — Septal leaflet — LVOT — Posterior leaflet

P A / S / Septum

Figure 6-11 In the PSAX view (left) the leaflet closest to the aorta is always the anterior or septal and never the posterior leaflet. Near the right ventricular (RV) free wall, the posterior or anterior leaflet may be seen but never the septal leaflet. The anterior leaflet was depicted if a single leaflet was seen on the 2D image (Panel A with corresponding MPR result to the right). The anterior-posterior combination was noted if two leaflets were seen with a central coaptation point together with the aortic valve (Panel B with corresponding MPR result to the right). When the 2D plane transected below the aortic valve, in the area of the left ventricular outflow tract or interventricular septum, and the aortic valve was not seen throughout the cardiac cycle, the leaflets imaged were the septal and posterior leaflets (Panel C with corresponding MPR result to the right). (Reprinted from Addetia K, Yamat M, Mediratta A, et al. Comprehensive two-dimensional interrogation of the tricuspid valve using knowledge derived from three-dimensional echocardiography. *J Am Soc Echocardiogr* 2019;29(1):74-82. Copyright © 2016 American Society of Echocardiography. With permission.)

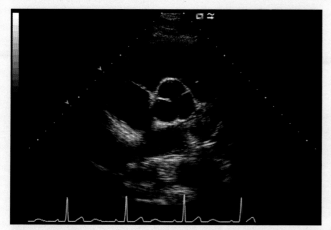

Figure 6-12 From this PSAX view, the infundibulum is seen anterior to the aortic valve, which is located in the center of the image. The pulmonary valve and main pulmonary artery are seen on the right side of the image and the tricuspid valve and right atrium are seen on the left side of the image.

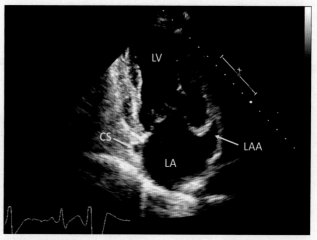

Figure 6-13 From this apical 2-chamber view, the left atrial appendage (LAA) and coronary sinus (CS) can be identified. LA, left atrium; LV, left ventricle.

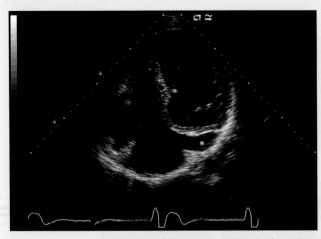

Figure 6-14 The coronary sinus (*) is seen by tilting the face of the probe posteriorly.

Table 6-1.

Anatomical Planes	Adult Echocardiography Planes
Sagittal	Parasternal long-axis Apical long-axis
Coronal (frontal)	Apical 4-chamber Subcostal 4-chamber
Transverse (or axial or short-axis)	Parasternal short-axis Subcostal short-axis

acquire the PLAX view, the probe is positioned left of the sternum in the patient's third to fifth intercostal space with the probe index marker directed toward the patient's right shoulder. Therefore, the ultrasound beam is oriented to the long axis of the left ventricle with the scan plane running parallel along an imaginary line joining the right shoulder and the left hip.

13. **Answer: C.** Acquiring images for the apical 4-chamber view is best achieved when the patient is in left lateral decubitus position. The probe is placed at the apex of the heart. Finding the point of maximal impulse (PMI), near the midaxillary line, is helpful in identifying the correct position. The probe index marker should be pointed to the patient's left side, down toward the bed, which will place it in the 3-o'clock position.

14. **Answer: B.** Standard anatomical nomenclature that is used to describe body planes is not generally used to describe 2D echocardiographic imaging planes in adults. Instead, 2D echocardiographic nomenclature is usually described with respect to the way in which the imaging plane transects the heart itself. However, in pediatric and 3D echocardiography, anatomical nomenclature is commonly used. Therefore, it is important for the sonographer to be aware of the similarities between these anatomical and 2D imaging planes (**Table 6-1**).

The anatomical coronal (or frontal) plane is a vertical plane that divides anterior from posterior; hence, echocardiographic coronal views divide the heart into anterior and posterior. The apical 4-chamber view is an example of an echocardiographic coronal view; therefore, answer B is correct.

Answers A and D are not correct. The anatomical axial and transverse plane, also referred to as the short-axis plane, is a horizontal plane that divides superior from inferior; therefore, the echocardiographic transverse views divide the heart into superior and inferior. Examples include parasternal and subcostal short-axis views.

Answer C is not correct. The anatomical sagittal plane is a vertical plane that divides right from left; therefore, corresponding echocardiographic views divide the heart into right and left. Examples include parasternal and apical long-axis views.

KEY POINTS
▶ Imaging planes that divide the heart into right and left are long-axis or sagittal imaging planes.
▶ Imaging planes that divide the heart into anterior and posterior are 4-chamber or coronal imaging planes.
▶ Imaging planes that divide the heart into superior and inferior are short-axis or transverse imaging planes.

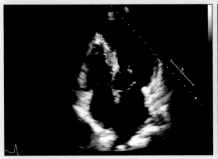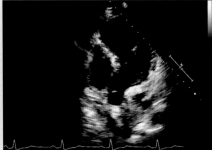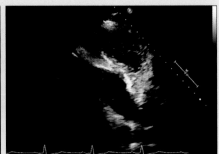

Figure 6-15 From the apical 4-chamber view (left), panning anteriorly brings the left ventricular outflow tract and aorta into view (middle) and panning even more anteriorly may bring the right ventricular outflow tract and main pulmonary artery into view (right).

15. **Answer: A.** Acquiring images for the subcostal view is best achieved when the patient is lying supine. The probe should be positioned just below the xiphoid process (inferior part of sternum). The probe is held in the horizontal position with the index marker directed toward the left side of the patient (at about 3 o'clock). On the image display, the heart is seen centrally with the apex pointed toward the right side of the image and the atria to the left; the liver is seen anterior and to the left of the heart on the image.

TEACHING POINT

Remember that the index marker indicates the edge of the imaging plane and this edge is always displayed to the right of the 2D sector. Therefore, when this marker is pointed toward the patient's left, these structures will appear to the right on the image display. So, while the apex of the heart is anatomically located on the left side, it will be displayed on the right side of the image. Likewise, the liver, which is a right-sided organ, will be displayed on the left of the image.

16. ▶ **Answer: D.** The two-dimensional (2D) sector is a wedge-shaped box with a top, a bottom, and two sides. Based on the probe rotation (direction of the index marker) and the probe angle/tilt, the anatomic orientation can be determined. From the subcostal 4-chamber view, anterior structures such as the liver and right heart chambers appear to the top of the image sector, posterior structures such as the left heart chambers appear to the bottom of the image sector, superior structures such as the atria appear to the left of the image sector, and inferior structures such as the ventricles appear to the right of the image sector (**Video 6-1**).

17. **Answer: C. Figure 6-1** is a parasternal long-axis view. The structures numbered 1 to 3 are: 1 = noncoronary cusp of the aortic valve (ncc), 2 = anterior mitral valve leaflet (amvl), and 3 = posterior wall of the LV (PW). The posterior wall of the left ventricle is also known as the inferolateral wall. Other structures seen include the LV cavity, left atrial (LA) cavity, a portion of the right ventricle (RV), aortic root (Ao), right coronary cusp of the aortic valve (rcc), interventricular septum (IVS), and posterior mitral valve leaflet (pmvl) (**Figure 6-16**). Observe that there is continuity between the anterior aortic wall and the IVS as well as between the posterior aortic wall and the amvl.

18. **Answer: C.** The RVIT can be obtained from the parasternal long-axis view of the left ventricle with a slight counterclockwise rotation and medial angulation underneath the sternum, and inferior tilt (face of the probe tilted toward the right hip). This view can be used to assess the right atrium (RA), the RV, and the tricuspid valve. Occasionally, the coronary sinus and inferior vena cava may also be seen draining into the RA.

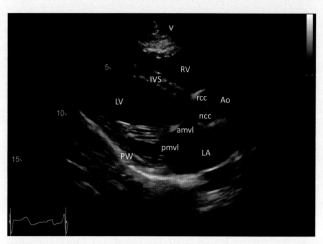

Figure 6-16

19. **Answer: B.** Using landmarks like the coronary sinus and the left atrial appendage (LAA) in this apical 2-chamber view allows better understanding of wall delineation. The coronary sinus is an inferior structure and the LAA is an anterior structure (see **Figure 6-13** from the answer outline for Question 8). Therefore, the left ventricular (LV) wall associated with the coronary sinus is the inferior wall. The anterior wall (answer A) is the LV wall closest to the LAA; in this view, this is the wall opposite to the inferior LV wall. The inferolateral wall (answer C) and the posterior wall (answer D) are the same and are seen in the apical long-axis, parasternal long-axis, and parasternal short-axis views.

20. **Answer: A.** Frame rate is the number of images that are displayed per second and is measured as frames/second (f/s) or Hertz (Hz). As frame rate increases, so does temporal resolution. A high temporal resolution is important to enable the accurate display of rapidly moving structures. Frame rate is directly related to the depth of the image. With increased depth, the frame rate decreases as a longer processing time is required to create the image. Likewise, when the image sector is widened, there are more scan lines to be written and processed, and therefore, the frame rate is reduced. Using multiple focal zones may also decrease the frame rate, thus reducing temporal resolution. Gain is a useful tool that can enhance the 2D exam by amplifying the receive signal but does not affect frame rate.

    Therefore, frame rate and temporal resolution are optimized by (1) decreasing the image depth, (2) narrowing the sector width, and (3) using a single focus. Preprocessing zooming (write-zoom) also increases the frame rate as the width of the image is narrower than a full sector image.

21. **Answer: B.** The transducer frequency should be as high as possible for the best spatial resolution. However, the use of high frequencies increases attenuation and reduces depth penetration. In larger

patients, greater depth penetration is required and therefore a lower transducer frequency is also required.

The amplitude of received ultrasound signals is very small. Amplification of these signals is achieved by increasing the gain. In larger patients being scanned at deeper image depths, increasing overall gain and time gain compensation (TGC) is required to enhance returning signals from the far field.

Adjusting the dynamic range (affected by the "compression" control on some machines), which represents the ratio between the highest and lowest received echo amplitudes, affects the number of shades of gray displayed on the 2D image. Increasing the dynamic range increases the range of echo intensities displayed, resulting in a softer image with less contrast. Decreasing the dynamic range results in a more black and white image with greater contrast, which may be beneficial in larger, more technically difficult patients.

Power is the rate at which energy is transferred and describes the magnitude of the ultrasound pulse, which in turn affects the brightness of the image. Therefore, increasing power may also improve images in larger patients. However, caution is required as increasing power increases the potential for occurrence of biological effects. Optimizing images by using controls that do not increase output power (e.g., gain, time gain compensation, transducer frequency, and dynamic range) are encouraged before resorting to increasing the output power.

22. **Answer: C.** The LVOTd is measured in mid-systole using an inner-edge-to-inner-edge method, perpendicular to the long-axis of the aorta. For LVOT stroke volume calculations, the LVOTd should be measured at the same level as where the pulsed-wave Doppler sample volume is placed to measure the LVOT velocity time integral. As flow acceleration may occur at the aortic annulus level, the American Society of Echocardiography (ASE) recommends that the LVOTd be measured approximately 3 to 10 mm from the aortic valve plane (aortic annulus) in this situation. Measurement of the LVOTd at the annulus is also acceptable. One of the advantages of measuring the LVOTd at the annulus is a higher measurement reproducibility owing to the clear anatomic landmarks of the hinge point of the right coronary cusp anteriorly and the mitral-aortic curtain posteriorly. Accordingly, in the 2017 ASE recommendations on the echocardiographic assessment of aortic valve stenosis, it is stated that there is no general consensus on the LVOTd measurements as many laboratories measure the diameter routinely at the annulus level, whereas others measure more apically in the LVOT.

The LVOTd measurement is the only aortic measurement that involves use of the inner-edge-to-inner-edge method at mid-systole. All other aortic measurements (trans-sinus diameter at the sinuses of Valsalva, sinotubular junction, and proximal ascending aorta) should be made at end-diastole using the leading-edge-to-leading-edge method. Although different modalities such as multidetector computed tomography and cardiac magnetic resonance imaging may use other methods (for example, inner-edge-to-inner-edge or outer-edge-to-outer-edge), the ASE and European Association of Cardiovascular Imaging writing committee for multimodality imaging of thoracic aorta diseases recommend the leading-edge-to-leading-edge convention for echocardiographic measurements of the aortic root and aorta.

23. **Answer: A.** In **Figure 6-4**, the caliper placement for each measurement is correct and measurements correctly performed perpendicular to the long axis of the aorta; however, all measurements are made in mid-systole. The aortic root at the sinus of Valsalva, sinotubular junction, and the ascending aorta should all be measured at end-diastole using the leading-edge-to-leading-edge method. The aortic root diameter is measured as the maximum diameter of the sinus and the sinotubular junction should be made at the junction of the distal sinuses and origin of the tubular aorta. It is also important to note that the optimal ascending aortic diameter may be acquired by moving the transducer to a higher parasternal window and closer to the sternum.

24. **Answer: D.** The interventricular septum (IVS), LV, and posterior wall (PW) should be measured at end-diastole, perpendicular to the long axis of the LV at a level just below the mitral valve leaflet tips (**Figure 6-17**). The parasternal long-axis view should demonstrate the chamber along its center axis to maximize the dimension, with the papillary muscles out of plane, if possible. End-diastole is identified as

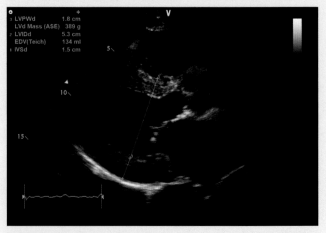

Figure 6-17

the frame at or immediately after mitral valve leaflet closure. In the case of poor visualization of the mitral valve, end-diastole may be identified as the peak of the R wave of the electrocardiogram.

The calipers should be positioned at the interface of the compacted myocardium of the interventricular septum and a line extended perpendicular to the long axis of the LV to the inner border of the compacted myocardium of the posterior wall.

25. **Answer: E.** Although the ASE guidelines recommend measuring the LV linear diameters just apical to the mitral valve leaflet tips, this is not the case when there is a septal bulge (sigmoid septum). Measurements performed at the base of the LV (as described in the answer outline for Question 24) will not only overestimate the IVS but will also underestimate the LV diastolic and systolic linear dimensions. In these cases where there is isolated thickening of the IVS, it is recommended that measurements be performed just apical to the septal bulge with the measurements perpendicular to the long axis of the LV. Answers A and B are incorrect as set 1 and set 2 measurements are too far distal. Answer C is incorrect; although the measurements are performed just apical to the septal bulge, the IVS measurement is not perpendicular to the long axis of the LV. Answer D is incorrect as set 4 measurements are measured at the level of the septal bulge.

26. **Answer: C.** The ASE recommends using a dedicated apical 4-chamber view to measure RA volume, which should be calculated using single-plane area-length or disk summation techniques. Measurements are performed at end-systole and the derived RA volume indexed to the body surface area (BSA). To calculate the RA volume, the RA area is traced at the blood-tissue interface from annulus to annulus and the RA length is measured from the mid-point of the tricuspid annulus to the middle of the superior RA wall (**Figure 6-18**). The normal range for two-dimensional right atrial volume is 25 + 7 mL/m² in men and 20.5 + 6 mL/m² in women. Answer A is not correct since there is a lack of established normal values for RA areas. Answer B is not correct as RA size appears to be gender dependent; therefore, consideration of the RA volume indexed for the BSA as well as the patient gender is required. Answer D is not correct since there is only one apical view that allows visualization of the RA; thus, the biplane method of disks is not possible.

27. **Answer: D.** The right ventricle (RV)-focused apical 4-chamber view is the recommended view by the ASE to measure the RV. This view is achieved by rotating the transducer counterclockwise and angling the probe face medially from the apical 4-chamber view while keeping the maximal RV area present (**Figure 6-19**). It is important to ensure that the LV apex is at the center of the scanning sector, while displaying the largest basal RV diameter. RV measurements are performed at end-diastole. The basal diameter is measured as the maximal transverse diameter in the basal third of the RV and the mid-cavity linear dimension is made at the level of the LV papillary muscles. A diameter >41 mm at the base and >35 mm at the midlevel in the RV-focused apical 4-chamber view indicate dilation. The modified apical 4-chamber view can also be used to evaluate RV size. Due to the complex geometry of the RV, multiple views should be used to assess RV size and function, but the RV-focused apical 4-chamber view is the view recommended to measure RV size.

28. **Answer: D.** The ASE recommends using the subcostal 4-chamber view to measure RV wall thickness. RV wall thickness is measured at end-diastole or at the peak of the R wave of the electrocardiogram, below the tricuspid annulus at a distance approximating the length of the anterior tricuspid leaflet (when it would be fully open) and perpendicular to the RV free wall (**Figure 6-20**). It is important to avoid trabeculae, papillary muscles, and epicardial fat.

While the parasternal and apical views may be used to measure the RV wall thickness, measurements from the subcostal view are more accurate. From the parasternal views, the RV is in very close proximity to the chest wall; therefore, reverberation artifacts in the near field may obscure the epicardial border of the anterior RV wall. From the apical views, RV wall thickness is measured across the width of the ultrasound beam in the lateral imaging plane and lateral resolution is generally poorer than the axial resolution.

29. **Answer: B.** From the PLAX view, the right ventricular outflow tract (RVOT) proximal diameter is measured at end-diastole from the anterior RV wall to the interventricular septal-aortic junction (**Figure 6-21A**). This measurement may also be performed in the parasternal short-axis (PSAX) view from the anterior RV wall to the aortic valve (**Figure 6-21B**).

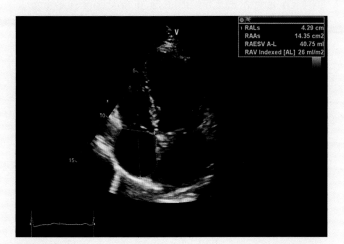

RALs	4.29 cm
RAAs	14.35 cm2
RAESV A-L	40.75 ml
RAV Indexed [AL]	26 ml/m2

Figure 6-18

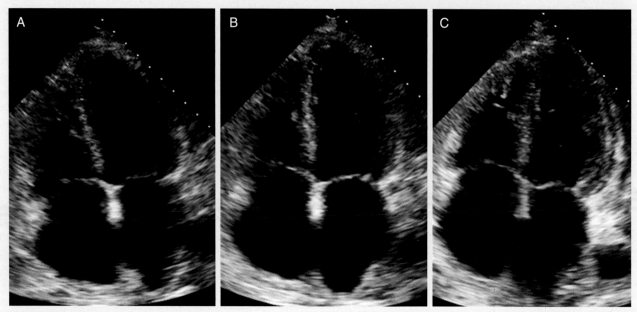

Figure 6-19 A, RV-focused view; B, Apical 4-chamber view; C, Modified apical 4-chamber view. (Reprinted with permission from Klein AL, Asher CR. *Clinical Echocardiography Review: a Self-Assessment Tool.* 2nd ed. Philadelphia, PA: Wolters Kluwer; 2017.)

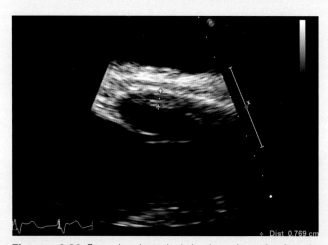

Figure 6-20 Zoomed subcostal 4-chamber view showing the measurement of the RV wall thickness.

The distal RVOT diameter (answer A) is measured from the PSAX view at the great vessel or pulmonary artery bifurcation view as the linear traverse dimension just proximal to the pulmonary valve (**Figure 6-21B**). The basal RV (answer C) and the mid-RV (answer D) are measured from the RV-focused apical 4-chamber view.

30. **Answer: B.** The IVC dimensions are performed from the subcostal view. Measurements are made perpendicular to the long axis of the IVC, just proximal to the junction of the hepatic veins, and approximately 1 to 2 cm proximal to the ostium of the RA. Answer A is incorrect since the measurement is too distal to the RA. Answer C is incorrect as this measurement is into the hepatic vein, thus overestimating the IVC diameter. Answer D is incorrect as this measurement is at the ostium of the RA.

It is important to minimize translation of the IVC with respiratory variation or with a patient "sniff" as this can give a false assumption of IVC collapse, especially on a one-dimensional M-mode trace. Imaging the IVC in a short-axis plane can demonstrate if the IVC translates out of the imaging plane during inspiration (**Figure 6-22**).

31. **Answer: A.** Left atrial volumes should be measured at end-systole from the apical 2-chamber and 4-chamber views using the biplane method of disks. When tracing the LA border, the confluences of the pulmonary veins and LA appendage with the left atrium should be excluded. The atrioventricular interface should be represented by the mitral annulus plane and not by the tip of the mitral leaflets (**Figure 6-23A**); that is, the LA area is traced from annulus to annulus and not into the mitral funnel.

TEACHING POINT

The LA length can be used as a reference for accuracy with the difference in lengths between the apical 4-chamber and apical 2-chamber views being within 5 mm. It is important to note that the view that represents the maximal LA volume will vary and minor adjustments should be made to ensure the largest LA volume is seen (**Figures 6-23B** and **6-23C**).

32. **Answer: D.** The ASE recommends calculating LV volumes using the biplane method of disks summation technique. It is important to include the papillary muscles and trabeculae as part of the volume. Similar to left atrial volumes, there should be <10% difference in LV lengths between the apical 4- and apical 2-chamber views. With laboratories with experience in 3D echocardiography, when image

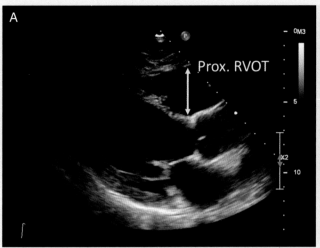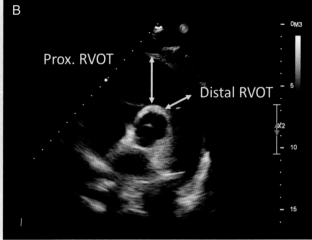

Figure 6-21 Measurements of the proximal RVOT (Prox. RVOT) and the distal RVOT dimensions. The proximal RVOT can be measured from the PLAX and PSAX views (A and B). The distal RVOT is measured from the PSAX view (B).

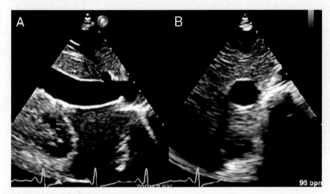

Figure 6-22 2D biplane or X-plane image of the IVC; A, Long axis of the IVC. B, Short axis of the IVC.

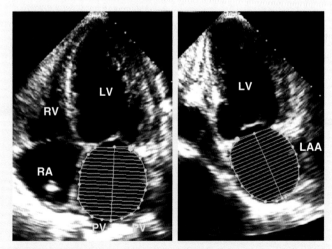

Figure 6-23A Left atrial border tracing. In the optimized left atrial (LA) acquisitions from the apical 4- and 2-chamber views (left and right images, respectively), the confluences of the pulmonary veins (PV), and left atrial appendage (LAA) should be excluded. The atrioventricular interface should be represented by the mitral annulus plane and not by the tip of the mitral leaflets. LV, left ventricle, RA, right atrium, RV, right ventricle. (Reprinted with permission from Klein AL, Asher CR. *Clinical Echocardiography Review: A Self-Assessment Tool.* 2nd ed. Philadelphia, PA: Wolters Kluwer; 2017.)

quality permits, 3D measurement of LV volumes is recommended. It is also recommended that LV size and volumes be indexed to BSA to allow comparison among individuals with different body sizes. The Teichholz method for calculating LV volumes from LV linear dimensions is no longer recommended for clinical use. The Teichholz formula for volumes assumes that the LV is a fixed geometric shape such as a prolate ellipsoid, which does not apply in a variety of cardiac pathologies.

> **TEACHING POINT**
>
> The area-length method can be very useful in estimating LV volumes when there is significant foreshortening of the LV apex or if only one apical view is visualized. The area-length method assumes a bullet-shaped ventricle. Via this method, the mid-LV cross-sectional area is traced from the parasternal short-axis view and the LV length is measured from the midpoint of the annular plane to the apex in the apical 4-chamber view (**Figure 6-24**). The LV volume (LVV) is calculated as:
>
> $$LVV = (0.85 \times A^2) \div L$$
>
> where A = area and L = length.

33. **Answer: C.** The mitral and tricuspid annular measurements are made at maximal valve opening in early diastole, approximately two to three frames after the end of the T wave on the electrocardiogram. Calipers are placed at the insertion points of the leaflets into the ventricular myocardium, using the inner-edge-to-inner-edge method. This measurement, along with the velocity time integral, can be used to calculate the stroke volume. Stroke volume calculations at the mitral and tricuspid annulus can be utilized to estimate regurgitant volumes of the mitral and tricuspid valves.

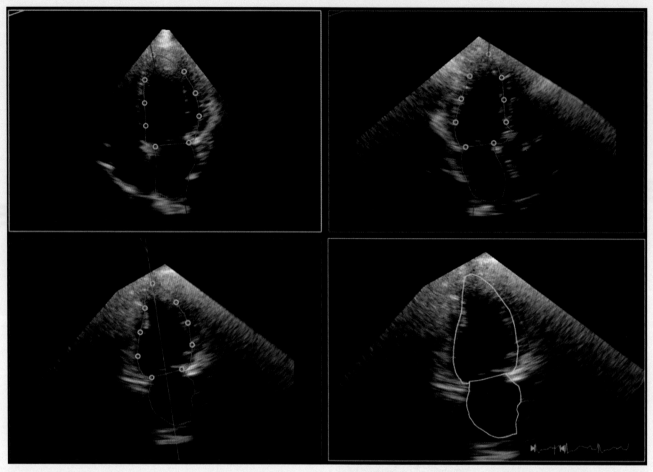

Figure 6-23B This 3D image illustrates how the image is appropriately optimized for the LV, but the LA length is shortened in the apical 4-chamber view (top left) compared to the apical 2-chamber view (bottom left).

34. ▶ **Answer: D.** The LVEF is calculated from the LV end-diastolic volume (LVEDV) and the LV end-systolic volume (LVESV) as:

$$\text{LVEF}(\%) = \left[(\text{LVEDV} - \text{LVESV}) \div \text{LVEDV}\right] \times 100$$

As previously discussed, the ASE recommends the calculation of LV volumes via the biplane method of disks summation (modified Simpson's) technique.

The area-length method (answer A) may be employed when the method of disks summation is not possible due to significant foreshortening of the LV apex or if only one apical view is visualized.

Estimation of LV volumes from linear measurements as in the Teichholz method (answer B) and the modified Quinones method (answer C) are not recommended due to geometric assumptions that may be invalid in the setting of regional wall motion abnormalities. Furthermore, if the base of the heart is hyperdynamic but the mid to apical segments are akinetic, as seen with takotsubo cardiomyopathy (**Video 6-2**), the calculated LVEF using the Teichholz and/or modified Quinones methods will be normal or hyperdynamic. This highlights the importance of volumetric measurements for the LVEF calculation.

35. Answer: B. LV mass is an important risk factor for and a strong predictor of cardiovascular events. It can be calculated from M-mode, 2D, and 3D echocardiographic images. All LV mass measurements should be made at end-diastole. M-mode and 2D echocardiography–derived linear measurements of the LV wall thickness and LV diastolic diameter rely on geometric formulas to calculate the volume of the LV myocardium. LV mass can also be calculated via 2D echocardiography using either the area-length or truncated ellipsoid techniques. As the linear and other 2D methods calculate the LV mass using different equations and different assumptions, the normal ranges for LV mass differ accordingly.

Answer A is a true statement. As for many chamber measurements, the LV mass should also be indexed to the BSA. However, there is controversy as to whether the LV mass should be indexed to height, weight, or the BSA.

Answer C is a true statement since in a normally shaped LV, both M-mode and 2D echocardiographic formulas may be used to calculate LV mass. However, in patients with basal septal hypertrophy, the linear methods may overestimate the true LV mass due to the thickest region of the LV being a part of the calculation. Furthermore, in these cases, the

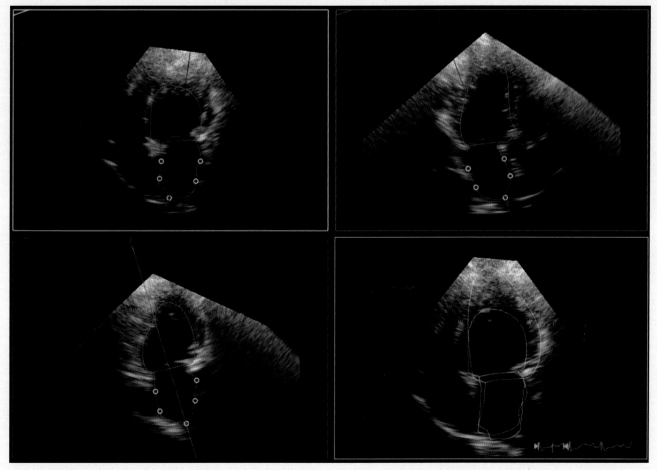

Figure 6-23C This 3D image illustrates how the image is appropriately optimized for the LA at the expense of the LV. Observe that in both the apical 4-chamber view (top left) and the apical 2-chamber view (bottom left), the LA length is not foreshortened.

area-length method, which uses mid-ventricular measurements, underestimates LV mass, because the thickest part of the IVS is not included.

Answer D is a true statement. 3D echocardiography is the only method that measures LV mass directly. LV mass normal value ranges from 3D echocardiography have not yet been established.

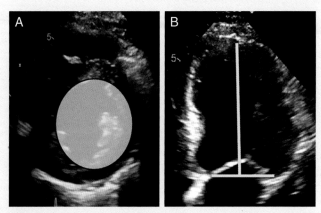

Figure 6-24 Area-length measurements. A, Parasternal short-axis view at end-diastole measuring the LV area, B, Apical 4-chamber view measuring end-diastolic LV length.

36. **Answer: B.** The regional wall motion score index (RWMSI) is calculated by dividing the total regional LV wall motion score by the total number of LV wall segments. The ASE recommends using the 17-segment model to assess myocardial perfusion and the 16-segment model for routine studies assessing wall motion. The scoring system for each segment is as follows: normal = 1, hypokinetic (reduced thickening) = 2, akinetic (absent or negligible thickening) = 3, and dyskinetic (systolic thinning or outward systolic expansion) = 4.

In the patient described, all four apical segments are akinetic so would score 3 and the remaining 12 segments are normal so would score 1. That would give a value of 12 (4 × 3) for the akinetic apical segments and a value of 12 (12 × 1) for normal segments with a total value of 24. As there are 16 segments, the RWMSI = 24 ÷ 16 = 1.5.

37. **Answer: C.** The RV FAC is a measurement of global, rather than regional, RV systolic function. Therefore, answer C is the incorrect statement.

RV FAC is a measurement performed in an apical 4-chamber view that includes visualization of the

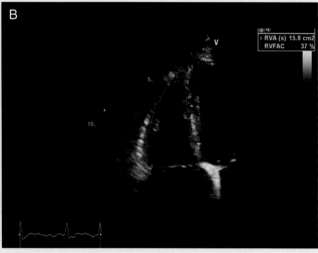

Figure 6-25 Measurement of the RV FAC. A, End-diastolic RV area. B, End-systolic RV area. The RV FAC is 37%.

entire RV in both diastole and systole. The RV area is measured at end-diastole and end-systole, making sure the diastolic and systolic measurements include the trabeculae within the RV cavity (**Figure 6-25**). From the RV end-diastolic area (RVEDA) and the RV end-systolic area (RVESA), the RV FAC is calculated as:

$$RV\ FAC(\%) = \left[(RVEDA - RVESA) \div RVEDA\right] \times 100$$

An RV FAC <35% is considered to be abnormal.

When tracing the RV areas, it is important to make sure the apex and the RV free wall are included within the sector. Measurement limitations include suboptimal image quality of the RV and the fact that RV FAC neglects the contribution of the right ventricular outflow tract to the overall RV systolic function.

38. **Answer: E.** Indexed to the BSA, a mildly dilated LA is 35 to 41 mL/m², a moderately dilated LA is 42 to 48 mL/m², and a severely LA dilated is >48 mL/m². Based on the measurements shown, the LA is severely dilated. However, looking at the accuracy of measurements, the pulmonary veins and LA appendage are correctly excluded, and the atrioventricular interface is correctly represented by the mitral annulus plane and not by the tip of the mitral leaflets, but the difference in LA lengths between the apical 4-chamber and apical 2-chamber views is greater than 5 mm.

In **Figure 6-7**, the apical 2-chamber view (right) shows a foreshortened LA. The LA length in this view is 5.38 cm versus a LA length of 6.10 cm in the apical 4-chamber view. The difference between the two is 0.72 cm or 7.2 mm; this exceeds the recommended cutoff of <5 mm.

Figure 6-26 shows a better window for the apical 2-chamber view, optimized for the LA. The LA length is now 6.06 cm (<5 mm from the apical 4-chamber view) and the indexed LAV is now calculated at 49 mL/m².

39. **Answer: B.** The ascending aorta is measured at end-diastole using the leading-edge-to-leading-edge method. It is recommended to report the ascending aortic diameter as an indexed value. In a male patient, a normal proximal ascending aorta is 1.5 + 0.2 cm/m². Measurements exceeding ± 1.96 standard deviations are classified as abnormal. Therefore, a proximal ascending aortic diameter >1.9 cm/m² is considered abnormal.

In this case, the indexed proximal ascending aorta is 1.95 cm/m² (3.9 cm ÷ 2.0 m²); therefore, the ascending aorta is dilated. Lastly, it does not matter what the indication is for the echocardiogram, the ascending aorta should be measured routinely on all examinations. In the case of an existing aortic aneurysm, imaging from a right parasternal window often visualizes more of the ascending aorta than does imaging from the standard left parasternal window.

40. **Answer: C.** The LVOTd is used to calculate the LVOT cross-sectional area (CSA_{LVOT}) using the equation:

$$CSA_{LVOT} = \pi \times r^2 \qquad (1)$$

or

$$CSA_{LVOT} = 0.785 \times D^2 \qquad (2)$$

where r is the LVOT radius and D is the LVOTd.

The aortic valve area (AVA) is then calculated from the CSA_{LVOT}, the LVOT velocity time integral (VTI_{LVOT}), and the VTI across the stenotic aortic valve (VTI_{AV}) using the following equation:

$$AVA = \left(CSA_{LVOT} \times VTI_{LVOT}\right) \div VTI_{AV} \qquad (3)$$

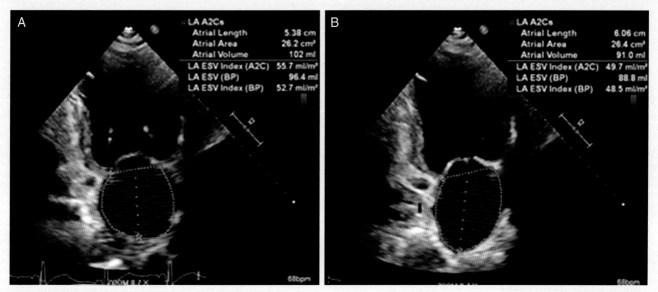

Figure 6-26 A, Apical 2-chamber view with foreshortened LA. B, Apical 2-chamber view optimized for the LA; observe that the LA is elongated compared with figure A.

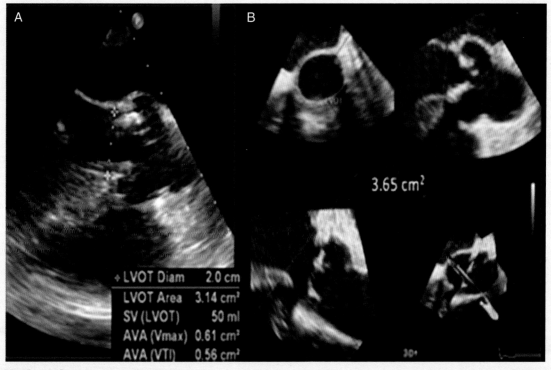

Figure 6-27 2D and 3D transesophageal echocardiographic measurements of the LVOT diameter are shown. A, Mid-esophageal LVOTd measurement is 2.0 cm, yielding an LVOT area of 3.14 cm²; B, 3D multiplanar reconstruction (MPR) view of the actual LVOT area in the same patient, yielding a CSA of 3.65 cm².

As the product of the $CSA_{LVOT} \times VTI_{LVOT}$ is equal to the stroke volume across the LVOT (SV_{LVOT}), the AVA can also be calculated as:

$$AVA = SV_{LVOT} \div VTI_{AV} \qquad (4)$$

Based on these equations, if the LVOTd is overestimated, then the SV_{LVOT} will be overestimated, the AVA will be overestimated, and the AS severity will be underestimated. Therefore, answer C is correct.

The table below summarizes the effects of overestimation and underestimation of the LVOTd on the CSA_{LVOT}, the SV_{LVOT}, the AVA, and the AS severity:

LVOTd	CSA$_{LVOT}$	SV$_{LVOT}$	AVA	As Severity
Underestimated	Underestimated	Underestimated	Underestimated	Overestimated
Overestimated	Overestimated	Overestimated	Overestimated	Underestimated

It is also important to note that the LVOTd is squared in order to calculate the CSA (Equation 2). Furthermore, 3D echocardiography shows that the LVOT is not a true circle and is often ellipsoid or irregular in shape. Therefore, if the LVOTd is measured a millimeter too large or too small, it can significantly alter the AVA calculation. For example, the CSA of an LVOTd of 2.0 cm equals a CSA of 3.12 cm^2, but if the LVOT is measured 1 mm larger at 2.1 cm, then the CSA is 3.46 cm^2. When 3D echocardiography is available, a true CSA of the LVOT can be traced as seen in **Figure 6-27**.

Acknowledgments: The authors thank and acknowledge the following contributions from Wendy Tsang MD, MSc, and Roberto M. Lang, MD (Chapter 4, Assessment of Chamber Quantification) in Clinical Echocardiography Review: A Self-Assessment Tool, 2nd ed., edited by Allan L. Klein, Craig R. Asher, 2017.

SUGGESTED READINGS

Addetia K, Yamat M, Mediratta A, et al. Comprehensive two-dimensional interrogation of the tricuspid valve using knowledge derived from three-dimensional echocardiography. *J Am Soc Echocardiogr.* 2016;29(1):74-82.

Anderson B. *Echocardiography: The Normal Examination and Echocardiographic Measurements.* 3rd ed. Echotext Pty Ltd; 2017:chaps 2 and 9.

Baumgartner H, Hung J, Bermejo J, et al. Recommendations on the echocardiographic assessment of aortic valve stenosis: a focused update from the European Association of Cardiovascular Imaging and the American Society of Echocardiography. *J Am Soc Echocardiogr.* 2017;30(4):372-392.

Goldstein SA, Evangelista A, Abbara S, et al. Multimodality imaging of diseases of the thoracic aorta in adults. From the American Society of Echocardiography and the European Association of Cardiovascular Imaging: endorsed by the Society of Cardiovascular Computed Tomography and Society for Cardiovascular Magnetic Resonance. *J Am Soc Echocardiogr.* 2015;28(2):119-182.

Lang RM, Badano LP, Mor-Avi V, et al. Recommendations for cardiac chamber quantification by echocardiography in adults: an update from the American Society of Echocardiography and the European Association of Cardiovascular Imaging. *J Am Soc Echocardiogr.* 2015;28(1):1-39.

Mitchell C, Rahko PS, Blauwet LA, et al. Guidelines for performing a comprehensive transthoracic echocardiographic examination in adults: recommendations from the American Society of Echocardiography. *J Am Soc Echocardiogr.* 2019;32(1):1-64.

Rudski LG, Lai WW, Afilalo J, et al. Guidelines for the echocardiographic assessment of the right heart in adults: a report from the American Society of Echocardiography endorsed by the European Association of Echocardiography, a registered branch of the European Society of Cardiology, and the Canadian Society of Echocardiography. *J Am Soc Echocardiogr.* 2010;23(7):685-713.

M-Mode Echocardiography

Contributors: Margaret M. Park, BS, ACS, RDCS, RVT and Maryellen H. Orsinelli, RN, RDCS

✪✪ Question 1

A 50-year-old woman presents to the emergency room (ER) complaining of increasing dyspnea over the last several weeks. On physical examination, systolic and diastolic murmurs are heard at the apex. The M-mode trace across the mitral valve (**Figure 7-1**) suggests the presence of:

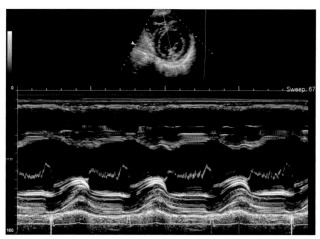

Figure 7-1

    A. Acute aortic regurgitation.
    B. Chronic aortic regurgitation.
    C. Chronic mitral regurgitation.
    D. Mitral stenosis.

✪✪ Question 2

A 29-year-old woman was referred to the Cardiology clinic because of a murmur. An echocardiogram was ordered to assess valve function. The M-mode trace of the aortic valve (**Figure 7-2**) suggests:

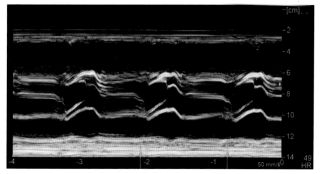

Figure 7-2

    A. A normal aortic valve.
    B. Aortic stenosis.
    C. Aortic insufficiency.
    D. A bicuspid aortic valve.

✪ Question 3

This 65-year-old man was admitted with increasing dyspnea on exertion and 3$^+$ pitting edema. The M-mode trace of the inferior vena cava (IVC) demonstrates an IVC with and without a "sniff" maneuver (**Figure 7-3**). Based on the current American Society of Echocardiography (ASE) guidelines, the estimated right atrial pressure (RAP) is:
    A. 3 mm Hg.
    B. 5 mm Hg.
    C. 8 mm Hg.
    D. 15 mm Hg.

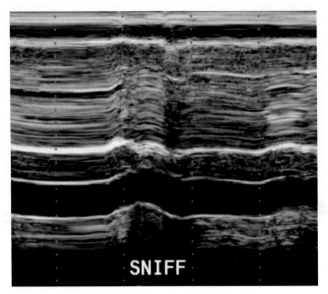

Figure 7-3

A. Axial
B. Temporal
C. Lateral
D. All the above

✪✪ Question 4

This 57-year-old woman with breast cancer was admitted with new-onset shortness of breath. She had previously been treated with chemotherapy. Chest x-ray showed an enlarged cardiac silhouette. A stat echocardiogram was ordered. The M-mode trace in **Figure 7-4** suggests:

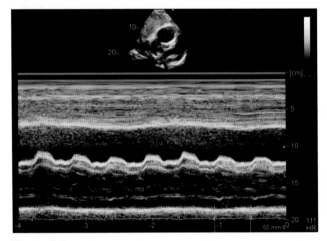

Figure 7-4

  A. Mitral stenosis.
  B. An enlarged right ventricle (RV) and no chamber collapse.
  C. RV chamber collapse consistent with cardiac tamponade.
  D. Left ventricular (LV) enlargement and dysfunction.

✪✪✪ Question 5

Which of the following image resolutions is superior in M-Mode echocardiography compared to two-dimensional (2D) echocardiography?

✪✪ Question 6

A 36-year-old man presents with shortness of breath and a heart murmur that increases in intensity with Valsalva maneuver. An M-mode trace of the mitral valve (**Figure 7-5A**) and aortic valve (**Figure 7-5B**) was obtained. The most likely diagnosis is:

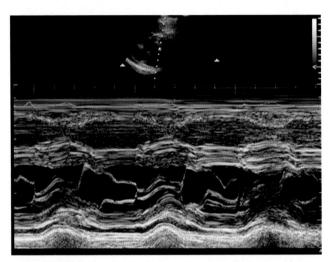

Figure 7-5A

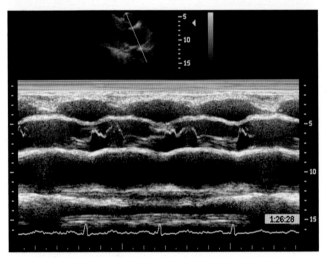

Figure 7-5B

  A. Mitral stenosis.
  B. Mitral valve prolapse.
  C. Aortic stenosis.
  D. Hypertrophic obstructive cardiomyopathy.
  E. B and C.

✪✪ Question 7

The M-mode trace in **Figure 7-6** was recorded from the apical 4-chamber view in a 62-year-old woman with complaints of dyspnea, mild lower leg edema, and fatigue. Which statement regarding this patient is likely to be true?

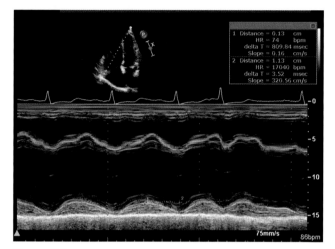

Figure 7-6

    A. RV function is likely impaired.
    B. Paradoxical septal motion is present.
    C. There is RV dilatation.
    D. Tricuspid annular thickening is present.

✪ Question 8

Which of the following statements about M-mode echocardiography is false?
    A. M-mode is a one-dimensional or "ice pick" ultrasound approach.
    B. Current M-mode has a temporal resolution of ~100 pulses per second.
    C. M-mode is a convenient way to record multiple cardiac cycles.
    D. M-mode echocardiography provides complementary hemodynamic information.

✪ Question 9

Which abnormality is identified in the M-mode trace shown in **Figure 7-7**?
    A. Left atrial myxoma
    B. Moderate mitral stenosis
    C. Flail posteromedial papillary muscle
    D. Reverberation artifact from a mechanical valve

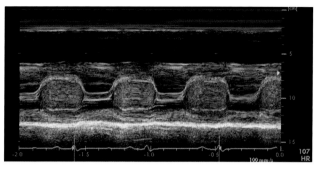

Figure 7-7

✪✪✪ Question 10

A 19-year-old soccer player with bradycardia and a systolic murmur on auscultation has an echocardiogram. His LV ejection fraction is 58% by the Simpson biplane method. The M-mode trace of the mitral valve (**Figure 7-8**) demonstrates:

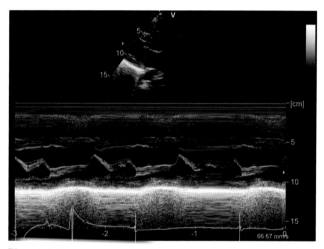

Figure 7-8

    A. An abnormal E-F slope.
    B. Delayed mitral valve closure.
    C. An L-wave indicating normal LV end-diastolic pressure.
    D. An L-wave indicating abnormal LV end-diastolic pressure.

✪✪✪ Question 11

The linear method for calculating LV mass (LVM) is based on M-mode end-diastolic measurements of the LV internal dimension (LVID), posterior wall thickness (PWT), and IVS thickness (IVST). The equation for this calculation is:

$$LVM(g) = 1.04\left(\left(LVID + PWT + IVST\right)^3 - LVID^3\right) \times 0.8 + 0.6$$

In this equation, what does the value 1.04 represent?
- **A.** A correction factor
- **B.** A constant for LV muscle volume
- **C.** A constant for LV epicardial volume
- **D.** A constant for the specific gravity of muscle

✪✪✪ Question 12

The M-mode trace of the left ventricle in **Figure 7-9** was acquired on an elderly patient with a history of coronary artery disease and recent tricuspid valve replacement. The contractility of the LV apex was normal. Using the measurements provided on this trace, the calculated fractional shortening (FS) and LV ejection fraction (EF) via the simplified Quinones method are:
- **A.** FS = 28%; EF = 55%.
- **B.** FS = 38%; EF = 48%.
- **C.** FS = 15%; EF = 28%.
- **D.** FS = 48%; EF = 28%.

✪✪ Question 13

Based on the M-mode recording in Question 12 (**Figure 7-9**), which of the following statements accurately describes the IVS motion?

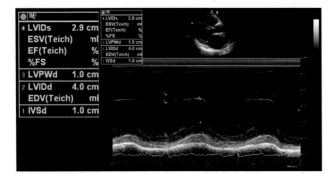

Figure 7-9

- **A.** Normal IVS wall motion
- **B.** Diastolic IVS shudder
- **C.** Paradoxical IVS wall motion
- **D.** Classic left bundle branch block IVS motion
- **E.** C or D

✪✪✪ Question 14

This M-mode is taken from the study of a 59-year-old man who presents with severe heart failure symptoms (**Figure 7-10**). On auscultation you would expect to hear:

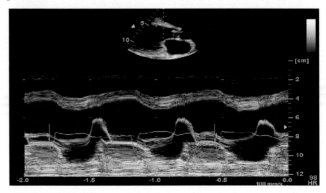

Figure 7-10

- **A.** An opening snap.
- **B.** Rales.
- **C.** An apical systolic murmur.
- **D.** A holodiastolic murmur.

✪✪✪ Question 15

The M-mode trace shown in **Figure 7-11** was acquired from a 42-year-old man with a history of palpitations and presyncope. On physical examination, he has a widely persistent split of the second heart sound. Which of the following statements regarding the findings on this M-mode trace is correct?

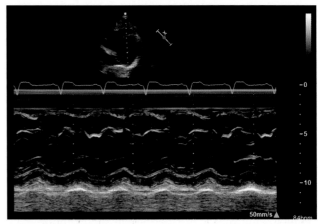

Figure 7-11

- **A.** Findings are normal.
- **B.** Findings are consistent with left bundle branch block (LBBB).
- **C.** Findings are consistent with right bundle branch block (RBBB).
- **D.** Findings are consistent with Wolff-Parkinson-White (WPW) syndrome.

✪✪ Question 16

Which portion of the mitral valve cycle labeled in **Figure 7-12** is most helpful in identifying abnormalities of LV diastolic pressure?

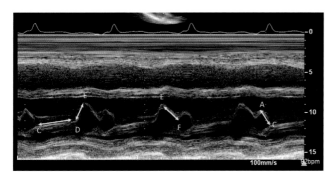

Figure 7-12

  A. D-E excursion
  B. E-F slope
  C. A-C mid to late diastole
  D. C-D closure line during systole

✪ Question 17

A 52-year-old man has complaints of dyspnea upon exertion and irregular heart rhythm. The M-mode trace shown in **Figure 7-13** is most consistent with:

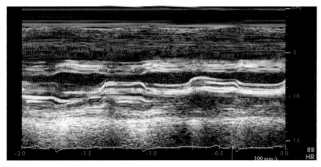

Figure 7-13

  A. Rheumatic mitral stenosis.
  B. Myxomatous mitral valve disease.
  C. Left atrial myxoma.
  D. Severe mitral annular calcification.

✪ Question 18

A 41-year-old woman comes to the emergency room with marked shortness of breath and complaints of a "heavy chest." The M-mode trace shown in **Figure 7-14** is consistent with:

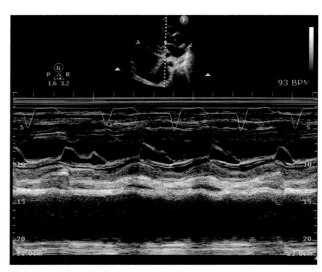

Figure 7-14

  A. A large pericardial effusion.
  B. Pericardial thickening and pleural effusion.
  C. Pleural effusion.
  D. Pericardial thickening and pericardial effusion.

✪✪ Question 19

The M-mode features seen in **Figure 7-15** are associated with:

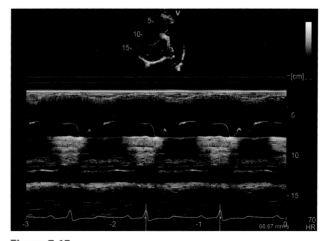

Figure 7-15

  A. Severe valvular pulmonic stenosis.
  B. Severe pulmonary hypertension.
  C. Acute pulmonary embolism.
  D. Normal pulmonary valve motion.
  E. B and C.

✪✪✪ Question 20

A 34-year-old man with a history of shortness of breath with exercise and difficulty walking up hills or climbing stairs presents for an echocardiogram. Which best describes the findings displayed in the M-mode traces acquired from the parasternal short-axis view (**Figure 7-16A**) and from the parasternal long-axis view (**Figure 7-16B**)?

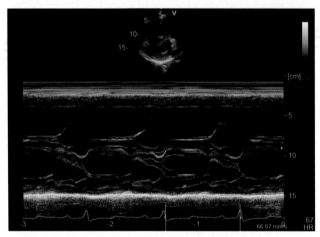

Figure 7-16A

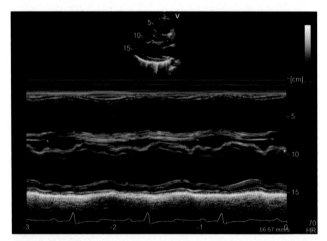

Figure 7-16B

A. A dilated RV, prominent moderator band, and normal mitral and tricuspid valves

B. A dilated LV, an LV tendon, and normal mitral and tricuspid valves

C. Ebstein anomaly with RV enlargement and abnormal IVS motion

D. RV enlargement with an RV mass and normal mitral and tricuspid valves

✪✪✪ Question 21

A 60-year-old man presents with increasing dyspnea and palpitations. The physical examination reveals an apical systolic murmur. This M-mode trace recorded from the parasternal long-axis view (**Figure 7-17**) is most consistent with:

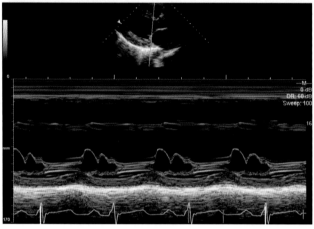

Figure 7-17

A. Reduced LV systolic function and a marked elevation in LV filling pressures (LVFP).

B. Reduced LV systolic function and elevated LV end-diastolic pressure (LVEDP).

C. A dilated LV and mitral valve prolapse.

D. A dilated LV with acute aortic regurgitation.

✪✪ Question 22

Which of the following M-mode findings is not an indicator of a low cardiac output?

A. Tapered closure of the aortic valve

B. An increased mitral E point-septal separation

C. A decreased aortic root amplitude

D. An increased LV end-diastolic dimension

ANSWERS

1. Answer: B. This M-mode trace is consistent with chronic aortic regurgitation (AR). The M-mode trace demonstrates a dilated left ventricle (LV) and diastolic fluttering of the anterior mitral leaflet due to the direction of the AR jet toward the anterior mitral valve leaflets during diastole. Answer A is not correct. With acute AR, diastolic fluttering of the mitral valve may be seen; however, the LV would not be dilated. Answer C is not correct. While chronic mitral regurgitation can lead to a dilated LV, it would not result in the fluttering of the anterior mitral valve leaflet. Answer D is not correct since in mitral stenosis, the LV would not be dilated. The E-F slope seen in this example is also not suggestive of the reduced E-F slope seen with mitral stenosis.

2. **Answer: D.** This M-mode trace is characteristic of a bicuspid aortic valve (BAV). The closure line of the aortic valve in diastole is eccentric, rather than equidistant from the anterior and posterior aortic walls. The eccentricity index (EI) may be calculated as:

$$EI = (0.5 \times AoD) \div DCLD \quad (1)$$

where AoD is the aortic lumen diameter and DCLD is the diastolic closure line distance.

The DCLD is defined as the minimum distance from the aortic valve closure line to the nearest aortic wall. A normal EI value is 1 as the closure line should be in the center of the aortic lumen.

In this case, the aortic lumen diameter is 3.0 cm and the DCLD is 0.75 cm (**Figure 7-18A**); therefore,

$$EI = (0.5 \times 3.0) \div 0.75 = 1.5 \div 0.75 = 2 \quad (2)$$

Values greater than 1.3 to 1.5 are suggestive of a bicuspid aortic valve, as is demonstrated in this example. The parasternal short-axis view of the aortic valve acquired in systole (**Figure 7-18B**) demonstrates two rather than three aortic cusps with only two commissural attachments to the aortic root at 10 o'clock and 4 o'clock.

This M-mode trace is not aortic stenosis (answer B) because the valve opens well. While patients with a bicuspid valve can have aortic regurgitation (AR), the presence of AR (answer C) cannot be determined from this M-mode tracing.

3. **Answer: D.** The vertical depth between the orange dots on the M-mode trace is 1 cm. The IVC is dilated (approximately 2.2 cm) and does not collapse with inspiratory sniff. Current ASE guidelines recommend using the IVC size and dynamic changes with an inspiratory "sniff" for the estimation of the RAP. This estimate of RAP should be used in estimation of the pulmonary artery pressures, rather than assuming a constant RAP for all patients. Furthermore, specific values of RAP, rather than ranges, should be estimated (**Table 7-1**).

The IVC diameter should be measured from a long-axis view of the IVC acquired from the subcostal window with the patient in the supine position. For accuracy, this measurement is made perpendicular to the IVC long axis.

4. ▶ **Answer: C.** The right ventricle (RV) is small and compressed by the large pericardial effusion. In addition, there is RV collapse in diastole (**Figure 7-19**, red arrow) consistent with cardiac tamponade. This is appreciated better on the real-time image (**Video 7-1**).

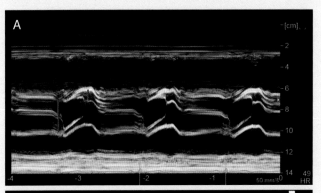
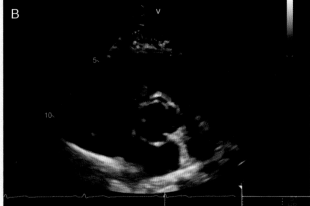

Figure 7-18 A, The red line on the left is the aortic lumen diameter (AoD) and the shorter red line on the right is the diastolic closure line distance (DCLD). B, Parasternal short-axis view of the aortic valve acquired in systole demonstrates two (anterior and posterior) rather than three aortic cusps with only two commissural attachments to the aortic root seen at 10 o'clock and 4 o'clock.

Answer A is not correct since the mitral valve opens widely. Answer B is not correct; however, this effusion is so large, and the RV is collapsed and therefore the fluid collection could be mistaken for the RV. Answer D is not correct as the LV is not dilated and while the posterior wall motion is not well defined, the interventricular septum (IVS) thickens normally making significant LV dysfunction unlikely.

5. **Answer: B.** The temporal resolution of M-Mode echocardiography is superior to that of 2D echocardiography. M-mode sampling rates are typically in the range of 1000 Hz, while 2D sampling rates typically range from 30 to 100 Hz. The higher sampling rate of M-mode allows for the better assessment of rapidly moving structures. In addition, M-mode traces have superior interface definition and have the ability to display multiple beats on a single trace, which is especially useful in the evaluation of timing of events and for the identification of respiratory changes and variations. Axial resolution (answer A) is similar between M-mode and 2D imaging since axial resolution is a function of transducer frequency, which is similar in the two techniques. Lateral resolution (answer C) is similar in 2D imaging as in the M-mode technique as the beam width along the scan line is the same.

Table 7-1. Inferior Vena Cava (IVC) Size and Collapsibility for the Estimation of Right Atrial Pressure (RAP)

Range	IVC Diameter (cm)	IVC Collapsibility With Sniff (%)	Estimated RAP (mm Hg)
Normal	≤2.1	>50	3
High	>2.1	<50	15
Intermediate*	≤2.1	<50	8
	>2.1	>50	8

*When there are no secondary signs of increased RAP, the RAP can be downgraded to 3 mm Hg; when the IVC collapses < 35% and there are secondary signs of increased RAP, then the RAP can be upgraded to 15 mm Hg. Secondary signs of an elevated RAP include a restrictive tricuspid inflow filling profile, a tricuspid E/e' ratio > 6, or a hepatic venous systolic filling fraction > 55%.

6. **Answer: D.** The mitral valve M-mode trace demonstrates systolic anterior motion (SAM) of the mitral valve leaflets (**Figure 7-20A**, arrow). In addition, the IVS is thickened. The aortic valve M-mode trace demonstrates mid-systolic closure of the valve (**Figure 7-20B**, arrow), which is related to a decreased stroke volume at the time of dynamic obstruction. These features are all consistent with hypertrophic obstructive cardiomyopathy (HOCM). **Figure 7-20C** demonstrates the 2D-directed linear measurements of the IVS, posterior wall, and LV cavity (IVS measures 1.6 cm).

Answer A is not correct since the mitral valve opens widely in diastole; thus, this is not mitral stenosis. Answer B is not correct. In mitral valve prolapse, the leaflets will be displaced posteriorly in systole. Answer C is not correct. While the IVS may be thickened in aortic stenosis, the aortic valve in this case opens widely, making aortic stenosis unlikely.

7. **Answer: A.** Measurement of the tricuspid annular plane systolic excursion (TAPSE) is demonstrated on the M-mode trace in **Figure 7-6**. TAPSE is properly acquired with the M-mode cursor aligned perpendicular to the tricuspid annulus. TAPSE is measured as the longitudinal distance or excursion of the

TV lateral annulus between end-diastole and peak systole and is a measure of RV longitudinal fiber shortening during systole. TAPSE in this subject was measured as 1.13 cm or 11.3 mm. A value < 16 mm is consistent with impaired RV function. TAPSE is not only determined by RV systolic function but also appears to be dependent upon LV systolic function; therefore, false abnormal results may occur when there is significant LV systolic dysfunction despite normal RV systolic function. Furthermore, TAPSE may be falsely normal when there is tethering of an akinetic RV segment to an actively contracting RV segment and may overestimate RV contractility when there is severe tricuspid regurgitation. Due to the complexity in evaluating RV systolic function, no single measure of RV systolic function should be relied upon, rather multiple methods of assessing RV systolic function should be evaluated and compared. Color M-mode may assist in the analysis of TAPSE (**Figure 7-21**).

8. **Answer: B.** 2D M-mode methods have a temporal resolution of approximately 1000 pulses per second. Therefore, Answer B is false. Early dedicated M-mode echocardiography had a sampling rate of approximately 2000 pulses per second.

Answer A is a true statement. M-mode traces are produced from a single ultrasound beam; therefore, M-mode provides a one-dimensional or "ice pick" view of cardiac structures moving over time. Answer C is a true statement as M-mode traces allow the display of multiple cardiac cycles. Answer D is a true statement since M-mode can provide complementary information to Doppler hemodynamic findings due to its ability to record very rapid and/or subtle motions. For example, the degree of left ventricular outflow tract (LVOT) obstruction in a patient with HOCM can be predicted based on the motion of the mitral valve during systole.

9. ▶ **Answer: A.** This M-mode trace illustrates a left atrial (LA) myxoma prolapsing through the mitral orifice during diastole (**Figure 7-22**). The tumor appears as a mass of echoes posterior to the mitral valve during diastole, occurring just

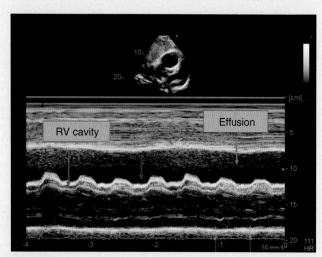

Figure 7-19

after the initial opening of the mitral valve, which is indicated by the slight echo-free space posterior to the anterior mitral leaflet at the onset of diastole (solid red arrow in **Figure 7-22**). A time lag exists between the initial diastolic opening of the valve and the suction of the tumor mass into the mitral orifice. The real-time motion of the tumor is shown in **Video 7-2**.

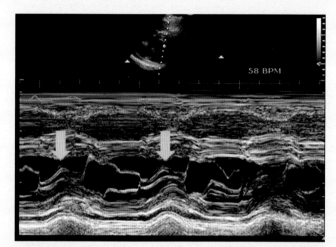

Figure 7-20A

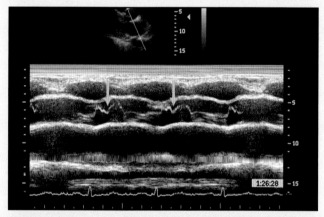

Figure 7-20B

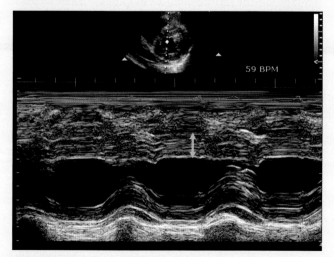

Figure 7-20C

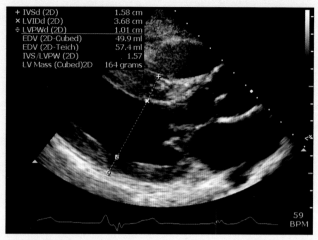

Figure 7-20D

Answer B is not correct. Although the mitral EF slope is diminished from the obstructing tumor, the posterior leaflet does appear to move normally (dotted yellow arrow in **Figure 7-22**), and the anterior leaflet is not significantly thickened. These findings are inconsistent with mitral stenosis. Answer C is not correct. In the case of a flail posteromedial papillary muscle, erratic movement of the papillary muscle would be seen in both systole and diastole. Answer D is not correct. Echo artifacts from a mechanical prosthetic valve would appear thicker and more linear and ladder-like in appearance.

10. **Answer: C.** An L-wave is recorded when there is middiastolic flow across the mitral valve (**Figure 7-23**, arrow). An L-wave may be seen in relatively bradycardic patients with normal hearts. Note that both the IVS and the LV posterior wall display normal thickness. A pathologic L-wave (answer D) is related to markedly abnormal LV relaxation in the setting of elevated LV filling pressures. This may be seen in patients with

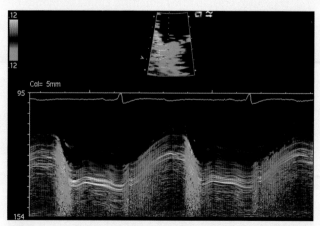

Figure 7-21 This is a zoomed view of the lateral tricuspid annulus showing color M-mode for TAPSE. Color M-mode aids in the identification of end-diastole and peak systole. In this example, the blue/red interface identifies end-diastole and the red/blue interface identifies peak systole.

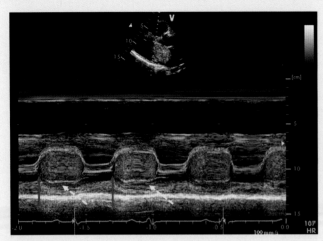

Figure 7-22

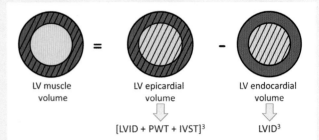

Figure 7-24

STEPS TO CALCULATING THE LV MASS

Step 1: Calculate the total LV epicardial volume: $(LVID + IVST + PWT)^3$

Step 2: Calculate LV endocardial volume: $(LVID)^3$

Step 3: Calculate LV muscle volume: (LV epicardial volume − LV endocardial chamber volume) or (Step 1 value − Step 2 value)

Step 4: Calculate LV mass: LVM (g) = ((1.04 × LV muscle volume) × 0.8) + 0.6

Step 5: Calculate the indexed LV mass: ILVM (g/m^2) = LVM ÷ BSA

increased LV wall thickness such as in LV hypertrophy. This finding on an M-mode trace is equivalent to the finding of an L-wave recorded on a spectral Doppler waveform of transmitral inflow and/or on the tissue Doppler trace acquired at the mitral annulus. Answer A is not correct since the mitral EF slope appears normal. Answer B is not correct as mitral valve closure appears to occur normally at the onset of systole as indicated by the timing on the ECG.

11. **Answer: D.** 1.04 represents the constant for specific gravity of muscle (g/mL). The values of 0.8 and 0.6 are constant correction factors. The LV mass is derived from the LV muscle volume and the specific gravity of muscle. LV muscle volume is equal to the total ventricular volume contained within the epicardial boundaries of the ventricle (epicardial volume) minus the chamber volume contained by the endocardial surfaces (endocardial volume) (**Figure 7-24**). The LV mass is then calculated by multiplying the LV muscle volume by the specific gravity of muscle. As for many chamber measurements, the LV mass should also be adjusted to the BSA. However, there is controversy as to whether the LV mass should be indexed to height, weight, or the BSA.

12. **Answer: A.** The fractional shortening (FS) is calculated from the LV internal dimension at end-diastole (LVIDd) and the LV internal dimension at end-systole (LVIDs):

$$FS(\%) = \left[(LVIDd - LVIDs) \div LVIDd\right] \times 100 \quad (1)$$

In this patient, the LVIDd is 4.0 cm and the LVIDs is 2.9 cm; therefore, the FS is:

$$FS(\%) = \left[(4.0 - 2.9) \div 4.0\right] \times 100 = 28\% \quad (2)$$

Calculation of the EF via the simplified Quinones method is more challenging. Using this method, three parameters are required (1) LVIDd, (2) LVIDs, and (3) the contractility of the apex. The EF is then derived from this equation:

$$EF(\%) = \left\{\left[(1 - \Delta D^2) \times \Delta L\right] + \Delta D^2\right\} \times 100 \quad (3)$$

where ΔD^2 is the square of the minor axis and ΔL is the apical contractility.

ΔD^2 is derived from the LVIDd and LVIDs:

$$\Delta D = (LVIDd^2 - LVIDs^2) \div LVIDd^2 \quad (4)$$

%ΔL can be evaluated subjectively by observing the contractility of the LV apex such that: normal apical contraction = 0.15, hypokinetic apical contraction = 0.05, akinetic apical contraction = 0, dyskinetic apical contraction −0.05, and frankly dyskinetic apical contraction = −0.10.

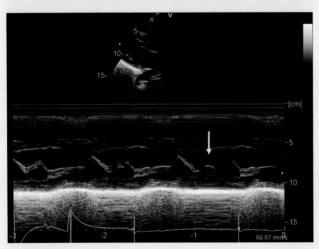

Figure 7-23

In this patient, the LVIDd is 4.0 cm and the LVIDs is 2.9 cm; therefore, the ΔD^2 is:

$$\Delta D = \left(4.0^2 - 2.9^2\right) \div 2.9^2 = 0.47 \qquad (5)$$

Apical contractility is normal; therefore, %ΔL is 0.15. Hence, the Quinones's EF is:

$$
\begin{aligned}
EF(\%) &= \left\{\left[(1-0.47)\times 0.15\right]+0.47\right\}\times 100 \\
&= \left\{\left[0.53\times 0.15\right]+0.47\right\}\times 100 \\
&= \left\{0.0795+0.47\right\}\times 100 \\
&= 55\% \qquad (6)
\end{aligned}
$$

TEACHING POINT

While it is possible to estimate the LVEF via the Quinones method (and the Teichholz method), the preferred method for estimating the LVEF is via the 2D Simpson biplane method (biplane method of disks) or via 3D LV volumes.

13. Answer: C. Paradoxical IVS motion is identified as diastolic flattening of the IVS and a rounded contour in systole with motion toward the RV. Systolic thickening of the IVS still occurs. Paradoxical IVS motion is associated with conditions in which there is RV volume overload.

Answer A is not correct. When there is normal IVS motion, the IVS moves anteriorly as the LV fills during diastole and following the onset of systole, the IVS moves rapidly posteriorly (**Figure 7-25A**). This is not seen in this case where the IVS moves posteriorly in diastole and anteriorly in systole. Answer B is not correct. A diastolic shudder or septal bounce is a characteristic feature of constrictive pericarditis. In this instance, there is a brisk septal shudder due to rapid filling in early diastole (**Figure 7-25B**). A septal shudder is not demonstrated in the M-mode trace provided. Answer D is not correct. When there is a left bundle branch block (LBBB) or RV pacing, there is a prominent downward (posterior) motion of the IVS in early systole (a septal "beak"), followed by a gradual anterior motion of the IVS toward the

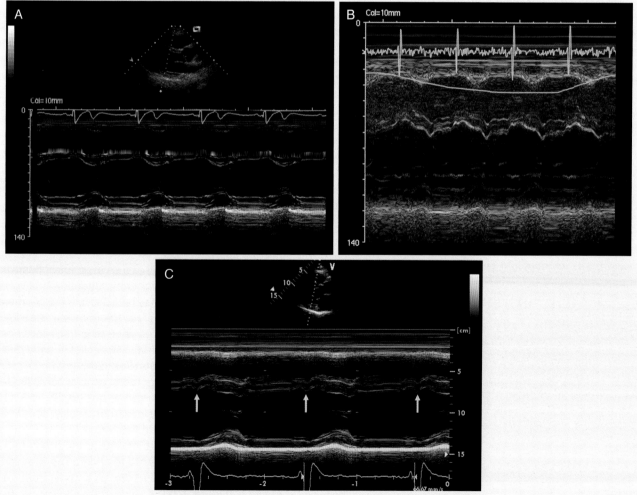

Figure 7-25 A, Normal IVS motion. B, Diastolic shudder of the IVS seen in a case of constrictive pericarditis. C, Abnormal motion of the IVS with LBBB with an early systolic downward (posterior) motion of the IVS (arrows).

RV during systole, and then an exaggerated early diastolic dip (**Figure 7-25C**).

After open heart surgery, there is prominent translation of the heart that can give the appearance of paradoxical septal motion.

14. **Answer: B.** The M-mode shows a classic example of early mitral valve closure, which is pathognomonic of acute severe aortic regurgitation (AR). There is also LV dilation and a generous E point-septal separation. Early closure of the mitral valve is caused by the rapid rise of LV diastolic pressure to equal left atrial pressure. Answer D is not correct, as the murmur will not be holodiastolic since there is rapid equilibration of the LV and aortic diastolic pressures. Patients with acute severe AR are likely to have evidence of elevated LV filling pressure and rales. Rales are abnormal lung sounds characterized by discontinuous crackling or rattling sounds; they have been compared to cellophane being crumbled.

Answer A is not correct since an opening snap is heard in patients with rheumatic mitral stenosis with pliable leaflets. This is not the echocardiogram of such a patient. Answer C is not correct as an apical systolic murmur implies the presence of mitral regurgitation and there is no suggestion that this patient has coexisting mitral regurgitation.

15. **Answer: D.** Findings are consistent with WPW syndrome. The pertinent finding on the M-mode trace (**Figure 7-26**) is an inward movement of the posterior wall (solid white arrow) prior to thickening of the IVS (dotted white arrow). This occurs because of preexcitation of the left posterior lateral wall prior to excitation of the IVS due to a left posterolateral accessory pathway of WPW. On physical examination with a left-sided pathway, there is early closure of the aortic valve and therefore persistent splitting of the second heart sound. In contrast, with a right-sided accessory pathway, there is early closure of the pulmonary valve, which results in paradoxical splitting of the second heart sound.

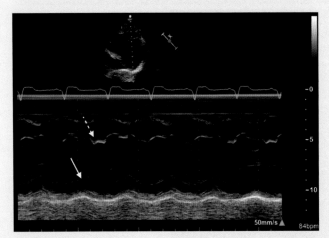

Figure 7-26

Answer A is not correct as the IVS motion is clearly abnormal. Answer B is not correct since with a LBBB, there is an initial posterior displacement of the septum, followed by a gradual anterior displacement during ventricular ejection; during ejection the posterior wall moves anteriorly as well. Answer C is not correct as RBBB causes no specific abnormalities of IVS motion.

16. **Answer: C.** This M-mode was recorded from a parasternal view at the level of the mitral valve leaflet tips. The anterior and posterior leaflets move away from each other as the valve opens in diastole in a mirrored pattern. The E point indicates early diastolic filling. The D-E distance or D-E amplitude marks the maximum anterior motion of the mitral valve in the beginning of ventricular diastole. The slope between the E and F points indicates rapid early ventricular filling with the normal E-F slope ranging from 70 to 150 mm/s. This slope is prolonged when there is mitral stenosis. The A-C line represents the period of time between atrial contraction (A) and the final closure position of the mitral valve (C point). On the mitral valve M-mode trace, a prolonged A-C slope (or the presence of a b-bump or atrial shoulder) is consistent with elevated LV end-diastolic pressure.

17. **Answer: A.** The classic M-mode findings of mitral stenosis include a reduced mitral valve E-F slope, thickened anterior and posterior leaflets, anterior motion of the posterior leaflet (due to commissural fusion and "pulling" of the posterior by the larger anterior leaflet), bright echoes indicating leaflet calcification, a reduced D-E leaflet excursion, and a diminished or absent A wave. These features are seen on **Figure 7-13**.

Answer B is not correct. Although a myxomatous mitral valve may display thickened leaflets, the D-E excursion and E-F slope would likely be within normal range and the posterior mitral valve leaflet would not move anteriorly during systole. If there is coexistent leaflet prolapse, systolic posterior displacement or dipping of the mitral valve leaflets may be seen.

Answer C is not correct as a LA myxoma appears as a mass of echoes posterior to the anterior mitral valve leaflet. When the myxoma prolapses into the LA, there is a slight time delay before the myxoma is sucked toward the LV. This appears as an echo-free space posterior to the anterior mitral valve leaflet in early diastole; this is not displayed on this trace. Answer D is not correct. In cases of severe mitral annular calcification, the anterior leaflet excursion is not usually reduced and the posterior leaflet does not display abnormal anterior motion as seen in this trace.

18. **Answer: C.** In this M-mode trace, there is a large echo-free space posterior to the heart. The descending aorta (DA) is noted at the LA-LV posterior wall junction (**Figure 7-27**). A pericardial effusion would

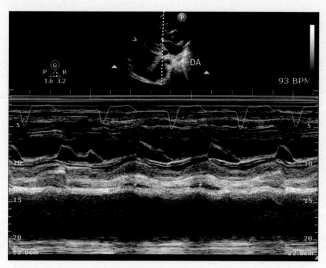

Figure 7-27

lie above (anterior to) the DA, and an echo-free space below (posterior) the DA is consistent with fluid in the left pleural cavity. The small echo-free space noted in this image in systole (the * in **Figure 7-27**) is not pericardial effusion. A close inspection of the 2D image above the M-mode trace reveals that the M-mode cursor is cutting across the DA. A pericardial space seen only in systole represents normal pericardial fluid. A true trivial-to-small pericardial effusion (<100 mL) seen posteriorly would appear as an echo-free space in systole and diastole <1 cm in size. Furthermore, a pericardial effusion will taper at the atrioventricular (AV) grove, while a pleural effusion will appear posterior to the AV groove and the LA. A pericardial effusion does not change with respiration, while a pleural effusion may.

19. **Answer: B.** This M-mode trace of the pulmonic valve acquired from the parasternal short axis view shows classic features associated with severe pulmonary hypertension (**Figure 7-28**). This includes midsystolic notching or "flying W sign" (gold arrow) and diminished "a wave" (blue arrow). The "a-wave"

on the pulmonary valve M-mode trace reflects atrial contraction. Normally, with atrial contraction, there is a small increase in the RV end-diastolic pressure (RVEDP), which pushes on the pulmonary valve to create this "a-wave." However, when there is pulmonary hypertension, the PA diastolic pressures are elevated, so atrial contraction has little or no impact on the pulmonary valve motion. Midsystolic notching on the pulmonary valve M-mode is a fairly specific finding of severe pulmonary hypertension and usually elevated pulmonary vascular resistance. Answer A is not correct. In severe pulmonic stenosis, the "a-wave" is preserved and often exaggerated. Answer C is not correct since the "flying W" sign is not usually present in acute pulmonary embolism as pulmonary artery pressures do not usually exceed 50 mm Hg. Answer D is not correct as this trace shows midsystolic notching and an absent "a-wave," which are not normal features of a normal pulmonary valve M-mode trace.

20. **Answer: A.** This gentleman has chronic, severe idiopathic pulmonary arterial hypertension. His RV end-diastolic diameter measures >5.0 cm based on the vertical depth markers at the right of the trace. A prominent moderator band is commonly seen in chronic conditions of RV pressure overload, creating the thick band of echoes seen above the IVS (see **Figure 7-16B**). Although there is slightly prolonged mitral valve closure (A-C slope), the tricuspid and mitral valves otherwise appear normal.

Answer B is not correct since the LV in these images is not dilated (<5.0 cm in diameter based on the vertical depth markers at the right of the trace).

Answer C is not correct. In Ebstein anomaly, it is common to record both the mitral and tricuspid leaflets with M-mode from the parasternal views. In this anomaly, the tricuspid valve will display exaggerated motion and late closure (**Figure 7-29A**). A mitral-to-tricuspid valve closure time difference >30 ms is highly suggestive of Ebstein anomaly. In this patient, the mitral and tricuspid valves close almost simultaneously at the QRS (**Figure 7-29B**).

21. **Answer: B.** This M-mode trace demonstrates a "b-bump" on the mitral valve (**Figure 7-30**, arrow) which has also been referred to as the "a-c shoulder." This finding is consistent with an elevated LVEDP. There is also increased mitral E point-septal separation (EPSS), which is measured as the distance between the most posterior point of the IVS during systole and the E point of the anterior mitral valve leaflet in the same cardiac cycle. This finding is consistent with a decreased stroke volume and impaired LV systolic function.

Answer A is not correct since it cannot be concluded from this trace alone that there is a marked elevation in LVFP. LVFP includes LVEDP and mean LA pressure (mLAP). It is important to note that LVEDP

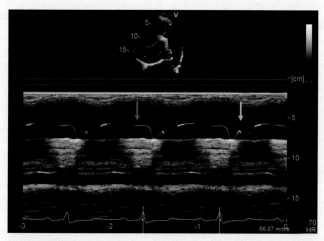

Figure 7-28

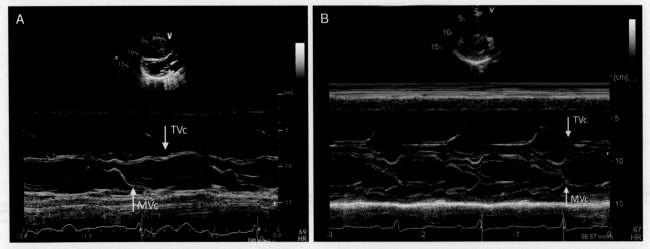

Figure 7-29 A, Ebstein anomaly. Observe that tricuspid valve closure (TVc) is much later than mitral valve closure (MVc). B, In Figure 7-16A, mitral valve closure (MVc) and tricuspid valve closure (TVc) occur almost simultaneously.

and mLAP are not the same. For example, when the LVEDP is elevated, the mLAP may be normal or elevated.

Answer C is not correct. While mitral valve prolapse (MVP) with regurgitation could account for the dyspnea and the systolic murmur, in **Figure 7-17**, the mitral valve closes normally with no posterior displacement of the leaflets in systole.

Answer D is not correct. Based on the vertical depth markers to the left of the trace, the LV measures approximately 6 cm. However, with acute aortic regurgitation, the LV would not be dilated. In addition, there is no diastolic fluttering of the anterior mitral leaflet, which can be seen with aortic regurgitation.

22. **Answer: D.** Although a dilated LV may exist in a low cardiac output state, a dilated LV alone does not indicate low cardiac output. For example, a dilated LV as seen in chronic, severe aortic regurgitation often demonstrates hyperdynamic function and normal cardiac output.

Tapered closure of the aortic valve (answer A) and a decreased aortic root amplitude (answer D)

are clues to a reduced cardiac output (**Figure 7-31A**). With a reduced cardiac output, decreased motion of the aortic root during systole occurs due to decreased pulmonary venous return into the LA (or a decreased stroke volume) while tapered closure of the valve during systole occurs due to an inability of the LV to maintain constant flow through the valve over the

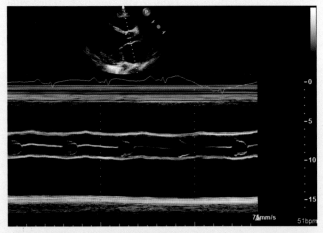

Figure 7-31A

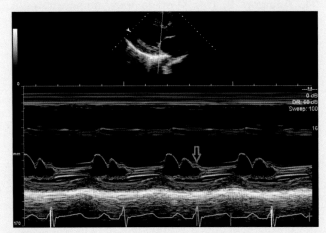

Figure 7-30

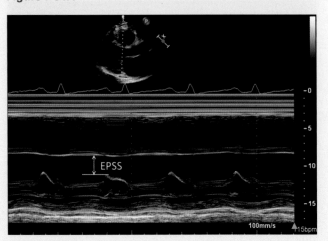

Figure 7-31B

systolic period. An increased mitral E point-septal separation (answer C) is a sign of a reduced cardiac output (**Figure 7-31B**). The mitral E point-septal separation (EPSS) is measured as the distance between the most posterior point of the IVS during systole and the E point of the anterior mitral valve leaflet in the same cardiac cycle. A normal EPSS is ≤ 5.5 mm. When there is a reduced cardiac output, the EPSS increases due to an anterior displacement of the IVS as the LV dilates, and reduced opening of the mitral valve because of decreased transmitral flow into the LV.

Acknowledgments: The authors thank and acknowledge the contributions from Gerard P. Aurigemma, MD, and Dennis A. Tighe, MD (Chapter 3, M-mode) in *Clinical Echocardiography Review: A Self-Assessment Tool,* 2nd Edition, edited by Allan L. Klein, Craig R. Asher, 2017.

SUGGESTED READINGS

Anderson B. *Echocardiography: The Normal Examination and Echocardiographic Measurements.* 3rd ed. Brisbane: Echotext Pty Ltd; 2017:chaps 4 and 10.

Feigenbaum H. Role of M-mode technique in today's echocardiography. *J Am Soc Echocardiogr.* 2010;23:240-257.

Kerut EK. The mitral L-wave: a relatively common but ignored useful finding. *Echocardiography.* 2008;25(2):548-550.

La CS, Han L, Oh JK, Yang H, Ling LH. The mitral annular middiastolic velocity curve: functional correlates and clinical significance in patients with left ventricular hypertrophy. *J Am Soc Echocardiogr.* 2008;21(2):165-170.

Lang RM, Badano LP, Mor-Avi V, et al. Recommendations for cardiac chamber quantification by echocardiography in adults: an update from the American society echocardiography and the European association of cardiovascular imaging. *J Am Soc Echocardiogr.* 2015;28:1-39.

Reynolds T. *The Echocardiographer's Pocket Reference.* 2nd ed. Phoenix: Arizona Heart Institute; 2000.

Spectral Doppler Examination

Contributors: Sally J. Miller, BS, RDCS, RT(R) and Natalie F. A. Edwards, M Cardiac Ultrasound, B Ex Sci, ACS

✪ Question 1

On a pulsed-wave (PW) Doppler spectral display, what is demonstrated on the horizontal axis?
   A. The pulse's time of flight to and from the reflector
   B. The velocity of the interrogated blood flow
   C. The depth of the produced reflection
   D. The timing and duration of the blood flow

✪✪ Question 2

A transthoracic echocardiogram is performed on a 48-year-old male with hypertrophic obstructive cardiomyopathy (HOCM). By two-dimensional (2D) imaging, significant systolic anterior motion (SAM) of the anterior mitral valve leaflet (AMVL) is identified. A pulsed-wave (PW) Doppler waveform is obtained by placing the sample volume near the area of greatest contact between the AMVL and the basal interventricular septum in the apical 4-chamber view. What information might be obtained from this Doppler trace?
   A. An accurate measurement of the peak velocity of the obstructive blood flow
   B. Identification of multiple obstructive areas within the left ventricle (LV)
   C. Confirmation of obstructive flow in the location of the sample volume
   D. An accurate measurement of stroke volume

✪✪✪ Question 3

Due to the patient's large body habitus, the pulsed-wave (PW) Doppler sample volume for mitral inflow interrogation is located at a depth of 15 cm. The peak mitral E

wave velocity is 1.5 m/s which results in aliasing of the signal. Adjustment of the transducer frequency is one method that can be employed to avoid aliasing and to resolve higher velocities. Which of the following statements regarding changing the transducer frequency to avoid aliasing is correct?
   A. Decreasing the transducer frequency decreases the Doppler frequency shift.
   B. Decreasing the transducer frequency increases the Nyquist limit.
   C. Increasing the transducer frequency decreases the Doppler frequency shift.
   D. Increasing the transducer frequency increases the Nyquist limit.
   E. None of the above

✪ Question 4

Which of the following statements is TRUE regarding the use of high pulse repetition frequency (PRF)?
   A. High PRF uses multiple sample volumes to obtain high velocities without aliasing, while eliminating the advantage of range resolution.
   B. High PRF places a single sample volume at the deepest possible depth in the field of view in an attempt to detect all velocities within the path of the beam.
   C. High PRF uses multiple sample volumes with range ambiguity, when attempting to interrogate very low blood flow velocities at shallow depths.
   D. High PRF is synonymous with continuous-wave (CW) Doppler.

✪ Question 5

Which of the following statements best describes what is being displayed in the Doppler image below (**Figure 8-1**)?

A. The velocity of blood flow prior to leaving the left ventricle (LV)

B. The velocity of blood flow after passing through the aortic valve

C. All velocities of blood flow from the apex of the LV to the aorta

D. All velocities of blood flow from the apex of the LV to the left atrium (LA)

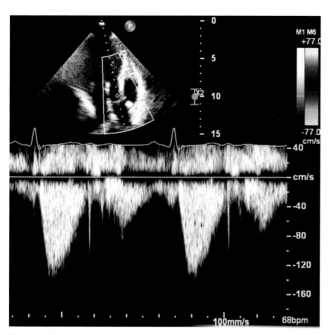

Figure 8-1

✪✪ Question 6

Which of the following statements is true regarding tissue Doppler imaging (TDI) when compared to conventional pulsed-wave (PW) Doppler?

A. The optimal TDI setting will display lower-velocity Doppler shifts to demonstrate the slow motion of tissue, rather than the higher velocities of blood flow.

B. The optimal TDI setting will display higher-velocity Doppler shifts to demonstrate the vigorous motion of the tissue, rather than the lower velocities of blood flow.

C. The optimal TDI setting will demonstrate both tissue motion velocities as well as blood flow velocities.

D. The optimal TDI setting would be the same setting used for conventional PW Doppler to interrogate blood flow.

✪✪ Question 7

Which of the following incident angles will result in the most accurate Doppler frequency shift?

A. 20°

B. 60°

C. 90°

D. 180°

✪ Question 8

Applying the simplified Bernoulli equation to the peak velocity of a continuous-wave (CW) Doppler trace of the aortic valve outflow will permit the measurement of:

A. Left ventricular (LV) stroke volume.

B. LV systolic pressure.

C. Aortic transvalvular mean pressure gradient.

D. Aortic transvalvular maximum instantaneous pressure gradient.

✪✪ Question 9

Which of the sample volume placements shown below in **Figures 8-2A** to **8-2D** would result in the optimal transmitral inflow pulsed-wave (PW) Doppler trace for the measurement of the peak E and A velocities in the evaluation of diastolic function?

A. Figure 8-2A

B. Figure 8-2B

C. Figure 8-2C

D. Figure 8-2D

✪✪ Question 10

The pulmonary venous pulsed-wave (PW) Doppler waveform shown in **Figure 8-3A** was obtained as part of a left ventricular diastolic function assessment. The sonographer was unsatisfied with the results and moved the sample volume, resulting in a more optimal Doppler trace as shown in **Figure 8-3B**. Which of the following images, shown in **Figures 8-4A** to **8-4D**, most likely demonstrates the new location of the sample volume?

A. Figure 8-4A

B. Figure 8-4B

C. Figure 8-4C

D. Figure 8-4D

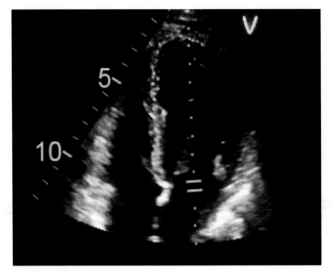

Figure 8-2A

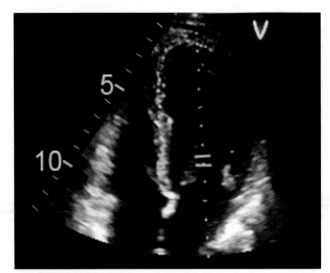

Figure 8-2B

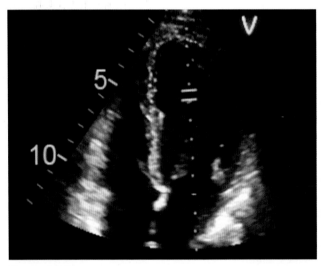

Figure 8-2C

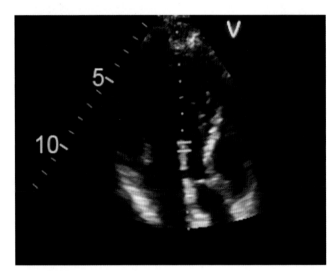

Figure 8-2D

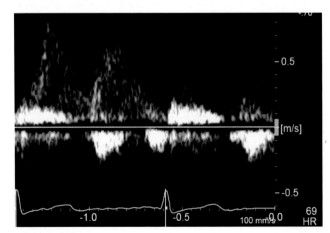

Figure 8-3A

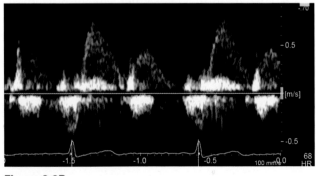

Figure 8-3B

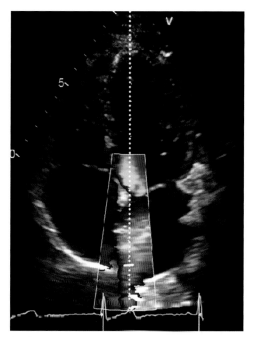

Figure 8-4A

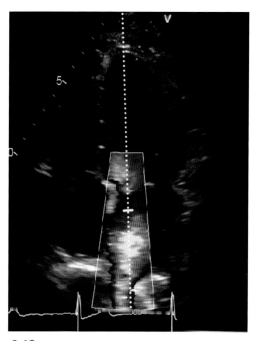

Figure 8-4C

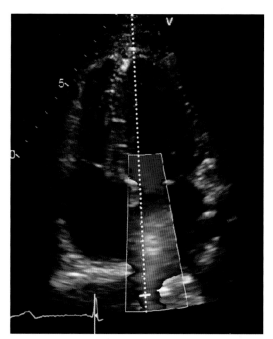

Figure 8-4B

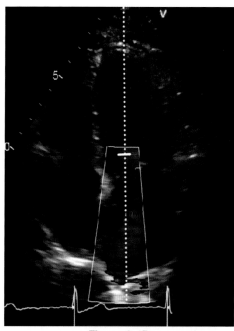

Figure 8-4D

✪ Question 11

Which of the following statements best describes the appropriate sample volume placement to obtain accurate tissue Doppler imaging (TDI) traces of the lateral tricuspid valve annulus?

A. A 5 to 10 mm sample volume is placed at the tricuspid valve annulus or slightly into the basal right ventricular (RV) myocardium in the apical 4-chamber view, aligned parallel with the motion of the tricuspid annulus.

B. A 5 to 10 mm sample volume is placed at the tricuspid valve annulus or slightly into the right atrial (RA) wall in the apical 4-chamber view, aligned parallel with the motion of the tricuspid annulus.

C. A 1 to 3 mm sample volume is placed near the tricuspid valve leaflets in the apical 4-chamber view, aligned parallel to the tricuspid inflow.

D. A 1 to 3 mm sample volume is placed in the tricuspid valve annulus from any imaging view as alignment is not as important for tissue velocity measurements as it is for blood flow.

✪ Question 12

What part of the cardiac cycle is being measured in the pulsed-wave (PW) Doppler trace shown in **Figure 8-5**?

A. Transmitral inflow early diastolic filling time
B. Left ventricular (LV) ejection time
C. Isovolumic relaxation time
D. Isovolumic contraction time

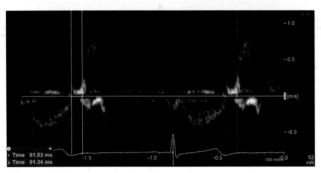

Figure 8-5

✪✪ Question 13

The pulsed-wave Doppler waveforms displayed in **Figure 8-6** were obtained from the right supraclavicular imaging window to interrogate the flow of the superior vena cava (SVC) in a 21-year-old female with normal cardiac pressures. The Doppler trace indicated by the arrow demonstrates:

A. Antegrade flow into the right atrium (RA) during the period of time the tricuspid valve is open.
B. Antegrade flow into the left atrium (LA) occurring as a result of left ventricular systole.
C. Antegrade flow into the RA occurring as a result of RA relaxation.
D. Retrograde flow from the RA to the SVC as a result of RA contraction.

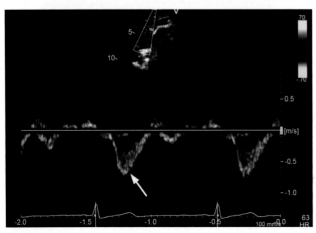

Figure 8-6

✪ Question 14

Which of the following pulsed-wave (PW) Doppler traces of the left ventricular outflow tract (LVOT) shown in the figures below (**Figures 8-7A** to **8-7D**) was most likely obtained using the recommended sample volume placement?

A. Figure 8-7A
B. Figure 8-7B
C. Figure 8-7C
D. Figure 8-7D

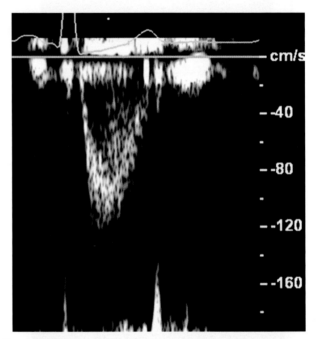

Figure 8-7A

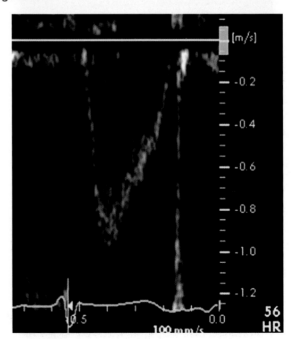

Figure 8-7B

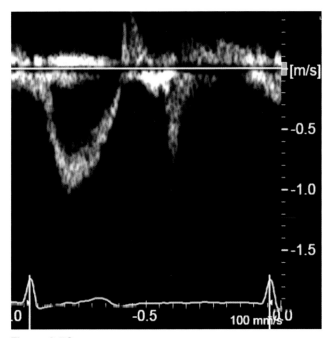

Figure 8-7C

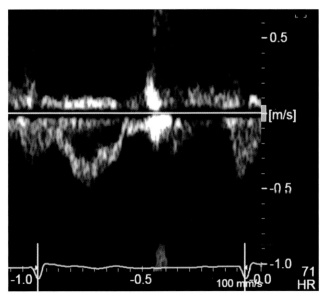

Figure 8-7D

C. The flow shown during diastasis is normal forward flow continuing from the left atrium (LA) to the left ventricle (LV) following early rapid filling due to inertia.

D. The flow shown during diastasis is referred to as the "L-wave" and represents prolonged relaxation of the left ventricle, resulting in an LA-LV pressure gradient continuing into middiastole.

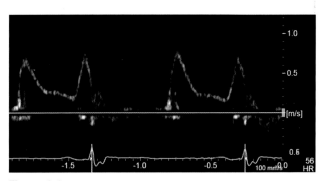

Figure 8-8

✪✪✪ Question 15

What is the significance of the flow during diastasis, which is demonstrated in **Figure 8-8**?

A. The flow shown during diastasis is referred to as a "J-wave" and represents blood being directed toward the left ventricular outflow tract (LVOT) during atrial contraction.

B. The flow shown during diastasis is referred to as the "B-bump" and represents elevated left ventricular end diastolic pressure due to high left atrial pressure causing a delayed closure of the mitral valve.

✪ Question 16

Which of the following best describes the recommended acquisition of a pulsed-wave (PW) Doppler waveform of the right ventricular outflow tract (RVOT)?

A. A 1 to 2 mm sample volume is placed approximately 2 cm proximal to the pulmonary valve.

B. A 1 to 2 mm sample volume is placed 0.5 to 1 cm distal to the pulmonary valve.

C. A 4 to 5 mm sample volume is placed approximately 2 cm distal to the pulmonary valve.

D. A 4 to 5 mm sample volume is placed 0.5 to 1 cm proximal to the pulmonary valve.

✪✪ Question 17

A transthoracic echocardiogram is ordered on a 39-year-old male for palpitations and a midsystolic click. He was found to have anterior leaflet mitral valve prolapse with moderate mitral regurgitation (MR). With regard to acquisition of a continuous-wave (CW) Doppler waveform of this patient's mitral regurgitation, the CW Doppler signal will most likely align best from:

A. The apical 4-chamber view and be most dense in mid-to-late systole.

B. An off-axis imaging window and be most dense in mid-to-late systole.

C. The apical 4-chamber view and be most dense in early systole.

D. The parasternal short-axis view and be most dense in mid-to-late diastole.

✪✪ Question 18

The pulsed-wave (PW) Doppler waveform of the abdominal aorta shown in **Figure 8-9** is a(n):

- **A.** Normal abdominal aortic tracing of a healthy 18-year-old female patient.
- **B.** Abnormal abdominal aortic tracing of a 72-year-old male with severe aortic stenosis.
- **C.** Abnormal abdominal aortic tracing of a 35-year-old female with severe coarctation of the aorta.
- **D.** Abnormal abdominal aortic tracing of a 48-year-old male with severe aortic regurgitation.

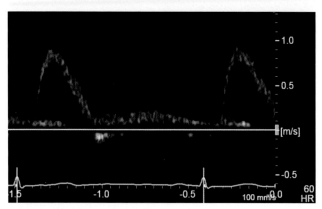

Figure 8-9

✪✪✪ Question 19

▶ A transthoracic echocardiogram was ordered for a 67-year-old female with shortness of breath. She has a history of breast cancer and has previously received radiation to the chest. The image in **Video 8-1** and Doppler spectra in **Figure 8-10** were obtained. Which of the following best describes the echocardiographic findings?

- **A.** Confirmation of constrictive pericarditis
- **B.** Restrictive cardiomyopathy with restrictive physiology
- **C.** Translational motion resulting in indeterminate interpretation
- **D.** Chronic obstructive pulmonary disease (COPD)

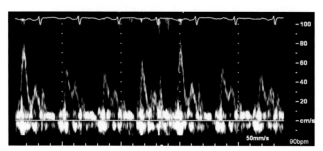

Figure 8-10

✪ Question 20

When obtaining a pulsed-wave (PW) Doppler tracing of laminar blood flow, the optimal Doppler tracing should demonstrate a narrow spectral band that represents the modal velocity. The modal velocity of a PW Doppler tracing:

- **A.** Is the highest velocity of blood flow, represented by the peak velocity.
- **B.** Represents the low-level velocities that are primarily affected by tissue motion.
- **C.** Is the densest part of the Doppler waveform, representing the velocity of the majority of the red blood cells within the sample volume.
- **D.** Is the faintly filled-in center of the Doppler waveform, representing the range of velocities within the sample volume.

✪✪ Question 21

The continuous-wave (CW) Doppler waveforms of pulmonary regurgitation (PR) in **Figures 8-11A** and **8-11B** were obtained on a 28-year-old female patient. Color Doppler imaging revealed only mild PR. Which of the following statements best describes the findings of the PR CW Doppler spectra?

- **A.** **Figure 8-11B** demonstrates a higher end-diastolic velocity than **Figure 8-11A**, indicating the Doppler cursor was more parallel to flow in **Figure 8-11A**.
- **B.** **Figures 8-11A** and **8-11B** demonstrate severe PR, suggesting the color Doppler imaging assessment was inaccurate.
- **C.** **Figures 8-11A** and **8-11B** contradict each other and do not demonstrate the same pressure gradients and severity of regurgitation.
- **D.** The variations in **Figures 8-11A** and **8-11B** are expected in the assessment of PR.

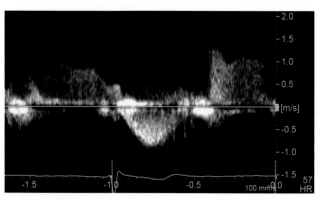

Figure 8-11A

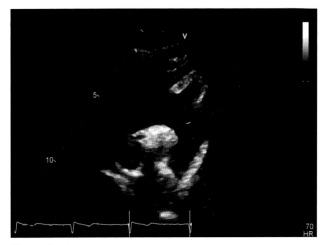

Figure 8-11B

⭐⭐ Question 23

A 19-year-old male was found to have a bicuspid aortic valve during a transthoracic echocardiogram. What error is occurring in the continuous-wave (CW) Doppler interrogation from the suprasternal notch image demonstrated in **Figure 8-13**?

    A. A CW Doppler signal from the suprasternal notch in the setting of a bicuspid aortic valve would be unnecessary.

    B. The CW Doppler cursor should be moved to align with the descending thoracic aorta.

    C. The CW Doppler cursor should be moved to align with right pulmonary artery.

    D. There is no error occurring with the CW Doppler placement in this view.

⭐ Question 22

Figure 8-12 demonstrates a tissue Doppler imaging (TDI) trace acquired at the mitral valve lateral annulus. What is represented by the arrow?

    A. Movement of the mitral annulus away from the apex during early diastole

    B. Movement of the mitral annulus toward the apex during early diastole

    C. Movement of the mitral annulus away from the apex during atrial contraction

    D. Movement of the mitral annulus toward the apex during systole

Figure 8-13

⭐ Question 24

A 68-year-old male was referred for echocardiography prior to undergoing coronary artery bypass grafting. The corresponding mitral inflow pulsed-wave (PW) Doppler waveform and tissue Doppler imaging (TDI) traces from the septal and lateral mitral annulus are displayed in **Figures 8-14A** to **8-14C**. From these data, the calculated E/A and average E/e′ ratio are:

    A. E / A = 0.8; E / e′ = 6.5.

    B. E / A = 1.25; E / e′ = 0.61.

    C. E / A = 0.8; E / e′ = 6.2.

    D. E / A = 1.25; E / e′ = 5.7.

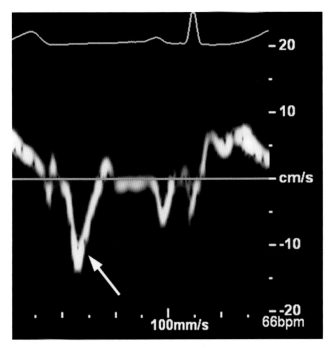

Figure 8-12

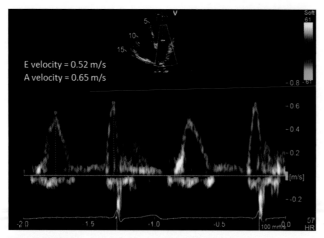

Figure 8-14A

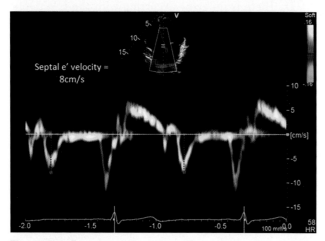

Figure 8-14B

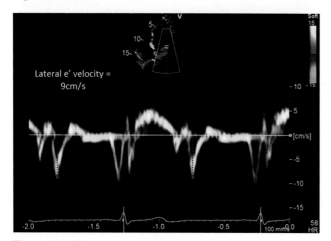

Figure 8-14C

✪✪✪ Question 25

▶ An 83-year-old male patient with a history of coronary artery bypass was referred for assessment of aortic stenosis. The patient's body surface area was 1.66 m², heart rate was 75 bpm, and the blood pressure was 102/60 mm Hg during the echocardiogram. The left ventricle was severely dilated (left ventricular end-diastolic volume index = 132 mL/m²) with poor systolic function (ejection fraction = 15%).

The 2D appearances of the aortic valve were consistent with severe aortic stenosis (**Video 8-2**); however, the Doppler findings were consistent with moderate aortic stenosis. From the data provided (**Figures 8-15A** and **8-15B**), the calculated stroke volume index confirming low flow, low gradient severe aortic stenosis is:

A. 27 mL/m².
B. 13 mL/m².
C. 35 mL/m².
D. 16 mL/m².

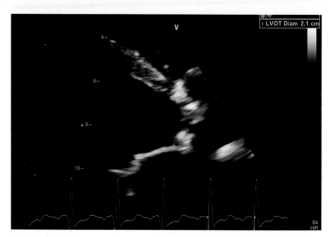

Figure 8-15A

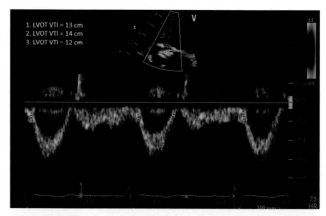

Figure 8-15B

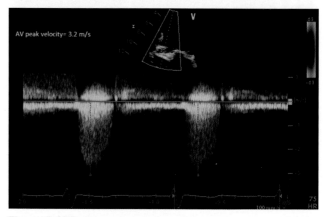

Figure 8-15C

✪ Question 26

A 26-year-old male patient with a history of tetralogy of Fallot repair and subsequent surgical pulmonary valvotomy presented for yearly review. The right ventricle was severely dilated with preserved systolic function, and there was no residual pulmonary stenosis (peak velocity through the valve of 1.3 m/s and mean gradient of 4 mm Hg). The septal tricuspid valve leaflet appeared mildly tethered resulting in a coaptation defect and subsequent grade 3/4 tricuspid regurgitation (TR). From the corresponding images (**Figures 8-16A** and **8-16B**), the calculated right ventricular systolic pressure (RVSP) is:

A. 21 mm Hg.
B. 38 mm Hg.
C. 26 mm Hg.
D. 31 mm Hg.

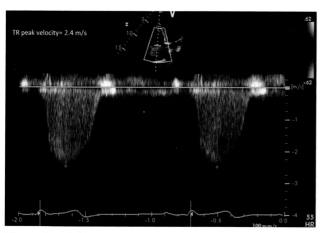

Figure 8-16A

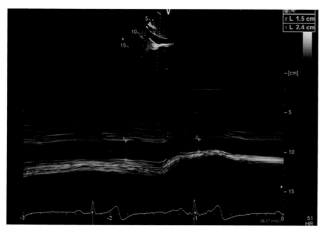

Figure 8-16B

✪✪ Question 27

A 57-year-old male was referred for assessment of left ventricular function following a recent coronary artery bypass graft. The patient had a history of a small membranous ventricular septal defect (VSD) with left to right shunting. The corresponding continuous-wave Doppler trace across the VSD is shown in **Figure 8-17**. The blood pressure was 150/76 mm Hg at the time of the echocardiographic study. Based on the data provided, the calculated right ventricular systolic pressure (RVSP) is:

A. 20 mm Hg.
B. 127 mm Hg.
C. 117 mm Hg.
D. 30 mm Hg.

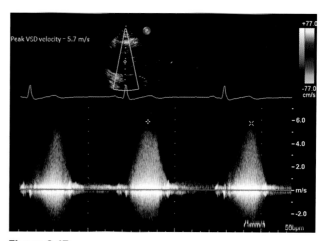

Figure 8-17

✪✪ Question 28

A 16-year-old female patient was referred for assessment of a dilated left ventricle (LV). The patient's blood pressure was 98/60 mm Hg with a heart rate of 60 bpm during the echocardiogram. On 2D imaging, the LV was severely dilated (LV end-diastolic volume index = 122 mL/m^2) with preserved systolic function. Color Doppler of the main pulmonary artery revealed a patent ductus arteriosus (PDA) with flow throughout the cardiac cycle (**Figure 8-18**). Based on the data provided, the calculated pulmonary artery systolic pressure (PASP) is:

A. 79 mm Hg.
B. 30 mm Hg.
C. 93 mm Hg.
D. 21 mm Hg.

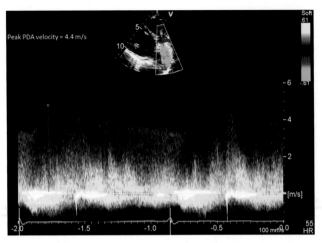

Figure 8-18

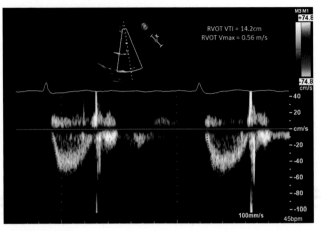

Figure 8-19B

✪✪ Question 29

A 73-year-old patient with a history of hemoptysis and long-standing hypertension was referred for echocardiography to assess for pulmonary hypertension. The right ventricle was moderately dilated with preserved systolic function and color Doppler revealed grade 3/4 tricuspid regurgitation (TR). The spectral Doppler traces of TR and from the right ventricular outflow tract (RVOT) are shown (**Figures 8-19A** and **8-19B**). The inferior vena cava was normal in size with less than 50% collapse as the patient sniffed. Based on the information provided, pulmonary vascular resistance (PVR) in Wood units (WU) is estimated at:

A. 4.8 WU.
B. 2.1 WU.
C. 4.0 WU.
D. 1.6 WU.

✪✪✪ Question 30

A 49-year-old male patient was referred for day 1 assessment post Amplatzer device occlusion of a patent ductus arteriosus (PDA). The left ventricle (LV) was severely dilated (indexed LV end-diastolic volume = 110 mL/m^2) with mildly reduced global systolic function (ejection fraction = 42%). From the images provided in **Figures 8-20A** and **8-20B**, the estimated myocardial performance index (MPI) for the LV is:

A. 0.30.
B. 0.43.
C. 3.3.
D. 2.30.

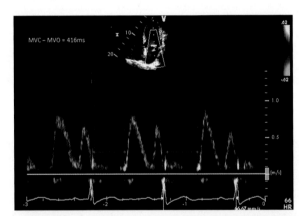

Figure 8-20A

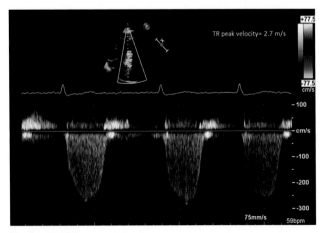

Figure 8-19A

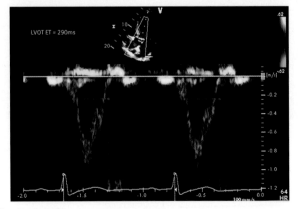

Figure 8-20B

✪ Question 31

Observe the tissue Doppler imaging (TDI) trace acquired from the right ventricle (RV) (**Figure 8-21**). Based on the information shown on this trace, the estimated myocardial performance index (MPI) for the RV is:

A. 0.51.
B. 0.02.
C. 0.64.
D. 1.57.

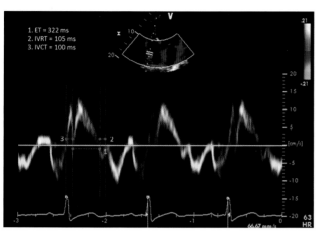

Figure 8-21

✪✪✪ Question 32

A 17-year-old male patient with a history of dilated cardiomyopathy presented for an echocardiogram. The left ventricle was severely dilated with severe systolic dysfunction and the right ventricle was severely dilated with moderate systolic dysfunction. From the corresponding pulsed-wave (PW) Doppler trace acquired from the right ventricular outflow tract (RVOT) (**Figure 8-22**), the estimated mean pulmonary artery pressure (mPAP) is:

A. 59 mm Hg.
B. 99 mm Hg.
C. 57 mm Hg.
D. Not accurate due to sinus tachycardia.

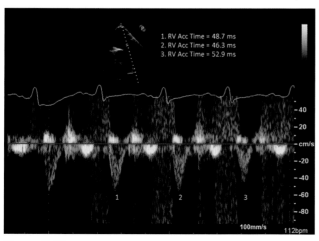

Figure 8-22

✪ Question 33

A 19-year-old male patient was referred for assessment of rheumatic aortic valve disease. In the corresponding pulsed-wave Doppler trace through the aortic valve (**Figure 8-23**), what is the spectral Doppler artifact represented by the arrows?

A. Beam width artifact
B. Range ambiguity artifact
C. Spectral aliasing artifact
D. Mirror artifact

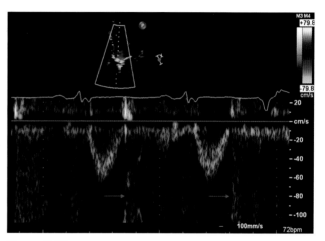

Figure 8-23

✪ Question 34

With reference to the artifact present in the previous question (**Figure 8-23**), which statement is correct with regards to how this phenomenon occurs?

A. The incident angle between the ultrasound beam and direction of blood flow is 90°, leading to flow signals both above and below the zero-velocity baseline.
B. The pulsed-wave Doppler sample volume is placed too close to the aortic valve.
C. The transducer frequency is too low for the velocity of the jet.
D. The velocity of the blood flow jet has exceeded one-half of the pulse repetition frequency.

✪✪ Question 35

With reference to **Figure 8-23** from the previous question, in order to avoid this type of artifact, the potential options are to:

- A. Use a lower transducer frequency, shift the zero-velocity baseline, decrease the sample volume depth, increase the number of sample volumes, and change from pulsed-wave (PW) to continuous-wave (CW) Doppler.
- B. Use a higher transducer frequency, decrease the spectral Doppler gain, increase the Doppler wall filter, shift the zero-velocity baseline, increase the sample volume depth, increase the number of sample volumes, and change from PW to CW Doppler.
- C. Use a higher transducer frequency, shift the zero-velocity baseline, increase the sample volume depth, increase the number of sample volumes, and change from PW to CW Doppler.
- D. Use a lower transducer frequency, decrease the spectral Doppler gain, decrease the Doppler wall filter, shift the zero-velocity baseline, increase the sample volume depth, increase the number of sample volumes, and change from PW to CW Doppler.

✪✪ Question 36

In the corresponding spectral Doppler profile of the pulmonary vein (**Figure 8-24**), what is the artifact that is present?

- A. Mirror artifact due to strong reflector
- B. Aliasing artifact
- C. Range ambiguity artifact
- D. "Cross-talk" mirror artifact

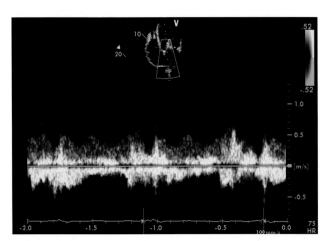

Figure 8-24

✪✪ Question 37

A 20-year-old male was referred for assessment of a possibly thrombosed mechanical mitral valve replacement (MVR). On 2D imaging, the posteromedial occluder failed to open normally due to thrombus formation; this resulted in a mean pressure gradient of 13 mm Hg and mitral valve area of 0.8 cm². In the corresponding spectral Doppler profile through the MVR, obtained from the apical 4-chamber view (**Figure 8-25**), the waveform below the zero-velocity baseline during diastole, represented by the arrow, is representative of:

- A. Significant mitral regurgitation.
- B. Spectral aliasing artifact.
- C. Mild aortic regurgitation.
- D. Mirror artifact.

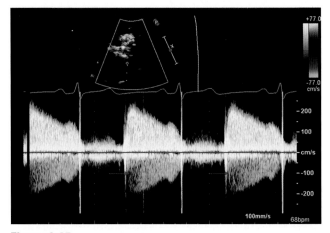

Figure 8-25

✪✪ Question 38

Isovolumic relaxation time (IVRT), the time interval from aortic valve closure to mitral valve opening, is used as an indicator of LV diastolic dysfunction. What type of spectral Doppler artifact is occurring and what ultrasound assumption is violated to enable this measurement?

- A. Beam width artifact; violated assumption is that all Doppler shifts are detected from within the central ultrasound beam.
- B. Slice thickness artifact; violated assumption is that all Doppler shifts are detected from within the central ultrasound beam.
- C. Mirror artifact; violated assumption is that all Doppler shifts arise from anatomical real structures only.
- D. Refraction artifact; violated assumption is that all Doppler shifts arise from anatomical real structures only.

ANSWERS

1. **Answer: D.** The horizontal axis of the PW Doppler spectral display demonstrates the timing and duration of the blood flow. The duration of a blood flow velocity waveform can be measured on the horizontal axis, and when paired with an electrocardiogram (ECG) recording, the timing of the blood flow in relation to the cardiac cycle can be identified.

   Answers A and C are not correct. The pulse's time of flight to and from the reflector determines the depth from which the produced reflection originates. The depth is not directly displayed on the PW Doppler spectral display; however, by use of the sample volume placement, range gating is used with PW Doppler to allow only the information from a specific depth to be displayed within the spectral display. Answer B is not correct. The velocity of the blood flow is displayed on the vertical axis.

TEACHING POINTS

The PW Doppler spectral display relies on information received from the sample volume. The location of the sample volume is chosen by the sonographer, and the ultrasound system will only process the information received by the transducer for a limited period of time and another signal will not be emitted until the transducer has received signals returning from the sample volume location. The time delay from the transmit pulse to the sampling of the echo signal is determined from the range equation:

$$T = (2 \times D) \div c$$

where T = time (s), D = sample volume depth, and c = propagation speed through soft tissue (1540 m/s).

The pulse repetition frequency (PRF), which is the number of pulses emitted per second, determines when the next signal is emitted. The information is then displayed demonstrating the velocities on the vertical axis and the timing and duration on the horizontal axis.

2. **Answer: C.** PW Doppler is capable of providing range resolution, which is the ability to know the exact depth at which the produced Doppler frequency shift was created. Obstructive flow will result in an increase in blood flow velocity. Recall that the maximum velocity that can be unambiguously detected and displayed by PW Doppler is limited by the sampling rate (or pulse repetition frequency [PRF]), and this is referred to as the Nyquist limit. Therefore, on a PW Doppler spectrum of obstructive flow due to HOCM, the velocity will most likely exceed the Nyquist limit, resulting in aliasing. While the peak velocity will not be able to be accurately obtained, the waveform will demonstrate increased flow velocity in the specific location of the sample volume. Also, in the setting of HOCM, the dynamic obstruction will result in a "dagger-shaped", late-peaking velocity waveform. Therefore, although the

full waveform may not be resolved, the late peak in velocity indicates dynamic outflow tract obstruction.

   Answer A is not correct. In the setting of HOCM with significant SAM, the peak velocity of the obstructive flow would most likely be higher than what is capable of being measured by PW Doppler (without the use of high PRF), as described earlier. Answer B is not correct. PW Doppler is capable of finding the location of multiple obstructions within the LV when the sample volume is placed in multiple different locations. However, a PW sample volume placed in only one location, as described above, will only obtain Doppler information from that specific location. Answer D is not correct. A PW Doppler waveform may be used in the calculation of stroke volume; however, velocities should be obtained from the same location at which the left ventricular outflow tract (LVOT) diameter was measured. Also, in the setting of LVOT obstruction, an accurate measurement of stroke volume cannot be obtained as blood flow is no longer laminar through the LVOT.

KEY POINTS

PW Doppler has the ability of "range gating," which is based on the range equation as previously described (see answer outline for Question 1).

The ultrasound system will only process information received during the period of time that correlates with the depth of the selected sample volume placement.

PW Doppler is also limited by the Nyquist limit, which is the maximum Doppler frequency shift (and, therefore, maximum velocity) that can be unambiguously displayed and measured by PW Doppler. The Nyquist limit (NL) is expressed as:

$$NL = PRF \div 2$$

where PRF = pulse repetition frequency.

If the velocity of the measured blood flow is producing a Doppler frequency shift exceeding this limit, the artifact of aliasing will be created rendering it impossible to accurately obtain the maximum velocity without the use of high PRF or continuous-wave Doppler.

NOTE: The Nyquist limit is not the maximum velocity, rather it determines the maximum velocity in combination with other factors.

3. **Answer: A.** As discussed previously (see answer outline for Question 2), the Nyquist limit is the maximum Doppler frequency shift that can be unambiguously displayed and measured by PW Doppler. Importantly, the Nyquist limit is not the maximum velocity; it determines the maximum velocity in combination with other factors. When this limit is exceeded, aliasing occurs. It therefore determines the maximum velocity that can be displayed unambiguously. The Nyquist limit (NL) is one-half of the sampling rate or pulse repetition frequency (PRF):

$$NL = PRF \div 2 \qquad (1)$$

The PRF is determined by the sample volume depth. For example, the greater the sample volume depth, the lower the PRF and the lower the Nyquist limit. Importantly, the Nyquist limit is not directly affected by the transducer frequency, and therefore, answers B and D are incorrect.

The Doppler frequency shift is the difference between the received frequency and the transmitted (transducer) frequency. The Doppler frequency shift (Δf) is expressed by the Doppler equation:

$$\pm\Delta f = \left(2 \times f_t \times V \times \cos\theta\right) \div c \qquad (2)$$

where 2 = double Doppler shift, f_t = transmitted frequency, V = velocity of blood flow, θ = intercept angle between the ultrasound beam and blood flow, and c = propagation speed through soft tissue.

To avoid aliasing of the signal, the Doppler frequency shift needs to be less than the Nyquist limit. It can be appreciated from equation (2) that if all other variables remain constant and the transmitted frequency (f_t) is decreased, the resultant Δf will decrease. Therefore, answer A is correct. This concept can be further explained by considering the Practical Example below.

PRACTICAL EXAMPLE

Given a Nyquist limit of 5000 Hz, a peak velocity of 1.5 m/s, an incident angle of 0° (cos θ = 1), and a transducer frequency of 3.5 MHz, the Δf is calculated as:

$$\begin{aligned} \pm\Delta f &= \left(2 \times f_t \times V \times \cos\theta\right) \div c \\ &= (2 \times 3.5 \times 10^6 \times 1.5 \times 1) \div 1540 \\ &= 6818\,\text{Hz} \end{aligned}$$

At this transducer frequency, the Δf exceeds the Nyquist limit of 5000 Hz. Therefore, a peak velocity of 1.5 m/s will not be unambiguously displayed (that is, aliasing will occur).

Using the same variables as above but with a transducer frequency of 2.5 MHz, the Δf is calculated as:

$$\begin{aligned} \pm\Delta f &= (2 \times 2.5 \times 10^6 \times 1.5 \times 1) \div 1540 \\ &= 4870\,\text{Hz} \end{aligned}$$

At this transducer frequency, the Δf is less than the Nyquist limit of 5000 Hz. Therefore, a peak velocity of 1.5 m/s can be unambiguously displayed (that is, aliasing is avoided).

NOTE: Baseline shift may also be employed to avoid aliasing. Moving the zero-velocity baseline up or down effectively increases the maximum velocity in one direction (toward or away flow) at the expense of the velocity in the other direction.

4. **Answer: A.** High PRF is used in an attempt to eliminate aliasing on the pulsed-wave (PW) Doppler trace when the Doppler frequency shift created by the blood flow velocity being interrogated exceeds the Nyquist limit. Recall that the Nyquist limit is equal to one-half the PRF and the PRF is determined by the sample volume depth. By using multiple sample volumes, the PRF is increased. The ultrasound system will determine the PRF from the shallowest depth, while still evaluating frequency shifts from the other sample volumes at deeper depths. By doing this, the frequency shift from deeper depths can be displayed without aliasing. However, by doing this, the advantage of range resolution will be lost; that is, the exact origin of the frequency shift is no longer known as all signals from all sample volumes return to the transducer at the same time and are, therefore, superimposed on top of one another.

Answer B is not correct. High PRF Doppler settings use multiple sample volumes at various depths. Answer C is not correct. Low blood flow velocities at shallow depths would be easily obtained by conventional settings of PW Doppler using a single sample volume. A shallow depth would result in a higher PRF giving a higher Nyquist limit. The higher the Nyquist limit, the less likely it is that aliasing will occur. When interrogating very low blood flow velocities, aliasing would be even less likely to exceed the higher Nyquist limit. Answer D is not correct. Although the use of high PRF settings are an alternative to CW Doppler as a way of obtaining higher velocity signals, these terms are not interchangeable. CW Doppler interrogates Doppler shifts along the entirety of the beam, whereas high PRF settings interrogate Doppler shifts from specific sample volume locations.

KEY POINTS

High PRF can be used to resolve blood flow velocities from PW Doppler when the sample volume is placed at a depth that results in a low PRF and a subsequent low Nyquist limit. The high PRF setting uses multiple sample volumes, resulting in an increase in the Nyquist limit. This will allow the display of blood flow velocities on the spectral Doppler waveform without aliasing; however, there will be range ambiguity similar to that which occurs with CW Doppler.

5. **Answer: C.** **Figure 8-1** demonstrates a continuous-wave (CW) Doppler waveform with the cursor aligned through the aortic valve. CW Doppler is not gated to a specific location, but rather displays all returning echo information from the entirety of the beam path. While the primary purpose of this alignment may be to demonstrate the blood flow across the aortic valve, the continuous nature of the CW Doppler will record Doppler shifts from the entire LV

as well as into the aorta. The advantage of CW Doppler is that the velocity of the displayed waveform is not limited by the Nyquist limit and high-velocity flow can be displayed accurately. Due to the fact CW Doppler is continuously sending and receiving ultrasound simultaneously by use of two separate crystals, the ultrasound system does not have to wait to receive a signal before sending another, as is necessary with PW Doppler. Therefore, the limitations of PW Doppler due to the pulse repetition frequency (PRF) and the Nyquist limit are irrelevant. The disadvantage, however, is that the exact location of the Doppler signal is unknown, as all Doppler frequency shifts along the beam path are being detected and displayed.

Answers A and B are not correct. Although the blood flow prior to leaving the LV and blood flow passing through the aorta are both being displayed within the Doppler waveform, this Doppler spectrum includes blood flow through the LV, valve, aorta, and anything else within the path of the beam. PW Doppler would be necessary to isolate blood flow from a specific location only.

Answer D is not correct. The alignment of the Doppler cursor is clearly shown from the LV apex through the aortic valve (in the apical long-axis view) and does not align with the LA.

KEY POINTS
CW Doppler utilizes two separate crystals, one to send the Doppler signal and one to receive. Because the sending and receiving can be done simultaneously, CW Doppler is not limited by PRF and is therefore capable of accurately displaying higher-velocity blood flow without aliasing. The disadvantage of CW Doppler is range ambiguity, meaning the exact location of the Doppler signal is unknown. It is important to realize the echoes constituting the CW Doppler signal could be a result of Doppler shifts throughout the entirety of the beam.

6. **Answer: A.** TDI, also known as Doppler tissue imaging (DTI), is a form of PW Doppler and has the advantage of range resolution, meaning the exact location of the Doppler shift can be identified. Both conventional PW Doppler and TDI can display received Doppler shifts from a moving target. Conventional PW Doppler is used to measure blood flow velocities, where TDI optimizes the PW Doppler settings to display the velocities of tissue motion. Two important differences between PW Doppler and TDI should be noted. First, blood flow velocities are usually much higher than tissue velocities. Although blood flow velocities within the venous system may be as low as 10 cm/s, normal arterial blood flow could be as high as 150 cm/s. Tissue motion is much slower than blood flow, with the typical velocities ranging from 1 to 20 cm/s. Secondly, as tissue is a much stronger reflector of the Doppler signal compared

with blood (approximately 40 dB higher than blood flow signals), the signal produced by tissue motion will typically have higher amplitudes (displayed as brightness) than blood flow. Therefore, proper optimization of the conventional PW Doppler waveform for blood flow involves filtering out the low-velocity, high-amplitude signals from valves and wall motion ("wall noise") by using a high-pass filter; the velocity scale is set to display higher velocities. Proper optimization for TDI involves optimizing the low-velocity signals by filtering out the high-velocity, low-amplitude signals created by the blood flow; this is achieved using a low-pass filter. The velocity scale is then set to display lower velocities, and the Doppler gain is also reduced to optimize these signals.

Answer B is not correct. TDI can be used to measure the motion of the annulus which often may be described as having vigorous motion; however, even if the annulus has vigorous motion with what would be considered a high velocity for tissue, it would still be a much lower velocity than what would result from blood flow. Answer C and D are not correct. Conventional PW Doppler and TDI are based on the same pulsed Doppler principle; however, the optimal setting for each would be different as discussed above.

KEY POINTS
Conventional PW Doppler and TDI are based on the same PW Doppler principle; however, the machine settings must be optimized differently.
▶ With conventional PW Doppler, the higher velocity, lower amplitude blood flow is optimized by setting the spectral Doppler velocity scale higher and by filtering out the low-velocity, high-amplitude signals from valves and wall motion (high-pass filter).
▶ With TDI, the lower velocity, higher amplitude tissue motion is optimized by decreasing the spectral Doppler velocity scale and by filtering out the high-velocity, low-amplitude signals created by the blood flow (low-pass filter).

Because these are both based on a Doppler principle, alignment is essential to ensure the accurate display of velocities. When using conventional PW Doppler, the alignment should be parallel with the blood flow, and when using TDI, the alignment should be parallel with the tissue motion.

7. **Answer: D.** The angle of incidence between the ultrasound beam and blood flow direction is one of the most common causes of significant error when obtaining a Doppler signal in both pulsed-wave and continuous-wave Doppler. To obtain the optimal angle of incidence the ultrasound beam should be aligned parallel to the blood flow being interrogated.

Based on the Doppler equation below, it can be appreciated that the incident angle between the ultrasound beam and blood flow direction may significantly affect the frequency shift (Δf):

$$\pm \Delta f = \left(2 \times f_t \times V \times \cos\theta\right) \div c$$

where 2 = double Doppler shift, f_t = transmitted frequency, V = velocity of blood flow, θ = intercept angle between the ultrasound beam and blood flow, and c = propagation speed through soft tissue.

For example, any angle of incidence other than parallel will result in an underestimation in velocity. If blood flow is moving parallel with the beam toward the transducer, the angle of incidence will be 0° resulting in a $\cos\theta$ of 1. If the blood flow is moving parallel with the beam away from the transducer, the angle of incidence will be 180° resulting in a $\cos\theta$ of −1. An angle of incidence of 0° will result in the most accurate positive Doppler shift, and an angle of incidence of 180° will result in the most accurate negative Doppler shift.

Answer A is not correct. Although an angle of incidence 20° or less is considered to be within a reasonable error (<6%) and will not make a significant impact on the calculated velocity, any angle other than parallel will result in an underestimation of blood flow velocity. Answer B is not correct. Based on the Doppler equation an angle of 60° will result in an error to the calculated velocity of 50%. Answer C is not correct. Based on the Doppler equation the cosine of a 90° angle is 0. This will result in a 100% error, and no Doppler shift will be detected.

KEY POINTS

An accurate velocity will only be calculated when the blood flow is parallel with the sound beam. An incident angle of 0° (blood flow parallel toward the transducer) or an incident angle of 180° (blood flow parallel away from the transducer) are the only incident angles that will not result in an error of underestimation. An incident angle of <20° will result in an error of <6% and is generally considered to be within a reasonable percentage of error as to not cause a significant underestimation of velocity. The further the incident angle is away from parallel, the larger the error will be. At a 90° angle of incidence, the Doppler shift will be undetected, causing a 100% error in velocity. The use of angle correction to account for the error in alignment, which may be applicable in vascular imaging, is not recommended in echocardiography.

8. **Answer: D.** The simplified Bernoulli equation is the equation used to convert a measured velocity (V) into a pressure gradient (ΔP):

$$\Delta P = 4V^2$$

When this equation is applied to only the peak velocity of a waveform, the maximum instantaneous pressure gradient will be calculated. The maximum instantaneous gradient of the CW Doppler trace of the aortic valve outflow represents the maximum instantaneous pressure difference between the LV and the aorta during systole (during LV ejection).

Answer A is not correct. The left ventricular outflow tract (LVOT) stroke volume (SV_{LVOT}) is derived from the LVOT cross-sectional area (CSA_{LVOT}) and the LVOT velocity time integral (VTI_{LVOT}):

$$SV_{LVOT} = CSA_{LVOT} \times VTI_{LVOT}$$

The CSA_{LVOT} is derived from the LVOT diameter measured in midsystole, and the VTI_{LVOT} is derived from the PW Doppler waveform acquired from the LVOT.

Answer B is not correct. The aortic valve peak velocity represents the pressure difference between the LV and the aorta during systole, not the LV systolic pressure. In the absence of aortic stenosis or LVOT obstruction, the LV systolic pressure will be equal to the systolic systemic blood pressure. Answer C is not correct. To calculate the aortic mean gradient, the CW Doppler waveform needs to be traced and the simplified Bernoulli equation is then applied to the peak velocity at equal time intervals throughout the entire waveform. The mean gradient is a representation of the average pressure difference between the two areas throughout the entire time period of the Doppler waveform (systole).

KEY POINTS

The simplified Bernoulli equation is used routinely in echocardiography to calculate a pressure gradient (ΔP) from a blood flow velocity (V):

$$\Delta P = 4V^2$$

When the simplified Bernoulli equation is applied to the peak Doppler-derived velocity, the maximum instantaneous gradient can be calculated. This represents the maximum change in pressure between two areas at a specific time point of the cardiac cycle. When the Doppler waveform is traced, the peak velocity at equal time intervals is measured. Applying the simplified Bernoulli equation to each of these velocities and then averaging the pressure gradients will calculate the mean pressure gradient, representing the average change in pressure between two areas during a specific timing of the cardiac cycle.

9. **Answer: B.** According to the American Society of Echocardiography (ASE) 2016 Recommendations for the Evaluation of Left Ventricular Diastolic Function by Echocardiography, the PW Doppler sample

volume for the acquisition of the mitral E and A waves should be 1 to 3 mm in size and placed between the mitral leaflet tips in the apical 4-chamber view. Color Doppler imaging is also recommended to assure proper alignment with transmitral inflow and obtain the most accurate velocity. The sample volume placement at the tips of the mitral valve leaflets will result in the highest E velocity of the mitral inflow waveform. A continuous-wave (CW) Doppler cursor directed through the mitral valve may assist in finding the highest E velocity, assuming no other high-peaking blood flow signals are within the path of the beam.

Answer A is not correct. Sample volume placement at the level of the annulus assesses the blood flow prior to going through the valve and will not yield accurate peak velocities of the mitral E and A waves. This sample volume placement is ideal for measuring the mitral annular velocity time integral for mitral annular stroke volume calculation. Sample volume placement toward the mitral annulus, but not at the annulus, is also recommended for the measurement of the mitral A duration. Answer C is not correct. The sample volume is placed too far toward the apex of the left ventricle (LV). A sample volume placed too far away from the mitral valve leaflet tips will result in lower velocities and may alter the profile of the Doppler signal. Answer D is not correct. The sample volume is placed between the mitral valve and aortic valve in the apical long-axis view. This would be the ideal sample volume placement for the measurement of isovolumic relaxation time. However, as the ultrasound beam is not aligned parallel to mitral inflow, it would not produce the most accurate velocity information.

TEACHING POINTS

When assessing diastolic function, peak mitral E and A wave velocities should be obtained by placing a 1 to 3 mm PW Doppler sample volume at the tips of the mitral valve leaflets in the apical 4-chamber view. Color Doppler imaging can help align the beam parallel to flow, particularly in the setting of LV dilation, where the inflow will be more laterally displaced. Doppler cursor alignment should always be parallel to flow to assure maximum velocities are obtained by eliminating the angle error. A CW Doppler cursor directed through the mitral valve may assist in finding the highest E velocity, assuming no other high-peaking blood flow signals are within the path of the beam.

10. **Answer: B.** The American Society of Echocardiography recommends that the sample volume be placed 1 to 2 cm into the right upper pulmonary vein in the apical 4-chamber view for optimal acquisition of velocity waveforms. The original spectral Doppler tracing (**Figure 8-3A**) demonstrated very little flow during atrial reversal. The high-amplitude (bright), low-flow velocities shown during atrial contraction are most likely due to wall motion (wall noise). However, it is important not to increase the low-velocity wall filter too much during acquisition as the atrial reversal flow is typically a very low velocity. By moving the sample volume into the pulmonary vein 1 to 2 cm, the flow from atrial reversal will be better detected.

Answer A is not correct. Although the sample volume is placed within the flow from the pulmonary veins, the sample volume is within the left atrium (LA). In this location the systolic and diastolic flows may be easily detected but this does not represent pulmonary venous flow and flow reversal with atrial contraction into the pulmonary vein is missed. Moving the sample volume to be located within the pulmonary vein will allow for detection of this flow. Answer C is not correct. The location of the sample volume is just proximal to the mitral valve. This location is too far away from the pulmonary vein to accurately represent flow from the pulmonary vein. Answer D is not correct. The location of the sample volume is distal to the mitral valve. This location would represent the pattern of flow moving through the mitral valve rather than from the pulmonary vein.

TEACHING POINTS

In the normal setting, blood flow from the pulmonary veins into the LA appears as antegrade flow during systole and early diastole, with retrograde flow occurring in late diastole as a result of atrial contraction. To optimally obtain all components of the Doppler signal, the PW Doppler sample volume should be placed 1 to 2 cm into the pulmonary vein. Color Doppler imaging is useful in visualizing the pulmonary venous flow for proper placement. In some pathological conditions, portions of the pulmonary venous flow could be absent or reversed from the normal profile (e.g., the absence of atrial reversal in the setting of atrial fibrillation, or reversal of systolic flow in the setting of severe mitral regurgitation). If the sample volume is not properly positioned, the pulmonary venous flow could be misinterpreted.

11. **Answer: A.** A larger sample volume size is beneficial when performing TDI to ensure that the annulus is covered during systole and diastole. TDI measurements represent systolic and diastolic properties of the ventricle and should be placed within the annulus and basal portion of the ventricle. Although this is a measurement of tissue motion rather than blood flow, Doppler is always angle dependent. In the case of TDI, it is the tissue motion to which the beam should be parallel.

Answer B is not correct. The sample volume should not be placed in the right atrium as this would not reflect the systolic and diastolic properties of the ventricle. Answers C and D are not correct. A small sample volume size is not recommended for tissue Doppler. The Doppler alignment is significant and needs to be parallel to annular motion, not blood flow.

KEY POINTS

TDI is a form of pulsed-wave Doppler and is therefore angle dependent. To obtain an accurate velocity, the TDI cursor must be in line with the motion of the tissue being interrogated. In some situations, this may result in additional angulation of the 2D image to align the Doppler cursor properly. Larger sample volumes sizes are used for TDI to ensure that the annulus is covered over systole and diastole.

12. **Answer: C.** The measurement is made along the horizontal axis of the PW Doppler spectral display, which corresponds with a measurement of time. In correlation with the electrocardiogram tracing at the bottom of the display, the measurement is being made during a time period immediately following the T wave, which represents ventricular repolarization. On the Doppler display, the measurement is being made from the end of the left ventricular outflow tract (LVOT) trace (aortic valve closure) to the beginning of the mitral inflow trace (mitral valve opening). After the aortic valve closes, the LV pressure decreases. When the LV pressure drops below left atrial pressure, the mitral valve will open. This period of time, where both the mitral and aortic valves are closed and there is a decrease in LV pressure without a change in LV volume, is referred to as isovolumic relaxation time (IVRT). The PW Doppler sample volume (or continuous-wave [CW] Doppler beam) must be positioned between the mitral and aortic valves from the apical long-axis or apical 5-chamber views, so that the flow through each valve can be superimposed on a single spectral Doppler display.

Answer A is not correct. The mitral inflow early diastolic filling time is represented by the E wave on the mitral inflow spectral Doppler display. Early filling begins with the opening of the mitral valve and ends with the equalization of pressures during diastasis. This is represented by the positive waveform (above the zero-velocity baseline) in early diastole on the spectral display.

Answer B is not correct. LV ejection time occurs from the time the aortic valve opens until the aortic valve closes. This period of time is represented by the negative waveform (below the baseline) during systole on the spectral display. Answer D is not correct. Isovolumic contraction time (IVCT) is the period of time between mitral valve closure and aortic valve opening. During this period of time, the LV pressure is increasing without a change in LV volume. On the spectral Doppler display this time is represented by the end of the A wave of the mitral inflow Doppler waveform until the beginning of the LVOT Doppler trace.

TEACHING POINTS

The IVRT is the period of time between aortic valve closure and mitral valve opening. During this time interval, both the aortic and mitral valves are closed, and LV pressure is decreasing without a change in LV volume. To obtain this Doppler signal for measurement, both the aortic outflow and mitral inflow velocity waveforms must be displayed simultaneously. To do this, the PW Doppler sample volume (or the CW Doppler beam) must be positioned between the flow of both valves using either the apical long-axis or apical 5-chamber view. An accurate measurement of velocity cannot be made from this location as the cursor is likely not parallel to either flow, but an accurate timing can be captured and measured.

13. **Answer: C.** From the right supraclavicular imaging window, the normal flow in the SVC is moving away from the transducer toward the RA during systole and diastole and is therefore, represented as a negative waveform (below the zero-velocity baseline) on the spectral display. With atrial contraction, flow is directed toward the transducer and is therefore, represented as a positive waveform (above the baseline) on the spectral display. In correlation with the electrocardiogram (ECG) tracing, the flow indicated by the arrow is occurring during ventricular systole. This timing occurs immediately following atrial contraction, so in the normal setting the atria would be relaxing, allowing blood to easily flow forward into the RA.

Answer A is not correct. Antegrade flow into the RA during the period of time the tricuspid valve is open would occur during ventricular diastole, which occurs after the T wave on the ECG. In the normal setting, this diastolic flow would also appear below the baseline on the spectral Doppler display. In **Figure 8-6**, this flow is shown immediately following the flow indicated by the arrow. Answer B is not correct. In the normal setting, blood flow from the SVC would not be connected to the LA. Answer D is not correct. Retrograde flow into the SVC as a result of atrial contraction occurs following the P wave on the ECG and is represented as flow above the baseline on the spectral Doppler display.

14. **Answer: B.** The LVOT PW Doppler waveform should be obtained from the apical 5-chamber or apical long-axis view, aligned parallel with flow. The sample volume should be placed approximately 0.5 cm proximal to the aortic valve in the center of the LVOT. The signal should display a thin spectral band with a distinct closing click at the end of flow. If the sample volume is placed too close to the valve, as in

Figure 8-7A, there will be spectral broadening of the waveform as well as an opening click at the beginning of systolic flow. If the sample volume is placed too far from the valve, as in **Figure 8-7C**, there will not be an opening or closing click and the velocity will most likely be reduced. **Figure 8-7D** is not correct as this signal demonstrates flow from the LVOT as well as transmitral inflow, indicating the sample volume was located between the mitral and aortic valves, and is not parallel to either flow.

15. **Answer: D.** Diastasis refers to the period of diastole after early rapid filling, prior to atrial contraction. As the heart rate increases, diastasis shortens. In the presence of a first-degree atrioventricular block, diastasis can be eliminated, fusing the mitral E and A waves. The spectral Doppler waveform in **Figure 8-8** demonstrates an abnormally high velocity of flow during diastasis. During diastasis, the left atrial and left ventricular pressures are equalizing, and there should be only low-velocity flow, if any, moving across the valve prior to atrial contraction. In the setting of prolonged relaxation of the LV into middiastole plus an elevated left atrial pressure, a resultant pressure gradient from the LA to the LV continuing into middiastole will be present. While this flow may be present with bradycardia, a flow velocity greater than 0.2 m/s should be considered significant and is referred to as the "L-wave."

Answer A is not correct. The "J-wave" is a spectral Doppler finding of the LVOT signal and occurs in late diastole rather than during diastasis. The "J-wave" will appear as presystolic flow in the LVOT as a result of a strong atrial contraction pushing blood into the LV and toward the LVOT. Answer B is not correct. The "B-bump" is an M-mode finding that occurs during late diastole, demonstrating an additional opening motion of the mitral valve following the opening from atrial contraction due to high left atrial pressure. A "B-bump" on M-mode is representative of elevated left ventricular end-diastolic pressure (LVEDP). Answer C is not correct. It is not unusual to see very low-velocity flow during diastasis, particularly in the setting of a slow heart rate. After early rapid filling, there may be some very low-velocity forward flow across the mitral valve simply due to inertia; however, the flow should have a velocity of less than 0.2 m/s.

16. **Answer: D.** As recommended by the American Society of Echocardiography (ASE), a 4 to 5 mm sample volume should be placed 0.5 to 1 cm proximal to the pulmonary valve within the RVOT. The Doppler alignment should be parallel to flow, resulting in a thin spectral band with a closing click. If a closing click is not present, the sample volume should be moved slightly closer to the valve.

Answer A is not correct as the sample volume is too small and placed too far from the valve. Answers B and C are not correct. The sample volume should be placed proximal to the pulmonary valve, within the RVOT, not distal to the valve.

TEACHING POINTS

The PW Doppler waveform of the RVOT can be obtained from the parasternal short-axis view at the level of the aorta, or from the parasternal long-axis view of the RVOT. The ASE recommends a sample volume size of 4 to 5 mm placed 0.5 to 1 cm proximal to the pulmonary valve in the center of the RVOT. The waveform should display a thin spectral band and usually includes a closing click. The PW Doppler RVOT trace can be used for multiple measurements of right heart hemodynamics and needs to be optimized for accurate measurements and calculations.

17. **Answer: B.** In the setting of anterior leaflet mitral valve prolapse (MVP), the MR jet will be posteriorly directed. The eccentric direction of the regurgitant jet will lead to difficult parallel alignment to flow; therefore, an off-axis imaging window is usually necessary to ensure parallel alignment to the eccentric jet. In the setting of MVP, the mitral valve initially closes at end diastole and remains closed during early systole. The valve then prolapses back into the left atrium during mid-to-late systole. The MR is usually not holosystolic, but rather begins when prolapse occurs in midsystole. Therefore, the CW Doppler waveform will show essentially no flow during early systole with an abrupt start to the flow at midsystole, as demonstrated in Figure 8-26, occasionally demonstrating a click on the Doppler signal

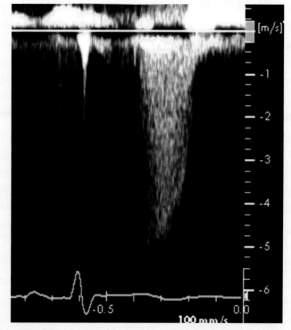

Figure 8-26

when the prolapse begins. The Doppler spectrum will be most dense in mid-to-late systole.

Answers A and C are not correct. The apical 4-chamber view will primarily be used in the setting of MR due to bileaflet prolapse or malcoaptation secondary to annular dilation where a centrally directed MR jet is most likely. The regurgitant flow of MVP will not be present in early systole.

Answer D is not correct. The parasternal short-axis view of the mitral valve is ideal for detecting the location, timing, and number of jets in the setting of MR; however, parallel Doppler alignment may be difficult. Also, the flow of MR would not be occurring during diastole.

18. **Answer: A.** This PW Doppler tracing demonstrates normal flow in the abdominal aorta from a healthy young patient. The velocity waveform obtained from the abdominal aorta should have a steep acceleration slope following the QRS complex with a slightly flatter deceleration slope ending near the T wave. It is common to also see very low-velocity flow throughout diastole just above the zero-velocity baseline.

Answer B is not correct. In the setting of severe aortic stenosis, the abdominal aortic velocity waveform will have a slow, delayed acceleration slope demonstrating parvus tardus downstream from the stenosis. Answer C is not correct. In the setting of coarctation of the aorta, the abdominal aortic velocity trace will demonstrate a continued pressure gradient throughout systole and diastole, with continued forward flow throughout diastole. Answer D is not correct. In the setting of severe aortic regurgitation, holodiastolic flow reversal may occur and can be demonstrated in the descending thoracic aorta as well as the abdominal aorta. If holodiastolic flow reversal is present in the abdominal aorta, this is consistent with severe aortic regurgitation.

19. **Answer: C.** The mitral inflow Doppler signal displayed in **Figure 8-10** demonstrates what appears to be respiratory variation similar to what would be expected in the setting of constrictive pericarditis. However, when viewing the apical 4-chamber view in **Video 8-1**, it is clear that there is extreme translational cardiac motion due to respiration. With each breath, the patient's heart is moving enough to result in the sample volume placement being in a significantly different position throughout the acquisition. Sample volume placement is extremely important when interrogating the transmitral inflow. Changing the location of the sample volume can result in different E-wave velocities as well as changing the overall profile of the waveform. In the assessment of constrictive pericarditis, it is necessary to have the patient breathing throughout the acquisition to assess for respiratory variation; however, the breathing should be shallow. When the translational motion of the heart is extreme enough to cause this much variation in the sample volume placement, the displayed information may not be interpretable to confirm constrictive pericarditis.

Answer A is not correct. The patient history is suspicious for the presence of constrictive pericarditis; however, with the extreme translational motion of the heart, constrictive pericarditis would not be able to be confirmed. Other parameters would need to be taken into consideration, as the assessment of constrictive pericarditis should include multiple parameters and not rely on transmitral inflow alone.

Answers B and D are not correct. Although the appearance of the Doppler signal could be suggestive of either of these options, again with the extreme translational motion due to the patient's breathing, other parameters would need to be interrogated.

20. **Answer: C.** When obtaining a PW Doppler signal, the blood flow is sampled from one particular location. If the blood flow is laminar, the majority of the red blood cells within that sample volume will be traveling at approximately the same velocity. The denseness of the Doppler signal corresponds with the quantity of red blood cells. A PW Doppler signal of laminar flow should demonstrate a thin dense line of velocities (narrow spectral band) with an open center to the tracing (spectral window). The dense line represents the modal velocity. Within the blood flow, there will be higher and lower velocities; however, the signal will be optimized to eliminate these and accentuate the velocities representing the majority of the flow. If the spectral window within the modal velocity of the waveform appears to be filled in, the blood flow might not be laminar, or the waveform has not been optimized to eliminate weaker signals.

KEY POINTS

The modal velocity of a PW Doppler tracing is represented by a thin bright line of velocities (narrow spectral band) representing the velocity of the majority of red blood cells within the flow being interrogated. Proper optimization of a PW Doppler signal may include increasing reject to eliminate weaker signals and/or increasing output power to improve the signal-to-noise ratio. However, it is important to be aware that an increase in output power will also increase patient exposure. In accordance with the ALARA principle, exposure should be kept **A**s **L**ow **A**s **R**easonably **A**chievable.

21. **Answer: D.** Both waveforms are consistent with mild PR based on the fainter density of the signal, as well as the plateau of velocity throughout diastole, indicating a slow equalization of pressure.

There are only slight variations in these two PR CW Doppler profiles, one of those being the difference in end-diastolic velocity, which is due to respiratory variation. It is common to see respiratory variation in Doppler signals on the right side of the heart. As blood returns to the heart from outside of the thoracic cavity, the decrease of intrathoracic pressure upon inspiration increases the pressure gradient and venous return to the heart. Therefore, the slight variations of these two waveforms are most likely due to normal respiratory variation rather than technical factors of Doppler acquisition. Respiratory changes would not be expected to be observed on the left side of the heart in the normal setting due to the flow originating within the intra-thoracic cavity and the same pressure changes in the chambers receiving the blood flow. However, the normal expectations of respiratory variation or luck of variation will be altered in certain pathological settings.

Answer A is not correct. If this were an error in Doppler alignment, the Doppler signal that is more parallel to flow would demonstrate the higher velocity. Answer B is not correct. In the setting of severe PR, the CW Doppler signal would be denser, representing a larger volume of regurgitant flow, and the pressure half-time would be very short, representing the rapid equalization of pressures. Early termination of the PR signal may also be seen with severe PR and very high RV end-diastolic pressures. Answer C is not correct. Even though the gradient represented by the CW Doppler spectra varies slightly, these waveforms are both consistent with mild PR.

22. **Answer: A.** TDI of the mitral valve lateral annulus demonstrates the motion of the annulus throughout the cardiac cycle. During diastole the mitral annulus will move away from the apex in two parts: early diastole and during atrial contraction. During systole the annulus will move toward the apex with contraction of the ventricle. The proper acquisition of the TDI traces is from an apical 4-chamber view aligned with the motion of the annulus. With the transducer being located near the apex, movement away from the apex (during diastole) will be displayed below the zero-velocity baseline, and movement toward the apex (during systole) will be above the baseline.

23. **Answer: B.** In the setting of a bicuspid aortic valve (BAV), coarctation of the aorta should be excluded as there is strong association of coarctation and bicuspid aortic valves (approximately 50% of cases of coarctation of the aorta will also have a BAV). Coarctation of the aorta most commonly occurs in the location of the aortic isthmus; the portion of the aorta distal to the left subclavian artery and proximal to the ligamentum arteriosum. The alignment of the

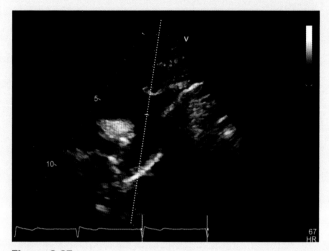

Figure 8-27

CW Doppler cursor in **Figure 8-13** will not accurately assess the portion of the aorta where the obstruction of blood flow from the coarctation would most likely occur. The 2D image and Doppler alignment should be adjusted to interrogate the flow going toward the distal portion of the descending aorta as shown in **Figure 8-27**.

24. **Answer: C.** The E/A ratio is calculated using the following equation:

$$E/A = E\,velocity \div A\,velocity \qquad (1)$$

From the data provided, the E/A ratio is:

$$E/A = 0.52 \div 0.65 = 0.8 \qquad (2)$$

The mitral valve (MV) E- (peak modal velocity in early diastole after the T wave on the electrocardiogram [ECG]) and A wave (peak modal velocity in late diastole after the P wave on the ECG) velocities are obtained from an apical 4-chamber view with the PW Doppler sample volume (1-3 mm) placed between the mitral valve leaflet tips. The mitral inflow *E/A* ratio in conjunction with the deceleration time of the mitral E wave are used to identify normal or abnormal diastolic filling patterns.

The E/e′ ratio is calculated using the following equation:

$$E/e' = E\,velocity \div e'\,velocity \qquad (3)$$

The mitral E velocity is 0.52 m/s or 52 cm/s. The E/e′ at the septal annulus is:

$$E/e' = 52 \div 8 = 6.5 \qquad (4)$$

The E/e′ at the lateral annulus is:

$$E/e' = 52 \div 9 = 5.8 \qquad (5)$$

Therefore, the average E/e′ ratio is:

$$E/e' = (6.5 + 5.8) \div 2 = 6.2 \qquad (6)$$

The MV E velocity is obtained and measured as above. The e′ velocity is obtained using TDI from the apical 4-chamber view with a sample volume size of 5 to 10 mm. Both septal and lateral aspects of the annulus are interrogated so an average E/e′ can be calculated. The E/e′ ratio can be used to predict LV filling pressures. An average E/e′ ratio <8 usually indicates normal LV filling pressures, whereas an average E/e′ >14 has high specificity for increased LV filling pressures. The E/e′ ratio is not accurate in patients with heavy mitral annular calcification, mitral valve and/or pericardial diseases.

25. **Answer: A.** The stroke volume index (SVi) is calculated using the following equation:

$$SVi = SV \div BSA \qquad (1)$$

where SV = stroke volume through the left ventricular outflow tract (LVOT) and BSA = body surface area.

The stroke volume is calculated as:

$$SV = CSA_{LVOT} \times VTI_{LVOT} \qquad (2)$$

where $CSA_{LVOT} = (0.785 \times LVOT\ diameter^2)$ and VTI_{LVOT} = velocity time integral across the LVOT.

Based on the data provided, the SVi is:

$$SVi = \left[(0.785 \times 2.1^2) \times 13\right] \div 1.66 = 27 mL/m^2 \qquad (3)$$

A stroke volume index <35 mL/m² confirms a low flow state.

26. **Answer: B.** Estimation of RVSP from the TR velocity waveform is performed using the following equation:

$$RVSP = 4 V_{TR^2} + RAP \qquad (1)$$

where RVSP = right ventricular systolic pressure (mm Hg); V_{TR} = peak systolic TR velocity (m/s); RAP = right atrial pressure (mm Hg).

The peak velocity of TR reflects the systolic pressure difference between the right ventricle and right atrium. If the RAP is estimated, then it is possible to calculate the RVSP. RAP may be estimated from the inferior vena cava (IVC) size and collapsibility index (IVCCI):

$$IVCCI = \left[(IVC_{max} - IVC_{min}) \div IVC_{max}\right] \times 100 \qquad (2)$$

In this example, the IVC measures 2.4 and 1.5 cm when the patient sniffs. Therefore, the IVCCI is derived as:

$$IVCCI = \left[(2.4 - 1.5) \div 2.4\right] \times 100 = 38\% \qquad (3)$$

Therefore, because the IVC is dilated (>2.1 cm) and collapses <50%, the RAP is estimated to be 15 mm Hg. Therefore, with a peak TR velocity of 2.4 m/s, the resultant RVSP is estimated as:

$$RVSP = (4 \times 2.4^2) + 15 = 23 + 15 = 38 mmHg \qquad (4)$$

Note: The RVSP will be slightly higher than the pulmonary artery systolic pressure (PASP), as there is mild pulmonary stenosis.

27. **Answer: A.** The RVSP can be estimated in the presence of a VSD. The peak systolic velocity across this defect is used to estimate the pressure difference between the left and right ventricles during systole. If the LV systolic pressure is known (assumed to be equal to the systolic blood pressure [SBP] in the absence of LVOT obstruction or aortic stenosis), the RVSP can be calculated using the following formula:

$$RVSP = SBP - 4V_{VSD^2} \qquad (1)$$

In this example, the RVSP is estimated as:

$$RVSP = 150 - (4 \times 5.7^2) = 150 - 130 = 20 mmHg \qquad (2)$$

28. **Answer: D.** The PASP can be estimated from a continuous-wave Doppler waveform obtained through a PDA and from the estimation of the systolic blood pressure (SBP). In the presence of a PDA, a continuous pressure gradient usually exists between the aorta and pulmonary artery. The systolic component of the PDA reflects the systolic pressure gradient between the aorta and pulmonary artery. If the systolic aortic pressure is known (assumed to be equal to the SBP in the absence of coarctation of the aorta), the PASP can be estimated using the equation:

$$PASP = SBP - 4V_{PDA^2} \qquad (1)$$

In this example, the peak systolic velocity of the PDA jet is measured at 4.4 m/s (with a pressure gradient between the descending aorta and pulmonary artery in systole of 77 mm Hg). Therefore, assuming the SBP is 98 mmHg, the estimated PASP is calculated as:

$$PASP = 98 - (4 \times 4.4^2) = 98 - 77 = 21 mmHg \qquad (2)$$

29. **Answer: B.** A commonly used formula for calculating PVR, expressed in Wood units (WU), from spectral Doppler is:

$$PVR = V_{TR} \div VTI_{RVOT} \times 10 + 0.16 \qquad (1)$$

Based on the data provided for this case, PVR is estimated as:

$$PVR = 2.7 \div 14.2 \times 10 + 0.16 = 2.1\,WU \qquad (2)$$

The peak RVOT velocity and the estimated right atrial pressure (from the size and collapsibility of the IVC) are not required for calculation of the PVR. A normal PVR value is <1.5 WU. The hemodynamic definition of pulmonary arterial hypertension is a mean pulmonary artery pressure >25 mm Hg at rest with a pulmonary capillary wedge pressure, left atrial pressure or left ventricular end-diastolic pressure ≤ 15 mm Hg, and a PVR >3 WU.

30. **Answer: B.** The MPI reflects global myocardial performance and incorporates elements of both diastole and systole. This index is useful in the assessment of conditions where systolic and diastolic dysfunction coexist. The formula for calculation is:

$$MPI = (IVRT + IVCT) \div ET \qquad (1)$$

where IVCT = isovolumic contraction time; IVRT = isovolumic relaxation time; ET = ejection time.

Using spectral Doppler, the MPI for the left heart is measured from the transmitral inflow profile as the time interval between two mitral inflow waveforms or as the duration of the mitral regurgitant waveform. Ejection time is measured from the beginning to the end of the left ventricular outflow tract (LVOT) velocity waveform. The IVCT is the time interval between mitral valve closure and aortic valve opening and the IVRT is the time interval between aortic valve closure and mitral valve opening. The time interval between mitral valve closure and mitral valve opening (MVc-MVo) is equivalent to IVRT + ET + IVCT (**Figure 8-28**); therefore, MVC-MVo minus ET is equal to IVRT + IVCT:

$$MPI = ([MVc - MVo] - ET) \div ET \qquad (2)$$

In this case the MPI, is calculated as:

$$MPI = (416 - 290) \div 290 = 0.43 \qquad (3)$$

For the left heart, a normal MPI derived via the pulsed-wave Doppler method as above is <0.4.

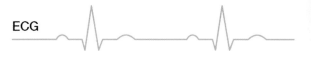

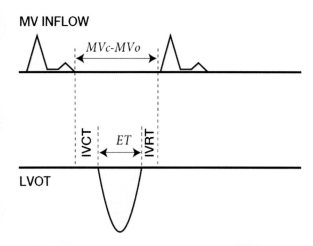

ECG

MV INFLOW

MVc-MVo

IVCT

ET

IVRT

LVOT

Figure 8-28 (Adapted with permission by Echotext Pty Ltd, from Anderson B. Doppler assessment of ventricular systolic function. In: *Echocardiography: The Normal Examination and Echocardiographic Measurements.* 3rd ed. Australia: Echotext Pty Ltd; 2017:285, chap 14.)

31. **Answer: C.** As previously described, the formula for calculating the MPI is:

$$MPI = (IVRT + IVCT) \div ET \qquad (1)$$

where IVCT = isovolumic contraction time; IVRT = isovolumic relaxation time; ET = ejection time

From the TDI trace, IVCT is the time interval between the end of the a′ velocity and the onset of the s′ velocity, the ejection time is the duration of the s′ velocity, and the IVRT is the time interval between the end of the s′ velocity and the onset of the next e′ velocity. Therefore, in this case, the RV MPI is derived as:

$$MPI = (105 + 100) \div 322 = 0.64 \qquad (2)$$

It is important to note that measurement of the MPI derived by the TDI method provides a measurement at one site of the ventricle only. Therefore, this regional MPI may not reflect the overall ventricular function. Furthermore, as the systolic intervals are longer and diastolic intervals are shorter via TDI, the normal values are slightly higher than those obtained via the pulsed-wave (PW) Doppler method. A normal RV MPI obtained by the PW Doppler method is ≤0.44 and obtained by the TDI method is ≤0.55.

32. **Answer: A.** The right ventricular acceleration time (RVAT) has been found to correlate with the mean pulmonary artery pressure (mPAP). The RVAT is the

time interval from the onset of flow to peak systolic flow. When pulmonary artery pressure and pulmonary vascular resistance are high the peak will occur earlier, shortening the RVAT. In severe pulmonary hypertension, there may be a midsystolic notch in the outflow signal, also reflecting a high afterload. The RVAT is measured using PW Doppler with the sample volume placed within the RVOT. An RVAT greater than 120 ms is associated with normal pulmonary artery pressures, while less than 100 ms is highly suggestive of pulmonary hypertension. When the patient has a heart rate between 60 and 100 bpm, the mPAP can be calculated using the formula:

$$mPAP = 79 - (0.45 \times RVAT) \qquad (1)$$

When the RVAT is 120 ms or less, an alternative formula should be used:

$$mPAP = 90 - (0.62 \times RVAT) \qquad (2)$$

Therefore, in this case, the mPAP is estimated as:

$$mPAP = 90 - (0.62 \times 49.5) = 59 \, mmHg \qquad (3)$$

Answer D is not correct. While heart rates outside of the normal range (<60 or >100 bpm) may reduce the accuracy of estimating the mPAP by this technique, when the mPAP exceeds 25 mm Hg, RVAT is accurate even in tachycardia (Parasuraman et al., 2016).

33. **Answer: C.** This is an example of a spectral Doppler aliasing artifact, which is the most common artifact seen in Doppler ultrasound. This patient has grade 2/4 aortic regurgitation (AR). During diastole, an ambiguous Doppler signal is displayed both above and below the zero-velocity baseline. Since AR is directed toward the transducer from the apical window, this signal should be displayed above the baseline. However, as the velocity has exceeded the Nyquist limit, this velocity has "wrapped around" and is displayed ambiguously both above and below the baseline.

34. **Answer: D.** Spectral Doppler aliasing occurs when the Nyquist limit has been exceeded, resulting in a "wrap-around" effect with waveforms displayed both above and below the zero-velocity baseline. As previously described, the maximal Doppler shift is limited by the Nyquist limit, which equals half the pulse repetition frequency (PRF). The sampling rate of Doppler signals should be twice that of the highest frequency contained within the signal, so that at least two samples are taken within each cycle. When the

blood flow velocity is high, the PRF may not be high enough to sample the returning frequencies at twice per cycle and therefore misses some of the Doppler shifts and results in misinterpretation of the velocities. If the perceived returning frequency is lower than the transmitted frequency, it is plotted below the baseline as a negative Doppler shift even though it may be a higher positive Doppler shift. This results in a wrap-around of the displayed Doppler signal.

35. **Answer: A.** Use a lower transducer frequency, shift the zero-velocity baseline, decrease the sample volume depth, increase the number of sample volumes, and change from PW to CW Doppler. Using a higher frequency transducer has a greater potential for aliasing since the Doppler shift is dependent on the transducer frequency according to the Doppler equation (see answer outline for Question 3). For any given velocity, higher-frequency transducers create higher Doppler shifts while lower-frequency transducers create lower Doppler shifts. When this is taken into context with the pulse repetition frequency (PRF) and Nyquist limit, lower frequency transducers are less likely to create a Doppler shift that exceeds the Nyquist limit. Shifting the baseline increases the maximum velocity in one direction at the expense of the velocity in the other direction. The maximum velocity (V_{max}) that can be unambiguously displayed can be increased by decreasing the sample volume depth (D) according to the equation:

$$V_{max} = c^2 \div (8 \times f_t \times \cos\theta \times D)$$

where c = propagation speed through soft tissue, f_t = transmitted frequency, and θ = intercept angle between the ultrasound beam and blood flow.

By increasing the number of sample volumes, the PRF is increased ("high PRF") to deliberately use range ambiguity to increase the maximum velocity that can be measured. Unlike PW Doppler, CW Doppler does not have sampling limitations due to the constant emission of ultrasound but is limited by range ambiguity.

36. **Answer: C.** This is an example of a range ambiguity artifact. The sample volume has been positioned in the right upper pulmonary vein, but when the scale is increased, the machine has converted to high pulse repetition frequency (PRF) and placed an additional sample volume at the level of the papillary muscles. The resultant trace is the "sum" of the flows in the pulmonary vein and within the mid-left ventricular cavity. Range ambiguity Doppler artifacts are most commonly seen when interrogating pulmonary venous flow. In this instance, the sample volume is deep into the image, leading to a decrease in the PRF and a subsequent reduction

in the Nyquist limit. To overcome this, the velocity scale can be increased by increasing the PRF as well as the number of sample volumes (high PRF mode). The disadvantage however is that the exact origin of the Doppler shift is unknown, and this can lead to a range ambiguity artifact. In high PRF, the transducer emits a pulse to a second, shallower sample volume before the signal is received from the first deeper sample volume and as a result signals from the initial pulse as well as signals from the most recently sent pulse arrive at the transducer at the same time and both signals are superimposed on top of one another.

37. **Answer: D.** In this example the signal below the zero baseline during diastole is representative of a mirror artifact caused from "cross-talk." The mitral inflow appears to occur both above and below the baseline. Spectral Doppler mirror artifacts result in the duplication or mirror image of Doppler shifts on the opposite side of the baseline to the actual unidirectional flow. This artifact appears as a symmetric signal of somewhat less intensity than the actual flow signal, and in the opposite direction. Mirror artifacts are produced by: (1) interaction with a strong reflector; (2) an incident angle near 90°; or (3) "cross-talk" between the forward and reverse channels.

Answer A is not correct as mitral regurgitation occurs during systole when the mitral valve is closed, whereas this waveform occurs during diastole. Answer B is not correct as spectral aliasing occurs when the Nyquist limit is exceeded with the resultant waveform wrapping around such that velocities appear both above and below

the baseline. Answer C is not correct as aortic regurgitation would appear above the baseline during diastole when interrogated from the apical 4-chamber view.

38. **Answer: A.** Beam width artifacts occur due to the nature of the Doppler beam. Therefore, when a strong Doppler signal adjacent to the central beam is detected, it will be superimposed on the spectral trace as though it has originated from the center of the main beam. For example, if both the mitral inflow and LVOT signals are detected by the central beam, there is simultaneous display of both signals (**Figure 8-29**). This Doppler beam width artifact enables the measurement of the IVRT. Beam width artifacts can also have undesirable effects and may hinder the distinction between aortic stenosis from mitral regurgitation.

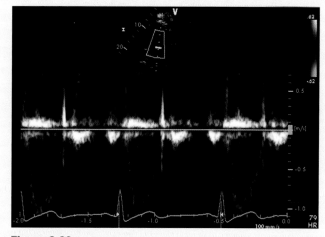

Figure 8-29

SUGGESTED READINGS

Ahmed M, Aurigemma GP. Doppler echocardiography: the normal antegrade flow patterns. In: Lang RM, Goldstein SA, Kronzon I, Khandheria BK, Mor-Avi V, eds. *ASE's Comprehensive Echocardiography*. 2nd ed. Philadelphia: Elsevier Saunders; 2016: chap 10.

Anavekar NS, Oh JK. Doppler echocardiography: a contemporary review. *J Cardiol*. 2009;54(3):347-358.

Anderson B. *Basic principles of spectral Doppler*. In: *Echocardiography: The Normal Examination and Echocardiographic Measurements*. 3rd ed. Brisbane, Australia: Echotext Pty Ltd; 2017:chap 5.

Anderson B. The spectral Doppler examination. In: *Echocardiography: The Normal Examination and Echocardiographic Measurements*. 3rd ed. Brisbane, Australia: Echotext Pty Ltd; 2017:chap 6.

Anderson B. Technical quality. In: Lang RM, Goldstein SA, Kronzon I, Khandheria BK, Mor-Avi V, eds. *ASE's Comprehensive Echocardiography*. 2nd ed. Philadelphia: Elsevier Saunders; 2016:chap 7.

Edelman S. *Understanding Ultrasound Physics*. 4th ed. Woodlands, Texas: E.S.P. Ultrasound; 2012.

Eidem BW, O'Leary PW. Quantitative methods in echocardiography-basic techniques. In: Eidem BW, O'Leary PW, Cetta F, eds. *Echocardiography in Pediatric and Adult Congenital Heart Disease*. 2nd ed. Philadelphia: Wolters Kluwer Health; 2015:chap 3.

Foley DA. Physics of ultrasound. In: Oh JK, Kane GC, Seward JB, Tajik AJ, eds. *The Echo Manual*. 4th ed. Philadelphia, PA and Rochester, MN: Wolters Kluwer; 2019:chap 27.

Gill R. *The Physics and Technology of Diagnostic Ultrasound. A Practitioner's Guide*. Sydney, Australia: High Frequency Publishing; 2012.

Kremkau FW. Physics and instrumentation. In: Lang RM, Goldstein SA, Kronzon I, Khandheria BK, Mor-Avi V, eds. *ASE's Comprehensive Echocardiography*. 2nd ed. Philadelphia: Elsevier Saunders; 2016:chap 3.

Mitchell C, Rahko PS, Blauwet LA, et al. Guidelines for performing a comprehensive transthoracic echocardiographic examination in adults: recommendations from the American Society of Echocardiography. *J Am Soc Echocardiogr*. 2019;32(1):1-64.

Nagueh SF, Smiseth OA, Appleton CP, et al. Recommendations for the evaluation of left ventricular diastolic function by echocardiography: an update from the American Society of Echocardiography and the European Association of Cardiovascular Imaging. *J Am Soc Echocardiogr*. 2016;29(4):277-314.

Oh JK, Miranda WR. Doppler echocardiography and color flow imaging: comprehensive noninvasive hemodynamic assessment. In: Oh JK, Kane GC, Seward JB, Tajik AJ, eds. *The Echo Manual*. 4th ed. Philadelphia, PA and Rochester, MN: Wolters Kluwer; 2019:chap 4.

Otto C. Principles of echocardiographic image acquisition and doppler analysis. In: *Textbook of Clinical Echocardiography*. 6th ed. Philadelphia: Elsevier; 2018:chap 1.

Otto C. Normal anatomy and flow patterns on rransthoracic echocardiography. In: *Textbook of Clinical Echocardiography*. 6th ed. Philadelphia: Elsevier; 2018:chap 2.

Quinones MA, Otto CM, Stoddard M, Waggoner A, Zoghbi WA. Recommendations for quantification of Doppler echocardiography: a report from the Doppler quantification task force of the nomenclature and Standards Committee of American Society of Echocardiography. *J Am Soc Echocardiogr*. 2002;15(2):167-184.

Villarraga HR, Kane GC, Oh JK. Tissue doppler and strain imaging. In: Oh JK, Kane GC, Seward JB, Tajik AJ, eds. *The Echo Manual*. 4th ed. Philadelphia, PA and Rochester, MN: Wolters Kluwer; 2019:chap 5.

Young R, O'Leary PW. Principles of cardiovascular ultrasound. In: Eidem BW, O'Leary PW, Cetta F, eds. *Echocardiography in Pediatric and Adult Congenital Heart Disease*. 2nd ed. Philadelphia: Wolters Kluwer Health; 2015:chap 1.

Color Doppler Examination

Contributors: Bonita Anderson, DMU (Cardiac), MAppSc (Medical Ultrasound), ACS and Alicia Armour, MA, BS, RDCS

✪ Question 1

Which of the following statements regarding the basic principles of color Doppler imaging is false?
- **A.** Color Doppler imaging is based on pulsed-wave Doppler principles.
- **B.** Color Doppler imaging displays mean velocity information.
- **C.** The value displayed at the top and bottom of the color bar is the Nyquist limit.
- **D.** The black region in the center of the color bar indicates the absence of flow.

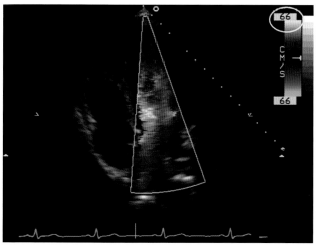

Figure 9-1

✪ Question 2

In **Figure 9-1**, the numerical value in the yellow circle indicates:
- **A.** The maximum color Nyquist limit of blood flow velocity toward the transducer.
- **B.** The maximum mean blood flow velocity toward the transducer.

- **C.** The maximum velocity at which color aliasing will occur.
- **D.** The maximum mean velocity at which turbulent flow will be identified.

✪ Question 3

In **Figure 9-2**, the green color added to the color bar indicates:
- **A.** A greater disparity in Doppler shifts.
- **B.** Frequency aliasing at high pulse repetition frequencies.
- **C.** High Doppler shifts exceeding the Nyquist limit.
- **D.** Parabolic blood flow.
- **E.** All of the above.

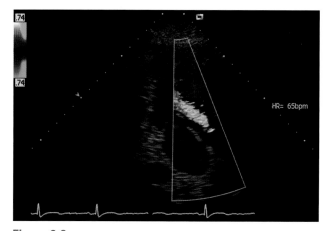

Figure 9-2

✪ Question 4

The color pattern characterizing turbulent flow in the color Doppler image (**Figure 9-3**) can be described as:
- A. Disorganized.
- B. Variance.
- C. Diverse.
- D. Mosaic.
- E. All of the above.

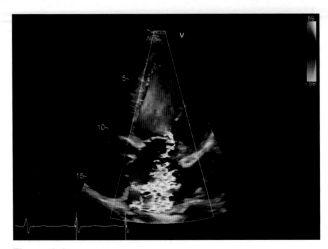

Figure 9-3

✪✪ Question 5

Aliasing on the color Doppler image is typically reduced by:
- A. Increasing the angle between the ultrasound beam and direction of flow.
- B. Decreasing the color velocity scale.
- C. Shifting the baseline away from the direction of flow.
- D. Increasing the depth of the image.

✪✪ Question 6

The color Nyquist limit (color velocity scale) may be increased by:
- A. Shortening the color box length.
- B. Narrowing the color box width.
- C. Using a higher transducer frequency.
- D. Decreasing the wall filter.
- E. All of the above.

✪ Question 7

Which is decreased with color Doppler imaging?
- A. Contrast resolution
- B. Temporal resolution
- C. Spatial resolution
- D. All of the above

✪✪ Question 8

▶ Observe **Video 9-1**, which was acquired from a subcostal 4-chamber view. Which of the following will improve the color Doppler interrogation of the interatrial septum?
- A. Decreasing color gain
- B. Increasing wall filter
- C. Decreasing color velocity scale
- D. Increasing transducer frequency
- E. All of the above

✪ Question 9

For the interrogation of regurgitant jets, the recommended standard for color Doppler settings is a high color gain and a color Nyquist limit set:
- A. Between 45 and 65 cm/s.
- B. Between 50 and 70 cm/s.
- C. Between 60 and 80 cm/s.
- D. Between 70 and 90 cm/s.
- E. As high as possible.

✪ Question 10

Compared to angiography as the gold standard, color Doppler echocardiography generally:
- A. Overestimates the severity of regurgitation.
- B. Underestimates the severity of regurgitation.
- C. Correlates well with the severity of regurgitation.

✪✪✪ Question 11

Which of the following will not increase regurgitant jet area?
- A. A slit-like orifice imaged along the long axis of the orifice
- B. Higher Nyquist limit
- C. Higher transducer frequency
- D. Lower pulse repetition frequency (PRF)
- E. Multiple orifices

✪✪✪ Question 12

Jet momentum is a major overall determinant of the regurgitant jet size. The simplified equation for expressing momentum (M) is written as:

    A. $M = A \times v$.
    B. $M = A \times Q$.
    C. $M = Q \times v$.
    D. $M = A \times Q \times v$.

where A is the effective orifice area, v is the velocity, and Q is flow rate.

✪✪✪ Question 13

Assuming there are mitral regurgitant (MR) and tricuspid regurgitant (TR) color Doppler jets of equal size with equal momentum: if the MR jet has a peak velocity of 550 cm/s and a flow rate of 110 mL/s and the TR jet has a peak velocity of 275 cm/s, what is the TR flow rate?

    A. 55 mL/s
    B. 220 mL/s
    C. 440 mL/s
    D. 605 mL/s

✪✪ Question 14

▶ Observe two images acquired from the same patient with mitral regurgitation (**Videos 9-2A** and **9-2B**). **Video 9-2B** is better optimized because in **Video 9-2A** the:

    A. Color velocity scale is set too low.
    B. Color gain is set too low.
    C. Color wall filters are set too high.
    D. Color wall filters are set too low.

✪✪ Question 15

▶ Observe two transesophageal images acquired from the same patient with mitral regurgitation (**Videos 9-3A** and **9-3B**). What color Doppler control was changed between **Videos 9-3A** and **9-3B**?

    A. Color wall filter
    B. Color map
    C. Color gain
    D. Color baseline

✪✪ Question 16

▶ Observe two transesophageal video/images performed on a patient with mitral regurgitation (**Videos 9-4A** and **9-4B** and **Figures 9-4A** and **9-4B**). The severity of mitral regurgitation (MR) appears more significant in **Video 9-4B**/**Figure 9-4B** compared with **Video 9-4A**/**Figure 9-4A**. The likely reason for this is that the:

    A. Color gain was increased between clips 9-4A and 9-4B.
    B. Color velocity scale was decreased between clips 9-4A and 9-4B.
    C. Patient's blood pressure increased between clips 9-4A and 9-4B.
    D. Patient's blood pressure decreased between clips 9-4A and 9-4B.

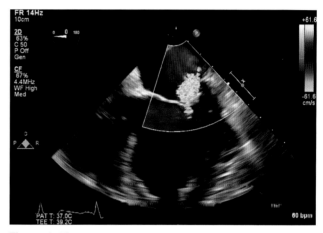

Figure 9-4A

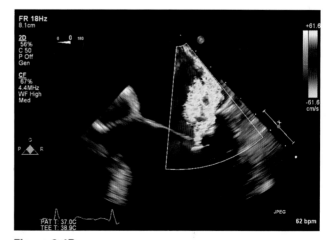

Figure 9-4B

✪ Question 17

When there is significant valvular regurgitation, blood flow converges toward the regurgitant orifice forming hemispheric shells of:

A. Increasing velocity and decreasing surface area.

B. Decreasing velocity and increasing surface area.

C. Increasing momentum and decreasing surface area.

D. Decreasing momentum and increasing surface area.

✪✪ Question 18

To increase the size of a hemisphere proximal to a narrowed orifice, the color Doppler baseline should:

A. Be shifted away from the direction of flow.

B. Be shifted toward the direction of flow.

C. Remain as is and decrease the color Nyquist limit.

D. A and C.

E. B and C.

✪✪ Question 19

The vena contracta (VC) can be used in the assessment of the severity of a regurgitant lesion. Which of the following statements regarding the VC is false?

A. The VC is slightly smaller than the anatomic regurgitant orifice.

B. The VC is an indirect measurement of the effective regurgitant orifice.

C. The VC is not strongly influenced by the color Nyquist limit.

D. The VC is best measured when the ultrasound beam is oriented parallel with flow.

E. The VC is independent of flow rate and driving pressure.

✪ Question 20

From the apical 4-chamber view, which pulmonary vein will show blue flow into the left atrium?

A. Left lower pulmonary vein

B. Left upper pulmonary vein

C. Right lower pulmonary vein

D. Right upper pulmonary vein

✪ Question 21

▶ Observe **Video 9-5** which was acquired from an apical 4-chamber view. The red flow seen lateral to the left atrium is:

A. Abnormal extracardiac flow from an extracardiac structure.

B. Normal flow from an aberrant right pulmonary vein.

C. Normal flow from the left lower pulmonary vein.

D. Normal flow from the left upper pulmonary vein.

E. Normal flow within the descending aorta.

✪✪✪ Question 22

▶ Observe **Video 9-6**, which was acquired from an apical 4-chamber view. In the same patient, the estimated pulmonary artery pressure was 93 mm Hg and the pulmonary vascular resistance (PVR) was 5 Wood units. Based on the images provided, the red flow into the left atrium most likely represents:

A. Prominent coronary sinus flow.

B. Obstructed right pulmonary venous flow into the left atrium.

C. Normal right pulmonary venous flow into the left atrium.

D. A patent foramen ovale with right-to-left shunting.

✪✪ Question 23

▶ Observe **Video 9-7**, which was acquired from an apical 4-chamber view. This color Doppler image, recorded from the abdominal aorta subcostal view, is consistent with:

A. Normal flow.

B. Severe aortic regurgitation.

C. Coarctation of the aorta.

D. Aortic dissection.

✪✪ Question 24

▶ Observe **Video 9-8**, which was acquired from an apical long-axis view. Based on this color Doppler image, the mitral regurgitant (MR) continuous-wave Doppler trace will show:

A. An MR velocity less than 3 m/s.

B. A V-wave cutoff sign of the MR signal.

C. An early systolic MR jet.

D. Diastolic MR.

✪✪ Question 25

Color Doppler M-mode incorporates both color Doppler imaging and M-mode. Therefore, color Doppler M-mode provides information about:

   A. Depth, time, velocity, and motion.
   B. Time, depth, velocity, and direction.
   C. Time, distance, flow, and direction.
   D. Velocity, motion, distance, and direction.

✪✪ Question 26

The color Doppler M-mode trace shown in **Figure 9-5** is characteristic of:

   A. Diastolic and systolic mitral regurgitation.
   B. Ischemic mitral regurgitation.
   C. Mitral valve prolapse.
   D. Severe mitral regurgitation.

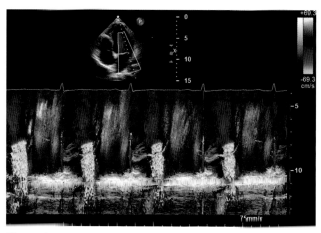

Figure 9-5

✪✪✪ Question 27

The color Doppler M-mode trace shown in **Figure 9-6** is most characteristic of:

   A. Abnormal left ventricular relaxation.
   B. Elevated left ventricular filling pressures.
   C. Restrictive left ventricular filling.
   D. All the above.

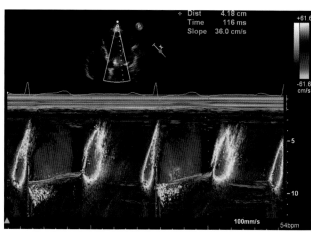

Figure 9-6

✪✪✪ Question 28

The color Doppler M-mode trace shown in **Figure 9-7** was acquired in the descending aorta from the suprasternal notch view. This trace is most consistent with:

   A. Coarctation of the aorta or a patent ductus arteriosus.
   B. Coarctation of the aorta or severe aortic regurgitation.
   C. A patent ductus arteriosus or severe aortic regurgitation.
   D. A patent ductus arteriosus only.
   E. Severe aortic regurgitation only.

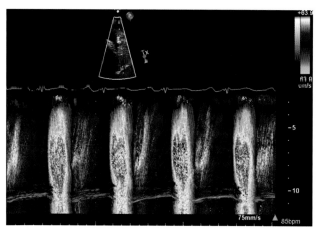

Figure 9-7

✪✪ Question 29

Figure 9-8 was acquired from the suprasternal notch window; the black region at the top of the aortic arch indicates:

   A. The absence of flow.
   B. The absence of a Doppler shift.
   C. Where flow changes direction.
   D. A and C.
   E. B and C.

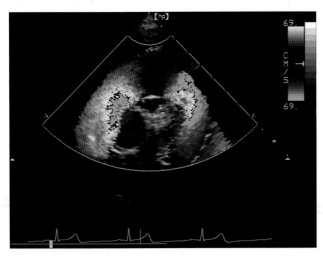

Figure 9-8

✪✪ Question 30

▶ Observe **Video 9-9**, which was acquired from a zoomed apical 2-chamber view. This color Doppler artifact adjacent to the left atrium is:

A. Ghosting.
B. Mirror.
C. Reverberation.
D. Waterfall.

ANSWERS

1. **Answer: D.** The black region in the center of the color bar indicates the absence of a detectable Doppler shift. Color Doppler imaging detects velocity (Doppler shifts) rather than flow. Hence, the black region in the center of the color bar indicates a zero Doppler shift rather than the absence of flow. Therefore, answer D is a false statement.

   Answer A is a true statement. Color Doppler is a form of pulsed-wave Doppler imaging that uses multiple sample volumes along multiple scan lines to record the Doppler shift.

   Answer B is a true statement. To create a color Doppler image, the machine must rapidly measure Doppler shifts in a large number of sample volumes within the color box at the same time. As a result, only the mean (or average) Doppler shifts are calculated.

   Answer C is a true statement. The velocity values displayed at the top and bottom of the color bar indicate the blood velocity at the Nyquist limit for forward and backward flow. Because color Doppler is based on pulsed-wave Doppler principles, the maximum possible Doppler shifts that can be correctly measured and displayed are limited by the Nyquist limit, which is equal to one-half the pulse repetition frequency (PRF).

2. **Answer: B.** The numerical values on the color Doppler bar represent the maximum **mean** blood flow velocity toward (top) and away from (bottom) the transducer. Therefore, answer B is correct.

   Answer A is incorrect. The numerical values on the color bar represent maximum **mean** blood flow velocity or the maximum mean color Nyquist limit of blood flow velocity.

   Answer C is incorrect. Color aliasing occurs when the maximum **mean** velocity exceeds the color Nyquist limit.

   Answer D is incorrect as turbulent flow is identified by a color mosaic pattern of "flow" which occurs when there is a greater variation of Doppler shifts or blood flow velocities within the color box.

3. **Answer: A.** Shades of green are traditionally used to display a greater disparity or variation in Doppler shifts. This is commonly referred to as color variance. A color variance map may be used to identify turbulent flow. With this type of flow, there is a greater variation in blood flow velocities, which produces a larger range of Doppler shifts and greater spectral broadening. Therefore, answer A is correct.

   Frequency aliasing tends to occur at low pulse repetition frequencies; therefore, answer B is incorrect.

   High Doppler shifts exceeding the Nyquist limit will result in aliasing but unless flow is turbulent, color variance will be absent; therefore, answer C is incorrect.

   Parabolic blood flow is a form of laminar (nonturbulent) flow. This type of flow shows minimal variation in the Doppler shifts; hence, color variance is not seen when there is parabolic flow. Therefore, answer D is incorrect.

   Answer E is incorrect based on the explanations above.

TECHNICAL TIP

The display of the color variance map is variable depending on the ultrasound machine being used. For example, green may be used to "tag" turbulent flow in both directions (**Figure 9-9A**) or yellow may be used to "tag" turbulent forward flow while green is used to "tag" turbulent backward flow (**Figure 9-9B**).

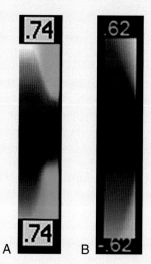

Figure 9-9

4. **Answer: D.** The color pattern characterizing turbulent flow in color Doppler imaging can be described as mosaic. This term refers to the display of a "mosaic" of reds, blues, yellows, and cyan in the turbulent area.

5. **Answer: C.** Aliasing occurs when the Doppler shifts exceed the Nyquist limit, which is one-half the pulse repetition frequency (PRF). Shifting the baseline away from the direction of flow will effectively increase the velocity range in the direction of forward flow (**Figure 9-10**); hence, this may reduce color aliasing in the direction of forward flow. Therefore, answer C is correct.

Increasing the angle between ultrasound beam and direction of flow can also reduce aliasing by decreasing the measured Doppler shift. However, this is not ideal as velocity information will be "underestimated"; therefore, answer A is incorrect. Decreasing the color velocity scale will result in

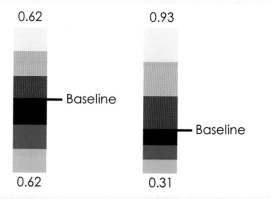

Figure 9-10 This schematic illustrates how shifting the color baseline changes the color velocity scale (Nyquist limit). On the left, the color baseline is set to the center and the Nyquist limit has the same value of 0.62 cm/s at the top and bottom of the color bar. On the right, the color baseline is shifted downward resulting in a decrease in the color Nyquist limit at the bottom of the color bar to 0.31 cm/s and a corresponding increase in the color Nyquist limit at the top to 0.93 cm/s.

aliasing occurring at lower Doppler shifts; therefore, answer B is incorrect. Imaging at an increased depth will decrease the PRF and increase aliasing; therefore, answer D is incorrect.

Other methods that can be employed to reduce color aliasing include decreasing the image depth, shortening the color box, and/or increasing the color velocity scale.

6. **Answer: A.** As stated previously, the color Nyquist limit is equal to one-half the pulse repetition frequency (PRF). In color Doppler imaging, the PRF is essentially determined by the length and depth of the color box (and the overall imaging depth). For example, longer color boxes and color boxes placed deeper into the image tends to lower the PRF and therefore will lower the color Nyquist limit. Conversely, shortening the color box (and placing the color box shallower on the image) will increase the color Nyquist limit; therefore, answer A is correct.

Answer B is incorrect since narrowing the color box width will increase the frame rate and improve the temporal resolution but will not increase the color Nyquist limit.

Answer C is incorrect as decreasing, not increasing, the transducer frequency will increase the color Nyquist limit. That is, lower frequency transducers can resolve higher velocities compared with higher frequency transducers, so a lower frequency transducer will increase the color Nyquist limit compared with a higher frequency transducer.

Answer D is incorrect since decreasing the wall filter simply enhances the detection of low velocity flow and will not increase the color Nyquist limit.

7. **Answer: B.** Temporal resolution refers to the ability of the ultrasound machine to accurately distinguish the time between two dynamic events. Temporal resolution is equal to the inverse of frame rate; for example, 20 frames/second corresponds to 1/20 second = 0.05 seconds = 50 ms. The creation of color Doppler images increases the processing time, so the frame rate and hence the temporal resolution is decreased; therefore, answer B is correct.

Contrast resolution refers to the ability to differentiate subtle differences in echogenicity between structures and to display those structures as being different, while spatial resolution is the ability of the ultrasound machine to detect structures that are anatomically separate and to display them as such; both are not affected by color Doppler imaging. Therefore, answers A, C, and D are all incorrect.

8. ▶ **Answer: C. Video 9-1** shows underfilling of the color box. This may occur when the color gain is set too low, when the color velocity scale is set too high, and/or when the wall filter is set too high. The aim of color Doppler interrogation of the interatrial septum is to exclude (or confirm) the presence of flow

across a patent foramen ovale or atrial septal defect. Typically, this flow, if present, will be low velocity. Therefore, to enhance the detection of low velocity flow, the first step would be to increase the color gain to the point just below color speckling and then if the color box remains underfilled, the next step would be to decrease the color velocity scale. Decreasing (not increasing) the wall filter may also be attempted to enhance the detection of low velocity flow. Increasing the transducer frequency will also effectively decrease the color velocity scale; however, the simplest method for enhancing the color Doppler image to detect low-velocity flow is to decrease the color velocity scale (see **Video 9-10**). Therefore, answer C is correct.

KEY POINT
When there is underfilling of the color box despite an adequate color gain optimization, the color velocity scale should be decreased until there is adequate filling of the color box. The effect of decreasing the color velocity scale to enhance the detection of low-velocity flow is illustrated in **Figure 9-11**. Observe that the color bar on the left shows the color velocity scale set to 60 cm/s. It can be appreciated that the range of colors assigned for the detection of low-velocity flow (30 cm/s) is relatively small. By decreasing the color velocity scale to 30 cm/s as shown in the color bar on the right, the full range of colors is now "devoted" to the detection of low-velocity flow.

9. **Answer: B.** According to the 2017 ASE Recommendations for Noninvasive Evaluation of Native Valvular Regurgitation, the standard technique for interrogating regurgitant jets is to use a Nyquist limit of 50 to 70 cm/s and a high color gain that just eliminates random color speckle from nonmoving regions.

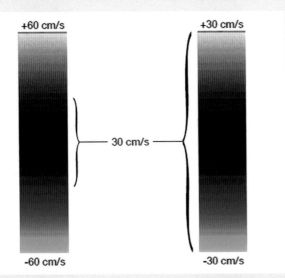

Figure 9-11 Reproduced with permission by Echotext Pty Ltd, from Anderson B. *Basic principles of colour flow doppler imaging*. In: *Echocardiography: The Normal Examination and Echocardiographic Measurements*. 3rd ed. Australia: Echotext Pty Ltd; 2017:132, chap 7.

10. **Answer: A.** Color Doppler imaging detects velocity (or Doppler shifts) rather than flow volume. For example, when a regurgitant jet enters the receiving chamber, it will displace blood cells already within this receiving chamber. If these blood cells reach minimal velocity, they will create detectable Doppler shifts. Therefore, in these circumstances, the color regurgitant jet will include the regurgitant volume as well as the blood volume already within the receiving chamber that has been displaced or "moved" by the regurgitant jet. This is referred to as the "billiard ball effect" (**Figure 9-12**).

11. **Answer: B.** A lower Nyquist limit, rather than a higher Nyquist limit, increases the jet area. A lower Nyquist limit reduces the velocity scale thereby emphasizing lower velocities and will therefore make the jet appear larger. Furthermore, as explained in the answer outline for Question 10, blood cells in the receiving chamber that are displaced by the regurgitant jet may reach the minimal velocity to create a detectable Doppler shift and will therefore be included within the color regurgitant jet.

Answer A is incorrect since a slit-like regurgitant orifice, imaged along the thin, long shape of the orifice, increases jet area. Answer C is incorrect as a higher transducer frequency increases the Doppler shift frequency, which increases the likelihood of aliasing at a given blood flow velocity. This effectively reduces the highest detectable velocities (Nyquist limit) and the lowest detectable velocities, making jets appear larger. Answer D is incorrect. Recall that the Nyquist limit is equal to one-half the PRF. Therefore, a lower PRF means a lower Nyquist limit and this reduces the velocity scale emphasizing lower velocities and making the jet appear larger. Other determinants of regurgitant jet size are listed in **Table 9-1**.

12. **Answer: C.** The simplified equation for momentum (M) is given by.

$$M = Q \times v \qquad (1)$$

where Q is flow rate (cm³/s), v is velocity (cm/s). The units for M are cm⁴/s².

Furthermore, since the flow rate (Q) is equal to $A \times v$, M (cm⁴/s²) can also be expressed as:

$$M = A \times v^2 \qquad (2)$$

where A is area (cm²) and v is velocity (cm/s).

13. **Answer: B.** Two jets of equal size should have equal momentum; that is, $M_1 = M_2$ where M_1 = momentum of jet 1 and M_2 = the momentum of jet 2. Since $M = Q \times v$, then:

$$Q_1 \times v_1 = Q_2 \times v_2$$

where Q_1 is the flow rate of jet 1, v_1 is the peak velocity of jet 1, Q_2 is the flow rate of jet 2, and v_2 is

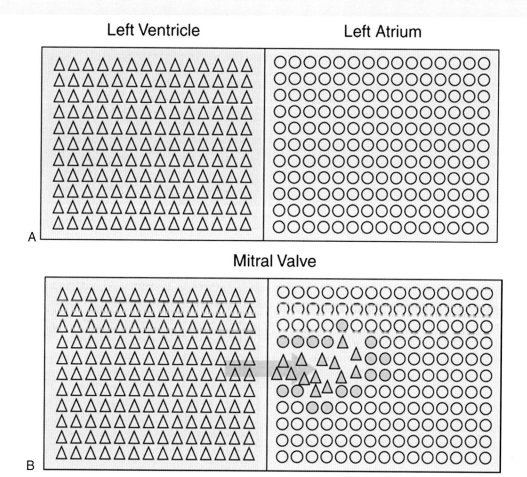

Figure 9-12 This is a schematic depiction of mitral regurgitation, with the triangles representing blood within the left ventricle and the circles indicating left atrial blood. B, Mitral regurgitation (MR) is demonstrated by some of the triangles moving through the orifice into the left atrium (filled triangles). Observe that this regurgitant volume displaces the left atrial blood (filled circles). Because these filled circles are moving and if they reach minimal velocity they will create detectable Doppler shifts. As the machine cannot distinguish between the MR volume (the filled triangles) and the displaced left atrial blood (the filled circles), the filled triangles and filled circles are all incorporated into the color Doppler regurgitant jet, thus overestimating the true mitral regurgitant volume. (Reprinted with permission from Feigenbaum H, Armstrong WF, Ryan T, eds. *Feigenbaum's Echocardiography*. 7th ed. Philadelphia, PA: Wolters Kluwer Health/Lippincott Williams & Wilkins; 2010.)

Table 9-1. Factors That Increase or Reduce the Color Doppler Jet Area

Increase Jet Area	Reduce Jet Area
Higher momentum	Lower momentum
Larger regurgitant orifice area	Smaller regurgitant orifice area
Higher velocity (greater pressure gradient)	Lower velocity (lower pressure gradient)
Higher entrainment of flow	Chamber constraint/wall-impinging jet
Lower Nyquist limit	Higher Nyquist limit
Higher Doppler gain	Lower Doppler gain
Far-field beam widening	Far-field attenuation/attenuation by an interposed ultrasound-reflecting structure
Slit-like regurgitant orifice, imaged along the thin, long shape of the orifice	
Multiple orifices	

Reprinted from Zoghbi WA, Adams D, Bonow RO, et al. Recommendations for noninvasive evaluation of native valvular regurgitation. a report from the American Society of Echocardiography developed in collaboration with the Society for Cardiovascular Magnetic Resonance. *J Am Soc Echocardiogr*. 2017;30(4):303-371. Copyright © 2017 by the American Society of Echocardiography. With permission.

the peak velocity of jet 2. Therefore, if the v_2 is half v_1, then the Q_2 will be double that of Q_1. Based on the information provided, if the TR velocity of 275 cm/s is half that of the MR velocity of 550 cm/s and the MR flow rate is 110 mL/s, then the TR flow rate would need double to 220 mL/s for the momentum to be equal. Therefore, answer B is correct.

14. **Answer: A.** In **Video 9-2A** (left), the color velocity scale, as displayed at the top and bottom of the color bar, is set too low at 38.5 cm/s; therefore, answer A is correct.

    Answer B is incorrect since the color gain, displayed under CF at the left of the image, is the same in both clips (it is at 75%).

    Answers C and D are incorrect since the wall filter (WF) is the same setting for both clips (it is set to high).

KEY POINT

The color velocity scale can significantly affect the color regurgitant jet area. Observe how the severity of mitral regurgitation appears greater in **Video 9-2A** (left) compared with **Video 9-2B** (right) where the color velocity scale is correctly set between 50 and 70 cm/s (65.9 cm/s).

15. **Answer: D.** Comparing **Videos 9-3A** and **9-3B**, it can be appreciated from the color bar that the color baseline was shifted upward (toward the direction of the mitral regurgitant jet into the left atrium). The color Nyquist limit at the top of the color bar in **Video 9-3B** (right) is now set to 33.5 cm/s; therefore, answer D is correct.

    Answer A is incorrect since the wall filter (WF) setting is set on high in both examples (**Videos 9-3A** and **9-3B**.

    Answer B is incorrect since the color map appears the same with respect to the depiction of colors on the color bar.

    Answer C is incorrect since the color gain strength is the same setting for both clips (it is 59%).

TECHNICAL POINTS

Shifting the color baseline in the direction of the MR jet is frequently employed to increase the size of the proximal isovelocity surface area (PISA) radius. Shifting the color baseline also increases the size of the regurgitant jet area and creates color aliasing of the regurgitant jet. Color aliasing occurs when the mean velocity exceeds the color Nyquist limit. In **Video 9-3B** the mean velocity of the MR jet toward the transducer exceeds the forward Nyquist limit of 33.5 cm/s; this results in color aliasing of the MR jet (the color of the MR jet changes from primarily red to primarily blue). In **Video 9-3B**, the jet area also increases in size because the jet velocity is greater than the minimally detectible velocity of 33.5 cm/s. In addition, if blood cells displaced by the regurgitant jet reach minimal velocity, they will create detectable Doppler shifts and be incorporated into the jet area, thus increasing the area of the jet.

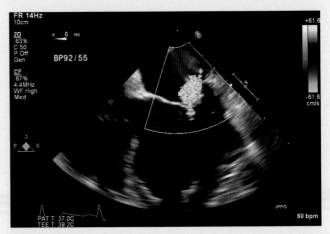

Figure 9-13A

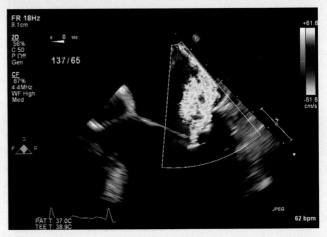

Figure 9-13B

16. **Answer: C.** Answers A and B are incorrect as the color gain and color velocity scale in **Figure 9-4A/Video 9-4A** and **Figure 9-4B/Video 9-4B** are unchanged at 67% and 61.6 cm/s, respectively. Therefore, the patient's blood pressure must have changed between the acquisition of these clips. Since the severity of MR appears to have increased, it can be assumed that the driving pressure of the MR jet, or systolic blood pressure (BP), has been increased; therefore, answer C is correct. In fact, **Figure 9-4A/Video 9-4A** were acquired at a baseline BP of 92/55 mm Hg (**Figure 9-13A**) and **Figure 9-4B/Video 9-4B** were acquired at a pharmacologically augmented BP of 137/65 mm Hg (**Figure 9-13B**).

KEY POINT

A regurgitant jet may appear larger by increasing the driving pressure across the valve (higher momentum) or may appear smaller by decreasing the driving pressure across the valve (lower momentum). Therefore, it is important that the blood pressure is recorded at the time of the study, particularly for left heart lesions and when the study is performed in the intraoperative setting or on a sedated patient.

17. **Answer: A.** When there is significant valvular regurgitation, blood flow converges toward the narrowed regurgitant orifice. Flow accelerates in

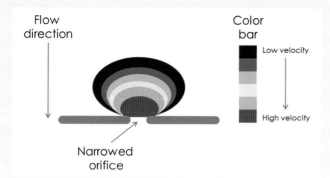

Figure 9-14 This schematic illustrates the changes in the color hemispheric shells and the velocity of each shell as flow converges toward a narrowed orifice. Flow direction and color velocities according to the color bar are shown. Observe that as the color velocity increases (moves from low to high), the hemispheric shells decrease in surface area.

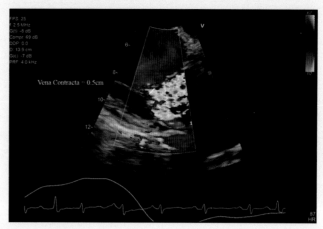

Figure 9-15

a laminar manner forming a series of concentric, roughly hemispheric shells of uniform velocity (isovelocities). As flow advances closer to the narrowed orifice, the area of each hemispheric shell decreases and the velocity of each shell increases. Color Doppler imaging has the ability to visually display this effect (**Figure 9-14**). This concept forms the main principle of the proximal isovelocity surface area (PISA) technique for estimating the size of a narrowed orifice.

18. ▶ **Answer: E.** The hemisphere proximal to a narrowed orifice may be increased by (1) shifting the baseline in the direction of flow or (2) simply decreasing the color Nyquist limit or color velocity scale which effectively decreases the aliasing velocity. In the case of baseline shift, since the flow rate proximal to the narrowing is constant, when the Nyquist limit (color velocity scale) is decreased, the cross-sectional area of the hemisphere must be increased to maintain the same flow rate (**Video 9-11**). By decreasing the color Nyquist limit, the entire color Doppler image is affected. Therefore, most operators prefer shifting the baseline.

19. **Answer: D.** As axial resolution is superior to lateral resolution, the VC is best measured when the ultrasound beam is oriented perpendicular to flow. For example, in mitral regurgitation (MR), the VC is best measured from the parasternal long-axis view where the MR jet is aligned perpendicular to the ultrasound beam, so the VC is then measured along the scan line (**Figure 9-15**). Therefore, answer D is a false statement.

Answer A is a true statement. As flow passes through a restricted orifice, it narrows downstream from this orifice; this is the VC. As a result, the VC is slightly smaller than the anatomic regurgitant orifice. Answers B, C, and E are also true statements.

20. ▶ **Answer: A.** From the apical 4-chamber view, it is possible to image all four pulmonary veins as they drain into the left atrium. Flow from the right upper, right lower, and left upper pulmonary veins

is typically directed toward the transducer and therefore flow is color-coded red. Flow from the left lower pulmonary vein is usually directed away from the transducer and therefore flow is color-coded blue (**Video 9-12**). This normal venous flow should not be confused with abnormal flow or fistulous flow into the left atrium.

21. **Answer: E.** This is normal flow within the descending aorta. Recall that from this view, the descending aorta is often seen lateral to the left atrium. Observe how the flow appears in systole only, which is also consistent with aortic flow; normal venous flow is continuous, so would be seen throughout the cardiac cycle.

22. **Answer: D.** This patient has pulmonary arterial hypertension, based on an increased pulmonary artery pressure of 93 mm Hg and an elevated PVR of 5 Wood units. There is also marked dilatation of the right atrium and right ventricle. The interatrial septum is bowing right-to-left and right-to-left shunting across the interatrial septum is noted, most likely via a patent foramen ovale. Therefore, answer D is correct.

Answer A is not correct since the coronary sinus is not seen in this image. The coronary sinus is visualized with posterior tilting and coronary sinus flow would be directed into the right atrium and therefore, would appear as low-velocity, blue flow.

Answers B and C are unlikely to be correct. Right pulmonary veins are usually better visualized with more anterior tilting; that is, from an apical 5-chamber view.

23. ▶ **Answer: C.** This color Doppler image shows continuous, red flow toward the transducer, which is most consistent with a severe coarctation of the aorta where there is a persistent forward pressure gradient across the narrowing over both systole and diastole. Therefore, answer C is correct.

Answer A is not correct. From the subcostal view, normal flow in the abdominal aorta occurs in systole, and as flow is toward the transducer, it is color-encoded red (**Video 9-13A**). Occasionally, low-velocity diastolic forward flow may also be noted.

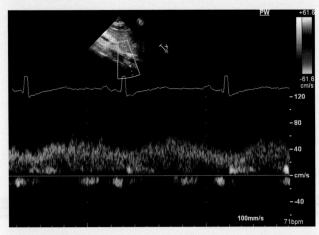

Figure 9-16

Answer B is not correct. With severe aortic regurgitation, pan-diastolic flow reversal may be noted within the abdominal aorta. This appears as blue flow away from the transducer during diastole (**Video 9-13B**).

KEY POINT

Continuous flow toward the transducer within the abdominal aorta is characteristic of a severe coarctation of the aorta. On color Doppler imaging, this appears as continuous, red flow toward the transducer (see **Video 9-7**). On pulsed-wave Doppler, this appears as a continuous, "damped" flow profile with velocities appearing above the zero-velocity baseline (**Figure 9-16**).

24. **Answer: D.** This color Doppler image shows diastolic mitral regurgitation (MR). Therefore, answer D is correct. **Figure 9-17** shows the continuous-wave Doppler trace from this patient. Observe that there is a low-velocity MR signal below the zero-velocity baseline prior to the R wave on the ECG (arrows); this is diastolic MR. Trace systolic MR is also noted. Diastolic MR occurs when the left ventricular (LV)

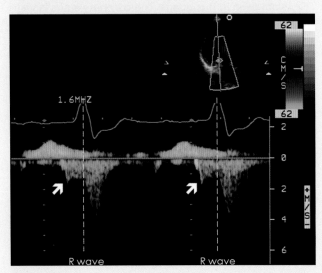

Figure 9-17

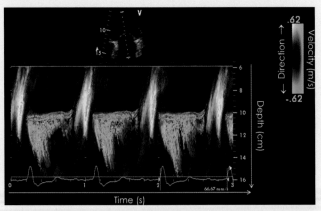

Figure 9-18 This is a CDM trace through the mitral valve acquired from a zoomed apical 4-chamber view in a patient with mitral regurgitation. Time is indicated on the x-axis and depth is indicated on the y-axis. As diastolic forward flow is directed toward the transducer, flow appears red with the various shades of red indicating the mean velocity of flow. The bright blue flow in late diastole indicates color aliasing where the mean velocity has exceeded the color Nyquist limit. Mitral regurgitation (MR) is directed away from the transducer and therefore appears blue. Furthermore, as MR is turbulent, flow appears green and mosaic.

end-diastolic pressure exceeds the left atrial (LA) pressure resulting in retrograde flow from the LV, across the open mitral valve, into the LA. Diastolic MR may be seen in certain conduction abnormalities such as heart blocks and with acute, severe aortic regurgitation.

25. **Answer: B.** Color Doppler M-mode (CDM) provides information about time, depth (or distance), velocity, and direction. Time is displayed on the horizontal or x-axis, depth is displayed on the vertical or y-axis, velocity is represented by the color shade on the color bar, and direction is also reflected on a color Doppler bar such that flow toward the transducer is color-coded red and flow away from the transducer is color-coded blue (**Figure 9-18**).

TEACHING POINT

Color Doppler M-mode (CDM) enables the rapid and careful evaluation of time-related events that may not be readily appreciated on the 2D or color Doppler images alone. CDM is also useful in the assessment of left ventricular diastolic function.

26. **Answer: C.** This color Doppler M-mode (CDM) trace is characteristic of mitral valve prolapse (MVP). MVP tends to occur in mid-to-late systole and therefore mitral regurgitation (MR) also occurs in mid-to-late systole. On the CDM trace, the MR jet is of short duration occurring in mid-to-late systole (**Figure 9-19**).

Answer A is not correct as there is no evidence of diastolic MR. As discussed in the answer outline for Question 24, diastolic MR occurs when the left ventricular (LV) end-diastolic pressure exceeds the left atrial (LA) pressure resulting in retrograde flow from the LV, across the open mitral valve, into the LA.

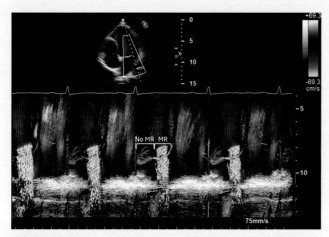

Figure 9-19

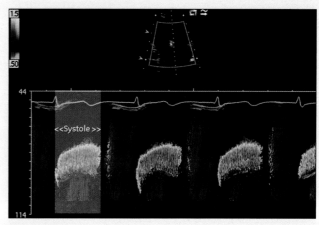

Figure 9-22

Answer D is not correct. This CDM trace shows mid-to-late systolic MR. Therefore, as MR is confined to the latter half of systole, this would not be considered severe. **Figure 9-22** shows a CDM trace of severe MR where the MR jet occurs over the entire systolic period; color baseline shift has also been used to increase the size of the proximal isovelocity surface area (PISA) radius.

27. **Answer: A.** This color Doppler M-mode trace shows the measurement of the flow propagation velocity (Vp) as blood flow propagates from the mitral annulus toward the LV apex. It is measured along the early diastolic slope of the first aliased velocity (red-blue interface) from the level of the mitral annulus to 4 cm into the left ventricular cavity. The Vp is directly related to LV relaxation; therefore, when LV relaxation is impaired, the Vp is slowed. In the example shown, the Vp (slope) is 36 cm/s, which is decreased (<45 cm/s is abnormal). Therefore, answer A is correct.

When there are elevated left ventricular filling pressures or restrictive left ventricular filling, the Vp will also be slowed, but this is because there is an underlying impairment of LV relaxation (that is, the Vp is slowed and will remain slowed across all diastolic dysfunction stages).

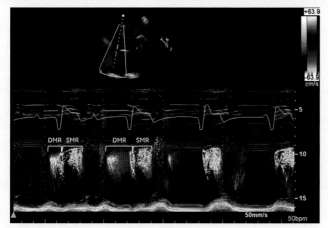

Figure 9-20

KEY POINT

Across all stages of diastolic dysfunction, there is an underlying impairment of LV relaxation, resulting in a decrease in flow propagation velocity (Vp) throughout.

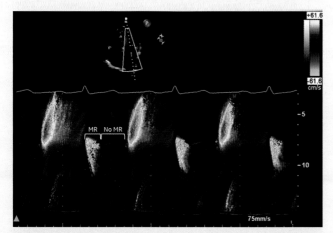

Figure 9-21

On the CDM trace, MR is therefore seen during diastole (before the onset of the R wave on the ECG). **Figure 9-20** shows an example of diastolic MR and systolic MR acquired from a patient in complete heart block.

Answer B is not correct. On the CDM trace with ischemic MR, one might expect to see early systolic MR (**Figure 9-21**). Early systolic MR may also be seen when there is a left bundle branch block and in acute, severe MR.

28. **Answer: C.** This color Doppler M-mode (CDM) trace shows pan-diastolic flow reversal in the descending aorta (red flow toward the transducer during diastole) (**Figure 9-23**). Pan-diastolic (or holodiastolic) flow reversal occurs when there is an "outlet" of flow from the aorta to a lower-pressure chamber or structure during diastole. Most commonly, pan-diastolic flow reversal is seen with severe aortic regurgitation where there is flow from the aorta to the left ventricle (LV) during diastole (aortic diastolic pressure exceeds the LV diastolic pressure).

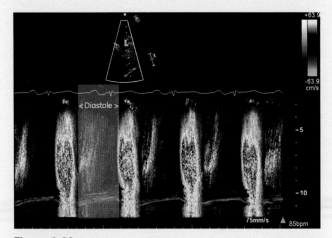

Figure 9-23

Pan-diastolic flow reversal may also be seen when there is a patent ductus arteriosus where there is diastolic shunting of blood from the higher-pressure aorta to the lower-pressure pulmonary artery. As previously discussed (see answer outline for Question 23), when there is a severe coarctation of the aorta, there is a persistent forward pressure gradient across the narrowing over both systole and diastole; thus, the CDM trace would not display diastolic flow reversal. Therefore, answer C is correct.

TEACHING POINT

Normally, flow within the descending aorta is predominantly systolic, although a small amount of retrograde, early diastolic flow can be recorded occasionally. On the CDM trace, this will appear as systolic blue flow (often aliased) away from the transducer and early diastolic red flow toward the transducer (**Figure 9-23**). Early diastolic retrograde flow occurs during the first third of diastole only (**Figure 9-24**).

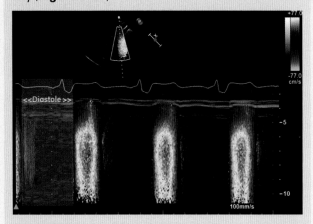

Figure 9-24

Pan-diastolic (holodiastolic) flow reversal within the descending aorta is considered a specific sign of severe aortic regurgitation. However, pan-diastolic flow reversal may also be seen when there is a diastolic pressure gradient between the aorta and a lower-pressure chamber. Examples include arteriovenous fistulas, ruptured sinus of Valsalva, or patent ductus arteriosus.

29. **Answer: B.** The black region at the top of the aortic arch occurs because blood flow is directly perpendicular to the ultrasound beam and therefore, no Doppler shifts are detected. As described earlier (see answer outline for Question 1), color Doppler imaging detects velocity (Doppler shifts) rather than flow. Hence, areas of black indicate a zero Doppler shift and not the absence of flow or a change in flow direction. Therefore, answer B is correct.

30. ▶ **Answer: A.** The artifact adjacent to the left atrium appears as transient "flashes" of low-velocity flow. This is most characteristic of a ghosting (or flash) artifact; therefore, answer A is correct. This artifact is produced by motion of the left atrial wall that is creating detectable Doppler shifts, which then results in the appearance of color on the image display. Importantly, this artifact does not relate to "real flow." Ghosting artifacts may be avoided or eliminated by increasing the wall filters and/or color velocity scale.

Answer B is not correct. Mirror artifacts are created when the ultrasound beam reflects off a highly reflective interface resulting in the duplication or mirror image of a structure that lies in front of the mirror interface. Color mirror artifacts may also occur when there is a duplication of Doppler shifts within the mirrored structure. Hence, on the color Doppler image, "flow" within the real structure and within the mirrored structure will be seen simultaneously. In **Video 9-9**, the artifact lateral to the left atrium is not a mirror of left atrial flow. This can be better appreciated on the frozen image (**Figure 9-25**). Observe that on this still frame image, there is no color within the left atrium (LA); therefore, the color artifact lateral to the LA cannot be a mirror artifact.

Answer C is not correct since color reverberation artifacts would appear as a "streak" of color and this is not seen on the provided video.

Answer D is not correct. Waterfall artifacts are characteristic of some left ventricular assist devices (LVADs). These artifacts are similar to color

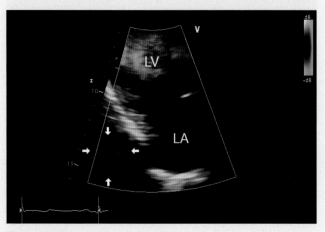

Figure 9-25

reverberation artifacts where there is a continuous streak of artifact that often originates near the left ventricular apex (**Video 9-14**).

Acknowledgments: The authors thank and acknowledge Victor Mor-Avi, MD, Rajesh Jaganath, MD, Lynn Weinert, MD, and Jim D. Thomas, MD, for their inspiration based on "Chapter 1 Physics: Fundamentals of Ultrasound Imaging and Instrumentation" in *Clinical Echocardiography Review: A Self-Assessment Tool, 2nd ed.,* edited by Allan L. Klein, Craig R. Asher, 2017. Additional thanks to Dr James D. Thomas, MD for his wisdom regarding the "physics" of jet momentum.

SUGGESTED READINGS

Anderson B. Basic principles of colour doppler imaging. In: *Echocardiography: The Normal Examination and Echocardiographic Measurements*. 3rd ed. Brisbane: Echotext Pty Ltd; 2017:chap 7.

Anderson B. The colour doppler examination. In: *Echocardiography: The Normal Examination and Echocardiographic Measurements*. 3rd ed. Brisbane: Echotext Pty Ltd; 2017:chap 8.

Edelman S. *Understanding Ultrasound Physics*. 3rd ed. Woodlands, TX: Knowledge Masters, Inc.; 2005.

Evans DH, Jensen JA, Nielsen MB. Ultrasonic colour Doppler imaging. *Interface Focus*. 2011;1:490-502.

Feigenbaum H, Armstrong WF, Ryan T, eds. *Feigenbaum's Echocardiography*. 7th ed. Philadelphia, PA: Lippincott Williams & Wilkins; 2010.

Klein AL, Asher CR. *Clinical Echocardiography Review. A Self-Assessment Tool*. 2nd ed. Philadelphia, PA: Wolters Kluwer; 2017.

Kisslo JK, Adams DB, Belkin RN. *Doppler Color Flow Imaging*. New York, NY: Churchill Livingstone; 1988.

Stevenson JG. The development of color Doppler echocardiography: innovation and collaboration. *J Am Soc Echocardiogr*. 2018;31(12):1344-1352.

Zoghbi WA, Adams D, Bonow RO, et al. Recommendations for noninvasive evaluation of native valvular regurgitation: a report from the American Society of Echocardiography developed in collaboration with the Society for Cardiovascular Magnetic Resonance. *J Am Soc Echocardiogr*. 2017;30(4):303-371.

Hemodynamics

Contributors: Bonita Anderson, DMU (Cardiac), MAppSc (Medical Ultrasound), ACS and Richard A. Palma, BS, ACS, RCS, RDCS

✪ Question 1

The relationship between pressure difference, resistance, and volumetric flow rate is described by:
- **A.** Bernoulli's law.
- **B.** The continuity principle.
- **C.** Poiseuille's law.
- **D.** The Doppler effect.

✪ Question 2

Which of the following equations correctly describes the relationship between volumetric flow rate (Q), pressure difference (ΔP), and resistance (R)?
- **A.** $Q = \Delta P \times R$
- **B.** $Q = \Delta P \div R$
- **C.** $Q = \Delta P \div R^2$
- **D.** $Q = R \div \Delta P$

✪ Question 3

The resistance to flow is determined by several variables and may be increased when the:
- **A.** Length of the vessel is decreased.
- **B.** Viscosity of blood is decreased.
- **C.** Flow rate is increased.
- **D.** Radius of the vessel is increased.

✪✪ Question 4

Assuming a constant flow rate, a decrease in a vessel diameter by one-half will result in a pressure increase at that point of:
- **A.** 2-fold.
- **B.** 4-fold.
- **C.** 16-fold.
- **D.** 32-fold.

✪✪✪ Question 5

Assuming a constant flow rate and a pressure gradient across an aortic valve of 6 mm Hg, what will the pressure gradient be if the aortic valve area (AVA) decreases by one-half?
- **A.** 12 mm Hg
- **B.** 24 mm Hg
- **C.** 48 mm Hg
- **D.** 96 mm Hg

✪✪ Question 6

The Bernoulli equation is used to estimate pressure gradients from Doppler velocities. This equation consists primarily of three components. Which of the following is NOT a component of this equation?
- **A.** Hydraulic resistance
- **B.** Convective acceleration
- **C.** Flow acceleration
- **D.** Viscous friction

✪ Question 7

Underestimation of pressure gradients may occur when various components of the simplified Bernoulli equation ($\Delta P = 4V^2$) are ignored or assumed. Which of the following statements is false regarding the potential underestimation of pressure gradients?

A. Underestimation of pressure gradients may occur in long (>10 mm), narrow (<0.10 cm^2) tubular obstructions at very low flow rates.

B. Underestimation of pressure gradients may occur in severe anemia.

C. Underestimation of pressure gradients may occur in some prosthetic valves as resistance to flow impedes flow dynamics.

D. Underestimation of pressure gradients may occur when there is nonparallel alignment between the Doppler beam and blood flow direction

✪ Question 8

Which of the following might lead to an overestimation of a pressure gradient by application of the simplified Bernoulli equation?

A. Ignoring significant viscous friction

B. Ignoring significant flow acceleration

C. Assuming the velocity proximal to a narrowing is insignificant

D. All the above

✪ Question 9

The peak Doppler velocities are acquired just downstream from the narrowed orifice. This region is referred to as the:

A. Constraining orifice.

B. Proximal flow convergence zone (or radius).

C. Nyquist orifice.

D. Vena contracta.

✪✪ Question 10

In aortic stenosis, the pressure gradient derived at cardiac catheterization is usually lower than the Doppler-derived pressure gradient because:

A. The catheter pressure gradient measures the pressure gradient between the peak left ventricular (LV) and the peak aortic systolic pressures.

B. The catheter pressure gradient measures the pressure gradient after rapid pressure recovery.

C. The catheter pressure gradient does not account for the cardiac output at the peak systolic pressure points.

D. The catheter pressure gradient is derived from LV and aortic systolic pressures measured at the same point in time.

✪✪✪ Question 11

The phenomenon of rapid pressure recovery (RPR) may explain significant discrepancies between Doppler-derived pressure gradients and catheter-derived pressure gradients when there is:

A. Aortic stenosis with ascending aorta less than 30 mm in diameter.

B. Hypertrophic nonobstructive cardiomyopathy.

C. Congenital valvular pulmonary stenosis.

D. A bioprosthetic valve in the aortic position.

✪✪ Question 12

Pressure gradients derived from Doppler velocities are flow dependent. Hence, transvalvular velocities may be increased in the absence of significant valvular stenosis. Which of the following scenarios does not result in increased velocities in the absence of significant valvular stenosis?

A. Increased transaortic velocities in the presence of severe aortic regurgitation

B. Increased transtricuspid velocities in the presence of severe pulmonic regurgitation

C. Increased transmitral velocities in early pregnancy

D. Increased transpulmonary velocities in the presence of a ventricular septal defect

✪✪ Question 13

The right atrial pressure (RAP) is required for the estimation of several intracardiac pressures. Which of the following does not require the RAP in the estimation of the stated intracardiac pressure?

A. The right ventricular systolic pressure (RVSP) from the peak tricuspid regurgitant (TR) velocity

B. The pulmonary artery end-diastolic pressure (PAEDP) from the peak end-diastolic pulmonary regurgitant (PR) velocity

C. The mean pulmonary artery pressure (mPAP) from the peak early diastolic PR velocity

D. The RVSP from the peak ventricular septal defect (VSD) velocity

✪✪ Question 14

The hepatic venous systolic filling fraction (SFF), which is derived from the systolic velocity time integral (VTI_S) and the diastolic velocity time integral (VTI_D), can be used to estimate right atrial pressure. The equation for calculating the SFF is expressed as:

A. $SFF = \left[(VTI_S + VTI_D) \div VTI_S\right] \times 100$
B. $SFF = \left[(VTI_S + VTI_D) \div VTI_D\right] \times 100$
C. $SFF = \left[VTI_S \div (VTI_S + VTI_D)\right] \times 100$
D. $SFF = \left[VTI_D \div (VTI_S + VTI_D)\right] \times 100$

✪ Question 15

Which of the following is NOT indicative of an elevated right atrial pressure (RAP)?

A. Hepatic venous systolic filling fraction of 60%
B. Inferior vena cava (IVC) of 2.2 cm with a 40% inspiratory collapse
C. Interatrial septum persistently bowing right-to-left from the apical 4-chamber view
D. Tricuspid E to e' ratio of 8

✪✪ Question 16

Estimation of the mean pulmonary artery pressure (mPAP) from the peak early diastolic pulmonary regurgitant (PR) velocity assumes that:

A. The square of the early diastolic PR velocity has a quadratic relationship to the mPAP, which is measured in early diastole.
B. The early diastolic PR velocity corresponds to the dicrotic notch on the PA pressure trace, which correlates to the mPAP.
C. The early diastolic PR velocity at the closure of the pulmonary valve approximates one-third of the pulmonary artery pressure, which is equivalent to the mPAP.
D. The peak early diastolic PR velocity reflects the right ventricular-to-right atrial mean pressure gradient, which also correlates to the mPAP.

✪ Question 17

Right ventricular acceleration time (RVAT) can be used to estimate the mean pulmonary artery (mPAP) pressure. Which of the following statements is false?

A. RVAT is measured by either pulsed-wave or continuous-wave Doppler.
B. RVAT is measured from the onset of the right ventricular outflow tract (RVOT) signal to the peak of the RVOT signal.
C. RVAT for estimating the mPAP is only valid if the heart rate is between 60 and 100 bpm.
D. An RVAT greater than 130 ms is usually associated with a normal mPAP.

✪ Question 18

In a normal heart, the velocity time integral (VTI) is lowest at the:

A. Left ventricular outflow tract.
B. Mitral annulus.
C. Right ventricular outflow tract.
D. Tricuspid annulus.

✪✪ Question 19

The aortic valve area (AVA) can be derived from various two-dimensional and spectral Doppler measurements. Which of the following equations CANNOT be used to calculate the aortic valve area (AVA)?

A. $AVA = SV_{LVOT} \div VTI_{AV}$
B. $AVA = (CSA_{LVOT} \times VTI_{LVOT}) \div VTI_{AV}$
C. $AVA = (\pi \times LVOTd^2 \times VTI_{LVOT}) \div VTI_{AV}$
D. $AVA = (LVEDV - LVESV) \div VTI_{AV}$
E. $AVA = (CSA_{LVOT} \times V_{LVOT}) \div V_{AV}$

where CSA_{LVOT} = cross-sectional area of the left ventricular outflow tract (LVOT), LVEDV = left ventricular end-diastolic volume, LVESV = left ventricular end-systolic volume, LVOTd = LVOT diameter, SV_{LVOT} = stroke volume (SV) across the LVOT, VTI_{LVOT} = velocity time integral (VTI) across the LVOT, VTI_{AV} = VTI across the aortic valve (AV).

✪ Question 20

When calculating the mitral valve area (MVA) by the continuity equation, the derived MVA will be:

A. The same size as the anatomical MVA.
B. The functional, not the anatomical MVA.
C. Slightly smaller than the anatomical MVA.
D. Slightly larger than the anatomical MVA.

✪✪ Question 21

The following images were acquired from a 36-year-old female patient with rheumatic mitral valve stenosis and no significant mitral or aortic regurgitation. Based on the data provided in **Figure 10-1A to 10-1D**, which statement is false?

A. The cardiac output is 5.4 L/min.

B. The mitral deceleration time is 602 ms.

C. The MVA by the pressure half-time is 1.3 cm^2.

D. The mitral valve area (MVA) cannot be calculated by the continuity equation as there is no measurement of the mitral annulus.

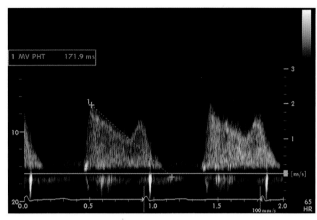

Figure 10-1D

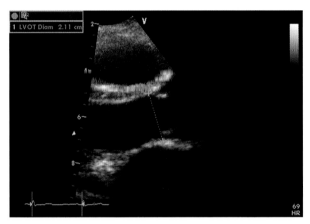

Figure 10-1A

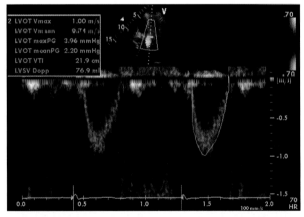

Figure 10-1B

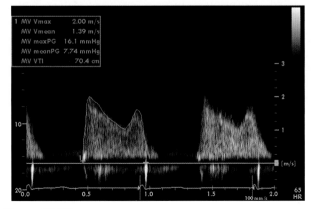

Figure 10-1C

✪✪ Question 22

The images provided in **Figure 10-2A to 10-2C** were acquired from a 65-year-old male patient with a body surface area of 1.82 m^2 and a resting heart rate of 56 bpm. The aortic valve was trileaflet and there was no aortic regurgitation. Based on the measurements shown in these figures, which of the following statements is false?

A. The corrected maximum aortic pressure gradient is 3 mm Hg.

B. The stroke volume is 54 mL.

C. The cardiac output is 5.6 L/min.

D. The cardiac index is 3.1 L/min/m^2.

E. The aortic valve area is 3.3 cm^2.

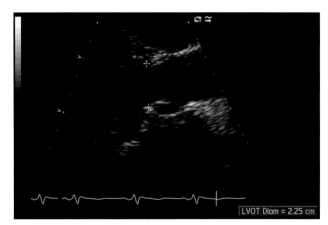

Figure 10-2A

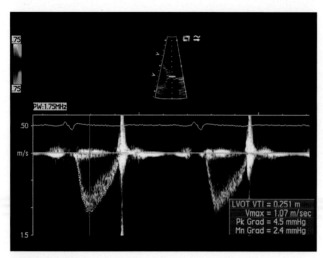

Figure 10-2B

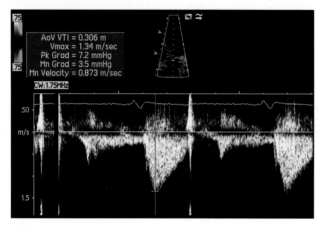

Figure 10-2C

✪✪ Question 23

An 84-year-old female patient has a transthoracic echocardiogram following an ST-elevation myocardial infarction. The tricuspid and pulmonary valves were structurally normal and mild pulmonic regurgitation (PR) was noted. Based on the continuous-wave spectral Doppler tracing of the PR jet (**Figure 10-3**) and the real-time image of the inferior vena cava (**Video 10-1**), which of the following statements is true?

A. Right atrial pressure (RAP) is estimated at 8 mm Hg.

B. Pulmonary artery end-diastolic pressure is approximately 22 mm Hg.

C. Pulmonary artery end-diastolic pressure is approximately 15 mm Hg.

D. Mean pulmonary artery pressure is estimated at 7 mm Hg plus the RAP.

E. Mean pulmonary artery pressure is estimated at 23 mm Hg minus the RAP.

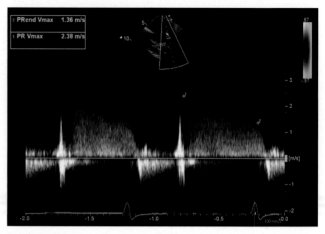

Figure 10-3

✪✪ Question 24

A 57-year-old female patient is referred for a transthoracic echocardiogram to assess the hemodynamic significance of a secundum atrial septal defect (ASD). The tricuspid and pulmonary valves were structurally normal and there was grade 1/4 tricuspid regurgitation present. Based on this information and the images provided in **Figure 10-4A to 10-4E** and **Video 10-2**, which of the following statements is false?

A. The Qp:Qs shunt ratio is approximately 2.4:1.

B. The systemic stroke volume is approximately 141 mL.

C. The shunt volume is approximately 6.4 L/min.

D. The right ventricular systolic pressure is approximately 32 mm Hg.

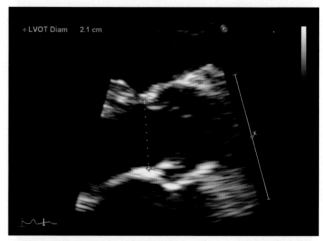

Figure 10-4A

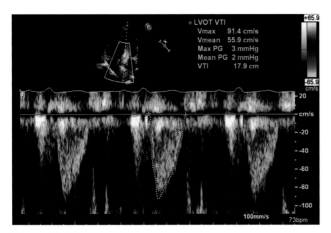

Figure 10-4B

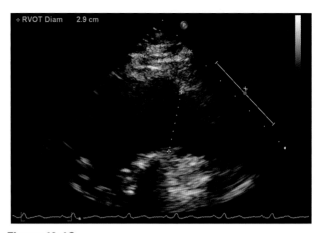

Figure 10-4C

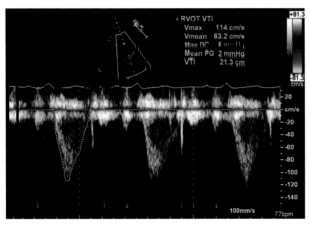

Figure 10-4D

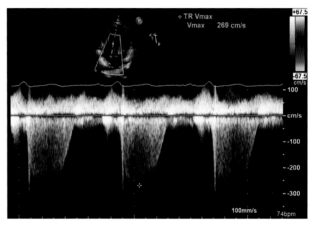

Figure 10-4E

✪✪ Question 25

Based on the data in **Table 10-1**, which statement is correct?

- **A.** The corrected peak transaortic velocity is 2.1 m/s.
- **B.** The corrected maximum transaortic pressure gradient is 18 mm Hg.
- **C.** The corrected Doppler velocity ratio/index is 0.20.
- **D.** The corrected mean transaortic pressure gradient is 28 mm Hg.

Table 10-1.

Left ventricular outflow tract (LVOT) peak velocity	1.5 m/s
LVOT mean pressure gradient	7 mm Hg
LVOT velocity time integral	32 cm
Aortic valve (AV) peak velocity	3.6 m/s
AV mean pressure gradient	35 mm Hg
AV velocity time integral	77 cm

✪✪ Question 26

The images provided were acquired from a 47-year-old woman with a dilated cardiomyopathy, an ejection fraction of 30%, and a blood pressure of 110/86 mm Hg. **Video 10-3** is a zoomed parasternal short-axis view of the aortic valve level, **Figure 10-5A** is the pulsed-wave Doppler trace across the left ventricular outflow tract (LVOT), and **Figure 10-5B** is the continuous-wave Doppler waveform of the mitral regurgitant (MR) jet. Based on the data provided, the estimated left atrial pressure (LAP) is closest to which value?

- **A.** 5 mm Hg
- **B.** 10 mm Hg
- **C.** 15 mm Hg
- **D.** 20 mm Hg

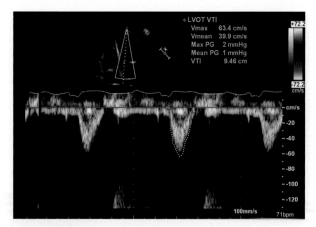

Figure 10-5A

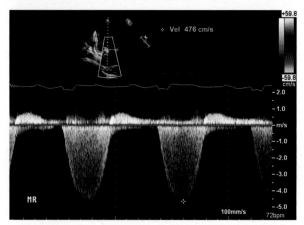

Figure 10-5B

✪✪ Question 27

Observe the pulsed-wave Doppler trace of transmitral inflow (**Figure 10-6A**) and the continuous-wave Doppler trace of mitral regurgitation (**Figure 10-6B**) acquired in a patient with a blood pressure of 120/80 mm Hg. What is the most likely diagnosis?

A. Significant aortic stenosis
B. Significant aortic regurgitation
C. Significant mitral regurgitation
D. Acute pulmonary embolism

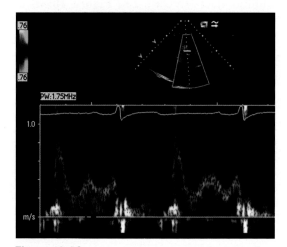

Figure 10-6A

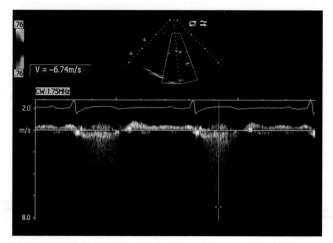

Figure 10-6B

✪✪ Question 28

A 26-year-old male patient is referred for a transthoracic echocardiogram to assess the severity of mitral regurgitation (MR). Based on the images provided in **Figure 10-7A** and **10-7B**, which of the following statements is true?

A. Vena contracta of the MR jet is expected to be less than 0.7 cm.
B. Effective regurgitant orifice area of MR is approximately 0.50 cm².
C. Instantaneous flow rate across the mitral valve is approximately 224 mL/s.
D. MR severity is moderate (grade II).
E. Mitral regurgitant volume is approximately 52 mL per beat.

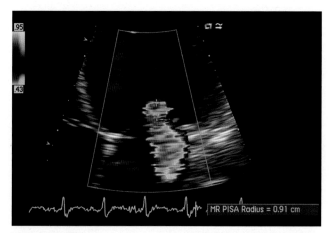

Figure 10-7A

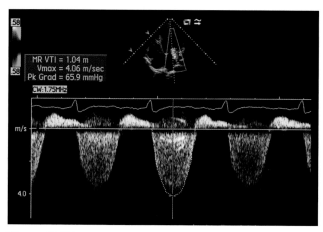

Figure 10-7B

✪✪✪ Question 29

A 59-year-old male patient with aortic stenosis is referred for a transthoracic echocardiogram. There was no mitral stenosis and grade 1/4 mitral regurgitation, and the blood pressure was 118/74 mm Hg. The continuous-wave Doppler trace recorded across the aortic valve (**Figure 10-8**) is shown below.

Based on the data shown in **Figure 10-8**, it can be concluded that:

A. The pressure half-time (PHT) is consistent with severe aortic regurgitation (AR).

B. The left ventricular systolic pressure (LVSP) is 179 mm Hg.

C. The aortic valve area (AVA) calculated using the continuity equation will not be accurate because there is AR present.

D. The left ventricular end-diastolic pressure (LVEDP) is estimated at 25 mm Hg.

E. All the above are correct.

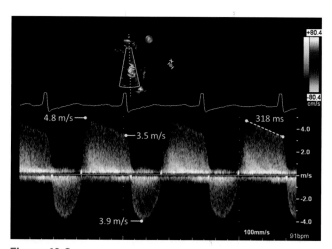

Figure 10-8

✪✪ Question 30

A 73-year-old man is referred for a transthoracic echocardiogram for the assessment of aortic regurgitation (AR) severity. All other cardiac valves are structurally normal with no significant regurgitation and there is no intracardiac shunt present. Based on the data provided in **Figure 10-9A to 10-9E**, which statement is true?

A. The cardiac output is 6.9 L/min.

B. The aortic effective regurgitant orifice area is 0.23 cm².

C. The aortic regurgitant volume is 59 mL.

D. The aortic regurgitant fraction is 59%.

E. There is severe AR.

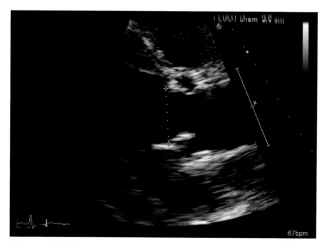

Figure 10-9A

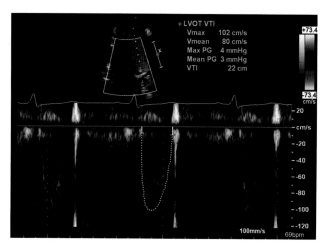

Figure 10-9B

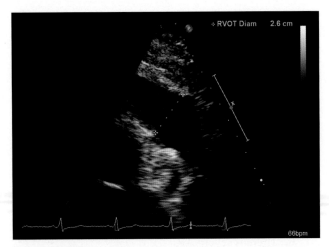

Figure 10-9C

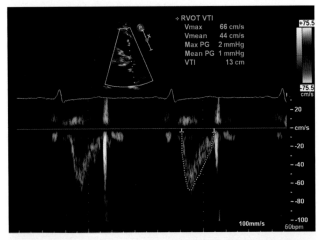

Figure 10-9D

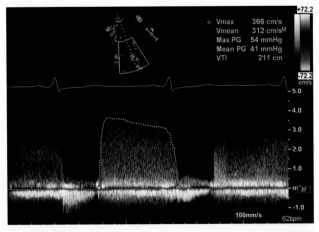

Figure 10-9E

✪✪✪ Question 31

A 30-year-old male patient was referred for a transthoracic echocardiogram following an aortic valve replacement (23 mm bileaflet mechanical ATS) and an attempted closure of a perimembranous ventricular septal defect (VSD). The blood pressure was 116/70 mm Hg, the tricuspid and pulmonary valves were structurally normal, and no significant valvular regurgitation was detected. Based on the images provided (**Figure 10-10A to 10-10F**), which of the following statements is false?

- **A.** The aortic valve replacement (AVR) effective orifice area of 1.4 cm² is overestimated.
- **B.** There is a residual VSD with a Qp:Qs shunt ratio of 1.6:1.
- **C.** There is a residual VSD with a significant elevation in the right ventricular systolic pressure (RVSP).
- **D.** The pulmonic flow rate is 7.8 L/min.

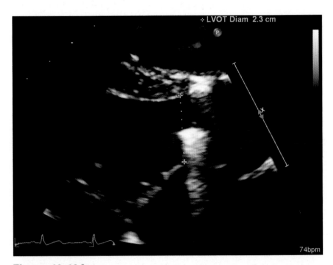

Figure 10-10A

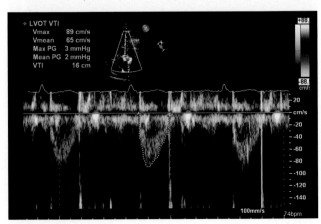

Figure 10-10B

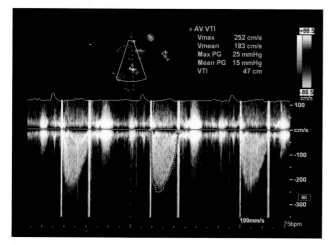

Figure 10-10C

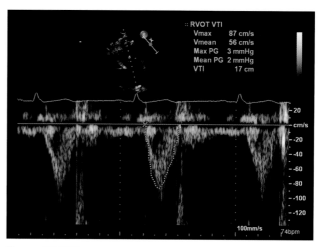

Figure 10-10E

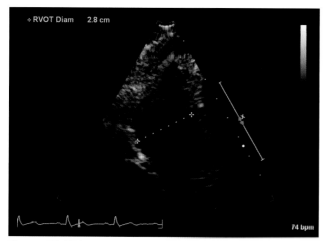

Figure 10-10D

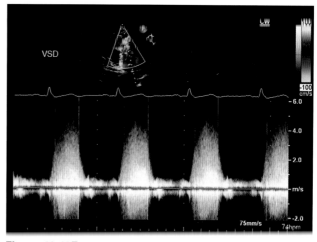

Figure 10-10F

⭐ Question 32

Based on the measurements shown in **Figure 10-11**, which of the following is true?

A. Left ventricular (LV) systolic function is normal.

B. LV systolic function is abnormal.

C. Left ventricular filling pressures (LVFP) are elevated.

D. A and C.

E. B and C.

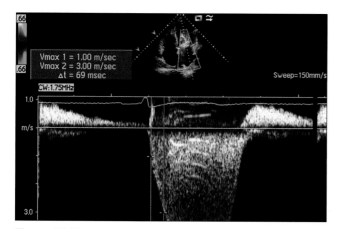

Figure 10-11

✪✪✪ Question 33

The following images were acquired from a 77-year-old female patient with a 33 mm St. Jude mitral valve replacement (MVR). The pulmonary valve was structurally normal with mild pulmonary regurgitation. Based on the data provided in **Figure 10-12A to 10-12D**, all of the following statements are true except:

A. The right ventricular systolic pressure (RVSP) is estimated at 76 mm Hg.

B. Mean pulmonary artery pressure (mPAP) is estimated at 50 mm Hg.

C. The tricuspid effective regurgitant orifice area (EROA) is 0.4 cm^2.

D. Tricuspid regurgitant volume is 49 mL.

E. The mitral valve area by pressure half-time is 2.1 cm^2.

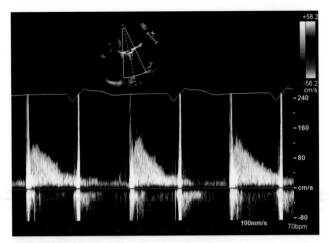

Figure 10-12A

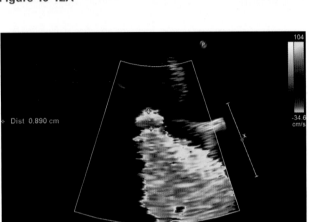

Figure 10-12B

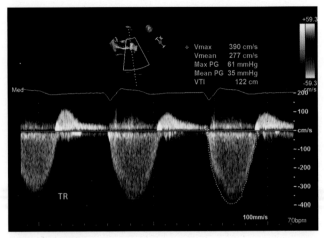

Figure 10-12C

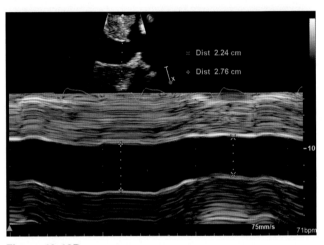

Figure 10-12D

✪✪✪ Question 34

▶ The images provided were acquired from a 79-year-old female patient with a systolic murmur and left ventricular hypertrophy on the electrocardiogram (ECG). The blood pressure was 112/73 mm Hg and the left atrial pressure (LAP) was estimated at 10 mm Hg. **Video 10-4** is an apical 4-chamber view and **Figure 10-13** is continuous-wave Doppler trace of mitral regurgitation (MR). Based on this information, which of the following statements is true:

A. The peak left ventricular outflow tract (LVOT) velocity will exceed the peak MR velocity.

B. The MR profile is consistent with mitral valve prolapse.

C. The aortic valve M-mode trace will show early systolic closure.

D. The maximal instantaneous LVOT pressure gradient is 89 mm Hg.

E. The left ventricular systolic pressure (LVSP) is 190 mm Hg.

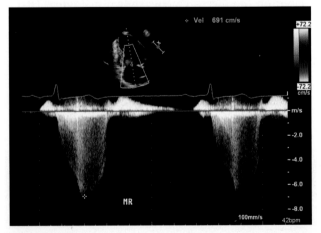

Figure 10-13

✪✪ Question 35

Table 10-2 lists the findings of a 76-year-old female patient who was admitted to the coronary care unit with unstable angina and shortness of breath. There was no history of prior cardiac surgery or other cardiac interventional procedures.

Table 10-2.

Heart rate in sinus rhythm	70 bpm
Blood pressure	90/50 mm Hg
Pulmonary artery wedge pressure (PAWP) by Swan-Ganz catheter	34 mm Hg
Left ventricular ejection fraction (LVEF)	38%
Mitral regurgitation (MR) grade	Mild

Which of the following transmitral inflow profiles is the most likely in this patient?

  A. Figure 10-14A
  B. Figure 10-14B
  C. Figure 10-14C
  D. Figure 10-14D
  E. Figure 10-14E

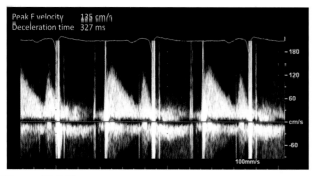

Figure 10-14A

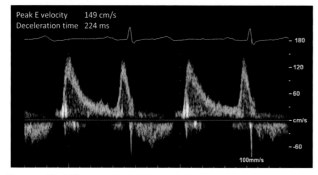

Figure 10-14B

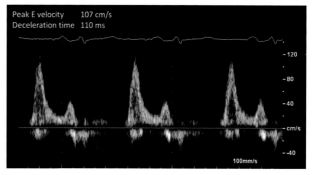

Figure 10-14C

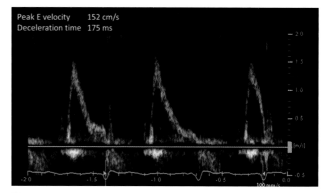

Figure 10-14D

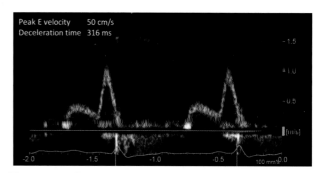

Figure 10-14E

✪✪ Question 36

A 30-year-old female patient was referred for a transthoracic echocardiogram for the investigation of a cardiac murmur. Mitral regurgitation (MR) was noted on this study. In addition, the left atrial pressure was estimated at 10 mm Hg and no aortic stenosis was present. The proximal isovelocity surface area (PISA) of the MR jet (**Figure 10-15A**) and the continuous-wave Doppler tracing across the mitral valve (**Figure 10-15B**) were acquired from the apical 4-chamber view. Based on the information provided, it can be concluded that:

  A. The patient was hypertensive at the time of this study.
  B. The mitral regurgitant fraction is 45%.

C. The regurgitant volume is indicative of mild (Grade I) MR.

D. The effective regurgitant orifice area reflects the severity of mitral regurgitation (MR).

E. The etiology of mitral regurgitation (MR) cannot be determined from this information alone.

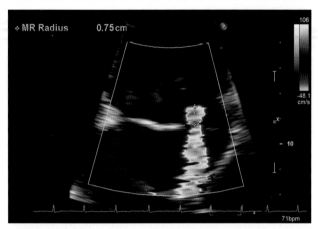

Figure 10-15A

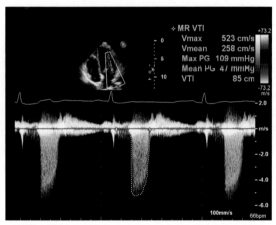

Figure 10-15B

✪✪✪ Question 37

Observe the three spectral Doppler traces provided of continuous-wave Doppler across the pulmonary valve (**Figure 10-16A**), continuous-wave Doppler of tricuspid regurgitation (**Figure 10-16B**), and pulsed-wave Doppler of the hepatic vein (**Figure 10-16C**). The blood pressure was 96/60 mm Hg. Based on these traces, which of the following statements is false?

A. The right atrial pressure is elevated.

B. There is moderate pulmonary stenosis.

C. There is pulmonary hypertension.

D. There will be systolic and diastolic flattening of the interventricular septum.

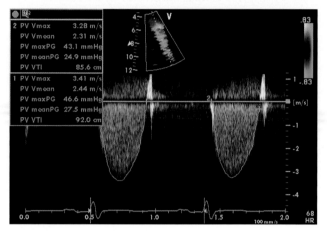

Figure 10-16A

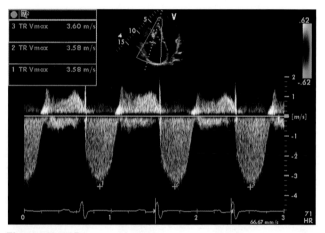

Figure 10-16B

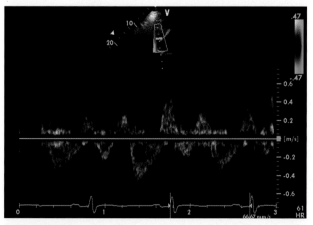

Figure 10-16C

✪✪✪ Question 38

A 36-year-old woman with a murmur is referred for a transthoracic echocardiogram. The study revealed a patent ductus arteriosus (PDA), structurally normal intracardiac valves, mild tricuspid regurgitation, and no significant pulmonary or aortic regurgitation. **Table 10-3** lists the additional findings of this study.

Based on this information, which of the following statements is true?

Table 10-3.

Left ventricular outflow tract (LVOT) diameter	2.6 cm
LVOT velocity time integral (VTI)	23 cm
Right ventricular outflow tract (RVOT) diameter	2.3 cm
RVOT VTI	12 cm
Heart rate	65 bpm
Right ventricular systolic pressure (RVSP)	35 mm Hg
Blood pressure	125/84 mm Hg

A. The PDA systolic velocity will be approximately 2.9 m/s.
B. The ratio of pulmonic to systemic blood flow (Qp:Qs) is less than 1.
C. Systemic blood flow (Qs) is 7.9 L/min.
D. The right heart chambers will be dilated.
E. None of the above.

ANSWERS

1. **Answer: C.** Poiseuille's law for fluids describes the relationship between pressure difference (ΔP), resistance (R), and volumetric flow rate (Q):

$$Q = \Delta P \div R$$

Therefore, answer C is correct.

Answer A is incorrect since Bernoulli's law describes the relationship between pressure difference (or pressure gradients) and velocity.

Answer B is incorrect since the continuity principle is based on the conservation of mass. This principle explains why velocities at the stenosis must be greater than the velocities proximal and distal to the stenosis in order to maintain flow.

Answer D is incorrect since the Doppler effect describes the assumed change in frequency or wavelength that occurs due to relative motion between the wave source, the receiver of the wave, and the reflector of the wave.

TECHNICAL TIP

Sometimes Poiseuille's law is referred to as Ohm's law. The principles for both laws are similar in that Ohm's law describes electric current flow while Poiseuille's law describes fluid flow. The degree of "flow" for each of these laws is determined by voltage drop (Ohm's law) or pressure drop (Poiseuille's law) and resistance (both laws).

2. **Answer: B.** As previously described, Poiseuille's law for fluids describes the relationship between pressure difference (ΔP), resistance (R), and volumetric flow rate (Q) and is expressed by the equation:

$$Q = \Delta P \div R \qquad (1)$$

Therefore, answer B is correct.

This equation may be translated to determine systemic vascular resistance (SVR) and pulmonary vascular resistance (PVR). For instance, SVR is derived from: (1) the pressure difference across the systemic circulation from its beginning to its end (the difference between the mean arterial pressure [mAP] and the central venous pressure [CVP]) and (2) the cardiac output (CO), which is equivalent to the volumetric flow rate:

$$SVR = (mAP - CVP) \div CO \qquad (2)$$

PVR is derived from: (1) the pressure difference across the pulmonary circulation from its beginning to its end (the difference between the mean pulmonary arterial pressure [mPAP] and the pulmonary capillary wedge pressure [PCWP]) and (2) the cardiac output (CO), which is equivalent to the volumetric flow rate:

$$\left[PVR = (mPAP - PCWP) \div CO\right] \qquad (3)$$

KEY POINT

Understanding Poiseuille's law, which describes the relationship between pressure difference, resistance, and volumetric flow rate, aids in the understanding of how the systemic vascular resistance and the pulmonary vascular resistance can be derived by echocardiography.

3. **Answer: D.** Resistance to flow is determined by the viscosity of blood (η), the radius of the vessel lumen (r), and the length of the vessel (L) and is expressed by the following equation:

$$R = [8 \times L \times \eta] \div [\pi \times r^4] \qquad (1)$$

Because the $8 \div \pi$ is a constant, this relationship may be simplified to:

$$R \infty [L \times \eta] \div r^4 \qquad (2)$$

Therefore, answer D is correct as it can be appreciated that resistance to flow will be increased as the radius increases.

Answers A and B are incorrect as a decrease in either of these variables will decrease resistance (see Equations (1) and (2)). Answer C is incorrect as the flow rate is determined by the pressure difference and resistance to flow, and therefore, changes to the flow rate do not affect the resistance to flow.

TEACHING POINT

As previously described, volumetric flow rate (Q) is determined by the pressure difference (ΔP) and the resistance (R) and this relationship is expressed by Poiseuille's law:

$$Q = \Delta P \div R \qquad (1)$$

Resistance to flow is determined by the viscosity of blood (η), the radius of the vessel lumen (r), and the length of the vessel (L) and is expressed by the following equation:

$$R = [8 \times L \times \eta] \div [\pi \times r^4] \qquad (2)$$

Thus, by substituting Equation (2) for resistance in Equation (1), flow rate (Q) can be derived as:

$$Q = (\Delta P \times [\pi \times r^4]) \div [8 \times L \times \eta] \qquad (3)$$

Since the viscosity of blood and the length of vessels within the cardiovascular system do not change, the primary determinant of the flow rate (Q) is the pressure difference (ΔP) and the radius of the vessel (r).

4. **Answer: C.** As previously discussed (see answer outline for Question 2), the relationship between flow rate (Q), pressure difference or gradient (ΔP), and resistance (R) is expressed as:

$$Q = \Delta P \div R \qquad (1)$$

Resistance to flow is derived from the viscosity of blood (η), the radius of the vessel lumen (r), and the length of the vessel (L):

$$R \infty [L \times \eta] \div r^4 \qquad (2)$$

Since the viscosity of blood and the length of vessels within the cardiovascular system do not change, resistance to flow is inversely proportional to the r^4:

$$R \infty 1 \div r^4 \qquad (3)$$

Furthermore, as changes in diameter (d) and radius (r) are directly proportional to each other ($d = 2r$; therefore $d \propto r$), diameter can be substituted for radius:

$$R \infty 1 \div d^4 \qquad (4)$$

Accounting for these associations, the relationship between Q, ΔP, and diameter can be expressed as:

$$Q \infty \Delta P \times d^4 \qquad (5)$$

It is apparent from this relationship that if the Q remains constant, then the primary determinant of the ΔP is the diameter:

$$\Delta P = 1 \div d^4 \qquad (6)$$

Since the diameter is raised to the fourth power, if the diameter is halved, then ΔP would need to increase 16-fold to maintain the same flow rate. For example, if the diameter is 1 cm then:

$$\Delta P = 1 \div d^4 = 1 \div 1^4 = 1 \qquad (7)$$

If the diameter is halved to 0.5 cm then:

$$\Delta P = 1 \div d^4 = 1 \div 0.5^4 = 16 \qquad (8)$$

Therefore, answer C is correct.

5. **Answer: B.** As previously discussed, if the flow rate (Q) remains constant, the primary determinant of the ΔP can be expressed as:

$$\Delta P = 1 \div d^4 \qquad (1)$$

Since the diameter is raised to the fourth power, if the diameter is halved, the pressure gradient would need to increase 16-fold to maintain the same flow rate. However, halving the cross-sectional area (CSA) is not the same as halving the diameter. CSA can be derived from the diameter as:

$$CSA = 0.785 \times d^2 \quad (2)$$

Rearranging this equation for the diameter, then:

$$d = \sqrt{(CSA \div 0.785)} \quad (3)$$

By substituting the diameter in Equation (3) for the diameter in Equation (1), then:

$$\Delta P = 1 \div \left[\sqrt{(CSA \div 0.785)} \right]^4 \quad (4)$$

Equation (4) can be further simplified as:

$$\Delta P = 1 \div (CSA \div 0.785)^2 \quad (5)$$

Since the CSA is squared if the CSA is halved, the pressure gradient would need to increase 4-fold to maintain the same flow rate. For example, if the CSA is 0.785 cm^2 then:

$$\Delta P = 1 \div (0.785 \div 0.785)^2 = 1 \div 1^2 = 1 \quad (6)$$

If the CSA is halved to 0.3925 cm^2 then:

$$\Delta P = 1 \div (0.3925 \div 0.785)^2 = 1 \div 0.5^2 = 4 \quad (7)$$

Therefore, answer B is correct. If the pressure gradient is 6 mm Hg and the AVA decreases by one-half, the resultant pressure gradient will be 24 mm Hg (6 × 4 = 24).

KEY POINT
By decreasing the cross-sectional area by one-half and to maintain a constant flow rate, the pressure gradient must increase to a value four times the original pressure gradient.

6. **Answer: A.** Hydraulic resistance refers to the resistance to flow which is determined by the viscosity of blood (η), the radius of the vessel lumen (r), and the length of the vessel (L). Hence, answer A (hydraulic resistance) is not a component of the Bernoulli equation.

The three primary components of the Bernoulli equation include (1) convective acceleration, which occurs whenever there is a change in the cross-sectional area of flow, (2) flow acceleration, which refers to the pressure drop required to overcome inertial forces between two points, and (3) viscous friction, which refers to the loss of velocity due to friction between blood cells and vessel walls between two points:

$$\Delta P = \frac{1}{2}\rho \left(V_2^2 - V_1^2 \right) + \rho \int_1^2 \frac{d\bar{v}}{dt} \times d\bar{s} + R\left(\bar{\eta}\right)$$

$$\frac{\text{Pressure}}{\text{difference}} = \frac{\text{coversion}}{\text{accelaration}} + \frac{\text{flow}}{\text{acceleration}} + \frac{\text{viscous}}{\text{friction}}$$

where ΔP = the pressure difference between 2 points, V_1 = velocity at proximal location, V_2 = velocity at distal location; ρ = density of blood, dv/dt = change in velocity over the change in time, ds = distance over which pressure decreases, R = viscous resistance in the vessel, η = viscosity.

7. **Answer: B.** Overestimation, rather than underestimation, of the pressure gradient may occur when there is severe anemia (hemoglobin <8.0 g/dL). In these instances, the blood viscosity is reduced, so estimating the pressure gradient via $4V^2$ will overestimate the pressure gradient. Hence, answer B is the false statement.

Answer A is a true statement. Viscous forces may become significant in the presence of long (>10 mm), narrow (<0.10 cm^2) tubular obstructions at very low flow rates (Reynolds number <500). Hence, ignoring this component of the Bernoulli equation will result in an underestimation of the pressure gradient.

Answer C is a true statement. In some types of prosthetic valves (especially mechanical valves), a greater increase in flow acceleration may be required to open the valve. As flow acceleration is ignored in the simplified form of the Bernoulli equation, the pressure gradient will be underestimated.

Answer D is a true statement. Nonparallel alignment of the ultrasound beam with flow will result in an underestimation of the peak velocity and thus an underestimation of the pressure gradient.

KEY POINTS
Using the simplified Bernoulli equation ($\Delta P = 4V^2$) may underestimate pressure gradients in certain clinical situations and in some types of prosthetic valves. Parallel alignment of the Doppler beam with blood flow direction is crucial in avoiding underestimation of the peak velocity and therefore underestimation of the pressure gradient. For this reason, multiple windows and off-axis imaging should be used to ensure parallel alignment. Color Doppler is especially useful for finding the correct parallel alignment in normal scanning positions and for off-axis images.

8. **Answer: C.** The simplified Bernoulli equation estimates the pressure gradient based on the peak velocity (V) across a narrowing:

$$\Delta P = 4V^2 \qquad (1)$$

In the setting of an elevated velocity proximal to a narrowing (V_1), using the simplified Bernoulli equation, which assumes that V_1 is insignificant, will overestimate the pressure gradient. Therefore, answer D is correct.

Answers A and B are incorrect because when viscous friction and/or flow acceleration are significant and are ignored, the pressure gradient will be underestimated.

KEY POINT

When V_1 becomes significant, the maximum and mean pressure gradients must be corrected by using the "expanded" Bernoulli equation:

$$\Delta P = 4\left(V_2^2 - V_1^2\right) \qquad (1)$$

where V_2 is the velocity at the narrowing and V_1 is the velocity proximal to the narrowing.

Mathematically, Equation (1) is the same as:

$$\Delta P = \left(4V_2^2\right) - \left(4V_1^2\right) \qquad (2)$$

Therefore, corrected pressure gradients can be derived by simply subtracting the proximal pressure gradient from the pressure gradient across the narrowing.

V_1 becomes significant when this velocity is ≥1.2 m/s. Examples of clinical situations where V_1 is significant include aortic stenosis with a high output state, significant aortic regurgitation, or coexistent left ventricular outflow tract obstruction, and in coarctation of the aorta.

9. **Answer: D.** As flow passes through a narrowed orifice, it streamlines and narrows. The narrowest region downstream from a narrowed orifice is referred to as the vena contracta (**Figure 10-17**). Therefore, answer D is correct.

Answer A is incorrect since the constraining orifice is the narrowed orifice, which is usually at the valvular level.

Answer B is incorrect since the proximal flow convergence zone (or radius) is the region proximal to, not downstream from, a narrowed orifice; this region is most commonly used in the assessment of valvular regurgitation.

Answer C is incorrect. The Nyquist *orifice* is a fictitious term. The Nyquist *limit* is the term used to describe the maximum Doppler shift that can be unambiguously displayed before aliasing occurs.

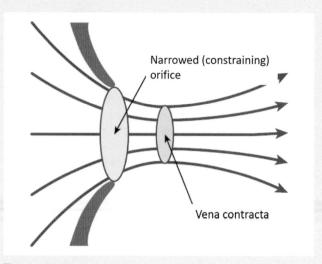

Narrowed (constraining) orifice

Vena contracta

Figure 10-17

10. **Answer: A.** As illustrated in **Figure 10-18**, the pressure gradient derived at cardiac catheterization in aortic stenosis is usually lower than the Doppler-derived pressure gradient. This is because the cardiac catheterization pressure gradient measures the pressure difference between the peak left ventricular (LV) pressure and the peak aortic pressure; this is referred to as the peak-to-peak (P2P) pressure gradient. The Doppler-derived pressure gradient measures the maximum instantaneous pressure gradient (MIPG) between the peak LV pressure and the aortic pressure at that same instant in time. Hence, the catheter-derived P2P pressure gradient is usually lower than the Doppler-derived MIPG.

Answer B is incorrect. As the name suggests, rapid pressure recovery refers to a rapid recovery of pressure downstream from the stenotic valve. Hence, the pull-back catheter pressure gradient, measuring the pressure drop between the LV and the proximal aorta, may be significantly less than the Doppler-derived pressure gradient measured from the peak aortic velocity at the vena contracta. However, this phenomenon is not common.

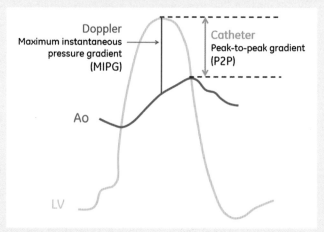

Doppler
Maximum instantaneous pressure gradient (MIPG)

Catheter
Peak-to-peak gradient (P2P)

Ao

LV

Figure 10-18

Answer C is incorrect as the cardiac output does not directly influence the systolic pressure gradient between the LV and aorta when compared with the Doppler-derived pressure gradient.

Answer D is incorrect. As previously described, the catheter pressure gradient is derived from the peak LV and the peak aortic systolic pressures, which do not occur at the same point in time (aortic pressure peaks *after* the LV pressure).

KEY POINT

In aortic stenosis, the Doppler-derived maximum instantaneous gradient often exceeds the catheter-derived peak-to-peak pressure gradient. Therefore, the two measurements should not be used synonymously.

11. **Answer: A.** As the name suggests, rapid pressure recovery (RPR) refers to the rapid recovery of pressure after flow has passed through a narrowed orifice. As illustrated in **Figure 10-19A**, in the normal situation, pressure gradually recovers downstream from the narrowest orifice. The pressure gradients derived by Doppler are acquired from the peak velocity recorded within the vena contracta (green circle number 1), while the catheter-derived pressure is obtained further downstream from the vena contracta (blue circle number 2). It can be appreciated that while the Doppler-derived gradient will be higher than the catheter-derived gradient, they will not be too dissimilar. When there is RPR as illustrated in **Figure 10-19B**, the pressure downstream from the vena contracta recovers very quickly; hence, the catheter-derived pressure gradient (blue circle number 2) will be much lower than the Doppler-derived gradient (green circle number 1). RPR occurs when there is a tunnel-like obstruction to flow and has been reported in patients with aortic stenosis with an ascending aorta less than

30 mm in diameter. Therefore, answer A is the correct choice.

Answer B is incorrect since RPR is not seen in hypertrophic *nonobstructive* cardiomyopathy but may be seen in hypertrophic *obstructive* cardiomyopathy.

Answer C is incorrect since RPR is not seen in congenital valvular pulmonary stenosis. RPR, however, may be seen in a subpulmonary tunnel.

Answer D is incorrect. RPR does not occur in bioprosthetic valves. RPR has been reported in small bileaflet prosthetic valves and ball-cage valves.

KEY POINTS

Rapid pressure recovery (RPR) is a complex concept that may result in an apparent overestimation of the Doppler-derived pressure gradients when compared with the catheter-derived pressure gradients. RPR is seen in tunnel-like obstructions and in certain types of prosthetic valves such as ball-cage and bileaflet mechanical valves. Recognition of this phenomenon is important to avoid overestimating the severity of an obstruction or mistaking high prosthetic valve gradients for prosthetic valve obstruction.

12. **Answer: B.** Transtricuspid velocities are not increased in the presence of severe pulmonic regurgitation (PR). In the presence of severe PR, the transpulmonary velocities would be increased as flow across the valve includes normal forward flow plus the PR volume. Therefore, answer B is correct.

Answer A is incorrect since the presence of severe aortic regurgitation (AR) often increases the transaortic velocities as flow across the valve includes normal forward flow plus the AR volume.

Answer C is incorrect as increases in transmitral velocities are noted in pregnancy due to a significant increase in the cardiac output. In particular, the peak transmitral *E* velocity increases up to 13%

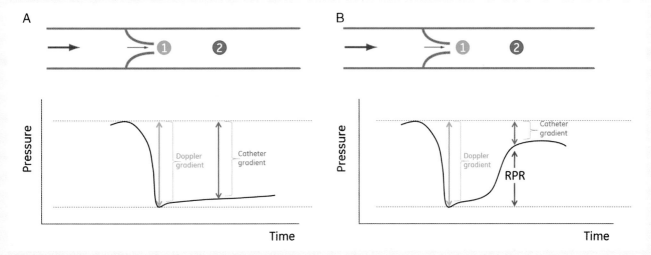

Figure 10-19

during the first trimester and remains at the high end of normal throughout pregnancy while the peak transmitral A velocity increases maximally in the third trimester (Mesa et al., 1999).

Answer D is incorrect since the presence of a ventricular septal defect (VSD) often increases the transpulmonary velocities as flow across the valve includes normal forward flow plus the VSD volume flow.

13. **Answer: D.** The peak VSD velocity occurs in systole and this reflects the difference between the left ventricular systolic pressure (LVSP) and RVSP:

$$\Delta P_{VSD} = 4V_{VSD^2} = LVSP - RVSP \quad (1)$$

In the absence of aortic stenosis or LV outflow tract obstruction, the systolic LV pressure is assumed to be the same as the systolic blood pressure (SBP), so Equation (1) can be rewritten as:

$$4V_{VSD^2} = SBP - RVSP \quad (2)$$

Therefore, the RVSP can then be estimated by rearranging Equation (2):

$$RVSP = SBP - 4V_{VSD^2} \quad (3)$$

Hence, Answer D is correct as the estimation of the RVSP from a VSD velocity does not require an estimation of the RAP.

Answers A-C all require an estimation of the RAP to calculate the stated intracardiac pressure. The TR velocity (V_{TR}) reflects the difference between the RVSP and the RAP:

$$\Delta P_{TR} = 4V_{TR^2} = RVSP - RAP \quad (4)$$

Therefore, if the RAP is estimated or known, then Equation (4) can be rewritten as:

$$RVSP = 4V_{TR^2} + RAP \quad (5)$$

The PR end-diastolic velocity (V_{PR-ED}) reflects the difference between the pulmonary artery end-diastolic pressure (PAEDP) and the RV end-diastolic pressure (RVEDP):

$$\Delta P_{PR-ED} = 4V_{PR-ED^2} = PAEDP - RVEDP \quad (6)$$

In the absence of tricuspid stenosis, it can be assumed that the RVEDP is the same as the RAP; hence, Equation (6) becomes:

$$4V_{PR-ED^2} = PAEDP - RAP \quad (7)$$

Therefore, if the RAP is estimated or known, then Equation (7) can be rewritten as:

$$PAEDP = 4V_{PR-ED^2} + RAP \quad (8)$$

The mPAP can also be estimated from the peak PR early-diastolic velocity (V_{PR-EaD}) and the RAP as:

$$mPAP = 4V_{PR-EaD^2} + RAP \quad (9)$$

14. **Answer: C.** The hepatic venous systolic filling fraction (SFF) is derived from the velocity time integral of the systolic and diastolic hepatic venous signals and is expressed as:

$$SFF = VTI_s \div (VTI_s + VTI_D) \times 100 \quad (1)$$

Therefore, answer C is correct. This SFF can also be simplified by measuring just the peak systolic velocity (V_S) and the peak diastolic velocity (V_D):

$$SFF = V_s \div (V_s + V_D) \times 100 \quad (2)$$

15. **Answer: A.** The hepatic venous systolic filling fraction (SFF) is derived from the velocity time integral (or peak velocities) of the systolic and diastolic hepatic venous signals and is expressed by either of the equations below:

$$SFF = VTI_s \div (VTI_s + VTI_D) \times 100 \quad (1)$$

$$SFF = V_s \div (V_s + V_D) \times 100 \quad (2)$$

where VTI_S is the systolic velocity time integral, VTI_D is the diastolic velocity time integral, V_S is the peak systolic velocity, and V_D is the peak diastolic velocity. As RAP increases, the pressure gradient between the hepatic veins and the RA decreases, thus lowering the forward systolic flow. As a result, the SFF decreases as RAP increases. A SFF less than 55% predicts an elevated RAP. Hence, answer C is correct as a hepatic venous SFF of 60% suggests a normal RAP.

Answer B is incorrect since a dilated IVC (>2.1 cm) that collapses less than 50% is indicative of an elevated RAP.

Answer C is incorrect as persistent bowing of the interatrial septum from right-to-left suggests that the RAP is consistently higher than the left atrial pressure (LAP). This contrasts with a normal RAP where the interatrial septum bows slightly left-to-right because the LAP is normally slightly higher than the RAP.

Answer D is incorrect since a tricuspid *E*/*e*' ratio greater than 6 predicts a mean RAP greater than 10 mm Hg.

While the IVC size and collapsibility index are most commonly used to estimate RAP, secondary indices such as the hepatic venous SFF and the tricuspid *E*/*e*' ratio may also be useful in confirming the presence or absence of elevated RAP. For example, in intermediate cases where the IVC is dilated but collapses more than 50% or when the IVC is of normal size but collapses less than 50%, the absence or presence of secondary indices of elevated RAP can be used to downgrade RAP to normal or upgrade RAP to high.

16. **Answer: B.** The dicrotic notch on the pulmonary arterial (PA) pressure tracing reflects the closure of the pulmonary valve and the end of right ventricular (RV) ejection. The pulmonary pressure at this point also corresponds to the mPAP (Figure 10-20). The peak early diastolic velocity occurs after closure of the pulmonary valve (PV); hence, the peak early diastolic velocity can be used to estimate the pressure gradient at PV closure, or at the dicrotic notch. Therefore, as the PA pressure at the dicrotic notch reflects the mPAP, it follows that the PR velocity at early diastole will also reflect the mPAP. Hence, answer B is correct. Furthermore, adding the RAP to this derived pressure improves the correlation between the actual mPAP and the Doppler-estimated mPAP.

17. **Answer: A.** Right ventricular acceleration time (RVAT) is acquired using pulsed-wave Doppler with a 3 to 5 mm sample volume placed within the right ventricular outflow tract. Pulsed-wave Doppler (PWD) rather than continuous-wave Doppler was used during validation studies comparing RVAT with mPAP. Therefore, answer A is correct as estimation of the RVAT by either pulsed-wave or continuous-wave Doppler is the false statement.

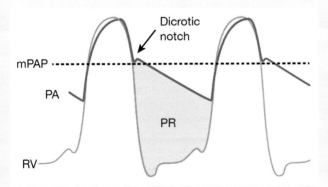

Figure 10-20 Reproduced with permission by Echotext Pty Ltd, from Anderson B. *Doppler haemodynamic calculations.* In: Echocardiography: The Normal Examination and Echocardiographic Measurements. 3rd ed. Australia: Echotext Pty Ltd; 2017:227, chap 11.

Answer B is a true statement. RVAT is measured as the time interval between the onset of the RVOT signal and the peak velocity point of the RVOT signal.

Answer C is a true statement. Estimation of the mPAP via the RVAT is only valid between heart rates of 60 and 100 bpm. Heart rates faster than 100 bpm may shorten the RVAT. However, it has been shown that with an mPAP greater than 25 mm Hg, increases in heart rate have no significant effect on acceleration time.

Answer D is a true statement. An RVAT greater than 130 ms is usually associated with a normal mPAP, while an RVAT less than 105 ms is highly suggestive of pulmonary hypertension.

18. **Answer: D.** Recall that the stroke volume (SV) is derived from the VTI and the cross-sectional area (CSA) of the valve:

$$SV = CSA \times VTI$$

In the normal heart, the SV across all four valves will be the same. Therefore, if the SV is constant, as the CSA decreases, the VTI must increase and as the CSA increases, the VTI must decrease. As the tricuspid annulus has the largest CSA, it will have the smallest VTI. Hence, answer D is correct.

19. **Answer: C.** The AVA is calculated from the continuity equation assuming that the stroke volume at the LVOT (SV_{LVOT}) is the same as the stroke volume across the aortic valve (SV_{AV}).

$$SV_{AV} = SV_{LVOT} \tag{1}$$

As previously shown, stroke volume (SV) may be derived from the cross-sectional area (CSA) and the velocity time integral (VTI):

$$SV = CSA \times VTI \tag{2}$$

Therefore, Equations (1) and (2) can be combined and expressed as:

$$CSA_{AV} \times VTI_{AV} = CSA_{LVOT} \times VTI_{LVOT} \tag{3}$$

If the CSA_{LVOT}, the VTI_{LVOT}, and VTI_{AV} are measured, then this equation can be rearranged to calculate the CSA_{AV} which is the AVA:

$$AVA = (CSA_{LVOT} \times VTI_{LVOT}) \div VTI_{AV} \tag{4}$$

As the SV is equal to CSA × VTI (Equation (2)), the AVA can also be derived as:

$$AVA = SV_{LVOT} \div VTI_{AV} \tag{5}$$

The SV can also be estimated from the LVEDV and LVESV as:

$$SV = LVEDV - LVESV \qquad (6)$$

Therefore, the AVA can also be calculated as:

$$AVA = (LVEDV - LVESV) \div VTI_{AV} \qquad (7)$$

Furthermore, because the flow duration through the LVOT and across the aortic valve are the same, the AVA can also be derived by substituting the peak LVOT and AV velocities for the LVOT and AV VTI; hence, Equation (4) may be rewritten as:

$$AVA = (CSA_{LVOT} \times V_{LVOT}) \div V_{AV} \qquad (8)$$

CSA is calculated as:

$$CSA = \pi \times r^2 \qquad (9)$$

where r = radius. Remembering that the radius is simply the diameter (d) divided by 2, then:

$$CSA = \pi \times (d \div 2)^2 \qquad (10)$$

Therefore, by substituting CSA_{LVOT} in Equation (4) for CSA derived by Equation (6)

$$AVA = \left(\pi \times (LVOTd \div 2)^2 \times VTI_{LVOT}\right) \div VTI_{AV} \qquad (11)$$

Therefore, answer C is correct as the equation shown cannot be used to calculate the aortic valve area (AVA) because the LVOTd is not divided by 2. The other equations in answers A, B, D, and E can be used to estimate the AVA.

KEY POINTS

Calculation of the AVA is based on the continuity principle and this assumes that the stroke volume of the LV or through the LVOT is the same as the stroke volume across the aortic valve. The SV through the LVOT can be estimated from the LVOT CSA and VTI, while the SV of the LV can be estimated from the LV end-diastolic and end-systolic volumes. However, as 2D echocardiography tends to underestimate LV volumes, the best method for calculating the stroke volume of the LV (LVOT) is via the CSA and VTI method.

The AVA can also be derived from the peak velocities across the LVOT and AV; this is often referred to as the V_{max} method. However, the most correct method for calculating the AVA is by using the VTIs across the LVOT and AV; this is the VTI method.

TECHNICAL TIPS

The units for the diameter and VTI measurements should be in cm. Hence, the units for SV will be cm^3 or cc or mL and the units for valve areas will be cm^2.

The CSA can also be derived from the diameter as:

$$CSA = 0.785 \times d^2 \qquad (1)$$

This is explained mathematically as follows:

$$
\begin{aligned}
CSA &= \pi \times (d \div 2)^2 \\
&= 3.14 \times (d \div 2)^2 \\
&= 3.14 \times (d^2 \div 2^2) \\
&= (3.14 \div 2^2) \times d^2 \\
&= (3.14 \div 4) \times d^2 \\
&= 0.785 \times d^2
\end{aligned}
$$

20. Answer: C. The MVA derived from the continuity equation is the effective orifice area (EOA), which is calculated at the vena contracta. As previously illustrated in **Figure 10-17**, the vena contracta is located downstream from the constraining orifice or anatomical orifice area. Therefore, answer C is correct since the EOA derived from the continuity equation will be slightly smaller than the anatomical orifice area.

KEY POINT

Hemodynamic methods such as the continuity equation provide an estimation of the effective orifice area (EOA). The EOA is measured downstream from the anatomical orifice area at the vena contracta. As a result, the EOA will be slightly smaller than the true anatomical valve area.

21. Answer: D. In the absence of significant mitral or aortic regurgitation, it can be assumed that the stroke volume across the mitral valve (SV_{MV}) will be the same as the stroke volume through the left ventricular outflow tract (SV_{LVOT}):

$$SV_{MV} = SV_{LVOT} \qquad (1)$$

As previously shown, stroke volume (SV) may be derived from the cross-sectional area (CSA) and the velocity time integral (VTI):

$$SV = CSA \times VTI \qquad (2)$$

Therefore, Equations (1) and (2) can be combined and expressed as:

$$CSA_{MV} \times VTI_{MV} = CSA_{LVOT} \times VTI_{LVOT} \qquad (3)$$

If the CSA_{LVOT}, the VTI_{LVOT}, and VTI_{MV} are measured, then this equation can be rearranged to calculate the CSA_{MV}, which is the MVA:

$$MVA = (CSA_{LVOT} \times VTI_{LVOT}) \div VTI_{MV} \qquad (4)$$

Therefore, answer D is the false statement since the mitral annulus measurement is not required to calculate the MVA by the continuity equation.

Answer A is a true statement as the cardiac output is 5.4 L/min. The cardiac output (CO) can be estimated from the SV_{LVOT} and the heart rate (HR):

$$CO = (SV_{LVOT} \times HR) \div 1000 \qquad (5)$$

The SV_{LVOT} is calculated by multiplying the cross-sectional area, which is derived from the LVOT diameter ($LVOT_d$), by the $LVOT_{VTI}$. Hence, the SV_{LVOT} in this patient is:

$$SV = (0.785 \times 2.11^2) \times 21.9 = 76.5 \, mL \qquad (6)$$

Hence, the CO in this patient is:

$$CO = (76.5 \times 70) \div 1000 = 5.4 \, L/min \qquad (7)$$

Answer B is a true statement as the mitral deceleration time is 602 ms. The mitral deceleration time (DT) can be calculated from the pressure half-time (PHT) as the PHT is 29% of the DT:

$$DT = PHT \div 0.29 \qquad (8)$$

Hence, the DT in this patient is:

$$DT = 174.7 \div 0.29 = 602 \, ms \qquad (9)$$

Answer C is a true statement as MVA by the pressure half-time is 1.3 cm². The MVA by PHT is calculated as:

$$MVA = 220 \div PHT \qquad (10)$$

Hence, the MVA via PHT in this patient is:

$$MVA = 220 \div 174.7 = 1.3 \, cm^2 \qquad (11)$$

Calculations related to this question are summarized in **Table 10-4**.

Table 10-4.

Parameter	Value	Comment
SV (mL)	76.5	Estimated from the LVOT diameter and VTI
CO (L/min)	5.4	Estimated from the SV and HR
MV DT (ms)	602	Estimated from the MV DT
MVA by PHT (cm²)	1.3	Estimated from the PHT

22. **Answer: A.** Correction of the aortic pressure gradients (maximum and mean) is only required when the left ventricular outflow tract (LVOT) velocity exceeds 1.2 m/s. In this patient, the LVOT peak velocity is 1.07 m/s (**Figure 10-2B**). Therefore, correction of the maximum aortic pressure gradient is not required, so answer A is the false statement.

Answer B is a true statement. Stroke volume (SV) is derived from the cross-sectional area (CSA) and the velocity time integral (VTI) of the left ventricular outflow tract (LVOT):

$$SV = CSA_{LVOT} \times VTI_{LVOT} \qquad (1)$$

CSA_{LVOT} can be derived from the LVOT diameter ($LVOT_d$) using one of the equations below:

$$CSA = \pi \times (LVOT_d \div 2)^2 \qquad (2)$$

$$CSA = 0.785 \times LVOT_d^2 \qquad (3)$$

In this patient, the SV is:

$$SV = (0.785 \times 2.25^2) \times 25.1 = 100 \, mL \qquad (4)$$

Answer C is a true statement. Cardiac output (CO) is derived from the SV and the heart rate (HR):

$$CO = (SV \times HR) \div 1000 \qquad (5)$$

In this patient, the CO is:

$$CO = (100 \times 58) \div 1000 = 5.8 \, L/min \qquad (6)$$

Answer D is a true statement. Cardiac index (CI) is derived from the CO and the body surface area (BSA):

$$CI = CO \div BSA \qquad (7)$$

In this patient, the CI is:

$$CI = 5.6 \div 1.82 = 3.1 \, L/min/m^2 \qquad (8)$$

Answer E is a true statement. As previously discussed, the aortic valve area (AVA) is calculated from the continuity equation:

$$AVA = SV_{LVOT} \div VTI_{AV} \qquad (9)$$

In this patient, the AVA is:

$$AVA = 100 \div 30.6 = 3.3 \, cm^2 \qquad (10)$$

Calculations related to this question are summarized in **Table 10-5**.

Table 10-5.

Parameter	Value	Comment
SV (mL)	100	Estimated from the LVOT diameter (cm) and VTI (cm)
CO (L/min)	5.6	Estimated from the SV (mL) and HR (bpm)
CI (L/min/m²)	3.1	Estimated from the CO (L/min) and BSA (m²)
AVA (cm²)	3.3	Estimated from the SV (mL) and AV VTI (cm)

23. Answer: B. As previously described (see answer outline for Question 13), the pulmonary artery end-diastolic pressure (PAEDP) can be estimated from the peak pulmonary regurgitant end-diastolic velocity (V_{PR-ED}) and the right atrial pressure (RAP):

$$PAEDP = 4V_{PR-ED^2} + RAP \qquad (1)$$

The RAP can be estimated from the maximum expiratory inferior vena cava (IVC) size and the IVC collapsibility index (IVCCI). The IVCCI is derived as:

$$IVCCI = \left[(IVC_{max} - IVC_{min}) \div IVC_{max}\right] \times 100 \qquad (2)$$

In this patient, the maximum IVC size is 2.38 cm and the minimum IVC diameter with inspiration is 1.7 cm (**Video 10-1**); thus, the IVCCI is calculated as:

$$IVCCI = \left[(2.6 - 1.7) \div 2.6\right] \times 100 = 35\% \qquad (3)$$

As the IVC is dilated (>2.1 cm) and collapses less than 50%, the estimated RAP is at least 15 mm Hg. Once RAP is known, the PAEDP can be estimated from the peak V_{PR-ED} of 1.36 m/s and the estimated RAP:

$$PAEDP = \left(4 \times 1.36^2\right) + 15 = 22 \text{ mm Hg (or greater)} \qquad (4)$$

Therefore, answer B is correct.

Answer A is incorrect because RAP in this patient is at least 15 mm Hg as demonstrated earlier.

Answer C is incorrect since the PAEDP is estimated as 22 mm Hg or greater as demonstrated earlier (see Equation (4)).

Answers D and E are incorrect. As previously described (see answer outline for Question 13), mean pulmonary artery pressure (mPAP) can be

estimated from the peak PR early diastolic velocity (V_{PR-EaD}), measured at 2.38 m/s, plus the RAP:

$$mPAP = 4V_{PR-EaD^2} + RAP \qquad (5)$$

In this patient, the peak PR early diastolic velocity is 1.36 m/s. Hence, the mPAP is estimated as:

$$mPAP = \left(4 \times 2.38^2\right) + 15 = 38 \text{ mm Hg (or greater)} \qquad (6)$$

Calculations related to this question are summarized in **Table 10-6**.

Table 10-6.

Parameter	Value	Comment
IVCCI (%)	35	Estimated from the maximum and minimum IVC dimensions (cm)
RAP (mm Hg)	15	Estimated from the IVC size and IVCCI
PAEDP (mm Hg)	22	Estimated from the PR end-diastolic velocity (m/s) and RAP (mm Hg)
mPAP (mm Hg)	38	Estimated from the PR early diastolic velocity (m/s) and RAP (mm Hg)

24. Answer: C. For an ASD, the shunt volume is derived as the difference between the pulmonic stroke volume (SV_p) and the systemic stroke volume (SV_s):

$$\text{Shunt volume} = SV_p - SV_s \qquad (1)$$

SV_p may be derived from the right ventricular outflow tract diameter (RVOTd) and right ventricular outflow tract VTI (VTI_{RVOT}):

$$SV_p = \left(0.785 \times RVOT_d^2\right) \times VTI_{RVOT} \qquad (2)$$

In this patient, the RVOTd is 2.9 cm (**Figure 10-4C**) and the VTI_{RVOT} is 21.3 cm (**Figure 10-4D**):

$$SV_p = \left(0.785 \times 2.9^2\right) \times 21.3 = 141 \text{ mL} \qquad (3)$$

SV_s is derived from the left ventricular outflow tract diameter (LVOTd) and left ventricular outflow tract VTI (VTI_{LVOT}):

$$SV_s = \left(0.785 \times LVOT_d^2\right) \times VTI_{LVOT} \qquad (4)$$

In this patient, the LVOTd is 2.1 cm (**Figure 10-4A**) and the VTI_{LVOT} is 17.9 cm (**Figure 10-4B**):

$$SV_s = \left(0.785 \times 2.1^2\right) \times 17.9 = 62 \text{ mL} \qquad (5)$$

Hence, the shunt volume is:

$$\text{Shunt volume} = 141 - 62 = 79 \text{ mL} \qquad (6)$$

The shunt flow rate is measured in L/min and is derived as the difference between the pulmonic flow rate (Qp) and the systemic flow rate (Qs). The Qp and Qs are derived from the pulmonic and systemic stroke volumes and the heart rate.

The Qp in this patient is:

$$Qp = \left(141 \times 77\right) \div 1000 = 10.9 \text{ L/min} \qquad (7)$$

where 141 is the pulmonic stroke volume (Equation (3)), and 77 is the heart rate recorded on the RVOT spectral Doppler trace (**Figure 10-4D**).

The Qs in this patient is:

$$Qs = \left(62 \times 73\right) \div 1000 = 4.5 \text{ L/min} \qquad (8)$$

where 62 is the systemic stroke volume (Equation (4)), and 73 is the heart rate recorded on the LVOT spectral Doppler trace (**Figure 10-4B**).

The shunt flow rate is the difference between the Qp and the Qs, therefore:

$$\text{Shunt flow rate} = 10.9 - 4.5 = 6.4 \text{ L/min} \qquad (9)$$

Therefore, answer C is the false statement. Importantly, the shunt volume is measured as the shunt flow per beat, while the shunt flow rate is measured as the shunt flow per minute.

Answer A is a true statement as the Qp:Qs shunt ratio is 2.4:1. As previously shown, the Qp in this patient is 10.9 L/min and the Qs is 4.5 L/min; hence:

$$Qp:Qs = 10.9 \div 4.5 = 2.4:1 \qquad (10)$$

Answer B is a true statement as the systemic stroke volume is approximately 62 mL, as previously shown (Equation (5)).

Answer D is a true statement. The right ventricular systolic pressure (RVSP) is derived as:

$$RVSP = 4 \times V_{TR^2} + RAP \qquad (11)$$

where V_{TR} is the peak tricuspid regurgitant (TR) velocity and RAP is the right atrial pressure, which can be estimated from the IVC size and collapsibility index. The peak TR velocity was 2.69 m/s (**Figure 10-4E**). **Video 10-2** shows the IVC and while measurements

Table 10-7.

Parameter	Value	Comment
SV_p (mL)	141	Stroke volume to the lungs; estimated from the RVOT diameter (cm) and VTI (cm)
SV_s (mL)	62	Stroke volume to the body; estimated from the LVOT diameter (cm) and VTI (cm)
Qp (L/min)	10.9	Estimated from the SV_p (mL) and HR (bpm)
Qs (L/min)	4.5	Estimated from the SV_s (mL) and HR (bpm)
Shunt flow rate (L/min)	6.4	Estimated from the Qp (L/min) and Qs (L/min)
Qp:Qs	2.4:1	Estimated from the Qp (L/min) and Qs (L/min)
RVSP (mm Hg)	32	Estimated from the peak TR velocity (m/s) and RAP (mm Hg)

are not shown, the IVC appears small and collapses with inspiration; thus, the RAP is normal at 3 mm Hg. Therefore,

$$RVSP = 4 \times \left(2.69^2\right) + 3 = 32 \text{ mm Hg} \qquad (12)$$

Calculations related to this question are summarized in **Table 10-7**.

TECHNICAL TIP

While the most correct method for calculating the Qp:Qs is to estimate the volumetric flow rate as shown above in Equations (7) and (8) (Question 24), often the Qp:Qs is calculated based on the systemic and pulmonary stroke volumes alone (SV_p:SV_s). This simplified calculation assumes that the heart rate is the same when each of these stroke volumes is calculated.

25. **Answer: D.** The maximum and mean pressure gradients should be corrected whenever the proximal velocity exceeds 1.2 m/s. In this instance, the expanded Bernoulli equation is used to calculate the corrected pressure gradient (ΔP_c):

$$\Delta P_c = 4\left(V_2^2 - V_1^2\right) \qquad (1)$$

where V_2 is the peak velocity across the narrowing and V_1 is the peak velocity proximal to the narrowing. Mathematically, this equation is the same as:

$$\Delta P_c = \left(4 \times V_2^2\right) - \left(4 \times V_1^2\right) \qquad (2)$$

Hence, the corrected mean pressure gradients ($m\Delta P_c$) are simply derived by subtracting the proximal mean pressure gradient ($m\Delta P_1$) from the mean pressure gradient across the narrowing ($m\Delta P_2$):

$$m\Delta P_c = m\Delta P_2 - m\Delta P_1 \qquad (3)$$

In this patient, $m\Delta P_1$ is the LVOT mean pressure gradient of 7 mmHg and the $m\Delta P_2$ is the AV mean pressure gradient of 35 mm Hg; therefore, the corrected mean transaortic pressure gradient ($m\Delta P_c$) is:

$$m\Delta P_c = 35 - 7 = 28 \text{ mm Hg} \qquad (4)$$

Therefore, answer D is correct.

Answer A is incorrect as the transaortic velocity is not corrected when there is an increase in the proximal velocity. Rather it is the maximum and mean pressure gradients that are corrected as demonstrated above.

Answer B is incorrect. The corrected maximum transaortic pressure gradient ($m\Delta P_c$) is derived using Equation (1) as:

$$\Delta P_c = 4\left(3.6^2 - 1.5^2\right) = 4\left(12.96 - 2.25\right)$$
$$= 4 \times 10.71 = 43 \text{ mm Hg} \qquad (5)$$

Alternatively, the corrected maximum transaortic pressure gradient can be derived using Equation (2) as:

$$\Delta P_c = \left(4 \times 3.6^2\right) - \left(4 \times 1.5^2\right)$$
$$= 52.84 - 9 = 43 = \text{mm Hg} \qquad (6)$$

Answer C is incorrect. The Doppler velocity ratio or index (DVI) is derived from the peak LVOT velocity (V_{LVOT}) and peak AV velocity (V_{AV}) or from the velocity time integrals across the LVOT and AV (VTI_{LVOT} and VTI_{AV}, respectively):

$$DVI = V_{LVOT} \div V_{AV} \qquad (7)$$

$$DVI = VTI_{LVOT} \div VTI_{AV} \qquad (8)$$

In this patient, using the peak LVOT and AV velocities, the DVI is:

$$DVI = 1.5 \div 3.6 = 0.42 \qquad (9)$$

Using the VTI across the LVOT and AV, the DVI is:

$$DVI = 32 \div 77 = 0.42 \qquad (10)$$

Calculations related to this question are summarized in **Table 10-8**.

Table 10-8.

Parameter	Value	Comment
Corrected mean AV ΔP (mm Hg)	28	Estimated from the mean AV and LVOT pressure gradients (mm Hg)
Corrected maximum AV ΔP (mm Hg)	43	Estimated from the maximum AV and LVOT pressure gradients (mm Hg)
DVI (unitless)	0.42	Estimated from the AV and LVOT peak velocities (m/s) or VTIs (cm)

26. **Answer: D.** Using the simplified Bernoulli equation, the peak MR velocity (V_{MR}) can be used to determine the pressure difference between the left ventricle (LV) and the left atrium (LA) during systole:

$$4V_{MR^2} = LVSP - LAP \qquad (1)$$

where LVSP is the left ventricular systolic pressure and LAP = left atrial pressure.

In the absence of aortic stenosis or left ventricular outflow tract (LVOT) obstruction, it can be assumed that the LVSP is the same as the systolic blood pressure (SBP); hence Equation (1) becomes:

$$4V_{MR^2} = SBP - LAP \qquad (2)$$

Therefore, if the SBP is known, Equation (2) can be rewritten as:

$$LAP = SBP - 4V_{MR^2} \qquad (3)$$

In this patient, the aortic valve does not appear stenotic (**Video 10-3**) and there is no significant LVOT obstruction (**Figure 10-5A**). Therefore, it can be assumed that the SBP is the same as the LVSP. The SBP is 110 mm Hg and the peak MR velocity is 4.76 m/s; hence, the LAP can be estimated as:

$$LAP = 110 - \left(4 \times 4.76^2\right) = 19 \text{ mm Hg} \qquad (4)$$

Therefore, answer D is correct.

27. **Answer: A.** As previously described, the peak mitral regurgitant velocity (V_{MR}) reflects the pressure difference between the left ventricle (LV) and the left atrium (LA) during systole:

$$4V_{MR^2} = LVSP - LAP \qquad (1)$$

where LVSP is the left ventricular systolic pressure and LAP = left atrial pressure.

By rearranging Equation (1), the LVSP can be estimated from the peak MR velocity and an estimation of the LAP:

$$LVSP = 4V_{MR^2} + LAP \qquad (2)$$

The peak MR velocity is 6.74 m/s (**Figure 10-6B**). The transmitral inflow profile (**Figure 10-6A**) shows a prominent L-wave, indicating an increase in the LAP. Hence, assuming an LAP of 15 mm Hg, the estimated LVSP is:

$$LVSP = 4V_{MR^2} + LAP = (4 \times 6.74^2) + 15$$
$$= 181 + 15 = 196 \text{ mm Hg} \qquad (3)$$

Given that the patient's SBP is 120 mm Hg and LVSP estimated at 196 mm Hg, there is a difference of 76 mm Hg between the LV and the aorta during systole:

$$\Delta P_{LV-Aorta} = LVSP - SBP = 196 - 120 = 76 \text{ mm Hg} \qquad (4)$$

This suggests the presence of aortic stenosis or LVOT obstruction. Therefore, answer A is correct.

Answer B is incorrect. Aortic regurgitation occurs during diastole and this does not affect the MR velocity, which occurs during systole.

Answer C is incorrect. The peak MR velocity is not directly related to the severity of MR; it simply reflects the systolic pressure gradient between the LV and LA.

Answer D is incorrect. With acute pulmonary embolism, the systolic blood pressure may drop. In this instance, the LV to LA pressure gradient during systole will decrease and the MR velocity will be lower.

TECHNICAL TIPS

The LV-to-aorta pressure gradient described in the answer outline for Question 27 is equivalent to the peak-to-peak pressure gradient (see the answer outline in Question 10 and **Figure 10-18**).

In the absence of aortic stenosis or LVOT obstruction and in the setting of a normal LAP, the peak MR velocity is typically around 5 m/s. For example, assuming a SBP of 120 mm Hg and a LAP of 7 mm Hg, then the MR velocity is 5.2 m/s:

$$4V_{MR^2} = 120 - 7 = 113 \text{ mm Hg}$$

$$V_{MR^2} = (113 \div 4) = 28.25$$

$$V_{MR} = \sqrt{28.25} = 5.2 \text{ m/s}$$

28. Answer: D. MR severity is based on the criteria listed in **Table 10-9A**.

The effective regurgitant orifice area (EROA) via the proximal isovelocity surface area (PISA) technique can be calculated using the following equation:

$$EROA = (2\pi \times r^2 \times V_N) \div V_{max} \qquad (1)$$

where r is the PISA radius, V_N is the color aliasing velocity (color Nyquist limit) at which PISA radius is measured, and V_{max} is the maximum velocity of the regurgitant jet.

In Equation (1), the expression $2 \times \pi \times r^2 \times V_N$ represents instantaneous flow rate (IFR):

$$IFR = 2\pi \times r^2 \times V_N \qquad (2)$$

Equation (1) can then be expressed as:

$$EROA = IFR \div V_{max} \qquad (3)$$

The regurgitant volume (R_{Vol}) is calculated as:

$$R_{Vol} = EROA \times VTI_{RJ} \qquad (4)$$

where VTI_{RJ} is the velocity time integral (VTI) of the regurgitant jet.

In this patient, the IFR is calculated as:

$$IFR = 6.28 \times 0.91^2 \times 43 = 224 \text{ mL/s} \qquad (5)$$

where 0.91 is the PISA radius and 43 is the color Nyquist limit taken as the bottom value from the color bar and converted to cm/s (**Figure 10-7A**).

The EROA is calculated as:

$$EROA = 224 \div 406 = 0.6 \text{ cm}^2 \qquad (6)$$

Table 10-9A.

	Grade I	Grade II	Grade III	Grade IV
VC-width (cm)	<0.3	Intermediate		≥0.7
RV (mL)	<30	30-44	45-59	≥60
RF (%)	<30	30-39	40-49	≥50
EROA (cm²)	<0.20	0.20-0.29	0.30-0.39	≥0.40

Reprinted from Zoghbi WA, Adams D, Bonow RO, et al. Recommendations for noninvasive evaluation of native valvular regurgitation. A report from the American Society of Echocardiography developed in collaboration with the Society for Cardiovascular Magnetic Resonance. *J Am Soc Echocardiogr.* 2017;30(4): 303-371. Copyright © 2017 by the American Society of Echocardiography. With permission.

where 224 is the IFR (mL) calculated above and 406 is the peak MR velocity converted to cm/s (**Figure 10-7B**).

The R_{Vol} is calculated as:

$$R_{Vol} = 0.6 \times 104 = 62 \, mL \qquad (7)$$

where 0.6 is the EROA (cm²) calculated above and 104 is the VTI of the MR jet converted to cm (**Figure 10-7B**).

Therefore, answer C is correct since the instantaneous flow rate across the mitral valve is approximately 224 mL/s (see Equation (5)).

Answer A is incorrect. The calculations above indicate the presence of severe MR since the EROA is ≥0.40 cm² (it is 0.60 cm²) and the R_{Vol} is ≥60 mL (it is 62 mL). The vena contracta in severe mitral regurgitation is ≥ 0.7 cm.

Answer B is incorrect as the EROA of MR is approximately 0.60 cm² (see Equation (6)).

Answer D is incorrect because mitral regurgitation is severe as previously stated.

Answer E is incorrect because the regurgitant volume (R_{Vol}) in this patient is 62 mL per beat (see Equation (7)).

Calculations related to this question are summarized in **Table 10-9B**.

TECHNICAL TIP

For the PISA calculations, the units should be in cm or cm/s. If the units are displayed in m or m/s, to convert to cm or cm/s simply move the decimal place back two spaces or multiply by 100.

---

29. **Answer: D.** The blood pressure and the measurements provided in **Figure 10-8** is tabled in **Table 10-10**.

The AR end-diastolic velocity (V_{AR-ED}) reflects the pressure gradient (equal to $4V^2$) between the diastolic blood pressure (DBP) and the LVEDP:

$$4V_{AR\_ED^2} = DBP - LVEDP \qquad (1)$$

By rearranging Equation (1), the LVEDP can be estimated as:

$$LVEDP = DBP - 4V_{AR\_ED^2} \qquad (2)$$

Table 10-9B.

Parameter	Value	Comment
MR IFR (mL/s)	224	Estimated from the PISA radius (cm) and color Nyquist limit (cm/s)
MR EROA (cm²)	0.6	Estimated from the IFR (mL/s) and the peak MR velocity (cm/s)
MR R_{Vol} (mL)	62	Estimated from the EROA and the MR VTI

Table 10-10.

Blood pressure	118/74 mm Hg
AR peak early diastolic velocity	4.8 m/s
AR end-diastolic velocity	3.5 m/s
Peak transaortic velocity	3.9 m/s
AR pressure half-time	318 ms

In this patient:

$$LVEDP = 86 - (4 \times 3.5^2) = 74 - 49 = 25 \, mm \, Hg \qquad (3)$$

Therefore, answer E is correct.

Answer A is incorrect. In AR, the Doppler velocity spectrum represents the pressure gradient between the aorta and left ventricle (LV) during diastole. The decline of this slope, as reflected by the PHT, can be used as an indicator of AR severity. For example, the shorter the PHT, the more severe the AR. A PHT of <200 ms suggests severe AR. In this patient, the PHT is 318 ms and this value alone does not indicate severe AR.

Answer B is incorrect. As previously stated, the left ventricular systolic pressure (LVSP) is assumed to be the same as the systolic blood pressure (SBP) in the absence of aortic stenosis or LVOT obstruction. Therefore, one may assume that the LVSP could be estimated by adding the peak transaortic pressure gradient to the systolic blood pressure (SBP). However, the peak transaortic velocity reflects the maximum instantaneous pressure gradient (MIPG) between the LVSP and the aortic pressure at the same instant in time (see **Figure 10-18** in Question 10). As a result, the LVSP estimated as SBP + MIPG in a patient with aortic stenosis would be overestimated.

Answer C is incorrect since the continuity equation can be used to calculate the AVA in patients with or without aortic regurgitation. As previously discussed, the AVA can be derived as:

$$AVA = (CSA_{LVOT} \times VTI_{LVOT}) \div VTI_{AV} \qquad (4)$$

In patients with AR, there is an increase in forward flow from the LV into the aorta due to an increase of the LV stroke volume caused by the additional AR volume. However, this increase equally affects the flow through the LVOT and the AV during systole and this will be reflected in a proportional increase in VTI_{LVOT} and VTI_{AV}. As the ratio of the two VTIs remains the same, the calculated AVA will not be affected by the presence of aortic regurgitation.

Answer E is incorrect based on the explanations above.

Table 10-11A.

	Grade I	Grade II	Grade III	Grade IV
RV (mL)	<30	30-44	45-59	≥60
RF (%)	<30	30-39	40-49	≥50
EROA (cm²)	<0.10	0.10-0.19	0.20-0.29	≥0.30

Reprinted from Zoghbi WA, Adams D, Bonow RO, et al. Recommendations for noninvasive evaluation of native valvular regurgitation: a report from the American Society of Echocardiography developed in collaboration with the Society for Cardiovascular Magnetic Resonance. *J Am Soc Echocardiogr.* 2017;30(4):303-371. Copyright © 2017 by the American Society of Echocardiography. With permission.

30. **Answer: B.** AR severity is based on the criteria listed in **Table 10-11A.**

The regurgitant volume (R_{Vol}) can be derived as the difference between the stroke volume across the incompetent valve (SV_{IV}) and the stroke volume across a competent valve (SV_{CV}):

$$R_{Vol} = SV_{IV} - SV_{CV} \qquad (1)$$

Since the stroke volume is derived from the cross-sectional area (CSA) and the velocity time integral (VTI), R_{Vol} can be estimated as:

$$R_{Vol} = (CSA_{IV} \times VTI_{IV}) - (CSA_{CV} \times VTI_{CV}) \qquad (2)$$

where CSA_{IV} is the CSA of the regurgitant valve annulus, VTI_{IV} is the VTI at the regurgitant valve annulus, CSA_{CV} is the CSA of the competent valve annulus, and VTI_{CV} is the VTI at the competent valve annulus.

The regurgitant fraction (RF) is the percentage of the total stroke volume that regurgitates or leaks through an incompetent valve and is expressed as:

$$RF = (R_{Vol} \div SV_{IV}) \times 100 \qquad (3)$$

The effective regurgitant orifice area (EROA) is derived from the R_{Vol} and the VTI across the incompetent valve (VTI_{IV}) and is expressed as:

$$EROA = R_{Vol} \div VTI_{IV} \qquad (4)$$

In this patient, the R_{Vol} is calculated as:

$$R_{Vol} = (0.785 \times 2.6^2 \times 22) - (0.785 \times 2.6^2 \times 13)$$
$$= 117 - 69 = 48 \, mL \qquad (5)$$

where the LVOT diameter is 2.6 cm (**Figure 10-9A**), the LVOT VTI is 22 cm (**Figure 10-9B**), the RVOT diameter is 2.6 cm (**Figure 10-9C**), and the RVOT VTI is 13 cm (**Figure 10-9D**).

The RF is calculated as:

$$RF = (48 \div 117) \times 100 = 41\% \qquad (6)$$

where 48 is the R_{Vol} (mL) and 117 is the LVOT stroke volume (mL) as calculated above.

The EROA is calculated as:

$$EROA = 48 \div 211 = 0.23 \, cm^2 \qquad (7)$$

where 48 is the R_{Vol} (mL) calculated above and 211 is the VTI of the AR jet (**Figure 10-9E**). Therefore, answer B is correct since EROA is 0.23 cm²s (Equation (7)).

Answer A is incorrect. As previously described, the cardiac output (CO) can be estimated from the stroke volume across the LVOT (SV_{LVOT}) and heart rate (HR):

$$CO = (SV_{LVOT} \times HR) \div 1000 \qquad (8)$$

However, in the setting of AR, the SV_{LVOT} cannot be used to estimate the CO as not all the blood ejected into the LVOT during systole travels to the body; some leaks back into the left ventricle during diastole. Therefore, when there is AR, the CO needs to be estimated from a competent valve. In this patient, the CO can be estimated from the stroke volume across the RVOT (SV_{RVOT}) and heart rate (HR):

$$CO = (SV_{RVOT} \times HR) \div 1000 \qquad (9)$$

In this patient, the CO is:

$$CO = (69 \times 59) \div 1000 = 4.1 L/min \qquad (10)$$

where 69 is the SV_{RVOT} (mL) and 59 is the heart rate recorded on the RVOT spectral Doppler trace (**Figure 10-10D**).

Answer C is incorrect as the R_{Vol} is 48 mL (see Equation (4)).

Answer D is incorrect as the RF is 41% (see Equation (5)).

Answer E is incorrect. The calculations above indicate the presence of moderately severe AR (grade III) as the R_{Vol} is between 45 and 59 mL (it is 48 mL), the RF is between 40% and 49% (it is 41%), and the EROA is between 0.20 and 0.29 cm² (it is 0.23 cm²).

Calculations related to this question are summarized in **Table 10-11B.**

Table 10-11B.

Parameter	Value	Comment
CO (L/min)	224	Due to presence of AR, estimated from the RVOT diameter (cm) and VTI (cm)
AR R_{Vol} (mL)	62	Estimated from the LVOT diameter (cm) and VTI (cm) and the RVOT diameter (cm) and VTI (cm)
AR RF	41	Estimated from the AR R_{Vol} (mL) and the LVOT stroke volume (mL)
AR EROA (cm²)	0.6	Estimated from the AR R_{Vol} (mL) and the AR VTI (cm)

31. Answer: A. Calculation of the aortic valve area (AVA) is based on the continuity equation assuming that flow proximal to the narrowing is the same as the flow across the narrowing. In aortic valve replacement, the effective orifice area (EOA) is calculated from the left ventricular outflow tract (LVOT) stroke volume (SV) and the AVR velocity time integral (VTI):

$$EOA = SV_{LVOT} \div AVR_{VTI} \quad (1)$$

Based on the measurements shown, the EOA is calculated as:

$$EOA = \left(0.785 \times 2.3^2 \times 16\right) \div 47 = 66 \div 47 = 1.4\,cm^2 \quad (2)$$

However, there is a residual perimembranous VSD present. Therefore, the overall stroke volume through the aortic valve will be less than the stroke volume across the LVOT as some of the LVOT stroke volume will be shunted across the VSD into the right ventricle. Thus, the assumption that the stroke volume at the LVOT is the same as the stroke volume across the aortic valve is violated. As a result, the EOA will be overestimated:

$$\downarrow EOA = SV_{LVOT} \div \downarrow AVR_{VTI} \quad (3)$$

Therefore, answer A is correct.

Answer B is incorrect because the Qp:Qs is calculated at 1:6:1. The echocardiographic formula to calculate volumetric flow (Q) is:

$$Q = CSA \times VTI \times HR \quad (4)$$

where CSA is the cross-sectional area, VTI is velocity time integral, and HR is the heart rate.

The Qp is the pulmonic flow rate which is derived from the right ventricular outflow tract diameter (RVOTd) and VTI (VTI$_{RVOT}$). In this patient, the RVOTd is 2.8 cm (**Figure 10-10D**), the VTI$_{RVOT}$ is

17 cm (**Figure 10-10E**), and the heart rate is 74 bpm; thus, the Qp is calculated as:

$$Qp = \left[\left(0.785 \times 2.8^2\right) \times 17 \times 74\right] \div 1000 = 7.8\,L/min \quad (5)$$

The Qs is the systemic flow rate which is derived from the LVOT diameter (LVOTd) and VTI (VTI$_{LVOT}$). In this patient, the LVOTd is 2.3 cm (**Figure 10-10A**), the VTI$_{LVOT}$ is 16 cm (**Figure 10-10B**), and the heart rate is 74 bpm; thus, the Qs is calculated as:

$$Qs = \left[\left(0.785 \times 2.3^2\right) \times 16 \times 74\right] \div 1000 = 4.9\,L/min \quad (6)$$

The Qp:Qs is then simply derived as the ratio of the Qp and the Qs:

$$Qp : Qs = 7.8 \div 4.9 = 1.6 \quad (7)$$

Answer C is incorrect as the continuous-wave Doppler trace across the VSD (**Figure 10-10F**) shows a high velocity close to 5 m/s. Using the simplified Bernoulli equation, this indicates that the LV-to-RV pressure gradient is approximately 100 mm Hg:

$$\Delta P = 4V^2 = 4 \times 5^2 = 100\,mm\,Hg \quad (8)$$

As previously discussed (see answer outline for Question 13), the RVSP can be estimated from the systolic blood pressure (SBP) and the peak VSD velocity (V_{VSD}):

$$RVSP = SBP - 4V_{VSD}^2 \quad (9)$$

In this patient, the RVSP is estimated as:

$$RVSP = 116 - 100 = 16\,mm\,Hg \quad (10)$$

where 116 is the SBP (mm Hg) and 100 is the estimated LV-to-RV pressure gradient derived from the peak VSD velocity (see Equation (8)).

Answer D is incorrect. The pulmonic flow rate is equivalent to the Qp. As shown previously, the Qp (pulmonic flow rate) is 7.8 L/min (see Equation (5)).

Calculations related to this question are summarized in **Table 10-12**.

32. Answer: B. The measurement shown is the *dP/dt*, which is the change in pressure (*dP*) over the change in time (*dt*) during the isovolumic contraction phase of the cardiac cycle, measured from the mitral regurgitant (MR) continuous-wave Doppler trace. The time taken for the LV to generate a pressure rise is directly related to myocardial contractility; for example, with normal contractility the LV can rapidly generate a pressure rise, while with impaired contractility the LV takes a longer time to generate a similar pressure rise. The dP/dt has no relationship with the LVFP.

Table 10-12.

Parameter	Value	Comment
Qp (L/s)	7.8	Stroke volume from the lungs; estimated from the RVOT diameter (cm) and VTI (cm)
Qs (L/s)	4.9	Stroke volume from the body; estimated from the LVOT diameter (cm) and VTI (cm)
Qp:Qs	1.6:1	Estimated from the Qp and Qs
RVSP (mm Hg)	16	Estimated from the SBP (mm Hg) and the peak VSD velocity (m/s)

The dP/dt is calculated from the time difference (Δt) between the MR velocity at 1 m/s and the MR velocity at 3 m/s:

$$dP/dt = \left[(4 \times 3^2) - (4 \times 1)^2 \right] \div \Delta t$$
$$= [36 - 4] \div \Delta t$$
$$= 32 \div \Delta t \tag{1}$$

In this patient, the dP/dt is:

$$dP/dt = 32 \div 0.069 = 464 \, \text{mm Hg/s} \tag{2}$$

where 0.069 is Δt converted from ms to seconds.

A normal dP/dt is >1200 mm Hg/s while a dP/dt < 800 mm Hg/s is consistent with severe LV systolic function. Therefore, answer B is correct since the dP/dt is <800 mm Hg/s (it was 464 mm Hg/s) and because there is no relationship between the dP/dt and LVFP.

33. **Answer: E.** As previously described, the mitral valve area (MVA) can be derived from the pressure half-time (PHT) using the equation:

$$MVA = 220 \div PHT \tag{1}$$

The PHT in this patient is 104 ms (**Figure 10-12A**). Using Equation (1), the MVA is:

$$MVA = 220 \div 104 = 2.1 \, \text{cm}^2 \tag{2}$$

However, several studies have shown that the MVA calculated via the PHT in prosthetic valves tends to be grossly overestimated. Therefore, the MVA cannot be estimated using the PHT when there is an MVR; therefore, answer E is correct as this is not a true statement.

Answer A is a true statement. Recall that the RVSP is derived from the peak tricuspid regurgitant velocity (V_{TR}) and the right atrial pressure (RAP):

$$RVSP = 4V_{TR}^2 + RAP \tag{3}$$

The peak TR velocity is 390 cm/s or 3.9 m/s (**Figure 10-12C**). As previously described, the RAP can be estimated from the maximal expiratory dimension of the inferior vena cava (IVC) and the IVC collapsibility index (IVCCI) (see answer outline for Question 23, Equation (4)). In this patient, the maximum IVC size is 2.76 cm and the minimum IVC diameter with inspiration is 2.24 cm and the IVCCI is 19%:

$$IVCCI = \left[(2.76 - 2.24) \div 2.76 \right] \times 100 = 19\% \tag{4}$$

As the IVC is dilated (>2.1 cm) and collapses less than 50%, the estimated RAP is at least 15 mm Hg. Thus, the RVSP is:

$$RVSP = (4 \times 3.9^2) + 15 = 61 + 15$$
$$- 76 \, \text{mm Hg (or greater)} \tag{5}$$

Answer B is a true statement. The mPAP can be estimated from the mean TR pressure gradient (which reflects the RV-to-RA mean systolic gradient) and the RAP. This is based on the concept that if the RVSP can be derived from the peak TR pressure gradient plus RAP, then the mPAP can be estimated in a similar function using the mean TR pressure gradient plus RAP. The mean TR pressure gradient is 35 mm Hg (**Figure 10-12C**) and the estimated RAP is at least 15 mm Hg as described above; thus, the mPAP is:

$$mPAP = 35 + 15 = 50 \, \text{mm Hg (or greater)} \tag{6}$$

Answer C is a true statement. The EROA via the proximal isovelocity surface area (PISA) technique can be calculated using the following equation:

$$EROA = (2\pi \times r^2 \times V_N) \div V_{max} \tag{7}$$

In this patient, the PISA radius is 0.89 cm and the color Nyquist limit in the direction of the TR jet (bottom of the color bar) is 34.6 cm/s (**Figure 10-12B**) and the peak TR velocity is 390 cm/s (**Figure 10-12C**); thus, the EROA is:

$$EROA = (2\pi \times 0.89^2 \times 34.6) \div 390$$
$$= 172 \div 390 = 0.44 \, \text{cm}^2 \tag{8}$$

Answer D is a true statement. As previously described, the regurgitant volume (R_{Vol}) via the PISA technique can be derived from the EROA and the VTI across the regurgitant jet (VTI$_{RJ}$):

$$R_{Vol} = EROA \times VTI_{RJ} \tag{9}$$

In this patient, the EROA is 0.44 cm² (see Equation (8)) and the VTI of the TR jet is 122 cm (**Figure 10-12C**); thus, the R_{Vol} is:

$$R_{Vol} = 0.44 \times 122 = 54 \text{ mL} \qquad (10)$$

Calculations related to this question are summarized in **Table 10-13**.

KEY POINT

When there is an MVR, the MVA or the effective orifice area (EOA) cannot be derived from the PHT. In the absence of significant mitral regurgitation, the EOA for prosthetic mitral valves should be calculated via the continuity equation using the stroke volume from either the left ventricular or the right ventricular outflow tracts (the latter may be used when there is significant aortic regurgitation).

Table 10-13.

Parameter	Value	Comment
IVCCI (%)	19	Estimated from the maximum and minimum IVC dimensions (cm)
RAP (mm Hg)	15	Estimated from the IVC size and IVCCI
RVSP (mm Hg)	76	Estimated from the peak TR velocity (m/s) and RAP (mm Hg)
mPAP (mm Hg)	50	Estimated from the mean PR pressure gradient (mm Hg) and RAP (mm Hg)
TR EROA (cm²)	0.44	Estimated from the PISA radius (cm), color Nyquist limit (cm/s), and the peak TR velocity (cm/s)
TR R_{Vol} (mL)	54	Estimated from the EROA (cm²) and the VTI of the TR jet (cm)

34. **Answer: D.** This patient has hypertrophic obstructive cardiomyopathy (HOCM) as evident by asymmetric septal hypertrophy and systolic anterior motion (SAM) of the anterior mitral leaflet (**Video 10-4**). SAM of the anterior mitral leaflet in HOCM leads to (1) dynamic left ventricular outflow tract (LVOT) obstruction and (2) MR. The resultant pressure gradients across the LVOT and of the MR jet peak late in systole. As previously discussed, the LVSP can be estimated from the peak MR velocity and an estimation of the LAP:

$$LVSP = 4V_{MR^2} + LAP \qquad (1)$$

In this patient, the peak MR velocity is 6.91 m/s (691 cm/s) and the LAP is given as 10 mm Hg; thus, the LVSP is estimated as:

$$LVSP = \left(4 \times 6.91^2\right) + 10 = 191 + 10 = 201 \text{ mm Hg} \quad (2)$$

The maximal instantaneous LVOT pressure gradient (ΔP_{LVOT}) can be estimated as the difference between the LVSP and the systolic blood pressure (SBP):

$$\Delta P_{LVOT} = LVSP - SBP \qquad (3)$$

In this patient, the maximal instantaneous LVOT pressure gradient is:

$$\Delta P_{LVOT} = 201 - 112 = 89 \text{ mm Hg} \qquad (4)$$

Therefore, answer D is correct.

Answer A is incorrect because even in the presence of aortic stenosis (AS) or LVOT obstruction (LVOTOB), the peak MR velocity will always be higher than the peak AS velocity or the peak velocity across the LVOTOB (**Figure 10-21A**). This is because the MR velocity reflects the pressure difference between the LV and the LA during systole while the AS/LVOTOB velocity reflects the pressure difference between the LV and the aorta (Ao) during systole.

Answer B is incorrect because in mitral valve prolapse (MVP) the MR jet is characteristically absent in early systole. This is because MR associated with MVP usually commences in mid-systole; thus, the MR jet associated with MVP is often mid-late systolic only. In this patient, the MR jet commences at the onset of systole as indicated by the QRS complex on the ECG (see **Figure 10-13**). An example of an MR jet seen with MVP is shown in **Figure 10-21B**; observe how the MR jet does not commence until mid-systole and well past the onset of the QRS complex.

Answer C is incorrect. In HOCM, LVOTOB is dynamic such that the degree of obstruction progressively increases during systole with maximum obstruction occurring at or just after mid-systole. This may result in mid-systolic closure or notching of the aortic valve, which is best appreciated on the M-mode trace (see **Figure 10-21C** acquired from this patient). Early systolic closure of the aortic valve is more characteristic of a fixed, rather than a dynamic, LVOT obstruction. When there is fixed LVOTOB, as in the case of discrete subaortic stenosis caused by a subaortic membrane, aortic valve closure occurs earlier in systole and remains in a near closure position for the remainder of systole.

Answer D is incorrect since the estimated LVSP is 201 mm Hg (see Equation (2)).

Calculations related to this question are summarized in **Table 10-14**.

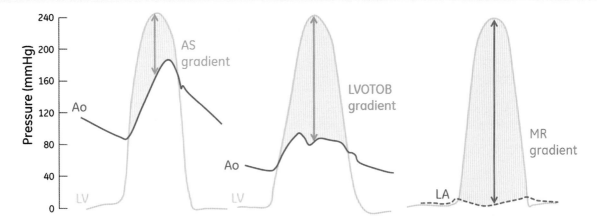

Figure 10-21A

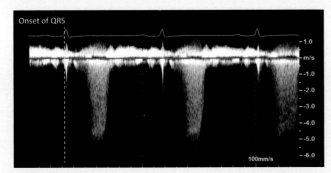

Figure 10-21B

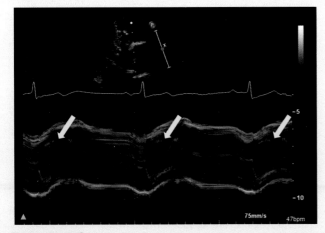

Figure 10-21C

Table 10-14.

Parameter	Value	Comment
LVSP (mm Hg)	201	Estimated from the peak MR velocity (m/s) and LAP
LVOT ΔP (mm Hg)	89	Estimated from the LVSP and systolic blood pressure

35. **Answer: C.** The five transmitral inflow patterns presented in Question 35 were as follows:
    A. Mitral inflow from a patient with mechanical mitral valve (note the vertical lines representing the opening and closing clicks of the prosthetic disks)
    B. Grade II diastolic dysfunction (pseudonormal pattern; moderate elevation in LAP)
    C. Restrictive filling pattern (grade III diastolic dysfunction; marked elevation in LAP)
    D. Mitral inflow in a patient with atrial fibrillation
    E. Abnormal relaxation pattern (grade I diastolic dysfunction; normal LAP)

    Since the patient has a normal native mitral valve and was in normal sinus rhythm at the time of the study, patterns A and D do not belong to this patient.

    A PAWP, which is synonymous with the pulmonary capillary wedge pressure, of 34 mm Hg is markedly elevated. Of the three remaining patterns, only the restrictive filling (pattern C) is consistent with a marked elevation in the PAWP. Therefore, answer C is correct.

36. **Answer: C.** As previously described, the effective regurgitant orifice area (EROA) via the PISA technique can be calculated from the PISA radius (r), the color Nyquist limit (V_N), and the peak regurgitant jet velocity (V_{max}):

$$EROA = \left(2\pi \times r^2 \times V_N\right) \div V_{max} \quad (1)$$

In this patient, the PISA radius is 0.75 cm at a color Nyquist limit of 48.1 cm (**Figure 10-15A**) and the peak MR velocity is 523 cm/s (**Figure 10-15B**); thus, the EROA is:

$$EROA = \left(2\pi \times 0.75^2 \times 48.1\right) \div 523$$
$$= 170 \div 523 = 0.33 \text{ cm}^2 \quad (2)$$

The regurgitant volume (R_{Vol}) is calculated as:

$$R_{Vol} = EROA \times VTI_{MR} \quad (3)$$

where VTI_{MR} is the velocity time integral (VTI) of the regurgitant jet.

In this patient, the EROA is 0.33 cm² (Equation (2)) and the VTI of the MR jet is 83 cm; thus, the R_{Vol} is:

$$R_{Vol} = 0.33 \times 83 = 27 \text{ mL} \quad (4)$$

The MR severity can be graded based on the values shown in **Table 10-9A** (answer outline for Question 28). In this patient, there is discordance of the MR severity based on the EROA and the R_{Vol}. The EROA of 0.33 cm² indicates moderately severe (0.30-0.39 cm²) regurgitation while the R_{Vol} of 27 mL indicates mild MR (<30 mL). The EROA assumes that the regurgitant orifice is maintained over systole (holosystolic). However, in this case, MR commences in mid-systole; thus, because MR is not holosystolic, the R_{Vol} rather than the EROA should be used to grade MR severity. Therefore, answer C is correct and answer D is incorrect.

Answer A is incorrect. As previously described (see answer outline for Question 27), the left ventricular systolic pressure (LVSP) can be estimated from the peak MR velocity and the LAP and in the absence of aortic stenosis or LVOT obstruction, the LVSP is synonymous with the systolic blood pressure (SBP); thus:

$$SBP = 4V_{MR}^2 + LAP \quad (5)$$

In this patient, the peak MR velocity is 5.16 m/s (516 cm/s), the LAP is given as 10 mm Hg and there is no aortic stenosis; thus, the SBP (LVSP) is estimated as:

$$SBP = \left(4 \times 5.16^2\right) + 10 = 107 + 10 = 117 \text{ mm Hg} \quad (6)$$

As this SBP is within normal range, the patient was not hypertensive at the time of this study.

Answer B is incorrect since the regurgitant fraction cannot be calculated from the provided data as the forward stroke volume across a competent valve is not provided for this patient.

Answer E is incorrect. As stated earlier, the MR jet commences in mid-systole and this is a characteristic feature of mitral valve prolapse (MVP). Hence, the likely etiology of MR in this patient is MVP.

Calculations related to this question are summarized in **Table 10-15**.

Table 10-15.

Parameter	Value	Comment
MR EROA (cm²)	0.33	Estimated from the PISA radius (cm), color Nyquist limit (cm/s), and the peak MR velocity (cm/s)
MR R_{Vol} (mL)	27	Estimated from the EROA and the MR VTI
SBP (mm Hg)	117	Estimated from the peak MR velocity and LAP

KEY POINT

When MR is holosystolic, both the effective regurgitant orifice area (EROA) and regurgitant volume (R_{Vol}) should be concordant with the MR severity. However, in patients with MVP with a mid-late systolic onset of MR, there will be discordance between the EROA and the R_{Vol}. In this situation, the EROA via PISA will overestimate the severity of MR. This is because the EROA assumes that the regurgitant orifice is maintained over the entire systolic period; however, in MVP with a mid-late systolic onset of MR, MR only occurs after mid-systole. Therefore, the mitral R_{Vol} is a better parameter for determining MR severity in these patients.

37. **Answer: C.** The right ventricular systolic pressure (RVSP) can be estimated from the peak tricuspid regurgitant (TR) velocity (V_{TR}) and the right atrial pressure (RAP):

$$RVSP = 4V_{TR}^2 + RAP \quad (1)$$

In this patient, the peak TR velocity is averaged at 3.22 m/s (**Figure 10-16B**). The RAP can be estimated from the hepatic venous Doppler trace (**Figure 10-16C**) by estimating the systolic filling fraction (SFF). As previously discussed (see answer outline for Question 14), the SFF can be calculated from the peak systolic velocity (V_S) and the peak diastolic velocity (V_D):

$$SFF = V_S \div \left(V_S + V_D\right) \times 100 \quad (2)$$

In this patient, the estimated peak systolic velocity is 0.25 m/s and the peak diastolic velocity is 0.5 m/s (**Figure 10-22A**); thus, the SFF is:

$$SFF = 0.25 \div \left(0.25 + 0.5\right) \times 100 = 33\% \quad (3)$$

As the SFF is <55%, the RAP is elevated (at least 15 mm Hg). Therefore, the estimated RVSP in this patient is:

$$RVSP = \left(4 \times 3.22^2\right) + 15 = 41 + 15$$

$$= 56 \text{ mm Hg} \left(\text{or greater}\right) \quad (4)$$

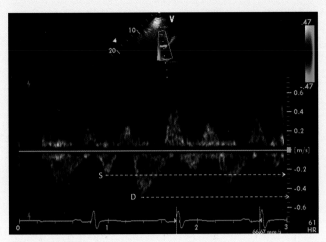

Figure 10-22A

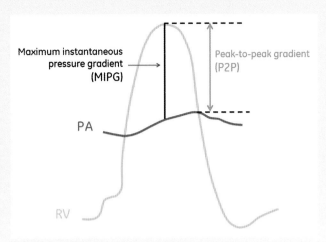

Figure 10-22C

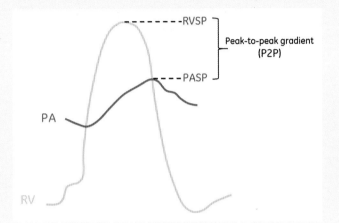

Figure 10-22B

In the absence of pulmonic stenosis (PS) or right ventricular outflow tract (RVOT) obstruction (RVO-TOB), the RVSP is assumed to be the same as the pulmonary artery systolic pressure (PASP). However, in this patient, there is moderate PS as the pulmonary valve gradient is between 36 and 64 mm Hg (it is averaged at 45 mm Hg). In this instance, the difference between the RVSP and the PASP will be the peak-to-peak (P2P) pressure gradient across the pulmonary valve (**Figure 10-22B**):

$$\Delta P_{P2P} = RVSP - PASP \qquad (5)$$

By rearranging Equation (5), the PASP can be estimated as:

$$PASP = RVSP - \Delta P_{P2P} \qquad (6)$$

According to Silvilairat et al. the Doppler pressure gradient that correlates best with the P2P pressure gradient in PS is the mean PS pressure gradient. Hence, Equation (6) can be expressed as:

$$PASP = RVSP - m\Delta P_{PV} \qquad (7)$$

where $m\Delta P_{PV}$ is the mean pressure gradient across the pulmonary valve.

In this patient, the RVSP is estimated as 56 mm Hg (Equation (4)) and the averaged mean pressure gradient across the pulmonary valve is 26 mm Hg (**Figure 10-16A**); therefore, the estimated PASP is:

$$PASP = 56 - 26 = 30 \ mm \ Hg \qquad (8)$$

As this PASP is <40 mm Hg, the PASP is normal so answer C is a false statement.

Answer A is a true statement. As explained earlier, the RAP is elevated based on the hepatic venous Doppler trace and estimated SFF.

Answer B is a true statement since the peak pulmonary valve gradient is between 36 and 64 mm Hg (it is averaged at 45 mm Hg; see **Figure 10-15A**).

Answer D is a true statement. As explained earlier, the RVSP is elevated and thus right ventricular pressure overload is present. This will result in the flattening of the interventricular septum in systole and diastole. In the parasternal short-axis view, the left ventricular contour becomes D-shaped rather than circular in both systole and diastole.

Calculations related to this question are summarized in **Table 10-16**.

Table 10-16.

Parameter	Value	Comment
SFF (%)	33	Estimated from the hepatic venous peak systolic and diastolic velocities
RAP (mm Hg)	15	Estimated from the SFF
RVSP (mm Hg)	56	Estimated from the PISA radius (cm), color Nyquist limit (cm/s), and the peak MR velocity (cm/s)
PASP (mm Hg)	30	Estimated from the RVSP and mean ΔP across the pulmonary valve

In the absence of RVOTOB or PS, the RVSP and PASP are virtually equal. However, when there is PS or RVOTOB, the RVSP will be higher than the PASP. In this situation, the PASP is equal to the RVSP minus the peak-to-peak (P2P) pressure gradient across the RVOT or pulmonary valve. In most situations, the Doppler equivalent of the P2P is the mean pulmonary valve pressure gradient ($m\Delta P_{PV}$), so the PASP can be calculated as:

$$PASP = RVSP - m\Delta P_{PV} \qquad (1)$$

In cases of critical PS, due to "flattening" of the pulmonary artery pressure waveform, the maximal instantaneous pressure gradient (MIPG) more closely correlates with the P2P (**Figure 10-22C**); thus, the PASP can be estimated as:

$$PASP = RVSP - MIPG \qquad (2)$$

38. **Answer: E.** In the presence of a PDA, the systolic velocity reflects the pressure difference between the aorta and the pulmonary artery during systole. Therefore, if the systolic blood pressure (SBP) is known, the pulmonary artery systolic pressure (PASP) can be estimated as:

$$PASP = SBP - \Delta P_{PDA} \qquad (1)$$

where ΔP_{PDA} is the peak systolic velocity across the PDA.

In the absence of pulmonary stenosis or RVOT obstruction, the RVSP is assumed to be the same as the PASP; thus, Equation (1) can be expressed as:

$$RVSP = SBP - \Delta P_{PDA} \qquad (2)$$

Rearranging this equation, the ΔP_{PDA} can be solved as:

$$\Delta P_{PDA} = SBP - RVSP \qquad (3)$$

In this patient, the RVSP is 35 mm Hg and the SBP is 125 mm Hg; thus, ΔP_{PDA} is:

$$\Delta P_{PDA} = 125 - 35 = 90 \text{ mm Hg} \qquad (4)$$

The peak systolic PDA velocity can then be resolved as:

$$4V_{PDA}^2 = 90 \text{ mm Hg} \qquad (5)$$

$$V_{PDA}^2 = (90 \div 4) = 22.5 \qquad (6)$$

$$4V_{PDA}^2 = 90 \text{ mm Hg} \qquad (7)$$

Therefore, answer A is incorrect.

In a PDA, there is shunting of blood from the descending aorta to the proximal left pulmonary artery. Hence, the Qp (pulmonary venous flow rate) is derived from the LVOT stroke volume, which reflects the amount of flow returning from the lungs proximal to the PDA, and the Qs (systemic venous flow rate) is derived from the RVOT stroke volume, which reflects the amount of flow returning from the body downstream from the PDA.

As previously describe, the volumetric flow (Q) is calculated as:

$$Q = CSA \times VTI \times HR \qquad (8)$$

where CSA is the cross-sectional area, VTI is velocity time integral, and HR is the heart rate.

In this patient, the LVOT diameter is 2.6 cm, the LVOT VTI is 23 cm, and the heart rate is 65 bpm; thus, the Qp is calculated as:

$$Qp = \left[\left(0.785 \times 2.6 \right) \times 23 \times 65 \right] \div 1000 = 7.9 \text{ L/min} \qquad (9)$$

The RVOT diameter is 2.3 cm, the RVOT VTI is 12 cm, and the heart rate is 65 bpm; thus, the Qs is calculated as:

$$Qs = \left[\left(0.785 \times 2.3 \right) \times 12 \times 65 \right] \div 1000 = 3.3 \text{ L/min} \qquad (10)$$

The Qp:Qs is:

$$Qp : Qs = 7.9 \div 3.3 = 2.4 \qquad (11)$$

Therefore, answers B and C are incorrect as the Qp:Qs is 2.4 and the Qs is 3.3 L/min.

Answer D is incorrect. There is a significant shunt across the PDA (Qp:Qs > 1.5:1). As a result, there is significant shunting of blood from the descending aorta to the pulmonary artery. This increases the stroke volume to the lungs which then returns through the pulmonary veins to the left atrium and to the left ventricle. This increase in volume to the left heart results in dilatation of the left heart chambers, not the right heart chambers.

Therefore, answer E is correct as all other answers are false statements.

Calculations related to this question are summarized in **Table 10-17**.

Table 10-17.

Parameter	Value	Comment
PDA systolic velocity (m/s)	4.7	Estimated from the SBP (mm Hg) and the RVSP (mm Hg)
Qp (L/s)	7.9	Stroke volume from the lungs proximal to the PDA; estimated from the LVOT diameter (cm) and VTI (cm)
Qs (L/s)	3.3	Stroke volume from the body downstream from the PDA; estimated from the RVOT diameter (cm) and VTI (cm)
Qp:Qs	2.4:1	Estimated from the Qp and Qs

KEY POINT

In the presence of a PDA, the Qp is calculated from the LVOT (flow returning from the lungs) and the Qs is calculated from the RVOT (flow returning from the body). This is in contrast to the Qp:Qs calculations for an atrial septal defect or a ventricular septal defect whereby the Qp is calculated from the RVOT (flow to the lungs) and the Qs is calculated from the LVOT (flow to the body).

Acknowledgments: The authors thank and acknowledge Muhamed Saric, MD, PhD, and Itzhak Kronzon, MD, for their inspiration based on Chapter 8 Doppler and Hemodynamics in *Clinical Echocardiography Review: A Self-Assessment Tool,* 2nd ed., edited by Allan L. Klein, Craig R. Asher; 2017.

SUGGESTED READINGS

Abbas AE, Fortuin FD, Schiller NB, Appleton CP, Moreno CA, Lester SJ. Echocardiographic determination of mean pulmonary artery pressure. *Am J Cardiol.* 2003;92(11):1373-1376.

Aduen JF, Castello R, Lozano MM, et al. An alternative echocardiographic method to estimate mean pulmonary artery pressure: diagnostic and clinical implications. *J Am Soc Echocardiogr.* 2009;22(7):814-819.

Anderson B. Basic principles of spectral Doppler. In: *Echocardiography: The Normal Examination and Echocardiographic Measurements.* 3rd ed. Brisbane, Australia: Echotext Pty Ltd; 2017a:chap 5.

Anderson B. Doppler haemodynamic calculations. In: *Echocardiography: The Normal Examination and Echocardiographic Measurements.* 3rd ed. Brisbane, Australia: Echotext Pty Ltd; 2017b:chap 11.

Anderson B. Doppler valve area calculations. In: *Echocardiography: The Normal Examination and Echocardiographic Measurements.* 3rd ed. Brisbane, Australia: Echotext Pty Ltd; 2017c:chap12.

Anderson B. Doppler quantification of regurgitation lesions. In: *Echocardiography: The Normal Examination and Echocardiographic Measurements.* 3rd ed. Brisbane, Australia: Echotext Pty Ltd; 2017d:chap 13.

Augustine DX, Coates-Bradshaw LD, Willis J, et al. The British Society of Echocardiography Education Committee. Echocardiographic assessment of pulmonary hypertension: a guideline protocol from the British Society of Echocardiography. *Echo Res Pract.* 2018;5(3):G11-G24.

Baumgartner H, Hung J, Bermejo J, et al. Recommendations on the echocardiographic assessment of aortic valve stenosis: a focused update from the European Association of Cardiovascular Imaging and the American Society of Echocardiography. *J Am Soc Echocardiogr.* 2017;30(4):372-392.

Feigenbaum H. Role of M-mode technique in today's echocardiography. *J Am Soc Echocardiogr.* 2010;23(3):240-257; 335-337.

Geske JB, Cullen MW, Sorajja P, Ommen SR, Nishimura RA. Assessment of left ventricular outflow gradient: hypertrophic cardiomyopathy versus aortic valvular stenosis. *JACC Cardiovasc Interv.* 2012;5(6):675-681.

Mesa A, Jessurun C, Hernandez A, et al. Left ventricular diastolic function in normal human pregnancy. *Circulation.* 1999;99(4):511-517.

Parasuraman S, Walker S, Loudon BL, et al. Assessment of pulmonary artery pressure by echocardiography – A comprehensive review. *Int J Cardiol Heart Vasc.* 2016;12:45-51.

Rudski LG, Lai WW, Afilalo J, et al. Guidelines for the echocardiographic assessment of the right heart in adults: a report from the American Society of Echocardiography endorsed by the European Association of Echocardiography, a registered branch of the European Society of Cardiology, and the Canadian Society of Echocardiography. *J Am Soc Echocardiogr.* 2010;23(7):685-713.

Silvilairat S, Cabalka AK, Cetta F, Hagler DJ, O'Leary PW. Echocardiographic assessment of isolated pulmonary valve stenosis: which outpatient Doppler gradient has the most clinical validity? *J Am Soc Echocardiogr.* 2005;18(11):1137-1142.

Yoganathan AP, Cape EG, Sung HW, Williams FP, Jimoh A. Review of hydrodynamic principles for the cardiologist: applications to the study of blood flow and jets by imaging techniques. *J Am Coll Cardiol.* 1988;12(5):1344-1353.

Zoghbi WA, Adams D, Bonow RO, et al. Recommendations for noninvasive evaluation of native valvular regurgitation: a report from the American Society of Echocardiography developed in collaboration with the Society for Cardiovascular Magnetic Resonance. *J Am Soc Echocardiogr.* 2017;30(4):303-371.

Left Ventricular Systolic Function

Contributors: Ashlee Davis, BS, ACS, RDCS and Ashley Woolf, BS, RDCS

✪ Question 1

Visual assessment of the left ventricular ejection fraction (LVEF) from limited acoustic windows is sometimes required (e.g., in an emergency). What is/are the potential limitation(s) of visual LVEF?
  A. Inability to interrogate multiple imaging planes simultaneously
  B. Image quality
  C. Extremes of heart rate
  D. Experience of the reviewer
  E. All of the above

✪ Question 2

Which statement about stroke volume (SV) is true?
  A. A decrease in afterload will decrease SV.
  B. As left ventricular end-diastolic volume (LVEDV) increases, SV increases.
  C. As LVEDV increases, SV decreases.
  D. Preload has no effect on SV.

✪✪ Question 3

Which statement regarding the mechanism of the respiratory pump and its effect on preload is correct?
  A. Expiration decreases pressure in the right ventricle, which increases preload.
  B. Inspiration draws blood into the left ventricle by decreasing left ventricular end-diastolic pressure.
  C. Inspiration decreases intrathoracic pressure and increases abdominal pressure, which pushes blood toward the right atrium.
  D. Inspiration increases intrathoracic pressure and decreases abdominal pressure, which pushes blood toward the right atrium.

✪ Question 4

Which of the following does not influence left ventricular afterload?
  A. Aortic impedance
  B. Left ventricular volume and pressure
  C. Pulmonary artery pressure
  D. Viscosity of blood
  E. None of the above

✪✪✪ Question 5

A 68-year-old man was admitted to the hospital with shortness of breath and lower extremity edema. An echocardiogram was ordered. **Table 11-1** includes some of the findings of this study. Which of the following statements can be extrapolated from this information?
  A. The left ventricular ejection fraction (LVEF) is normal.
  B. The myocardial performance index (MPI) is abnormal.
  C. There is a restrictive filling pattern.
  D. There is severe mitral regurgitation (MR).
  E. All of the above.

Table 11-1.

LVEDV	259 mL
IVCT	0.08 s
E/e′	10
LVET	0.2 s
IVRT	0.113 s

IVCT, isovolumic contraction time; IVRT, isovolumic relaxation time; LVET, left ventricular ejection time; LVEDV, left ventricular end-diastolic volume.

✪✪✪ Question 6

▶ The image provided in **Video 11-1** is an example of tissue motion annular displacement (TMAD). Which of the following statements regarding this technique is false?

    A. There is a correlation between TMAD and left ventricular ejection fraction.

    B. TMAD is derived from speckle tracking echocardiography.

    C. TMAD is equivalent to the mitral annular displacement (MAD).

    D. TMAD is highly angle-dependent.

✪✪ Question 7

According to the 2015 Chamber Quantification Guidelines from the American Society of Echocardiography (ASE), which method is recommended for accurate and reproducible left ventricular (LV) volumetric measurements?

    A. 2D area-length method

    B. 2D modified Simpson biplane method

    C. 3D echocardiography

    D. Teichholz method

✪✪✪ Question 8

A 68-year-old male patient is admitted to the hospital for shortness of breath and peripheral edema. The echocardiogram showed moderate mitral regurgitation (MR). The blood pressure was 120/65 mm Hg, the peak MR velocity measured 5.2 m/s, and the time duration between the peak MR velocity at 1 m/s and at 3 m/s was measured at 0.032 s. Based on these measurements, what is the dP/dt?

    A. 100 mm Hg/s

    B. 163 mm Hg/s

    C. 1000 mm Hg/s

    D. 3000 mm Hg/s

    E. dP/dt cannot be calculated from the information provided

✪✪ Question 9

A female patient presents for an echocardiogram at 35 weeks gestation. Her study shows an increased left ventricular end-diastolic volume (LVEDV) resulting in increased stroke volume (SV). This is an example of which principle?

    A. Frank-Starling

    B. Kussmaul

    C. Laplace

    D. McConnell

✪ Question 10

Which of the following equations are used to calculate the left ventricular (LV) stroke volume (SV)?

    A. SV = CSA × VTI

    B. SV = LVEDV − LVESV

    C. SV = LVEDV ÷ LVESV

    D. Both A and B

    E. Both A and C

where CSA is cross-sectional area; LVEDV is left ventricular end-diastolic volume; LVESV is left ventricular end-systolic volume; VTI is velocity-time integral.

✪✪ Question 11

Which of the following will not result in an underestimation of the cardiac index (CI)?

    A. Nonparallel alignment of the pulsed-wave (PW) Doppler cursor with flow in the left ventricular outflow tract (LVOT)

    B. Underestimation of the LVOT diameter

    C. Placement of the PW Doppler sample volume too close to the aortic valve

    D. Overestimation of the patient's height

    E. All of the above

✪✪ Question 12

How is fractional shortening (FS) calculated?

    A. FS= ((LVEDD − LVESD) ÷ LVEDD) × 100

    B. FS= ((LVEDV − LVESV) ÷ LVEDV) × 100

    C. FS= (SV × HR) ÷ 100

    D. FS= (SV ÷ LVEDV) × 100

where LVEDD is left ventricular end-diastolic dimension; LVEDV is left ventricular end-diastolic volume; LVESD is left ventricular end-systolic dimension; LVESV is left ventricular end-systolic volume; SV is stroke volume.

✪✪ Question 13

Which of the following is not a limitation of fractional shortening (FS)?

    A. FS is derived from measurements performed in one dimension.

    B. FS is inaccurate when there are linear measurement errors.

    C. FS is not reliable in the setting of globally reduced left ventricular function.

    D. FS is not reliable in the setting of regional wall motion abnormalities.

✪ Question 14

Which of the following statements is/are true of tissue Doppler imaging (TDI) s′ velocities?

A. Velocities are dependent on the incident angle between sampling site and myocardial motion.

B. Velocities are unable to detect radial and circumferential motion from apical views.

C. Velocities can be affected by translation and myocardial tethering.

D. Velocities sample a small segment that is assumed to reflect the entire ventricle.

E. All of the above.

✪✪ Question 15

When calculating the myocardial performance index (MPI), which of the following will not have an effect on the accuracy of this calculation for the evaluation of global left ventricular (LV) function?

A. Arrhythmias

B. Quality of Doppler signals

C. Two-dimensional (2D) image quality

D. Tissue Doppler imaging (TDI) method

✪✪ Question 16

Which statement about ventricular contractility is true?

A. A decrease in contractility reduces stroke volume (SV) and increases end-systolic volume (ESV).

B. A decrease in contractility increases SV and decreases EDV.

C. An increase in contractility reduces SV and decreases ESV.

D. An increase in contractility increases SV and decreases EDV.

✪ Question 17

_____ is the volume of blood pumped by the heart per minute.

A. Cardiac index

B. Cardiac output

C. Ejection fraction

D. Stroke volume

✪ Question 18

All the following can affect left ventricular ejection fraction (LVEF) except:

A. Aortic stenosis.

B. Loading conditions.

C. Mitral regurgitation.

D. Tricuspid regurgitation.

✪ Question 19

In which phase of the cardiac cycle does the left ventricle reach its the smallest volume?

A. Diastolic ejection phase

B. Isovolumic contraction

C. Rapid ejection phase

D. Reduced ejection phase

✪✪ Question 20

A 45-year-old man presents with moderate aortic stenosis. Given the information provided in **Figures 11-1A** and **11-1B**, what is the cardiac output?

A. 4.5 L/min

B. 4.7 L/min

C. 5.8 L/min

D. 6.0 L/min

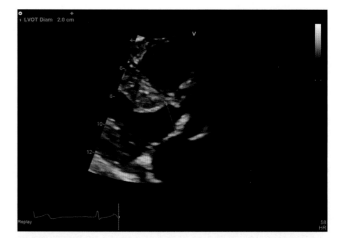

Figure 11-1A

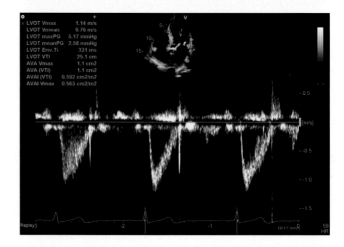

Figure 11-1B

✪ Question 21

Which of the following influences the stroke volume (SV)?

A. Preload
B. Afterload
C. Contractility
D. All of the above

✪✪ Question 22

A 35-year-old woman presents with sudden onset of dyspnea and pulmonary edema. She underwent bedside transthoracic echocardiography, which revealed hyperdynamic left ventricular systolic function, a normal aortic valve, and mitral regurgitation. The following data in **Table 11-2** were obtained from the echocardiogram. Based on these data, which of the following statements is true?

A. Left ventricular (LV) systolic function is normal.
B. LV systolic function is markedly diminished.
C. The rate of pressure rise in the left ventricle is 1600 mm Hg/s.
D. Both A and C.
E. Both B and C.

Table 11-2.

BP	95/50 mm Hg
HR	120 bpm
Peak MR velocity	4.0 m/s
Time interval from onset of MR to jet velocity of 1 m/s	5 ms
Time interval from onset of MR to jet velocity of 3 m/s	25 ms

BP, blood pressure; HR, heart rate; MR, mitral regurgitation.

✪✪✪ Question 23

The change in left ventricular (LV) function attributable to cell therapy is sought in a postinfarct patient. Which of the following echocardiographic measures is the most feasible marker of myocardial contractility?

A. dP/dt measured from the mitral regurgitant (MR) jet
B. Ejection fraction
C. Myocardia performance index (MPI)
D. Systolic strain
E. Systolic strain rate

✪✪ Question 24

When compared with two-dimensional based strain, the biggest disadvantage of tissue Doppler imaging (TDI)-based strain is:

A. Angle dependency.
B. Low sensitivity to signal noise.
C. The inability to determine both strain and strain rate.
D. Susceptibility to tethering.

✪✪✪ Question 25

In left ventricular (LV) torsion:

A. Basal twisting is the main component of LV systolic torsion.
B. During systole, the basal segments of the LV myocardium rotate counterclockwise.
C. During ejection, the apical segments rotate counterclockwise.
D. During ejection, the basal segments of the LV myocardium rotate counterclockwise.

✪✪✪ Question 26

Left ventricular (LV) strain has been proposed as a simple quantitative tool for assessing LV function. Which of the following is associated with reduced strain, irrespective of myocardial status?

A. Decreased afterload
B. Decreased preload
C. Decreased heart rate
D. All of the above
E. None of the above

CASE 1

The data provided in **Table 11-3** include parameters acquired during an echocardiogram.

Table 11-3.

LVOT diameter	20 mm
LVIDd	4.5 cm
LVIDs	2.5 cm
LVOT VTI	15 cm
AV VTI	30 cm
HR	75 bpm
BSA	1.7 m²

AV, aortic valve; bpm, beats per minute; BSA, body surface area; HR, heart rate; LVIDd, left ventricular internal dimension at end-diastole; LVIDs, left ventricular internal dimension at end-systole; LVOT, left ventricular outflow tract; VTI, velocity-time integral.

⚙ Question 27

Based on the data provided in **Table 11-3**, the stroke volume (SV) is:

A. 47.1 mL
B. 470 mL
C. 94.2 mL
D. 942 mL

⚙ Question 28

Based on the data provided in **Table 11-3**, the cardiac output (CO) is:

A. 7.0 L/min
B. 3.5 L/min
C. 3500 L/min
D. 7000 mL/min

⚙⚙ Question 29

Based on the stroke volume (SV) and cardiac output (CO) calculated in the two prior questions for this case (1), what can be stated about these values?

A. SV is normal and CO is abnormal.
B. SV is abnormal and CO is normal.
C. Both SV and CO are normal.
D. Both SV and CO are abnormal.

CASE 2

A 45-year-old female patient presents to the echocardiography lab for routine surveillance while on chemotherapy for breast cancer. According to the American Society of Echocardiography (ASE) and the European Association of Cardiovascular Imaging (EACVI) guidelines for imaging during and after cancer therapy, calculation of left ventricular ejection fraction (LVEF) is recommended. The following left ventricular (LV) volumes were measured by 2D echocardiography: end-diastolic volume (EDV) of 130 mL and an end-systolic volume (ESV) of 60 mL.

⚙ Question 30

Based on the data provided for this case (2), which of the following numbers represents the closest LVEF?

A. 35%
B. 45%
C. 55%
D. 65%

⚙ Question 31

Based on the data provided for this case (2), what is the stroke volume (SV)?

A. 53 mL
B. 70 mL
C. 190 mL
D. SV cannot be derived based on the limited information provided

⚙⚙ Question 32

According to the ASE/EACVI guidelines, the definition of cancer therapeutics–related cardiac dysfunction (CTRCD) is a:

A. Decrease in the left ventricular ejection fraction (LVEF) >10%, to a value <53%.
B. Decrease in the LVEF >15%, to a value below the normal reference value for patient gender.
C. Decrease in the left ventricular ejection fraction (LVEF) >10%, to a value <53% and a concurrent decrease in global longitudinal strain (GLS) by >15%.
D. Decrease in the LVEF >15%, to a value below the normal reference value for patient gender and/or a decrease in GLS by >10%.

ANSWERS

1. **Answer: E.** Visual LVEF should not be considered the "standard of care." The LVEF is derived from left ventricular (LV) volumes measured at end-diastole and end-systole. From these volumes the LVEF is then derived. Current guidelines recommend the calculation of LV volumes by the biplane method of disks summation technique (modified Simpson method) or by three-dimensional (3D) echocardiography when possible. Accuracy and reproducibility are especially important when the echocardiographic LVEF may be a component of major decisions, such as suitability for implantable defibrillator or cardiac resynchronization devices.

   However, although quantitation is accepted as the preferred method, this may not be achievable under all circumstances. As in other qualitative assessments in echocardiography, the inexperience of the reviewer and suboptimal image quality are potential limitations to the "eyeball" assessment of LVEF. Extremes of heart rate can make the assessment challenging and the evaluation of LV function from multiple views (tomographic approach) is crucial in the postinfarct ventricle.

TEACHING POINT

Although quantitation is accepted as the preferred method, potential problems with respect to spatial and temporal resolution need to be considered. Concerns about spatial resolution can be addressed by appropriate depth and zoom; LV opacification should be considered if two or more myocardial segments are inadequately visualized. Temporal resolution is an issue to the extent that the time course of contraction is neglected by assessment of only end-diastolic and end-systolic images, and global strain or similar parameters may help address this.

2. **Answer: B.** Preload, or the degree of myocardial distension prior to shortening, has a direct effect on SV. A greater stretch, or preload, leads to a greater force of contraction and an increased SV; therefore, answer B is correct. Answer A is incorrect because as the afterload (the force against which the ventricle is acting to eject blood) decreases, SV increases. This is especially true when contractility is impaired; this is the rationale for the need for afterload-reducing medications. Answer C is incorrect because as the LVEDV increases, so does SV. Answer D is incorrect as preload, or the degree of myocardial distension prior to shortening, has a direct effect on SV as previously stated.

3. **Answer: C.** Preload is affected by two main pumps, the respiratory pump and the skeletal muscle pump. The respiratory pump affects preload in the following way: intrathoracic pressure decreases during inspiration and abdominal pressure increases, which pushes blood toward the right atrium. The skeletal muscle pump affects preload in the following way: muscles in the legs squeeze the deep veins pushing blood back toward the heart.

4. **Answer: C.** Afterload is the resistance the ventricle faces as it ejects blood. Aortic impedance, viscosity of blood, left ventricular volume and pressure, as well as mass of blood in the aorta, all have an effect on left ventricular afterload. For example, an increase in blood viscosity leads to an increase in resistance and therefore an increase in afterload. Aortic impedance is determined by the resistance of the aorta and the compliance of this vessel; for example, increased resistance or decreased compliance will increase aortic impedance leading to an increase in afterload.

Afterload can also be defined as ventricular wall stress during systole. Wall stress is calculated using Laplace law:

$$\sigma = \left(P \times r\right) \div \left(2 \times h\right)$$

where σ = wall stress, P = ventricular transmural pressure, r = radius, h = wall thickness.

From this equation, it can be appreciated that when the radius of the ventricle increases (i.e., the ventricle dilates and volume increases), wall stress increases and therefore afterload increases. Likewise, as the pressure in the ventricle increases, wall stress increases, and afterload increases.

Pulmonary artery pressure does not affect left ventricular afterload. High pulmonary artery pressure, or pulmonary hypertension, affects the right side of the heart, as it has to work harder to pump blood to the lungs.

5. **Answer: B.** The MPI, also known as Tei index or the index of myocardial performance (IMP), is a Doppler-derived index used to assess global ventricular function. Systolic dysfunction results in a prolongation of the pre-ejection isovolumic contraction time (IVCT) and a shortening of the ejection time (ET), while both systolic and diastolic dysfunction cause abnormal myocardial relaxation, which prolongs the IVRT. This index is derived from the sum of the isovolumic times divided by the ejection time (**Figure 11-2**). In this example, the MPI is greater than 0.4, which is abnormal:

$$\begin{aligned} MPI &= \left(IVRT + IVCT\right) \div ET \\ &= \left(0.113 + 0.08\right) \div 0.2 \\ &= 0.965 \end{aligned}$$

6. **Answer: D.** Tissue motion annular displacement (TMAD) is derived from speckle tracking echocardiography and is equivalent to the mitral annular dis-

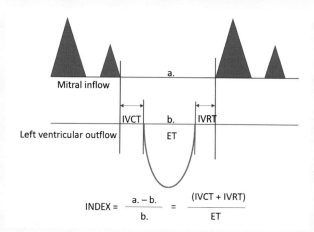

Figure 11-2

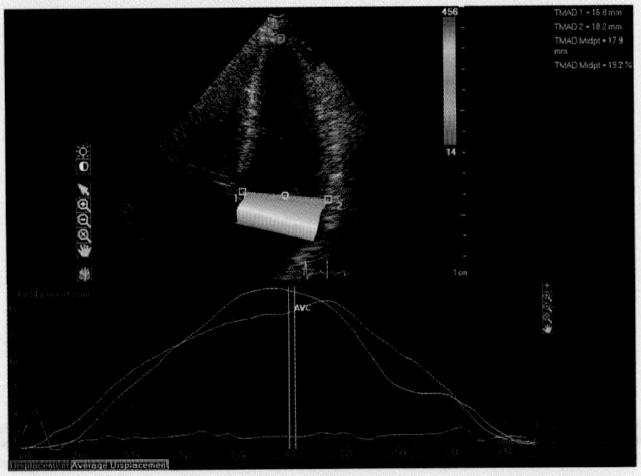

Figure 11-3 TMAD. Points are selected at the medial (1) and lateral (2) mitral valve annulus and LV apex (square). The points are automatically tracked through the cardiac cycle, producing two curves representing displacement of the medial and lateral points of the mitral valve annulus over time. Color kinesis demonstrates mitral annular displacement over the cardiac cycle. Values are generated for maximum displacement of the medial (TMAD1), lateral (TMAD2), and midpoint of the mitral valve annulus (TMAD Midpoint in mm), and displacement of the midpoint as a percentage of left ventricular length at end-diastole (TMAD Midpoint as %). AVC = aortic valve closure.

placement (MAD) that can be derived via M-mode (similar to the tricuspid annular plane systolic excursion or TAPSE). TMAD has been demonstrated to correlate with left ventricular ejection fraction. An advantage of this technique is that it is angle-independent; therefore, answer D is the false statement. TMAD is measured by selecting three points: at the lateral margin of the mitral valve annulus, at the medial margin of the mitral valve annulus, and at the left ventricular apex (**Figure 11-3**). A normal TMAD is >12 mm.

7. **Answer: C.** LV volumes are important for determining LV size and for calculating LV ejection fraction. As 3D echocardiographic LV volume measurements do not rely on geometric assumptions and are more accurate and reproducible compared to other methods listed, 3D echocardiographic measurements should be used when available and when there is good image quality.

    The 2D area-length method (answer A) is an alternative method to calculate LV volumes when apical endocardial definition precludes accurate tracing. However, this method assumes that the LV is bullet shaped and this assumption does not always hold true. The modified Simpson biplane method (answer B) is commonly used for 2D echocardiographic LV volume calculations and this is the recommended 2D method for estimating LV volumes. The Teichholz method (answer D) estimates LV volumes from LV linear dimensions assuming a fixed geometric LV shape (prolate ellipsoid). As this assumption does not apply in a variety of cardiac pathologies, this method for calculating LV volumes is no longer recommended for clinical use.

8. **Answer: C.** The dP/dt refers to the change in pressure (dP) over the change in time (dt) during the isovolumic contraction phase of the cardiac cycle. This is measured from the MR continuous-wave Doppler trace as the time difference (Δt) between the MR velocity at 1 m/s and the MR velocity at 3 m/s. Using the simplified Bernoulli equation, the pressure difference between 1 m/s and 3 m/s is 32 mm Hg:

$$\Delta P \text{ at } 3\,\text{m/s} = \left(4 \times 3^2\right) = 36\,\text{mm Hg}$$

$$\Delta P \text{ at } 1\,\text{m/s} = \left(4 \times 1^2\right) = 4\,\text{mm Hg}$$

$$\Delta P \text{ between } 3 \text{ and } 1\,\text{m/s} = 36 - 4 = 32\,\text{mm Hg} \qquad (1)$$

Therefore, the dP/dt is:

$$\text{d}P/\text{d}t = \Delta P \text{ between } 3 \text{ and } 1\,\text{m/s} \div \Delta t$$

$$= 32 \div 0.032$$

$$= 1000\,\text{mm Hg/s} \qquad (2)$$

A normal left ventricular (LV) dP/dt is >1200 mm Hg/s while a dP/dt <800 mm Hg/s is consistent with severe LV systolic function.

9. **Answer: A.** The Frank-Starling principle states that the heart is able to change its force of contraction in response to changes in venous return. In pregnancy, the mother's venous return increases, which results in an increase in the LVEDV. With this change in LVEDV, the muscle fibers stretch, creating increased preload. The increased preload results in an increase in the force of ventricular contraction and SV.

    The Kussmaul sign (answer B) refers to the absence of normal jugular vein collapse or a paradoxical rise in the jugular column due to impaired venous return to the right heart on inspiration. This sign is classically seen in constrictive pericarditis or restrictive cardiomyopathy but can be seen in some subjects with heart failure with reduced ejection fraction. The Laplace law (answer C) describes the relationship between the tension or wall stress, intracavity pressure, radius, and thickness of a thinned-walled sphere; this law explains why a dilated ventricle requires more tension to generate the same pressure as a normal ventricle. The McConnell sign (answer D) describes the presence of akinesis of the right ventricular (RV) middle free wall with preserved contractility or sparing of the RV apex. This sign has a high accuracy for diagnosing massive pulmonary embolism.

10. **Answer: D.** SV is the amount of blood pumped by the heart per beat and is measured in mL. SV can be calculated either by the 2D/Doppler method as CSA x VTI (answer A) or from left ventricular end-diastole and end-systolic volumes as LVEDV − LVESV (answer B). As previously described,

current guidelines recommend the calculation of left ventricular volumes by the biplane method of disks summation technique (modified Simpson method) or by 3D echocardiography when feasible.

For the 2D/Doppler method, the CSA is derived from the left ventricular outflow tract (LVOT) diameter and the VTI is derived from the pulsed-wave Doppler trace of the LVOT.

11. **Answer: C.** The CI is calculated as the cardiac output (CO) measured in L/min divided by the body surface area (BSA) measured as m^2:

$$CI\left(L/min/m^2\right) = CO \div BSA \qquad (1)$$

Cardiac output (CO) is derived from the stroke volume (SV) measured in mL and the heart rate (HR) measured as beats per minute.

$$CO\left(L/min\right) = \left(SV \times HR\right) \div 1000 \qquad (2)$$

The SV can be measured from the LVOT cross-sectional area of the LVOT (CSA_{LVOT}) measured in cm^2 and the LVOT velocity-time integral (VTI_{LVOT}) measured in cm:

$$SV\left(mL\right) = CSA_{LVOT} \times VTI_{LVOT} \qquad (3)$$

Placement of the PW Doppler sample volume too close to the aortic valve will result in an overestimation of the LVOT VTI and therefore an overestimation of the SV, CO, and CI as per Equations (1) to (3). Therefore, this answer is correct.

Nonparallel alignment of the PW Doppler cursor with flow in the LVOT (answer A) will result in an underestimation of the LVOT VTI and therefore an underestimation of the SV, CO, and CI as per Equations (1) to (3). Underestimation of the LVOT diameter (answer B) will result in an underestimation of the CSA of the LVOT and therefore an underestimation of the SV, CO, and CI as per Equations (1) to (3). Overestimation of the patient's height will result in an overestimation of the BSA and therefore an underestimation of the CI as per Equation (1).

12. **Answer: A.** FS is the percentage of change in left ventricular (LV) cavity dimension with systole. It is typically calculated from 2D or M-mode linear LV measurements acquired from the parasternal long-axis or parasternal short-axis views at end-diastole and end-systole. These measurements are obtained just distal to the mitral leaflet tips and perpendicular to the long axis of the left ventricle. It is current practice to measure the LV dimensions at the blood-tissue interfaces from the basal septum to the basal inferolateral wall. It is important to obtain good-quality, non-foreshortened images and accurate measurements to calculate FS. A normal FS is 27% to 45%. FS evaluates only basal contractility and therefore is not a reliable method for the evaluation of LV function in the setting of regional wall motion abnormalities.

13. **Answer: C.** FS can be accurately calculated in the setting of reduced global (symmetrical) systolic function.

One of the major limitations of FS is that it is a one-dimensional measurement that assumes all of the wall segments are contracting equally. Therefore, this calculation does not reflect overall left ventricular (LV) systolic function in the setting of regional wall motion abnormalities beyond the anterior septal and inferolateral walls. This is due to the potential change in shape and size of the left ventricle that can occur in the setting of regional wall motion abnormalities. As FS is calculated from linear LV measurements, any errors in these measurements will result in an inaccurate FS calculation.

14. **Answer: E.** TDI enables the measurement of longitudinal myocardial velocities. The TDI measurements are most commonly obtained from the apical views. Measurement of the peak s′ velocity reflects the systolic longitudinal shortening of the ventricle and therefore may provide an estimation of left ventricular (LV) systolic function. There are several limitations to using s′ as a measure of LV systolic function. The most significant disadvantage is that only a localized segment is sampled, and it is assumed that this small segment represents the entire ventricle. Proper placement of the sample volume is also important as well as the incident angle between the sampling site and myocardial motion. TDI from the apical views only detects longitudinal motion and not radial or circumferential myocardial motion. Translation and myocardial tethering can also affect this measurement. TDI is not able to distinguish between actively contracting myocardium and passive myocardial motion.

15. **Answer: C.** As previously described, the MPI is a Doppler-derived index used to assess global ventricular function (see answer outline for Question 5). Therefore, 2D image quality does not directly affect the accuracy of the MPI calculation. As measurements used to calculate MPI are derived from the spectral Doppler signal, this index can be useful to determine left ventricular systolic function when an estimation of ejection fraction is not possible.

Arrhythmias (answer A) affect the accuracy of the MPI calculation when MPI is derived via pulsed-wave Doppler. As previously shown in **Figure 11-2**, MPI can be calculated from the time interval between the mitral valve closure to the next mitral valve opening, and the ejection time measured from the left ventricular outflow tract trace. Therefore, as measurements are not performed on the same cardiac cycle, the accuracy may be affected by changes in the cycle lengths due to arrhythmias and/or heart rate fluctuation. The quality of Doppler signals (answer B) influences the accuracy of this calculation since the MPI is derived from spectral Doppler signals.

The TDI-derived MPI is calculated from TDI signals acquired at a single mitral annular site and by measuring the isovolumic contraction and relaxation times and the ejection time (duration of the s′ velocity). Therefore, as the TDI-derived MPI provides a measurement of the MPI at one site of the ventricle only, this is a measurement of the regional MPI and this index, therefore, may not reflect the overall LV function.

16. **Answer: A.** Contractility, also known as inotropy, describes the inherent strength of the ventricular muscle and its ability to shorten or contract with systole. A change in ventricular contractility causes an altered rate of ventricular pressure rise, thereby affecting SV and ESV. For example, when contractility (inotropy) increases, the SV increases and the ESV decreases. Conversely, a decrease in contractility (inotropy) reduces SV and increases ESV.

17. **Answer: B.** Cardiac output is the amount of blood the heart pumps in 1 minute, and it is dependent on the heart rate, contractility, preload, and after-load. Cardiac output (CO) is derived from the stroke volume (SV) measured in mL and the heart rate (HR) measured as beats per minute:

$$CO\left(L/min\right) = \left(SV \times HR\right) \div 1000$$

Cardiac index (answer A) is the cardiac output indexed to the body surface area. Ejection fraction (answer C) is the percentage of the ventricular end-diastolic volume that is ejected with systole. Stroke volume (answer D) is the amount of blood pumped by the heart per beat.

18. **Answer: D.** Tricuspid regurgitation does not have a direct effect on LVEF. In cases of aortic stenosis (answer A), increased afterload may reduce LVEF. In some cases of mitral regurgitation (answer C), increased preload and decreased afterload can increase LVEF. Therefore, loading conditions (answer D) can have either a positive or negative effect on LVEF depending on the circumstances.

19. **Answer: D.** There are seven phases to the cardiac cycle (**Figure 11-4**). The reduced ejection phase (phase 4) occupies the latter portion of systole and results in the smallest left ventricular volume. This phase marks the beginning of ventricular repolarization as depicted by the onset of the T wave on

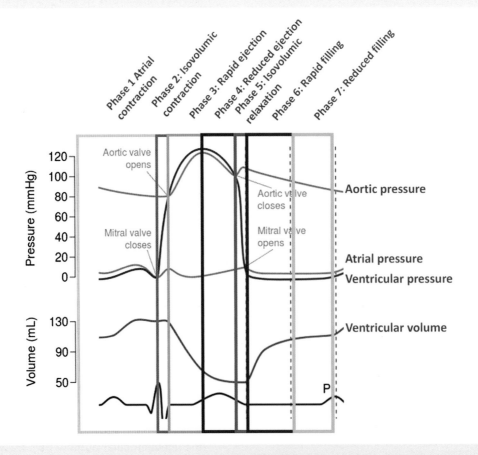

Figure 11-4

the electrocardiogram. Repolarization leads to a rapid decline in ventricular pressures and hence the reduced rate of ejection. However, some forward flow of blood continues secondary to remnant kinetic (or inertial) energy from the previous rapid ejection phase. This reduced ejection phase usually lasts for approximately 15% of the cardiac cycle.

20. **Answer: B.** As previously described, the cardiac output (CO) is derived from the stroke volume (SV) measured in mL and the heart rate (HR):

$$CO\left(L/min\right) = \left(SV \times HR\right) \div 1000 \qquad (1)$$

The SV can be measured from the cross-sectional area of the left ventricular outflow tract (CSA_{LVOT}) measured in cm^2 and the LVOT velocity-time integral (VTI_{LVOT}) measured in cm:

$$SV\left(mL\right) = CSA_{LVOT} \times VTI_{LVOT} \qquad (2)$$

CSA_{LVOT} is derived from the LVOT diameter ($LVOT_d$):

$$CSA_{LVOT}\left(cm^2\right) = 0.785 \times LVOT_{d^2} \qquad (3)$$

Combining the above three equations, the CO is derived from:

$$CO\left(L/min\right) = \left(0.785 \times LVOT_{d^2} \times VTI_{LVOT} \times HR\right) \div 1000 \qquad (4)$$

Therefore, based on the measured $LVOT_d$ in **Figure 11-1A** and the measured VTI_{LVOT} and heart rate shown in **Figure 11-1B**, the CO is:

$$CO\left(L/min\right) = \left(0.785 \times 2.0^2 \times 25.1 \times 59\right) \div 1000$$

$$= \left(4650\right) \div 1000$$

$$= 4.7 \qquad (5)$$

21. **Answer: D.** Preload, afterload, and contractility all influence the end-diastolic volume (EDV) and end-systolic volume (ESV). Therefore, as SV is derived from the EDV and ESV, these factors ultimately influence SV as well. For example, an increase in preload increases the EDV, which increases the SV, while a decrease in preload decreases the EDV, which decreases the SV. A decrease in afterload decreases ESV and increases SV, and an increase in afterload increases ESV and decreases SV. An increase in inotropy decreases the ESV and increases the SV while a decrease in inotropy increases the ESV and decreases the SV.

22. **Answer: D.** As previously described, from the MR signal the dP/dt can be calculated as the time difference (Δt) between the MR velocity at 1 m/s and the MR velocity at 3 m/s measured in seconds (s). Using the simplified Bernoulli equation, the pressure difference between 1 m/s and 3 m/s is 32 mm Hg. Therefore, the dP/dt is:

$$dP/dt\left(mm\ Hg/s\right) = 32 \div \Delta t \qquad (1)$$

In this example, the Δt is:

$$\Delta t = 25\,ms - 5\,ms = 20\ ms \qquad (2)$$

Converting this interval from milliseconds to seconds:

$$\Delta t = 20\,ms = 0.02\ s \qquad (3)$$

Therefore, the dP/dt is:

$$dP/dt\left(mm\ Hg/s\right) = 32 \div 0.02$$

$$= 1600\ mm\ Hg/s \qquad (4)$$

A dP/dt >1200 mm Hg/s is consistent with normal LV systolic function while a value <800 mm Hg/s would indicate markedly diminished LV systolic function. Therefore, as the dP/dt is 1600 mm Hg/s, answer D is correct.

23. **Answer: E** Contractility is a term that is often misused to describe systolic function. In fact, this parameter describes systolic function independent of loading. Changes in cardiac function can be attributed to alterations in contractility if heart rate, conduction velocity, preload, and afterload are held constant. Strain rate is a load-independent contractility marker that corresponds to the dP/dt. In contrast, ejection fraction, strain, and the MPI are load-dependent. Although LV dP/dt can be measured from the MR jet, this is restricted to when an MR signal is available and may be compromised in severe MR, as the calculation assumes that left atrial pressure is zero.

24. **Answer: A.** TDI-derived strain, like all Doppler techniques, is sensitive to alignment. Answer B is incorrect as the comparison of adjacent TDI velocities is extremely sensitive to signal noise. Answer C is incorrect since the instantaneous gradient of velocity, along a sample length, may be quantified by performing a regression calculation between the velocity data from adjacent sites along the scan line, and this instantaneous data may then be combined to generate a strain rate curve. Integration of this curve provides instantaneous data on deformation (strain). Answer D is incorrect since TDI is not susceptible to tethering to adjacent tissue, as the myocardial motion is measured relative to the adjacent myocardium and not relative to the transducer.

25. **Answer: C.** The LV myocardium has a spiral architecture with myocardial fibers that vary in orientation depending on where in the myocardium they are located. Fiber direction is predominantly longitudinal in the endocardial region, transitioning into a circumferential direction in the midwall and becoming longitudinal again over the epicardial surface. In addition to radial and longitudinal deformation, there is torsional deformation of the LV during the cardiac cycle due to the helical orientation of the myocardial fibers. During isovolumic contraction (Phase 1), the apex shows a brief clockwise rotation and the base a short counterclockwise rotation. During ejection (phase 2), the direction of the rotation changes to counterclockwise at the LV apex and clockwise at the LV base, respectively. Ventricular torsion and untwisting are essential for normal ventricular function.

26. **Answer: B.** Strain can be considered as an analog of regional ejection, as it reflects shortening from the beginning to the end of systole. Reduced preload, which is associated with reduced LV cavity size, will reduce strain, reflecting the lower position of the ventricle on the Frank-Starling curve as well as the lower deformation of an already empty LV cavity. Conversely, reduction of afterload is associated with increased strain, reflecting the lower impedance to LV ejection. Higher heart rate is associated with a reduction of LV filling and reduced strain. These observations are important in understanding the strain and strain rate response to dobutamine stress. Strain rate (which is time dependent) shows a linear increment with dobutamine, whereas strain increases initially but decreases toward peak dose, as the stroke volume falls at higher heart rates.

27. **Answer: A.** SV can be measured from the cross-sectional area of the left ventricular outflow tract (CSA_{LVOT}) measured in cm² and the LVOT velocity-time integral (VTI_{LVOT}) measured in cm:

$$SV\left(mL\right) = CSA_{LVOT} \times VTI_{LVOT} \qquad (1)$$

CSA_{LVOT} is derived from the LVOT diameter ($LVOT_d$):

$$CSA_{LVOT}\left(cm^2\right) = 0.785 \times LVOT_{d^2} \qquad (2)$$

Combing the above equations, the SV is derived from:

$$SV\left(mL\right) = \left(0.785 \times LVOT_{d^2}\right) \times VTI_{LVOT} \qquad (3)$$

Therefore, based on the data in **Table 11-3**, the $LVOT_d$ is 20 mm and the VTI_{LVOT} is 15 cm. To calculate the SV using Equation (3), the $LVOT_d$ needs to first be converted to cm (i.e., 2.0 cm). Therefore, the SV is:

$$SV = \left(0.785 \times 2.0^2\right) \times 15$$
$$= 47.1 mL \qquad (4)$$

28. **Answer: B.** As previously described, the CO is derived from the stroke volume (SV) measured in mL and the heart rate (HR):

$$CO\left(L/min\right) = \left(SV \times HR\right) \div 1000 \qquad (1)$$

The SV calculated in Question 27 is 47.1 mL. The heart rate from **Table 11-3** is 75 bpm; therefore, the CO is:

$$CO = \left(47.1 \times 75\right) \div 1000$$
$$= 3.5 L/min \qquad (2)$$

29. **Answer: D.** The normal values for SV are 70 to 100 mL and the normal values for CO are 4 to 8 L/min. Both SV and CO values in this case example are abnormal.

30. **Answer: C.** The LVEF from 2D LV volumes is calculated as:

$$LVEF\left(\%\right) = \left[\left(EDV - ESV\right) \div EDV\right] \times 100 \qquad (1)$$

Based on the data provided, the LVEF is:

$$LVEF = \left[\left(130 - 60\right) \div 130\right] \times 100$$
$$= 54\% \qquad (2)$$

31. **Answer: B.** As previously described SV can be calculated by either the 2D/Doppler method or from the left ventricular end-diastole and end-systolic volumes as:

$$SV\left(mL\right) = EDV - ESV \qquad (1)$$

Based on the data provided, the SV is:

$$SV = 130 - 60$$
$$= 70 mL \qquad (2)$$

32. **Answer: A.** Highly effective chemotherapeutic agents may cause CTRCD. For this reason, a careful evaluation of left ventricular (LV) systolic function is required. CTRCD is defined as a decrease in the LVEF of >10% points, to a value <53% (normal

reference value for 2D echocardiography) and this decrease should be confirmed on repeated studies. Accurate calculation of LVEF should be done with the best method available in the echocardiography laboratory (ideally 3D echocardiography). However, if 3D echocardiography is not available, the biplane modified Simpson technique is the method of choice. The early detection of subclinical LV dysfunction using GLS has also been advocated when there is no significant change in the LVEF. In cases where the baseline GLS is available, a relative percentage decrease of >15% compared with baseline is likely to be of clinical significance.

Acknowledgments: The authors thank and acknowledge the contributions from Muhamed Saric, MD, PhD, and Itzhak Kronzon, MD (Chapter 8 Doppler and Hemodynamics), Juan Carlos Plana Gomez, MD (Chapter 9 Tissue Doppler and Strain), and Thomas H. Marwick, MD, PhD (Chapter 12 Systolic Function Assessment) in Clinical Echocardiography Review: A Self-Assessment Tool, 2nd ed., edited by Allan L. Klein, Craig R. Asher, 2017.

SUGGESTED READINGS

Anderson B. Ventricular size and systolic function. In: *A Sonographer's Guide to the Assessment of Heart Disease*. Brisbane, Australia: Echotext Pty Ltd; 2014:chap 2.

Armstrong W, Ryan T. Evaluation of systolic function of the left ventricle. In: *Feigenbaum's Echocardiography*. 8th ed. Philadelphia: Wolters Kluwer; 2019:chap 5.

DeCara JM, Toledo E, Salgo IS, Lammertin G, Weinert L, Lang RM. Evaluation of left ventricular systolic function using automated angle-independent motion tracking of mitral annular displacement. *J Am Soc Echocardiogr*. 2005;18(12):1266-1269.

Lang RM, Badano LP, Mor-Avi V, et al. Recommendations for cardiac chamber quantification by echocardiography in adults: an update from the American Society of Echocardiography and the European Association of Cardiovascular Imaging. *J Am Soc Echocardiogr*. 2015;28(1):1-39.

Larsen CM, Vanden Bussche CL, Mankad S. Principles of measuring chamber size, volume and hemodynamic assessment of the heart. In: Nihoyannopoulos P, Kisslo J, eds. *Echocardiography*. 2nd ed. Switzerland: Springer; 2018:chap 6.

Plana JC, Galderisi M, Barac A, et al. Expert consensus for multimodality imaging evaluation of adult patients during and after cancer therapy: a report from the American Society of Echocardiography and the European Association of Cardiovascular Imaging. *J Am Soc Echocardiogr*. 2014;27(9):911-939.

Porter TR, Shillcutt SK, Adams MS, et al. Guidelines for the use of echocardiography as a monitor for therapeutic intervention in adults: a report from the American Society of Echocardiography. *J Am Soc Echocardiogr*. 2015;28(1):40-56.

CHAPTER 12

Left Ventricular Diastology

Contributors: Daniel P. Bourque, MS, RCS, Bryan Doldt, BS, RDCS, and Jeffrey C. Hill, BS, ACS

✪✪ Question 1

Which of the following variables is not useful in predicting an elevated left atrial pressure (LAP)?

A. Averaged mitral E/e′ ratio >14
B. Left atrial end-systolic volume index >34 mL/m²
C. Peak tricuspid regurgitant velocity >2.8 m/s
D. Septal e′ velocity >7 cm/s

✪ Question 2

Which of the following pressures is consistent with an elevated left ventricular end-diastolic pressure (LVEDP)?

A. 10 mm Hg
B. 13 mm Hg
C. 17 mm Hg
D. 8 mm Hg

✪✪✪ Question 3

The best echocardiographic finding that differentiates restrictive cardiomyopathy from constrictive pericarditis is the:

A. Mitral inflow pattern.
B. Pulmonary venous flow pattern.
C. Atrial size.
D. Inferior vena cava (IVC) size.
E. Early diastolic mitral annular medial velocity.

✪ Question 4

Which of the following technical considerations is not recommended when measuring left atrial (LA) volumes?

A. Exclude left atrial appendage
B. Exclude mitral annular tenting area

C. Trace into the pulmonary vein orifice
D. Trace the LA at end-systole

✪ Question 5

The E/e′ ratio is used to estimate:

A. Mean left atrial pressure (LAP).
B. Mean right atrial pressure (RAP).
C. Pulmonary artery systolic pressure (PASP).
D. Right ventricular systolic pressure (RVSP).

✪✪✪ Question 6

Which of the following statements is true regarding pulmonary venous spectral Doppler?

A. An atrial reversal (AR) duration < mitral inflow A duration indicates an increased LV end-diastolic pressure (LVEDP).
B. A peak AR velocity >35 cm/s suggests elevated left ventricular (LV) filling pressures.
C. The systolic (S) wave is related to LV relaxation.
D. The systolic to diastolic ratio (S/D) provides an accurate estimation of LV filling pressures in patients with preserved and reduced systolic function.
E. Pulmonary venous AR flow can be obtained in only 50% of patients.

✪✪ Question 7

Which of the Doppler variables is not seen in a patient with an advanced restrictive cardiomyopathy?

A. An isovolumic relaxation time (IVRT) of 45 ms
B. Mitral E/A ratio of 2.8
C. Mitral E-wave deceleration time of 180 ms
D. Septal and lateral e′ velocities of 3 and 4 cm/s

✪✪ Question 8

Which of the following statements is true regarding the estimation of left ventricular (LV) filling pressures in patients with atrial fibrillation?

A. A short deceleration time in patients with a normal ejection fraction (EF) correlates with elevated PCWP.

B. A septal E/e′ ≥11 correlates well with elevated pulmonary capillary wedge pressure (PCWP).

C. An increased left atrial size (>34 mL/m²) will reflect chronically elevated LV filling pressures.

D. The peak diastolic pulmonary venous velocity will reflect left atrial pressure.

E. It is impossible to estimate PCWP since there is no mitral A wave and the variability in cycle length precludes any accurate estimation.

✪✪✪ Question 9

Which of the following measurements best correlates with an elevated left ventricular end-diastolic pressure (LVEDP)?

A. Left atrial (LA) end-systolic volume index >34 mL/m²

B. Mitral E-wave velocity <50 cm/s

C. Pulmonary venous atrial reversal (AR) velocity >35 cm/s

D. Right ventricular systolic pressure (RVSP) <20 mm Hg

E. Both A and C

✪✪✪ Question 10

Which of the following resting echocardiographic findings is an indicator for diastolic stress testing in a symptomatic patient?

A. Mitral E/A = 0.8; E/e′ = 10; peak tricuspid regurgitation (TR) velocity = 2.7 m/s

B. Mitral E/A = 1.4; E/e′ = 8; peak TR velocity = 2.2 m/s

C. Mitral E/A = 1.9; E/e′ = 15; peak TR velocity = 3.2 m/s

D. Mitral E/A = 2.2; E/e′ = 19; peak TR velocity = 3.8 m/s

✪✪ Question 11

In the event that only the lateral or septal e′ velocity is available, what value of E/e′ ratios can be used to accurately predict elevated left ventricular (LV) filing pressures?

A. Lateral E/e′ >6; septal E/e′ >7

B. Lateral E/e′ >8; septal E/e′ >5

C. Lateral E/e′ >9; septal E/e′ >9

D. Lateral E/e′ >13; septal E/e′ >15

✪✪ Question 12

When performing pulsed-wave (PW) Doppler imaging in the apical 4-chamber view to acquire mitral annular velocities, which of the following is true?

A. Angulation of up to 40° between the ultrasound beam and the plane of cardiac motion is acceptable.

B. In general, the velocity scale should be set at ~30 cm/s above and below the zero-velocity baseline.

C. Spectral recordings are ideally obtained during inspiration and measurements should reflect the average of three consecutive cardiac cycles.

D. The PW Doppler sample volume should be positioned at or 1 cm within the septal and lateral insertion sites of the mitral leaflets.

E. The PW Doppler sample volume should be small enough (usually 2-3 mm) to evaluate the longitudinal excursion of the mitral annulus in both systole and diastole.

✪ Question 13

Mitral E-wave deceleration time is defined as the:

A. Measurement of the duration of the mitral E-wave velocity.

B. Time required for the peak E-wave velocity to decrease to zero.

C. Duration of time between the peak mitral E-wave and A-wave velocities.

D. Time required for the peak E-wave velocity to decrease by 29%.

✪✪✪ Question 14

Color Doppler M-mode (CMM) echocardiography provides information on flow propagation (Vp) and is relatively independent of which of the following?

A. Cardiac output

B. Heart rate

C. Left atrial size

D. Left ventricular (LV) compliance

E. Loading conditions

✪✪✪ Question 15

What is the strongest determinant of mitral deceleration time?

- **A.** Left atrial (LA) mechanical function
- **B.** Left ventricular (LV) operating stiffness
- **C.** Left ventricular end-diastolic pressure (LVEDP)
- **D.** Ejection fraction
- **E.** LA reservoir function

✪ Question 16

Which of the following mitral E-wave velocity changes occurs in a patient with pericarditis and constrictive physiology?

- **A.** Increase in the mitral E-wave velocity is seen during inspiration.
- **B.** Decrease in the mitral E-wave velocity is seen during shallow breathing.
- **C.** Increase in the mitral E-wave velocity is seen at end-expiration.
- **D.** Increase in the mitral E-wave velocity is seen during early expiration.

✪✪✪ Question 17

In patients with dilated cardiomyopathy, the pulsed-wave (PW) Doppler mitral inflow profile correlates with which of the following?

- **A.** Left ventricular (LV) filling pressures and functional class, but not prognosis
- **B.** Prognosis, but not LV filling pressures or functional class
- **C.** LV filling pressures, functional class, and prognosis, but less so than does LV ejection fraction
- **D.** LV filling pressures, functional class, and prognosis better than does LV ejection fraction
- **E.** LV filling pressures, functional class, and prognosis, but to a lesser degree than in patients with LV ejection fraction >50%

✪✪ Question 18

Which statement is most correct with respect to the application of the Valsalva maneuver in the assessment of diastolic function?

- **A.** In cardiac patients, a decrease of ≥50% in E/A ratio is highly specific for increased left ventricular (LV) filling pressures.
- **B.** The lack of reversibility in E/A ratio with Valsalva in patients with advanced diastolic dysfunction indicates irreversible restrictive physiology and implies a very poor prognosis.

- **C.** The Valsalva maneuver is a sensitive and specific way to differentiate normal from stage 1 diastolic function.
- **D.** The Valsalva maneuver should be used in every patient when assessing diastolic function.

✪✪ Question 19

Which of the following statements best describes Grade II (moderate) diastolic dysfunction?

- **A.** Mitral E/A ratio of 0.8, E/e' ratio of 9, peak tricuspid regurgitant (TR) velocity of 4.1 m/s, LA volume index (LAVi) of 30 mL/m²
- **B.** Mitral E/A ratio of 1.4, E/e' ratio of 17, peak TR velocity of 3.1 m/s, LAVi of 68 mL/m²
- **C.** Mitral E/A ratio of 1.9, E/e' ratio of 5, peak TR velocity of 2.1 m/s, LAVi of 22 mL/m²
- **D.** Mitral E/A ratio of 0.5, E/e' ratio of 9, peak TR velocity of 2.6 m/s, LAVi of 28 mL/m²

✪✪ Question 20

A 35-year-old male athlete complains of exercise intolerance. An echocardiogram shows normal left ventricular (LV) systolic function (ejection fraction of 60%) and no valvular dysfunction. Based on the pulsed-wave Doppler recording of his mitral inflow pattern in **Figure 12-1**, which additional echocardiographic parameter, is most helpful in confirming whether his symptoms should be attributed to elevated LV filling pressures?

- **A.** Left atrial volume index of 34 mL/m²
- **B.** The presence of mild concentric LV hypertrophy
- **C.** Tissue Doppler early diastolic velocity of the mitral annulus of 6 cm/s
- **D.** Prolonged diastolic filling time
- **E.** Indexed LV end-diastolic volume of 80 mL/m²

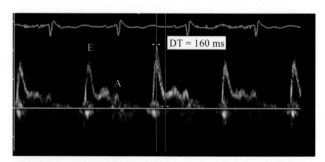

Figure 12-1 DT, deceleration time.

✪✪✪ Question 21

A 59-year-old man with a history of sleep apnea, hypertension, and hyperlipidemia presents to the emergency room with shortness of breath, edema and chest pain. Based on echocardiographic findings listed in **Table 12-1**, left ventricular (LV) diastolic function is:

A. Normal.
B. Grade I.
C. Grade II.
D. Grade III.
E. Cannot be determined.

Table 12-1.

LVEF	60%-65%
Mitral E-wave velocity	48 cm/s
E/A ratio	1.1
Averaged E/e′ ratio	7
LAVi	36 mL/m²
Pulmonary venous	S-wave > D-wave
Peak TR velocity	Inadequate
Linear LVMi	168 g/m²

LAVi, left atrial volume index; LVEF, left ventricular ejection fraction; LVMi, left ventricular mass index; TR, tricuspid regurgitant.

✪✪ Question 22

Which label on **Figure 12-2**, acquired in a patient with a left bundle branch block and myocardial disease, correctly identifies the peak e′ velocity?

A. A
B. B
C. C
D. None of the above

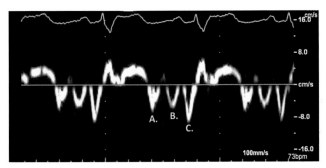

Figure 12-2

✪✪ Question 23

A 61-year-old woman with ischemic cardiomyopathy is referred for cardiac resynchronization therapy. Just before implantation of her biventricular device, she undergoes transthoracic echocardiography. Six months later, a new echocardiogram is obtained. Based on the data in **Table 12-2** and **Figures 12-3A** and **12-3B**, which statement is correct?

A. Left ventricular (LV) relaxation has improved.
B. LV filling pressures are decreased.
C. Left atrial contractility has increased.
D. LV stiffness has increased.
E. There is less dyssynchrony.

Table 12-2.

Baseline	6-Month Follow-up
E = 78 cm/s	E = 111 cm/s
A = 72 cm/s	A = 28 cm/s
E/A = 1.1	E/A = 3.6
DT = 180 ms	DT = 126 ms
Vp = 28 cm/s	Vp = 25 cm/s

DT, deceleration time; Vp, flow propagation.

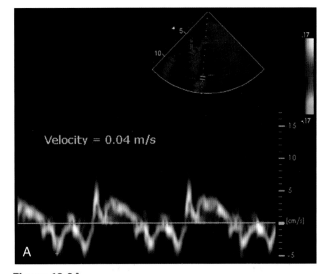

Figure 12-3A

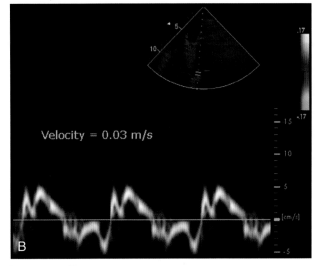

Figure 12-3B

✪✪ Question 24

A 76-year-old woman presents to the echocardiography laboratory with a history of hypertension, diabetes mellitus, New York Heart Association functional class III heart failure, and lower extremity edema. Based on echocardiographic findings listed in **Table 12-3**, left ventricular (LV) diastolic function is:

A. Normal.
B. Grade I.
C. Grade II.
D. Grade III.
E. Indeterminate.

Table 12-3.

LVEF	25%-30%
Mitral E-wave velocity	1.26 m/s
DT	128 ms
E/A ratio	2.6
E/A ratio with Valsalva	2.3
Averaged E/e′ ratio	20
LAVi	56 mL/m²
Pulmonary vein velocities	S-wave < D-wave
Peak TR velocity	3.9 m/s
Linear LVMi	130 g/m²

DT, mitral deceleration time; LAVi, left atrial volume index; LVEF, left ventricular ejection fraction; LVMi, left ventricular mass index; TR, tricuspid regurgitant.

✪ Question 25

In **Figure 12-4**, what is most likely affecting the quality of the tissue Doppler tracing in this patient with suboptimal image quality?

A. Overall gain
B. Doppler angle of incidence
C. Sample volume placed below the annulus
D. Mitral annual calcification is present

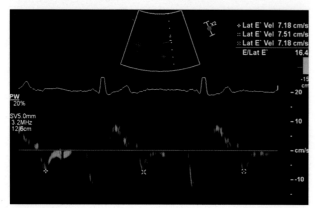

Figure 12-4

✪ Question 26

The mitral inflow pattern shown in **Figure 12-5** should be considered abnormal for which of the following patients?

A. A 41-year-old man with normal ejection fraction (EF) and moderate pulmonary hypertension
B. A 46-year-old woman with a bicuspid aortic valve and moderately severe aortic insufficiency
C. A 28-year-old athlete complaining of atypical chest pain
D. A 37-year-old obese woman complaining of shortness of breath
E. A 65-year-old man with a normal ejection fraction and left atrial enlargement

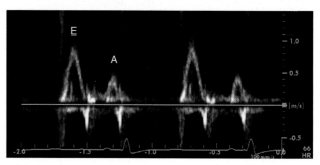

Figure 12-5

✪✪ Question 27

⏵ A 55-year-old man with a history of metabolic syndrome and known obstructive three-vessel coronary artery disease presents to the echocardiography laboratory for preoperative evaluation. His echocardiogram demonstrates moderately to severely reduced ejection fraction (EF), moderate left atrial (LA) enlargement, and no significant mitral regurgitation (**Video 12-2**). The tricuspid regurgitant jet was inadequate for measurement. Based on the Doppler findings in **Figures 12-6A** to **12-6E** diastolic function is:

A. Grade I.
B. Grade II.
C. Grade III (reversible).
D. Grade III (irreversible).
E. Indeterminate due to conflicting data.

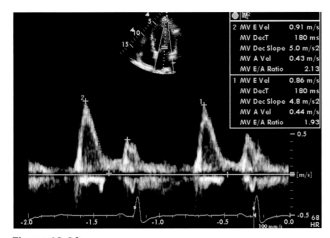

Figure 12-6A

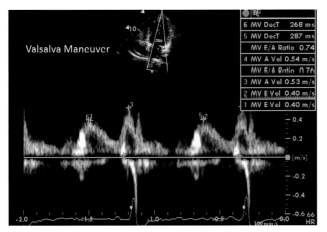

Figure 12-6B

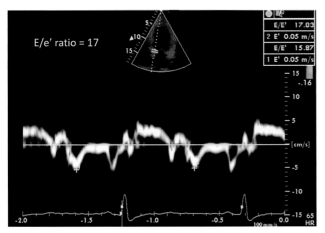

Figure 12-6C

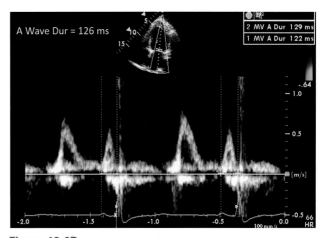

Figure 12-6D

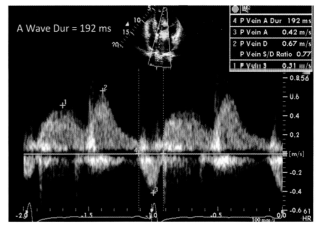

Figure 12-6E

⭐ Question 28

What did the sonographer adjust to improve the quality and consistency of the e′ velocity waveforms between the traces shown in **Figures 12-7A** and **12-7B**?

- **A.** Increased the Doppler gain
- **B.** Obtained traces during apnea
- **C.** Decreased the Doppler gain
- **D.** Repositioned the sample volume toward the atrium

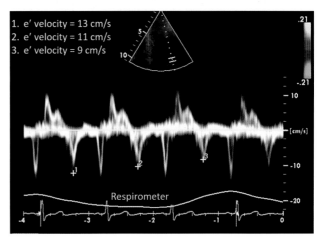

Figure 12-7A

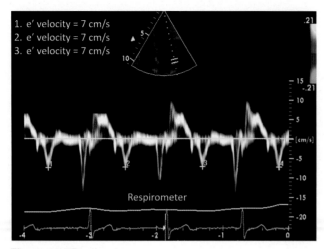

Figure 12-7B

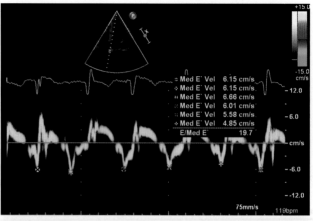

Figure 12-8B

✪✪ Question 29

The spectral Doppler traces shown in **Figures 12-8A** and **12-8B** were acquired in a patient with atrial fibrillation, mild mitral regurgitation, mild pulmonary hypertension, and severe left atrial enlargement. Based on this information, left ventricular (LV) filling pressures are most likely:

   A. Low.
   B. Normal.
   C. High.
   D. Inconclusive.

✪✪ Question 30

The mitral inflow pattern shown in **Figure 12-9** is by itself suggestive of elevated left ventricular (LV) filling pressures if:

   A. The patient has an ejection fraction (EF) of 25%.
   B. The patient has an EF of 60%.
   C. The patient has a dilated left atrium and a prior history of paroxysmal atrial fibrillation.
   D. The patient has mitral valve prolapse and moderately severe mitral regurgitation (MR).
   E. The maximal velocity of the tricuspid regurgitant jet is 3.5 m/s.

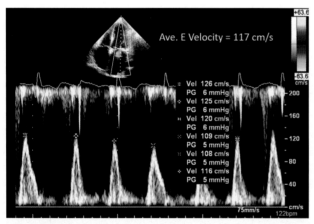

Figure 12-8A

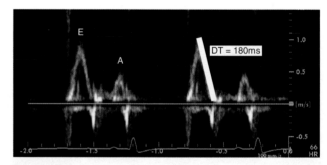

Figure 12-9

✪✪✪ Question 31

The absence of diastasis on the trace shown in **Figures 12-10A** and **12-10B**, acquired in this patient with a displayed heart rate of 77 bpm, is due to:

   A. Prolongation of the isovolumic relaxation time.
   B. Elevation of the left atrial pressure.
   C. First-degree heart block.
   D. A high heart rate (heart rate of 77 bpm is incorrectly displayed).

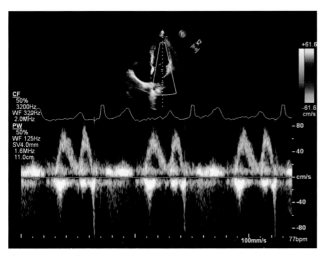

Figure 12-10A

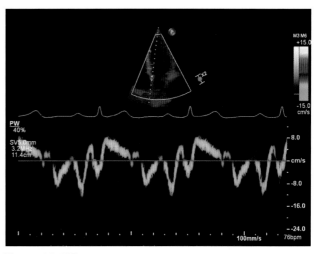

Figure 12-10B

✪✪✪ Question 32

The Doppler findings in **Figures 12-11A and 12-11B** are most likely to be found in which clinical scenario?

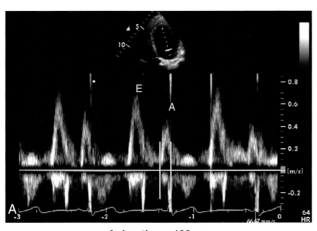

A duration = 100 ms
Mitral inflow

Figure 12-11A

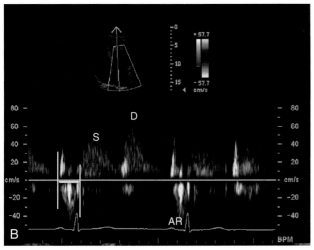

AR duration = 180 ms
Pulmonary venous flow

Figure 12-11B

A. A 35-year-old male athlete

B. A 40-year-old man with asymptomatic newly diagnosed hypertrophic cardiomyopathy

C. A 50-year-old woman with significant mitral regurgitation

D. A 50-year-old woman with atrial fibrillation

E. A 60-year-old man with advanced hypertensive heart disease

✪✪ Question 33

In the absence of conventional diastolic measurements, which of the following secondary measurements can aid in the diagnosis of Grade I diastolic dysfunction in a patient with left atrial (LA) enlargement and myocardial disease?

A. Pulmonary venous D wave > S wave

B. Color M-mode Vp slope >50 cm/s

C. Isovolumic relaxation time (IVRT) >100 ms

D. Decrease in mitral E/A ratio >0.5 during Valsalva maneuver

CASE 1

A 66-year-old man with a history of nonischemic cardiomyopathy and New York Heart Association (NYHA) functional class IV heart failure underwent cardiac resynchronization therapy (CRT) in 2011. Pulsed-wave Doppler of his mitral inflow and tissue Doppler imaging at the septal (medial) mitral annulus were recorded pre-implantation of the CRT device (**Figures 12-12A** and **12-12B**). The patient's peak tricuspid regurgitant (TR) velocity was 3.4 m/s. Postimplantation, the patient was classified as a "responder" to CRT with a reduction in his NYHA classification from class IV to class I. Several follow-up echocardiograms were performed thereafter. The abovementioned echocardiographic data were re-recorded in 2014 as seen in **Figures 12-12C** and **12-12D**. The patient's peak TR velocity had decreased to 2.3 m/s.

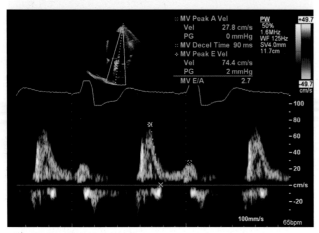

Figure 12-12A

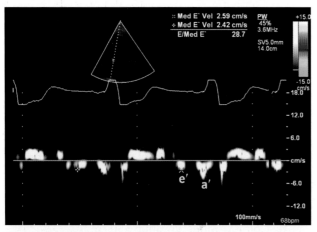

Figure 12-12B

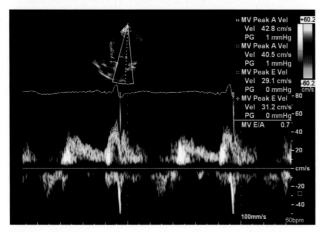

Figure 12-12C

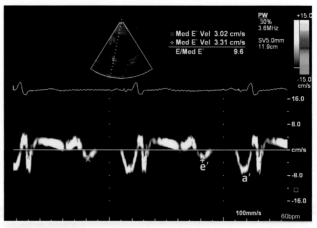

Figure 12-12D

⭐ Question 34

What changes, if any occurred to this patient's diastolic function?

- **A.** Diastolic function worsened
- **B.** Diastolic function did not change
- **C.** Diastolic function improved slightly
- **D.** Diastolic function improved significantly

CASE 2

A 67-year-old man recently diagnosed with multiple myeloma has been complaining of worsening dyspnea. His medical history is otherwise remarkable only for hyperlipidemia and prior tobacco abuse. Physical examination is notable for a 2/6 systolic ejection murmur at the left lower sternal border. No S3 or S4 is audible. Neck veins are mildly elevated at 10 cm. There is mild lower extremity pitting edema. The electrocardiogram is remarkable for relatively low voltages. In addition, there are Q waves present in the anteroseptal precordial leads. An abdominal fat pad biopsy confirms the diagnosis of amyloidosis (type AL) with apple-green birefringence under a polarized light microscope after staining with Congo red.

⭐⭐ Question 35

In patients with more advanced stages of amyloidosis, a combined relaxation abnormality and a mild increase in left atrial pressure (LAP) will result in which of the following?

- **A.** Grade I diastolic dysfunction (impaired relaxation)

B. Grade II diastolic dysfunction (pseudonormalized)
C. Decreasing pulmonary venous atrial reversal (AR) velocity
D. Decreasing left ventricular end-diastolic pressure (LVEDP)

CASE 3

A 70-year-old male patient has had a biventricular pacemaker inserted. He does not notice much improvement in his shortness of breath and an atrioventricular (AV) optimization echocardiogram is requested to assess post-implantation diastolic filling. Mitral valve (MV) inflow patterns at different paced AV delays are obtained from a baseline setting of 130 ms through 300 ms as shown in **Figure 12-13**.

✪✪✪ Question 36

Based upon the echocardiographic data, which of the following statements can be made about this patient's diastology?

A. A grade I left ventricular (LV) diastolic filling pattern represents a desirable result after AV optimization.
B. Assessment of the degree of mitral regurgitation is not relevant during AV optimization.
C. Baseline AV delay settings here appear to be optimal.
D. Diastolic filling times are independent of AV delay settings.
E. The relative contributions of "passive" (E wave) versus "active" (A wave) diastolic filling are independent of AV delay settings.

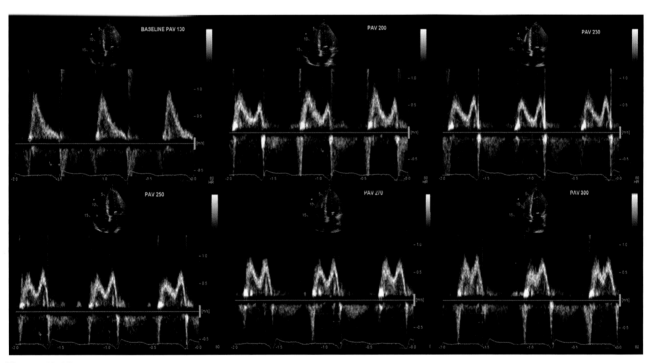

Figure 12-13

ANSWERS

1. **Answer: D.** The septal e' velocity by itself represents the rate of left ventricular (LV) relaxation only and does not estimate LV filling pressures. However, when combined with the peak mitral E-wave velocity, the E/e' ratio can be useful in estimating LAP. According to the 2016 American Society of Echocardiography Recommendations for the Evaluation of Diastolic Function, answers A, B, and C are not correct because when combined, those three variables are associated with elevated LAP (**Figure 12-14**).

2. **Answer: C.** LVEDP is considered abnormal when it is >15 mm Hg. Note that the term "left ventricular filling pressures" can refer to four different pressures that are measured by different methods. The LVEDP and left ventricular (LV) pre-A pressures can be measured via left heart catheterization by advancing a catheter across the aortic valve into the left ventricle (**Figure 12-15**). The LVEDP, as it is named, is the pressure recorded at end-diastole, just before mitral valve closure. The LV pre-A pressure is the LV pressure just prior

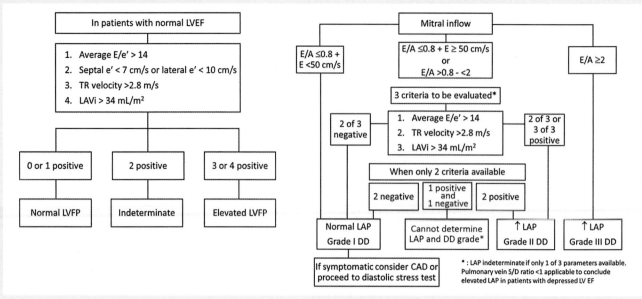

Figure 12-14 Modified algorithms for estimation of left ventricular filling pressure (LVFP) and grading LV diastolic function. **Left:** For patients with a normal left ventricular ejection fraction (LVEF). **Right:** For patients with elevated LVFP based on left algorithm, patients with depressed LVEF, and patients with myocardial disease and normal LVEF. This would usually apply to a patient with coronary artery disease and wall motion abnormalities, LV hypertrophy, or cardiomyopathy. Also note for patients with a depressed LVEF, a pulmonary vein S/D ratio <1 may suggest elevated LAP. CAD, coronary artery disease; DD, diastolic dysfunction; E/A, ratio of peak mitral E-wave velocity over peak mitral A-wave velocity; E/e′, ratio of peak mitral E-wave velocity over tissue Doppler early diastolic annular velocity; TR, tricuspid regurgitation; LAP, left atrial pressure; LAVi, left atrial volume indexed to body surface area; pulmonary vein S/D, ratio of pulmonary venous systolic velocity over pulmonary venous diastolic velocity. (Modified from Nagueh SF, Smiseth OA, Appleton CP, et al. Recommendations for the evaluation of left ventricular diastolic function by echocardiography: an update from the American Society of Echocardiography and the European Association of Cardiovascular Imaging. *J Am Soc Echocardiogr.* 2016;29(4):277-314. Copyright © 2016 American Society of Echocardiography. With permission; and Reprinted with permission from Oh JK, Assessment of diastolic function. In: Oh JK, Kane GC, eds. *The Echo Manual.* 4th ed. Philadelphia, PA: Wolters Kluwer; 2019:chap 8.)

to the A wave on the left atrial pressure (LAP) trace; this pressure is a surrogate for the mean LAP and precedes the LVEDP. The pulmonary capillary wedge pressure (PCWP) and the mean LAP can be measured via right heart catheterization. The PCWP is measured by wedging a catheter into a small pulmonary arterial branch; this pressure is also a surrogate for the mean LAP. The mean LAP is measured via an interatrial septal puncture; the direct measurement of the LAP via this technique is rarely performed.

Echocardiographic variables such as the E/e′ ratio correlate with PCWP, mean LAP, and LV pre-A-wave

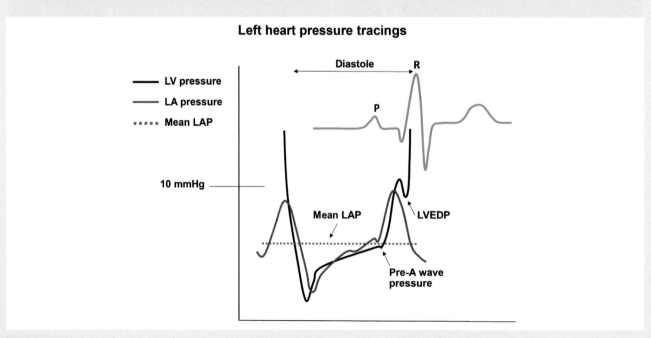

Figure 12-15

pressure, while the mitral A-wave duration compared to pulmonary venous atrial reversal (AR) wave duration, along with the peak pulmonary venous AR velocity, correlates with the LVEDP.

3. **Answer: E.** Differentiating restrictive cardiomyopathy from constrictive pericarditis by echocardiography can be challenging. A mitral septal early diastolic (e′) velocity ≥8 cm/s has been shown to be highly accurate in differentiating patients with constrictive pericarditis from those with restrictive cardiomyopathy, a point that was highlighted in the 2016 ASE/EACVI guideline document in an algorithmic form (**Figure 12-16**). In particular, the presence of a normal annular e′ velocity in a patient referred with a heart failure diagnosis should raise suspicion of pericardial constriction. The presence of grade 1 filling or absence of IVC dilatation makes a diagnosis of constriction/restriction unlikely. Respirophasic ventricular septal shift is an echocardiographic correlate of ventricular interdependence whereby one ventricle fills at the expense of the other and is generally present in constriction.

Apart from 2D features that give clues to the differentiation of diseases, tissue Doppler imaging (TDI) can provide important specific information. In patients with restrictive cardiomyopathy, myocardial relaxation (e′) will be severely impaired, whereas patients with constriction usually have preserved mitral annular vertical excursion. Of note, the lateral annular e′ velocity could be decreased if the constrictive process involves the lateral mitral annulus. **Figures 12-17A** and **12-17B** illustrate typical tissue Doppler tracings from a patient with constrictive pericarditis as opposed to a patient with restrictive cardiomyopathy.

4. **Answer: C.** The LA volume measurement is an important parameter that is considered in evaluation of left ventricular diastolic function (see **Figure 12-14**). Therefore, accurate LA volume measurements are essential. When performing LA volume measurements, the sonographer should avoid tracing into the pulmonary vein orifice, as this may overestimate LA volumes. A straight line should be drawn across the mitral annulus to exclude the mitral annular tenting area. Measurements should

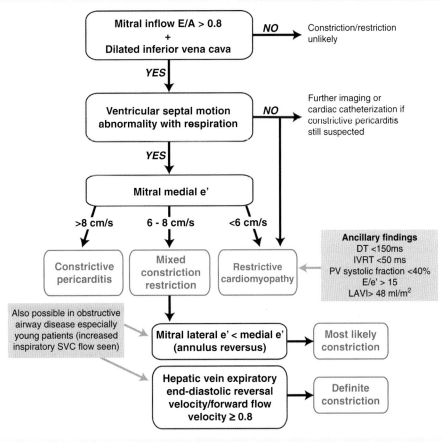

Figure 12-16 Algorithm comparing constrictive pericarditis and restrictive cardiomyopathy. Note that restriction is associated with elevated E/A ratio, short deceleration time, and decreased mitral annular velocity (<6 cm/s). E/A = ratio of peak mitral flow velocity of the early filling wave over peak mitral flow velocity of the late filling wave due to atrial contraction; mitral medial e′ = tissue Doppler early diastolic mitral annular velocity; DT = deceleration time; IVRT = isovolumic relaxation time; E/e′ = ratio of peak mitral flow velocity of the early filling wave over tissue Doppler early diastolic annular velocity; PV = pulmonary vein; LAVI = left atrial volume index; SVC = superior vena cava. (Reprinted from Nagueh SF, Smiseth OA, Appleton CP, et al. Recommendations for the evaluation of left ventricular diastolic function by echocardiography: an update from the American Society of Echocardiography and the European Association of Cardiovascular Imaging. *J Am Soc Echocardiogr.* 2016;29:277-314, Copyright 2016, with permission from Elsevier.)

Constrictive pericarditis

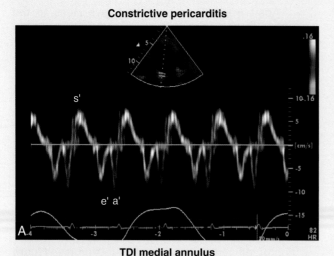

TDI medial annulus

Figure 12-17A

Restrictive cardiomyopathy

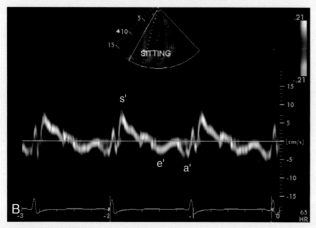

Figure 12-17B

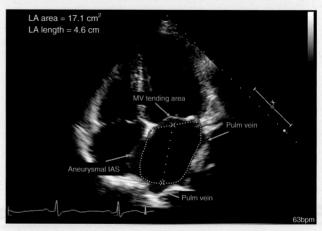

Figure 12-18 The left atrial (LA) area is traced to exclude the mitral valve (MV) tenting area, pulmonary (Pulm) vein and an aneurysmal interatrial septum (IAS) as depicted by the red zones. The LA length is measured from the center of the mitral annulus to the center of the superior LA wall.

be made at end-ventricular systole, which should correlate with the largest LA volume, preceding mitral valve opening. In addition, if the LA appendage is visualized in the apical 2-chamber view, it should be excluded as well (**Figure 12-18**).

TECHNICAL TIP

In some instances, the sonographer may encounter an aneurysmal interatrial septum (IAS). Including tracing of the IAS aneurysm is not recommended when measuring LA volumes due to the transient movement of the IAS during the cardiac cycle. In the event LA pressure is elevated at the time of the echocardiogram, the IAS may be displaced toward the right atrium. In this instance, when tracing the LA volume, a straight line across the IAS is recommended (see **Figure 12-18**).

5. **Answer: A.** The peak mitral E-wave velocity divided by the peak tissue Doppler e' velocity has been validated as a reliable index for the estimation of mean LAP. Mean RAP assessment (answer B) requires visualization of the inferior vena cava (IVC) and is estimated based on IVC size and inspiratory collapse. PASP (answer C) is equal to RVSP (answer D)

in the absence of right ventricular outflow tract obstruction or pulmonary valve stenosis. The estimation of the PASP and RVSP requires measurement of the peak tricuspid regurgitant velocity and an estimation of the RAP (as above).

6. **Answer: B.** The pulmonary venous AR velocity may increase with age, but an AR velocity >35 cm/s is usually consistent with elevated LV filling pressures, particularly at end-diastole. Answer A is incorrect as AR duration greater than (not less than) the mitral inflow A duration indicates an increased LVEDP. In particular, an AR-A duration >30 ms is consistent with an elevated LVEDP. Answer C is incorrect since it is the pulmonary venous D wave that is related to LV relaxation. Young and healthy individuals can therefore exhibit large D waves, indicating forceful elastic recoil of the left ventricle rather than high left atrial pressure. The pulmonary venous S wave is related to LV contractility, atrial function, atrial pressure, and mitral regurgitation. Answer D is incorrect as the S/D ratio is not very reliable for assessment of LV filling pressures in patients with an overall normal systolic function. ARdur-Adur >30 ms is a more robust marker of elevated LVEDP in this group of patients. Answer E is incorrect as the pulmonary venous AR flow can be obtained in more than 70% of patients. A commercially available ultrasound enhancing agent (contrast) injection can help enhance the Doppler tracing.

7. **Answer: C.** A mitral E-wave deceleration time of 180 ms is normal and is not typically seen in a patient with an advanced restrictive cardiomyopathy. In these patients, left ventricular (LV) compliance is decreased and the LV filling pressures are markedly elevated; as a result, the mitral deceleration time is usually shortened. Answers A and B are classic findings in a patient with myocardial disease and are suggestive of highly elevated LV filling pressures.

The markedly reduced tissue Doppler velocities (answer D) represent the extent of myocardial disease. Note that an E/A ratio of 2.8 would meet the criteria for restrictive filling and thus a shortened E-wave deceleration time would also be present.

8. **Answer: B.** Although sometimes challenging, an estimate of LV filling pressures can be obtained in patients with atrial fibrillation using the E/e′ ratio (with the septal e′). Different studies have shown good correlations between LV filling pressures and various Doppler indices in patients with atrial fibrillation. For example, E/e′ ≥11 predicts an LVEDP ≥15 mm Hg, and a mitral deceleration time <150 ms in the presence of LV systolic dysfunction, or the pulmonary venous diastolic deceleration time of ≤220 ms, is associated with higher LV filling pressures (**Table 12-4**).

9. **Answer: C.** A pulmonary venous AR velocity >35 cm/s is highly sensitive and specific for increased LVEDP (>15 mm Hg). An RVSP of <20 mm Hg is normal and does not typically correlate with an elevated LVEDP. A mitral E-wave velocity <50 cm/s is indicative of low filling pressures and most likely a normal LVEDP. Although an LA end-systolic volume index >34 mL/m² may indicate elevated filling pressures, like most measurements, it

alone cannot predict elevated left ventricular (LV) filling pressures. Additional echocardiographic findings are often needed to support elevated LV filling pressures at the time of the study.

TECHNICAL TIPS

In order to capture the peak pulmonary venous AR velocity more accurately, the sonographer should position the pulsed-wave Doppler sample volume at least 1 cm into the right upper pulmonary vein. Blood flow into the left atrium (LA) from this vein is typically most parallel, thus improving the accuracy of the peak Doppler velocity measurements. The use of color Doppler imaging may improve visualization of the pulmonary venous flow entering the LA.

10. **Answer: A.** Diastolic stress testing is indicated in patients with Grade I (mild) diastolic dysfunction and symptoms of dyspnea at rest or on exertion that cannot be explained by the results of a baseline (resting) echocardiogram. An increase in the mitral E/A ratio, E/e′ ratio, and peak TR velocity may reflect an abnormal increase in left ventricular (LV) filling pressures during the diastolic stress test. Conversely, it is atypical to see a significant rise in the abovementioned parameters in patients with normal diastolic function

Table 12-4. Assessment of LV Filling Pressures in Special Populations

Disease/Condition	Echocardiographic Measurements and Cutoff Values for Elevated LV Filling Pressures
1. Atrial fibrillation	Peak acceleration rate of mitral E velocity (≥1900 cm/s²), IVRT (≤65 ms), DT of pulmonary venous diastolic velocity (<220 ms), E/Vp ratio (≥1.4), and septal E/e′ ratio (≥11).
2. Sinus tachycardia	Mitral inflow pattern with predominant early LV filling in patients with EF <50%, IVRT ≤70 ms is specific (79%), systolic filling fraction ≤40% is specific (88%), lateral E/e′ >10 (a ratio >12 has highest specificity of 96%).
3. Hypertrophic cardiomyopathy	Lateral E/e′ (≥10), AR-A (≥30 ms), pulmonary artery pressures (>35 mm Hg), and LA volume (≥34 mL/m²).
4. Restrictive cardiomyopathy	DT (<140 ms), mitral E/A (>2.5), IVRT (<50 ms has high specificity), and septal E/e′ (>15)
5. Noncardiac pulmonary hypertension	Lateral E/e′ can be applied to determine whether a cardiac etiology is the underlying reason for the increased pulmonary artery pressures (cardiac etiology: E/e′ >10, noncardiac etiology: E/e′ is <8)
6. Mitral stenosis	IVRT (<60 ms has high specificity), IVRT/TE-e′ (<4.2), mitral A velocity (>1.5 m/s)
7. Mitral regurgitation	AR-A (≥30 ms), IVRT (<60 ms has high specificity), and IVRT/TE-e′ (<5.6) may be applied for the prediction of LV filling pressures in patients with MR and normal EF, whereas average E/e′ (>15) is applicable only in the presence of a depressed EF.

A, peak mitral flow velocity of the late filling wave due to atrial contraction; AR-A, the time difference between duration of pulmonary venous flow and mitral inflow during atrial contraction; DT, deceleration time; E, peak mitral flow velocity of the early filling wave; E/e′, ratio of peak mitral flow velocity of the early filling wave over tissue Doppler early diastolic annular velocity; EF, ejection fraction; E/Vp, ratio of peak mitral flow velocity of the early filling wave over flow propagation velocity by color M-mode; IVRT, isovolumic relaxation time; LAVI, left atrial volume index; TE-e′, the time difference between the onset of e′ velocity compared with onset of mitral E velocity.

Reprinted from Nagueh SF, Smiseth OA, Appleton CP, et al. Recommendations for the evaluation of left ventricular diastolic function by echocardiography: an update from the American Society of Echocardiography and the European Association of Cardiovascular Imaging. *J Am Soc Echocardiogr.* 2016;29:277-314, Copyright 2016, with permission from Elsevier.

during exercise. A mitral E/A ratio of 0.8, E/e' ratio of 10, and peak TR velocity of 2.7 m/s (answer A) would be consistent with mild diastolic dysfunction at rest. These findings should alert the clinician that LV filling pressures may abnormally increase during exertion in this patient, particularly the peak TR velocity. Diastolic stress testing is not indicated for patients with suspected elevated filling pressures at rest, as seen in answers C and D. The echocardiographic data in answer B is consistent with normal LV filling pressures. Diastolic stress testing is considered abnormal when all of the following three conditions are met: (1) average E/e' >14 with exercise, (2) peak TR velocity >2.8 m/s with exercise, and (3) baseline septal e' velocity is <7 cm/s or lateral e' velocity <10 cm/s. The results are normal when average (or septal) E/e' ratio is <10 at rest and with exercise and peak TR velocity is <2.8 m/s at rest and with peak exercise.

11. **Answer: D.** According to the 2016 American Society of Echocardiography Recommendations for the Evaluation of Diastolic Function, it is recommended to average both septal and lateral E/e' ratios when calculating the E/e' ratio. However, it is recognized that at times only the lateral e' or septal e' velocity is available and clinically valid. For example, in a patient with significant mitral annular calcification or akinetic wall segments, the e' velocity at the affected annulus should not be used in the calculation of the E/e' ratio and the estimation of LV filling pressures. The two ratios in answer D are consistent with elevated LV filling pressures, whereas the E/e' ratios in answers A to C are too low and would categorize patients incorrectly.

12. **Answer: D.** The PW Doppler sample volume should be positioned at or 1 cm within the septal and lateral insertion sites of the mitral leaflets and adjusted as necessary (usually 5-10 mm) to cover the longitudinal excursion of the mitral annulus in both systole and diastole. This contrasts with a sample volume size of 1 to 3 mm at the mitral valve tips for optimal PW Doppler assessment of mitral inflow, and a sample volume of 2 to 3 mm placed >0.5 cm into the pulmonary vein for optimal recording of pulmonary venous flow. Attention should be directed to Doppler spectral gain settings because annular velocities have high signal amplitude. Most current ultrasound systems have tissue Doppler presets for the proper velocity scale and Doppler wall filter settings to display the annular velocities. In general, the velocity scale should be set at ~20 cm/s above and below the zero-velocity baseline, although lower settings may be needed when there is severe left ventricular dysfunction, and annular velocities are markedly reduced (scale set to 10-15 cm/s). Minimal angulation (<20°) should be present between the ultrasound beam and the plane of cardiac motion.

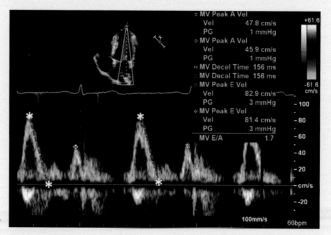

Figure 12-19

13. **Answer: B.** Mitral E-wave velocity represents the early rapid filling of the left ventricle or phase 2 of diastole. Measurement of the E-wave deceleration time is made by placing the caliper at the peak E velocity and extrapolating to the zero-velocity Doppler baseline (as indicated by the red dashed line in **Figure 12-19**). Measurement of the mitral E-wave duration, as well as the duration of time between the peak mitral E- and A-wave velocities, is not a useful parameter for the assessment of diastolic function. The time required for the peak E-wave velocity to decrease by 29% (answer D) is the pressure half-time, which is used to calculate mitral valve area in patients with mitral stenosis.

14. **Answer: E.** CMM echocardiography provides a spatiotemporal map of blood distribution within the heart with a typical temporal resolution of 5 ms, a spatial resolution of 300 microns, and a velocity resolution of 3 cm/s. CMM can be used to measure intraventricular pressure gradients over time as blood flow propagates from the mitral annulus toward the LV apex. In sinus rhythm, two waves are seen. The first wave corresponds to early diastolic filling and is determined by the rate of relaxation and the diastolic suction of the left ventricle; the second wave corresponds to atrial contraction. The flow propagation (Vp) is measured during early diastole from the mitral annulus to a distance of 4 cm into the LV cavity (**Figures 12-20A** and **12-20B**). A normal Vp is ≥50 cm/s. The Vp is inversely related to LV relaxation; therefore, when LV relaxation is impaired (or prolonged), the Vp is slowed. This parameter is relatively independent of loading conditions. E/Vp ≥2.5 predicts a pulmonary capillary wedge pressure >15 mm Hg. However, Vp has limited incremental value to e' velocity for assessing myocardial relaxation; it is not included in the most recent recommendations for the routine assessment of LV diastolic function.

15. **Answer: B.** E-wave deceleration time is mostly influenced by the operating stiffness of the left ventricle. Changes in LV compliance (i.e., the relationship

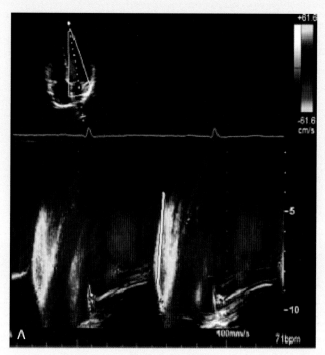

Color M-mode

Figure 12-20A

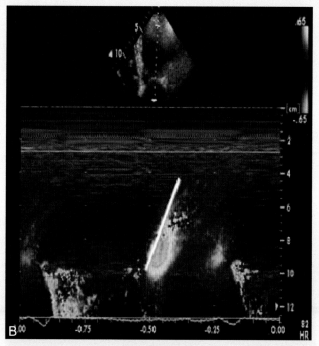

Color M-mode

Figure 12-20B

between LV pressure and volume) and also changes in ventricular relaxation or early (instead of late) diastolic ventricular pressures will affect the deceleration time (**Figure 12-21**). LA mechanical function and ejection fraction are not or are only weakly and indirectly correlated with deceleration time.

16. ▶ **Answer: D.** In a patient with pericardial disease and constrictive physiology, enhanced ventricular interdependence (i.e., a significant

leftward shift of the ventricular septum during inspiration) may be present due to sudden changes in ventricular volume and pressure during normal respiration (**Video 12-1**). With inspiration, there is exaggerated leftward shift of the interventricular septum due to pericardial restraint, resulting in an abnormal increase of flow across the tricuspid valve; just the opposite is seen in the mitral E-wave velocity during early expiration (**Figures 12-22A** and **12-22B**).

During inspiration (answer A), normally there is little or no change in the mitral E-wave velocity and <25% change in the tricuspid E-wave velocity. As for answers B and C, changes in the mitral (or tricuspid) E-wave velocity are not typically seen during shallow breathing, and no changes should be observed during end-expiratory apnea.

TECHNICAL TIPS

When assessing patients with suspected pericardial disease, the sonographer should activate the ultrasound system's respirometer to allow for evaluation of changes in mitral and tricuspid E-wave velocities during the respiratory cycle. It is also important to be aware of additional echocardiographic variables that can aid in the diagnosis of constrictive pericarditis. These variables include comparison of the e′ velocities (measured by tissue Doppler imaging [TDI]) of the septal and lateral aspects of the mitral annulus; normally, the peak TDI e′ velocity recorded at the septal annulus should be slightly lower than that of the lateral annulus in the apical 4-chamber view. However, in patients with pericardial disease and pericardial restraint, the inverse of the TDI peak e′ velocities may be observed. This finding has been referred to as "annulus reversus" and occurs because the lateral annulus is tethered by adherent pericardium. In addition, the evaluation of inferior vena cava (IVC) changes is important in patients with suspected pericardial disease. In a patient with advanced pericarditis and constrictive physiology, IVC plethora and noncollapse is seen during normal respiration (**Figure 12-22C**). This is indicative of increased right atrial pressure. Lastly, pulsed-wave Doppler interrogation of hepatic vein flow can assist in the diagnosis of constrictive pericarditis and will demonstrate prominent early diastolic flow reversal (**Figure 12-22D**).

17. **Answer: D.** In patients with dilated cardiomyopathies, the PW Doppler mitral inflow profile correlates better with LV filling pressures, functional class, and prognosis than does LV ejection fraction. Patients with impaired LV relaxation are the least symptomatic, while a short isovolumic relaxation time, short mitral deceleration time and increased E/A ratio characterize advanced diastolic dysfunction, increased left atrial pressure, and a worse functional class. This restrictive filling pattern is associated with a poor prognosis, especially if it persists after preload reduction. Likewise, a pseudonormal or restrictive filling pattern associated with acute myocardial

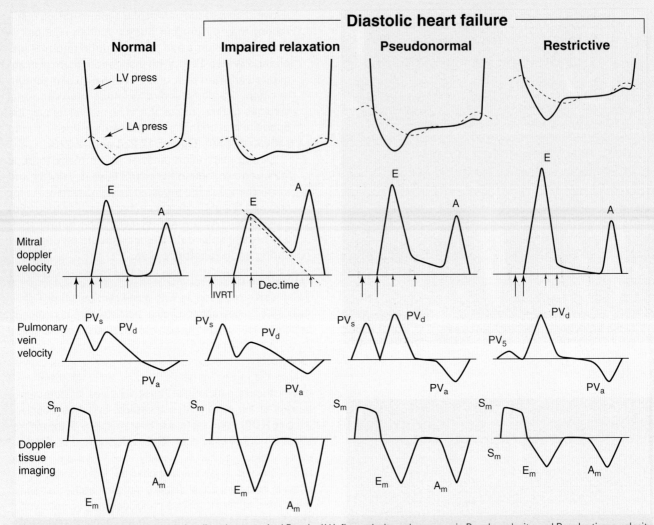

Figure 12-21 LV and LA pressures during diastole, transmitral Doppler LV inflow velocity, pulmonary vein Doppler velocity, and Doppler tissue velocity. IVRT indicates isovolumic relaxation time; Dec. time, e-wave deceleration time; E, early LV filling velocity; A, velocity of LV filling contributed by atrial contraction; PVs, systolic pulmonary vein velocity; PVd, diastolic pulmonary vein velocity; PVa, pulmonary vein velocity resulting from atrial contraction; S_{m}, annular myocardial velocity during systole; E_{m}, annular myocardial velocity during early filling; and A_{m}, annular myocardial velocity during filling produced by atrial contraction. (Reprinted with permission from Zile MR, Brutsaert DL. New concepts in diastolic dysfunction and diastolic heart failure: part I: diagnosis, prognosis, and measurements of diastolic function. *Circulation.* 2002;105(11):1387-1393.)

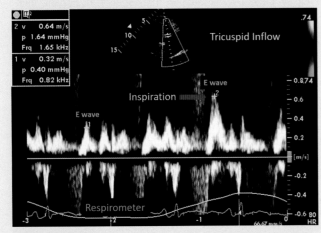

Figure 12-22A

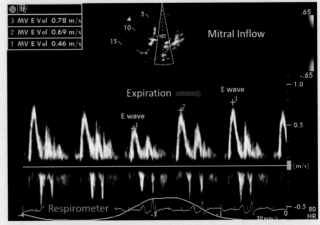

Figure 12-22B

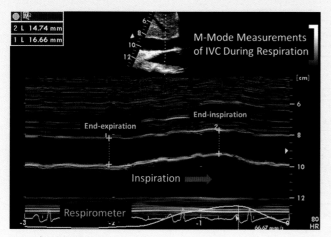

Figure 12-22C

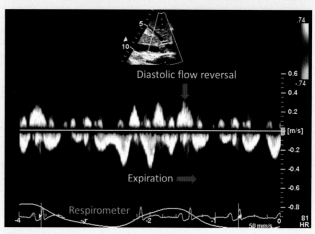

Figure 12-22D

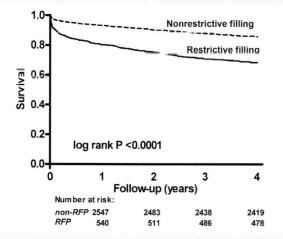

Figure 12-23 Event-free survival in patients with restrictive and nonrestrictive filling patterns. (Reprinted with permission from Meta-Analysis Research Group in Echocardiography [MeRGE] AMI Collaborators, Møller JE, Whalley GA, Dini FL, et al. Independent prognostic importance of a restrictive left ventricular filling pattern after myocardial infarction: an individual patient meta-analysis: meta-Analysis Research Group in Echocardiography Acute Myocardial Infarction. *Circulation.* 2008;117(20):2591-2598.)

Pattern	Baseline	Valsalva	Assessment
Normal			Normal
Stage 1A			Normal filling pressures
Stage 1B			↑LV A wave, ↑EDP
Stage 2			Pseudonormal
Stage 3			Reversible restrictive
Stage 4			Irreversible restrictive

Figure 12-24

infarction indicates an increased risk of heart failure, unfavorable LV remodeling, and increased cardiovascular mortality, irrespective of ejection fraction (**Figure 12-23**). In addition to dilated cardiomyopathy, deceleration time has also been shown to be an important predictor of survival in restrictive cardiomyopathy (e.g., cardiac amyloidosis).

18. **Answer: A.** In cardiac patients, a decrease of ≥50% in E/A ratio with application of the Valsalva maneuver is highly specific for increased LV filling pressure. However, a smaller magnitude of change does not always indicate normal diastolic function. One major limitation of the Valsalva maneuver is that not everyone is able to perform this maneuver adequately and it is not standardized. The Valsalva maneuver is performed by forceful expiration (about 40 mm Hg) against a closed nose and mouth. A decrease of 20 cm/s in mitral peak E velocity is usually considered an adequate effort in patients

without restrictive filling. Lack of reversibility with Valsalva is imperfect as an indicator that the diastolic filling pattern is irreversible. In a busy clinical laboratory, the Valsalva maneuver can be reserved for patients in whom diastolic function assessment is not clear after mitral inflow and annulus velocity measurements. The Valsalva is obviously of little use in patients with stage 1 diastolic dysfunction but is useful to differentiate stage 2 diastolic function from normal (**Figure 12-24**).

19. **Answer: B.** Mitral E/A ratio of 1.4 is considered normal; however, this might also be categorized as "pseudonormal" in the presence of additional echocardiographic variables that are consistent with elevated left ventricular (LV) filling pressures. An E/e' ratio of 17 (>14), a peak TR velocity of 3.1 m/s (>2.8 m/s), and a LAVi of 68 mL/m² (>34 mL/m²) are all highly suggestive of elevated LV filling pressures. Values in answer A are most consistent with normal LV filling pressures; however, the TR velocity, when converted to pressure, is 67 mm Hg. This finding is

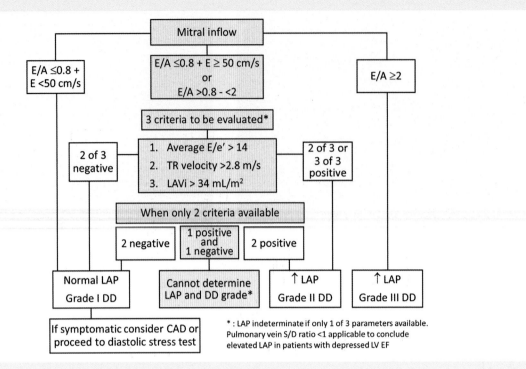

Figure 12-25

consistent with significant pulmonary hypertension and additional clinical correlation should be considered. For answer C, although the E/A ratio is high (>1.5), all other values are within normal range, suggesting normal filling pressures. The high E/A ratio in this case is likely due to normal early rapid filling into a left ventricle with normal relaxation. As for answer D, all values are consistent with normal LV filling pressures.

20. **Answer: C.** Athletes not uncommonly have resting bradycardia, mild concentric hypertrophy, and/or mild chamber dilatation due to increased pressure and volume loads related to sustained increases in activity. An early diastolic velocity of the mitral annulus derived by tissue Doppler echocardiography (e') < 8 cm/s is, however, a markedly abnormal finding especially in a 35-year-old person. Combinations of other findings that suggest elevated LV filling pressures are summarized in an algorithmic form in **Figure 12-14** (answer outline for Question 1).

21. **Answer: B.** The 2016 ASE Recommendations for the Assessment of Diastolic Function guidelines include two algorithms for the evaluation of LV diastolic function. The first algorithm is used for patients with a normal LVEF as a starting point to determine if the patients have diastolic dysfunction or not. The second algorithm is used for patients with established diastolic dysfunction based on the first algorithm, subjects with a depressed LVEF, or subjects with myocardial disease and normal LVEF (see **Figure 12-14**). This patient's medical history of sleep apnea, hypertension, and an increased LV mass (index value > 115 g/m²) suggests pathologic

changes of the myocardium even though the LVEF is normal and therefore, the estimation of LV filling pressures and grading LV diastolic function is based on the second algorithm. Based on this algorithm, the first parameter to consider is the mitral inflow E/A ratio. Because the E/A ratio is between 0.8 and 2 (was 1.1), three additional variables are required to properly categorize diastolic function. This includes the averaged E/e', the LAVi, and the TR velocity. The averaged E/e' ratio does not exceed 14 (was 7), the TR velocity is inadequate, and the LAVi exceeds 34 mL/m² (was 36 mL/m²). Therefore, based on the algorithm where there are two criteria available and one is positive, and one is negative, diastolic function grade cannot be determined (**Figure 12-25**). However, an important clue to possibly normal LV filling pressures is the low mitral E-wave velocity. The 2016 ASE guidelines suggest that a low E-wave velocity (≤50 cm/s) is most consistent with normal LV filling pressures. The pulmonary vein signal is also systolic dominant (S > D), further supporting normal LV filling pressures. Based on the findings the patient does not meet criteria for elevated LV filling pressures and thus has grade I (mild) diastolic dysfunction.

22. **Answer: B.** The peak e' velocity occurs after the isovolumic period. **Figure 12-26** shows the peak s' velocity which appears above the zero-baseline between aortic valve opening (AVO) and aortic valve closure (AVC). The peak s' velocity correlates with ventricular systolic contraction or coiling during "mechanical systole." In patients with myocardial disease, the isovolumic relaxation time (IVRT)

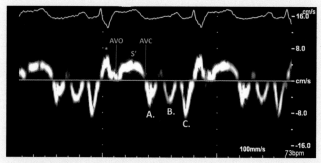

Figure 12-26

increases as a result of slowing of ventricular relaxation. Because of this, the first waveform detected below the zero-velocity baseline is most always the IVRT velocity (labeled A). In addition, a faint Doppler signal can be seen above baseline as well, preceding the e′ velocity (B). Waveform C represents the atrial contraction velocity (or a′ velocity), which coincides with the timing of the P wave on the electrocardiogram. Lastly, electrical conduction disturbances such as a bundle branch block prolong the QRS complex, increasing the time from mitral valve closure to aortic valve opening (i.e., increasing the isovolumic contraction time [IVCT]). This can be seen as a prominent positive velocity to the left of the s′ velocity (*).

23. **Answer: D.** Note that color M-mode Vp and tissue Doppler e′ are essentially unchanged. A higher 6-month E/e′ ratio and E/Vp ratio both indicate increased LV filling pressures. A lower A-wave velocity indicates reduced left atrial contractility. The shorter deceleration time indicates increased LV operating stiffness. The association between tissue

Doppler e′ and LV relaxation has been observed in both animal and human studies.

24. **Answer: D.** Based on the algorithms outlined in the 2016 ASE Recommendations for the Assessment of Diastolic Function guidelines, assessment of diastolic function in this patient with a depressed LVEF starts with the mitral E/A ratio. As the E/A ratio exceeds 2, there is Grade III (severe) diastolic dysfunction (**Figure 12-27**). The increased mitral E-wave velocity, in the presence of severely reduced systolic function, is most likely due to an increased driving pressure from the left atrium (LA) to the left ventricle. Other evidence of increased LA pressure includes a short E-wave deceleration time (<140 ms), E/A ratio >1.5, E/e′ ratio >14, and a significantly increased LAVi. Furthermore, in this patient there was little change in the E/A ratio during the Valsalva maneuver, further classifying the mitral inflow pattern as "stage 4" irreversible restrictive filling. The pulmonary venous D-wave velocity > S-wave velocity, in the setting of a depressed LVEF, further supporting elevated left ventricular (LV) filling pressures. In addition, there is significant pulmonary hypertension present. It would be highly unlikely for this patient to have normal pulmonary pressures in the presence of severe LV diastolic dysfunction and highly elevated LV filling pressures. Lastly, the LV mass, although increased, suggests pathologic changes of the myocardium, but this does not support elevated LV filling pressures.

25. **Answer: A.** Although the overall gain is not typically adjusted when assessing tissue Doppler imaging (TDI), in the event of suboptimal image quality,

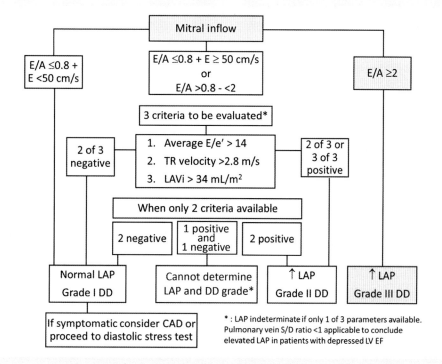

Figure 12-27

particularly at the annular level, the sonographer may be required to increase the overall gain to improve the TDI signal. Although the measurements made appear to be the same, the Doppler signal is faint and may result in an underestimation of the e' velocity, resulting in overestimating the E/e' ratio. Mitral annular calcification (MAC) is commonly encountered in the echocardiography laboratory. However, recent data suggest the e' velocity and the calculation of the E/e' ratio is unreliable in the assessment of filling pressures in patients with moderate to severe MAC.

TECHNICAL TIPS

Systematic approach to the assessment of TDI e' velocities:
- Position the sample volume (SV) as perpendicular as possible to annulus; this may require tilting the 2D image slightly left or right.
- Have the patient take a small breath in or breath out; reposition the SV at the annulus.
- Activate the TDI preset.
- Doppler sweep speed and velocity scale should be adjusted to allow for clear visualization of the e' velocity.
- The TDI signals should be clear with minimal spectral broadening; peak velocities above and below the zero-velocity baseline should be clearly delineated. In addition, there should be minimal background noise on the Doppler display.
- If the signal is faint, increase the gain until optimal.
- All measurements should be made during apnea.

26. **Answer: E.** Cutoff values for differentiating a normal from an abnormal mitral inflow profile in patients with a normal EF should consider multiple parameters such as the e' velocity, E/e' ratio, indexed left atrial (LA) volume, and the peak tricuspid regurgitation velocity (see **Figure 12-14** for further explanation on estimation of filling pressures in patients with normal EF). In this case, the E/A ratio is almost 2 and this, combined with an increase in LA size in a 65-year-old man is suggestive of elevated left ventricular filling pressures.

27. **Answer: C.** Based on the algorithms outlined in the 2016 ASE Recommendations for the Assessment of Diastolic Function guidelines, assessment of diastolic function in this patient with a depressed left ventricular EF starts with the mitral E/A ratio. As the E/A ratio equals 2 (**Figure 12-6A**), there is Grade III (severe) diastolic dysfunction. The reason for the increased mitral E-wave velocity is an increased "driving pressure" from the left atrium to the left ventricle in early diastole, in the face of diminished myocardial disease. The Valsalva maneuver was correctly performed in this patient, demonstrating significant decreases in the mitral E-wave velocity (88 to 40 cm/s), mitral E-wave deceleration time (180 to 278 ms), and mitral E/A ratio (2.0-0.75)

(**Figure 12-6B**); these findings indicate reversible restrictive filling and therefore, answer C is correct.

Other findings consistent with elevated left ventricular (LV) filling pressures include an averaged E/e' ratio of 17, a pulmonary venous S/D ratio <1, a pulmonary venous atrial reversal (AR) velocity of 42 cm/s, and a difference between the pulmonary venous AR duration and the mitral A-wave duration of 66 ms. A pulmonary venous AR velocity >35 cm/s and an AR-A duration >30 ms are highly sensitive and specific for elevated LV end-diastolic pressure.

Lastly, observe the high-quality Doppler tracings that demonstrate clear peaks, slopes, and durations, which may improve the accuracy during the assessment of diastolic function.

28. **Answer: B.** The sonographer recorded and measured traces at the lateral annulus during normal respiration in **Figure 12-7A**. Note the significant changes in the peak e' velocity as the patient began to inspire, as seen on the respirometer trace. In **Figure 12-7B**, the sonographer asked the patient to take a small breath in and hold it; placed the sample volume at the annulus and recorded the traces. Observe the improvement in the consistency between the peak e' velocities in **Figure 12-7B**.

29. **Answer: C.** The E/e' ratio is high in this patient. It has been proposed that a septal E/e' ratio >11 can be used to accurately predict elevated LV filling pressures in patients with atrial fibrillation. The E/e' ratio in this patient is 19.7. See **Table 12-4** for additional parameters that may be used to identify elevated LV filling pressures in patients with atrial fibrillation.

TECHNICAL TIP

When assessing patients with atrial fibrillation, multiple measurements should be made and averaged as seen in **Figures 12-8A** and **12-8B**. Note that up to six measurements were made for each parameter.

30. **Answer: A.** The mitral inflow pattern can be used with relative accuracy to assess filling pressures in patients with depressed LV systolic function. In this population, changes in the inflow pattern will reflect changes in preload (e.g., due to volume overload or changes in medical therapy). Confusion between normal and pseudonormal filling should be easily avoided since diastolic function is intrinsically abnormal in the presence of advanced systolic dysfunction (i.e., diastolic dysfunction precedes systolic dysfunction).

In contrast, additional information is needed in the presence of preserved EF as this Doppler pattern could equally represent normal or pseudonormal filling. As mentioned earlier, the sonographer should assess the tissue Doppler-derived e', Vp obtained by color Doppler M-mode, left atrial (LA) volume, and the effect of a Valsalva maneuver to detect an underlying relaxation abnormality in the case of pseudonormal filling. Left atrial dilatation can merely represent atrial remodeling independent of filling pressures in the setting of atrial fibrillation. Moderate and severe MR usually leads to an elevation of peak E velocity, representing the increased flow rate during diastole with a normal deceleration time. However, particularly with chronic MR, the left atrium will dilate and the increased LA compliance may be sufficient to maintain filling pressures at a normal level. Finally, a high velocity tricuspid regurgitant jet may be suggestive of (but is not specific for) elevated left-sided filling pressures. Many other conditions may lead to pulmonary hypertension in the presence of normal diastolic function.

31. **Answer: C.** This patient is in first-degree heart block with a PR interval of 242 ms. A normal PR interval is <200 ms. With prolongation of the PR interval, atrial contraction occurs before early filling has been completed; as a result, fusion of the mitral E-wave and A-wave and early closure of the mitral valve may occur. An additional consequence of first-degree heart block is the shortening of diastolic filling time and absence of diastasis as seen in this patient. Normally the mitral valve should close on, or about the R wave on the electrocardiogram (ECG) (vertical dotted line in **Figure 12-28A**). In the same patient, the tissue Doppler imaging trace demonstrated early termination of the a′ velocity as seen in **Figure 12-28B**.

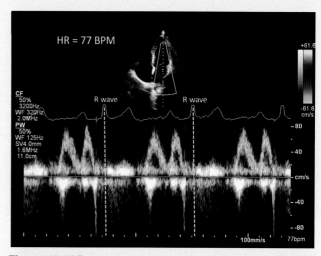

Figure 12-28A

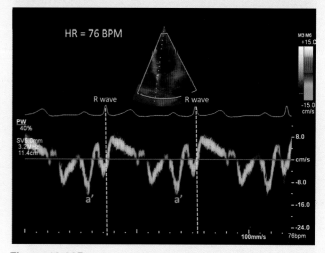

Figure 12-28B

TECHNICAL TIP

One of the first adjustments the sonographer should make prior to starting the echocardiogram is optimization of the ECG. The ECG gain should be increased until all electrical signals (i.e., P wave, QRS complex, and T wave) are well displayed. This can aid in the identification of arrhythmias such as atrial fibrillation as seen in Question 29.

32. **Answer: E.** The Doppler findings demonstrate a large (>30 ms) difference between the duration of the mitral A-wave velocity and the duration of the late diastolic pulmonary venous flow reversal (AR) velocity, suggesting elevated left ventricular end-diastolic pressure (LVEDP). This is usually seen in patients with grade I or grade II diastolic dysfunction, so that the most likely answer is the 60-year-old man with advanced hypertensive heart disease. A waves will be absent if atrial fibrillation is present. Reversal or at least blunting of the S wave would be expected if significant mitral regurgitation is present. Pulmonary venous inflow velocities are influenced by age: normal young subjects aged <40 years usually have prominent D velocities (reflecting their mitral E waves); the S/D ratio increases with increasing age. AR velocities also typically increase with age but usually do not exceed 35 cm/s without increased LVEDP.

33. **Answer: C.** Grade I or mild diastolic dysfunction includes prolongation of the rate of left ventricular (LV) relaxation, resulting in an increase of the IVRT >100 ms. Note that patients with normal filling pressures typically display a normal IVRT of <70 ms. Color M-mode Vp slope >50 cm/s is considered normal in most patients. Conversely, patients with LA enlargement, elevated LV filling pressures, and myocardial disease will most likely demonstrate a pulmonary vein D wave > S wave. Lastly, a significant decrease in the mitral E/A ratio (>0.5) during a Valsalva maneuver may also support elevated LV filling pressure and would be more typical of grade 2 diastolic dysfunction.

TECHNICAL TIPS

When attempting to measure IVRT, pulsed-wave or continuous-wave Doppler is used and the cursor should be positioned between the left ventricular outflow tract and mitral inflow in either the apical 5-chamber or apical long-axis view. Sweep speed should be set between 100 and 150 mm/s and filters can be increased to exclude the Doppler baseline artifact. Onset of the demarcation points reflected by aortic valve closure and mitral valve opening should be clearly visualized (**Figure 12-29A**). Close attention should be paid to the vertical closing "click" artifact of aortic valve closure and mitral valve opening. In addition, too slow of a sweep speed may underestimate the IVRT as seen in **Figure 12-29B**, top.

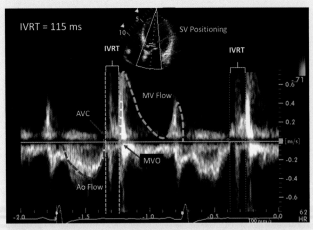

Figure 12-29A

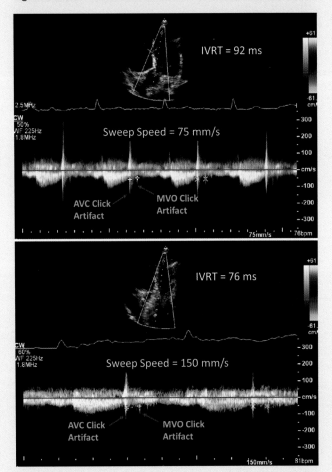

Figure 12-29B

34. **Answer: D.** This patient's diastolic function improved significantly from grade III (severe) to grade I (mild). Mitral inflow preimplantation demonstrated an E/A ratio of 2.7, E-wave deceleration time of 90 ms, consistent with grade III (restrictive filling); E/e' ratio was 29, consistent with markedly elevated LV filling pressures. Postimplant mitral inflow demonstrated a low E-wave velocity of 30 cm/s, E/A ratio of 0.7, and E/e' ratio of 10. These findings are consistent with grade I diastolic dysfunction. Although there appears to be no significant increase in the e' velocity, there was a

significant increase in the a' velocity, which is most likely reflecting an improvement of atrial mechanical function. In addition, the peak TR jet decreased significantly from 3.4 to 2.3 m/s respectively. These additional findings support a significant reduction in filling pressures and improvement in diastolic function.

35. **Answer: B.** In most, if not all cardiac diseases, as with cardiac amyloidosis, the initial diastolic dysfunction stage is impaired relaxation. With disease progression, continued impaired relaxation ultimately results in mild to moderate increases in LAP that can cause the mitral inflow velocity pattern to appear similar to a normal filling ("pseudonormal") pattern. The E/A ratio is typically 1 to 1.5 and the E-wave deceleration time is usually between 160 and 220 ms. The best way to identify a grade II diastolic dysfunction or pseudonormal filling pattern is by demonstrating impaired myocardial relaxation by average E/e' >14, tricuspid regurgitant velocity >2.8 cm/s, and left atrial volume index >34 mL/m² (see **Figure 12-14**) as per the 2016 ASE diastology guidelines. In patients with known systolic dysfunction or abnormally increased wall thickness, a normal E/A ratio suggests that increased LAP is masking abnormal relaxation. By decreasing preload (via the Valsalva maneuver), one may unmask the impaired left ventricular (LV) relaxation by causing a decrease in the E/A ratio by 0.5 or more and reversal of the E/A ratio. In addition, color M-mode of mitral inflow can determine rate of flow propagation into the left ventricle, and with worsening diastolic function, myocardial relaxation is always impaired and flow propagation is slow even when LAP and mitral E velocity are increased. Cardiac amyloidosis is characterized by regional variations in longitudinal strain with relative "apical sparing." This pattern is an easily recognizable, accurate, and reproducible method of differentiating cardiac amyloidosis from other causes of LV hypertrophy (**Figure 12-30**).

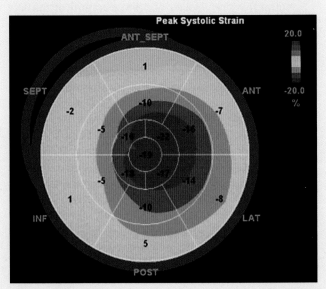

Figure 12-30

KEY POINTS

▶ Deceleration time is an important prognostic factor in patients with cardiac amyloidosis.

▶ Grade II diastolic dysfunction ("pseudonormal" pattern) represents a moderate stage of diastolic dysfunction, combining mildly to moderately elevated left atrial pressures, and an LV relaxation abnormality.

▶ A relative "apical sparing" longitudinal strain pattern is an easily recognizable, accurate, and reproducible method of differentiating cardiac amyloidosis from other causes of LV hypertrophy.

36. **Answer: B.** As shown in **Figure 12-31A**, the baseline AV delay in this patient was set so short that there was inadequate time to see an A wave (systolic contraction was initiated too early). Increasing the AV delay to 250 ms delayed the onset of systolic contraction enough to reveal an "optimal" A wave. AV delay settings above 250 ms resulted in delay of systolic contraction to the point that passive filling compromised the A wave, resulting in E-A fusion. This is further characterized in **Figure 12-31B**. The presence of severe mitral regurgitation means that a desirable result of a grade I LV diastolic filling pattern is not likely to be achieved.

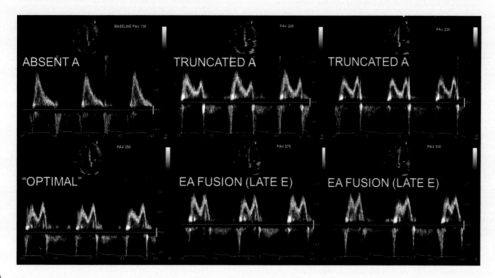

Figure 12-31A

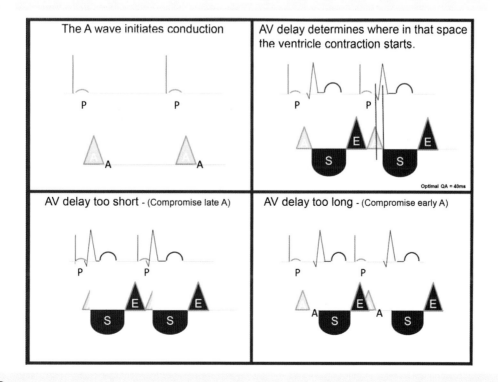

Figure 12-31B

Acknowledgments: We want to thank Bonita Anderson and Margaret (Koko) Park for including us in this interactive and contemporary textbook. It is an honor to be included in such a publication that we believe is one of the most educational echocardiography textbooks to date. In addition, we would like to recognize the outstanding contributions of the original work by Patrick Collier, MD, PhD, Andrew O. Zurick III, MD, David Verhaert, MD, and Allan L. Klein, MD (Chapter 13 Diastology in Clinical Echocardiography Review: A Self-Assessment Tool, 2nd ed., edited by Allan L. Klein, Craig R. Asher, 2017) that provided the foundation in writing this chapter.

SUGGESTED READINGS

Anderson B. Ventricular diastolic function. In: *A Sonographer's Guide to the Assessment of Heart Disease.* 1st ed. Brisbane: Echotext Pty Ltd; 2014:chap 3.

Collier P, Zurick AO III, Verhaert D, Klein AL. Diastology. In: Klein AL, Asher CR, eds. *Clinical Echocardiography Review: A Self-Assessment Tool.* 2nd ed. Philadelphia, PA: Wolters Kluwer; 2017:chap 13.

Ha JW, Oh JK, Ling LH, Nishimura RA, Seward JB, Tajik AJ. Annulus paradoxus: transmitral flow velocity to mitral annular velocity ratio is inversely proportional to pulmonary capillary wedge pressure in patients with constrictive pericarditis. *Circulation.* 2001;104(9):976-978.

Hill JC, Palma RP. Doppler tissue imaging for the assessment of left ventricular diastolic function: a systematic approach for the sonographer. *J Am Soc Echocardiogr.* 2005;18(1):80-88.

Lang RM, Badano LP, Mor-Avi V, et al. Recommendations for cardiac chamber quantification by echocardiography in adults: an update from the American Society of Echocardiography and the European Association of Cardiovascular Imaging. *J Am Soc Echocardiogr.* 2015;28(1):1-39.

Nagueh SF, Kopelen HA, Quinones MA. Assessment of left ventricular filling pressures by Doppler in the presence of atrial fibrillation. *Circulation.* 1996;94(9):2138-2145.

Nagueh SF, Middleton KJ, Kopelen HA, et al. Doppler tissue imaging: a non-invasive technique for evaluation of left ventricular relaxation and estimation of filling pressures. *J Am Coll Cardiol.* 1997;30(6):1527-1533.

Nagueh SF, Smiseth OA, Appleton CP, et al. Recommendations for the evaluation of left ventricular diastolic function by echocardiography: an update from the American Society of Echocardiography and the European Association of Cardiovascular Imaging. *J Am Soc Echocardiogr.* 2016;29(4):277-314.

Oh JK. Assessment of diastolic function. In: Oh JK, Kane GC, eds. *The Echo Manual.* 4th ed. Philadelphia/Rochester: Wolters Kluwer and Mayo Foundation for Medical Education and Research; 2019:chap 8.

Ommen SR, Nishimura RA, Appleton CP, et al. Clinical utility of Doppler echocardiography and tissue Doppler imaging in the estimation of left ventricular filling pressures: a comparative simultaneous Doppler-catheterization study. *Circulation.* 2000;102(15): 1788-1794.

Rossvoll O, Hatle LK. Pulmonary venous flow velocities recorded by transthoracic Doppler ultrasound: relation to left ventricular diastolic pressures. *J Am Coll Cardiol.* 1993;21(7):1687-1696.

Systemic Hypertension

Contributors: Lisa A. Bienvenu, BS, ACS, RDCS and Jennifer L. Schaaf, BS, ACS, RDCS

✪✪ Question 1

According to the ACC/AHA Task Force on Clinical Practice Guidelines, blood pressure (BP) is categorized as normal, elevated, hypertension stage 1, and hypertension stage 2 based on the systolic blood pressure (SBP) and the diastolic blood pressure (DBP). Hypertension stage 1 is classified as _____ whereas hypertension stage 2 is considered _____.

- **A.** SBP 120 to 129 mm Hg and DBP <80 mm Hg; SBP 130 to 139 mm Hg or DBP 80 to 89 mm Hg
- **B.** SBP 130 to 139 mm Hg or DBP 80 to 89 mm Hg; SBP ≥140 mm Hg or DBP ≥90 mm Hg
- **C.** SBP ≥140 mm Hg or DBP ≥90 mm Hg; SBP >180 mm Hg and/or DBP >120 mm Hg
- **D.** SBP >180 mm Hg and/or DBP >120 mm Hg; SBP >200 mm Hg and/or DBP >130 mm Hg

✪ Question 2

According to the ACC/AHA Task Force on Clinical Practice Guidelines, which of the following blood pressures would be considered a hypertensive emergency when organ damage may be a result?

- **A.** 160/100 mm Hg
- **B.** 170/110 mm Hg
- **C.** 185/122 mm Hg
- **D.** 130/85 mm Hg

✪✪ Question 3

Hypertension may be classified as primary (or essential) hypertension or secondary hypertension. Which of the following is not a cause of secondary hypertension?

- **A.** A high-sodium diet
- **B.** Coarctation of the aorta
- **C.** Primary renal disease
- **D.** Primary aldosteronism
- **E.** Both C and D

✪✪ Question 4

Echocardiography is considered an important tool for periodic evaluation of patients with hypertension. Particularly, it is important to pay careful attention to the cardiac structures and compare serial studies to look for the progressive characteristics of hypertensive heart disease. Which of the following is a finding in a patient with hypertensive heart disease?

- **A.** Increased left ventricular (LV) mass index
- **B.** Left atrial (LA) dilatation
- **C.** LV diastolic dysfunction
- **D.** LV hypertrophy
- **E.** All of the above

✪✪✪ Question 5

Left ventricular hypertrophy (LVH) results in changes to the strain mechanics of the myocardium. In the case of early-stage hypertension, longitudinal strain _____ while radial strain _____.

- **A.** Remains intact, increases
- **B.** Increases, decreases
- **C.** Decreases, increases
- **D.** Decreases, decreases

✪✪ Question 6

A 22-year-old male college student was found unresponsive in the locker room and was taken to the hospital. A routine chest X-ray was performed. The findings suggested cardiomegaly, which triggered an order for an echocardiogram. **Table 13-1** includes some of the findings of this study. Given these findings, what is the diagnosis?

- **A.** Advanced stage amyloidosis
- **B.** Advanced stage sarcoidosis
- **C.** Athlete's heart
- **D.** Hypertrophic cardiomyopathy
- **E.** Primary hemochromatosis

Table 13-1.

ECG	Normal sinus rhythm
Indexed LVIDd	2.9 cm/m²
IVSd	1.7 cm
PWTd	1.7 cm
LVEF	65%
Diastolic function	Grade I
LV lateral e′ velocity	8 cm/s

IVSd, interventricular septal thickness at end-diastole; LV, left ventricle, LVEF, left ventricular ejection fraction; LVIDd, left ventricular internal dimension at end-diastole; PWTd, posterior wall thickness at end-diastole.

✪✪ Question 7

A 72-year-old woman presents for a routine echocardiogram. Her vital signs are a blood pressure of 138/88 mm Hg and a heart rate of 80 bpm. **Table 13-2** includes some of the measurements acquired during this study. Given these values, what is this patient's relative wall thickness (RWT)?

Table 13-2.

LVIDd	5.2 cm
LVIDs	3.2 cm
IVSd	1.1 cm
IVSs	1.3 cm
PWTd	1.3 cm
PWTs	1.5 cm
Indexed LVM	90 g/m²

IVSd, interventricular septal thickness at end-diastole; IVSs, interventricular septal thickness at end-systole; LVIDd, left ventricular internal dimension at end-diastole; LVIDs, left ventricular internal dimension at end-systole; LVM, left ventricular mass; PWTd, posterior wall thickness at end-diastole; PWTs, posterior wall thickness at end-systole.

- **A.** 0.28
- **B.** 0.42
- **C.** 0.50
- **D.** 0.56

✪✪ Question 8

Using the values given from the previous question, which left ventricular (LV) geometry class best defines this woman's heart?

- **A.** Normal
- **B.** Concentric remodeling
- **C.** Concentric hypertrophy
- **D.** Eccentric hypertrophy

✪✪ Question 9

An obese 49-year-old man with untreated hypertension is seen in the clinic and presents with shortness of breath. His blood pressure is 142/92 mm Hg and he has a heart rate of 90 bpm. The physician ordered an echocardiogram and **Table 13-3** includes some of the measurements acquired during this study. Given these values, what is this patient's relative wall thickness (RWT)?

- **A.** 0.28
- **B.** 0.47
- **C.** 0.49
- **D.** 0.52

Table 13-3.

LVIDd	5.1 cm
LVIDs	3.5 cm
IVSd	1.3 cm
IVSs	1.5 cm
PWTd	1.2 cm
PWTs	1.5 cm
Indexed LVM	122 g/m²

For abbreviations, see the legend of **Table 13-2**.

✪✪ Question 10

Using the values given from the previous question, which left ventricular (LV) geometry class best defines this man's heart?

- **A.** Normal
- **B.** Concentric remodeling
- **C.** Concentric hypertrophy
- **D.** Eccentric hypertrophy

✪✪ Question 11

Left ventricular hypertrophy (LVH) can be a direct result of all of the following except?

    A. Aortic vessel stiffness

    B. Aortic stenosis

    C. Cardiac amyloidosis

    D. Genetic hypertrophic cardiomyopathy

    E. None of the above

✪✪✪ Question 12

Which of the following statements regarding a hypertensive response to exercise (HRE) is false?

    A. An HRE is frequently observed in individuals without hypertension or other cardiovascular disease.

    B. An HRE is defined as a peak systolic blood pressure during exercise ≥210 mm Hg in men and ≥190 mm Hg in women.

    C. An HRE with associated regional wall motion abnormalities is indicative of significant coronary artery disease.

    D. An HRE is associated with an increased risk of future development of hypertension.

    E. None of the above.

✪ Question 13

Which one of the following echocardiographic images demonstrates the correct technique for measuring left ventricular mass (LVM)?

    A. Figure 13-1A

    B. Figure 13-1B

    C. Figure 13-1C

    D. Figure 13-1D

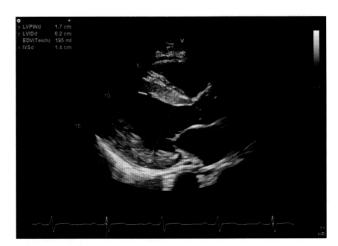

Figure 13-1A

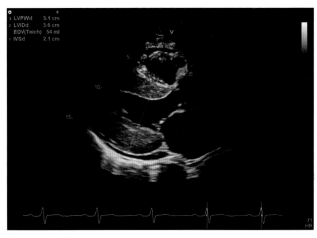

Figure 13-1B

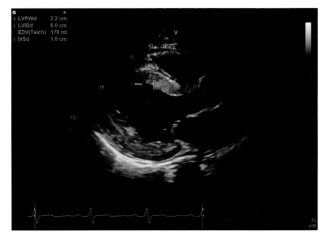

Figure 13-1C

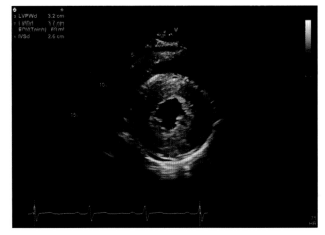

Figure 13-1D

✪ Question 14

Which of the following statements is true regarding normal values for left ventricular mass (LVM)?

    A. Normal values for LVM are not influenced by a patient's age.

    B. Gender has no influence on LVM measurement.

    C. Only height and weight influence measurement of LVM.

    D. Age, height, weight, gender, and ethnicity all influence normal values for LVM.

✪ Question 15

Based on the measurements listed in **Table 13-4**, what is the calculated value for left ventricular mass (LVM)?

    A. 616 grams (g)
    B. 458 g
    C. 472 g
    D. 204 g

Table 13-4.

LVIDd	6.2 cm
LVIDs	3.5 cm
IVSd	1.4 cm
IVSs	2.1 cm
PWd	1.7 cm
PWTs	2.8 cm

For abbreviations, see the legend of **Table 13-2**.

✪ Question 16

The normal values for left ventricular mass (LVM) derived from linear left ventricular (LV) measurements are:

    A. <95 g for women and <115 g for men.
    B. <95 g/m^2 for women and <115 g/m^2 for men.
    C. <115 g/m^2 for women and <95 g/m^2 for men.
    D. <115 g for women and <95 g for men.

✪✪ Question 17

A 70-year-old woman presents for an echocardiogram. The following information appears on the echocardiographic report: Moderately decreased left ventricular (LV) ejection fraction at 30% with regional wall motion abnormalities (mid-anteroseptal and mid-anterior wall akinesis and an aneurysmal apex). LV dimensions are listed in **Table 13-5**. What is the calculated value for LV mass (LVM)?

    A. 132 grams (g)
    B. 228 g
    C. 140 g
    D. Indeterminate

Table 13-5.

LVIDd	5.9 cm
LVIDs	5.0 cm
IVSd	0.7 cm
IVSs	1.1 cm
PWTd	0.6 cm
PWTs	0.8 cm

For abbreviations, see the legend of **Table 13-2**.

✪ Question 18

Which one of the following M-mode traces provides values that could be used to accurately calculate the left ventricular mass (LVM)?

    A. Figure 13-2A
    B. Figure 13-2B
    C. Figure 13-2C
    D. Figure 13-2D
    E. None of the above

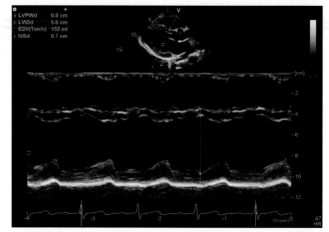

Figure 13-2A

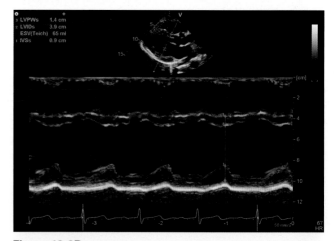

Figure 13-2B

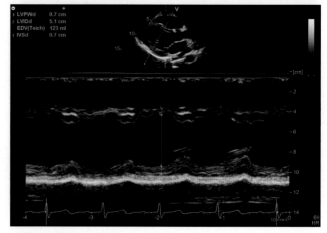

Figure 13-2C

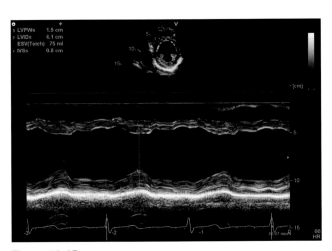

Figure 13-2D

A. Figure 13-3A
B. Figure 13-3B
C. Figure 13-3C
D. Figure 13-3D
E. None of the above

✪✪ Question 19

Which of the following statements regarding the calculation of left ventricular mass (LVM) via three-dimensional echocardiography (3DE) is false?

A. 3DE can directly measure myocardial volume and is therefore more accurate than 2D and linear LVM measurements.

B. The upper limit of normal for 3DE-indexed LVM in men is slightly smaller than the upper limit for 2D-indexed LVM.

C. 3DE tends to overestimate LVM compared with cardiac magnetic resonance (CMR) imaging in patients with cardiac disease.

D. 3DE for LVM calculations is able to account for regional variations in LV wall thickness.

✪✪ Question 20

Which one of the following images reflects the correct measurement of left ventricular (LV) wall thickness?

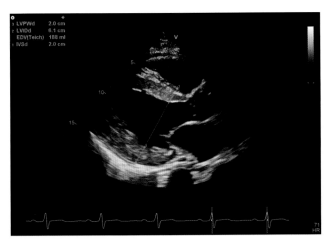

Figure 13-3A

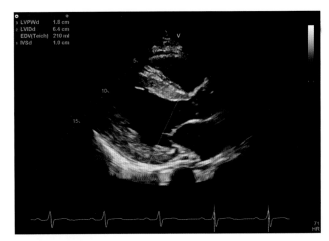

Figure 13-3B

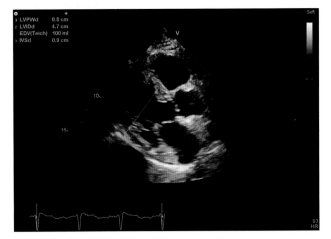

Figure 13-3C

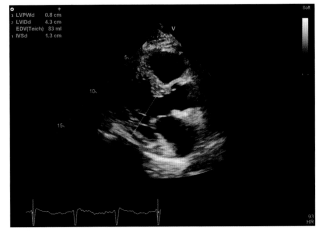

Figure 13-3D

✪✪✪ Question 21

▶ A 68-year-old man presents to the hospital with heart failure symptoms. The patient's past medical history is positive for multiple myeloma and his electrocardiogram (ECG) reveals low-voltage QRS complexes. An echocardiogram is ordered. Based on the images provided in **Video 13-1A-13-1F** and **Figure 13-4**, the most probable diagnosis for this patient is:

    A. Cardiac amyloidosis.
    B. Cardiac sarcoidosis.
    C. Hypertrophic cardiomyopathy.
    D. Systemic hypertension.
    E. Any of the above (more information is required).

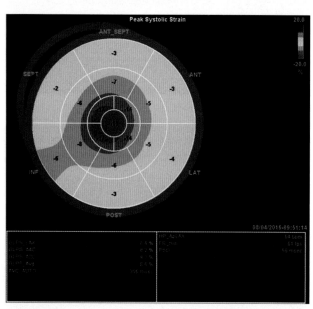

Figure 13-4

✪✪ Question 22

A 35-year-old woman with hypertension presents to the cardiology clinic for preoperative clearance from the fertility clinic. The patient was diagnosed with hypertension at the age of 21 years and was subsequently started on antihypertensive medications. Upon presentation to the cardiology clinic, left arm blood pressure (BP) is noted to be 158/80 mm Hg. Which of the following steps should be taken next?

    A. Since the patient is already on antihypertensive medications, she should be cleared for surgery. Her elevated BP is likely due to white coat syndrome.
    B. An echocardiogram should be ordered.
    C. The patient should be switched to a different antihypertensive medication.
    D. The patient's BP should be checked in both arms and both legs.
    E. Both B and D.

ANSWERS

1. **Answer: B.** Hypertension stage 1 is classified as SBP of 130 to 139 mm Hg or DBP of 80 to 89 mm Hg. Hypertension stage 2 is classified as SBP of ≥140 mm Hg or DBP of ≥90 mm Hg. A normal BP is SBP <120 mm Hg and DBP <80 mm Hg. An elevated BP is classified as SBP of 120 to 129 mm Hg and DBP of <80 mm Hg. Individuals with SBP and DBP in two categories should be designated to the higher BP category.

2. **Answer: C.** The previously used term "hypertensive crisis" has now been replaced by "hypertensive urgency" or "hypertensive emergency." Hypertensive urgency and emergency are differentiated by the absence or presence of new or worsening target organ damage, respectively. For both conditions, the classification based on the blood pressure is systolic blood pressure >180 mm Hg and/or a diastolic blood pressure >120 mm Hg.

3. **Answer: A.** In primary (or essential) hypertension, there is no identifiable cause. Secondary hypertension occurs because of an identifiable cause. There are numerous causes of secondary hypertension including primary renal disease (answer C), primary aldosteronism (answer D), obstructive sleep

apnea, pheochromocytoma, thyroid diseases, coarctation of the aorta (answer B), and various medications.

TEACHING POINT
The etiology of primary (or essential) hypertension remains unclear; however, there are a number of risk factors associated with its development including a high-sodium diet (answer A), advancing age, obesity, a family history, race, reduced nephron number, excessive alcohol consumption, and physical inactivity.

4. **Answer: E.** Hypertensive heart disease can be thought of as having a domino effect. LV hypertrophy is the result of a chronic increase in arterial resistance. The hypertrophied muscle results in increased LV mass, which inhibits normal LV relaxation, resulting in LV diastolic dysfunction. LA dilatation is a secondary result of LV diastolic dysfunction and elevated LV filling pressures.

5. **Answer: C.** In hypertensive heart disease with LVH, longitudinal strain decreases as a result of the increase in wall stress while the radial strain increases as a compensatory mechanism for longitudinal functional decline. As a result, the LV ejection fraction (LVEF) remains relatively unchanged. Ultimately, both longitudinal and radial strain decrease as the hypertensive disease progresses due to subendocardial fibrosis and this is concurrent with declining LVEF.

6. **Answer: D.** All given parameters are consistent with early stage hypertrophic cardiomyopathy. The indexed LVIDd is well within normal limits (normal 2.2-3.0 cm/m^2), there is a significant increase in LV wall thickness (>1.6 cm), LVEF is normal (normal 52%-72%), diastolic dysfunction is present, and the lateral e′ <10 cm/s.

    Advanced stage amyloidosis (answer A) presents with depressed LVEF, low normal to normal LVIDd, increased LV wall thickness, restrictive LV filling, and markedly reduced e′ velocities. Common echo findings for late stage sarcoidosis (answer B) are as follows: regional wall motion abnormalities, scarring/thinning of the LV wall, and dilated chambers with conduction abnormalities. Athlete's hearts (answer C) typically have an increase in LVIDd, an increased wall thickness but <1.6 cm, normal or supranormal diastolic function, and a preserved e′ ≥ 10 cm/s. Hearts in primary hemochromatosis (answer E) generally do not to exhibit left ventricular hypertrophy, rather, there is global systolic dysfunction and chamber dilatation.

7. **Answer: C.** The relative wall thickness (RWT) is calculated from the left ventricular internal dimension at end-diastole (LVIDd) and the posterior wall thickness at end-diastole (PWTd) as:

$$RWT = (2 \times PWTd) \div LVIDd \qquad (1)$$

Based on the measurements provided, the RWT is:

$$RWT = (2 \times 1.3) \div 5.2 = 0.50 \qquad (2)$$

The RWT may also be derived from the left ventricular internal dimension at end-diastole (LVIDd), the posterior wall thickness at end-diastole (PWTd), and the interventricular septal thickness at end-diastole (IVSd):

$$RWT = (IVSd + PWTd) \div LVIDd \qquad (3)$$

However, the recommended method is that described above in Equation (1); this is because the use of septal measurements will overestimate the RWT when there is a septal bulge.

8. **Answer: B.** The pattern of LV geometry is based on the calculated relative wall thickness (RWT) and the patient's LV mass indexed to the body surface area (BSA). Based on a normal or increased RWT and a normal or increased LV mass index, four patterns are identified (**Table 13-6**).

    In this female patient, concentric remodeling (answer B) is the correct answer because the RWT is above threshold of 0.42 (at 0.50) and the indexed LV mass via 2D linear measurements is normal (<95 g/m^2).

9. **Answer: B.** As previously described, the relative wall thickness is calculated from the left ventricular internal dimension at end-diastole (LVIDd) and the posterior wall thickness at end-diastole (PWTd) as:

$$RWT = (2 \times PWTd) \div LVIDd \qquad (1)$$

Based on the measurements provided, the RWT is:

$$RWT = (2 \times 1.2) \div 5.1 = 0.47 \qquad (2)$$

10. **Answer: C.** In this male patient, concentric hypertrophy (answer C) is the correct answer because the RWT is above threshold of 0.42 (at 0.47) and the indexed LV mass is >115 g/m^2 (at 122 g/m^2). See **Table 13-6**.

11. **Answer: C.** LVH refers to an increase in left ventricular wall thickness secondary to an increase in the thickness/size of cardiac myocytes, which is typically caused by a chronically increased workload of the left ventricle (LV). In cardiac amyloidosis, there is a significant increase in LV wall thickness, but this is due to the deposition of amyloid proteins between myocytes. Aortic vessel stiffness (answer A), or noncompliant vessels, may increase blood pressure (BP) and workload on the LV, resulting in LVH. This physiologic

Table 13-6. Patterns of LV Geometry

LV Geometry	Indexed LVM (g/m²)		RWT
	Men	**Women**	
Normal	≤115	≤95	≤0.42
Concentric hypertrophy	>115	>95	>0.42
Eccentric hypertrophy	>115	>95	≤0.42
Concentric remodeling	≤115	≤95	>0.42

cascade of the hypertension process is the most common cause of LVH. LVH is also a byproduct of aortic stenosis (answer B) and has a physiologic effect on the LV similar to that of hypertension. Long-standing outflow resistance of the stenotic valve increases afterload, resulting in LVH. Genetic hypertrophic cardiomyopathy (answer D) is an inherited disease where there is an abnormally thick left ventricular muscle, even with a BP that is within normal range.

12. **Answer: C.** Systolic blood pressure (SBP) normally rises with exercise as cardiac output increases in response to the increased oxygen demand. In some individuals, there is an abnormally exaggerated rise in SBP during exercise; this is known as a hypertensive response to exercise (HRE). All answer choices regarding an HRE are true statements except for answer C since an HRE can provoke global ventricular dysfunction or even regional wall motion abnormalities in the absence of angiographically significant coronary artery disease. In this case, the abnormally high afterload in the left ventricle triggers subendocardial ischemia, caused by the inability of the blood supply to keep up with the myocardial demand.

13. **Answer: A.** As is stated in the 2015 American Society of Echocardiography (ASE) Guidelines for Chamber Quantification, linear measurements of the left ventricle (LV) and its walls should be performed in the parasternal long-axis view, perpendicular to the long axis of the LV at end-diastole, and at or immediately below the level of the mitral valve leaflet tips. A 2D-guided M-mode approach can also be used; however, measurements from 2D images are preferred to avoid oblique sections of the LV. **Figure 13-1A** shows the correct measurement technique.

   Figure 13-1B (answer B) is incorrect as the measurements are incorrectly performed during systole; observe that the aortic valve is open. **Figure 13-1C** (answer C) is incorrect as measurements are performed at the mid-LV cavity level. **Figure 13-1D** (answer D) is incorrect since the measurements are performed from a parasternal short-axis view in mid-diastole; observe that the red vertical

electrocardiogram (ECG) marker is before the P wave of the ECG.

14. **Answer: D.** The 2015 American Society of Echocardiography Hypertension Guidelines state that normal values for LVM vary depending on age, height, weight, gender, and ethnicity. LVM is higher in men compared to women, LVM decreases with age, normal ranges of LVM can differ across races, with African Americans having higher values than white Americans and Hispanics, and Asian Americans having smaller values.

15. **Answer: C.** Left ventricular (LV) myocardial volume is calculated by subtracting the LV cavity volume (endocardial volume) from the volume enclosed within the LV epicardium (epicardial volume). This volume is then multiplied by the specific gravity of the myocardium to obtain LVM. The accepted formula for LVM calculation is:

$$LVM = 0.8 \times 1.04 \times \left[\left(LVIDd + IVSd + PWTd \right)^3 - \left(LVIDd \right)^3 \right] + 0.6 \tag{1}$$

where $(LVIDd + IVSd + PWTd)^3$ represents the LV epicardial volume, $LVIDd^3$ represents the LV endocardial volume, 1.04 is the specific gravity of muscle, and ($\times$ 0.8 + 0.6) is a "correction" factor.

Based on the values provided, the LVM is:

$$\begin{aligned} LVM &= 0.8 \times 1.04 \times \left[\left(6.2 + 1.4 + 1.7 \right)^3 - \left(6.2 \right)^3 \right] + 0.6 \\ &= 0.8 \times 1.04 \times \left[\left(9.3 \right)^3 - \left(6.2 \right)^3 \right] + 0.6 \\ &= 0.8 \times 1.04 \times \left[804 - 238 \right] + 0.6 \\ &= 0.8 \times 1.04 \times 566 + 0.6 \\ &= 471 + 0.6 \\ &= 472 \, g \end{aligned} \tag{2}$$

16. **Answer: B.** The indexing of LV mass allows comparisons in subjects with different body sizes. The most commonly accepted method for indexing the LVM is to the body surface area. However, others prefer to index the LVM to the height. Using the height raised to the allometric power of 2.7, the normal value for men is <48 g/ht$^{2.7}$ and for women is <44 g/ht$^{2.7}$.

17. **Answer: D.** As is stated in the 2015 American Society of Echocardiography Hypertension Guidelines, the following are limitations in the calculation of LVM using linear measurements:
   1. The "cube" formula is not accurate in patients with major distortions in LV geometry (e.g., apical aneurysm, or any condition where the 2:1 axis ratio requirement is not met).
   2. Because this formula involves cubing primary measurements, even small errors in these measurements may be magnified.

3. These measurements are insensitive to small changes in mass.

4. The measurements are highly dependent on imaging quality and observer expertise.

Therefore, as this patient has an apical aneurysm, the LVM cannot be calculated in this patient using linear LV measurements.

18. **Answer: E.** As discussed earlier, linear LVM measurements are acquired from the parasternal long-axis view at end-diastole. Measurements are performed perpendicular to the long axis of the left ventricle (LV) at or immediately below the level of the mitral valve leaflet tips. Via the M-mode approach, the M-mode cursor is placed just distal to the open mitral leaflet tips during diastole. End-diastole is identified as the onset of the QRS of the electrocardiogram (ECG). **Figure 13-2A** shows the closest measurement technique; however, it must be lined up with the R wave to be correct. **Figure 13-2B** (answer B) is incorrect as the measurements are performed during systole and LVM is calculated at end-diastole. **Figure 13-2C** (answer C) is incorrect as measurements are performed at the mid-LV cavity level and beyond the peak R wave of the ECG. **Figure 13-2D** (answer D) is incorrect since the measurements are performed from a parasternal short-axis view in systole and LVM measurements should be performed from the parasternal long-axis view at end-diastole.

19. **Answer: C.** Cardiac magnetic resonance imaging is considered the "gold standard" for the estimation of LVM. While the accuracy of LVM derived by 3DE is reportedly similar to CMR imaging, there is a tendency of 3DE to underestimate LVM in patients with cardiac disease. This primarily relates to difficulties in accurately tracing the LV epicardial border, particularly when the left ventricle is dilated.

Answer A is a true statement since 3DE is a direct measurement of LVM without geometrical assumptions about cavity shape and hypertrophy distribution and is therefore more accurate than 2D LVM measurements. Answer B is a true statement. In men, the upper limit of normal for 3DE-indexed LVM is 97 g/m^2 while the upper limit of normal for 2D-indexed LVM is 102 g/m^2. In women, the upper limits for normal for 3DE-indexed LVM and 2D-indexed LVM are similar at 90 g/m^2 and 88 g/m^2, respectively. Answer D is a true statement since 3DE has the advantage of being able to accommodate regional differences in wall thickness and therefore can provide the most accurate measurements of LV mass.

20. **Answer: C. Figure 13-3C** shows the correct method for measuring the interventricular septum (IVS) and the posterior LV wall thickness. The measurements in **Figure 13-3A** (answer A) are incorrect as the anterior caliper for the interventricular septum (IVS) has been placed too anteriorly. Including the right ventricle in the measurement of the IVS will lead to an overestimation of LV wall thickness. The measurements in **Figure 13-3B** (answer B) are incorrect. In patients with severe LV hypertrophy, the IVS should not be measured where it tapers as it approaches the aortic valve. This will lead to an underestimation of LV wall thickness. The measurements in **Figure 13-3D** (answer D) are incorrect. In cases of a sigmoid septum, the IVS should be measured just apical to the sigmoid septum to avoid overestimating LV wall thickness.

21. **Answer: A.** The echocardiogram reveals concentric increase in left ventricular (LV) wall thickness with a ground glass appearance, increased right ventricular wall thickness, biatrial enlargement with immobility, a small pericardial effusion, and valvular mitral and tricuspid regurgitation. The "bulls-eye" longitudinal strain plot (**Figure 13-4**) shows decreased strain in the basal and mid-wall segments with apical sparing, demonstrating a "cherry on top" pattern. All these findings in addition to the presenting symptoms of heart failure, low voltages on the ECG, and the patient history of multiple myeloma are indicative of a diagnosis of cardiac amyloidosis.

Answer B is incorrect. Cardiac sarcoidosis manifests as regional and global hypokinesis similar to ischemic and dilated cardiomyopathy; a common ECG finding with cardiac sarcoidosis is atrioventricular heart block. Answer C is incorrect. Although hypertrophic cardiomyopathy (HCM) reveals concentric LV hypertrophy, it generally exhibits asymmetric interventricular septal thickening and presents at a younger age. In addition, longitudinal strain is significantly attenuated in patients with HCM at the site of hypertrophy with less abnormal deformation elsewhere and does not display apical sparing. Answer D is incorrect. Although patients with systemic hypertension exhibit thickened walls, the endocardium does not have a ground glass appearance and while the left atrium may become enlarged later in the disease stage, biatrial enlargement with immobility is not seen. Furthermore, in hypertensive heart disease, the longitudinal strain may be mildly decreased but the bulls-eye pattern does not display apical sparing.

KEY POINTS

The strain "bulls-eye" plot is extremely valuable in differentiating among different causes of increased LV wall thickness. The "cherry on top" strain pattern is a characteristic finding of cardiac amyloidosis.

22. **Answer: E.** The fact that she developed hypertension at a young age is suspicious for coarctation of the aorta. Therefore, the patient should undergo an echocardiogram. In most patients with coarctation

of the aorta, the origin of the left subclavian artery is proximal to the coarctation, resulting in hypertension in both arms and a diminished BP in the legs. Less often, the origin of the left subclavian artery is just distal to the coarctation; therefore, the BP in the right arm will be higher than the BP in the left arm. Infrequently, both the right and left subclavian arteries originate below the area of coarctation, resulting in BPs that are equally decreased in all four extremities. Furthermore, if the origin of the right subclavian artery is anomalously located distal to the coarctation, comparing BP measurements between the right arm and leg may be misleading as they will be diminished to a similar degree. Therefore, the patient's blood pressure should also be taken in both arms and both legs.

SUGGESTED READINGS

Aurigemma GP. Quantitative evaluation of left ventricular structure, wall stress, and systolic function. In: Otto CM, ed. *The Practice of Clinical Echocardiography*. 5th ed. Philadelphia: Elsevier Saunders; 2017:chap 7.

Kim D, Ha JW. Hypertensive response to exercise: mechanisms and clinical implication. *Clin Hypertens*. 2016;22:17.

Lang RM, Badano LP, Mor-Avi V, et al. Recommendations for cardiac chamber quantification by echocardiography in adults: an update from the American Society of Echocardiography and the European Association of Cardiovascular Imaging. *J Am Soc Echocardiogr*. 2015;28(1):1-39.

Liu D, Hu K, Nordbeck P, Ertl G, Störk S, Weidemann F. Longitudinal strain bull's eye plot patterns in patients with cardiomyopathy and concentric left ventricular hypertrophy. *Eur J Med Res*. 2016;21(1):21.

Marwick TH, Gillebert TC, Aurigemma G, et al. Recommendations on the use of echocardiography in adult hypertension: a report from the EACVI and ASE. *J Am Soc Echocardiogr*. 2015;28(7):727-754.

Whelton PK, Carey RM, Aronow WS, et al. 2017 ACC/AHA/AAPA/ABC/ACPM/AGS/APhA/ASH/ASPC/NMA/PCNA guideline for the prevention, detection, evaluation, and management of high blood pressure in adults: a report of the American College of Cardiology/American Heart Association Task Force on Clinical Practice Guidelines. *J Am Coll Cardiol*. 2018;71(19):e127-e248.

Woo A. Hypertrophic cardiomyopathy: echocardiography in diagnosis and management of patients. In: Otto CM, ed. *The Practice of Clinical Echocardiography*. 5th ed. Philadelphia: Elsevier Saunders; 2017:chap 26.

CHAPTER 14

Right Ventricle

Contributors: Lanqi Hua, BS, ACS, RDCS, Jane E. Marshall, BS, RDCS, and
Leah Wright, BSc, DMU (Cardiac), PhD

✪✪✪ Question 1

▶ A 36-year-old woman with pulmonary arterial hypertension secondary to secundum atrial septal defect (ASD) presents for her annual assessment of right ventricular (RV) function. Based on the images provided (**Videos 14-1A** and **14-1B**), which of the following echocardiographically derived parameters is the best method to assess the RV function?

A. RV fractional area change (FAC)
B. RV global longitudinal strain (GLS)
C. RV index of myocardial performance (RIMP)
D. Three-dimensional (3D) RV volumes/ejection fraction (RVEF)
E. Tricuspid annular plane systolic excursion (TAPSE)

✪✪ Question 2

Which of the following parameters is least influenced by loading conditions when assessing right ventricular (RV) function?

A. 3D RV ejection fraction (RVEF)
B. RV fractional area change (FAC)
C. RV global longitudinal strain (GLS)
D. RV index of myocardial performance (RIMP)
E. Tricuspid annular plane systolic excursion (TAPSE)

✪✪ Question 3

The eccentricity index is a parameter used to quantitate the degree of right ventricular (RV) enlargement. Based on the data shown in **Figure 14-1**, which was obtained from a 78-year-old woman with history of pulmonary arterial hypertension, the eccentricity index is:

A. 0.5.
B. 0.8.
C. 1.3.
D. 2.0.
E. 2.1.

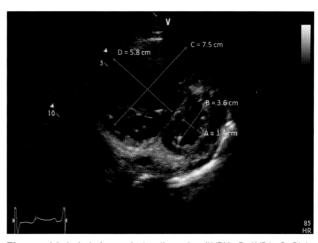

Figure 14-1 A, Left ventricular dimension (LVD)2, B, LVD1, C, Right ventricular dimension (RVD)2, D, RVD1.

✪✪ Question 4

▶ Based on the echocardiographic images provided (**Videos 14-2A** and **14-2B**), the findings are most likely due to:

A. 99% right coronary artery (RCA) occlusion.
B. Acute severe mitral regurgitation (MR).
C. Ebstein anomaly.
D. Mild pulmonary stenosis (PS).
E. Pulmonary artery hypertension (PAH).

✪✪ Question 5

Regarding right ventricular (RV) myocardial fiber arrangement, which of the following statements is false?

A. The mid-layer containing spiral fibers is responsible for the systolic twist motion.

B. Circumferentially oriented myofibers are located on the epicardial surface and are responsible for inward contraction (radial motion).

C. Epicardial circumferential oriented myofibers are components of the myofiber tracts that are shared with the left ventricle.

D. Longitudinally oriented myofibers are located in the deep (subendocardial) layer and are responsible for a base-to-apex motion (longitudinal motion).

✪✪ Question 6

Compared to the left ventricle (LV), which of the following statements regarding the right ventricle (RV) in a normal heart is false?

A. The RV has one-sixth of the muscle mass of the LV.

B. The RV cardiac output is less than the LV cardiac output.

C. The RV has multiple papillary muscles while the LV has two distinct papillary muscles.

D. The RV has chordal attachments from the tricuspid valve to the interventricular septum (IVS) while the LV has no chordal attachments to the IVS.

E. The RV inlet and outlet components are separated while there is continuity between the inlet and outlet components of the LV.

✪✪✪ Question 7

Which of the following statement(s) is/are incorrect?

A. Tricuspid inflow peak E velocity is a good indicator of right atrial (RA) pressure.

B. Tricuspid annular e′ velocity is a good indicator of right ventricular (RV) myocardial relaxation.

C. Tricuspid E/e′ ratio is a good indicator of RV myocardial relaxation and RV filling pressure.

D. Both A and C are incorrect.

E. Both B and C are incorrect.

✪✪ Question 8

Obstruction of which of the following coronary arteries is least likely to cause right ventricular (RV) ischemia?

A. Acute marginal artery

B. Conus artery

C. Obtuse marginal artery

D. Distal right coronary artery (RCA)

E. Posterior descending artery (PDA)

✪ Question 9

Which of the following transthoracic echocardiographic views is recommended for measurements of right ventricular (RV) size?

A. Apical 4-chamber view

B. RV-modified apical 4-chamber view

C. Parasternal RV inflow view

D. RV-focused apical 4-chamber view

E. Subcostal 4-chamber view

✪✪✪ Question 10

▶ Which of the following clinical presentations matches the echocardiographic findings shown in Videos 14-3A and 14-3B?

A. A 56-year-old man post right knee surgery presents to the emergency department (ED) after becoming acutely hypotensive and tachycardic when working with a physical therapist.

B. A 55-year-old man with history of portopulmonary hypertension and post liver transplant.

C. A 45-year-old man, with no significant past medical history, presents to the ED with syncope.

D. A 25-year-old woman with a past history of patent ductus arteriosus (PDA) ligation at 18 months of age presents to the ED with fever and chills.

✪✪ Question 11

A 78-year-old man with progressive shortness of breath has a transthoracic echocardiogram 5 days following coronary artery bypass surgery (grafts to the posterior descending artery and the left anterior descending and obtuse marginal coronary arteries). Echocardiographic findings included normal left ventricular (LV) size with a LV ejection fraction of 53%, mild mitral regurgitation, normal right ventricular (RV) size, mild tricuspid regurgitation (TR) with a TR velocity of 2.6 m/s, tricuspid annular plane systolic excursion (TAPSE) of 11 mm, tissue Doppler imaging (TDI) s′ velocity of 8 cm/s, RV fractional area change (FAC) of 40%, and no pericardial effusion. Based on these findings, his RV systolic function is most likely:

A. Mildly impaired.
B. Moderately impaired.
C. Severely impaired.
D. Within the limits of normal.

✪✪ Question 12

An echocardiographic study was performed on a 69-year-old man who presented to the emergency department with shortness of breath, chest pain, and history of hypertension and hyperlipidemia. On the tricuspid regurgitant (TR) spectral Doppler tracing, the peak TR velocity measured 3.5 m/s and the time duration between the peak velocity at 1 m/s and at 2 m/s was measured at 30 ms. What is the dP/dt?

A. 50 mm Hg/s
B. 400 mm Hg/s
C. 533 mm Hg/s
D. 1633 mm Hg/s
E. dP/dt cannot be calculated from the information provided

✪ Question 13

Based on 2015 guidelines from the American Society of Echocardiography (ASE), which of the following measurements is currently recommended for right ventricular (RV) two-dimensional (2D) global longitudinal strain (GLS)?

A. The average value of three segments of the RV free wall
B. The average value of six segments of the RV free wall and interventricular septum (IVS)
C. The highest value of the RV free wall
D. The highest value of the RV free wall and IVS

✪✪✪ Question 14

The term "athlete's heart" refers to the structural and electrical remodeling of the heart that occurs due to high exercise training levels. A 29-year-old avid cyclist presents with a history of two prior syncopal episodes. The transthoracic echocardiogram initially shows a dilated right ventricle (RV). Which of the following statements is true for differentiating between physiological and pathological changes in RV anatomy?

A. RV enlargement is training specific: rowers and cyclers (aerobic based) are more likely to show RV enlargement as compared to strength-based athletes; therefore, careful quantification of exercise levels is needed to determine if the individual is exercising enough to cause physiological remodeling.
B. RV enlargement occurs during endurance training but is explicitly linked to the increased load the left ventricle (LV) experiences; therefore, any right-sided remodeling is considered pathological.
C. Prominent trabeculation and RV regional abnormalities are suggestive of the presence of arrhythmogenic right ventricular cardiomyopathy (ARVC).
D. A and C.
E. All the above.

✪ Question 15

Tricuspid annular plane systolic excursion (TAPSE) was measured at 6 mm in a 47-year-old patient with cardiac amyloidosis (**Figure 14-2**). Which of the following statements is true?

A. The lower limit for preserved right ventricular (RV) function is 16 mm.
B. TAPSE represents the longitudinal function of the right ventricle.
C. TAPSE is an accurate assessment of global RV function.
D. A and B.
E. All of the above.

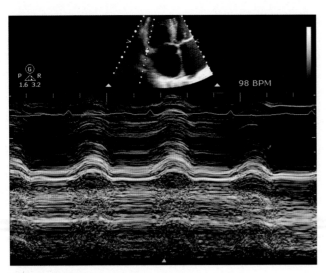

Figure 14-2

✪✪ Question 16

Which of the following echocardiographic findings is compatible with advanced right ventricular (RV) disease in patients with cardiac amyloidosis?

- **A.** A hepatic venous systolic velocity to diastolic velocity ratio of 1.2
- **B.** Deceleration time of tricuspid E velocity of 260 ms
- **C.** Increased inspiratory hepatic venous flow reversal with atrial contraction
- **D.** RV free wall thickness of 5 mm
- **E.** Tricuspid E/A ratio of 1

✪✪ Question 17

Which of the following echocardiographic findings is characteristic of patients with long-standing arrhythmogenic right ventricular dysplasia (ARVD)?

- **A.** Left ventricular ejection fraction (LVEF) of 26%
- **B.** Regional right ventricular (RV) dysfunction in the RV outflow tract (RVOT) and apical segments
- **C.** RV fractional area change (FAC) of 45%
- **D.** Tricuspid regurgitation (TR) velocity by continuous-wave Doppler of 3.6 m/s
- **E.** All of the above

✪✪✪ Question 18

Which of the following patient scenarios is compatible with the hepatic venous pulsed-wave (PW) Doppler signal shown in **Figure 14-3**?

- **A.** A 29-year-old woman with pulmonary hypertension and systemic venous congestion (right heart failure)
- **B.** A 49-year-old man with dilated cardiomyopathy and systemic venous and pulmonary venous congestion (right and left heart failure)
- **C.** A 55-year-old man with cardiac amyloidosis and lower extremity swelling
- **D.** A 65-year-old woman with hypertrophic cardiomyopathy and right ventricular (RV) hypertrophy
- **E.** Any of the above

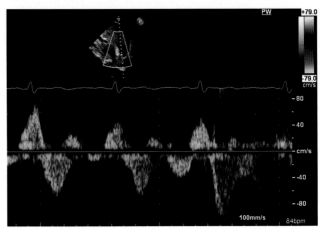

Figure 14-3

✪ Question 19

A 49-year-old woman presents with dyspnea on exertion. Based on the images provided (**Videos 14-4A** and **14-4B**), what is the diagnosis?

- **A.** Ebstein anomaly
- **B.** Carcinoid heart disease
- **C.** Rheumatic valvular disease
- **D.** None of the above

✪✪✪ Question 20

Which is true about this patient with pulmonary regurgitation (PR) (**Figure 14-4**)?

- **A.** The tricuspid E/A ratio is 0.6.
- **B.** Systolic reversal in the hepatic veins is present.
- **C.** Right ventricular (RV) stiffness is increased.
- **D.** Right ventricular end-diastolic pressure (RVEDP) is normal.

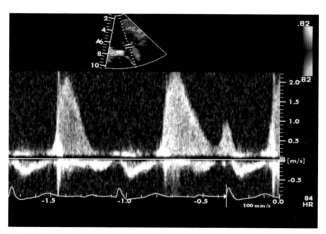

Figure 14-4

✪✪ Question 23

Which of the following is true about the continuous-wave (CW) Doppler signal obtained from the same patient as in Question 22 (**Figure 14-6**)?

A. Pulmonary vascular resistance is normal.

B. A transcatheter pulmonary valve replacement should be considered.

C. Diastolic flattening of the interventricular septum is likely present.

D. Right ventricular (RV) diastolic pressures are increased.

E. All of the above.

✪✪ Question 21

The sonographer is interrogating hepatic venous flow without a respirometer in a normal patient (**Figure 14-5**). Which of the following is true?

A. Inspiration is represented in part I and expiration is represented in part II.

B. Expiration is represented in part I and inspiration is represented in part II.

C. Inspiration is represented in part I and respiratory apnea is represented in part II.

D. Expiration is represented in part I and respiratory apnea is represented in part II.

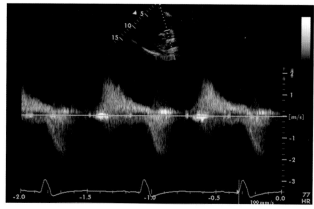

Figure 14-6

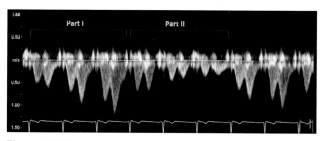

Figure 14-5

✪✪ Question 24

Which of the following is suggestive of pseudonormal right ventricular (RV) filling?

A. A tricuspid E/A ratio of 1 with an E/e′ ratio of 7 and systolic flow predominance in the hepatic veins

B. A tricuspid E/A ratio of 1.2 with an E/e′ ratio of 8 and diastolic flow predominance in the hepatic veins

C. A tricuspid E/A ratio of 1.8 with an E/e′ ratio of 10 and increased atrial systolic flow reversal in the hepatic veins

D. A tricuspid E/A ratio 1.5 with an E/e′ ratio of 6 and increased atrial systolic flow reversal flow in the hepatic veins

✪✪ Question 22

▶ The parasternal views in **Videos 14-5A** and **14-5B** were obtained from a 36-year-old man with lower extremity swelling. Which is true?

A. Right ventricular (RV) volumes are normal.

B. RV systolic pressure is increased.

C. Left ventricular (LV) ejection fraction is mild to moderately depressed.

D. There is a positive history of congenital heart disease.

E. B and C.

ANSWERS

1. **Answer: B.** Of the options listed, RV GLS is the best method for assessing RV function. This is because RV GLS is a measure of RV longitudinal myocardial function and is less load-dependent compared to the other listed parameters. This patient has a large ASD and significant tricuspid regurgitation as shown in the videos, which has markedly increased the preload. 3D RVEF is considered to be a true global measure of RV systolic function as it integrates both radial and longitudinal components of RV contraction as well as the contribution from the RV outflow tract (RVOT), with no geometric assumptions. However, because the 3D RVEF reflects the interaction between RV contractility and the RV loading conditions, it may overestimate RV systolic function in conditions with markedly increased preload such as with severe tricuspid regurgitation (TR) and a large ASD or it may underestimate RV performance when there is a high afterload such as in pulmonary thromboembolism and pulmonary hypertension.

   FAC (answer A) is derived from the RV diastolic area (RVDA) and the RV systolic area (RVSA):

$$FAC = \left[\left(RVDA - RVSA\right) \div RVDA\right] \times 100 \qquad (1)$$

   FAC is a measure of RV systolic function but neglects the contribution of the RVOT. RIMP (answer C) is a nonvolumetric measure of global RV function and is independent of the geometric shape of the right ventricle. RIMP is derived from the isovolumetric relaxation time (IVRT), the isovolumetric contraction time (IVCT), and the ejection time (ET) as:

$$RIMP = \left(IVRT + IVCT\right) \div ET \qquad (2)$$

   RIMP can be falsely low in conditions associated with elevated right atrial (RA) pressures, which will shorten the IVCT. This patient has moderate TR and a large ASD, which significantly increased the RA pressure. Therefore, RIMP is not the best method for the global RV function assessment. TAPSE (answer E) measures the displacement of the lateral tricuspid annulus during systole; therefore, this is a measurement of RV longitudinal function. As this measurement neglects the contribution of the RV free wall and the interventricular septum, it is not a true measure of RV function.

2. **Answer: C.** RV GLS is a noninvasive index of RV contractility. It is less confounded by heart motion and geometry changes, and less dependent on load than conventional RV function indices or 3D RVEF.

   As previously discussed, 3D RVEF (answer A) reflects the interaction between RV contractility and load; therefore, 3D RVEF overestimates RV systolic function in the setting of markedly increased preload, and underestimates RV systolic function when there is a high afterload. Other variables such as FAC (answer B), RIMP (answer D), and TAPSE (answer E) are also influenced by loading conditions.

3. **Answer: C.** There are two echocardiographic eccentricity indices: the LV eccentricity index (LVEI), which quantifies the abnormal interventricular septal (IVS) curvature in RV volume overload (when measured at end-diastole) and RV pressure overload (when measured at end-systole), and the RV eccentricity index (RVEI), which quantifies the RV geometry and the degree of RV dilatation. Both the LVEI and the RVEI are measured from a parasternal short-axis view at the level of the papillary muscles at either end-diastole or end-systole. For the LVEI, the LV cavity is measured parallel to the IVS (LVD2) and perpendicular to the IVS (LVD1). The LVEI is then calculated as:

$$LVEI = LVD2 \div LVD1 \qquad (1)$$

   For the RVEI, the RV cavity is measured parallel to the IVS (RVD2) and perpendicular to the IVS (RVD1). The RVEI is then calculated as:

$$RVEI = RVD2 \div RVD1 \qquad (2)$$

   As the question asks for the eccentricity index to quantitate the degree of RV enlargement, the RVEI is calculated from RVD2, which is 7.5 cm, and from RVD1, which is 5.8 cm; therefore, the RVEI is:

$$RVEI = 7.5 \div 5.8 = 1.3 \qquad (3)$$

4. **Answer: E.** The images provided demonstrate classic echocardiographic features of pulmonary arterial hypertension, which include significant right ventricular (RV) enlargement, right atrial enlargement, RV dysfunction, and a small pericardial effusion.

   A 99% RCA occlusion (answer A) is unlikely as the coronary flow to the RV occurs during both systole and diastole, and the RV has a thin wall. Therefore, the RV is less vulnerable to ischemia alone than it is to preload and afterload conditions. Acute severe MR (answer B) would cause acute pulmonary edema and an increase in pulmonary pressures, also called postcapillary pulmonary hypertension; however, there is typically no or only mild RV enlargement and RV systolic dysfunction. In Ebstein anomaly (answer C), a portion of the RV is "atrialized"; this is not seen in the images provided. Mild PS (answer D) would not cause severe RV enlargement and RV systolic dysfunction.

5. **Answer: A.** The myocardium of both the right and left ventricles consists of a complex 3D network of myofibers in a multiple helical arrangement. RV contraction is generated by a deep subendocardial layer of longitudinal fibers that cause a base-to-apex (longitudinal) motion, and a superficial layer of circumferential fibers that cause inward contraction (radial motion). The RV, however, lacks the mid-layer of spiral fibers that are present in the left ventricle (LV) that account for the LV twist motion. The interventricular septum also contributes to RV systolic function.

KEY POINTS

Three main mechanisms contribute to RV systolic function: (1) longitudinal base-to-apex shortening, (2) inward (radial) movement of the RV free wall, and (3) bulging of the IVS into the RV during LV contraction causing RV shortening in the anteroposterior direction.

6. **Answer: D.** While the RV is smaller than the LV, has one-sixth of the LV muscle mass, and pumps against approximately one-sixth of the resistance the LV encounters, the RV pumps the same cardiac output as the LV. This is because the RV and lungs are in series with the LV and systemic circulation. Therefore, the entire cardiac output of the LV must pass through the RV within the circuit. In cases where there is a significant intracardiac shunt, then the cardiac output of each ventricle is no longer the same.

7. **Answer: D.** The tricuspid peak E velocity (answer A) reflects a combination of myocardial relaxation and the RA-RV pressure gradient during diastole; hence, this velocity is not reflective of the RA pressure alone. Therefore, this answer is an incorrect statement. The tricuspid E/e′ ratio (answer C) is an indicator of RA pressure rather than an indicator of RV myocardial relaxation and RV filling pressure; therefore, this answer is an incorrect statement.

The tricuspid annular e′ velocity (answer B) reflects myocardial relaxation; therefore, this answer is a correct statement.

KEY POINTS

▶ The tricuspid E velocity reflects a combination of myocardial relaxation and RA-RV pressure gradient.

▶ The tricuspid annular e′ velocity reflects myocardial relaxation.

▶ When the tricuspid E velocity is divided by the e′, the subsequent E/e′ reflects the RA-RV pressure gradient, or the RA pressure, in isolation. Therefore, when elevated, the E/e′ is a sign of elevated RA pressure.

8. **Answer: C.** The blood supply of the RV varies according to the dominance of the coronary system. In a right-dominant system, which is found in the majority of individuals, the RCA supplies most of the RV. The RCA divides into smaller branches, including the right PDA, the acute marginal artery, and the conus artery. The lateral wall of the RV is supplied by the acute marginal branches of the RV, whereas the inferior RV wall and the inferoseptal region are supplied by the PDA, and the infundibulum derives its supply from the conus artery (**Figure 14-7**). The anterior wall of the RV and the anteroseptal region are supplied by branches of the left anterior descending coronary artery. The obtuse marginal artery (OMA) is a branch of the left circumflex coronary artery, which supplies most of the left atrium and the posterior and lateral left ventricular walls. Obstruction to the OMA would not cause RV ischemia; therefore, answer C is correct.

9. **Answer: D.** The comprehensive assessment of the RV requires a complete set of standardized views, which includes the parasternal long-axis, parasternal RV inflow, parasternal short-axis, apical 4-chamber, RV-focused apical 4-chamber, and subcostal views. Two-dimensional (2D) measurements of the RV are challenging due to the complex shape of the RV and its lack of right-sided anatomic landmarks to ensure optimization of the RV. To overcome these issues, it is recommended that the RV be measured from an RV-focused apical 4-chamber view. This view is obtained by moving the probe laterally and angling the probe face medially from the apical 4-chamber view, while maintaining the left ventricular (LV) apex in the center of the image sector, and rotating counterclockwise to ensure display of the largest RV basal diameter, the longest RV long axis, and the entire RV free wall (**Figure 14-8**).

The apical 4-chamber view (answer A) is not recommended for the measurement of RV size because there is considerable variation in how the RV is sectioned from this view, and therefore, there is also considerable measurement variability. The RV-modified apical 4-chamber view (answer B) is the opposite of the RV-focused view and is obtained by sliding medially and angling the probe face laterally from the apical 4-chamber view. This off-axis view may be used for the qualitative assessment of RV function and for improving the alignment of the ultrasound beam for the interrogation of tricuspid inflow and the tricuspid regurgitant Doppler jet. The parasternal RV inflow view (answer C) is useful for the assessment of anterior and inferior RV wall motion. The subcostal 4-chamber view (answer E) is the best view for measurement of RV wall thickness. Due to foreshortening and the oblique imaging angle, RV size measurements should not be performed from the RV-modified apical 4-chamber view, the parasternal RV inflow view, or the subcostal 4-chamber view.

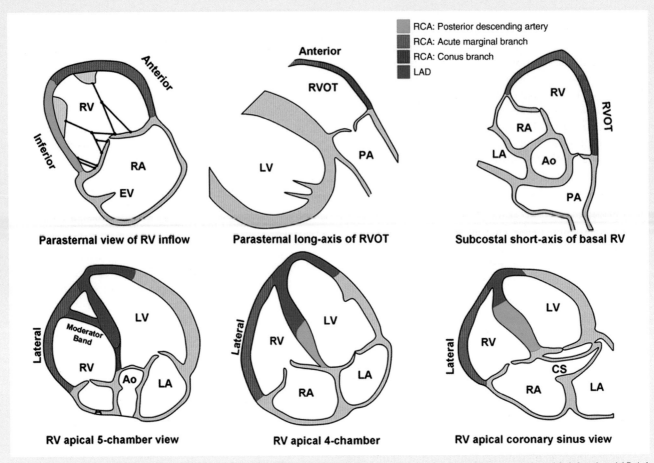

Figure 14-7 Segmental nomenclature of the right ventricular walls, along with their coronary supply. Ao, Aorta; CS, coronary sinus; LA, left atrium; LAD, left anterior descending artery; LV, left ventricle; PA, pulmonary artery; RA, right atrium; RCA, right coronary artery; RV, right ventricle; RVOT, right ventricular outflow tract. (Reprinted from Rudski LG, Lai WW, Afilalo J, et al. Guidelines for the echocardiographic assessment of the right heart in adults: a report from the American Society of Echocardiography endorsed by the European Association of Echocardiography, a registered branch of the European Society of Cardiology, and the Canadian Society of Echocardiography. *J Am Soc Echocardiogr.* 2010;23(7):685-713. Copyright © 2010 American Society of Echocardiography. With permission.)

10. ▶ **Answer: A.** The echocardiographic images show a regional pattern of right ventricular (RV) dysfunction, with akinesis of the mid-free wall and hypercontractility of the RV apex (**Figure 14-9**). This is a classic example of McConnell sign, which is a distinct echocardiographic feature of acute massive pulmonary embolism. **Video 14-6**, also acquired from this patient, shows a saddle pulmonary embolus. This patient presented with this event shortly following knee surgery and during the time-frame where patients are highly vulnerable for acute

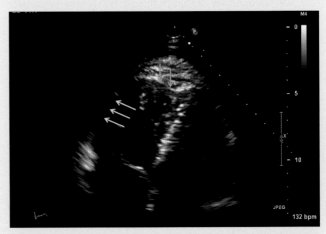

Figure 14-9 This is an RV-modified apical 4-chamber view from **Video 14-3B**, which was acquired in a patient with a massive pulmonary embolism. The end-systolic still frame image shows preserved contractility of the apical segment of the RV (green arrows) with dysfunction of the more basal portions (yellow arrows); this is the McConnell sign.

Figure 14-8

Table 14-1. Summary of RV Systolic Measurements and Normal/Abnormal Values

Parameter	Measurement in This Study	Normal Values
TAPSE (mm)	11	≥16
TDI s′ (cm/s)	8	≥10
FAC (%)	40	≥35

deep vein thrombosis and pulmonary embolism. The other patient presentations are not consistent with these echo findings.

11. **Answer: D.** The TAPSE, TDI s′ velocity and FAC for this study, as well as the normal and abnormal values for each, are listed in **Table 14-1**. In this patient, the values for TAPSE and TDI s′ are below normal. However, in postoperative patients, these measurements can appear low despite normal RV inward motion. Possible hypotheses to explain this reduction in RV performance detected along the long-axis include geometrical changes of the RV chamber (in association with interventricular septal paradoxical motion), intraoperative ischemia, extra-myocardial causes (pericardium, changes in fossa ovalis, and postoperative adherence of RV to the thoracic wall). Therefore, the FAC should be considered for the evaluation of RV systolic function. FAC was 40%, so the RV systolic function is within the limits of normal.

12. **Answer: B.** The peak positive dP/dt is a measurement of the rate of right ventricular (or left ventricular) pressure rise during isovolumic contraction. "dP" refers to the change in ventricular pressure, while "dt" refers to the change in time. The time taken for the ventricle to generate a pressure rise is directly related to myocardial contractility. The dP/dt is calculated from the time difference (Δt) between the TR velocity at 1 m/s and the TR velocity at 2 m/s:

$$dP/dt = \left[\left(4 \times 2^2\right) - \left(4 \times 1\right)^2\right] \div \Delta t$$
$$= \left[16 - 4\right] \div \Delta t$$
$$= 12 \div \Delta t \qquad (1)$$

In this patient, the time it took the TR velocity to increase from 1 to 2 m/s was 30 ms. Therefore, the dP/dt is:

$$dP/dt = 12 \div 0.030 = 400\,mm\,Hg/s \qquad (2)$$

where 0.030 is Δt converted from ms to seconds.

A dP/dt of more than 400 mm Hg/sec strongly predicts normal RV ejection fraction.

13. **Answer: A.** 2D speckle-tracking echocardiography can be used to measure RV GLS. RV GLS is measured from an RV-focused apical 4-chamber view as either the average of the three RV free wall and three IVS segments or the three RV free wall segments alone (**Figure 14-10**). The six-segment RV GLS, which includes the deformation of the IVS in its calculation, is heavily influenced by left ventricular function and is thus considered as less reliable for the assessment of RV function. Furthermore, the RV free wall segments alone, excluding the IVS, have been reported to have prognostic value in various disease states. Therefore, the recommended RV GLS is the average value of three segments of the RV free wall.

14. **Answer: D.** Physiological remodeling of the heart in response to exercise training, termed "athlete's heart," involves the enlargement of all four chambers of the heart. Severe enlargement should not be seen in a recreational athlete but would not be unusual in an athlete who participates at a competition level. Careful quantification of exercise levels is needed to determine where the patient fits within this context; thus, answer A is correct. During endurance exercise, the volume load is the same on the right and left heart chambers, hence remodeling of all four chambers will be seen, making answer B incorrect. Presence of prominent trabeculation and enlargement of the RV more than the LV may be found in an athlete with ARVC; thus, answer C is correct. In addition, RV regional wall motion abnormalities as well as isolated enlargement of the RV outflow tract may also aid in the differentiation of ARVC from athlete's heart. An awareness of moderator band tethering is important as this may occur, giving a false impression of wall motion abnormalities, leading to an incorrect diagnosis of ARVC.

15. **Answer: D.** The lower limit for preserved RV function is 16 mm; therefore, answer A is true. TAPSE measures the displacement of the lateral tricuspid annulus during systole, so this is a measurement of RV longitudinal function; therefore, answer B is true. As this measurement neglects the contribution of the RV free wall and the interventricular septum, it is not a true measure of global RV function. Therefore, answer C is a false statement.

16. **Answer: C.** With advanced RV disease in patients with cardiac amyloidosis, hepatic venous flow at is characterized by reduced forward systolic (S) flow, increased forward diastolic (D) flow, and greater inspiratory flow reversal with atrial contraction; therefore, answer C is correct. Answer A is incorrect as S forward flow is reduced and D forward flow is increased; thus, the S/D ratio is <1.

Answers B and E are incorrect since the tricuspid inflow shows a restrictive filling pattern with

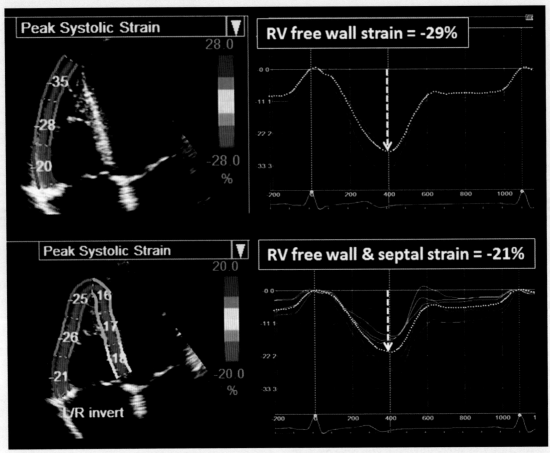

Figure 14-10 RV strain measurements from the RV-focused apical 4-chamber view. The upper panel demonstrates RV free wall strain whereby the three segments of the free wall alone are averaged. The lower panel demonstrates longitudinal strain averaged from six segments: three RV free wall and three IVS segments. (Reprinted from Lang RM, Badano LP, Mor-Avi V, et al. Recommendations for cardiac chamber quantification by echocardiography in adults: an update from the American Society of Echocardiography and the European Association of Cardiovascular Imaging. *J Am Soc Echocardiogr.* 2015;28(1): 1-39. Copyright © 2015 Elsevier. With permission.)

advanced RV disease. Therefore, the tricuspid inflow profile will display an E/A ratio >2.1 and a deceleration time <120 ms. Answer D is incorrect as a normal RV wall thickness is up to 5 mm and in cardiac amyloidosis with advanced RV disease, the RV free wall thickness is moderate to markedly thickened.

17. **Answer: B.** In ARVD, there are frequent abnormalities in RV regional and global function. The regional dysfunction is commonly noted in the RVOT, apex, and basal RV free wall, the so-called "triangle of dysplasia." RV dilatation and depressed global systolic function also occur, though not in all patients early on. In one study, dilatation of the RVOT was noted in all patients with ARVD and may occur as an isolated finding. Other abnormalities include an abnormally bright moderator band, RV sacculations (or diastolic outpouchings), aneurysm (systolic outpouchings), and trabecular derangements.

Answer A is not correct as the LVEF is characteristically normal in most patients with ARVD, although infrequently a left-sided cardiomyopathy may occur.

Answer C is not correct as a FAC of 45% is normal, and a depressed FAC is expected in patients with long-standing ARVD. Given the presence of RV systolic dysfunction, pulmonary artery pressures are usually normal and not elevated. Therefore, a peak TR velocity of 3.6 m/s, which indicates an elevation in the RV systolic pressure, is not consistent with ARVD; thus, answer D is not correct.

18. **Answer: D.** The hepatic venous PW Doppler trace shows a large atrial reversal (AR) signal above the zero-velocity baseline. Prominence of the AR velocity occurs when there is a forceful right atrial (RA) contraction, which may occur when there is tricuspid stenosis or RV hypertrophy. In the latter, a prominent AR velocity is caused by increased RV diastolic pressure and decreased compliance of the RV. This hemodynamic finding is compatible with answer D. Systemic venous congestion occurs with increased mean RA pressure and predominant diastolic forward flow in all other choices.

19. **Answer: B.** The apical 4-chamber view (**Video 14-4A**) demonstrates the presence of prominent thickening and retraction of septal and anterior tricuspid leaflets with the valve remaining in a fixed semi-open position throughout the cardiac cycle. This leads to severe tricuspid regurgitation (**Video 14-4B**). These features are characteristic findings of carcinoid heart disease. Ebstein anomaly (answer A) is characterized by apical displacement of the septal leaflet and an elongated anterior leaflet in that view. Rheumatic tricuspid valve disease (answer C) is usually accompanied by mitral valve rheumatic disease in patients with a history of rheumatic fever. The pathologic characteristic is commissural fusion of the leaflets with diffuse thickening and resultant stenosis and regurgitation.

20. **Answer: C.** The PR continuous-wave Doppler signal is steep, indicating rapid equilibration of pressure between the pulmonary artery (PA) and the right ventricle during diastole. When RV stiffness is increased, RV diastolic pressure rises rapidly leading to a PR signal that is similar to that seen in this case. This patient has increased RVEDP and right atrial pressure. In this case, the tricuspid inflow would be characterized by predominant early filling with an E/A ratio >1, and a steep deceleration time of tricuspid E velocity. Furthermore, the hepatic venous trace would show predominant forward flow in diastole (not systolic reversal).

21. **Answer: A.** Onset of inspiration is confirmed by an augmentation in forward flow velocities (part I) while onset of expiration is confirmed by a decrease in forward flow velocities (part II) and usually with an increase in diastolic flow reversal (although not seen in this example).

TEACHING POINT

With inspiration, the intrathoracic pressure decreases and there is a decrease in the right atrial (RA) and right ventricular (RV) pressures. The decrease in RA pressure results in increased blood flow from the inferior vena cava (IVC) and hepatic veins into the RA. Therefore, systolic and diastolic forward flow velocities increase with inspiration. During expiration, the opposite occurs. The intrathoracic pressure increases and there is an increase in the RA and RV pressures and a decrease in blood flow from the IVC and hepatic veins into the RA. Therefore, systolic and diastolic forward flow velocities decrease with expiration, and there is also a slight increase in reversal velocities with expiration.

22. **Answer: D.** The parasternal long-axis view (**Video 14-5A**) shows a left ventricle with normal size and function but a dilated right ventricle. The color Doppler image acquired from a parasternal

short-axis view at the level of the great vessels (**Video 14-5B**) shows some acceleration across the pulmonic valve in systole indicating increased systolic flow across the valve. However, the most important finding by color Doppler is the presence of severe pulmonary regurgitation. This lesion is common after surgery for the repair of tetralogy of Fallot and does not lead to increased RV systolic pressure.

23. **Answer: E.** The CW Doppler signal is indicative of severe pulmonary regurgitation (PR), and the small increase in velocity across the pulmonic valve is largely due to increased transvalvular flow, and not valve stenosis. Patients with severe PR have a steep rise in RV diastolic pressure that leads to rapid equalization of the pressure gradient between the pulmonary artery and the right ventricle in mid-to-late diastole, and therefore the CW Doppler PR signal shows a steep deceleration and short pressure half-time as in this case. Severe PR leads to increased RV diastolic, not systolic, pressures. Therefore, answer D is a true statement. Pulmonary vascular resistance is not elevated in patients with severe PR as the RV systolic pressures are usually normal; therefore, answer A is true. A transcatheter pulmonary valve replacement is a good option for patients with severe PR; therefore, answer B is true. Diastolic flattening of the interventricular septum (answer C) is an indicator of diastolic RV volume overload. RV diastolic volume overload is present in severe PR; therefore, this answer is true.

KEY POINTS

▸ Patients with significant PR have a dilated RV.

▸ Interventricular septal motion is characterized by an RV volume overload pattern, with a flat septum only in diastole.

▸ Color Doppler can be used to assess the severity of PR.

▸ Severe PR by CW Doppler shows rapid deceleration with short pressure half-time.

24. **Answer: B.** The grading of RV diastolic function may be divided into normal filling, impaired relaxation (mild diastolic dysfunction), pseudonormal filling (moderate diastolic dysfunction), and restrictive filling (severe diastolic dysfunction). A tricuspid E/A ratio <0.8 suggests impaired relaxation, a tricuspid E/A ratio of 0.8 to 2.1 with an E/e′ ratio >6 or diastolic flow predominance in the hepatic veins suggests pseudonormal filling, and a tricuspid E/A ratio >2.1 with deceleration time <120 ms suggests restrictive filling. Therefore, answer B is correct as a tricuspid E/A ratio of 1.2 with an E/e′ ratio of 8 and diastolic flow predominance in the hepatic veins suggests pseudonormal filling.

SUGGESTED READINGS

Appleton CP, Hatle LK, Popp RL. Superior vena cave and hepatic vein Doppler echocardiography in healthy adults. *J Am Coll Cardiol.* 1987;10(5):1032-1039.

Bhattacharyya S, Toumpanakis C, Burke M, Taylor AM, Caplin ME, Davar J. Features of carcinoid heart disease identified by 2- and 3-dimensional echocardiography and cardiac MRI. *Circ Cardiovasc Imaging.* 2010;3(1):103-111.

Genovese D, Mor-Avi V, Palermo C, et al. Comparison between four-chamber and right ventricular-focused views for the quantitative evaluation of right ventricular size and function. *J Am Soc Echocardiogr.* 2019;32(4):484-494.

Haddad F, Doyle R, Murphy DJ, Hunt SA. Right ventricular function in cardiovascular disease, Part II pathophysiology, clinical importance, and management of right ventricular failure. *Circulation.* 2008;117(13):1717-1731.

Haddad F, Hunt SA, Rosenthal DN, Murphy DJ. Right ventricular function in cardiovascular disease, Part I: anatomy, physiology, aging, and functional assessment of the right ventricle. *Circulation.* 2008;117(11):1436-1448.

Kohli P, Schiller N. The physiologic basis of right ventricular echocardiography. In: Lang RM, Goldstein SA, Kronzon I, Khandheria BK, Mor-Avi V, eds. *ASE's Comprehensive Echocardiography.* 2nd ed. Philadelphia: Elsevier Saunders; 2016:142-151.

Kovács A, Lakatos B, Tokodi M, Merkely B. Right ventricular mechanical pattern in health and disease: beyond longitudinal shortening. *Heart Fail Rev.* 2019;24(4):511-520.

Lang RM, Badano LP, Mor-Avi V, et al. Recommendations for cardiac chamber quantification by echocardiography in adults: an update from the American Society of Echocardiography and the European Association of Cardiovascular Imaging. *J Am Soc Echocardiogr.* 2015;28(1):1-39.

McConnell MV, Solomon SD, Rayan ME, Come PC, Goldhaber SZ, Lee RT. Regional right ventricular dysfunction detected by echocardiography in acute pulmonary embolism. *Am J Cardiol.* 1996;78(4):469-473.

Mor-Avi V, Lang R, Badano LP, et al. Current and evolving echocardiographic techniques for the quantitative evaluation of cardiac mechanics: ASE/EAE consensus statement on methodology and indications endorsed by the Japanese Society of Echocardiography. *J Am Soc Echocardiogr.* 2011;24(3):277-313.

Prior D. Differentiating athlete's heart from cardiomyopathies – the right side. *Heart Lung Circ.* 2018;27(9):1063-1071.

Rudski LG, Muraru D, Afilalo J, Lester SJ. Assessment of right ventricular systolic and diastolic function. In: Lang RM, Goldstein SA, Kronzon I, Khandheria BK, Mor-Avi V, eds. *ASE's Comprehensive Echocardiography.* 2nd ed. Philadelphia: Elsevier Saunders; 2016:151-161.

Ruski LG, Lai WW, Afilalo J, et al. Guidelines for the echocardiographic assessment of the right heart in adults: a report from the American Society of Echocardiography endorsed by the European Association of Echocardiography, a registered branch of the European Society of Cardiology, and the Canadian Society of Echocardiography. *J Am Soc Echocardiogr.* 2010;23(7):685-713.

CHAPTER 15

Pulmonary Hypertension

Contributors: Margaret M. Park, BS, ACS, RDCS, RVT and Evelina Petrovets, BASc, RDCS

★ Question 1

Which of the following statements is not true concerning pulmonary arterial hypertension (PAH)?

A. The classic signs and symptoms of PAH make it easy to diagnose the disease early on.

B. PAH is the result of obstructed pulmonary arterioles.

C. One of the causes of PAH is congenital heart disease.

D. The gold standard for the diagnosis of PAH is right heart catheterization.

E. PAH is also referred to as precapillary pulmonary hypertension.

★★ Question 2

A 72-year-old woman with shortness of breath presents for an echocardiogram. The tricuspid regurgitant (TR) continuous-wave Doppler profile is displayed in **Figure 15-1A**. The inferior vena cava (IVC) response to the sniff test is displayed in **Figure 15-1B**. The calculated right ventricular systolic pressure (RVSP) is:

A. 105 mm Hg.

B. 108 mm Hg.

C. 113 mm Hg.

D. 120 mm Hg.

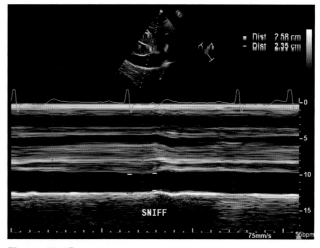

Figure 15-1A

Figure 15-1B

✪✪ Question 3

Results of an echocardiogram display a peak tricuspid regurgitant (TR) velocity of 4.0 m/s by continuous-wave Doppler, a dilated right ventricle (RV), no RV outflow tract (RVOT) obstruction or pulmonary stenosis, and a mitral E/e′ of 20. According to these findings, which of the following statements is correct?

   A. There is pulmonary arterial hypertension (PAH).
   B. There is postcapillary pulmonary hypertension.
   C. There is an increased right ventricular systolic pressure (RVSP), but the category of pulmonary hypertension cannot be determined.
   D. The presence or absence of pulmonary hypertension cannot be identified based on this limited information.

✪✪ Question 4

▶ A 70-year-old man with a history of cirrhosis is referred to the cardiology department with symptoms of significant dyspnea, abdominal distension, and ankle swelling. A clinical assessment and echocardiogram were performed. Based on **Figures 15-2A** to **15-2C** and **Video 15-1**, what is the most likely cause for pulmonary hypertension (PH) in this patient?

   A. Arrhythmogenic right ventricular dysplasia (ARVD)
   B. Portal hypertension
   C. Cardiac amyloidosis
   D. Ischemic cardiomyopathy

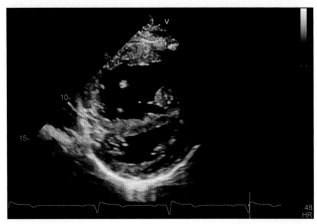

Figure 15-2A

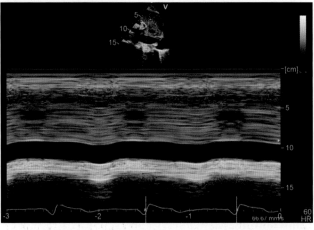

Figure 15-2B

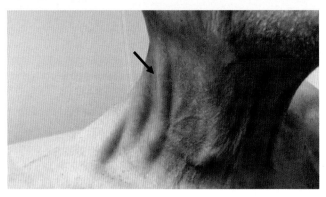

Figure 15-2C

✪✪ Question 5

Which of the following equations cannot be used to estimate mean pulmonary artery pressure (mPAP)?

   A. $mPAP = 79 - (0.45 \times RVAT)$
   B. $mPAP = 90 - (0.62 \times RVAT)$
   C. $mPAP = 4V_{PR\text{-}ED}^2 + RAP$
   D. $mPAP = \Delta P_{mTR} + RAP$

where ΔP_{mTR} is the mean pressure gradient of the tricuspid regurgitant signal, RAP is the right atrial pressure, RVAT is the right ventricular outflow tract acceleration time, and $V_{PR\text{-}ED}$ is the peak end-diastolic pulmonary regurgitant velocity.

✪✪✪ Question 6

All of the following are clinical and echocardiographic features associated with poor prognosis in pulmonary arterial hypertension (PAH) except:

   A. A pericardial effusion
   B. Right atrial (RA) enlargement
   C. Male >50 years of age
   D. Shortened QRS duration on the electrocardiogram

✪✪ Question 7

Which of the following diseases requires an annual echocardiogram as a screening measure for the potential development of pulmonary hypertension (PH)?

A. Obstructive sleep apnea (OSA) syndrome
B. Chronic obstructive pulmonary disease (COPD)
C. Prior acute pulmonary embolism (APE)
D. Sickle cell disease (SCD)

✪✪ Question 8

Which of the following is not true with respect to the estimation of right ventricular systolic pressure (RVSP) using the tricuspid regurgitant (TR) continuous-wave (CW) Doppler waveform?

A. Measurement of an incomplete CW Doppler envelope will underestimate the RVSP.
B. Measurement of "fringing" artifacts on the CW Doppler signal will overestimate the RVSP.
C. Measurements taken from "wide-open" TR jet will overestimate the RVSP.
D. Measurement of the highest velocity in atrial fibrillation will overestimate the RVSP.
E. All of the above statements are true.

✪✪✪ Question 9

Which of the following options correctly describes the chronological order for the development of Eisenmenger syndrome?

A. Left-to-right shunt, severe pulmonary hypertension (PH), right heart pressure > left heart pressure causing a right-to-left shunt, peripheral cyanosis
B. Peripheral cyanosis, left-to-right shunt, severe PH, right heart pressure > left heart pressure causing a right-to-left shunt
C. Left-to-right shunt, peripheral cyanosis, severe PH, right heart pressure > left heart pressure causing a right-to-left shunt
D. Severe PH, left-to-right shunt, peripheral cyanosis, right heart pressure > left heart pressure causing a right-to-left shunt

✪✪✪ Question 10

In patients with chronic obstructive pulmonary disease (COPD), the respiratory variation in spectral Doppler findings may mimic constrictive pericarditis (CP). Which of the following may differentiate between these two conditions?

A. In COPD the inspiratory variation in the transmitral E velocity is much greater than that seen in patients with CP.
B. In COPD the inspiratory variation in the transtricuspid E velocity is much less than that seen in patients with CP.
C. In COPD the superior vena cava (SVC) forward flow velocities are augmented with inspiration while in CP the SVC velocities show minimal variation.
D. B and C.
E. All of the above.

✪✪ Question 11

McConnell sign may be seen in cases of acute pulmonary embolism and in many different etiologies of acute cor pulmonale. The characteristic echocardiographic appearance of this sign is:

A. Isolated akinesis of the right ventricular (RV) apex.
B. A D-shaped left ventricle (LV) during systole from the parasternal short axis view.
C. A rocking motion of the RV due to a tethering effect from the LV.
D. Severe hypokinesis of the RV with relative sparing of the RV apex.

✪✪✪ Question 12

Which of the following echocardiographic variables favors pulmonary arterial hypertension (PAH) over pulmonary hypertension due to heart failure with a preserved ejection fraction (PH-HFpEF)?

A. Bowing of the interatrial septum from left to right
B. Delayed relaxation pattern on the transmitral inflow profile
C. Mitral E/e′ ratio with exercise >15
D. Echo-derived pulmonary vascular resistance (PVR) >3 Wood units

✪✪✪ Question 13

▶ A 19-year-old college hockey player experienced chest pains during a recent game. His physical examination was unremarkable. An electrocardiogram (ECG) shows normal sinus rhythm with a right bundle branch block. Based on the images provided (**Videos 15-2A** to **15-2E**), what is the likely diagnosis?

A. Patent foramen ovale (PFO)
B. Pulmonary veno-occlusive disease (PVOD)
C. Athlete's heart with an incidental PFO
D. Arrhythmogenic right ventricular dysplasia (ARVD) and a PFO

✪✪ Question 14

Figure 15-3 shows a parasternal short-axis view of the left ventricle (LV) acquired at the level of the papillary muscles. The index shown is often used to determine the presence of pulmonary arterial hypertension (PAH) in infants when there is no visible or only a weak tricuspid regurgitant signal present. The correct name for this index is the left ventricular _____ index.

   A. Sphericity

   B. Eccentricity

   C. D-shaped

   D. Tei Index

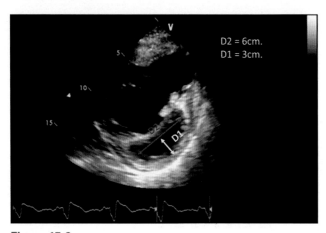

Figure 15-3

✪ Question 15

The left ventricular eccentricity index (LVEI) can be calculated from the measurements provided in **Figure 15-3**. What is the correct timing and calculated LVEI based on the measurements provided?

   A. At end-systole = 2.0

   B. At end-diastole = 2.0

   C. At end-systole = 0.5

   D. At end-diastole = 0.5

✪✪✪ Question 16

In patients with pulmonary hypertension, an agitated-saline bubble study is often ordered with the echocardiogram to determine if a patent foramen ovale (PFO) with right-to-left shunting is present. Which statement is not true regarding an agitated bubble saline study in these cases?

   A. A coexistent Eustachian valve can result in false-negative findings.

   B. Bubbles in the left atrium within 3 beats indicate an intracardiac shunt.

   C. Left ventricular diastolic dysfunction is a reason for a false-positive study.

   D. A Valsalva maneuver and cough should always be performed.

✪✪ Question 17

Which of the following echocardiographic findings is not an indirect sign of pulmonary hypertension (PH)?

   A. An increased "a wave" on the pulmonary valve M-mode trace

   B. Mid-systolic notching on the aortic valve M-mode trace

   C. Right ventricular outflow tract acceleration time (RVAT) of 90 ms

   D. Right ventricular wall thickness at end-diastole of 6 mm

   E. A and B

✪✪✪ Question 18

▶ Based on the information provided in **Figures 15-4A** to **15-4D** and **Video 15-3** acquired from a patient with chronic idiopathic pulmonary hypertension (PH), which statement regarding the right ventricle (RV) is correct?

   A. There is mild RV dilatation and normal systolic function.

   B. There is mild RV dilatation and mild systolic dysfunction.

   C. There is moderate RV dilatation and mild systolic dysfunction.

   D. There is moderate RV dilatation and moderate systolic dysfunction.

   E. There is severe RV dilatation and moderate systolic dysfunction.

✪✪✪ Question 19

All of the following contribute to increased vascular remodeling and resistance in pulmonary arterial hypertension (PAH) except:

   A. Vascular inflammation

   B. Overproduction of nitric oxide

   C. Intimal fibrosis

   D. Platelet dysfunction and thrombosis

   E. Vasoconstriction

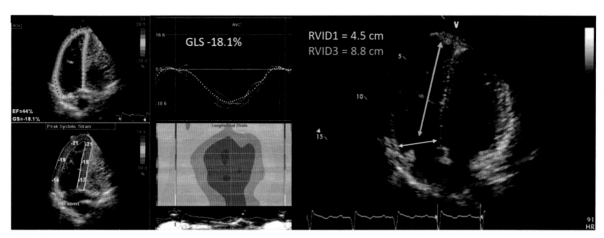

Figure 15-4A

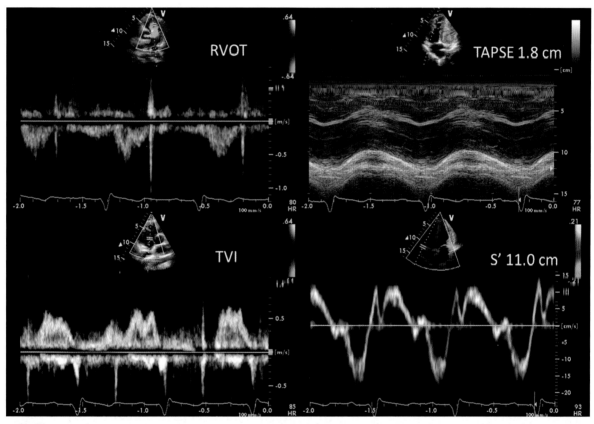

Figure 15-4B

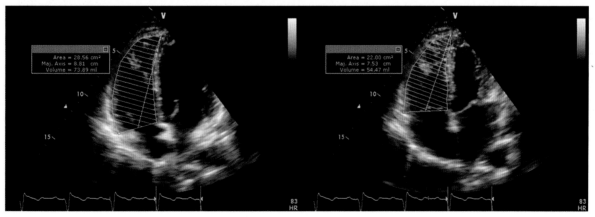

Figure 15-4C

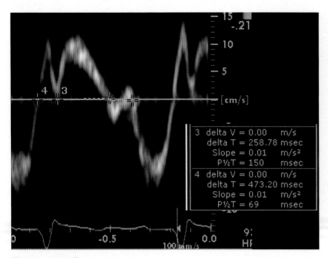

Figure 15-4D

✪✪✪ Question 20

Based on the information provided in **Figure 15-5**, the calculated pulmonary vascular resistance (PVR) is:

    A. 1.7.

    B. 2.0.

    C. 2.7.

    D. PVR cannot be calculated from this information alone.

✪✪✪ Question 21

A 35-year-old woman with a diagnosis of scleroderma is scheduled for a transthoracic echocardiogram. Patients with connective tissue disorders such as scleroderma have been shown to develop associated pulmonary arterial hypertension (SSc-PAH) and have worse survival rates in comparison to other idiopathic pulmonary arterial hypertension (IPAH) patients. Which feature on the echocardiogram is less likely to distinguish this patient with SSc-PAH and worsening right ventricular (RV) function from a patient with IPAH and no connective tissue disorder?

    A. RV volume overload pattern

    B. Pericardial effusion

    C. Left atrial dilatation

    D. Left ventricular diastolic dysfunction

    E. RVSP >30 mm Hg

✪✪ Question 22

Secondary echocardiographic indices of elevated right atrial pressure (RAP) that are predictive of adverse outcomes in patients with pulmonary arterial hypertension include all of the following except:

    A. A hepatic vein systolic filling fraction <55%.

    B. An inferior vena cava collapsibility index of <55%.

    C. A tricuspid valve inflow E/e′ >6.

    D. A right ventricular outflow tract acceleration time of <60 ms.

    E. A restrictive tricuspid inflow filling pattern.

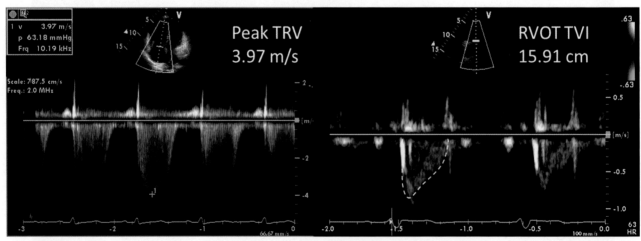

Figure 15-5

ANSWERS

1. **Answer: A.** Early in the disease, the signs and symptoms of PAH are often nonspecific or may be mistaken for other causes such as asthma, anxiety, or a lack of fitness. Therefore, PAH is usually not diagnosed until the level of disease is at least moderate and causes significant shortness of breath (SOB) with exertion, marked fatigue, and right heart failure. Answer B is a true statement. PAH is a disease of the blood vessels of the lungs meaning the vessels themselves become abnormal and narrowed, similar to atherosclerotic heart disease. The pulmonary arterioles and small vessels of the lungs eventually become so diseased that "pruning" of the pulmonary trunk occurs, making oxygen uptake and transport less efficient. This narrowing of the arterioles leads to an increase in pulmonary artery pressure, thus increasing the work of the right ventricle. If left untreated, this eventually leads to right heart failure and death. Answer C is a true statement. The World Health Organization (WHO) classifies pulmonary hypertension (PH) into five groups based upon the etiology (**Table 15-1**). Group 1 is the PAH group, which includes many causes, including congenital heart disease (CHD). For example, in CHD where there is an uncorrected left-to-right shunt, the persistent exposure of the pulmonary vasculature to increased blood flow and pressure may result in vascular remodeling and dysfunction. This leads to increased pulmonary vascular resistance (PVR) and increased pressures in the right heart. Answer D is a true statement as the gold standard for the diagnosis of PAH is right heart catheterization in which PAH is defined as a mean pulmonary artery pressure (mPAP) at rest >25 mm Hg, a pulmonary capillary wedge pressure (PCWP) ≤15 mm Hg and a PVR ≥3 Wood Units. Answer E is correct as PAH is also referred to as precapillary pulmonary hypertension (PH). The terms precapillary and postcapillary PH are based on the location of the etiology of PH. For example, conditions causing vascular changes on the arterial side of the pulmonary circulation (such as PAH etiologies) are referred to as precapillary, while conditions causing vascular changes on the venous side of the pulmonary circulation (such as left heart causes) are referred to as postcapillary.

2. **Answer: D.** The RVSP is calculated using the following equation where V_{TR} is the peak TR velocity measured in m/s and RAP is the right atrial pressure estimated from the IVC size and collapsibility with a sniff:

$$RVSP = 4V_{TR^2} + RAP \qquad (1)$$

In this case, the maximum IVC diameter is measured at 2.58 cm and the minimum IVC diameter with a sniff is 2.35 cm; therefore, the IVC collapsibility index (IVCCI) is 9%:

$$IVCCI = \left[(2.58 - 2.35) \div 2.58\right] \times 100 = 9\% \qquad (2)$$

Table 15-1. Clinical Classification of Pulmonary Hypertension

1. PAH
   - Idiopathic PAH
   - Heritable PAH
   - Drug- and toxin-induced PAH
   - PAH associated with:
     - Connective tissue disease
     - HIV infection
     - Portal hypertension
     - Congenital heart disease
     - Schistosomiasis
   - PAH long-term responders to calcium channel blockers
   - PAH with overt features of venous/capillaries (PVOD/PCH) involvement
   - Persistent PH of the newborn syndrome
2. PH due to left heart disease
   - PH due to heart failure with preserved LVEF
   - PH due to heart failure with reduced LVEF
   - Valvular heart disease
   - Congenital/acquired cardiovascular conditions leading to postcapillary PH
3. PH due to lung disease and/or hypoxia
   - Obstructive lung disease
   - Restrictive lung disease
   - Other lung disease with mixed restrictive/obstructive pattern
   - Hypoxia without lung disease
   - Developmental lung disorders
4. PH due to pulmonary artery obstructions
   - Chronic thromboembolic PH
   - Other pulmonary artery obstructions
5. PH with unclear and/or multifactorial mechanisms
   - Hematologic disorders
   - Systemic and metabolic disorders
   - Others
   - Complex congenital heart disease

HIV, human immunodeficiency virus; LVEF, left ventricular ejection fraction; PAH, pulmonary arterial hypertension; PCH, pulmonary capillary hemangiomatous; PH, pulmonary hypertension; PVOD, pulmonary veno-occlusive disease.

Reproduced from Simonneau G, Montani D, Celermajer DS, et al. Haemodynamic definitions and updated clinical classification of pulmonary hypertension. *Eur Respir J.* 2019;53(1). pii:1801913.

Using **Table 15-2**, the estimated RAP is assumed to be 15 mm Hg. Therefore, the estimated RVSP is:

$$RVSP = 4(5.13)^2 + 15 = 105.26 + 15 = 120.26 \, mm \, Hg \quad (3)$$

Rounding to the nearest whole number, the answer is D (120 mm Hg).

3. **Answer: B.** The peak TR velocity is 4.0 m/s which yields a right ventricular-to-right atrial pressure gradient (ΔP_{RV-RA}) of 64 mm Hg using the simplified Bernoulli equation:

$$\Delta P_{RV-RA} = 4V_{TR^2} = 4(4)^2 = 64 \, mm \, Hg \quad (1)$$

Hence, the RVSP is 64 mm Hg + right atrial pressure. In the absence of RVOT obstruction or pulmonary stenosis, there is pulmonary hypertension (PH) present; therefore, answer D is incorrect. As discussed in the answer outline for Question 1, the definition of PAH includes a pulmonary capillary wedge pressure (PCWP) ≤15 mm Hg. In this case, there is evidence of an increased PCWP based on a mitral E/e' of 20 (an E/e' >14 is consistent with an elevated left atrial [LA] pressure, which is equivalent to the PCWP; the ePLAR [see the following Teaching Point] is 0.2 m/s in this patient). Therefore, answer A is not correct. Answer B is correct since PH with an increased PCWP is characteristic of postcapillary PH. Left heart disease, such as heart failure with preserved ejection fraction (HFpEF), left ventricular systolic or diastolic dysfunction, ischemic cardiomyopathy, and aortic and mitral valve disease, can cause postcapillary PH due to backward transmission of elevated left-sided filling pressures into the pulmonary circulation; that is, the cause of PH relates to an elevation in pulmonary venous pressures. In contrast, diseases characterized by precapillary PH have elevated pulmonary artery pressure (PAP) in the setting of normal pulmonary venous pressures (**Table 15-1**).

TEACHING POINT

Precapillary PH may be differentiated from postcapillary PH based on the calculation of the echocardiographic pulmonary to left atrial ratio (ePLAR). This ratio is derived as:

$$ePLAR = V_{TR} \div E/e'$$

where V_{TR} is the peak TR velocity (m/s) and E/e' is the mitral E to septal e' ratio.

A normal ePLAR is approximately 0.30 m/s. Patients with postcapillary PH tend to have values of 0.25 m/s or lower and those with precapillary PH have values over 0.40 m/s.

4. **Answer: B.** There are multiple indirect echocardiographic signs of PH seen in this patient: **Figure 15-2A** and **Video 15-1** display a D-shaped left ventricle due to septal flattening caused by the increased pressures of the right ventricle (RV) that moves the interventricular septum to the left in systole, and **Figure 15-2B** displays a dilated inferior vena cava that does not collapse with sniff due to high right atrial pressure. **Figure 15-2C** is an image of the jugular veins, which have become distended due to backup of pressure from the superior vena cava. The patient history states that he has a history of cirrhosis, which is the most common cause of portal hypertension. As listed in **Table 15-1**, portal hypertension is a known cause of pulmonary arterial hypertension; therefore, answer B is correct. Other findings that are indicative of PH that should be looked for in this study include a tricuspid regurgitant continuous-wave Doppler jet greater than 3 m/s and bulging of the interatrial septal to the left due to an elevated right atrial pressure.

ARVD (answer A) is a genetic disorder characterized by fibrofatty infiltration of the RV myocardium, ventricular arrhythmias, sudden death, RV dilatation, and dysfunction leading to RV failure. PH is not commonly associated with ARVD. In addition to evidence of RV dilatation, other echocardiographic

Table 15-2. IVC Size and Collapsibility for the Estimation of RAP

Range	IVC Diameter (cm)	IVC Collapsibility with Sniff (%)	Estimated RAP (mm Hg)
Normal	≤2.1	>50	3
High	>2.1	<50	15
Intermediate[a]	≤2.1	<50	8
	>2.1	>50	8

[a]When there are no secondary signs of increased RAP, the RAP can be downgraded to 3 mm Hg; when the IVC collapses <35% and there are secondary signs of increased RAP, then the RAP can be upgraded to 15 mm Hg. Secondary signs of an elevated RAP include a restrictive tricuspid inflow filling profile, a tricuspid E/e' ratio >6, or a hepatic venous systolic filling fraction >55%.

findings of ARVD include regional RV akinesis, dyskinesis, aneurysm, and dilatation of the right ventricular outflow tract; none of these are evident based on the limited figures provided. Importantly, to assess for ARVD, one would need to evaluate the RV in multiple views. Cardiac amyloidosis (answer C) is a restrictive cardiomyopathy caused by abnormal protein deposits that lead to increased ventricular stiffness. PH with right-sided cardiac failure is a complication of amyloidosis. Characteristic echocardiographic findings of cardiac amyloidosis include increased thickness of the ventricular walls, normal-sized ventricles, normal ventricular function, biatrial dilatation, and a small pericardial effusion. Ischemic cardiomyopathy (answer D) may result in PH (PH due to heart failure with a reduced ejection fraction; see **Table 15-1**). Echocardiographic findings of ischemic cardiomyopathy include wall motion abnormalities; there are no obvious regional wall motion abnormalities present in this case.

5. **Answer: C.** The mPAP is calculated from the peak early diastolic pulmonary regurgitant (PR) velocity, not the end-diastolic velocity. The end-diastolic PR velocity is used to estimate the pulmonary artery end-diastolic pressure (PAEDP). The mPAP can be estimated from the RVAT, which is the time interval between the onset of flow to the peak systolic flow, measured from the pulsed-wave Doppler traced acquired at the RVOT. Both equations in answers A and B have been described for estimating the mPAP. When the RVAT is ≤120 ms, the equation in answer B performs better. The mPAP can be estimated from the mean pressure gradient of the tricuspid regurgitant (TR) signal. The mean TR pressure gradient, which reflects the systolic right ventricular-to-right atrial mean gradient, is derived by tracing the velocity-time integral of the TR signal. This calculation is analogous to the estimation of the pulmonary artery systolic pressure (PASP), or right ventricular systolic pressure, using the peak TR pressure gradient + RAP. Thus, if the peak TR pressure gradient + RAP estimates the PASP, then the mean TR gradient + RAP can estimate the mPAP.

6. **Answer: D.** Prolongation of the QRS duration, rather than shortening, suggests severe disease and is associated with poor outcomes. In advanced PAH, the compensatory right ventricular hypertrophy and damage of the myocardium of the right side of the heart leads to prolongation of the QRS duration.

   The presence of a pericardial effusion (answer A) is a predictor of mortality in patients with PAH. Patients with PAH and an associated pericardial effusion tend to have more severe PAH. The proposed mechanism for pericardial effusion in these patients is an increased right atrial pressure, which impairs venous and lymphatic drainage. RA enlargement (answer B) reflects the severity of right heart failure and predicts adverse outcomes in patients with severe PAH. There are no concrete data as to why increased age and male gender (answer C) have a poor prognosis, but it may be attributed to cardiopulmonary hemodynamic differences.

7. **Answer: D.** SCD is an inherited hemoglobinopathy. Adults with SCD most commonly develop pulmonary arterial hypertension (WHO group 1 classification) or pulmonary venous hypertension caused by heart failure with preserved ejection fraction (WHO group 2 classification). As the symptom recognition relating to the development of PH is often delayed, it is recommended that a baseline transthoracic echocardiogram be performed in asymptomatic children (ages 8-18 years) and in asymptomatic adults every 1 to 3 years. A peak tricuspid regurgitant velocity of ≥2.5 m/s is linked to an increased risk for mortality, suggesting a need for further evaluation. There are no requirements for annual echocardiographic screening for OSA syndrome, COPD, or APE.

8. **Answer: C.** When there is "wide-open" or "free" TR, measurement of the peak TR velocity is not accurate for the estimation of the RVSP. In this instance, the regurgitant orifice is not "restrictive" and there is equalization of the right ventricular (RV) and right atrial (RA) pressures. Therefore, the calculation of the RV-to-RA pressure gradient via the simplified Bernoulli equation is not valid. Incomplete CW Doppler (answer A) waveforms will underestimate the RVSP because the peak is not seen. "Fringing" (answer B) is due to transit-time artifact and/or overgaining of the CW signal; therefore, measurement of the TR velocity from these signals will overestimate the RVSP. Decreasing the Doppler gain, decreasing the dynamic range, and/or increasing the reject may eliminate this artifact and improve measurement accuracy. In patients with atrial fibrillation (answer D), any Doppler gradients must be averaged by measuring at least 3 to 5 consecutive cardiac cycles. Measuring only the highest velocity will overestimate the RVSP.

9. **Answer: A.** Eisenmenger syndrome often occurs in patients with large, nonrestrictive intracardiac or extracardiac communications, such as ventricular septal defects (VSDs), atrial septal defects (ASDs), atrioventricular septal defects, and patent ductus arteriosus (PDA). Eisenmenger syndrome is often seen and associated with a large VSD. The left-to-right shunt allows for high pulmonary blood flow, which, over time, leads to irreversible pulmonary vascular injury, increased pulmonary artery pressures and, ultimately, a reversal of the shunt to right-to-left. As a result, peripheral cyanosis develops, initially only on exertion, and later even at rest.

10. **Answer: C.** Answers A and B are not correct since the characteristic respiratory variations of the transmitral and transtricuspid E velocities

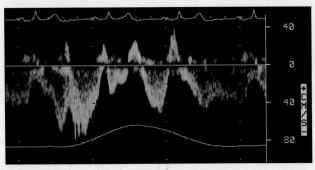

Figure 15-6A SVC Doppler profile typical of COPD showing a marked augmentation of the SVC forward flow velocities with inspiration.

associated with CP are also seen in patients with COPD. In COPD patients, the exaggerated respiratory variation of these velocities occurs due to exaggerated respiratory changes in the intrathoracic pressures. In this situation, the evaluation of the SVC flow profile can be useful to differentiate between COPD and CP patients. In patients with COPD the intrapleural pressure becomes more negative during inspiration. As a result, the right atrial pressure decreases more than usual, leading to augmentation of superior vena cava forward flow velocities ≥20 cm/s (**Figure 15-6A**). In patients with CP, the respiratory change in SVC velocities is minimal (**Figure 15-6B**).

11. ▶ **Answer: D.** The McConnell sign describes a characteristic pattern of generalized severe hypokinesis with relative sparing of the RV apex (**Video 15-4**). While this sign was initially thought to be specific for acute pulmonary embolism, it may also be seen in other etiologies of acute cor pulmonale such as sepsis, acute respiratory distress syndrome, and pulmonary hemorrhage, and may also be seen in patients with RV myocardial infarction. A suggested mechanism of the McConnell sign is localized ischemia of the RV free wall because of increased wall stress. However, strain studies now suggest that the RV apex is actually dysfunctional in the McConnell sign and only appears normal due to a tethering effect from the hyperdynamic LV apex. Nonetheless, this finding on echocardiography should raise the level of clinical suspicion for the diagnosis of acute pulmonary embolism.

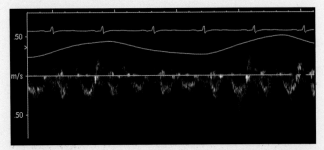

Figure 15-6B SVC Doppler profile typical of CP showing minimal variation in systolic forward flow velocities over the respiratory cycle.

12. **Answer: B.** There are several echocardiographic variables that may aid in the distinction between PAH versus PH-HFpEF (**Table 15-3**). A delayed or impaired relaxation pattern on the transmitral inflow trace is a common finding in patients with PAH. This occurs due to dilatation of the RV, a reduction in LV filling due to a decrease in RV output, and an abnormal shift of the IVS toward the LV.

Bowing of the IAS from left to right (answer A) favors PH-HFpEF over PAH, while a bowing of the IAS from right to left favors PAH over PH-HFpEF. A mitral E/e' ratio with exercise >15 (answer C) favors PH-HFpEF over PAH, while a mitral E/e' ratio with exercise <10 favors PAH over PH-HFpEF. The echo-derived PVR (answer D) is not helpful in distinguishing between PAH and PH-HFpEF.

13. **Answer: D.** As discussed earlier, ARVD or arrhythmogenic right ventricular cardiomyopathy (ARVC) is a genetic disorder characterized by fibrofatty infiltration of the right ventricular (RV) myocardium, ventricular arrhythmias, sudden death, RV dilatation, and dysfunction leading to RV failure. Echocardiographic features of this disease include RV morphologic abnormalities such as a hyperreflective moderator band, RV sacculations (or diastolic outpouchings), aneurysm (systolic outpouchings), and trabecular derangements (**Figure 15-7**). Other subtle abnormalities include a dilated RVOT (>32 mm at end-diastole) and reduced RV global longitudinal and regional strains. On the ECG, inverted T waves in the anterior leads, incomplete or complete right bundle branch block, and frequent epsilon waves in leads V_1 to V_3 are found. Early in the disease, RV size and function may present as normal. The left ventricle is usually not affected and will display normal function. In this case, an incidental finding of a PFO with a right-to-left shunt was found in an agitated saline study. Answer B, pulmonary venous occlusive disease (PVOD), also known as pulmonary venous sclerosis, obstructive disease of the pulmonary veins, or the venous form of primary pulmonary hypertension, is incorrect. PVOD is characterized by occlusion or narrowing of the pulmonary veins and venules by collagen-rich fibrous tissue. Pulmonary arterial hypertension (PAH) as a result of PVOD may not be distinguishable from other forms of PAH by echocardiography alone. A ventilation-perfusion (V/Q) scan can determine the probability of PVOD, and computed tomography can confirm its existence. Answer C is incorrect; the athlete's heart commonly shows increased wall mass, eccentric or concentric left ventricular hypertrophy, and an increase in ventricular dimensions. A PFO (answer A) is demonstrated in **Video 15-2E**. However, this was an incidental finding and by itself is not descriptive of ARVD.

Table 15-3. Echocardiographic Factors Favoring PAH Versus PH-HFpEF

Echo Variable	PAH	PH-HFpEF
Left atrial size	Normal	Enlarged
LV mass	Normal	Increased
RA/LA size ratio	RA >> LA	LA > RA
Intra-atrial septum	Bows to left	Bows to right
Mitral inflow pattern	Delayed relaxation pattern	Restrictive
Medial e'	Maybe low	Low
Lateral e'	Normal	Low
ePLAR (TRVmax/E/e')	>0.30	<0.30
E/e' with exercise	<10	>15
Echo-PVR	Not helpful in distinguishing mechanism	

From Kane GC, Chang S-A. Right heart assessment and pulmonary hypertension. In: Oh JK, Kane GC, eds. *The Echo Manual*. 4th ed. Wolters Kluwer and Mayo Foundation for Medical Education and Research; 2019:chap 9.

14. Answer. B. The left ventricular eccentricity index (LVEI) quantifies the abnormal interventricular septal (IVS) curvature in right ventricular (RV) pressure and volume overload states. This index is measured from a parasternal short-axis view at the level of the papillary muscles at either end-diastole or end-systole. The left ventricular (LV) cavity is measured parallel to the IVS (D2) and perpendicular to the IVS (D1). The LVEI is then calculated as:

$$LVEI = D2 \div D1$$

In an RV volume overload state, the end-diastolic LVEI will be increased due to diastolic septal flattening caused by RV volume overload while the end-systolic index remains normal. In a systolic pressure overload state, the end-systolic index will be increased due to systolic septal flattening caused by RV pressure overload while the end-diastolic index remains normal. In some cases of PAH, both RV volume and systolic pressure overloads exist, and the LVEI measured at both end-diastole and end-systole will be abnormal. An eccentricity index >1.2 is abnormal. For serial assessment, the 2D images and the electrocardiogram tracing should be clearly optimized to ensure that the same location in space and time (in the cardiac cycle) is used for accurate measurements.

The LV sphericity index (answer A) is a measurement related to ischemic mitral regurgitation. This index is derived from the biplane LV volume end-systolic volumes (measured from the apical 4-chamber and apical 2-chamber views) and from the LV end-systolic dimension (measured in the apical 4-chamber view). The LV D-shaped index (answer C) is a fictitious measurement. The LV Tei index (answer D) or myocardial performance index is a measure of global LV function. This index is derived from spectral Doppler time measurements as the ratio of the LV isovolumic relaxation and contraction times and the LV ejection time.

15. ▶ **Answer: B. Figure 15-3** shows the calculation of the LVEI at end-diastole based on the position of the red vertical marker on the electrocardiogram. As previously described, the LVEI is calculated as:

$$LVEI = D2 \div D1 \tag{1}$$

In **Figure 15-3**, D2 is 6 cm and D1 is 3 cm; therefore, the LVEI is:

$$LVEI = 6 \div 3 = 2 \tag{2}$$

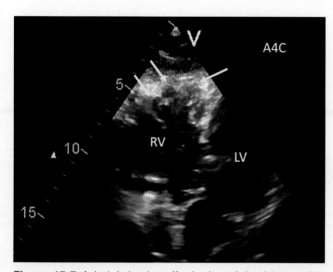

Figure 15-7 Apical 4-chamber off-axis view of the right ventricle focused to display the multiple small aneurysmal apical outpouchings (arrows) that may be seen in arrhythmogenic right ventricular cardiomyopathy.

This patient also has significant flattening of the interventricular septum during systole (**Video 15-5**) consistent with both right ventricular (RV) diastolic volume overload and RV systolic pressure overload and clinically had severe long-standing pulmonary arterial hypertension with a right ventricular systolic pressure over 75 mm Hg while on multiple specialty therapies.

16. **Answer: C.** In patients with pulmonary hypertension, the foramen ovale may be stretched open and when the right atrial (RA) pressure exceeds the left atrial (LA) pressure, then right-to-left shunting across the interatrial septum (IAS) is seen. However, left ventricular diastolic dysfunction with increased LA pressure can result in a false-negative study. In this setting, if the LA pressure remains higher than the RA pressure, then no right-to-left shunting will be seen across a PFO.

Answer A is correct. A large Eustachian valve directing venous return from the inferior vena cava to the interatrial septum may prevent the bubbles entering from the superior vena cava to cross over the IAS. Other potential causes for false-negative studies include an inadequate Valsalva maneuver, poor agitation of bubbles, inadequate opacification of the RA, or an inability to raise RA pressure as in LV diastolic dysfunction with increased LA pressure. Answer B is correct. Bubbles in the left atrium within 3 beats of contrast appearance in the right heart indicate an intracardiac shunt, while bubbles that appear in the left atrium after 3 to 5 beats are more consistent with an intrapulmonary or pulmonary arteriovenous shunt. Answer D is correct. Physiological maneuvers such as a Valsalva maneuver and cough should always be performed if the initial attempts for a positive study are not realized. The Valsalva strain must be held long enough for bubbles to fill the right atrium. The patient should be instructed to breathe in and hold the breath during the strain. The presence of a leftward shift of the IAS indicates the Valsalva maneuver was adequate and confirms that the RA pressure has exceeded the LA pressure.

17. **Answer: A.** An increased "a wave" on the pulmonary valve M-mode trace may be seen when there is severe pulmonary stenosis. When there is PH, the "a wave" on the pulmonary valve M-mode trace is usually absent due to a marked elevation in the pulmonary artery end-diastolic pressure. Answer B is incorrect since mid-systolic notching on the aortic valve M-mode trace may be seen in patients with PH. The mechanism of mid-systolic notching on the aortic valve in these cases is due to a low cardiac output with normal left ventricular (LV) size, a hyperdynamic interventricular septum, and distortion of LV geometry. Answer C is incorrect as an RVAT <100 ms is consistent with PH. The mechanism of a short RVAT is an increase in the pulmonary vascular resistance, which causes rapid acceleration of flow into the pulmonary artery in systole. Answer D is incorrect as an RV wall thickness of >5 mm is abnormal and would be consistent with RV hypertrophy secondary to PH.

18. **Answer: D.** Evaluation of RV size and systolic function is often difficult to determine when not clearly mild or severe in patients with PH. For example, some parameters may be discordant with the visual assessment. Therefore, several parameters for RV size and systolic function need to be evaluated carefully. In this patient, an RV chamber that is visually more than two-third the size of the left ventricle is consistent with moderate RV enlargement (**Figure 15-4A**, right). The internal RV diastolic dimension at the base of 4.5 cm (American Society of Echocardiography [ASE] normal range = 2.5-4.1 cm) and the internal RV length measured from the apex to the base of 8.8 cm (ASE normal range = 5.9-8.3 cm) indicate at least mild-to-moderate RV enlargement. Measurements of RV systolic function along with the normal and abnormal ASE-recommended values are summarized in **Table 15-4**. The tricuspid annular plane systolic excursion (TAPSE) and s' velocity measurements are discordant with the fractional area change (FAC), strain, and RV myocardial performance index (MPI). Based on the **Video 15-3**, the visual assessment of RV systolic function suggests moderate RV systolic dysfunction. Recall that the TAPSE and s' velocity are measurements of regional RV systolic function and may be normal when there is hyperdynamic left ventricular systolic function.

Table 15-4. Summary of RV Systolic Measurements and Normal/Abnormal Values

Parameter	Measurement in This Study	Normal Values	Abnormal Values[a]
TAPSE (mm)	18	24 ± 3.5	<17
FAC (%)	30	49 ± 7	<35
s' (cm/s)	11.5	14.1 ± 2.3	<9.5
RV MPI	.83	0.38 ± 0.08	>0.54
RV free wall strain (%)	−18.1	−29 ± 4.5	Less negative than −20

[a]Measurements exceeding ± 1.96 standard deviations (that is, the 95% confidence interval) are classified as abnormal.

19. **Answer: B.** There is an underproduction of nitric oxide in PAH, leading to a decrease in cellular function. Answer A, C, D, and E are all mechanisms in PAH that contribute to the obstructive remodeling of the pulmonary vascular bed, which is responsible for the increases in pulmonary vascular resistance and arterial pressure that eventually progress to right heart failure. Remodeling of the pulmonary vasculature in PAH is caused by an overgrowth of vascular cells (endothelial, smooth muscle cells, fibroblasts, mast cells) and by increased inflammation, which occludes the smaller precapillary vessels in the pulmonary vasculature by reducing the vessel lumen size. The pulmonary bed basically becomes "pruned" like a tree leaving mainly the larger trunk vessels. Reduced production of vasodilators and an overproduction of vasoconstrictors increase endothelial and smooth muscle cell proliferation (growth), and thus fibrosis and inflammation. The resultant product of this continuous cycle is remodeling of the pulmonary vascular bed and increasing vascular resistance.

20. **Answer: C.** PVR is calculated as:

$$PVR = (mPAP - PCWP) \div CO \qquad (1)$$

where mPAP is the mean pulmonary arterial pressure in mm Hg, PCWP is the pulmonary capillary wedge pressure in mm Hg, and CO is the cardiac output in liters per minute.

Several methods have been described for the echocardiographic estimation of PVR. Of these methods, the one that is most commonly employed is one that is based on substituting the peak tricuspid regurgitant velocity (V_{TR}) for the transpulmonary gradient (mPAP − PCWP) and using the right ventricular outflow tract velocity-integral (VTI_{RVOT}) as a surrogate for the right ventricular cardiac output:

$$PVR = (V_{TR} \div VTI_{RVOT}) \times 10 + 0.16 \qquad (2)$$

In this patient, the peak TR velocity is 3.97 m/s and the TVI_{RVOT} is 15.91 cm; therefore,

$$PVR = (3.97 \div 15.91) \times 10 + 0.16 = 2.7 \text{ WU} \qquad (3)$$

A simplified method for identifying if the PVR is normal or markedly elevated is based on the ratio of the V_{TR} and the VTI_{RVOT}. When this ratio is <0.175, then the PVR is likely normal. When this ratio is >0.275, then the PVR is likely markedly elevated (>6 WU).

21. **Answer: A.** Systemic sclerosis, also known as scleroderma, is a rare connective tissue disorder. Scleroderma contains a variable degree of systemic manifestations, including fibrosis (affecting multiple organs), telangiectasias, and abnormalities of the digestive system. The organs most frequently affected by scleroderma are the skin, gastrointestinal tract, lungs, kidneys, skeletal muscle, and pericardium. Patients with scleroderma frequently develop PAH and have worse outcomes than patients with other types of IPAH. Traditional hemodynamic measures of disease severity, such as cardiac index and right atrial pressure (RAP), both strongly predict survival in IPAH, but are weaker predictors of outcome in SSc-PAH. Echocardiographic measures are similar in both forms of PAH. Paul Hasson et al. and others examined demographic characteristics and hemodynamic, echocardiographic, and survival differences between patients with IPAH and with SSc-PAH. By echocardiography, both groups had a similar prevalence of right-sided chamber enlargement. However, left ventricular (LV) diastolic dysfunction was more common in patients with SSc-PAH despite normal LV systolic function, and left atrial dilation and size were also significantly more prevalent in the SSc-PAH group. Pericardial effusion was found to be nearly three times more prominent among patients with SSc-PAH than among patients with IPAH (34.7% vs. 13.2%; $P < .005$). The presence of pericardial effusion predicted a poor survival in both groups. Therefore, answer A, RV volume overload pattern, is least likely to differentiate outcomes in patients with SSc-PAH from those with IPAH.

22. **Answer: D.** True statements include answers A, B, C, and E, which are all indices that predict elevated RAP of at least 8 mm Hg and are associated with worse outcomes for patients with a diagnosis of PAH. A hepatic venous systolic filling fraction of less than 55% is predictive of a RAP greater than 8 mm Hg. An inferior vena cava collapsibility index of <50% usually indicates at least an intermediate level (8 mm Hg) of elevated RAP. A restrictive tricuspid inflow pattern is indicative of right ventricular (RV) diastolic dysfunction with increased filling pressures (RAP) and a tricuspid inflow E/e′ >6 has a high sensitivity and specificity for predicting a mean RAP >10 mm Hg. Answer D is a false statement, as a shortened RV acceleration time is commonly seen in acute pulmonary embolism and can be used to estimate mean pulmonary artery pressure.

SUGGESTED READINGS

Abbas AE, Franey LM, Marwick T, et al. Noninvasive assessment of pulmonary vascular resistance by Doppler echocardiography. *J Am Soc Echocardiogr*. 2013;26(10):1170-1177.

Baggen VJM, Driessen MMP, Post MC, et al. Echocardiographic Findings associated with mortality or transplant in patients with pulmonary hypertension: a systematic review and meta-analysis. *Neth Heart J*. 2016;24(6):374-389.

D'Alto M, Mahadevan VS. Pulmonary arterial hypertension associated with congenital heart disease. *Eur Respir Rev*. 2012;21(126):328-337.

Galiè N, Humbert M, Vachiery JL, et al. 2015 ESC/ERS Guidelines for the diagnosis and treatment of pulmonary hypertension: the Joint Task Force for the Diagnosis and Treatment of Pulmonary Hypertension of the European Society of Cardiology (ESC) and the European Respiratory Society (ERS): endorsed by: Association for European Paediatric and Congenital Cardiology (AEPC), International Society for Heart and Lung Transplantation (ISHLT). *Eur Heart J.* 2016;37(1):67-119.

Hassoun PM. The right ventricle in scleroderma (2013 Grover Conference Series). *Pulm Circ.* 2015;5(1):3-14.

Hopkins W, Rubin LJ. Treatment and prognosis of pulmonary arterial hypertension in adults (group 1). UpToDate Inc. https://www.uptodate.com. Accessed August 23, 2019.

Humbert M, Guignabert C, Bonnet S, et al. Pathology and pathobiology of pulmonary hypertension: state of the art and research perspectives. *Eur Respir J.* 2019;53(1). pii:1801887.

Kane GC, Chang S-A. Right heart assessment and pulmonary hypertension. In: Oh JK, Kane GC, eds. *The Echo Manual.* 4th ed. Philadelphia, PA & Rochester, MN: Wolters Kluwer; 2019:chap 9.

Lang RM, Badano LP, Mor-Avi V, et al. Recommendations for cardiac chamber quantification by echocardiography in adults: an update from the American Society Echocardiography and the European Association of Cardiovascular imaging. *J Am Soc Echocardiogr.* 2015;28(1):1-39.

McConnell MV, Solomon SD, Rayan ME, Come PC, Goldhaberc SZ, Lee RT. Regional right ventricular dysfunction detected by echocardiography in acute pulmonary embolism. *Am J Cardiol.* 1996;78(4):469-473.

Rudski LG, Lai WW, Afilalo J, et al. Guidelines for the echocardiographic assessment of the right heart in adults: a report from the American Society of Echocardiography endorsed by the European Association of Echocardiography, a registered branch of the European Society of Cardiology, and the Canadian Society of Echocardiography. *J Am Soc Echocardiogr.* 2010;23(7):685-713.

Scalia GM, Scalia IG, Kierle R, et al. ePLAR – the echocardiographic pulmonary to left atrial ratio – A novel non-invasive parameter to differentiate pre-capillary and post capillary pulmonary hypertension. *Int J Cardiol.* 2016;212:379-386.

Simonneau G, Montani D, Celermajer DS, et al. Haemodynamic definitions and updated clinical classification of pulmonary hypertension. *Eur Respir J.* 2019;53(1). pii:1801913.

Vaid U, Singer E, Marhefka GD, Kraft WK, Baram M. Positive predictive value of McConnel's sign on transthoracic echocardiography for the diagnosis of acute pulmonary embolism. *Am J Cardiol.* 1996;78(4):469-473.

Vonk MC, Sander MH, van den Hoogen FH, van Riel PL, Verheugt FW, van Dijk AP. Right ventricle Tei-index: a tool to increase the accuracy of non-invasive detection of pulmonary arterial hypertension in connective tissue diseases. *Eur J Echocardiogr.* 2007;8(5):317-321.

CHAPTER 16

Ischemic Heart Disease and Complications of Myocardial Infarctions

Contributors: Ashlee Davis, BS, ACS, RDCS and Laura T. Boone, BS, RDCS, RVT, RDMS, RT(R)

✪ Question 1

Which coronary artery lies in the left atrioventricular sulcus between the left atrium (LA) and left ventricle (LV)?

- A. Left circumflex coronary artery
- B. Left anterior descending coronary artery
- C. Posterior descending coronary artery
- D. Right coronary artery

✪ Question 2

In the majority of patients, the posterior descending artery (PDA) branches off the:

- A. Left anterior descending coronary artery.
- B. Left circumflex coronary artery.
- C. Left coronary artery.
- D. Right coronary artery.

✪ Question 3

Which of the following best describes myocardial ischemia?

- A. The deoxygenated myocardial blood supply does not meet the demand of the myocardium, resulting in a decrease in myocardial contractility and relaxation.
- B. The oxygenated myocardial blood supply does not meet the demand of the myocardium, resulting in a decrease in myocardial contractility and relaxation.
- C. There is a balance between the oxygenated myocardial supply and the demand, resulting in abnormal myocardial contractility and relaxation.
- D. There is an imbalance between the oxygenated myocardial supply and the demand, resulting in an increase in myocardial contractility and relaxation.

✪✪ Question 4

Which of the following represents the correct sequence of events in the ischemic cascade?

- A. Angina, regional wall motion abnormalities, ischemic electrocardiogram (ECG) changes, perfusion abnormality, diastolic dysfunction
- B. Ischemic ECG changes, perfusion abnormality, regional wall motion abnormalities, diastolic dysfunction, angina
- C. Perfusion abnormality, diastolic dysfunction, regional wall motion abnormalities, ischemic ECG changes, angina
- D. Angina, perfusion abnormality, regional wall motion abnormalities, diastolic dysfunction, ischemic ECG changes
- E. Regional wall motion abnormalities, perfusion abnormality, diastolic dysfunction, ischemic ECG changes, angina

✪ Question 5

Which of the following is most likely an atherosclerotic cause of coronary artery disease?

- A. Coronary plaque rupture
- B. Coronary artery spasm
- C. Aortic regurgitation
- D. Anomalous coronary artery

✪ Question 6

All of the following are within the spectrum of acute coronary syndromes (ACS) except:

- A. Non–ST-elevation myocardial infarction.
- B. Stable angina.
- C. ST-elevation myocardial infarction.
- D. Unstable angina.

✪ Question 7

Which of the following scenarios would most likely identify a patient with an acute myocardial infarction (AMI)?

A. Global ST-elevation with positional chest pain and slightly elevated troponin

B. Normal ST segment with epigastric pain and low troponin

C. ST-depression in lead II, III, and aVF with chest pain and low troponin

D. ST-elevation in leads V_1 and V_2 with chest pain and elevated troponin

✪ Question 8

Which coronary artery is indicated by the arrow in **Figure 16-1**?

A. Left anterior descending coronary artery

B. Left circumflex coronary artery

C. Posterior descending coronary artery

D. Right coronary artery

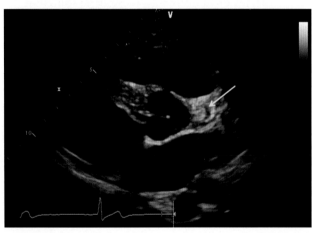

Figure 16-1

✪ Question 9

What level of the left ventricle (LV) is identified from the tips of the papillary muscles to the base of the papillary muscles?

A. Apical level

B. Basal level

C. Mid-level

D. Posterior level

✪ Question 10

The left ventricular wall segment depicted by the arrow in **Video 16-1** is the:

A. Anteroapical segment.

B. Apicolateral segment.

C. Apicoseptal segment.

D. Inferoapical segment.

✪ Question 11

The left ventricular (LV) wall segment depicted by the arrow in **Video 16-2** is the:

A. Basal anterolateral segment.

B. Basal anteroseptal segment.

C. Basal inferolateral segment.

D. Basal inferoseptal segment.

✪✪✪ Question 12

A 75-year-old male patient has a transthoracic echocardiogram (TTE) 12 months post an NSTEMI. Based on the images provided (**Video 16-3**), which coronary artery is most likely occluded?

A. Left anterior descending coronary artery

B. Left circumflex coronary artery

C. Left main coronary artery

D. Right coronary artery

✪ Question 13

A 65-year-old male patient has a transthoracic echocardiogram following an ST-segment myocardial infarction with unsuccessful lysis. Based on the images provided (**Video 16-4**), which coronary artery is most likely occluded?

A. Left anterior descending coronary artery

B. Left circumflex coronary artery

C. Posterior descending coronary artery

D. Right coronary artery

✪ Question 14

What term is used to describe the left ventricular wall motion depicted by the arrows in **Video 16-5**?

A. Akinetic

B. Aneurysmal

C. Dyskinetic

D. Hypokinetic

✪✪✪ Question 15

A patient presents for a stress echocardiogram. What is the wall motion score index (WMSI) if the mid and apical inferoseptal walls become hypokinetic immediately post exercise?

A. 0.88

B. 1.13

C. 17

D. 19

✪ Question 16

Which of the following methods for measuring left ventricular (LV) systolic function is often limited by foreshortening of the LV?

    A. 2D Doppler method for stroke volume

    B. 2D linear method

    C. 2D method of disks

    D. M-mode linear method

✪✪ Question 17

Which of the following pathologies may directly cause a reduction in coronary artery perfusion due to decreased diastolic pressure in the aorta?

    A. Aortic stenosis

    B. Aortic regurgitation

    C. Aortic dissection

    D. Aortic coarctation

    E. All the above

✪✪ Question 18

A 74-year-old woman presents to the emergency room with chest pain and weakness following a loved one's funeral. The electrocardiogram (ECG) showed evidence of T wave inversions of the anterior precordial leads and her cardiac catheterization study showed patent coronary arteries. What is the most likely diagnosis for this patient?

    A. Acute coronary syndrome

    B. Acute pericarditis

    C. Left apical infarct

    D. Takotsubo cardiomyopathy

✪✪✪ Question 19

▶ A 53-year-old truck driver presents to the emergency room with pleuritic chest pain and shortness of breath. A transthoracic echocardiogram is ordered. What is the most likely diagnosis based on the images provided (**Video 16-6**)?

    A. Acute pericarditis

    B. Acute pulmonary embolism

    C. Chronic pulmonary hypertension

    D. Right ventricular (RV) infarct

✪✪✪ Question 20

▶ A 73-year-old male patient presents with sudden ripping chest pain that is radiating to the neck. The physician orders a transthoracic echocardiogram. What is the most likely diagnosis based on the images provided (**Video 16-7**)?

    A. Acute coronary syndrome

    B. Ascending aortic aneurysm

    C. Ascending aortic dissection

    D. Ventricular septal rupture

✪✪✪ Question 21

▶ A systolic murmur is heard in a 67-year-old man, 3 days following a myocardial infarction. The transthoracic echocardiogram (TTE) taken from a subcostal view (**Figures 16-2A** and **16-2B** and **Videos 16-8A** and **16-8B**) shows:

    A. Congenital (muscular) ventricular septal defect (VSD).

    B. Congenital (perimembranous) VSD.

    C. Ischemic mitral regurgitation.

    D. Papillary muscle rupture.

    E. Postinfarct ventricular septal rupture (VSR).

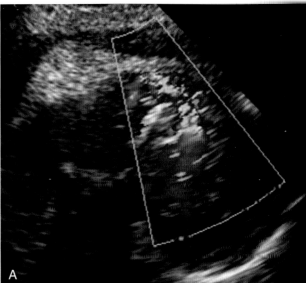

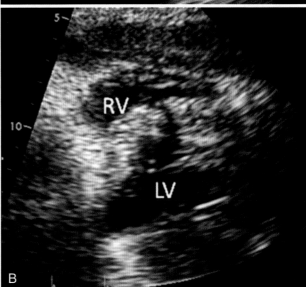

Figure 16-2A, B (Reprinted with permission from Klein AL, Asher CR. *Clinical Echocardiography Review: a Self-Assessment Tool.* 2nd ed. Philadelphia, PA: Wolters Kluwer; 2017.)

✪✪✪ Question 22

A patient, after inferior myocardial infarction, is thought on clinical grounds to have right ventricular (RV) infarction. Which parameter gives a reliable assessment of RV function?

A. 2D echocardiographic RV ejection fraction (EF)
B. RV free wall strain
C. Tricuspid annular plane displacement (TAPSE)
D. RV tissue Doppler imaging (TDI) s' velocity
E. None of the above is reliable

✪ Question 23

In which time frame is a mechanical complication such as papillary muscle rupture, ventricular septal rupture, or free wall rupture post–myocardial infarction (post--MI) most likely to occur?

A. 1 to 4 hours
B. 3 to 7 days
C. 1 to 3 months
D. 6 to 12 months

✪✪✪ Question 24

▶ A 67-year-old man with chest pain 5 days prior to presentation suddenly presents with shortness of breath and increasing fatigue. Upon arrival to the emergency room, the patient is found to have positive troponins, an elevated BUN (blood-urea-nitrogen) test, and a harsh holosystolic murmur. A transthoracic echocardiogram was ordered. Based on the images provided (**Video 16-9** and **Figure 16-3**), which coronary artery is the likely culprit?

A. Left main coronary artery
B. Left circumflex coronary artery
C. Left anterior descending coronary artery
D. Right coronary artery

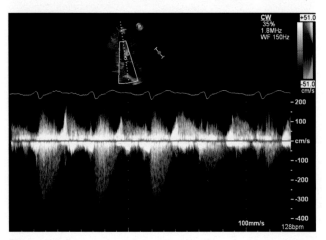

Figure 16-3

✪✪✪ Question 25

▶ A 56-year old woman with past medical history of hypertension, hyperlipidemia, and a 20-pack-per-year smoking history presents to the emergency room with shortness of breath and left shoulder and jaw pain. The electrocardiogram shows anterior ST-elevation. The patient is immediately taken to the cardiac catherization laboratory and the angiogram shows a severe blockage of the left anterior descending (LAD) coronary artery. From the post–cardiac catheterization echocardiographic images, acquired from the apical 4-chamber view (**Figure 16-4** and **Video 16-10**), what is the diagnosis?

A. Apical left ventricular (LV) aneurysm
B. Inferior pseudoaneurysm
C. Right ventricular (RV) infarction
D. Takotsubo cardiomyopathy

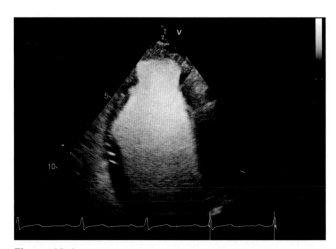

Figure 16-4

✪✪ Question 26

In the setting of a recent myocardial infarction (MI), a patient presents with elevated jugular venous pressure and hypotension. The electrocardiogram shows elevation of the ST segments in the right precordial leads. The patient undergoes cardiac catheterization, which shows blockage in the right coronary artery. What is the echocardiogram likely to show?

A. Global left ventricular (LV) dysfunction
B. Mitral regurgitation
C. Pulmonary hypertension
D. Right ventricular (RV) Infarction
E. All the above

⊙ Question 27

What is the name of the condition occurring several days to weeks after myocardial infarction (MI) that causes inflammation of the pericardium?

- **A.** Constrictive pericarditis
- **B.** Costochondritis
- **C.** Dressler syndrome
- **D.** Kawasaki disease

⊙⊙ Question 28

A 50-year-old man was admitted to the hospital following a myocardial infarction (MI) and underwent percutaneous coronary intervention (PCI). Twenty-four hours after his MI, the patient begins to complain of sharp chest pain that is exaggerated when he takes a deep breath. What is the likely source of this patient's symptoms?

- **A.** Aortic dissection
- **B.** Blockage of the coronary stent
- **C.** Pericarditis
- **D.** Recurrent MI
- **E.** Any of the above

⊙⊙⊙ Question 29

▶ The post–myocardial infarction complication that results from a cardiac rupture that is contained by adherent pericardium (**Figure 16-5** and **Video 16-11**) is known as:

- **A.** Diverticulum.
- **B.** Pseudoaneurysm.
- **C.** True aneurysm.
- **D.** Any of the above.

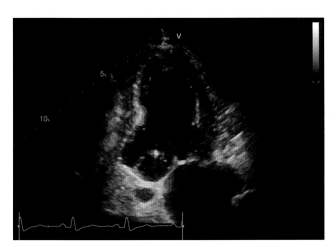

Figure 16-5

⊙ Question 30

Echocardiographically, which of the following differentiates a pseudoaneurysm from a true aneurysm of the left ventricle?

- **A.** Pseudoaneurysm has a narrow neck, while a true aneurysm does not have a discrete neck.
- **B.** Pseudoaneurysm has no blood flow while a true aneurysm has to-and-fro blood flow.
- **C.** True aneurysm has a narrow neck while a pseudoaneurysm does not have a discrete neck.
- **D.** True aneurysm has to-and-fro blood flow while a pseudoaneurysm has high-velocity turbulent blood flow.

⊙ Question 31

The three complications of an acute myocardial infarction with the highest mortality rates are:

- **A.** Acute mitral regurgitation, apical aneurysm, and free wall rupture.
- **B.** Apical aneurysm, free wall rupture, and papillary muscle rupture.
- **C.** Free wall rupture, ventricular septal rupture, and apical aneurysm.
- **D.** Free wall rupture, ventricular septal rupture, and papillary muscle rupture.

⊙ Question 32

Which papillary muscle is more susceptible to rupture following an acute myocardial infarction and why?

- **A.** Posteromedial (PM) papillary muscle due to a dual blood supply
- **B.** Anterolateral (AL) papillary muscle due to a singular blood supply
- **C.** PM papillary muscle due to a single blood supply
- **D.** AL papillary muscle due to a dual blood supply
- **E.** Each papillary muscle is equally susceptible to rupture

⊙⊙ Question 33

▶ A 67-year-old man presents for a 3-month follow-up echocardiogram after an acute myocardial infarction (AMI) post percutaneous coronary intervention (PCI) to the left anterior descending coronary artery. Based on the images provided (**Figure 16-6** and **Video 16-12**), what other pathology is seen in the image?

A. A pseudoaneurysm with thrombus
B. An apical akinesis and left ventricular (LV) thrombus
C. An apical rupture with right ventricular infarction
D. Papillary muscle dysfunction and an apical aneurysm

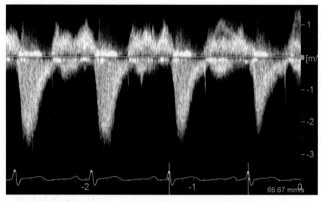

Figure 16-7

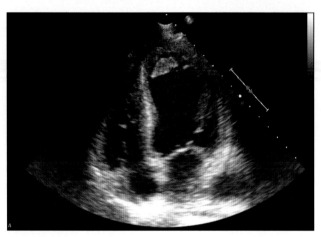

Figure 16-6

✪ Question 34

What is the complication that is seen in approximately 2% of post–myocardial infarction (post-MI) cases that can be catastrophic leading to hemopericardium and death from cardiac tamponade?

A. Post-pericardiotomy syndrome
B. Post–cardiac injury syndrome
C. Post–myocardial infarction syndrome
D. Post-myocardial free wall rupture

✪✪✪ Question 35

The continuous-wave (CW) Doppler waveform of mitral regurgitation (MR) shown in **Figure 16-7** was acquired from a patient following an acute myocardial infarction. Based on this profile, what can be ascertained?

A. The patient is hypertensive and in cardiogenic shock.
B. There is a marked elevation in left ventricular (LV) filling pressures due to diastolic dysfunction.
C. There is acute, severe MR because of papillary muscle rupture or dysfunction.
D. There is underfilling of the left ventricle with dynamic left ventricular outflow tract obstruction.
E. All of the above.

✪✪ Question 36

In a patient with a post–myocardial infarction ventricular septal rupture (VSR), the peak velocity across the VSR jet is 5 m/s, the blood pressure is 130/85 mm Hg, and the right atrial pressure is estimated at 15 mm Hg. Based on this information, the right ventricular systolic pressure (RVSP) is:

A. 30 mm Hg.
B. 45 mm Hg.
C. 100 mm Hg.
D. 110 mm Hg.

✪✪ Question 37

Which scenario of myocardial infarction (MI) is most likely to involve a post-MI ventricular septal rupture (VSR)?

A. Elderly female
B. Occlusion of the left anterior descending coronary artery
C. First MI with no collateral flow
D. Any of the above

✪✪✪ Question 38

Which of the following statements regarding post–myocardial infarction (post-MI) ventricular septal rupture (VSR) is most accurate?

A. Patients with an MI due to occlusion of a "wraparound" left anterior descending (LAD) coronary artery do not have an elevated risk of VSR.
B. The diagnosis of a VSR by transthoracic echocardiography (TTE) is established in less than 10% of cases.
C. The majority of VSRs rarely occur within 2 weeks post-MI.
D. VSR is seen with higher frequency in anterior MI compared with nonanterior MI.
E. With anterior MI, the defect is most commonly found in the apical septum, and with inferior MI, it most often occurs at the base.

ANSWERS

1. **Answer: A.** The left main coronary artery has two branches, the left anterior descending (LAD) coronary artery and the left circumflex (Cx) coronary artery. The Cx lies in the left posterior atrioventricular sulcus (or groove) and wraps around the left lateral side of the heart between the LA and LV. The LAD lies in the anterior interventricular sulcus that runs down the front of the heart between the two ventricles. The right coronary artery lies in the right atrioventricular sulcus and wraps around the right atrium and right ventricle posteriorly.

2. **Answer: D.** The posterior descending artery (PDA) branches off the right coronary artery (RCA) in the majority of people. In this instance, this is referred to as a right dominant circulation. A much smaller percentage of people have a left dominant circulation in which the PDA branches from the left circumflex coronary artery. Rarely, patients receive a posterior blood supply from branches of the RCA and the left circumflex coronary artery; this is called a co-dominant circulation. **Figure 16-8** illustrates right and left coronary arteries in a right dominant circulation.

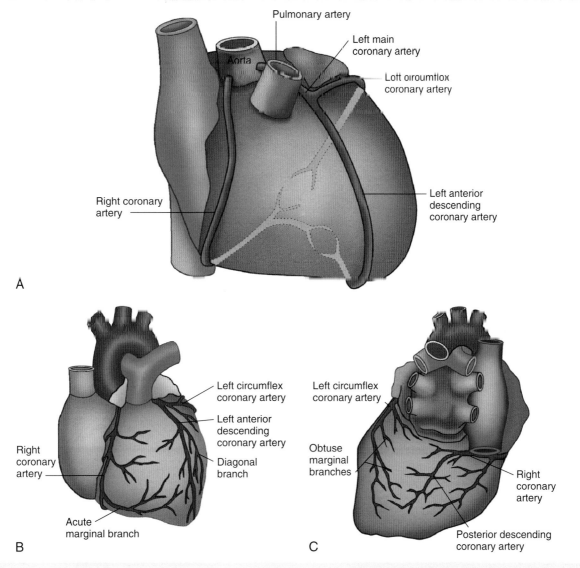

Figure 16-8 Schematic representation of the right and left coronary arteries demonstrating their orientation to one another. The left main coronary artery bifurcates into the left circumflex artery, which perfuses the lateral and posterior regions of the left ventricle (LV), and the left anterior descending artery, which perfuses the LV anterior wall, the anterior portion of the interventricular septum, and a portion of the anterior right ventricular (RV) wall. The right coronary artery (RCA) perfuses the right ventricle and variable portions of the posterior left ventricle through its terminal branches. The posterior descending artery most often arises from the RCA. B, Anterior view of the heart demonstrating the coronary arteries and their major branches. C, Posterior view of the heart demonstrating the terminal portions of the right and circumflex coronary arteries and their branches. (Reprinted with permission from Lemieux JE, Edelman ER, Strichartz GR, et al. Normal cardiac structure and function. In: *Pathophysiology of Heart Disease: A Collaborative Project of Medical Students and Faculty.* 6th ed. Philadelphia, PA: Wolters Kluwer; 2016:9, chap 1.)

3. **Answer: B.** Myocardial ischemia occurs when the oxygenated myocardial blood supply does not meet the demand of the myocardium, resulting in a decrease in myocardial contractility and relaxation. Myocardial ischemic patients at rest may be getting adequate coronary artery perfusion; however, these same patients may not have enough supply to adequately perfuse the myocardium during times of physical exertion.

4. **Answer: C.** The ischemic cascade is a series of pathophysiologic events caused by myocardial ischemia. Coronary artery disease causes a reduction in myocardial blood flow that leads to a supply-demand imbalance. This is followed by perfusion abnormalities, impaired left ventricular relaxation and compliance (diastolic left ventricular [LV] dysfunction), impaired myocardial contractility (systolic LV dysfunction or regional wall motion abnormalities), ECG changes (ST-segment changes), and lastly angina.

5. **Answer: A.** Depending on the severity of coronary artery disease, a patient may experience an acute myocardial infarction (AMI), unstable angina, or stable angina. A major cause for an AMI is a ruptured coronary artery plaque resulting in thrombosis of the coronary artery. Plaque and/or thrombosis limits the amount of flow through the vessel and therefore limits coronary artery perfusion. The following represent some nonatherosclerotic causes of myocardial ischemia or infarction: anomalous coronary origin and course, aortic regurgitation and stenosis, coronary artery spasm, coronary artery emboli, and coronary vasculitis.

6. **Answer: B.** ACS covers a spectrum of coronary artery diseases. Unstable angina represents the least severe type with only a partially occlusive thrombus and no myocardial necrosis. A non–ST-elevation myocardial infarction (NSTEMI) also has a partially occlusive thrombus but differs from unstable angina because it has myocyte necrosis. These two types of ACS are differentiated from each other by observing the cardiac biomarker results. Patients with negative biomarkers fall into the unstable angina category while patients with positive biomarkers are in the NSTEMI category. The final acute coronary syndrome is an ST-elevation myocardial infarction (STEMI), which involves a completely occlusive thrombus with myocyte necrosis. These patients will have an elevation of the ST-segment on their electrocardiogram along with positive cardiac biomarkers.

7. **Answer: D.** An ST-elevation myocardial infarction (STEMI) can be identified by ST-segment elevation in affected leads on the electrocardiogram (ECG) with positive cardiac biomarkers such as elevated troponin. ST-depression often represents myocardial ischemia and is often identified during stress testing. Global ST-elevation is when most or all ECG leads are affected. Global ST-elevation with or without elevated troponin most likely represents acute pericarditis.

8. **Answer: A.** The parasternal short-axis view at the level of the aortic valve is the best view for obtaining images of the coronary artery origins. The left main coronary artery (LMCA) arises from the left sinus of Valsalva at approximately the 4- to 5-o'clock position. The LMCA extends about 1 cm in length before bifurcating into the left anterior descending (LAD) and left circumflex (Cx) coronary arteries (**Figure 16-9**). The left Cx will course horizontally across the image around the lateral aspect of the left heart, while the LAD will course anteriorly on the image down the front of the heart. The right coronary artery (RCA) may be identified by tilting the probe slightly superiorly above the level of the aortic valve. The RCA originates at the anterior portion of the aorta at approximately 11 or 12 o'clock and then courses toward the right heart.

9. **Answer: C.** The LV is divided into three equal levels (**Figure 16-10**). The basal level is from the mitral valve annulus to the tips of the papillary muscles. The mid-level is from the tips of the papillary muscles to the base of the papillary muscles, and the apical level is from the base of the papillary muscles to the apex of the LV.

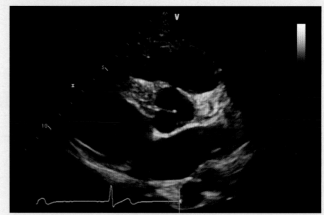

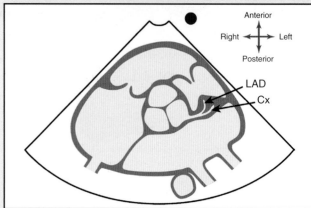

Figure 16-9 Origins of the left anterior descending (LAD) and the left circumflex (Cx) coronary arteries as seen from the PSAX view at the level of the aortic valve. (Adapted with permission by Echotext Pty Ltd, from Anderson B. The two-dimensional echocardiographic examination. In: *Echocardiography: The Normal Examination and Echocardiographic Measurements.* 3rd ed. Australia: Echotext Pty Ltd; 2017:43, chap 2.)

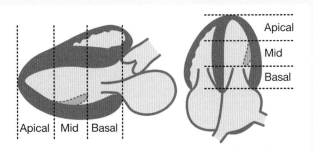

Figure 16-10 The three LV levels using the LV papillary muscles as anatomic landmarks. (Reproduced with permission by Echotext Pty Ltd, from Anderson B. The two-dimensional echocardiographic examination. In: *Echocardiography: The Normal Examination and Echocardiographic Measurements*. 3rd ed. Australia: Echotext Pty Ltd; 2017:166, chap 2.)

10. Answer: B. The left ventricle (LV) is divided into 17 segments based on anatomic landmarks. As previously described, the LV is first divided into basal, mid and apical levels. At each level the LV is then subdivided into segments. The basal and mid-levels are divided into 6 segments while the apical level is divided into 4 segments plus the apical cap, which is defined as the area of myocardium beyond the end of the LV cavity (**Figure 16-11**). In **Video 16-1**, the segment depicted by the arrow is the apicolateral segment.

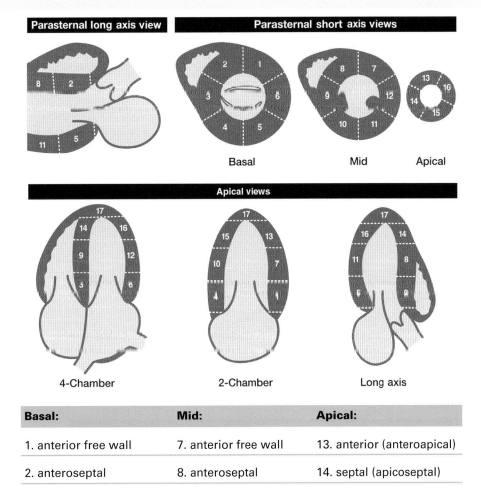

Basal:	Mid:	Apical:
1. anterior free wall	7. anterior free wall	13. anterior (anteroapical)
2. anteroseptal	8. anteroseptal	14. septal (apicoseptal)
3. inferoseptal *	9. inferoseptal *	15. inferior (inferoapical)
4. inferior *	10. inferior *	16. lateral (apicolateral)
5. inferolateral *	11. inferolateral *	17. apical cap
6. anterolateral	12. anterolateral	

*The basal inferolateral wall, basal inferior wall and basal inferoseptum may also be referred to as the posterobasal lateral wall, posterobasal wall and posterobasal ventricular septum, respectively.

Figure 16-11 The 17-segment model of the LV is illustrated based on the standard parasternal and apical echocardiographic views. (Reproduced with permission by Echotext Pty Ltd, from Anderson B. The two-dimensional echocardiographic examination. In: *Echocardiography: The Normal Examination and Echocardiographic Measurements*. 3rd ed. Australia: Echotext Pty Ltd; 2017:167, chap 2.)

11. **Answer: C.** As previously discussed in the answer outline for Question 10, the left ventricle is divided into 17 segments (see **Figure 16-11**). In **Video 16-2**, the segment depicted by the arrow is the basal inferolateral segment.

12. **Answer: D.** Recognition of the coronary blood supply to each individual segment of the 17-segment left ventricle aids in the identification of regional abnormalities across multiple segments (**Figure 16-12A**). In this patient there are regional wall motion abnormalities in the basal inferior wall and basal inferoseptal segments (**Figure 16-12B**), which is consistent with right coronary artery occlusion.

13. **Answer: A.** As previously discussed, the recognition of the coronary blood supply to each individual segment of the 17-segment left ventricle aids in the identification of regional abnormalities across multiple segments (see **Figure 16-12**). In this patient, there is an anteroapical infarct consistent with a left anterior descending coronary artery occlusion (**Figure 16-13**).

14. **Answer: A.** The motion of this segment is described as akinetic. The myocardial wall segments that receive adequate coronary artery perfusion normally thicken greater than 40% during systole. When myocardial wall segments are not receiving adequate coronary artery perfusion, they will present with regional wall motion abnormalities (RWMA).

The terms used to describe RWMA are hypokinetic, akinetic, and dyskinetic. Hypokinetic wall segments thicken less than 40% during systole. Akinetic wall segments demonstrate no visual thickening during systole. Dyskinetic wall segments demonstrate outward bulging in systole. Wall segments may be described as aneurysmal, which is a morphologic characterization of either an akinetic or dyskinetic wall displaying outward bulging throughout the cardiac cycle.

15. **Answer: B.** The wall motion score index (WMSI) is calculated by first scoring each left ventricular (LV) segment based on the degree of contractility as seen in **Table 16-1**. These scores are then summed to derive the total regional LV wall motion score, which is then divided by the total number of LV wall segments:

$$WMSI = \sum wall\ motion\ scores \div No.\ segments\ visualized \qquad (1)$$

The ASE recommends using the 17-segment model to assess myocardial perfusion and the 16-segment model for routine studies assessing wall motion. A perfect (or normal) score would be a value of 1. Any wall motion score index >1 would represent an abnormality. In this case, 2 of the 16 segments are hypokinetic and the other 14 segments can be assumed to be normal. Normal is

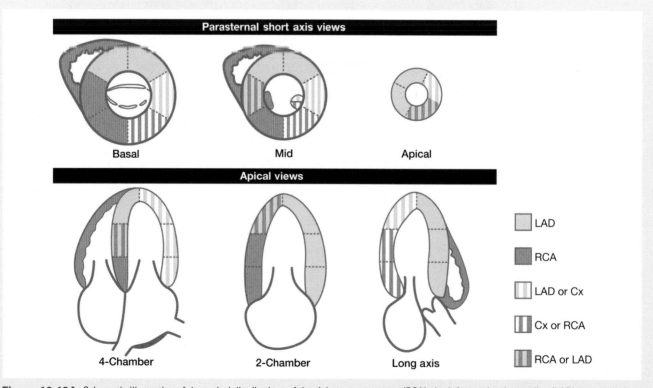

Figure 16-12A Schematic illustration of the typical distributions of the right coronary artery (RCA), the left anterior descending (LAD) coronary artery, and the left circumflex (Cx) coronary artery based on the standard echocardiographic views. Note that coronary arterial distribution is variable between individuals. (Reproduced with permission by Echotext Pty Ltd, from Anderson B. The two-dimensional echocardiographic examination. In: *Echocardiography: The Normal Examination and Echocardiographic Measurements.* 3rd ed. Australia: Echotext Pty Ltd; 2017:167, chap 2.)

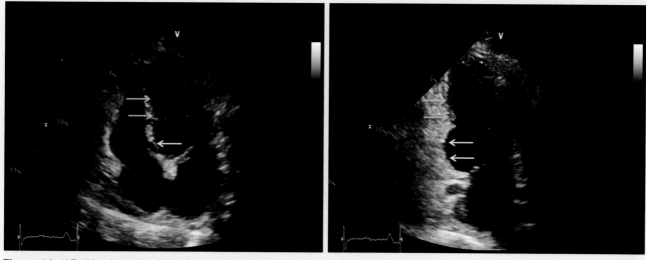

Figure 16-12B LV end-systolic still-frame images acquired from the apical 4-chamber view (left) and the apical 2-chamber view (right) show regional wall motion abnormalities in the right coronary artery (RCA) territory. In the apical 4-chamber view, there is dyskinesis of the basal inferior septum (yellow arrow) and normal motion of the more distal septal wall (blue arrows). A wall motion abnormality in the basal inferior septum is common in RCA occlusion as the proximal inferior septum is perfused by the RCA. In the apical 2-chamber view, there is dyskinesis of the basal inferior wall (yellow arrows) and normal motion of the more distal inferior wall segments (blue arrows)—see **Video 16-3** for real-time images.

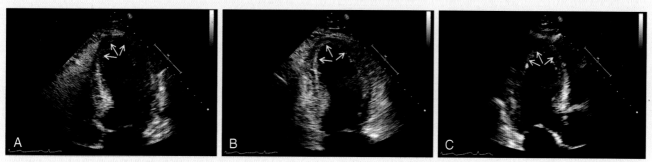

Figure 16-13 Left ventricular end-systolic still-frame images acquired from the apical 4-chamber view (A), the apical 2-chamber view (B), and the apical long-axis view (C) show regional wall motion abnormalities in the left anterior descending coronary artery territory (arrows)—see **Video 16-4** for real-time images.

Table 16-1. Wall Motion Contractility Grades

Grade	Contractility	Description
1	Normal	Systolic wall thickening >40%
2	Hypokinetic	Systolic wall thickening <40%
3	Akinetic	Absent systolic wall thickening and thin diastolic wall dimension
4	Dyskinetic	Outward bulging in systole and thin diastolic wall dimension

given a value of 1 and hypokinetic is given a value of 2; therefore, the WMSI is:

$$WMSI = [(2 \times 2) + (1 \times 14)] \div 16$$

$$= [4 + 14] \div 16 = 18 \div 16 = 1.13 \qquad (2)$$

16. **Answer: C.** The 2D method of disks or the modified Simpson biplane method is most often limited by foreshortening of the apical 4- and/or 2-chamber views. Foreshortening is recognized in the apical view when the LV appears short and squatty and/or when the apex squeezes toward the mitral valve. Foreshortening is also identified quantitatively by comparing the apical 4- and 2-chamber view ventricular lengths from the method of disks. The two lengths should not vary more than 10%. A variation >10% indicates foreshortening and the view yielding the shorter length is the foreshortened view. In this instance, foreshortening may be avoided by sliding down a rib space or two to obtain an elongated image.

The 2D Doppler method for stroke volume (answer A) is limited by nonparallel insonation angles, errors in LV outflow tract (LVOT) diameter measurements, and/or or LVOT velocity time integral (VTI) measurements. The 2D linear method (answer B) is most limited by regional wall motion abnormalities that are outside of the plane of measurement. The M-mode linear method (answer D) is most often limited by nonperpendicular alignment of the M-mode cursor with the long axis of the LV

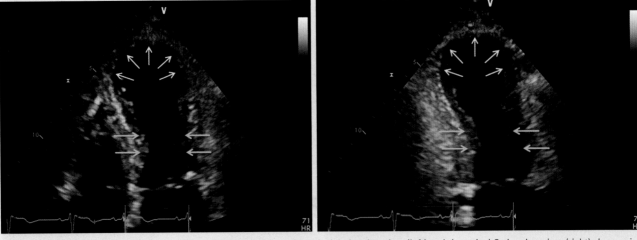

Figure 16-14A LV end-systolic still-frame images acquired from the apical 4-chamber view (left) and the apical 2-chamber view (right) show apical ballooning (yellow arrows). Basal LV segments are hyperdynamic (blue inward arrows)—see **Video 16-13A** and **16-13B** for real-time images.

and regional wall motion abnormalities that are outside of the M-mode region of interrogation.

17. **Answer: B.** Aortic regurgitation (AR) may cause angina due to a decrease in coronary artery perfusion. This occurs from decreased aortic pressure during diastole when a volume of blood is regurgitated back into the left ventricle instead of remaining in the aorta. This limits the amount of flow filling the coronary arteries during diastole creating a mismatch between the supply and demand of oxygenated myocardial blood flow. This imbalance causes the patient to experience angina.

Aortic dissection (answer B) can also cause angina if the coronary artery origins are directly involved in the dissection; for example, if the dissection flap obstructs the coronary artery orifice or if the dissection involves the aortic valve resulting in AR. In contrast to dissection, however, AR directly causes a decrease in diastolic aortic pressure, resulting in angina.

Aortic stenosis (answer A) and aortic coarctation (answer D) may also cause angina but in these instances, this is due to LV hypertrophy (LVH). LVH increases the overall mass of the LV, which increases the myocardial oxygen demand. At some point, the myocardial supply cannot meet the increased demand leading to myocardial ischemia and angina. Aortic stenosis may also reduce coronary artery perfusion due to reduced cardiac output.

18. ▶ **Answer: D.** Takotsubo cardiomyopathy often mimics acute coronary syndrome. This condition is typically seen in postmenopausal women following physical or emotional stress. Patients present with chest pain, acute ECG changes, and mildly positive cardiac biomarkers. These patients often undergo cardiac catheterization where there are no significant coronary artery lesions identified. The left ventriculogram during cardiac catheterization and the echocardiogram characteristically show apical ballooning with hypocontractility of the apical

segments and hypercontractility of the basal segments (**Figures 16-14A** and **16-14B** and **Videos 16-13A** to **16-13C**). Left ventricular (LV) function usually recovers within 3 days to 6 weeks.

19. **Answer: B.** In this case, the McConnell sign is present suggesting acute pulmonary embolism (**Figure 16-15**). Acute pulmonary embolism typically presents with chest pain that is pleuritic in nature, and shortness of breath. The patient may have recently had long hours of inactivity as seen with travel and/or illnesses. Echocardiography cannot exclude pulmonary embolism, but it can provide supporting evidence for the diagnosis. 2D echocardiographic signs include RV dilatation, impaired RV systolic function at the basal and/or mid segments with

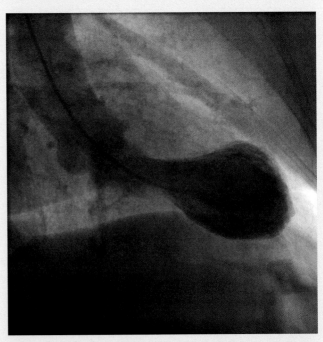

Figure 16-14B End-systolic still-frame image of the left ventriculogram showing LV apical ballooning.

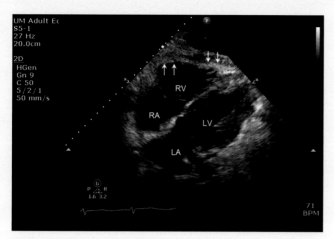

Figure 16-15 This subcostal image end-systolic frame shows preserved contractility of the apical segment of the right ventricle (downward arrows) with dysfunction of the more basal portions (upward arrows)—see **Video 16-6** for real-time images. This is referred to as the McConnell sign, which is a finding associated with acute pulmonary embolism. (Reprinted with permission from Armstrong W, Ryan T. *Feigenbaum's Echocardiography*. 8th ed. Philadelphia, PA. Wolters Kluwer, 2019.713.)

preserved apical systolic function (known as the McConnell sign), and spectral Doppler signs such as mid-systolic notching on the pulmonary valve

pulsed-wave Doppler trace and a short RV acceleration time ≤60 ms in addition to a tricuspid regurgitant (TR) pressure gradient ≤60 mm Hg (known as the "60/60 sign"). It is important to distinguish the features of acute pulmonary embolism from those of an acute coronary syndrome as the management of each condition is vastly different.

20. **Answer: C.** The patient in the figure has a Stanford type A aortic dissection (**Figure 16-16**). Patients usually present with an acute ripping or tearing type of chest pain that may radiate toward the neck and through to the back particularly in cases that involve the descending thoracic aorta. On echocardiography, the dissection, if seen, will appear as a thin mobile intimal flap inside of the aorta. In some cases of aortic root dissection, an intimal flap cannot be identified by echocardiography particularly in the aortic root, but it should be suspected if there is acute severe aortic regurgitation. Regional wall motion abnormalities must be evaluated for in cases of aortic root dissection to check for coronary artery involvement.

21. **Answer: E.** The development of a systolic murmur post–myocardial infarction (post-MI) may be due to mitral regurgitation (MR) or a VSR. In contrast to

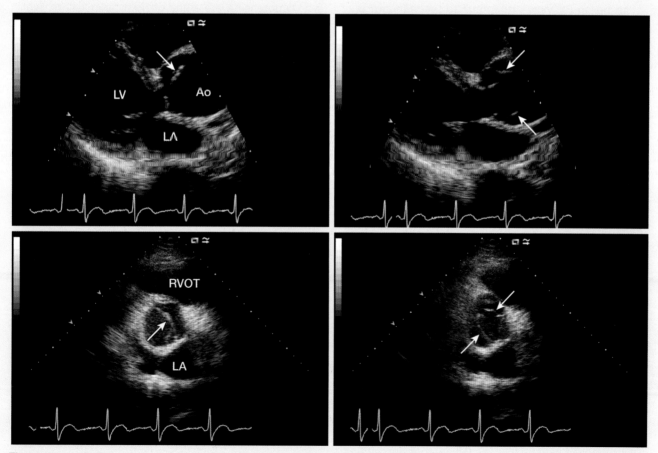

Figure 16-16 These images show a type A aortic dissection as viewed from the parasternal long-axis view (top) and a high parasternal short-axis view superior to the aortic valve (bottom). The left images are diastolic frames and the right images are systolic frames. Observe the linear echoes (arrows) within the aorta; on real-time imaging these linear echoes showed an independent and undulating motion, which is characteristic of a dissection flap. Ao = aorta; LA = left atrium; LV = left ventricle; RVOT = right ventricular outflow tract.

congenital VSDs, post-MI VSRs are identified within areas of wall motion abnormality and are often irregularly shaped. Cardiac magnetic resonance is an alternative diagnostic approach, but the defects are normally readily visualized by TTE. The use of 3D echocardiography may minimize the possibility of missing multiple defects, which may be important in planning device closure.

22. **Answer: E.** The diagnosis of RV infarction should be suspected with hemodynamic changes in a patient after an inferior myocardial infarction (MI), and echocardiography is confirmatory in a qualitative sense. Quantification of the degree of RV systolic function in these cases is problematic because the RV is a nongeometric chamber and 2D volumes are often underestimated as images are frequently off-axis. Even if the end-systolic and end-diastolic volumes are underestimated to the same degree, the 2D RVEF may vary according to the view used to perform this measurement. TAPSE, TDI s′, and strain reflect longitudinal displacement. Although these measurements offer a means of overcoming the geometric limitations of the EF calculation, they are regional measures that may be influenced by the site of the MI. Potentially, these measurements may be averaged over multiple segments using an RV view orthogonal to the standard apical 4-chamber view. The Tei index is also another method that can be used to assess RV function as it is independent of RV geometry; however, this measurement is not purely a measure of systolic function.

TEACHING POINT

RV systolic function is notoriously difficult to quantify. 3D echocardiography (3DE) may overcome issues related to the complex, crescentic, and irregular shape of the RV, and therefore, RV evaluation may become an important indication for 3DE.

23. **Answer: B.** 3 to 7 days is the most common time frame for a mechanical complication post-MI to occur. Mechanical complications occur due to "softening" of the necrotic tissue. Immediate complications post-MI occurring within minutes to hours may include arrhythmias, heart block, hypotension, and congestive heart failure.

24. **Answer: D.** This patient experienced a papillary muscle rupture due to blockage of the right coronary artery (RCA). This occurs most commonly in the setting of an inferior myocardial infarction because the RCA is usually the only vessel that supplies the posteromedial (PM) papillary muscle. The anterolateral papillary muscle is less likely to rupture because it is supplied with flow by the left anterior descending and left circumflex coronary arteries.

25. **Answer: A.** The diagnosis for this patient is LV apical aneurysm resulting from a weakening of the apical wall due to left anterior descending coronary artery occlusion. The echocardiographic characteristics of an LV aneurysm include an outpouching of the myocardium, a wide neck, and dyskinesis during systole. Complications include thrombus formation and embolization, congestive heart failure due to reduced LV ejection fraction, and ventricular arrhythmias. Treatments for apical aneurysm include anticoagulation to prevent thromboembolization and afterload reduction to reduce LV wall tension.

Answer B is not correct since an inferior pseudoaneurysm would not be seen in the apical 4-chamber view; it would be better seen in the apical 2-chamber view. Answer C is not correct as RV function is normal in this patient, which would rule out RV infarction. Answer D is not correct. While takotsubo cardiomyopathy (TTC) would have a similar appearance to an LV apical aneurysm with distal LV wall motion hypokinesis, the patient history and abnormal cardiac catheterization rule out TTC. Patients with TTC would likely have a normal cardiac catheterization.

26. **Answer: D.** The right coronary artery (RCA) supplies blood flow to the right ventricle and when occluded can cause an RV infarction. Jugular vein distention, peripheral edema, hepatomegaly, and hypotension are signs of right heart failure, which should be considered in this case.

Blockage to the RCA would not likely result in global LV dysfunction; therefore, answer A is not correct. Mitral regurgitation (answer B) could be caused by a blockage in the RCA in the setting of ruptured papillary muscle but would likely result in rapid pulmonary edema and a loud holosystolic murmur. Pulmonary hypertension (answer C) may result from chronic RV dysfunction but is not the first thought in the setting of a recent MI.

27. **Answer: C.** Dressler syndrome, also known as post–cardiac injury syndrome, and post–myocardial infarction syndrome, is the name for pericarditis that occurs days or weeks after a myocardial infarction and is caused by an inflammation of the pericardium. With improvements in the management of acute MI, this syndrome is infrequently seen. Patients with this syndrome may present with pleuritic pain and a low-grade fever. Upon clinical examination, a pericardial friction rub may be present. Treatment includes nonsteroidal anti-inflammatory medications.

Constrictive pericarditis (answer A) is caused by an adherent, inflamed, fibrotic, or calcified pericardium that limits diastolic filling of the heart and is most commonly caused from previous cardiac surgery, radiotherapy, and viral or idiopathic causes. Costochondritis (answer B) is a condition where the cartilage in the breastbone becomes inflamed, causing severe chest pain. Kawasaki disease (answer D), also known as mucocutaneous lymph node syndrome, is an acute, febrile vasculitis of childhood that affects medium-sized arteries, particularly the coronary arteries. Coronary artery involvement includes coronary artery aneurysms or ectasia.

28. **Answer: C.** While any of the options provided may be a complication following PCI, the clue is the type of chest pain. Chest pain that is exaggerated on deep inspiration is characteristic of pleuritic chest pain, which is one of the symptoms of acute pericarditis. Pericarditis (answer C) in acute MI is a complication seen in approximately 7% of patients. It is generally seen between 4 and 48 hours after the acute MI. This is not to be confused with Dressler syndrome, which is a late-onset pericarditis seen at least a week out from an acute MI. Blockage of a stent (answer B) or recurrent MI (answer D) are both possibilities but would likely present with nonpleuritic chest pain. Aortic dissection (answer A) is also a possible differential; however, the classic presentation would be stabbing or ripping back pain between the shoulder blades.

29. **Answer: B.** When left ventricular (LV) outpouchings are detected, the main differential diagnoses are pseudoaneurysm, aneurysm, and diverticulum. In the images provided and as stated in the question stem, there is a cardiac (free wall) rupture that is contained by adherent pericardium. This is referred to as a pseudoaneurysm; therefore, answer B is correct. Usually a free wall rupture (FWR) results in acute hemopericardium, cardiac tamponade, and death. However, sometimes the FWR is contained by pericardial adhesions that form a pseudoaneurysm (or false aneurysm). As pseudoaneurysms are lined only by pericardium, the risk of rupture is very high. Therefore, it is crucial that a pseudoaneurysm is identified.

True aneurysms (answer C) result from the weakening of an infarcted (necrotic) wall and the pulsatile force of ventricular contractions. As previously described, the echocardiographic characteristics of an LV aneurysm include an outpouching of the myocardium, a wide neck, and dyskinesis during systole. An LV diverticulum (answer B) also appears as an outpouching of the LV. An LV diverticulum contains endocardium, myocardium, and pericardium and displays normal contraction. Furthermore, most LV diverticula are found in the apex. **Table 16-2** summarizes the differences among these LV outpouchings.

30. **Answer: A.** A pseudoaneurysm typically has a small, discrete, narrow neck that then bulges out into a saccular aneurysm formation. This occurs due to myocardial rupture that is contained by the pericardial layer. In a true aneurysm, the endocardial, myocardial, and pericardial layers remain intact and all three layers are stretched. This typically creates a more uniform bulge without a discrete neck. Refer to Table 16-2.

31. **Answer: D.** Although all three are rare complications, free wall rupture, ventricular septal rupture, and papillary muscle rupture carry the highest mortality rates and are cardiovascular emergencies due to their extensive hemodynamic compromise. Each of these complications can be diagnosed on a transthoracic echocardiogram. When diagnosed, all three require immediate surgery.

32. **Answer: C.** The PM papillary muscle is more susceptible to rupture because it is supplied by only the posterior descending artery. The AL papillary muscle has dual blood supply (left anterior descending and left circumflex coronary arteries). Therefore, this papillary muscle is not as vulnerable to rupture; that is, if one of these coronary arteries becomes occluded, it has a backup blood supply from the other coronary artery.

Table 16-2. Differentiating Left Ventricular Outpouchings

Parameter	True Aneurysm	Pseudoaneurysm	Diverticulum
Lining	Endocardium, myocardium (scar), and pericardium	Pericardium	Endocardium, myocardium, and pericardium
Neck	Nondiscrete wide neck	Narrow neck	Variable
Mechanical and hemodynamic considerations	Bulges outward during systole increasing the size and causing stasis of blood flow	To-and-fro flow through the neck of pseudoaneurysm	Synchronous contractility
Cause	Infarction	Infarction with rupture of the left ventricle	Usually congenital
Likelihood of rupture	Rare	Common	Rare
Thrombus	Both true and pseudoaneurysms may be lined with thrombus		Possible, incidence unknown

33. **Answer: B. Figure 16-6** and **Video 16-11** show akinesis of the LV apex and distal septum and an apical LV thrombus. LV thrombus may form within 24 hours after an acute myocardial infarction. It forms adjacent to regional wall motion abnormalities due to endothelial damage and stagnant blood flow swirling from lack of adequate systolic thickening. LV thrombus has a potential risk of thromboembolism and ultimately stroke or acute arterial occlusions.

34. **Answer: D.** Free wall rupture, or cardiac rupture, post-MI most commonly results from a distinct tear in the myocardial wall, usually between the junction of the infarcted and normal muscle. While a rare complication, it can be a catastrophic event leading to cardiogenic shock and even death. Death generally occurs as a result of cardiac tamponade.

    Post–cardiac injury syndrome, post-pericardiotomy syndrome, and post–myocardial infarction syndrome (answers A, B, and C) are all synonymous terms used to describe pericarditis with or without a pericardial effusion resulting from injury of the pericardium. As previously mentioned, Dressler syndrome is another term used to describe this entity.

35. **Answer: C.** The CW Doppler MR waveform is dense and triangular; these features are consistent with severe MR. The dense MR Doppler signal indicates a large number of red blood cells. The triangular shape of the MR waveform indicates that there is a high left atrial (LA) pressure due to the large regurgitant volume filling the left atrium during systole, which causes pressures to equalize quickly between the left ventricle and left atrium. In addition, the MR velocity is <3 m/s, which suggests a low LV systolic pressure (hypotension) and/or a very high LA pressure. Based on these findings, there is most likely acute, severe MR because of papillary muscle rupture or dysfunction; therefore, answer C is correct.

    Answer A is not correct as the MR velocity is low; this is not consistent with hypertension where a high MR velocity would be expected. Answer B is not correct. While there is evidence of a marked increase in the LA pressure (or LV filling pressure),

this is due to severe MR rather than LV diastolic dysfunction. Answer D is not correct as it is not possible to make any conclusions regarding the degree of LV filling or the presence or absence of dynamic left ventricular outflow tract obstruction based on the MR velocity waveform alone.

36. **Answer: A.** The peak VSR velocity represents the pressure difference between left and right ventricles during systole. Therefore, the RVSP can be calculated from the peak VSR velocity (V_{VSR}) and the systolic blood pressure (SBP):

$$RVSP = SBP - 4V_{VSR}^2 \qquad (1)$$

The peak VSR velocity is 5 m/s and the SBP is 130 mm Hg; therefore:

$$RVSP = 130 - 4\left(5^2\right) = 130 - 100 = 30\,mm\,Hg \qquad (2)$$

37. **Answer: D.** An increased risk of VSR may be observed in patients with single-vessel disease (especially the left anterior descending coronary artery), extensive myocardial damage, and poor septal collateral circulation. VSR may also be seen in patients with multivessel coronary artery disease. VSR is also more common in elderly women who have not had a previous MI.

38. **Answer: E.** Answer A is incorrect since due to the nature of the septal blood supply, patients with an MI due to occlusion of a "wraparound" LAD appear to have an elevated risk of VSR. Answer B is incorrect as the diagnosis of a VSR can be established in up to 90% of cases with TTE. Answer C is incorrect since the majority of post-MI VSRs occur within the first week and may develop as early as the first 24 hours following an acute MI; VSR rarely occurs after 2 weeks post-MI. Answer D is incorrect since the frequency of VSR is equal in both anterior and nonanterior MI.

Acknowledgments: The authors thank and acknowledge the contributions from Thomas H. Marwick, MD, PhD (Chapter 12, Systolic Function Assessment) in *Clinical Echocardiography Review: A Self-Assessment Tool*, 2nd Edition, edited by Allan L. Klein, Craig R. Asher, 2017.

SUGGESTED READINGS

Anderson B. The two-dimensional echocardiographic examination. In: *Echocardiography: The Normal Examination and Echocardiographic Measurements*. 3rd ed. Brisbane, Australia: Echotext Pty Ltd; 2017:chap 2.

Anderson B. Two-dimensional echocardiographic measurements and calculations. In: *Echocardiography: The Normal Examination and Echocardiographic Measurements*. 3rd ed. Brisbane, Australia: Echotext Pty Ltd; 2017:chap 9.

Anderson B. Ischaemic heart disease. In: *A Sonographer's Guide to the Assessment of Heart Disease*. Brisbane, Australia: Echotext Pty Ltd; 2014:chap 5.

Armstrong W, Ryan T. The comprehensive echocardiographic examination. In: *Feigenbaum's Echocardiography*. 8th ed. Philadelphia: Wolters Kluwer; 2019:chap 4.

Armstrong W, Ryan T. Echocardiography and coronary artery disease. In: *Feigenbaum's Echocardiography*. 8th ed. Philadelphia: Wolters Kluwer; 2019:chap 15.

Lilly L. Normal cardiac structure and function. In: *Pathophysiology of Heart Disease: A Collaborative Project of Medical Students and Faculty*. Portland, OR: Wolters Kluwer; 2016:chap 1.

Lilly L. Ischemic heart disease. In: *Pathophysiology of Heart Disease: A Collaborative Project of Medical Students and Faculty*. Portland, OR: Wolters Kluwer; 2016:chap 6.

Lilly L. Acute coronary syndromes. In: *Pathophysiology of Heart Disease: A Collaborative Project of Medical Students and Faculty*. Portland, OR: Wolters Kluwer; 2016:chap 7.

Mankad SV, Oh JK. Coronary artery disease, acute myocardial infarction, takotsubo syndrome. In: Oh JK, Kane GC, Seward JB, Tajik AJ, eds. *The Echo Manual*. 4th ed. Philadelphia, PA & Rochester, MN: Wolters Kluwer; 2019:chap 17.

Porter TR, Mulvagh SL, Abdelmoneim SS, et al. Clinical applications of ultrasonic enhancing agents in echocardiography: 2018 American Society of Echocardiography guidelines update. *J Am Soc Echocardiogr*. 2018;31(3):241-274.

Nihoyannopoulos P, Kisslo J. Mechanical complications of myocardial infarction. In: *Echocardiography*. 2nd ed. London, UK: Springer; 2018:385-398:chap 19.

CHAPTER 17

Cardiomyopathies

Contributors: Christopher J. Kramer, BA, ACS, RDCS and Matt Umland, BS, ACS, RDCS

✪✪ Question 1

The diagnostic criteria for dilated cardiomyopathy (DCM) include:
- **A.** Left ventricular (LV) dilatation with normal LV ejection fraction (LVEF) (>52% or better).
- **B.** LV dilatation with mild reduction of LVEF (>50%).
- **C.** Normal ventricular size with severely reduced LVEF (<30%).
- **D.** LV dilatation with mild reduction of LVEF (<45%).

✪ Question 2

When assessing the maximal left ventricular (LV) chamber size from the parasternal long-axis scan plane, which two-dimensional (2D) echocardiographic measurement should be used?
- **A.** LV end-diastolic volume (LVEDV)
- **B.** LV end-systolic dimension (LVESD)
- **C.** LV end-diastolic dimension (LVEDD)
- **D.** LV end-systolic volume (LVESV)

✪ Question 3

The recommended and most accurate technique for evaluating left ventricular (LV) systolic function in dilated cardiomyopathy (DCM) is the:
- **A.** Linear dimension ejection fraction measurement.
- **B.** LV index of myocardial performance (LIMP).
- **C.** Mitral annular systolic velocity (s′).
- **D.** Volume ejection fraction measurement.

✪ Question 4

Figure 17-1 demonstrates which M-mode finding in this patient with dilated cardiomyopathy?

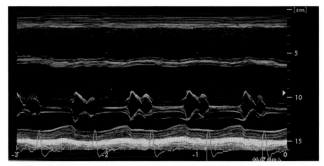

Figure 17-1

- **A.** Abrupt A-wave opening
- **B.** E-point-septal separation (EPSS)
- **C.** Normal right ventricular size
- **D.** Tapered opening of the mitral valve
- **E.** All of the above

✪✪ Question 5

Figure 17-2 demonstrates which M-mode finding in this patient with a dilated cardiomyopathy?
- **A.** Ascending aortic dissection
- **B.** Premature opening of the aortic valve
- **C.** Midsystolic notching of the aortic valve
- **D.** Tapered closure of the aortic valve
- **E.** All of the above

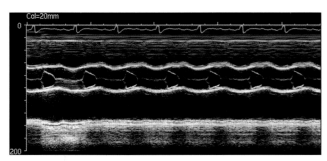

Figure 17-2

✪✪ Question 6

The right ventricle is commonly affected in patients with dilated cardiomyopathy (DCM). Which of the following indices shows an abnormal right ventricular (RV) function value?

A. Fractional area change (FAC) = 40%

B. Right ventricular index of myocardial performance (RIMP) = 0.32

C. Tricuspid annular plane systolic excursion (TAPSE) = 12 mm

D. Tricuspid annular systolic velocity (s′) = 12 cm/s

✪ Question 7

Figure 17-3 demonstrates which abnormal right ventricular (RV) function measurement?

A. Peak early diastolic (e′) velocity of 7 cm/s

B. Peak isovolumic contraction (IVC) velocity of 0.07 m/s

C. Peak systolic (s′) velocity of 7 cm/s

D. Tricuspid annular plane systolic excursion (TAPSE) of 7 cm

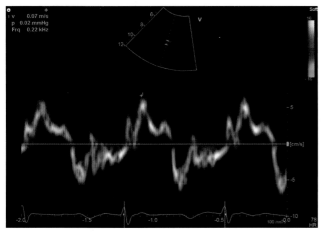

Figure 17-3

✪✪ Question 8

Which of the following equations is used to calculate the right ventricular index of myocardial performance (RIMP) by the spectral Doppler method?

A. $(\text{TVCOt} - \text{ET}_{\text{PV}}) \div \text{ET}_{\text{PV}}$

B. $(\text{TVOCt} - \text{ET}_{\text{PV}}) \div \text{ET}_{\text{PV}}$

C. $(\text{TRd} - \text{ET}_{\text{AV}}) \div \text{ET}_{\text{PV}}$

D. $(\text{TRd} - \text{ET}_{\text{PV}}) \div \text{ET}_{\text{AV}}$

where ET_{AV} = aortic valve ejection time; ET_{PV} = pulmonary valve ejection time; TRd = tricuspid regurgitation duration; TVCOt = tricuspid valve closure to tricuspid valve opening time; TVOCt = tricuspid valve opening to tricuspid valve closure time.

✪✪ Question 9

What is the primary mechanism for functional mitral regurgitation in a patient with dilated cardiomyopathy?

A. Annular dilatation and/or flail leaflets

B. Annular dilatation and/or malposition of the papillary muscles

C. Valve prolapse and/or malposition of the papillary muscles

D. Cleft valve leaflet, annular dilatation, and/or malposition of the papillary muscles

✪ Question 10

What is the effective regurgitant orifice area (EROA) criterion for severe mitral regurgitation (MR) in the setting of dilated cardiomyopathy (DCM)?

A. 0.2 to 0.29 cm²

B. >0.3 cm²

C. ≥0.4 cm²

D. B and C

✪ Question 11

▶ Echocardiography, including the use of an ultrasound enhancing agent (UEA), plays a key role in detection of thrombus in patients with dilated cardiomyopathy (DCM). The images shown in **Figure 17-4** and **Video 17-1** demonstrate which common UEA artifact?

A. Apical shadowing

B. Apical swirling

C. Attenuation

D. Foreshortening

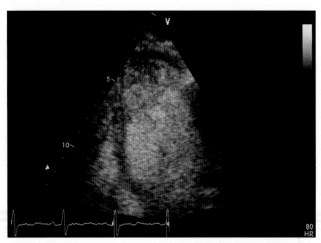

Figure 17-4

✪✪ Question 12

Which cardiomyopathy is characterized by nondilated ventricles with impaired ventricular filling?

A. Arrhythmogenic right ventricular cardiomyopathy
B. Dilated cardiomyopathy
C. Valvular cardiomyopathy due to aortic regurgitation
D. Restrictive cardiomyopathy
E. All of the above except B

✪ Question 13

Which infiltrative restrictive cardiomyopathy (RCM) is characterized by thickened valves, increased right and left ventricular wall thickness, a small pericardial effusion, normal left ventricular size (LV), normal systolic function, and an apical-sparing reduction in longitudinal strain?

A. Amyloidosis
B. Carcinoid heart disease
C. Glycogen storage disease
D. Hemochromatosis

✪ Question 14

Which restrictive cardiomyopathy (RCM) has the characteristic appearance of ventricular apical thrombus and possible involvement of the papillary muscles and tethering of the posterior mitral valve leaflet?

A. Amyloidosis
B. Fabry disease
C. Hypereosinophilic syndrome
D. Sarcoidosis

✪ Question 15

A characteristic 2D echocardiographic feature of restrictive cardiomyopathy is:

A. Biatrial enlargement.
B. Biventricular dilation in the early stages of the disease.
C. Fatty infiltration of the right ventricle apex.
D. Normal left ventricular (LV) wall thickness.
E. Both A and D.

✪✪ Question 16

A typical spectral Doppler finding in restrictive cardiomyopathy (RCM) is:

A. An increased pulmonary venous systolic velocity
B. Diastolic dysfunction
C. Hepatic venous flow reversal during systole
D. Increased forward flow during inspiration in the superior vena cava (SVC)
E. Both A and B

✪✪✪ Question 17

Which of the following spectral Doppler findings used to differentiate restrictive cardiomyopathy (RCM) from constrictive pericarditis (CP) is incorrect?

A. Respiratory variation in transmitral and transtricuspid inflow velocities is absent in RCM and usually present in CP.
B. Atrial reversal velocities on the hepatic venous velocity trace are increased with inspiration in RCM and increased with expiration in CP.
C. Mitral septal e' velocity is decreased with RCM and normal or increased with CP.
D. Mitral septal e' velocity is > lateral e' with RCM and the septal e' velocity is < lateral e' with CP.

✪✪ Question 18

Which of the following statements regarding arrhythmogenic right ventricular cardiomyopathy (ARVC) is false?

A. ARVC is an inherited cardiomyopathy.
B. A clinical manifestation of ARVC is ventricular arrhythmias and sudden death.
C. ARVC is characterized by fibrofatty infiltration of the ventricular myocardium.
D. The diagnosis of ARVC is a diagnosis of exclusion.

✪✪ Question 19

The characteristic electrocardiographic abnormality observed in patients with arrhythmogenic right ventricular cardiomyopathy (ARVC) is:
- **A.** Epsilon waves.
- **B.** First degree heart block.
- **C.** Giant negative T waves.
- **D.** Low-voltage QRS complexes.

✪ Question 20

Which of the following is an echocardiographic feature of arrhythmogenic right ventricular cardiomyopathy (ARVC)?
- **A.** Obstruction of the left ventricular outflow tract
- **B.** Rigid, fixed tricuspid valve leaflets in semi-open position
- **C.** Right ventricular regional akinesis
- **D.** Rigid pulmonary valve cusps causing stenosis
- **E.** All of the above except A

✪ Question 21

Which of the following is a characteristic echocardiographic finding associated with arrhythmogenic right ventricular cardiomyopathy (ARVC)?
- **A.** Hyperdynamic right ventricular (RV) systolic function
- **B.** Thickened RV free wall
- **C.** Thinned segmental RV wall
- **D.** Small (hypoplastic) right ventricle
- **E.** Both C and D

✪✪ Question 22

What is the effect that causes abnormal motion of the mitral valve leaflet(s) seen in **Figure 17-5**?
- **A.** Frank-Starling
- **B.** Poiseuille
- **C.** Laplace
- **D.** Venturi

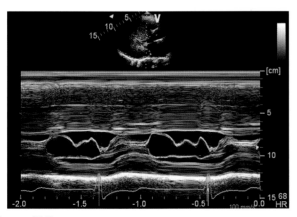

Figure 17-5

✪✪ Question 23

Differentiation between continuous-wave Doppler signals arising from left ventricular outflow tract (LVOT) obstruction and mitral regurgitation (MR) can be accomplished by considering the:
- **A.** Ejection times.
- **B.** Isovolumic periods.
- **C.** Diastolic filling.
- **D.** Velocity.

✪ Question 24

Which of the following best differentiates a fixed versus dynamic left ventricular outflow tract (LVOT) obstruction?
- **A.** Consideration of the peak velocity and pressure gradient
- **B.** Pulsed-wave Doppler mapping
- **C.** Use of the PEDOF transducer
- **D.** Use of provocative maneuvers

✪ Question 25

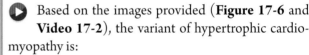 Based on the images provided (**Figure 17-6** and **Video 17-2**), the variant of hypertrophic cardiomyopathy is:
- **A.** Apical.
- **B.** Concentric.
- **C.** Obstructive.
- **D.** Sigmoid.

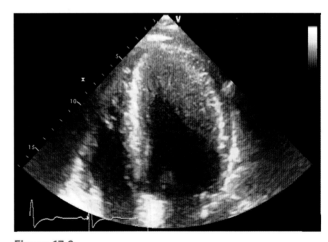

Figure 17-6

✪✪✪ Question 26

What are the pathophysiological changes that occur in maneuvers aimed to provoke gradients in patients with hypertrophic obstructive cardiomyopathy?

A. Increased preload, decreased afterload, or increased force of contraction

B. Decreased preload, decreased afterload, or increased force of contraction

C. Increased preload, increased afterload, or decreased force of contraction

D. Decreased preload, increased afterload, or decreased force of contraction

✪✪ Question 27

The echocardiographic criterion for the diagnosis of left ventricular noncompaction (LVNC) based on measurements of noncompacted (NC) and compacted (C) myocardium is:

A. An end-systolic NC/C ratio of >2.

B. An end-diastolic NC/C ratio <2.

C. An end-diastolic NC/(NC + C) ratio >0.5.

D. An end-systolic NC/(NC + C) ratio <0.5.

E. Both A and C.

✪✪ Question 28

The predominant areas of trabeculation seen in left ventricular noncompaction (LVNC) are at the _____ regions of the ventricle.

A. Mid-anterior, mid-inferior, and mid-lateral

B. Mid-lateral, mid-inferior, and apical

C. Basal lateral, mid-inferior, and apical

D. Mid-anterior, mid-inferior, and basal lateral

✪ Question 29

Which of the following is not a characteristic echocardiographic feature of apical hypertrophic cardiomyopathy?

A. Apical obliteration

B. Possible apical pouch

C. Thickened basal and mid-ventricular segments

D. Thickened middle to apical segments

✪ Question 30

All of the following are common causes of restrictive cardiomyopathy except:

A. Coronary artery disease.

B. Genetic abnormalities.

C. Connective tissue disorders.

D. Sarcoidosis.

✪✪✪ Question 31

In the setting of hypertrophic obstructive cardiomyopathy without a continuous-wave Doppler cursor directed through left ventricular outflow tract (LVOT), which of the following calculations can be used to identify the LVOT pressure gradient?

A. $LVSP - (MR_{PG} + LAP)$

B. $LVSP - DBP$

C. $(MR_{PG} - LAP) - SBP$

D. $(MR_{PG} + LAP) - SBP$

where DBP = diastolic blood pressure; LAP = left atrial pressure; LVSP = left ventricular systolic pressure; MR_{PG} = mitral regurgitant pressure gradient; SBP = systolic blood pressure.

✪✪✪ Question 32

The continuous-wave (CW) Doppler traces across the left ventricular outflow tract (LVOT) in **Figure 17-7** were acquired from a patient with hypertrophic obstructive cardiomyopathy. What is the most likely rationale for variance in the peak gradient between the trace on the left and the trace on the right?

A. Mitral regurgitation contaminates the signal on the left.

B. A postprandial effect is seen in the left signal.

C. The systolic blood pressure increased between the acquisition of traces.

D. The CW Doppler signal on the right is poorly aligned with the LVOT.

E. The left signal was acquired with the patient supine and the right signal was acquired with the patient standing.

✪ Question 33

What is the most likely cardiomyopathy displayed in **Figure 17-8**?

A. Arrhythmogenic right ventricular cardiomyopathy

B. Dilated

C. Hypertrophic

D. Infiltrative

E. Restrictive

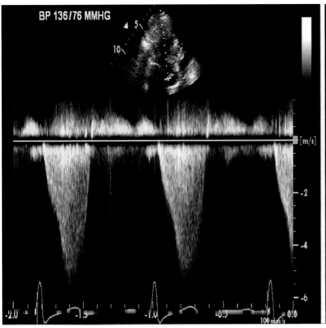
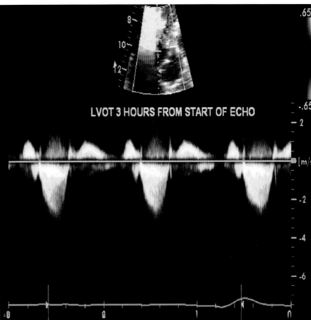

LVOT 3 HOURS FROM START OF ECHO

Figure 17-7

✪✪ Question 34

The leading cause of sudden cardiac death (SCD) in athletes younger than 35 years is a cardiomyopathy of which type?

- **A.** Arrhythmogenic right ventricular cardiomyopathy
- **B.** Dilated
- **C.** Hypertrophic
- **D.** Infiltrative
- **E.** Restrictive

✪✪ Question 35

Which of the following is considered a hallmark echocardiographic feature of Chagas cardiomyopathy?

- **A.** Left ventricular apical aneurysms
- **B.** Markedly increased biventricular wall thickness
- **C.** Diastolic dysfunction with a restrictive filling pattern
- **D.** Isolated thinning of the basal interventricular septum

✪✪✪ Question 36

What abnormality does the continuous-wave Doppler trace in **Figure 17-9**, acquired from an apical window, most likely represent?

- **A.** Mitral regurgitation
- **B.** Mitral valve prolapse
- **C.** Left ventricular outflow tract obstruction
- **D.** Apical hypertrophic cardiomyopathy with pouch

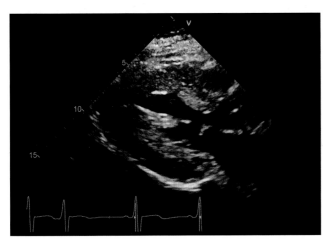

Figure 17-8

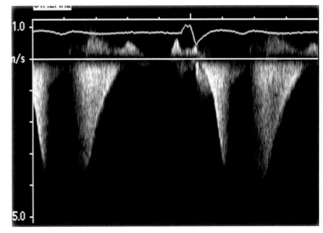

Figure 17-9

✪ Question 37

What abnormality does the continuous-wave (CW) Doppler trace in **Figure 17-10**, acquired from an apical window, most likely represent?

    A. Aortic stenosis

    B. Dynamic left ventricular outflow tract (LVOT) obstruction

    C. Fixed LVOT obstruction due to a subaortic membrane

    D. Mitral regurgitation (MR) secondary to mitral valve prolapse

    E. B or C

✪✪ Question 38

What is the most common characteristic feature utilized to differentiate athlete's heart from hypertrophic cardiomyopathy (HCM)?

    A. Chamber dimensions

    B. Diastolic function

    C. Gender

    D. Wall thickness

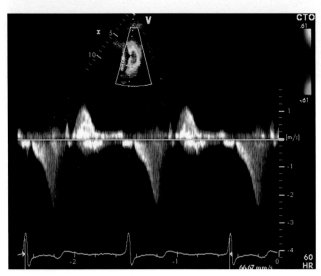

Figure 17-10

ANSWERS

1. **Answer: D.** Dilated cardiomyopathy is characterized by chamber enlargement and contractile dysfunction of the left ventricle in the absence of chronic LV volume and/or pressure overload. The diagnostic criteria include LV dilatation of greater than 112% of the predicted value corrected for age and the body surface area (BSA), with an LVEF less than 45% or a fractional shortening (FS) less than 25%.

2. **Answer: C.** The measurement to assess LV size from the parasternal long-axis scan plane is performed at end-diastole. At this point of the cardiac cycle, the left ventricle is at its largest, maximal dimension. The LV dimension or internal dimension is measured perpendicular to the LV long-axis, at the level of the mitral valve leaflet tips with the electronic calipers positioned between myocardial wall and cavity interface or blood-tissue interface (**Figure 17-11**). While

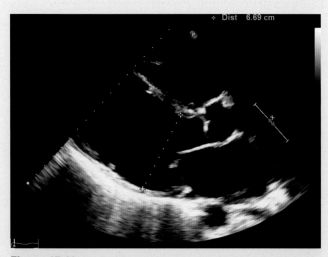

Figure 17-11

end-systolic measurements can also be considered for the degree of LV dilatation, at end-systole, the left ventricle is at its smallest size and therefore does not yield the maximal LV dimension. LV volumes may also be used for determining the degree of LV dilatation, but the recommended method for estimating LV volumes is the method of disks or from three-dimensional (3D) echocardiography and these measurements are performed from the apical views.

3. **Answer: D.** The recommended method for evaluating LV systolic function is the left ventricular ejection fraction (LVEF) derived from LV volumes acquired by 3D echocardiography or by applying the modified biplane Simpson's method of disks. Answers A-C may also be used to evaluate LV systolic function. The estimation of the LVEF via linear dimensions (answer A) is no longer recommended for clinical use as these measurements rely on geometric assumptions of LV shape which may not apply in DCM. The LIMP (answer D) incorporates both isovolumic and ejection time intervals in expressing global LV performance; however, this index is not the recommended method for assessing LV systolic function. The systolic annular velocity derived by tissue Doppler imaging (answer C) also provides a measurement of LV systolic function; however, this technique is prone to Doppler angle pitfalls. For example, if the path of the annulus is not in line with the Doppler cursor, the peak systolic velocity will be underestimated.

4. **Answer: B.** The M-mode tracing shows decreased mitral valve opening as well as an increased EPSS. These findings are consistent with a poor left ventricular ejection fraction and reduced stroke volume and cardiac output. The EPSS is a distance measurement that is perpendicular to the most posterior point of the interventricular septum (IVS) during systole and the early diastolic point (E point) of the anterior mitral valve leaflet during the same cardiac cycle (**Figure 17-12**). In systolic dysfunction, this distance increases due to a combination of the anterior displacement of the IVS as the left ventricular dimension increases/dilates, and a reduced opening

of the mitral valve due to decreased inflow into the left ventricle. A normal EPSS value is ≤5 mm.

5. **Answer: D.** The M-mode tracing shows a tapered or gradual closure of the aortic valve throughout systole (**Figure 17-13A**, arrows). This finding is consistent with reduced stroke volume, reduced cardiac output, and poor ejection fraction. Normally, the M-mode trace of the aortic valve shows a characteristic "box-shape" within the aortic root (**Figure 17-13B**).

6. **Answer: C.** DCM often affects both left and right ventricles. RV systolic function can be measured by many techniques. TAPSE is an M-mode measurement where the cursor is placed through the lateral tricuspid annulus, parallel to the motion of the annulus. TAPSE is the trough-to-peak systolic movement of the annulus and is measured from the end-diastolic (ED) point to the peak systolic (PS) point on the M-mode trace (**Figure 17-14**). Normal TAPSE measurements are >17 mm. Therefore, a TAPSE value of 12 mm is abnormal.

The s′ velocity (upward/positive peak systolic wave) is measured from the tissue Doppler imaging (TDI) trace with the sample volume placed within the lateral tricuspid annulus. The normal s′ velocity is >9.5 cm/s. The RIMP, like the left ventricular index of

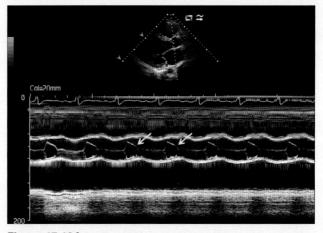

Figure 17-13A

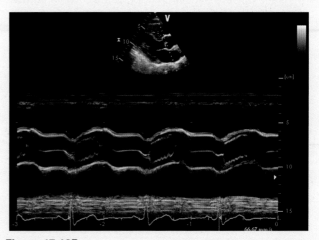

Figure 17-13B

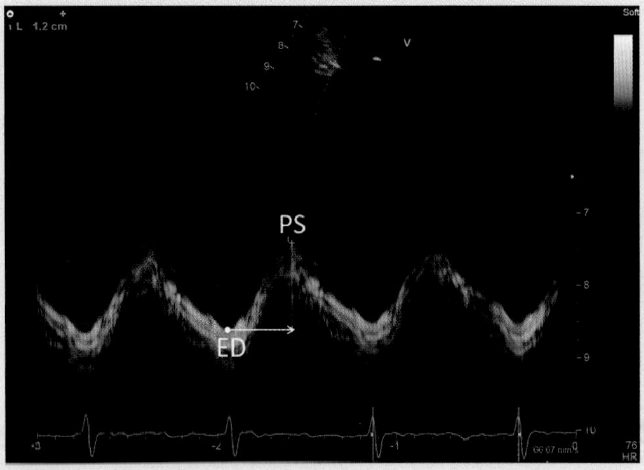

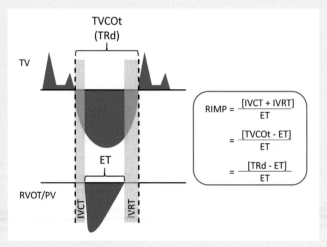

Figure 17-14

Figure 17-15

myocardial performance, incorporates both isovolumic and ejection time intervals and is calculated as the sum of the isovolumic contraction time and the isovolumic relaxation time divided by the ejection time. The RIMP can be calculated from the TDI trace or from the spectral Doppler traces of tricuspid inflow and RV outflow. The normal RIMP by spectral Doppler is <0.43 and by TDI is <0.54. Fractional area change is derived from the RV area traced at end-diastole and end-systole. The FAC calculation is similar to an ejection fraction calculation whereby the RV areas are substituted for the ventricular volumes. A normal FAC is >35%.

7. **Answer: C.** The measurement in **Figure 17-3** is performed on the tissue Doppler imaging (TDI) trace at the lateral tricuspid annulus and demonstrates a value of 0.07 m/s or 7 cm/s. The measurement shown is measured on the upward/positive peak systolic velocity; thus, this is the s' velocity. The normal s' wave measures >9.5 cm/s or >0.095 m/s.

   Both the peak e' velocity (answer A) and the peak IVC velocity (answer B) can be seen in **Figure 17-3**. The e' velocity represents the downward deflection in the trace during early diastole. The IVC velocity or spike is the upward deflection prior to the s' wave. Knowledge of the cardiac cycle can help in the assessment of the TDI signals and avoid potential measurement mistakes. TAPSE (answer D) is measured from an M-mode trace as the vertical distance between the end-diastolic trough and the systolic peak. A normal TAPSE measurement is >1.7 cm (17 mm).

8. **Answer: A.** The index of myocardial performance is calculated as:

$$IMP = (IVRT + IVCT) \div ET \qquad (1)$$

   where IMP = index of myocardial performance (unitless), IVCT = isovolumic contraction time (ms), IVRT = isovolumic relaxation time (ms), and ET = ejection time (ms).

Via the spectral Doppler method, the RIMP can by calculated from the time interval between tricuspid valve closure and the next tricuspid valve opening (TVCOt) or the duration of tricuspid regurgitation (TRd), and the ejection time (ET) measured from either the right ventricular outflow tract (RVOT) or pulmonary valve (PV) traces. TVCOt or the TRd is equivalent to [IVCT + ET + IVRT] (**Figure 17-15**). Therefore, [TVCOt − ET] or [TRd − ET] is the same as [IVCT + IVRT]. Thus,

$$RIMP = (TVCOt - ET) \div ET \qquad (2)$$

$$RIMP - (TRd - ET) \div ET \qquad (3)$$

   The normal value for RIMP via spectral Doppler is <0.43.

9. **Answer: B.** Annular dilatation and/or malposition of the papillary muscles leading to incomplete coaptation of the leaflets is the primary mechanism for functional mitral regurgitation (MR). Based on the Carpentier classification for functional MR, MR secondary to annular dilatation is functional type I MR (normal leaflet motion) and MR secondary to malposition of the papillary muscles is functional type IIIb (restricted leaflet motion during systole only). Valve prolapse and flail leaflets are examples of primary or organic causes of MR whereby MR occurs due to increased leaflet motion (Carpentier type II functional MR). A cleft mitral valve is another example of Carpentier type I functional MR.

10. **Answer: D.** In the setting of DCM or global remodeling, the assessment of secondary MR can be more challenging due to the often elliptical regurgitant orifice. In this instance, the EROA derived from the proximal isovelocity surface

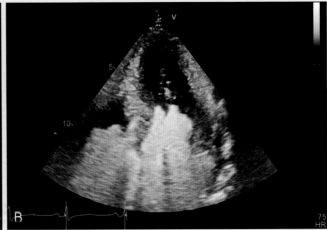

Figure 17-17 A, Diastolic frame. B, Systolic frame. Myocardial contrast images showing black, wedge-shaped thrombi within the apices of the left and right ventricles.

The use of ultrasound-enhancing agents can help delineate the ventricular shape and endocardial borders for better evaluation of thrombus or apical obliteration (**Video 17-4C** and **Figures 17-17A** and **17-17B**). HES can mimic apical hypertrophic cardiomyopathy with an appearance of the "ace of spades" presentation in the apical 4-chamber view.

Amyloidosis, Fabry disease, and sarcoidosis are all RCMs but have different echocardiographic features. The features associated with cardiac amyloidosis have been described previously (see answer outline for Question 13). Fabry disease is a storage-type RCM that mimics hypertrophic cardiomyopathy and not the apical variant of hypertrophic cardiomyopathy. Sarcoidosis is a multiorgan, inflammatory disorder characterized by granulomatous infiltration. Echocardiographic findings include regional wall thinning, wall motion abnormalities, systolic and diastolic dysfunction, reduced myocardial strain, and right ventricular, valvular, and pericardial involvement. The most common characteristic finding is thinning or aneurysm of the basal portion of the interventricular septum.

Apical 4-chamber images showing endocardial thickening with obliteration of the left and right ventricular apices caused by deposits of thrombus and eosinophils.

15. **Answer: A.** Restrictive cardiomyopathies are a group of heart muscle diseases that frequently look alike by echocardiography. They all have biatrial enlargement, normal or small LV cavity size, normal or increased LV wall thickness, preserved LV systolic function early in the disease (systolic dysfunction occurs in late stages), and abnormal diastolic function, frequently with a restrictive filling pattern. Biatrial dilatation occurs as a consequence of chronically elevated ventricular filling pressures.

16. **Answer: B.** RCM may be defined as any heart muscle disease that results in impaired ventricular filling with normal or reduced diastolic volumes of either or both ventricles with normal or near-normal systolic function. Therefore, the hallmark feature of RCM is abnormal diastolic function (grades I to III). Typical findings in RCM include reduced mitral annular tissue Doppler velocities (septal velocity e' <7 cm/s and a lateral e' <10 cm/s) and an increased average E/e' ratio (>14). As the disease process continues, the e' velocities will become less and less, making the E/e' ratio larger and larger.

Increased pulmonary venous systolic velocities (answer A) are seen in normal diastolic function. In abnormal restrictive filling, the pulmonary venous systolic velocity decreases as the filling pressure increases. Hepatic venous flow reversal during systole (answer C) is an important Doppler finding associated with severe tricuspid regurgitation. Increased forward flow during inspiration in the SVC (answer D) is an important Doppler characteristic when comparing constrictive pericarditis (CP) and chronic obstructive pulmonary disease (COPD). COPD can be a mimicker of CP but can be differentiated from CP by an increase in SVC forward flow during inspiration.

17. **Answer: D.** The characteristic clinical and pathophysiologic presentation of patients with RCM may be identical to that seen in patients with CP. Distinction between these two conditions is important as CP is a treatable cause of diastolic heart failure. All of the answers with the exception of answer D can be helpful in differentiating RCM from CP. In RCM, the septal e' velocity is ≤ lateral e' while in CP the septal e' velocity is > lateral e' with CP. In CP, the septal e' is normal or increased and the lateral e' is reduced due to lateral adhesion of the pericardium. When the

septal e′ exceeds lateral e′ velocity, this is referred to as "annulus reversus" (reverse of the normal situation where the septal e′ is < lateral e′ velocity).

KEY POINTS

In RCM, the septal e′ is decreased (<7 cm/s) due to an intrinsic decrease in myocardial relaxation. In contrast, the e′ is usually increased (≥9 cm/s) in CP because the longitudinal movement of the myocardium is enhanced due to the constricted radial expansion of the heart.

18. **Answer: D.** ARVC, formerly called arrhythmogenic right ventricular dysplasia (ARVD), is characterized by progressive loss of ventricular myocardium and fibrofatty infiltration. While the right ventricular myocardium is predominantly affected, left ventricular-dominant or biventricular forms are also recognized. ARVC is hereditary and is associated with mutations in genes encoding proteins of the intercalated disk. The disease classically manifests itself as ventricular arrhythmias or an episode of sudden death. The diagnosis of ARVC is based on the presence of major and minor criteria in six categories including global and/or regional dysfunction and structural alterations, tissue characterization, repolarization abnormalities on the electrocardiogram (ECG), depolarization/conduction abnormalities on the ECG, arrhythmias, and family history. The definitive diagnosis of ARVC requires two major criteria, or one major and two minor criteria, or four minor criteria from different categories.

The role of echocardiography in the diagnosis of ARVC is based on the identification of global or regional dysfunction and structural alterations to the right ventricle.

19. **Answer: A.** An epsilon wave is a small positive deflection or spike at the end of the QRS complex or buried within the QRS complex of the electrocardiogram (ECG) (**Figure 17-18**). The presence of an epsilon wave is a characteristic finding in ARVC and is a marker of delayed activation of the right ventricular free wall and outflow tract. The presence of an epsilon wave is one of the major diagnostic criteria for ARVC under the depolarization/conduction abnormalities in the ECG category; these waves are seen in 5% to 30% of patients with ARVC.

    Common causes for first-degree heart block (answer B) include myocarditis and acute myocardial infarction. Giant negative T waves (answer C) are seen in the apical variant of hypertrophic cardiomyopathy. Examples of low-voltage QRS complexes (answer D) across all leads of a 12-lead ECG include pericardial effusion or cardiac amyloidosis.

20. **Answer: C.** Echocardiographic findings of ARVC include regional right ventricular (RV) akinetic, dyskinetic or aneurysmal segments, and dilatation of the right ventricle, particularly the RV outflow tract. Other findings include increased echogenicity of the moderator band and abnormal trabeculations. Echocardiographic findings are variable and the use

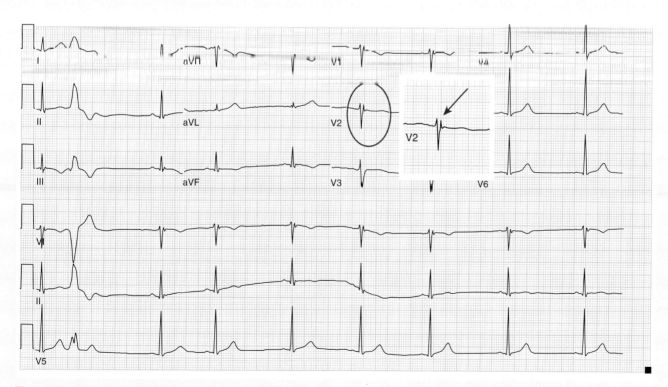

Figure 17-18 This 12-lead ECG shows an example of epsilon waves that are most notable in leads V1-V2 (arrow in zoomed insert).

RV Inflow View

V

RV

RA

A

B

45
HR

Figure 17-19 A, This cardiac magnetic resonance image demonstrates the fatty fibrous tissue and thinned myocardial wall (arrows). B, This image shows a thinned anterior wall of the right ventricle with a possible enhancement to the myocardium suggesting a fatty/fibrous tissue presence.

of other imaging techniques, such as cardiovascular magnetic resonance, may be more accurate for diagnosing ARVC.

Obstruction of the left ventricular outflow tract (answer A) is a finding in hypertension and hypertrophic cardiomyopathy patients. Both rigid, fixed tricuspid valve leaflets in semi-open position (answer B) and rigid pulmonary valve cusps causing stenosis (answer D) are findings in carcinoid heart disease patients.

21. **Answer: C.** As previously described, ARVC is anatomically characterized by fibrous or fibro-fatty replacement of myocardium. This results in myocardial thinning (**Figures 17-19A** and **17-19B**). The most commonly affected regions include the posterior and inferior areas of the right ventricular inflow tract adjacent to the tricuspid valve, the anterior infundibulum, and the apex, thus forming what is known as the "triangle of dysplasia."

22. **Answer: D.** The M-mode trace shows abnormal systolic anterior motion (SAM) of the mitral valve leaflets in a patient with hypertrophic obstructive cardiomyopathy (HOCM) (**Figure 17-20**, arrow). Several causes for mitral SAM have been proposed including the Venturi effect, malposition of the papillary muscles, drag forces, and displacement of the valve apparatus. The Venturi effect is described as a decrease in pressure when blood flows through a narrowing at a high velocity. This causes a suction effect. In HOCM, there is a narrowing of the left ventricular outflow tract (LVOT) due to increased thickness of the interventricular septum, which causes the anterior mitral leaflet and/or subvalvular apparatus to be displaced or "sucked" into the LVOT during systole.

23. **Answer: B.** Isovolumic periods are helpful in differentiating LVOT obstruction from MR on the

continuous-wave Doppler trace. The LVOT obstruction signal only occurs during the ejection time while MR is holosystolic, including the ejection time and the isovolumic periods (**Figure 17-21**).

24. **Answer: D.** Provocative maneuvers can assist in the differentiation between fixed and dynamic LVOT obstruction. With dynamic LVOT obstruction, the pressure gradient is dependent upon loading conditions and the contractile force of the left ventricle. Therefore, LVOT gradients can be provoked (or increased) by any maneuver that increases contractility, reduces left ventricular volume, and/or decreases resistance to left ventricular outflow. As such, the peak velocity arising from a dynamic LVOT obstruction increases with provocation while a fixed LVOT obstruction, as in the case of a subaortic membrane, will have no change in the peak velocity.

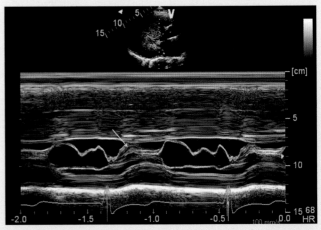

Figure 17-20 Systolic anterior motion of the mitral valve leaflet is demonstrated by the yellow arrow. Also observe the marked thickening of the interventricular septum.

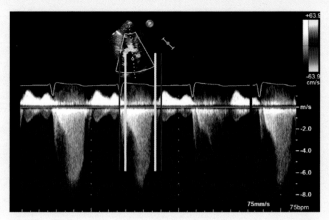

Figure 17-21 On the continuous-wave Doppler signal, both an LVOT obstruction signal and an MR signal are displayed. The LVOT signal includes the ejection time only (between the yellow lines). The duration of the MR signal (between the blue lines) is longer as this signal includes isovolumetric periods and the ejection time.

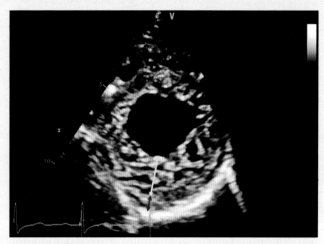

Figure 17-22 Yellow arrow shows the noncompacted myocardium and the purple arrow shows the compacted myocardium; measured at end-diastole.

The Valsalva maneuver is the most commonly utilized provocative maneuver. Other provocations include amyl nitrite inhalation, exercise, supine leg lifts, or rapid standing from a squatting position.

TEACHING POINT

PEDOF is the acronym for **P**ulsed **E**cho **DO**ppler **F**low velocity meter. This probe was originally used for pulsed-Doppler but was later developed exclusively for continuous-wave (CW) Doppler. This transducer is also known as the pencil probe, stand-alone probe, blind Doppler probe or the nonimaging CW Doppler probe.

25. **Answer: A.** The images provided demonstrate an apical hypertrophic cardiomyopathy. The apical variant typically presents as an "Ace of Spades" configuration in the standard 4-chamber view. The apical variant will present with thickened left ventricular walls in the apical segments with or without any basal segment thickening.

26. **Answer: B.** In some patients with hypertrophic obstructive cardiomyopathy, there may be no or only mild left ventricular outflow tract (LVOT) obstruction at rest. This is because the obstruction to flow across the LVOT is dynamic and is dependent upon loading conditions and the contractile force of the left ventricle. LVOT gradients can be provoked (or increased) by any maneuver that increases contractility, reduces left ventricular (LV) volume, and/or decreases resistance to LV outflow. In other words, the aim of provocative maneuvers is to decrease preload (reduce LV volume), decrease afterload (decrease resistance to LV outflow), or increase the force of LV contraction.

27. ⏵ **Answer: A.** LVNC is characterized by a thickened left ventricular wall consisting of two layers: a thin compacted epicardial layer and a thickened endocardial layer with numerous prominent trabeculae and deep intertrabecular recesses (noncompacted layer) (**Video 17-5**).

The ratio between the compacted (C) and non compacted (NC) layers is one of the criteria used to make the diagnosis of LVNC by echocardiography. An NC/C ratio >2 measured from a short-axis view at either end-systole (Jenni et al.) or end-diastole (Paterick et al.) are criteria for LVNC. Measurements at end-diastole are preferred by Paterick et al. as this timing was felt to better visualize the noncompacted portion that may be difficult to visualize at end-systole (**Figure 17-22**). Chin et al. defined LVNC as a ratio of C/(NC + C) < 0.5 assessed at end-diastole on short-axis or apical views.

The other criteria for LVNC include the presence of three or more trabeculations protruding from the left ventricular wall, apically to the papillary muscles, visible in a single image plane and evidence of flow within the intertrabecular spaces as seen by color Doppler (or ultrasound enhancing agents).

28. **Answer: B.** The areas of noncompaction are most commonly observed at the apex, the mid-inferior and the mid-lateral areas of the left ventricle. Importantly, at the apex the noncompacted myocardial layer is not always uniformly and evenly distributed. The noncompacted layer location may be regional, with the apicolateral wall segment most commonly involved. Awareness of the regional distribution of the noncompacted myocardium should lead to targeted imaging so that the diagnosis of LVNC is not missed.

29. **Answer: C.** The characteristic echocardiographic features of apical hypertrophic cardiomyopathy (HCM) include thickened middle to apical left ventricular segments, possible apical obliteration, and an apical pouch. The apical pouch usually presents at a later stage of apical HCM and is caused by cavity obstruction with continued high pressure in the apical region, which succumbs to the pressure and causes an outpouching.

30. **Answer: A.** Restrictive cardiomyopathies (RCM) incorporate a diverse group of myocardial diseases and may be defined as a myocardial disorder in which the heart muscle is structurally and functionally abnormal in the absence of coronary artery disease, systemic hypertension, valvular disease, or congenital heart disease. Therefore, coronary artery disease is not a cause of RCM. Potential secondary causes of RCM include infiltrative diseases such as amyloidosis, and storage diseases such as Gaucher disease, Fabry disease and hemochromatosis, inflammatory diseases such as sarcoidosis, and endomyocardial diseases such as endomyocardial fibrosis and hypereosinophilic syndrome.

31. **Answer: D.** The peak gradient derived from the mitral regurgitant (MR) signals represents the pressure difference between the left ventricle (LV) and left atrium (LA) during systole. Therefore, if the LA pressure is estimated or known, then the left ventricular systolic pressure (LVSP) can be estimated as:

$$LVSP = 4V_{MR^2} + LAP \qquad (1)$$

where $4V_{MR}^2$ = mitral regurgitant pressure gradient and LAP = left atrial pressure.

Then from the estimated LVSP and the systolic blood pressure (SBP), the LVOT gradient (ΔP_{LVOT}) can be estimated as:

$$\Delta P_{LVOT} = LVSP - SBP \qquad (2)$$

Therefore, answer D is correct since (MR$_{PG}$ + LAP) is the same as the LVSP. Hence, Equation (2) can also be written as:

$$\Delta P_{LVOT} = (MR_{PG} + LAP) - SBP \qquad (3)$$

32. **Answer: B.** As previously described, obstruction in hypertrophic obstructive cardiomyopathy (HOCM) is dynamic and, therefore, the degree of obstruction and resultant pressure gradient are dependent upon loading conditions and the contractile force of the left ventricle. Patients with HOCM can experience postprandial exacerbation following consumption of a meal. The effects of a meal on cardiovascular function are similar to those of an arterial vasodilator in that systemic vascular resistance falls, largely due to mesenteric vasodilatation, and a secondary increase in cardiac output occurs due to increased heart rate and stroke volume. Therefore, a postprandial rise in pressure gradient is due to a combination of increased contractility and decreased afterload.

33. **Answer: C.** Current American College of Cardiology and American Heart Association diagnostic criteria for hypertrophic cardiomyopathy (HCM) include a disease state characterized by unexplained left ventricular (LV) hypertrophy with a maximal LV wall thickness ≥15 mm. While asymmetric septal hypertrophy has long been recognized as a common feature of HCM, other morphologic variants of HCM include global/concentric hypertrophy, mid-ventricular hypertrophy with or without apical aneurysm, apical hypertrophy, and focal hypertrophy.

34. **Answer: C.** The incidence of SCD in young athletes (<35 years of age) ranges between 0.5 and 13 per 100,000. Studies have also shown a strong male preponderance for SCD, particularly in African American athletes who compete in sports with sudden movements and adrenergic surges such as football or basketball. When present, the most common structural heart diseases include hypertrophic cardiomyopathy, anomalous origin of a coronary artery, arrhythmogenic right/left ventricular cardiomyopathy, myocarditis, and coronary atherosclerosis.

35. **Answer: A.** Chagas disease, which is endemic in Latin American countries, is caused by a parasitic infection (*Trypanosoma cruzi*). Up to 30% of infected individuals eventually develop Chagas cardiomyopathy. This produces characteristic abnormalities such as biventricular enlargement, ventricular aneurysms, thinning of the ventricular wall, and thromboembolic complications. The hallmark of this disease is apical left ventricular aneurysms.

KEY POINT

Chagas cardiomyopathy has many clinical and imaging similarities to idiopathic dilated cardiomyopathy; however, one of the distinguishing hallmarks of Chagas disease is a left ventricular apical aneurysm.

36. **Answer: D.** Apical hypertrophic cardiomyopathy (HCM) initially presents with the "Ace of Spades" appearance with thickened apical wall segments. Often a middle-to-apical obstruction causes early obstruction in systole, increasing volume and pressure in the far apical segments. Over time this may cause a pouch in the apical region. The Doppler trace shown in **Figure 17-9** represents a case of apical HCM with pouch. On this trace, early systolic flow is seen (**Figure 17-23**, yellow arrow), followed by mid-ventricular cavity obstruction with no flow and then a high early diastolic velocity from the apex to base concurrent with the transmitral E wave (**Figure 17-23**, blue arrow). This paradoxical early diastolic flow is thought to represent blood trapped in the apical cavity in systole, which subsequently leaves the apex in early diastole when the ventricle begins to relax and dilate.

37. **Answer: B.** The CW Doppler trace shows classic dynamic LVOT obstruction, which is characterized by a late-peaking, dagger shape. This can easily be

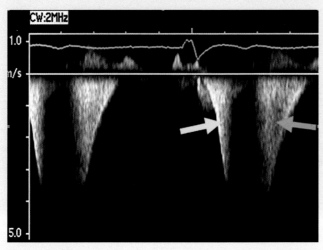

Figure 17-23

mistaken for aortic stenosis or MR. Aortic stenosis (answer A) would have a more mid-systolic peak with symmetry of both sides of the waveform. MR due to mitral valve prolapse (answer D) often peaks in mid-to-late systole. However, the signal shown terminates before the onset of mitral inflow. MR

traces are contiguous with mitral forward flow. CW Doppler traces associated with a fixed obstruction, as in the case of a subaortic membrane (answer C), display a peak velocity earlier in systole, similar to aortic stenosis signals.

38. **Answer: B.** Patients with HCM will have abnormal diastolic filling profiles, including decreased mitral annulus tissue Doppler velocities. Trained athletes will exhibit a normal or supranormal diastolic function with preserved mitral annulus tissue Doppler velocities.

    Chamber dimensions (answer B) may be useful as cardiac remodeling can result in increases in the left ventricular (LV) size, whereas patients with HCM tend to have a normal LV size (but may be increased at end stages). Gender (answer C) does have some value as highly trained female athletes rarely demonstrate LV wall thickness >11 mm. Therefore, multiple parameters need to be included in the assessment of HCM. Left ventricular wall thickness (answer D) tends to overlap with up to 2% of highly trained athletes having a septal thickness of 13 to 15 mm. The physiological upper limit of normal for a highly trained athlete, however, is 16 mm.

SUGGESTED READINGS

Afonso L, Bernal J, Bax J, Abraham T. Echocardiography in hypertrophic cardiomyopathy: the role of conventional and emerging. *JACC Cardiovasc Imaging.* 2008;1(6):787-800.

Acquatella H, Asch FM, Barbosa MM, et al. Recommendations for multimodality cardiac imaging in patients with Chagas disease: a report from the American Society of Echocardiography in Collaboration with the InterAmerican Association of Echocardiography (ECOSIAC) and the Cardiovascular Imaging Department of the Brazilian Society of Cardiology (DIC-SBC). *J Am Soc Echocardiogr.* 2018;31(1):3-23.

Chin TK, Perloff JK, Williams RG, Jue K, Mohrmann R. Isolated non-compaction of left ventricular myocardium. A study of eight cases. *Circulation.* 1990;82(2):507-513.

Geske JB, Oh JK. Cardiomyopathies. In: Oh JK, Kane GC, Seward JB, Tajik AJ, eds. *The Echo Manual.* 4th ed. Philadelphia, PA and Rochester, MN: Wolters Kluwer; 2019:chap 10.

Ha JW, Oh JK, Ling LH, et al. Annulus paradoxus: transmitral flow velocity to mitral annular velocity ratio is inversely proportional to pulmonary capillary wedge pressure in patients with constrictive pericarditis. *Circulation.* 2001;104(9):976-978.

Habib G, Bucciarelli-Ducci C, Caforio AL, et al. Multimodality imaging in restrictive cardiomyopathies: an EACVI expert consensus document in collaboration with the "Working Group on myocardial and pericardial diseases" of the European Society of Cardiology Endorsed by the Indian Academy of Echocardiography. *Eur Heart J Cardiovasc Imaging.* 2017;18(10):1090-1121.

Haugaa KH. Arrhythmogenic right ventricular cardiomyopathy, clinical manifestations, and diagnosis. *Europace.* 2016;18(7):965-972.

Jenni R, Oechslin E, Schneider J, Jost C, Kaufmann P. Echocardiographic and pathoanatomical characteristics of isolated left ventricular non-compaction: a step towards classification as a distinct cardiomyopathy. *Heart.* 2001;86(6):666-671.

Lang RM, Badano LP, Mor-Avi V, et al. Recommendations for cardiac chamber quantification by echocardiography in adults: an update from the American Society of Echocardiography and the European Association of Cardiovascular Imaging. *J Am Soc Echocardiogr.* 2015;28(1):1-39.

Maron B, Ommen S, Semsarian C, et al. Hypertrophic cardiomyopathy, present and future. *J Am Coll Cardiol.* 2014;64(1):83-99.

Mathew T, Williams L, Navaratnam G, et al. Diagnosis and assessment of dilated cardiomyopathy: a guideline protocol from the British Society of Echocardiography. *Echo Res Pract.* 2017;4(2):G1-G13.

Ommen SR, Seward JB, Tajik AJ. Clinical and echocardiographic features of hypereosinophilic syndromes. *Am J Cardiol.* 2000;86(1):110-113.

Paterick TE, Umland MM, Jan MF, et al. Left ventricular noncompaction: a 25-year odyssey. *J Am Soc Echocardiogr.* 2012;25(4):363-375.

Phelan D, Collier P, Thavendiranathan P, et al. Relative apical sparing of longitudinal strain using two-dimensional speckle-tracking echocardiography is both sensitive and specific for the diagnosis of cardiac amyloidosis. *Heart.* 2012;98(19):1442-1448.

Seward JB, Casaclang-Verosa G. Infiltrative cardiovascular diseases: cardiomyopathies that look alike. *J Am Coll Cardiol.* 2010;55(17):1769-1779.

Welch TD, Ling LH, Espinosa RE, et al. Echocardiographic diagnosis of constrictive pericarditis: Mayo Clinic criteria. *Circ Cardiovasc Imaging.* 2014;7(3):526-534.

CHAPTER 18

Diseases of Aorta

Contributors: Bharatbhushan Patel, RDCS, RDMS, RVS and Keith A. Collins, MS, RDCS

✪ Question 1

According to the recommendations of the American Society of Echocardiography (ASE), which of the following statements regarding measurements of the ascending aorta on an adult transthoracic echocardiogram (TTE) is true?

A. Measurements should be performed via two-dimensional (2D) or M-mode echocardiography in systole.

B. Measurements are performed from inner edge to inner edge at end-diastole.

C. Measurements should be interpreted when indexed to an individual's height and weight.

D. Measurements are best performed from the standard parasternal long-axis view.

✪ Question 2

On **Figure 18-1** of the aorta, which is the segment of the aorta marked by the letter "A"?

A. Abdominal aorta

B. Arch of aorta

C. Descending aorta

D. Ascending aorta

✪✪ Question 3

The three arteries labeled 1, 2 and 3 in **Figure 18-1** are:

A. 1 = Innominate, 2 = left common carotid, and 3 = left subclavian.

B. 1 = Left carotid, 2 = vertebral, and 3 = subclavian.

C. 1 = Vertebral, 2 = left common carotid, and 3 = right common carotid.

D. 1 = Left common carotid, 2 = right common carotid, and 3 = subclavian arteries.

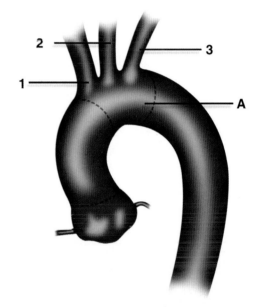

Figure 18-1 (Reprinted with permission from Grover F, Mack MJ. *Cardiac Surgery.* 1st ed. Philadelphia, PA: Wolters Kluwer; 2016.)

✪ Question 4

Which of the statements below for differentiating the abdominal aorta from the inferior vena cava (IVC) from the subcostal window is true?

A. The abdominal aorta has systolic pulsations and a more horizontal course compared to the IVC.

B. The course of the abdominal aorta is more vertical compared to the IVC, which courses more horizontally.

C. During normal respiration, the abdominal aorta does not vary in size while the IVC size increases with inspiration.

D. On pulsed-wave (PW) Doppler, the flow in the abdominal aorta is away from the transducer while IVC flow is continuous.

✪✪ Question 5

The type of aortic dissection shown in **Figure 18-2** is a:
A. Stanford A or DeBakey III.
B. Stanford B or DeBakey I.
C. Stanford A or DeBakey II.
D. Stanford A or DeBakey I.

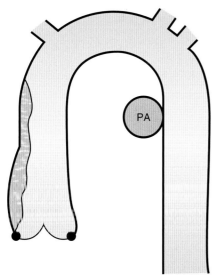

Figure 18-2 (Reprinted with permission from Armstrong WF, Ryan T. *Feigenbaum's Echocardiography*. 8th ed. Philadelphia, PA: Wolters Kluwer; 2019:629.)

✪ Question 6

Which of the following is the least likely cause of a thoracic aortic aneurysm (TAA)?
A. Connective tissue disorders
B. Hypertension
C. Atherosclerosis
D. Chronic dissection
E. Primary infection of the aorta

✪ Question 7

The most common site for the formation of a thoracic aortic aneurysm (TAA) is the:
A. Proximal ascending aorta.
B. Distal descending aorta.
C. Aortic arch.
D. All of the above.

✪✪ Question 8

A transesophageal echocardiogram (TEE) is performed on a patient with recent history of multiple ischemic lesions, identified on a computed tomography (CT) scan of the head. Based on **Figure 18-3** shown of the aortic arch, which statement best describes the finding?

A. There is a large aortic atheroma.
B. There is an intramural thrombus.
C. There is a heavily calcified atheromatous plaque.
D. There is a mural thrombus.

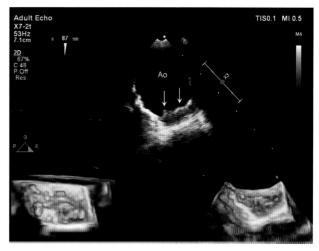

Figure 18-3 (Reprinted with permission from Armstrong WF, Ryan T. Diseases of the aorta. In: *Feigenbaum's Echocardiography*. 8th ed. Philadelphia, PA: Wolters Kluwer; 2019:643, chap 20.)

✪✪✪ Question 9

▶ A 77-year-old man has a transesophageal echocardiogram (TEE) for a suspected aortic dissection. Based on **Figure 18-4** and **Video 18-1**, which statement is most accurate regarding the descending aorta?
A. The images show the ostium of the right bronchial artery and an atheroma.
B. There is an intramural hematoma with a penetrating atherosclerotic lesion.
C. There is an intramural hematoma with a classic aortic dissection.
D. There is a focal thoracic aortic aneurysm with atheroma.

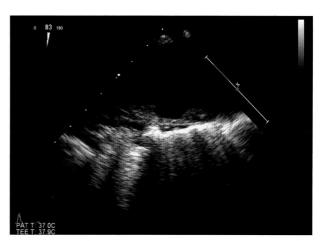

Figure 18-4 Long-axis image of the descending aorta.

✪✪ Question 10

▶ A 25-year-old woman with complex medical history (lupus nephritis, end-stage renal disease, Raynaud phenomenon, and hypertension) presents with increasing shortness of breath and a loud diastolic murmur. A transthoracic exam is quickly performed and shows a trileaflet aortic valve. Based on the transthoracic echocardiographic (TTE) images provided (**Video 18-2A** and **Video 18-2B**), what is the likely course of treatment?

A. Surgery for an aortic aneurysm and an aortic valve replacement for aortic regurgitation (AR) is required when the patient is more stable.

B. Surgery for an aortic root replacement with aortic valve sparing is required when the patient is more stable.

C. Urgent surgery for acute severe AR is required.

D. Urgent surgery is required to repair an acute aortic dissection with an aortic valve repair or replacement.

✪✪ Question 11

Which of the following statements regarding aortic aneurysms is true?

A. The majority of aortic aneurysms are saccular.

B. True aneurysms involve all three layers of the arterial wall.

C. True aneurysms only involve the intima and media.

D. Pseudoaneurysms occur due to focal rupture of the aortic wall that is contained by the pericardium.

E. Pseudoaneurysms of the aorta are more common than true aortic aneurysms.

✪ Question 12

Which of the following clinical signs of acute aortic dissection is least likely to occur?

A. Chest pain

B. Shoulder and lower back pain

C. Normal blood pressure in both upper extremities

D. Shortness of breath

✪✪ Question 13

Which of the following statements regarding a means to distinguish the true lumen from the false lumen in a patient with an aortic dissection is correct?

A. The true lumen is bigger in size than the false lumen.

B. The true lumen has slow flow and thrombosis.

C. The true lumen expands during systole.

D. The true lumen shows retrograde flow.

E. All the above.

✪✪✪ Question 14

Which of the following is not a common finding of Takayasu arteritis?

A. Aortic aneurysm of ascending aorta

B. Narrowing of the coronary artery ostia

C. Narrowing of cerebral branches with possible obstruction

D. Aortic dissection

E. B and D

✪✪ Question 15

As a young child, this patient with Turner syndrome underwent a surgical repair of aortic coarctation. She presents with uncontrolled hypertension and lower extremity pain. The spectral Doppler tracing in **Figure 18-5** shows:

A. Evidence of re-coarctation of aorta.

B. A poor Doppler tracing due to suboptimal Doppler alignment.

C. An uninterpretable Doppler signal without signals proximal to the coarctation repair site.

D. A Doppler pattern of aortic insufficiency.

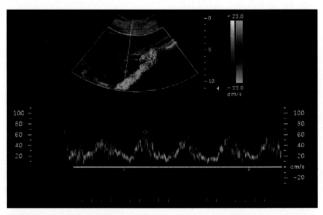

Figure 18-5 (Reprinted with permission from Klein AL, Asher CR. *Clinical Echocardiography Review: a Self-Assessment Tool.* 2nd ed. Philadelphia, PA: Wolters Kluwer; 2017.)

✪✪ Question 16

A 26-year-old woman with a bicuspid valve, trace aortic regurgitation (AR), and an episode of chest pain is referred from an outside hospital. What can be said regarding the continuous-wave (CW) Doppler tracing (**Figure 18-6**) obtained from the suprasternal notch?

A. The peak pressure gradient obtained by the simplified Bernoulli equation will equal the pressure gradient obtained at cardiac catheterization.

B. The peak pressure gradient obtained by the simplified Bernoulli equation will be less than that obtained at cardiac catheterization.

C. The peak pressure gradient obtained by the simplified Bernoulli equation will be greater than that obtained at cardiac catheterization.

D. The peak pressure gradient obtained by the simplified Bernoulli equation will equal the pressure gradient obtained at cardiac catheterization, with correction for the AR diastolic flow reversal.

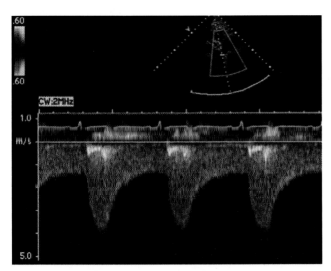

Figure 18-6 (Reprinted with permission from Klein AL, Asher CR. *Clinical Echocardiography Review: a Self-Assessment Tool.* 2nd ed. Philadelphia, PA: Wolters Kluwer; 2017.)

✪✪ Question 17

A 28-year-old asymptomatic man with a bicuspid aortic valve (BAV) is shown to have a dilated aortic root (**Figure 18-7**). In this patient, which statement is false?

A. The aortic arch is likely enlarged.

B. A coarctation of the aorta is highly probable.

C. Surgical intervention is indicated.

D. Marfan syndrome cannot be excluded.

E. B and D.

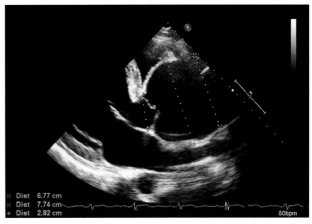

Figure 18-7

✪ Question 18

Marfan syndrome is commonly related to aortic disease. Which statement is correct?

A. Aortic aneurysms are more common in the region above the aortic root.

B. A descending aortic aneurysm without an ascending aortic aneurysm is rare.

C. Isolated abdominal aortic aneurysms are common.

D. An "onion bulb" appearance with dilatation of the aortic root, sinotubular effacement, and normal size ascending aorta is commonly seen.

✪✪✪ Question 19

A patient undergoing a transesophageal echocardiogram (TEE) is found to have an atheroma in the descending thoracic aorta measuring 11 mm in thickness (**Figure 18-8**). Based on the 2D echocardiographic appearances, this atheroma is graded as:

A. Grade 1.

B. Grade 2.

C. Grade 3.

D. Grade 4.

E. Grade 5.

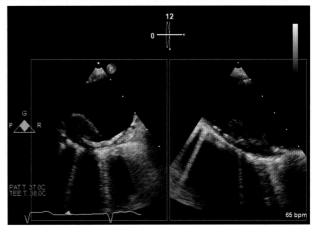

Figure 18-8

✪✪ Question 20

▶ A 67-year-old man presents to the emergency room with extreme dyspnea and chest pain. He reports emergent aortic valve replacement 3 years ago after type A dissection and recently, frequent fevers. A transesophageal echocardiogram (TEE) is performed with the following images: long-axis and short-axis biplane views (**Video 18-3A**), color Doppler short-axis view (**Video 18-3B**), biplane views with color Doppler at ascending aortic level (**Figure 18-9A**), and at the distal arch level (**Figure 18-9B**). Which statement best describes the findings of the TEE?

A. There is an abscess with thrombus, hematoma, and/or infection surrounding the ascending aorta.

B. There is a dissection flap with multiple fenestrations between the true and false lumens.

C. There is thrombosis within the false lumen at the level of the distal arch.

D. A and C.

E. All of the above.

✪✪✪ Question 21

▶ A 21-year-old woman with bipolar disease and unknown cardiac history except a murmur noted from her referring physician presents for a transthoracic echocardiogram (TTE). The TTE shows a mildly enlarged left ventricle (LV) with normal systolic function, normal right ventricular (RV) size and systolic function, and mild pulmonary hypertension. Based on the images provided (**Figure 18-10A** and **18-10B** and **Video 18-4A** and **18-4B**), which statement best describes the findings?

A. There is a right sinus of Valsalva aneurysm that has ruptured into the right atrium (RA).

B. There is a right coronary artery fistula with connection to the RA.

C. There is a Gerbode-type defect with shunting from the LV into the RA.

D. There is a dilated right coronary artery with an eccentric jet of tricuspid regurgitation.

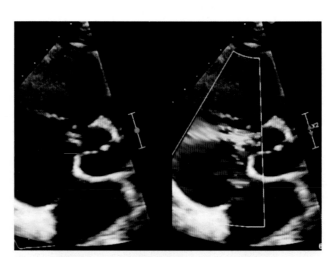

Figure 18-10A

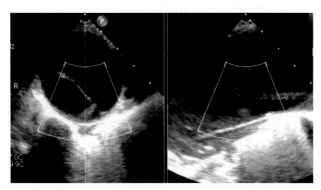

Figure 18-9A

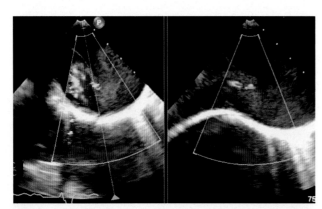

Figure 18-9B

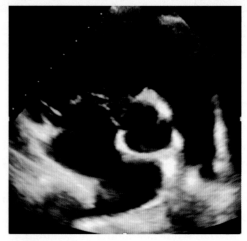

Figure 18-10B

⭐ Question 22

A 24-year-old male intravenous drug user presents to the emergency department. A transthoracic echocardiogram (TTE) reveals multiple mobile thrombi extending from the tricuspid valve to the right ventricular outflow tract (RVOT). This image obtained from the subcostal position (**Figure 18-11**) shows a mass in the abdominal aorta. This patient likely has:

A. An invasive tumor.

B. A large calcified atherosclerotic plaque.

C. A dissection of the abdominal aorta.

D. A large, occlusive aortic thrombus.

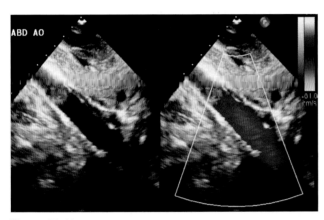

Figure 18-11

⭐⭐⭐ Question 23

A 60-year-old man with complex cardiac history of ischemic cardiomyopathy, coronary artery bypass grafts (CABG), a mitral valve ring and hyperlipidemia presents with syncope, fever, and shortness of breath. Due to poor image quality on the transthoracic examination, a transesophageal echocardiogram (TEE) was performed to assess for bacteremia. **Figure 18-12** was

obtained at the level of the upper descending thoracic aorta. This image most likely shows:

A. A complex atherosclerotic plaque.

B. An intramural hematoma (IMH) with intimal calcification.

C. A type B dissection with thrombus in the false lumen.

D. An IMH with a penetrating ulcer.

⭐⭐ Question 24

A thin 55-year-old man presents to the emergency department with chest pain and hypertensive crisis after cocaine use. A faint systolic flow murmur is heard. Echocardiographic images, with and without color Doppler, were obtained from the subcostal and suprasternal notch positions (**Figure 18-13**). Which statement best describes the findings?

A. There is a type B dissection with coarctation of the descending aorta.

B. There is a type B dissection, which begins in the proximal descending thoracic aorta and extends to the abdominal aorta.

C. There is a probable type A dissection, which cannot be seen from these images.

D. There is a type A dissection, which requires immediate surgery.

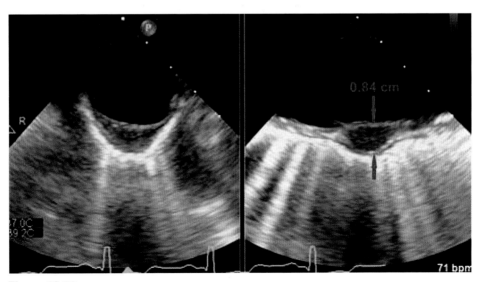

Figure 18-12

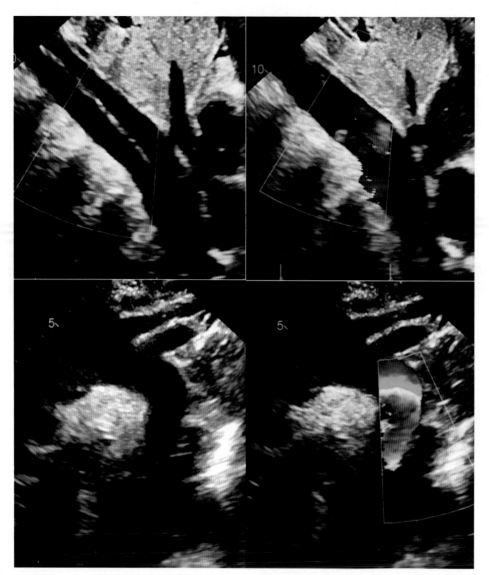

Figure 18-13 Top: Subcostal images. Bottom: Suprasternal images.

✪✪✪ Question 25

A 68-year-old man presents with atrial fibrillation, hypertension, heart failure with preserved ejection fraction (HFpEF), and a continuous, grade 2/6 left subclavicular murmur. **Figure 18-14** was acquired from the suprasternal notch position. Which additional finding would most support the need for intervention in this patient?

A. Dilated right ventricle (RV)
B. Bicuspid aortic valve (BAV)
C. Dilated left ventricle (LV)
D. QP:QS of 1.4
E. All of the above

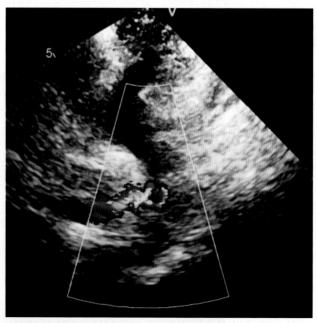

Figure 18-14

✪ Question 26

Which of the following correctly lists the sites of a sinus of Valsalva aneurysm (from most common to least common)?

- **A.** Right coronary sinus, noncoronary sinus, left coronary sinus
- **B.** Left coronary sinus, noncoronary sinus, right coronary sinus
- **C.** Right coronary sinus, left coronary sinus, noncoronary sinus
- **D.** Noncoronary sinus, right coronary sinus, left coronary sinus

✪✪ Question 27

Which of the following is a known cause of a sinus of Valsalva (SOV) aneurysm?

- **A.** Connective tissue disorders
- **B.** Infection
- **C.** Chest trauma
- **D.** Bicuspid aortic valve (BAV)
- **E.** All of the above

✪✪✪ Question 28

A 51-year-old woman with uncontrolled hypertension presents with a loud diastolic murmur. The transthoracic echocardiogram (TTE) shows moderate aortic regurgitation (AR) and an aortic root measuring 62 mm. Which statement best describes the abnormality shown in **Figure 18-15A to 18-15C?**

- **A.** There is a sinus of Valsalva (SOV) aneurysm arising from the right coronary cusp.
- **B.** There is an aortic root pseudoaneurysm mimicking an SOV aneurysm.
- **C.** There is an SOV aneurysm arising from the noncoronary cusp.
- **D.** There is a noncoronary SOV aneurysm that has ruptured.
- **E.** This SOV aneurysm is relatively benign and requires regular monitoring.

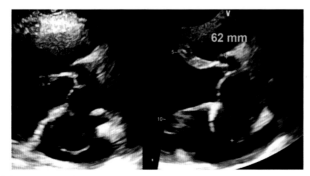

Figure 18-15A

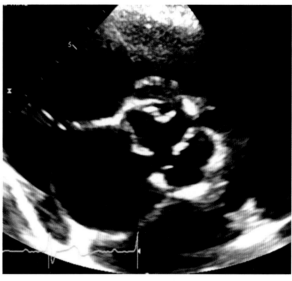

Figure 18-15B

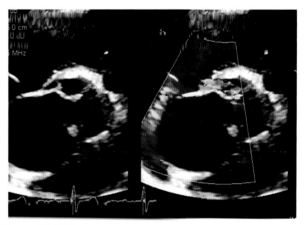

Figure 18-15C

✪ Question 29

The part of the aorta that is most vulnerable to blunt trauma is the:

- **A.** Abdominal aorta.
- **B.** Aortic isthmus.
- **C.** Aortic arch.
- **D.** Ascending aorta.
- **E.** Descending aorta.

✪✪✪ Question 30

Which of the following statements regarding a "bovine" aortic anomaly is correct?

- **A.** A bovine aorta is defined as the left subclavian artery arising from the innominate artery.
- **B.** A bovine aortic branching pattern is present in 1% of individuals.
- **C.** A bovine aorta is readily detectable from a standard parasternal long-axis image.
- **D.** A bovine aorta is defined as the left common carotid artery arising from a common origin with the innominate artery.

ANSWERS

1. **Answer: C.** In adults, aortic dimensions are strongly correlated to age, gender, and body surface area (BSA). Therefore, measurements should be interpreted when indexed to an individual's height and weight (see **Figure 18-16** showing normal thoracic aortic sizes by echocardiography).

   The ASE-recommended method for performing aortic measurements in adults is leading-edge-to-leading-edge, at end-diastole, and perpendicular to the long axis of the aorta. As the tubular ascending aorta is often not adequately visualized from a standard parasternal window, imaging of the ascending aorta is improved by moving the transducer closer to the sternum and up one or two intercostal spaces. The ascending aorta may be well visualized from right parasternal windows (second or third intercostal spaces), especially when the aorta is dilated. Correlation between computed tomography or magnetic resonance imaging of the ascending aortic dimensions is useful when TTE image quality precludes measurement.

   If alignment allows, M-mode may be used to measure the ascending aorta. However, 2D echocardiographic measurements of the aortic root are preferable to M-mode measurements, because cardiac motion may result in changes in the position of the M-mode cursor relative to the maximum diameter of the sinuses of Valsalva and this translational motion may result in systematic underestimation of the aortic root.

   Of note, in the pediatric population, the recommended method for aortic measurements is the inner edge to inner edge convention at mid-systole.

Since these adult and pediatric guidelines are not aligned, it is important to recognize measurement differences as pediatric patients transition to adults. Also, measurements made in systole may be 1 to 2 mm greater than those made in diastole for younger patients with compliant aortas.

KEY POINTS
The size of the aorta correlates well when indexed to the height and weight of the patient (BSA). In adults, the aorta is measured perpendicular to the long axis of the aorta at end-diastole, using leading-edge-to-leading-edge convention. In pediatric populations, the aorta is measured in mid-systole, via the inner edge to inner edge convention.

2. **Answer: B.** The aorta consists of five main anatomic segments: the aortic root, the tubular portion of the ascending aorta, the aortic arch, the descending thoracic aorta, and the abdominal aorta. The aortic arch extends from the innominate (brachiocephalic) to the left subclavian artery; the aortic arch gives rise to the three major head and neck vessels.

   The aortic root is the section of the aorta between the left ventricular outflow tract (LVOT) and the peripheral attachment of the aortic cusps to the sinotubular (ST) junction. The ascending aorta, which is approximately 5 cm in length, extends from the ST junction and terminates at the origin of the innominate artery. The descending thoracic aorta extends from the left subclavian artery to the diaphragm. The abdominal aorta extends from below the diaphragm to the bifurcation of the aorta into the common iliac arteries.

3. **Answer: A.** All three head and neck vessels arise from the aortic arch; these vessels include the innominate (brachiocephalic) artery (1 on **Figure 18-1**), the left common carotid artery (2 on **Figure 18-1**), and the left subclavian artery (3 on **Figure 18-1**).

TEACHING POINT
The innominate artery is also often referred to as the brachiocephalic trunk or brachiocephalic artery. This artery bifurcates into the right subclavian and right common carotid arteries.

4. **Answer: B.** The abdominal aorta courses more vertically compared to the IVC, which courses more horizontally (**Figure 18-17**). The abdominal aorta also shows systolic pulsations while the IVC size varies with respiration and decreases in size with inspiration. On the PW Doppler examination, aortic flow is systolic and directed toward the transducer while IVC flow is continuous with forward flow directed away from the transducer.

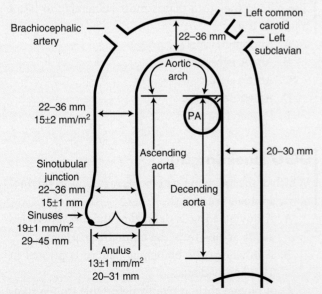

Brachiocephalic artery

Left common carotid

Left subclavian

22–36 mm

Aortic arch

PA

22–36 mm
15±2 mm/m²

Ascending aorta

20–30 mm

Sinotubular junction
22–36 mm
15±1 mm

Decending aorta

Sinuses
19±1 mm/m²
29–45 mm

Anulus
13±1 mm/m²
20–31 mm

Figure 18-16 (Reprinted with permission from Armstrong WF, Ryan T. *Feigenbaum's Echocardiography.* 8th ed. Philadelphia, PA: Wolters Kluwer; 2019:613.)

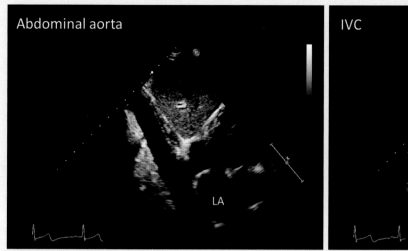
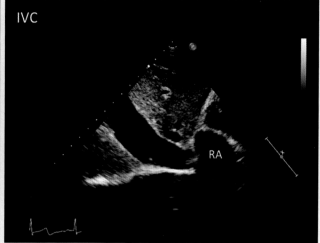

Figure 18-17 The abdominal aorta (left) courses vertically and passes posterior to the left atrium (LA). The IVC (right) courses more horizontally and drains into the right atrium (RA).

KEY POINTS

Differentiation of the abdominal aorta from the IVC can be made by recognition of the systolic pulsations of the aorta and the more vertical course of the aorta. The IVC can be identified based on its variation in size with respiration; it also has a more horizontal course compared to the aorta. In addition, the hepatic veins can usually be seen draining into the IVC and the IVC can be followed to confirm its drainage into the right atrium. On PW Doppler, the aortic flow is systolic and is directed toward the transducer, so flow appears above the zero baseline. IVC flow is continuous and forward flow is directed away from the transducer so appears below the zero baseline.

5. **Answer: C.** There are several classification systems developed to describe aortic dissection (**Table 18-1**). The two most commonly used are DeBakey type I, II, and III and Stanford type A and B. The DeBakey classification is based on location and extent of the aortic dissection, whereas the Stanford classification is based on whether the dissection is located in the proximal or distal aorta. The Svensson classification has classes 1 to 5 and is based on the pathophysiology of aortic syndrome. This patient has a Stanford A and DeBakey II dissection, as the ascending aorta alone is involved.

6. **Answer: E.** An aneurysm is defined as an enlargement to more than 1.5 times the normal dimension for that part of aorta. There are numerous etiologies for a TAA. Of these, aneurysmal formation from true primary bacterial infection of the ascending aortic wall is rare, and results from either an episode of bacterial endocarditis or from infection of a laminar clot within a previously formed aneurysm.

TAA due to connective tissue disorder (answer A) is common and occurs as a result of medial degeneration, which is characterized by disruption and loss of elastic fibers, increased deposition

Table 18-1. Classification of Aortic Dissection Involving the Thoracic Aorta

DeBakey Classification	Region of Aorta Involved
Type I	Ascending, arch +/− descending
Type II	Ascending only
Type IIIa	Descending (above diaphragm)
Type IIIb	Descending (below diaphragm)
Stanford Classification	**Region of Aorta Involved**
Type A	Ascending and/or arch +/− descending
Type B	Descending only (distal to left subclavian artery)
Svensson Classification	**Type of Aortic Syndrome**
Class 1	Classic intimal flap (two lumens)
Class 2	Intramural hematoma (no intimal tear or flap)
Class 3	Localized intimal flap (discrete/subtle dissection)
Class 4	Penetrating aortic ulcer
Class 5	Iatrogenic/posttraumatic

of proteoglycans, and loss of smooth muscle cells within the media. Aneurysmal aortic dilatation as a result of hypertension (answer B) occurs due to increased stress on the aortic lumen. TAAs are also associated with risk factors for atherosclerosis (answer C); atherosclerosis is a major cause of abdominal aortic aneurysm. A chronic dissection (answer D) can also lead to progressive aortic expansion; these aneurysms are frequently referred to as a "dissecting aneurysm" or "aneurysmal dissection."

Aortic dilatation is a nonspecific term that encompasses both ectasia and aneurysm. Ectasia is defined as aortic dilation up to 50% greater than the normal reference diameter, and aneurysm is defined as greater than 50% dilation. There are numerous etiologies for a TAA including at risk for atherosclerosis, connective tissue disorders, prior aortic dissection, chest trauma, bicuspid aortic valve, and aortic infection.

7. **Answer: A.** TAA can involve one or more aortic segments including the aortic root, ascending aorta, aortic arch, or descending aorta. Sixty percent of TAAs involve the aortic root and/or ascending tubular aorta, 40% involve the descending aorta, 10% involve the arch, and 10% involve the thoracoabdominal aorta.

8. **Answer: A.** The TEE image shown in **Figure 18-3** was recorded in the short-axis view of the arch of the aorta in a patient with moderate atheromatous involvement. The central figure is the 2D image in which complex atheroma is noted predominantly between 3 o'clock and 6 o'clock (*arrows*). The two insets are real-time three-dimensional images of the same area of the aorta more clearly demonstrating the diffuse nature of the complex atheroma with multiple protruding components and the suggestion of an ulcerated atheroma in the inset at the lower left.

By TEE, any irregular thickening of ≥2 mm is considered to be an atheroma.

While aortic thrombi may also form in areas of aortic aneurysm, they usually appear as mural, layered, and not pedunculated. The irregular surface is demonstrated with these 2D and 3D images. Nor does the mass appear to be intramural, as the edges are relatively distinct from the intima. This excludes answers B and D. While most sources of emboli from the aorta are related to complex atherosclerotic plaques, this mass appears bright but not significantly calcified. Therefore, answer C is incorrect.

9. **Answer: B.** A penetrating atherosclerotic or aortic ulcer (PAU) appears as a crater-like "pocket" or "divot" within the aortic wall. There is also an associated intramural hematoma that appears as a hypoechoic thickening of the aortic wall.

A PAU is one of the three conditions included in acute aortic syndromes (AAS); the other two conditions include aortic dissection and intramural hematoma (IMH). A PAU forms when an atherosclerotic lesion with ulceration penetrates the internal elastic lamina and allows hematoma formation within the media of the aortic wall. Consequences of a penetrating ulcer include a saccular aneurysm, pseudoaneurysm, aortic dissection, or aortic rupture. Clinically, PAU presents in a manner similar to that of aortic dissection. Risk factors for complications include the depth and diameter of the outpouching. A symptomatic penetrating ulcer is an acute aortic syndrome and surgery should be considered.

KEY POINTS

Penetrating aortic ulcers are characterized by:
1. Calcified plaque
2. Crater-like pouch
3. Complications that can include aortic dissection, saccular aneurysm, or aortic rupture

10. **Answer: D.** The image shown in **Video 18-2A** was acquired from the zoomed parasternal long-axis view and **Video 18-2B** was acquired from a high parasternal window. There is a type A aortic dissection with mobile anterior intimal flap. There is also significant aortic regurgitation (AR) present. A type A aortic dissection is a surgical emergency because of the high mortality rates associated with this condition. Therefore, urgent surgery is required to repair the acute aortic dissection and the aortic valve. Numerous aortic valve sparing procedures have been successfully performed with supracoronary aortic grafting; however, replacement of the aorta alone will not likely resolve aortic regurgitation in this setting. AR is common in the setting of a type A aortic dissection. The mechanisms for AR in a type A dissection include (1) incomplete closure of a normal aortic valve due to sinotubular junction (STJ) dilatation; (2) aortic valve prolapse due to extension of the dissection into the aortic root, which disrupts normal leaflet attachments to the aortic wall; (3) prolapse of the dissection flap through normal aortic valve leaflets, disrupting leaflet coaptation; (4) loss of annular support or tearing of the leaflets themselves may render the valve incompetent; and (5) associated primary valve abnormalities such as a bicuspid aortic valve (BAV).

TEE can accurately distinguish the mechanism of AR as well as the severity and aid the surgeon in determining the feasibility of repair. Computed tomography of the aorta can help define the part(s) of the aorta that are dissected and demonstrate blood flow between the false and true lumen.

KEY POINTS

▶ Type A aortic dissection is a surgical emergency.

▶ Aortic regurgitation (AR) is common in type A aortic dissections.

▶ Mechanisms of AR include annular dilatation, leaflet prolapse, flap prolapse into the left ventricular outflow tract, loss of annular support or tearing of leaflets, and primary valve abnormalities such as a BAV.

▶ Aortic valve sparing procedures are feasible in many patients with type A aortic dissection depending on the mechanism and severity of AR.

11. Answer: B. A true aneurysm involves all three layers of the arterial wall structure; this includes the tunica intima, tunica media, and tunica externa or tunica adventitia. Therefore, answer B is true and answer C is false. In aortic dissection, there is a tear in the aortic intima that enables blood to force its way between the other layers of the vessel wall, forming an intimal or dissection flap.

Answer A is false as most aortic aneurysms are fusiform. The morphologic types of aortic aneurysm include fusiform (spindle-shaped in which the walls of the aorta bulge outward symmetrically), saccular (spherical outpouching in which one wall of the aorta protrudes asymmetrically), and pseudoaneurysms (false aneurysm or contained rupture where there is a collection of blood and connective tissue outside the aortic wall). Answer D is false as pseudoaneurysms are contained either by the remaining adventitia or by surrounding mediastinal structures, not the pericardium. Answer C is false since a pseudoaneurysm of the aorta is rare and if present occurs at sites of penetrating atherosclerotic ulcers, due to blunt aortic injury, or as a complication of prior aortic surgery.

12. Answer: C. When there is an acute aortic dissection, there may be a blood pressure differential between arms due to a perfusion deficit to one arm caused by the dissection flap. As a result, there is a blood pressure difference between the upper extremities. Patients with aortic dissection very often present with shortness of breath with or without extreme chest pain. The pain may be felt in the shoulder or lower back.

The clinical triad for acute aortic dissection includes an abrupt onset of thoracic or abdominal pain with a sharp, tearing, and/or ripping character; a variation in pulse (absence of a proximal extremity or carotid pulse) and/or blood pressure (>20 mm Hg difference between the right and left arm); and mediastinal and/or aortic widening on chest radiograph.

13. Answer: C. The diagnostic hallmark of aortic dissection is a mobile dissection flap that separates the true and false lumens. The true and false lumens can be differentiated based on several echocardiographic finding (**Table 18-2**). **Video 18-6** shows several of these characteristics including the expansion of the true lumen toward the false lumen in systole and the expansion of the false lumen toward the true lumen in diastole.

Answer A is false as the false lumen is generally larger than the true lumen. Answer B is false since flow in the false lumen is generally more sluggish, resulting in spontaneous echo contrast (SEC) within the false lumen. The false lumen is prone to forming thrombus. Answer D is false as flow in the true lumen is antegrade and flow in the false lumen is retrograde. Examination along the entirety of the dissection is important to document the severity and emergent nature of the repair. Distinguishing the true and false lumens has implications regarding prognosis and management, particularly if the coronary arteries, great vessels, or peripheral vessels originate from the false lumen.

14. Answer: D. Takayasu arteritis is a chronic inflammatory disease of unknown etiology that primarily affects the proximal aorta and the ostia of major branches including the coronary arteries. The inflammatory process initially leads to granuloma formation and may result in fibrosis and thickening of vessel walls, stenosis, occlusion, thrombus formation, and aneurysmal changes. The diagnostic criteria include age of onset <40 years, intermittent claudication, diminished brachial pulse, subclavian or aortic bruit, systolic blood pressure variation of >10 mm Hg between the arms, and angiographic evidence of aortic or branch vessel stenosis. Aortic dissection in Takayasu arteritis is a rare complication.

Table 18-2. Echocardiographic Differentiation Between True and False Lumens

	True Lumen	False Lumen
Size	True < false	False > true
Pulsation	Systolic expansion, diastolic collapse	Diastolic expansion, systolic compression
Flow direction	Systolic antegrade flow	Systolic antegrade flow reduced or absent, or retrograde flow
Flow communication	From true to false lumen in systole	
Spontaneous echo contrast	Absent or low intensity	Common +/− pronounced
Thrombus	Minimal or none	Complete or partial

From Evangelista A, Flachskampf FA, Erbel R, et al. Echocardiography in aortic diseases: EAE recommendations for clinical practice. *Eur Heart J Cardiovasc Imaging.* 2010;11(8):645-658. Copyright © 2010 The Author. Adapted by permission of Oxford University Press; and Reprinted from Goldstein SA, Evangelista A, Abbara S, et al. Multimodality imaging of diseases of the thoracic aorta in adults from the American Society of Echocardiography and the European Association of Cardiovascular Imaging: endorsed by the Society of Cardiovascular Computed Tomography and Society for Cardiovascular Magnetic Resonance. *J Am Soc Echocardiogr.* 2015;28(2):119-182. Copyright 2015 by the American Society of Echocardiography. With permission.

15. **Answer: A. Figure 18-5** shows a pulsed-wave (PW) Doppler tracing acquired from the abdominal aorta that is consistent with re-coarctation of the aorta. The findings consistent with coarctation include low-velocity systolic flow that is continuous into diastole (diastolic tail). Answer B is incorrect. Even though the angle of insonation between the ultrasound beam and the abdominal aorta is not optimal, a normal PW Doppler profile of the abdominal aorta would show an early, rapid upstroke and downstroke and minimal flow during diastole. Answer C is incorrect. Although the velocity at the coarctation repair site is unknown, a very low cardiac output would be necessary to have such low systolic velocities, and this is not clinically compatible with this patient who is said to be hypertensive. Answer D is incorrect as IVC forward flow would be directed away from the transducer, so velocities would appear below the zero-velocity baseline.

16. **Answer: C.** The CW Doppler profile shown in **Figure 18-6** is consistent with coarctation of the aorta with a high-velocity systolic and diastolic flow (continuous flow, saw-tooth pattern). The simplified Bernoulli equation typically overestimates the peak gradient obtained at cardiac catheterization. This occurs because the pre-coarctation velocity is often elevated due to flow acceleration. However, using the "modified" or "expanded" Bernoulli equation ($\Delta P = 4 \, [V_2^2 - V_1^2]$), where the proximal velocity V_1 is accounted for, results in a good correlation between Doppler echocardiography and cardiac catheterization.

17. **Answer: B.** While a BAV is commonly associated with coarctation of the aorta, a coarctation of the aorta is not commonly associated with a BAV. For example, a BAV occurs in approximately 50% of cases of coarctation of the aorta, while coarctation of the aorta has been found in only 6% of patients with a BAV.

    Answer A is true as the aortic arch is commonly dilated. Frequently, dilatation of the aortic root and ascending aorta is seen in BAV-related aortopathy. The aortopathy of BAVs is due to both genetic predispositions and hemodynamic flow patterns. The aortic arch is commonly enlarged in patients with a BAV, particularly where there is diffuse dilatation of the sinus of Valsalva, sinotubular junction, and proximal ascending aorta. Answer C is true as operative intervention to repair the aortic sinuses or replace the ascending aorta is indicated in patients with a BAV if the diameter of the aortic sinuses or ascending aorta is greater than 5.5 cm. This is because these patients are at greater risk of an acute aortic dissection. Answer D is true as patients with Marfan syndrome may have a BAV.

18. **Answer: D.** Marfan syndrome is a systemic connective tissue disorder, characterized primarily by aortic

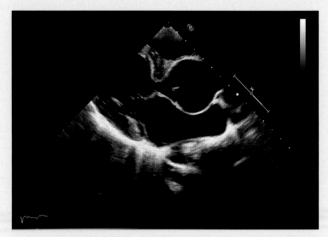

Figure 18-18 Onion-shaped aortic root dilatation as seen from a high parasternal long-axis view.

aneurysms and other cardiovascular, skeletal, and ocular abnormalities. The condition is caused by a genetic mutation in the FBN1 gene. A principal manifestation (major criterion) for diagnosis of Marfan syndrome is dilatation/aneurysms of the ascending aorta involving at least the sinuses of Valsalva. This is the most common site for aneurysm formation. The pattern of dilatation is often "onion-shaped" (**Figure 18-18**), although other variations have been observed. Dilatation/aneurysms of the aortic arch, descending thoracic, and thoracoabdominal aorta are also common and can develop in the absence of coexisting ascending aortic aneurysms. Isolated abdominal aortic aneurysms are relatively rare.

19. **Answer: D.** The normal intimal thickness is ≤ 1 mm. Any irregular thickening of ≥ 2 mm on TEE is considered an atheroma. Distinguishing intimal thickening from atheroma is not easy. Intimal thickening is usually diffuse, homogeneous, and without significant calcification. A grading system exists that classifies atheroma based on plaque thickness and the presence or absence of mobile or ulcerated components, assigning them a grade of 1 to 5 (**Table 18-3**). A descriptive scale may also be used, ranging from mild to complex. Based on the criteria listed in **Table 18-3**, the grade of atheroma in this case is grade 4.

20. **Answer: E.** The TEE images show significantly thickened tissue surrounding the aortic root. Antegrade flow in the distal aortic arch by color Doppler demonstrates the origin of the false lumen thrombosis. Further interrogation at various levels of the ascending aorta show multiple fenestrations between the false and true lumens (see **Video 18-3A** and **18-3B**). With TEE it may be possible to determine if the false lumen provides flow to aortic arch vessels thus compromising flow. With biplane imaging of the ascending aorta and pulling out to the arch, the TEE operator is able to follow the dissection flap from its origin, across the arch, and as it continues

Table 18-3. Grading System for Severity of Aortic Atheroma

Grade	Severity (Atheroma Thickness)	Description
1	Normal	Intimal thickness <2 mm
2	Mild	Mild intimal thickening (2-3 mm)
3	Moderate	Atheroma >3-5 mm (no mobile/ulcerated components)
4	Severe	Atheroma >5 mm (no mobile/ulcerated components)
5	Complex	Grade 2, 3, 4 plus mobile or ulcerated components

Reprinted from Goldstein SA, Evangelista A, Abbara S, et al. Multimodality imaging of diseases of the thoracic aorta in adults: from the American Society of Echocardiography and the European Association of Cardiovascular Imaging: endorsed by the Society of Cardiovascular Computed Tomography and Society for Cardiovascular Magnetic Resonance. *J Am Soc Echocardiogr.* 2015;28(2):119-182. Copyright © 2015 The American Society of Echocardiography. With permission.

in the descending aorta. Color flow imaging is then applied to show the connection(s) from true to false lumen. As previously discussed, the true lumen can be differentiated from the false lumen based on echocardiographic features (see **Table 18-2**).

21. **Answer: B.** In the still images (**Figure 18-10A and 18-10B**), the enlarged right coronary artery and the fistulous connection between the coronary artery and the RA are evident. Color Doppler interrogation confirms the fistulous communication to the RA (**Video 18-4A and 18-4B**).

Coronary fistulas are rare congenital heart malformations that result in a connection between one or more coronary arteries and a cardiac chamber or great vessel. In about half of cases, the fistula originates from the right coronary artery, in one-third from the left anterior descending (LAD) coronary artery, and in about one-fifth from the left circumflex coronary artery. The majority of coronary artery fistulas drain to the right side of the heart, more frequently into the RV, followed by drainage into the RA. This will cause volume overload into right heart structures and increase pulmonary vascular flow, similar to left-to-right shunt from an atrial septal defect (ASD).

Coronary fistulas are usually asymptomatic until the second decade of life. Occasionally a continuous murmur may be heard, or cardiomegaly may be accidentally detected by chest X-ray. Interventional catheterization techniques and surgery are both useful in closure of these vascular abnormalities.

22. **Answer: D.** The transthoracic image (**Figure 18-11**) depicts a large occlusive aortic mass in the abdominal aorta. Although most sources of emboli from the aorta are related to complex atherosclerotic plaques, large aortic thrombi may also occur. A majority of these thrombi develop in areas of diffuse atheromatous disease, but they may also occur in regions with minimal or no apparent atherosclerosis. An alternative etiology of aortic thrombus is an underlying thrombophilic state such as antiphospholipid antibody syndrome or malignancy. In this clinical scenario, the presence of multiple, mobile thrombi in the heart makes aortic thrombus more likely than alternatives such as invading tumor, vegetation, infection, or plaque. Treatment for aortic thrombi has not been well established although anticoagulant therapy is supported by some studies. If recurrent embolic events occur, surgical removal of the aortic thrombi may be necessary. Aortic thrombi do not predispose to aortic dissection although they may be seen at the site of traumatic aortic disruption. Aortic aneurysms may be a site for aortic thrombus formation but usually they appear as mural and layered rather than pedunculated.

23. ▶ **Answer: A.** The TEE X-plane echocardiographic image of the upper descending thoracic aorta depicts severe aortic atheromatous plaque of >5 mm. There are no apparent mobile components, with only minor outpouching (**Video 18-5**). Plaque size can be graded based on intimal or atheroma thickness (see **Table 18-3**).

An IMH is a possibility, as there is calcification on the edges, intimal calcium displacement on the video, and the mass appears homogeneous. However, an IMH refers to the presence of blood or hemorrhage within the media of the aortic wall but no intimal tear. IMH appears as a hypoechoic thickening of the aortic wall. It can be distinguished from atherosclerotic plaque by its smooth contours (in long and short axes) and homogeneous swelling below the intima. The irregular features on the periphery of this large mass make IMH a less likely answer. Answer C is incorrect since there is no evidence of a dissection flap. Answer D is also incorrect. As already described, the findings are not consistent with an IMH. Although there is minor outpouching of the aortic wall; other features consistent with a penetrating aortic ulcer such as a large calcified atheromatous plaque with a crater-like outpouching of the aortic wall are not seen in these images.

24. ▶ **Answer: B.** The images display a prominent dissection, which originates in the proximal descending aorta, close to the mid aortic arch. The true and false lumens are clearly visible in the descending thoracic aorta (see **Video 18-7**).

In the DeBakey classification, this would be type IIIa aortic dissection; in the Stanford classification, this is a type B aortic dissection (see **Tables 18-1**). The dissection in this case may or may not require immediate surgical intervention or thoracic endovascular aortic repair (TEVAR), depending on the hemodynamic stability of the patient.

25. **Answer: C.** The suprasternal notch color Doppler image shows flow from the upper descending aorta, distal to the left subclavian artery, to the pulmonary artery (PA), which is consistent with a patent ductus arteriosus (PDA). A PDA should be considered in any patient with a murmur of unknown cause. Several views can be utilized to detect a PDA, including the parasternal short-axis view with orientation toward the pulmonary artery bifurcation, the high left parasternal view (mostly used in pediatrics), and the suprasternal notch view (most sensitive view in adults). On color Doppler imaging, color flow is continuous as the pressure in the aorta exceeds the pressure in the PA throughout systole and diastole.

Interventions for ductal closure include percutaneous catheter occlusion and surgical ligation. The indications for closure are multifactorial. PDA closure is recommended for patients with a moderate or large PDA associated with symptoms of left-to-right shunting, clinical evidence of left-sided volume overload (that is, left atrial or LV enlargement), or mild to moderate pulmonary hypertension. Although QP:QS is often calculated during TTE when shunts are present, the accuracy is limited due to difficulties in measuring the right ventricular outflow tract diameter. A QP:QS shunt ratio of 1.5:1 indicates the presence of a hemodynamically significant shunt.

26. **Answer: A.** A sinus of Valsalva (SOV) aneurysm is a rare congenital anomaly where there is dilatation of a single sinus of Valsalva as a result of congenital weakening or absence of the media in one of the aortic sinuses. Due to the high aortic pressures, the weakened sinus gradually dilates and eventually forms an aneurysm. The most common location of a SOV aneurysm is the right coronary sinus (**Figure 18-19A**); the next most likely location is the noncoronary sinus (**Figure 18-19B**), followed by the left coronary sinus.

27. **Answer: E.** SOV aneurysm can be either congenital or acquired. Congenital SOV aneurysm causes are more common and include connective tissue diseases, such as Marfan syndrome and Ehlers-Danlos syndrome, and BAVs. Causes of acquired SOV aneurysms include infectious etiologies (such as syphilis, bacterial endocarditis, and tuberculosis), atherosclerosis, vasculitic diseases (such as Takayasu arteritis), chest trauma, and iatrogenic injury during aortic valve surgery. SOV aneurysm occurs more often in males, compared to females, by a factor of 3:1.

28. ▶ **Answer: C.** The TTE images of the aortic root demonstrate a large sinus of Valsalva aneurysm of the noncoronary cusp (see **Video 18-8**).

SOV aneurysms are not benign and have a high probability of rupture. Rupture of a right SOV aneurysm usually results in a fistulous communication between the aorta and the RV or RVOT, and less commonly between the aorta and the RA. Rupture of a noncoronary SOV aneurysm usually results in a fistulous communication between the aorta and the RA, and less commonly between the aorta and the RV. Left SOV aneurysms are rare; rupture of these aneurysms may occur with rupture into the LA, LV, and pericardium. On the Doppler examination, ruptured SOV aneurysms will show continuous flow. The color Doppler image in this case shows

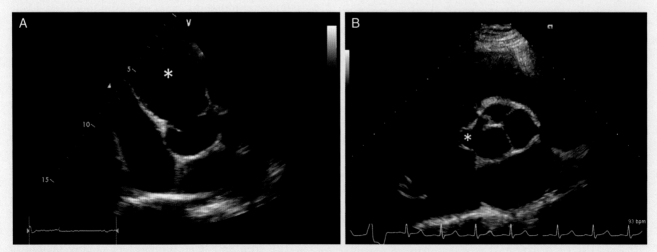

Figure 18-19 Parasternal short-axis views from two different patients showing a large right sinus of Valsalva aneurysm (A) and a noncoronary sinus of Valsalva aneurysm (B). The asterisk (*) marks the aneurysm.

diastolic flow from the central coaptation of the aortic leaflets, directed eccentrically. There is no communication from the noncoronary sinus of Valsalva into the RA.

KEY POINTS

1. Sinus of Valsalva aneurysms may be congenital or acquired.
2. SOV aneurysms are more predominant in males.
3. SOV aneurysms most commonly originate from right coronary sinus.
4. Rupture of a SOV aneurysm results in a fistulous communication between the aorta and another site.
5. The site of rupture and the resultant fistulous communication is dependent upon the origin of the SOV aneurysm.

29. **Answer: B.** Blunt trauma can result in traumatic aortic injuries such as aortic dissection, frank rupture, and complete transection. Blunt trauma may be caused by the rapid acceleration or deceleration of the body, which occurs most commonly during a motor vehicle accident. The most common site for traumatic aortic injury is the aortic isthmus because it is here that the ascending aorta and arch becomes relatively fixed to the thoracic cage by the pleural reflections, the intercostal arteries, and the left subclavian artery. Other sites of trauma include the ascending aorta, the aortic arch, the distal descending thoracic aorta, and the abdominal aorta.

30. **Answer: D.** A "bovine arch" refers to the anatomic variation where only two great vessels, instead of the normal three great vessels, originate from the aortic arch. In the most common configuration, the innominate artery and the left common carotid artery have a common origin (**Figure 18-20**). These aortic configurations occur in about 9% to 13% of individuals. The aortic arch and great vessels are not visualized from the standard parasternal window but can be best imaged from the suprasternal notch.

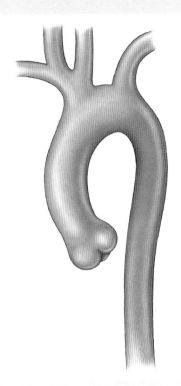

Figure 18-20

TEACHING POINT

The "bovine arch" that is used to describe a common anatomic variant of the human aortic arch branching is a misnomer, as the human variant has no resemblance to the bovine aortic arch. The aortic arch branching pattern found in cattle has a single brachiocephalic trunk originating from the aortic arch, which eventually splits into the bilateral subclavian arteries and a bicarotid trunk. In the human variant, the left common carotid artery has a common origin with the innominate artery

Acknowledgments: The authors thank and acknowledge the contributions from Gian M. Novaro, MD and Craig R. Asher, MD (Chapter 26 Aortic Diseases) in *Clinical Echocardiography Review: A Self-Assessment Tool*, 2nd Edition, edited by Allan L. Klein, Craig R. Asher, 2017.

SUGGESTED READINGS

Armstrong WF, Ryan T. *Feigenbaum's Echocardiography.* 8th ed. Philadelphia, PA: Lippincott Williams and Wilkins; 2019.

Evangelista A, Flachskampf FA, Erbel R, et al. Echocardiography in aortic diseases: EAE recommendations for clinical practice. *Eur J Echocardiogr.* 2010;11(8):645-658.

Goldstein SA, Evangelista A, Abbara S, et al. Multimodality imaging of diseases of the thoracic aorta in adults from the American Society of Echocardiography and the European Association of Cardiovascular Imaging: endorsed by the Society of Cardiovascular Computed Tomography and Society for Cardiovascular Magnetic Resonance. *J Am Soc Echocardiogr.* 2015;28:119-182.

Hiratzka LF, Bakris GL, Beckman JA, et al. 2010 ACCF/AHA/AATS/ACR/ASA/SCA/SCAI/STR/STS/SVM Guidelines for the diagnosis and management of patients with thoracic aortic diseases. Executive summary. *Circulation.* 2010;121:1544-1579.

Lang RM, Badano LP, Mor-Avi V, et al. Recommendations for cardiac chamber quantification by echocardiography in adults: an update from the American Society of Echocardiography and the European Association of Cardiovascular Imaging. *J Am Soc Echocardiogr.* 2015;28:1-39.

Lopez L, Colan SD, Frommelt PC, et al. Recommendations for quantification methods during the performance of a pediatric echocardiogram: a report from the pediatric measurements writing group of the American Society of Echocardiography pediatric and congenital heart disease council. *J Am Soc Echocardiogr.* 2010;23:465-495.

CHAPTER 19

Aortic Valve Disease

Contributors: Theresa A. Green, RDCS and Jason B. Pereira, MS, RCS

✪ Question 1

▶ In **Figure 19-1** and **Video 19-1**, a transthoracic echocardiogram (TTE) shows a parasternal short-axis (PSAX) view of a normal trileaflet aortic valve. The leaflets numbered 1 to 3 are:

A. 1 = LCC, 2 = NCC, 3 = RCC.
B. 1 = RCC, 2 = LCC, 3 = NCC.
C. 1 = NCC, 2, RCC, 3 = LCC.
D. 1 = RCC, 2 = NCC, 3 = LCC.

where LCC is the left coronary cusp, NCC is the non-coronary cusp, and RCC is the right coronary cusp.

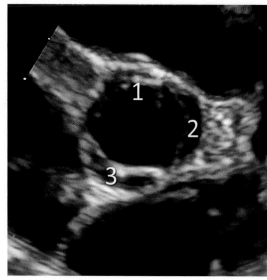

Figure 19-1

✪ Question 2

Which images in **Figure 19-2** labeled A to D show a bicuspid aortic valve (BAV)?

A. A and B
B. A, C, and D
C. B, C, and D
D. A and D
E. All of the above

✪✪ Question 3

▶ A 50-year-old woman with a chief complaint of chest pain, dyspnea on exertion, and a history of rheumatic fever is referred for a cardiology evaluation from her primary care physician. A transthoracic echocardiogram (TTE) is performed. Based on the images provided (**Video 19-2**), what is the likely etiology of the aortic stenosis?

A. Congenital bicuspid aortic valve (BAV)
B. Congenital unicuspid aortic valve
C. Rheumatic aortic valve (AV) disease
D. Senile degeneration of the AV

✪ Question 4

Several hemodynamic variables can be derived during the echocardiographic assessment of aortic stenosis (AS). Which of the three hemodynamic variables listed in **Table 19-1** are used to evaluate the severity of AS?

A. A, B, and C
B. A, B, and D
C. B, C, and E
D. A, C, and E
E. C, D, and E

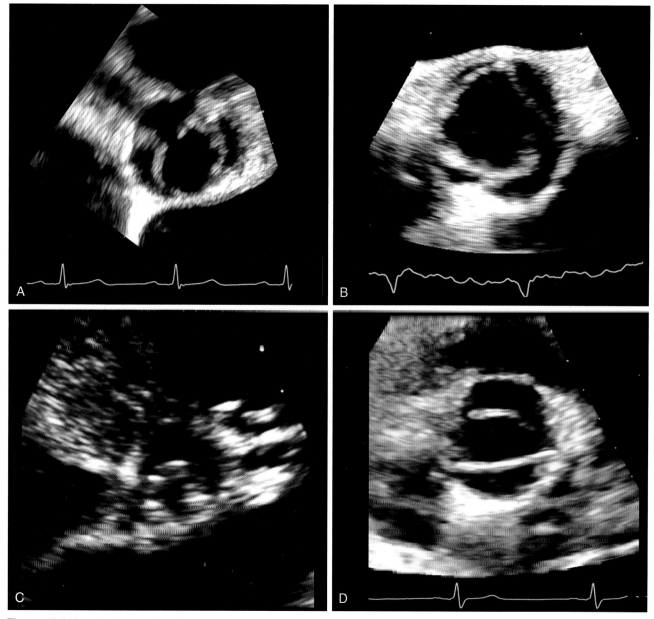

Figure 19-2 A and B: Transesophageal short-axis images. C and D: Parasternal short-axis images.

Table 19-1.

A. Aortic valve (AV) peak velocity

B. AV maximum gradient

C. AV mean gradient

D. AV velocity time integral (VTI)

E. AV area (AVA)

✪✪ Question 5

A patient undergoes a percutaneous balloon aortic valvuloplasty (PBAV). Transthoracic echocardiography (TTE) and cardiac catheterization (Cath) were used to evaluate the postprocedure aortic valve (AV) hemody-

namics. How does peak AV gradient by both techniques compare?

A. The peak pressure gradient acquired with TTE will be greater than the pressure gradient measured at cardiac Cath.

B. The peak pressure gradient acquired with TTE will equal the pressure gradient measured at cardiac Cath.

C. The peak pressure gradient acquired with TTE will be less than the pressure gradient measured at cardiac Cath.

D. The peak pressure gradient acquired with TTE has no relationship to the pressure gradient measured at cardiac Cath.

✪✪ Question 6

Which spectral Doppler measurement can be directly compared with the cardiac catheterization (Cath) hemodynamic measurement for aortic stenosis (AS) severity?

- **A.** Aortic maximum pressure gradient
- **B.** Aortic mean pressure gradient
- **C.** Peak instantaneous pressure gradient
- **D.** Peak to peak pressure gradient (P2P)

✪✪✪ Question 7

Based on the information provided in **Figure 19-3**, which of the following measurements/calculations have been overestimated?

- **A.** AVA and AoV Mean Grad
- **B.** AoV Peak Grad and AoV Mean Grad
- **C.** AVA, AoV Peak Grad and AoV Mean Grad
- **D.** All aortic measurements

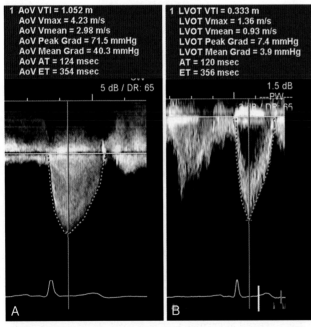

Figure 19-3 AoV is the aortic valve, LVOT is the left ventricular outflow tract, V_{max} is the maximum velocity, V_{mean} is the mean velocity, Peak Grad is the peak pressure gradient, Mean Grad is the mean pressure gradient, AT is the acceleration time, and ET is the ejection time. The aortic valve area (AVA) is 1.1 cm² (not shown).

✪✪✪ Question 8

Based on the data provided in **Table 19-2**, what are the corrected aortic valve (AV) maximum and mean pressure gradients?

- **A.** 66 and 38 mm Hg
- **B.** 72 and 40 mm Hg
- **C.** 74 and 42 mm Hg
- **D.** 72 and 42 mm Hg
- **E.** 66 mm Hg and cannot calculate the corrected mean pressure gradient

Table 19-2.

	AV	LVOT
V_{max} (m/s)	4.3	1.4
Peak gradient (mm Hg)	74	8
V_{mean} (m/s)	3.2	0.9
Mean gradient (mm Hg)	42	4
VTI (cm)	95	36
AT (ms)	120	100
ET (ms)	300	300

AT, acceleration time; ET, ejection time; LVOT, left ventricular outflow tract; V_{max}, maximum velocity; V_{mean}, mean velocity; VTI, velocity-time integral.

✪ Question 9

To calculate the aortic valve area (AVA) using the continuity equation, which of the following is required?

- **A.** Anatomical orifice area (AOA)
- **B.** Cardiac output (CO)
- **C.** Aortic valve (AV) and left ventricular outflow tract (LVOT) ejection times
- **D.** LVOT stroke volume and AV velocity time integral (VTI)
- **E.** All of the above

✪ Question 10

Which of the following measurements used to calculate the aortic valve area (AVA) by the continuity equation may cause the largest error when measured incorrectly?

- **A.** Left ventricular outflow tract (LVOT) peak velocity (V_{max})
- **B.** LVOT velocity time integral (VTI)
- **C.** LVOT diameter
- **D.** Aortic valve (AV) VTI

✪✪ Question 11

Which of the following spectral Doppler measurements listed below is the most common source of error in the calculation of the aortic valve area (AVA)?
  A. Aortic valve (AV) maximum velocity
  B. Left ventricular outflow tract (LVOT) peak gradient
  C. LVOT velocity time integral (VTI)

✪✪✪ Question 12

Based on the continuous-wave (CW) Doppler signals shown in **Figure 19-4**, which of the following statements is true?
  A. Signal A represents aortic stenosis (AS) because the jet starts during the isovolumic contraction period.
  B. Signal B represents mitral regurgitation (MR) and the patient has significant MR.
  C. Signal B represents AS because the jet has a shorter duration.
  D. Neither signal A or B is MR.
  E. Both signals represent AS and were acquired from slightly different windows.

✪✪ Question 13

Which of the following statements regarding aortic regurgitation (AR) is correct?
  A. A proximal isovelocity surface area (PISA) radius of 0.8 cm with an aliasing velocity of 40 cm/s and a peak aortic regurgitant velocity of 4 m/s is consistent with severe AR.
  B. A pressure half-time greater than 250 ms is consistent with severe AR.
  C. Vena contracta is best evaluated from the apical long-axis view.
  D. The use of the suprasternal notch window is not useful in the assessment of AR.

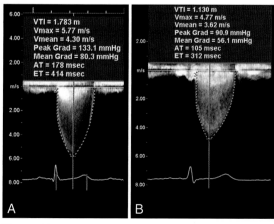

VTI = 1.783 m
Vmax = 5.77 m/s
Vmean = 4.30 m/s
Peak Grad = 133.1 mmHg
Mean Grad = 80.3 mmHg
AT = 178 msec
ET = 414 msec

VTI = 1.130 m
Vmax = 4.77 m/s
Vmean = 3.62 m/s
Peak Grad = 90.9 mmHg
Mean Grad = 56.1 mmHg
AT = 105 msec
ET = 312 msec

Figure 19-4

A 47-year-old man presents to the emergency department with vasovagal syncope. The physical exam is unremarkable except for a grade 2/6 systolic murmur best heard at the mid-left and upper right sternal edge. He has history of "spontaneous closure" of congenital ventricular septal defect (VSD). He undergoes a transthoracic echocardiogram (TTE) as part of the workup for syncope and cardiac murmur.

✪✪ Question 14

Which of these is most likely to be seen on the TTE?
  A. Atrial septal defect (ASD)
  B. Bicuspid aortic valve (BAV)
  C. Ebstein anomaly
  D. Patent ductus arteriosus (PDA)
  E. Any of the above

✪✪ Question 15

The aortic valve of the patient in Case 1 is shown in **Figure 19-5**. Which of the following best describes the morphology of the aortic valve?
  A. Unicuspid aortic valve (UAV)
  B. Trileaflet aortic valve with minor thickening
  C. Bicuspid aortic valve (BAV) type 2
  D. BAV type 1
  E. BAV type 0

A 58-year-old man with a body surface area (BSA) of 1.75 m^2 presents with shortness of breath and dizziness with exertion. He denies chest pain and has no cardiac history. **Table 19-3** includes some of the parameters measured during the transthoracic echocardiogram (TTE). His blood pressure at the time of the TTE was 117/62 mm Hg and the biplane left ventricular (LV) ejection fraction was 57%.

✪ Question 16

Using data provided in **Table 19-3**, what is the calculated aortic valve area (AVA)?
  A. 0.62 cm^2
  B. 0.71 cm^2
  C. 0.36 cm^2
  D. 1.0 cm^2

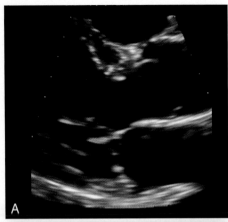

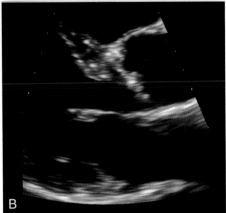

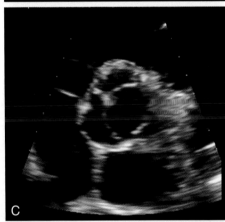

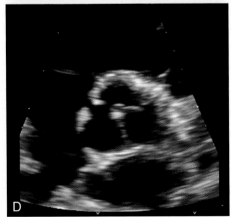

Figure 19-5 A and C: systolic frames; B and D: diastolic frames.

Table 19-3.

	AV	LVOT
VTI (cm)	93	21
V_{max} (m/s)	4.1	0.9
V_{mean} (m/s)	3.2	0.6
Peak gradient (mm Hg)	67	3
Mean gradient (mm Hg)	41	1
AT (ms)	120	100
ET (ms)	355	356
LVOT diameter (cm)	–	2.0
LVOT SV (mL)	–	66

AT, acceleration time; ET, ejection time; LVOT, left ventricular outflow tract; SV, stroke volume; V_{max}, maximum velocity; V_{mean}, mean velocity; VTI, velocity-time integral.

✪✪ Question 17

In Case 2, continuous-wave (CW) Doppler interrogation of the aortic valve from the apical window demonstrated a peak velocity greater than 4 m/s. Which of the following statements is true?

    A. CW Doppler interrogation should be attempted from the suprasternal notch.

    B. CW Doppler interrogation should be attempted from the right sternal edge.

    C. CW Doppler interrogation should be attempted from the right supraclavicular fossa.

    D. A, B, and C.

    E. No further CW Doppler interrogation is required.

✪✪✪ Question 18

Based on the answer for Question 16 and the data provided in **Table 19-3**, what is the correct classification of aortic stenosis (AS) severity presented in this case?

    A. Mild to moderate AS

    B. Moderate to severe AS

    C. Normal-flow, high-gradient (NF-HG) severe AS

    D. Paradoxical low-flow, low-gradient (LF-LG) severe AS

CASE 3

▶ An 88-year-old man with a body surface area of 1.83 m² presents to the emergency department with a history of heart failure with preserved ejection fraction (HFpEF). His chief complaint is worsening dyspnea on exertion, bilateral lower extremity edema, and fatigue. A transthoracic echocardiogram (TTE) was ordered for the assessment of HFpEF and aortic stenosis. **Videos 19-3A** to **19-3D** and **Table 19-4** show some of the images acquired and parameters measured during the examination. His blood pressure at the time of the TTE was 127/62 mm Hg and the biplane left ventricular ejection fraction (LVEF) was 27%.

✪✪✪ Question 19

Assuming all measurements in **Table 19-4** are accurate, what is the severity of the aortic stenosis (AS) presented in Case 3?

A. Low-flow, low-gradient (LF-LG) severe AS
B. Paradoxical low-flow, low-gradient (LF-LG) severe AS
C. Moderate AS
D. Mild-moderate AS

✪✪✪ Question 20

Which of the variables can help determine if the patient from Case 3 has severe aortic stenosis (AS)?

A. Aortic valve (AV) acceleration time (AT)
B. AV ejection time (ET)
C. Dimensionless index (DI)
D. Valvuloarterial impedance (Z_{VA})

CASE 4

▶ A patient with a body surface area (BSA) of 2.1 m² undergoes a transthoracic echocardiogram (TTE) to assess for aortic stenosis (AS) severity. **Videos 19-4A** to **19-4D** and **Table 19-5** show some of the images acquired and parameters measured during the examination. His blood pressure at the time of the TTE was 111/72 mm Hg and the biplane left ventricular ejection fraction (LVEF) was 51%.

✪✪✪ Question 21

Assuming all measurements in **Table 19-5** are accurate, what is the severity of the aortic stenosis (AS) presented in Case 4?

A. Low-flow, low-gradient (LF-LG) severe AS
B. Paradoxical low-flow, low-gradient (LF-LG) severe AS
C. Moderate AS
D. Mild-to-moderate AS

✪✪ Question 22

How many types of low-flow, low-gradient (LF-LG) severe aortic stenosis (AS) are there?

A. 1
B. 2
C. 3
D. 4

Table 19-4.

	AV	LVOT
VTI (cm)	90	13
V_{max} (m/s)	3.6	0.5
V_{mean} (m/s)	2.6	0.4
Peak gradient (mm Hg)	52	1
Mean gradient (mm Hg)	27	0.6
AT (ms)	133	120
ET (ms)	380	383
LVOT diameter (cm)	–	2.3
LVOT SV (mL)	–	54

AT, acceleration time; ET, ejection time; LVOT, left ventricular outflow tract; SV, stroke volume; V_{max}, maximum velocity; V_{mean}, mean velocity; VTI, velocity-time integral.

Table 19-5.

	AV	LVOT
VTI (cm)	56	12
V_{max} (m/s)	2.4	0.6
V_{mean} (m/s)	1.8	0.4
Peak gradient (mm Hg)	23	1
Mean gradient (mm Hg)	13	1
AT (ms)	116	83
ET (ms)	307	294
LVOT diameter (cm)	-	2.0
LVOT SV (mL)	-	38

AT, acceleration time; ET, ejection time; LVOT, left ventricular outflow tract; SV, stroke volume; V_{max}, maximum velocity; V_{mean}, mean velocity; VTI, velocity-time integral.

CASE 5

▶ A 60-year-old male patient with history of uncontrolled hypertension and tobacco use is initially brought to the emergency department with acute onset shortness of breath and left-sided chest pain. A transesophageal echocardiogram (TEE) was performed. **Figure 19-6A** and **19-6B** and **Videos 19-5A** to **19-5D** and **Table 19-6** show some of the images acquired and parameters measured during the examination. In addition, Doppler examination of the descending aorta revealed no holodiastolic flow reversal.

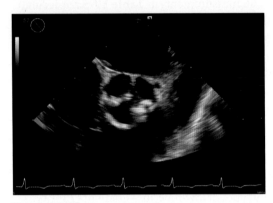

Figure 19-6A

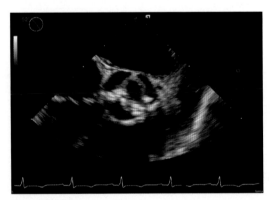

Figure 19-6B

Table 19-6.

LVEF (%)	20-25
AR VCW (cm)	0.44
AR PHT (ms)	296
AV V_{max} (m/s)	4.2
AV mean gradient (mm Hg)	46
DI	0.23

AR, aortic regurgitation; AV, aortic valve; DI, dimensionless index; LVEF, left ventricular ejection fraction; PHT, pressure half-time; V_{max}, maximum velocity; VCW, vena contracta width.

✪ **Question 23**

Based on the images provided, which type of aortic valve is seen?

    A. Bicuspid aortic valve (BAV)

    B. Rheumatic trileaflet aortic valve

    C. Trileaflet aortic valve

    D. Unicuspid aortic valve

✪✪ **Question 24**

Based on the images and data provided, what is the type and degree of aortic valve disease?

    A. Moderate aortic stenosis (AS) with severe aortic regurgitation (AR)

    B. Severe AS and moderate AR

    C. Severe AS and severe AR

    D. None of the above

CASE 6

▶ A 62-year-old man referred from primary care for a new murmur had a transthoracic echocardiogram (TTE) that showed significant valve disease and left ventricular (LV) dysfunction. The patient was followed up with a transesophageal echocardiogram (TEE). **Table 19-7** summarizes the findings of this study and **Figure 19-7A** and **19-7B** and **Videos 19-6A** to **19-6C** show some of the images acquired during the TEE.

✪✪ **Question 25**

What is the severity and main mechanism of the aortic regurgitation (AR) in this case?

    A. Severe AR with aortic cusp perforation

    B. Moderate AR with aortic cusp restriction

    C. Severe AR with aortic annulus dilatation and normal cusp motion

    D. Moderate AR with aortic cusp prolapse

    E. Severe AR with aortic valve prolapse

Table 19-7.

LV Size and Function	Severely dilated LVEF = 45%-50%
AR PISA radius (cm)	0.67
Aliasing velocity (m/s)	0.39
Peak AR velocity (m/s)	4.94
Aortic EROA (cm²)	0.22

AR, aortic regurgitation; EROA, effective regurgitant orifice area; PISA, proximal isovelocity surface area.

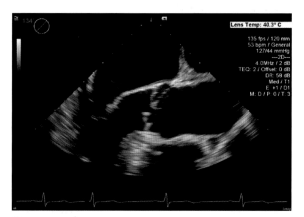

Figure 19-7A

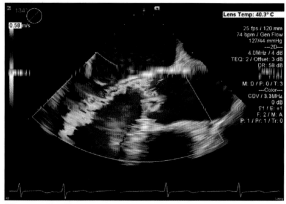

Figure 19-7B

Question 26

Based on the functional classification for aortic regurgitation (AR), the mechanism of AR in this case is:

A. Type I.
B. Type II.
C. Type III.
D. Type IV.

Question 27

Which of the following is the most likely cause for error in the calculation of the effective regurgitant orifice (EROA) in this case?

A. Reduced compliance of the aorta
B. Reduced compliance of the left ventricle
C. Eccentricity of the aortic regurgitant jet
D. A and C

CASE 7

A 46-year-old man with a history of substance abuse presents to the emergency department with cocaine-induced angina. The patient also complains of dyspnea and body aches. Representative images from the transthoracic echocardiogram are shown in **Videos 19-7A** to **19-7E** and **Figure 19-8**.

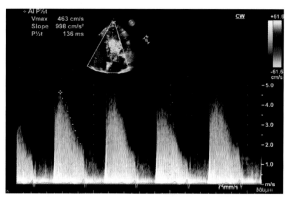

Figure 19-8

Question 28

What is the probable etiology of the mass (measured at 1.08 × 1.60 cm) in this patient?

A. Infectious vegetation
B. Myxoma
C. Papillary fibroelastoma
D. Paraganglioma
E. Rhabdomyoma
F. Thrombus

Question 29

What is the severity of aortic regurgitation (AR) in this patient?

A. Moderate central AR
B. Severe central AR
C. Moderate eccentric AR
D. Severe eccentric AR

CASE 8

▶ A 73-year-old male outpatient with family history of aortic aneurysms is referred for screening. Representative images from the transthoracic echocardiogram are shown in **Figure 19-9A** to **19-9C** and **Videos 19-8A** and **19-8B**. The aortic root was measured at 4.0 cm and the ascending aorta was measured at 4.2 cm.

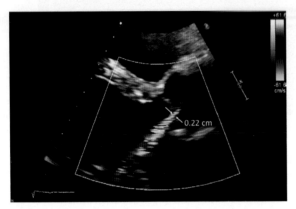

Figure 19-9A

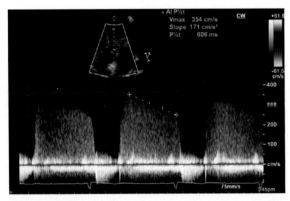

Figure 19-9B

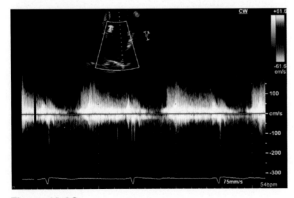

Figure 19-9C

✪ Question 30

Which of the following statements regarding the severity of aortic regurgitation (AR) is correct?

A. There is severe AR confirmed by the vena contracta width (VCW) and density of the AR spectral Doppler jet.

B. There is moderate eccentric AR based on the color and spectral Doppler profile.

C. There is moderate central AR confirmed by the VCW.

D. There is mild eccentric AR based on the color and spectral Doppler images.

✪✪ Question 31

Which of the following is the cause for contamination of the mitral continuous-wave Doppler signal (**Figure 19-9C**)?

A. Moderate eccentric aortic regurgitation (AR) directed posteriorly

B. Severe eccentric AR causing systolic anterior motion of the mitral valve

C. Mild eccentric AR directed posteriorly

D. Mild eccentric AR directed anteriorly

✪✪ Question 32

Which of the following statements regarding the measurement of the vena contracta width (VCW) in aortic regurgitation (AR) is true?

A. With eccentric jets, the VCW is measured perpendicular to the long axis of the jet, not the long axis of the outflow tract.

B. The VCW is measured from the color Doppler image with the Nyquist limit set to the highest possible level.

C. The VCW is equivalent to the effective regurgitant orifice area.

D. The VCW is the same as the AR color jet width or height.

E. All of the above.

CASE 9

▶ An 87-year-old presents with occasional chest pain. The patient is symptomatic with dizziness and syncope and is referred for a transcatheter aortic valve replacement (TAVR) evaluation and a transesophageal echocardiogram was requested. **Videos 19-9A** and **19-9B** and **Table 19-8** show some of the images acquired and parameters measured during the examination.

Table 19-8.

LV size and Function	Dilated LVEF = 40%-45%
AV peak velocity (m/s)	4.3
AV mean gradient (mm Hg)	46
AVA (cm²)	0.8
DI	0.22
AR VCW (cm)	0.52
AR PHT (ms)	423
AR R$_{Vol}$ (mL)	43

AR, aortic regurgitation; AV, aortic valve; AVA, aortic valve area; DI, dimensionless index; PHT, pressure half-time; R$_{Vol}$, regurgitant volume; VCW, vena contracta width.

⭐ Question 33

What is the type and severity of aortic valve disease?
- **A.** Severe aortic stenosis (AS) and moderate aortic regurgitation (AR)
- **B.** Moderate AS with mild AR
- **C.** Severe AS and severe AR
- **D.** Mild AS and moderate AR

⭐⭐ Question 34

What would be the appropriate management of this patient with aortic stenosis (AS) and aortic regurgitation (AR)?
- **A.** The AS and AR are moderate, and a follow-up echocardiogram can be obtained in 1 to 2 years.
- **B.** The AS is severe, but a "watchful waiting" strategy is appropriate and follow-up echocardiogram can be obtained in 6 months to 1 year to monitor the progression of the AR.
- **C.** The AS is severe, and the AR is moderate, the patient is symptomatic, and surgical or transcatheter aortic valve replacement is recommended.
- **D.** The AS is moderate, and the AR is severe, and a follow-up echocardiogram should be repeated in 6 months if the patient's symptoms continue.

⭐ Question 35

Which of the following is not a specific indicator of chronic severe aortic regurgitation (AR)?
- **A.** A vena contracta width (VCW) of 0.65 cm
- **B.** An AR pressure half-time (PHT) of 190 ms
- **C.** Prominent holodiastolic flow reversal in descending aorta
- **D.** A dilated left ventricle (LV) with normal function
- **E.** An aortic regurgitant volume (R$_{Vol}$) of 50 mL

ANSWERS

1. **Answer: B.** Leaflet 1 is the RCC because it is closest to the right ventricular outflow tract (RVOT); the right coronary ostium (R Ostium) is located adjacent to that leaflet (**Figure 19-10A** and **19-10B**). The other two leaflets are adjacent to the left atrium (LA). Leaflet 2 is the LCC because the left coronary ostia (L Ostium) is seen adjacent to it (**Figure 19-10A** and **19-10C**). Leaflet 3 is the NCC, which does not have a coronary ostium and is closest to the interatrial septum (IAS).

2. **Answer: D.** BAVs may have 0, 1, or 2 raphes, as seen in **Figure 19-11**. A raphe is defined as a seam or fibrous ridge between two leaflets (also known as a false commissure). A BAV is diagnosed from the PSAX view during systole by identifying the number of commissural attachments to the aortic root. **Figure 19-2A** has one raphe and two cusps, which makes this a type I BAV. **Figure 19-2B** has no raphe and four leaflets, which makes this a quadricuspid aortic valve (QAV). **Figure 19-2C** has no raphe with an eccentric orifice, which is classified as a unicuspid aortic valve (UAV). **Figure 19-2D** has no raphe, two sinuses instead of three, and has an anterior and posterior leaflet. This is a type 0 or a true BAV. Therefore, answer D is correct.

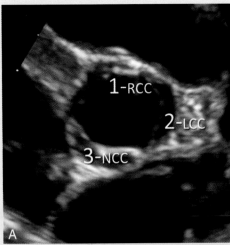

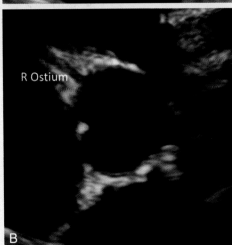

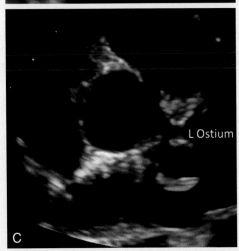

Figure 19-10 1 = right coronary cusp (RCC); 2 = left coronary cusp (LCC); 3 = noncoronary cusp (NCC).

3. **Answer: C.** Rheumatic aortic valve disease is typically characterized by commissural fusion and calcification resulting in a central, triangular orifice in systole. However, artifacts caused by calcification and poor acoustic windows make it difficult to visualize the distribution of calcium. Also, calcification in rheumatic AV disease may extend into the leaflet surface and annulus. This may make it difficult to differentiate from degenerative calcific aortic stenosis (AS). Therefore, additional information and echocardiographic clues are utilized to make the diagnosis of rheumatic AV disease. The following make rheumatic AV disease more likely: age <60 years old, history of rheumatic fever, and presence of valvular mitral stenosis (MS). Also, aortic regurgitation (AR) is more common in rheumatic AV disease and AS tends to be nonsevere. In this patient, who is 50 years old and has a past history of rheumatic fever, there is evidence of rheumatic MS with a characteristic hockey-stick appearance of the anterior mitral leaflet and at least moderate aortic and mitral regurgitation (**Figure 19-12**). Therefore, these findings are most consistent with rheumatic AS.

A BAV (answer A) is unlikely based on the clinical history and the associated finding of a hockey-stick appearance of the anterior mitral valve. However, in the parasternal short-axis (PSAX) view, the aortic valve appears functionally bicuspid with fusion between the right and left coronary cusps; fused commissures are commonly seen in rheumatic AS and should not be confused for a congenitally bicuspid AV. A congenital unicuspid aortic valve (answer B) is very rare; these valves are usually stenotic from birth. Senile degenerative AS (answer D) is unlikely as the patient is only 50 years of age.

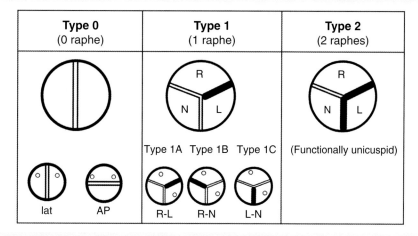

	Type 0 (0 raphe)	Type 1 (1 raphe)	Type 2 (2 raphes)

Type 1A   Type 1B   Type 1C

lat   AP

R-L   R-N   L-N

(Functionally unicuspid)

Figure 19-11 Classification of BAV based on the number of raphes and the spatial position. In type 0: there is no raphe; this is also sometimes referred to as a true BAV. In type 1: there is one raphe and in type 2 there are two raphes between the right and left and between the left and noncoronary cusps. For the type 0 BAV, the orientation of the free edge of the cusps can be either lateral (lat) with right and left cusps, or anteroposterior (AP) with anterior and posterior cusps. The type 1 BAV can also be subcategorized according to the position of the raphe. In type 1A (R-L), the raphe is between the right (R) and left (L) coronary cusps; in type 1B (R-N), the raphe is between right (R) and noncoronary (N) cusps; in type 1C (L-N), the raphe is between noncoronary (N) and left (L) cusps. The most common type is type 1A. A type 2 BAV is rare and has two raphe and two cusps; this is a functionally bicuspid valve. Prominent lines in schematic drawings represent a raphe and the circles represent the coronary ostia. (Adapted from Sievers HH, Schmidtke C. A classification system for the bicuspid aortic valve from 304 surgical specimens. *J Thorac Cardiovasc Surg* 2007;133(5):1226-1233. Copyright (C) 2007 The American Association for Thoracic Surgery. With permission.)

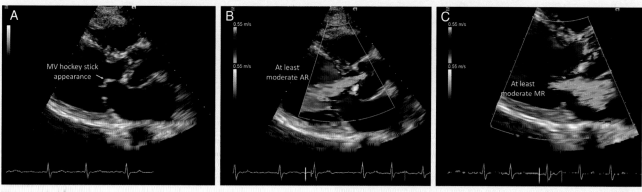

Figure 19-12

4. **Answer: D.** Hemodynamic severity is used to determine if a patient's symptoms are caused by a stenotic valve and how frequently the patient needs follow-up. Of all the indices listed in **Table 19-1**, the three that are recommended for routine clinical practice include: AV peak velocity, mean pressure gradient, and AVA. These are found to be good predictors of clinical outcomes. The current recommendations for hemodynamic classification of AS severity based on these variables are listed in **Table 19-9**. Other variables that may be considered include the AVA indexed to the body surface area and the velocity ratio or dimensionless index (DI), which is the peak velocity across the left ventricular outflow tract (LVOT) divided by the peak AV velocity.

5. **Answer: A.** Pressure gradients obtained by cardiac Cath are not truly physiologic because the gradient is derived from measurements of peak left ventricular (LV) systolic pressure (LVSP) and the peak ascending aortic pressure. Hence, the

term "peak to peak" (P2P) gradient. This systolic pressure gradient is generally measured as a pullback gradient between the left ventricle and the ascending aorta. As illustrated in **Figure 19-13A**, the peak LV pressure does not occur simultaneously with the peak aortic pressure; therefore, this is a nonphysiologic measurement. Conversely, the Doppler-derived pressure gradient measures the maximal instantaneous pressure gradient between the peak LVSP and the aortic pressure at that same point in systole (**Figures 19-13B** and **19-13C**). Hence, the term "instantaneous" pressure gradient is often used to describe this measurement. This is a physiologic measurement because it is actually the maximal pressure gradient generated across the AV during ventricular ejection. Therefore, a P2P gradient by cardiac Cath (50 mm Hg) and a peak gradient by Doppler (75 mm Hg) in the same patient are not comparable and should not be used interchangeably.

Table 19-9. Recommendations for Grading of AS Severity

	Aortic Sclerosis	Mild	Moderate	Severe
Peak velocity	≤2.5	2.6-2.9	3.0-4.0	≥4.0
Mean gradient (mm Hg)	-	<20	20-40	≥40
AVA (cm²)	-	>1.5	1.0-1.5	<1.0
Indexed AVA (cm²/m²)	-	>0.85	0.60-0.85	<0.6
Velocity ratio (or DI)	-	>0.50	0.25-0.50	<0.25

Reprinted from Baumgartner H, Hung J, Bermejo J, et al. Recommendations on the echocardiographic assessment of aortic valve stenosis: a focused update from the European Association of Cardiovascular Imaging and the American Society of Echocardiography. *J Am Soc Echocardiogr.* 2017;30(4):372-392. Copyright © 2017 by the American Society of Echocardiography. With permission.

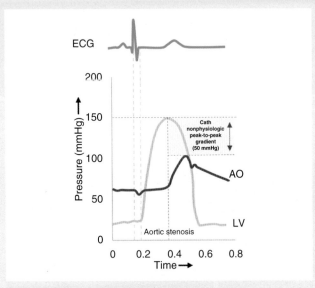

Figure 19-13A Cath P2P gradient.

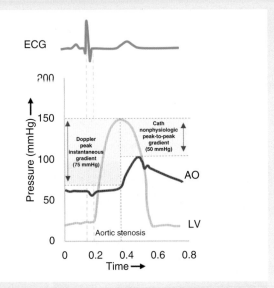

Figure 19-13C Comparison between the Cath P2P gradient and the Doppler pressure gradient.

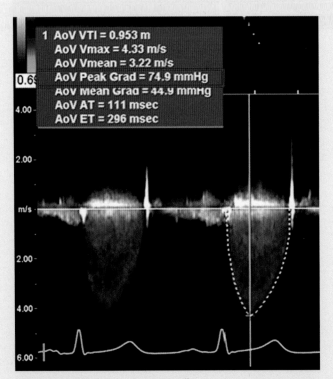

Figure 19-13B Doppler pressure gradient.

6. **Answer: B.** Via cardiac Cath, the mean AV gradient is usually measured by superimposing the left ventricular and aortic pressure curves and by then measuring the integrated gradient throughout the entire systolic ejection period (shaded portion in **Figure 19-14A**). The Doppler mean gradient is measured by tracing the continuous-wave (CW) Doppler spectrum (**Figure 19-14B**). Since both measurements are measuring the area under the curve (AUC) throughout the entire systolic ejection period, the mean gradient is comparable between both techniques. Thus, when assessing the severity of AS using pressure gradients by Cath and Doppler, it is best to compare the mean pressure gradients. Therefore, answer B is correct.

As discussed previously, the P2P by cardiac Cath and the peak instantaneous pressure gradient by Doppler (or the aortic maximum pressure gradient) are not comparable; therefore, answers A, C, and D are incorrect.

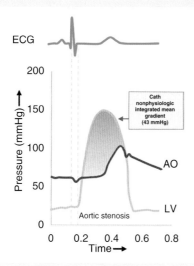

Figure 19-14A Cath mean pressure gradient is the shaded area between the LV and aortic pressure traces.

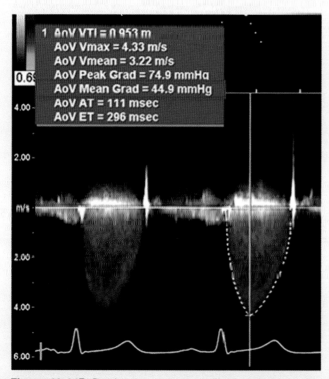

Figure 19-14B Doppler mean pressure gradient is derived by tracing the Doppler spectrum.

7. **Answer: B.** When the LVOT velocity is ≥1.2 m/s, the peak and mean aortic valve (AV) pressure gradients derived from the simplified Bernoulli equation will be overestimated. This is because the simplified Bernoulli equation ($\Delta P = 4\ V^2$) assumes that the proximal velocity (V_1) is insignificant. However, when the LVOT velocity (V_1) is increased, the AV pressure gradients must be corrected using the "expanded" or "modified" Bernoulli equation.

The accuracy of the AVA is unaffected because this calculation, derived from the continuity equation, accounts for the proximal LVOT velocity (V_1) and the distal AV velocity (V_2). The other AV measurements such as the velocity-time integral (area under the Doppler spectrum), ejection time (time interval between the onset and end of flow), and acceleration time (time interval between the onset of ejection to the time of peak AV velocity) are not affected by the LVOT velocity.

8. **Answer: A.** The maximum and mean pressure gradients should be corrected whenever the proximal velocity exceeds 1.2 m/s. In this instance, the expanded Bernoulli equation is used to calculate the corrected pressure gradient (ΔPc):

$$\Delta Pc = 4\left(V_2^2 - V_1^2\right) \qquad (1)$$

where V_2 is the peak velocity across the narrowing and V_1 is the peak velocity proximal to the narrowing.

Therefore, when the LVOT velocity ≥1.2 m/s, the AV maximum and mean pressure gradients may be corrected using the following equation:

$$\Delta Pc = 4\left(V_{AV^2} - V_{LVOT^2}\right) \qquad (2)$$

In this example, the peak V_{AV} is 4.3 m/s and the peak V_{LVOT} is 1.4 m/s; therefore, the corrected AV maximum pressure gradient (maxΔPc) is:

$$\max\Delta Pc = 4\left(4.3^2 - 1.4^2\right) = 4\left(18.49 - 1.96\right)$$
$$= 4 \times 16.53 = 66 \text{ mm Hg} \qquad (3)$$

Alternatively, the AV maximum pressure gradient may be corrected by simply subtracting the LVOT peak pressure gradient from the AV peak pressure gradient. This is because Equation (1) is mathematically the same as:

$$\Delta Pc = \left(4 \times V_2^2\right) - \left(4 \times V_1^2\right) \qquad (4)$$

Therefore, the corrected AV maximum pressure gradient (maxΔPc) is:

$$\max\Delta Pc = 74 - 8 = 66 \text{ mm Hg} \qquad (5)$$

Likewise, the corrected AV mean pressure gradient (mΔPc) can be derived by subtracting the LVOT mean pressure gradient from the AV mean pressure gradient as:

$$m\Delta Pc = 42 - 4 = 38 \text{ mm Hg} \qquad (6)$$

9. **Answer: D.** The AVA is calculated from the following equation:

$$AVA = (CSA_{LVOT} \times VTI_{LVOT}) \div VTI_{AV} \qquad (1)$$

where CSA_{LVOT} is the cross-sectional area (CSA) of the LVOT (derived from the LVOT diameter), VTI_{LVOT} is the LVOT VTI, and VTI_{AV} is the VTI across the AV.

The first part of this equation ($CSA_{LVOT} \times VTI_{LVOT}$) is the LVOT stroke volume (SV_{LVOT}); therefore, the AVA is calculated as:

$$AVA = SV_{LVOT} \div VTI_{AV} \qquad (2)$$

The AVA derived by this method is also known as the effective orifice area (EOA).

The AOA (answer A) is derived from a direct 2D or 3D planimetry of the AV when the leaflets are fully open. The EOA and the AOA are not the same as the EOA is calculated in the region where the jet is the narrowest and gradient highest, which is derived downstream from the true AOA. Therefore, the EOA is usually slightly smaller than the AOA. The cardiac output (answer B) and the AV and LVOT ejection times (answer C) are not required for the calculation of the AVA.

10. **Answer: C.** The LVOT diameter (LVOTd) is used to calculate the CSA of the LVOT via the following equation:

$$CSA = 0.785 \times LVOTd^2$$

Since the LVOT diameter is squared, small errors will cause large discrepancies in the calculated AVA. The LVOT diameter is measured from a zoomed parasternal long-axis (PLAX) view in midsystole, using an inner edge-to-inner edge method and parallel to the annulus, either at the annulus or approximately 3 to 10 mm from the aortic annulus. In patients where the LVOT is difficult to measure (e.g., sigmoidal septum or upper septal hypertrophy), measurement of the LVOT diameter 3 to 10 mm from the annulus may result in a significant underestimation of the diameter (**Figure 19-15A**). In these cases, the LVOT diameter should be measured at the aortic annulus since it has clear landmarks (leaflet insertion) (**Figure 19-15B**). The reported variability of the LVOT diameter measurement ranges from 5% to 8% compared to ~3% to 4% variability in spectral Doppler data.

Errors made in measuring the LVOT V_{max}, LVOT VTI, or AV VTI can also under- or overestimate the calculated AVA, but this is significantly less than the error caused by wrong LVOT diameter measurement.

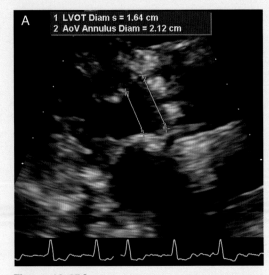

Figure 19-15A

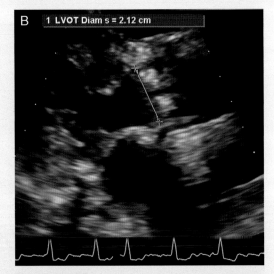

Figure 19-15B

11. **Answer: A.** Measurement of the AV maximum velocity (V_{max}) is the most common Doppler error in the calculation of AVA and assessment of aortic stenosis (AS) severity. Nonparallel alignment with the AS jet will result in an underestimation of V_{max}, while overestimation of V_{max} will occur when the Doppler gains are set too high. In **Figure 19-16**, nonparallel alignment is suggested by signals above and below the zero baseline and increased spectral spread of the AS jet is seen as the Doppler gains are set too high. The AS continuous-wave Doppler signal is optimized by interrogating the AS jet from multiple acoustic windows and accurate measurements are made by placing the caliper at the most intense portion of the signal, which can be clearly seen by optimizing the Doppler gain to reduce the spectral spread of the Doppler signal.

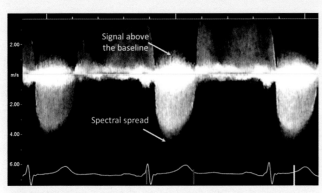

Figure 19-16

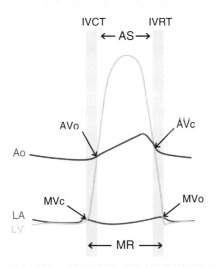

Figure 19-17A The MR signal is longer than the AS signal because it incorporates the isovolumic contraction time (IVCT) as well as the isovolumic relaxation time (IVRT). The IVCT is the time interval between mitral valve closure (MVc) and aortic valve opening (AVo) while the IVRT is the time interval between aortic valve closure (AVc) and mitral valve opening (MVo). Ao = aortic pressure trace; LA = left atrial pressure trace; LV = left ventricular pressure trace.

12. Answer: C. AS and MR may be present on the same study and distinguishing between the two

jets may be difficult, especially when using the nonimaging CW Doppler probe. Differentiation between these two signals is based on the duration of the signal and the peak velocity. The aortic signal commences when the AV opens, and the signal terminates when the AV closes while the MR waveform commences on mitral valve (MV) closure and continues until the MV opens again. Between MV closure and AV opening is the isovolumic contraction time (IVCT). During this time, the left ventricle (LV) is contracting, but the LV pressure is still below the aortic pressure, so the AV remains closed. When the LV pressure exceeds the aortic pressure, the AV opens and there is flow across the AV; this is ejection. The AV closes when the pressure in the LV falls below the aortic pressure, but the MV does not open until the LV pressure falls below the left atrial (LA) pressure. Therefore, there is a short time interval known as the isovolumic relaxation time (IVRT). Since MR commences on MV closure and continues until the MV reopening, the MR waveform incorporates both the IVCT and IVRT; therefore the duration of the MR signal is longer than that of AS (**Figure 19-17A**). In **Figure 19-4**, the duration or ejection time (ET) of signal A is 414 ms and the duration or ET of signal B is 312 ms; therefore, signal B is AS.

The second clue is the peak velocity of the Doppler signal. The AS V_{max} reflects the pressure gradient between the LV and aorta during systole. When there is severe AS, the V_{max} is between 4 and 5 m/s, and even in very severe AS the V_{max} does not usually exceed 6 m/s. The MR velocity reflects the pressure gradient between the LV and LA during systole. As the LV systolic pressure is usually much higher than the LA pressure, the MR peak velocity is typically between 6 to 8 m/s. When AS and MR coexist, the MR velocity will always be higher than the AS velocity (**Figure 19-17B**).

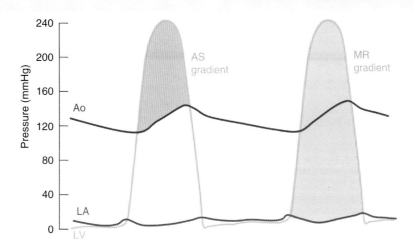

Figure 19-17B The MR gradient will always exceed the AS gradient and because the Doppler velocity reflects the pressure gradient, the MR velocity will always be higher than the AS velocity.

13. **Answer: A.** This question refers to the proximal isovelocity surface concept in calculating the effective regurgitant orifice area (EROA). According to the continuity equation, the flow converging to the valve must be equal to flow through the valve. As blood flow accelerates toward a narrowing orifice (in this case the regurgitant orifice), the spatial distribution of points in which the fluid has the same velocity (isovelocity surface) is approximated by a hemisphere.

    Based on this concept, one can transcribe the continuity equation as:

$$\text{Isovelocity flow} = \text{regurgitant flow} \qquad (1)$$

$$\text{Isovelocity area} \times V_N = EROA \times V_{max} \qquad (2)$$

where V_N is the aliasing velocity (Nyquist limit) and V_{max} is the maximum velocity of the regurgitant jet.

$$2\pi \times r^2 \times V_N = EROA \times V_{max} \qquad (3)$$

where r is the PISA radius.

    Rearranging this equation to calculate the EROA:

$$EROA = (2\pi \times r^2 \times V_N) \div V_{max} \qquad (4)$$

    Replacing the numbers, this becomes:

$$EROA = (2\pi \times 0.8^2 \times 40) \div 400 = 0.40 \text{ cm}^2 \qquad (5)$$

    Based on the values in **Table 19-10**, the severity of AR is severe.

Table 19-10. Quantitative Parameters for AR Severity

	Mild	Moderate		Severe
	Grade I	Grade II	Grade III	Grade IV
R_{Vol} (mL)	<30	30-44	45-59	≥60
RF (%)	<30	30-39	40-49	≥50
EROA (cm²)	<0.1	0.1-0.19	0.20-0.29	≥0.4

R_{Vol}, regurgitant volume; RF, regurgitant fraction; EROA, effective regurgitant orifice area.

Reprinted from Zoghbi WA, Adams D, Bonow RO, et al. Recommendations for noninvasive evaluation of native valvular regurgitation. A report from the American Society of Echocardiography developed in collaboration with the Society for Cardiovascular Magnetic Resonance. *J Am Soc Echocardiogr.* 2017;30(4):303-371. Copyright © 2017 by the American Society of Echocardiography. With permission.

A pressure half-time of less than 200 ms is consistent with severe AR; therefore, answer B is incorrect. The vena contracta is best measured in the parasternal long-axis view, as the measurement will be influenced by axial resolution, which is superior to lateral resolution. In the apical long-axis view, the vena contracta will be typically parallel to the ultrasonic beam, meaning the measurement will be less accurate by having to rely on the lateral resolution; therefore, answer C is incorrect. The suprasternal notch window allows pulsed-wave (PW) Doppler evaluation of flow reversal in the descending thoracic aorta; holodiastolic (pan-diastolic) flow reversals are suggestive of severe AR; therefore, answer D is incorrect.

14. **Answer: B.** A BAV is the most common congenital heart disease in the adult with a prevalence of 1% to 2%. BAV also occurs in men more often than women (3:1 ratio). The systolic timing of the murmur makes the diagnosis of PDA unlikely as the murmur associated with a PDA is a continuous, "machinery" murmur. Both ASD and Ebstein anomaly can cause a systolic murmur although at different locations (left upper and left lower sternal edge, respectively). Also, ASD occurs more commonly in women than men (2:1), while Ebstein anomaly is very rare (<1% of live births) and is more common in women than men. Lastly, BAV and ventricular septal defect are the two most common forms of congenital heart defect in the adult, with ASD coming in third. Thus, given the clinical picture, the most likely echocardiographic finding in this man is BAV.

15. **Answer: D.** As previously described, the classification of a BAV may be based on the number of raphes (see answer outline for Question 2 and **Figure 19-11**). Type 0 BAV has no raphe and two valve cusps. Type 1 BAV is the most common, and has one raphe and two valve cusps. Type 2 BAV is rare and has two raphes and two cusps. A unicuspid aortic valve is also rare and can present with two raphes as seen with type 2 BAV (unicommissural type) or as a single membrane-like leaflet with a central orifice and no apparent commissural attachment to the aortic root (acommissural type). A unicommissural unicuspid valve can lead to misdiagnosis of BAV. The diagnosis of a BAV and UAV is made from the parasternal short-axis view by identifying the number of commissural attachments to the aortic root.

    In this patient, there is a raphe between the right and left coronary cusps and only two commissural attachments to the aortic root (**Figure 19-18**); therefore, this is a type 1 BAV.

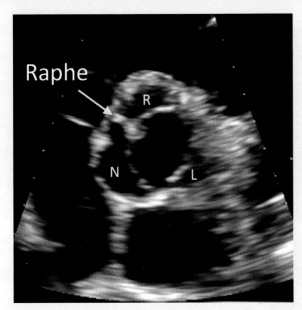

Figure 19-18

16. **Answer: B.** The AVA is calculated from the following equation:

$$AVA = (CSA_{LVOT} \times VTI_{LVOT}) \div VTI_{AV} \qquad (1)$$

where CSA_{LVOT} is the cross-sectional area (CSA) of the LVOT (derived from the LVOT diameter), VTI_{LVOT} is the LVOT VTI, and VTI_{AV} is the VTI across the AV.

The CSA is calculated from the LVOT diameter (LVOTd) as:

$$CSA = 0.785 \times LVOTd^2 \qquad (2)$$

Therefore, the AVA is calculated as:

$$AVA = \left(0.785 \times LVOTd^2 \times VTI_{LVOT}\right) \div VTI_{AV} \qquad (3)$$

Substituting the values from **Table 19-3** into this equation, the AVA is calculated as:

$$AVA = (0.785 \times 2.0^2 \times 21) \div 93 = 0.7\,cm^2 \qquad (4)$$

Alternatively, as the first part of Equation (3) ($CSA_{LVOT} \times VTI_{LVOT}$) is the LVOT stroke volume (SV_{LVOT}), the AVA can also be calculated as:

$$AVA = SV_{LVOT} \div VTI_{AV} \qquad (5)$$

Substituting the values from **Table 19-3** into this equation, the AVA is calculated as:

$$AVA = 66 \div 93 = 0.7\,cm^2 \qquad (6)$$

17. **Answer: D.** A peak velocity across the aortic valve ≥4.0 m/s is consistent with severe AS (see **Table 19-9**). However, even when the peak velocity (and resultant pressure gradients) reflect severe AS, it is important to rule out severe AS versus very severe or critical AS. Therefore, the interrogation with a nonimaging probe from three additional windows is important, because the true peak velocity may be present in any of the nonapical windows in up to 60% of patients with AS. These additional windows include the suprasternal notch, the right sternal border, and the right supraclavicular fossa (**Figure 19-19A**). Neglecting this could result in misclassification of the severity of AS in about 25% of the patients. Using the nonimaging probe, which has a small footprint, allows for better access between intercostal, suprasternal, and supraclavicular spaces.

18. **Answer: C.** The calculated AVA is 0.70 cm², which indicates severe AS (see **Table 19-9**). However, the AS severity should always be verified by checking the gradients, the flow status, and the LV ejection fraction (LVEF). In this case, the aortic valve (AV) maximum velocity and mean pressure gradient (PG) were 4.1 m/s and 43 mm Hg, respectively. These are consistent with the calculated aortic valve area of 0.70 cm² (severe AS). The flow status is derived from the stroke volume index (SVi), which is the stroke volume divided by the body surface area (BSA):

$$SVi = SV_{LVOT} \div BSA \qquad (1)$$

Normal SVi is >35 mL/m². In this case, the LVOT SVi was:

$$SVi = 66 \div 1.75 = 38\ mL/m^2 \qquad (2)$$

In addition, the LVEF was 57% (normal). Hence, this would be classified as normal-flow, high-gradient (NF-HG) severe AS.

Answers A and B are incorrect as all parameters are consistent with severe AS. Paradoxical low-flow, low-gradient (LF-LG) severe AS is a term used to describe LF-LG AS in the setting of a normal LVEF but a reduced forward stroke volume due to other causes. As the flow status is normal, this is not paradoxical LF-LG severe AS; therefore, answer D is not correct.

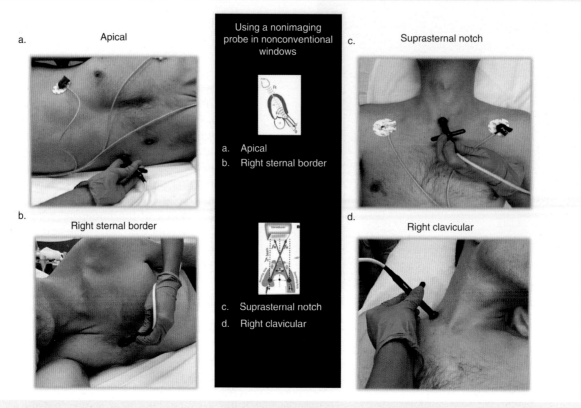

a. Apical

Using a nonimaging probe in nonconventional windows

a. Apical
b. Right sternal border

c. Suprasternal notch

b. Right sternal border

c. Suprasternal notch
d. Right clavicular

d. Right clavicular

Figure 19-19A

TEACHING TIP

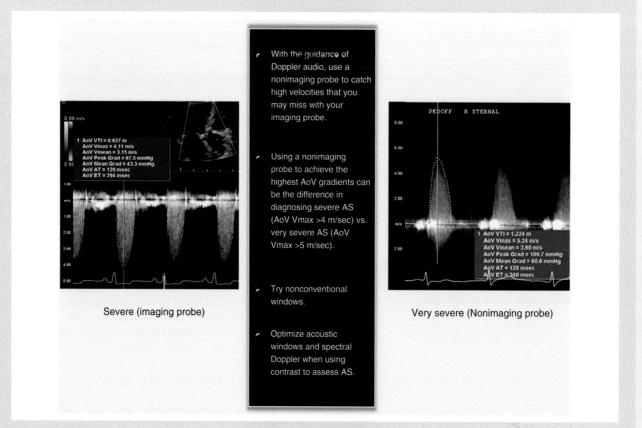

> With the guidance of Doppler audio, use a nonimaging probe to catch high velocities that you may miss with your imaging probe.

> Using a nonimaging probe to achieve the highest AoV gradients can be the difference in diagnosing severe AS (AoV Vmax >4 m/sec) vs. very severe AS (AoV Vmax >5 m/sec).

> Try nonconventional windows.

> Optimize acoustic windows and spectral Doppler when using contrast to assess AS.

Severe (imaging probe)

Very severe (Nonimaging probe)

Figure 19-19B offers tips for using the non-imaging CW Doppler probe in the assessment of aortic stenosis (AS).

KEY POINTS

▶ Transthoracic echocardiography is the best way to evaluate and assess AV disease and allows for a comprehensive hemodynamic evaluation of AS severity.

▶ Understand limitations and challenges of 2D and Doppler measurements and steps to reduce errors.

▶ Always interrogate AS signals from multiple windows using the nonimaging continuous-wave Doppler probe.

▶ AV hemodynamics are dependent on flow, so always pay attention to SV/SVi.

19. **Answer: A.** The visual assessment of the aortic valve (AV) shows that it has three leaflets that are calcified and restricted in motion. The calculated aortic valve area (AVA) is 0.60 cm², which indicates severe AS:

$$AVA = (0.785 \times 2.3^2 \times 13) \div 90 = 0.6 \text{ cm}^2 \quad (1)$$

The calculated AVA is probably correct because the valve is severely calcified and restricted. However, the AV V_{max} is 3.8 m/s and the mean PG is 27 mm Hg which are not consistent with severe AS. The discrepancy between the V_{max}, mean gradient and the AVA could be a result of measurement error or a low-flow state. Given that the measurements are said to be accurate, the flow status needs to be considered. As previously described, the stroke volume index (SVi) is calculated from the LVOT stroke volume and the body surface area (BSA). In this case, the SVi is:

$$SVi = 54 \div 1.83 = 30 \text{ mL/m}^2 \quad (2)$$

This is consistent with low flow across the AV, which explains the V_{max} <4 m/s and mean gradient <40 mm Hg in the setting of severe AS. When there is a low-flow status, the next step is to consider the LVEF to determine if this is LF-LG severe AS or paradoxical LF-LG severe AS. In this case, this is reduced at 27% (reduced). Therefore, there is LF-LG AS with a reduced LVEF.

Answer B is incorrect as in paradoxical LF-LG AS the LVEF is normal. Answers C and D are incorrect as the AVA is <1.0 cm² and this is not consistent with moderate or mild-moderate AS.

20. **Answer: C.** The DI or velocity ratio is simply a ratio of the LVOT V_{max} (or VTI) and the AV V_{max} (or VTI):

$$DI = LVOT_{Vmax/VTI} \div AV_{Vmax/VTI} \quad (1)$$

DI is useful when the LVOT diameter is unattainable or unreliable. Severe AS is suggested when the DI or velocity ratio is 0.25 or less (see **Table 19-9**), corresponding to a valve area 25% of normal. In this patient, the DI via V_{max} is:

$$DI = 0.5 \div 3.6 = 0.14 \quad (2)$$

And the DI via VTI is:

$$DI = 13 \div 90 = 0.14 \quad (3)$$

The Z_{VA} (or global hemodynamic load) is an index that reflects the total resistance to flow across the AV. This index is defined as the ratio of the estimated left ventricular systolic pressure (the sum of systolic blood pressure [SBP] and mean AV pressure gradient [mPG]) to the indexed stroke volume (SVi):

$$Z_{VA} = (SBP + mPG) \div SVi \quad (4)$$

This is most helpful in low-flow states ($Z_{VA} \geq 4.5$ mm Hg/mL/m² = severe AS). In this patient, the Z_{VA} is:

$$Z_{VA} = (112 + 27) \div 30 = 4.6 \text{ mm Hg/mL/m}^2 \quad (5)$$

The AV AT measures the time from the AV opening to the AV peak velocity. This is useful in identifying early versus late peaking AS jets. When the AS jet is late peaking (AT $\geq$120 ms), this indicates severe AS, and AT >100 ms is likely severe AS. The AT in this patient is 133 ms, which is consistent with severe AS.

The ejection time is the time from onset to end of systolic flow. This measurement by itself does not help to assess for AS severity. However, the AT/ET ratio can help evaluate AS severity. An AT/ET ratio $\geq$0.35 is able to identify severe AS with good accuracy. In this patient, the AT/ET ratio is:

$$AT/ET = 133 \div 380 = 0.35 \quad (6)$$

21. **Answer: B.** The visual assessment of the aortic valve (AV) shows that it has three leaflets that are calcified and restricted in motion. The calculated aortic valve area (AVA) is 0.7 cm², which indicates severe AS:

$$AVA = (0.785 \times 2^2 \times 12) \div 56 = 0.7 \text{ cm}^2 \quad (1)$$

The calculated AVA is probably correct because the valve is severely calcified and restricted. However, the AV V_{max} is 2.4 m/s and the mean PG is 13 mm Hg, which are not consistent with severe AS. The discrepancy between the V_{max}, mean gradient, and the AVA could be a result of measurement error or a low-flow state. Given that the measurements are said to be accurate, the flow status needs to be considered. As previously described, the SVi is calculated from the LVOT stroke volume and the BSA. In this case, the SVi is:

$$SVi = 38 \div 2.1 = 18 \text{ mL/m}^2 \qquad (2)$$

This is consistent with low flow across the AV, which explains the V_{max} <4 m/s and mean gradient <40 mm Hg in the setting of severe AS. When there is a low-flow status, the next step is to consider the LVEF to determine if this is LF-LG severe AS or paradoxical LF-LG severe AS. In this case, the LVEF is 51%, which is normal. Hence, this would be classified as severe LF-LG AS with normal LVEF, also called paradoxical LF-LG AS. This patient is referred for additional testing to rule out true severe AS versus pseudo-severe AS. But by considering the DI of 0.25 by V_{max} (0.21 by VTI), the Z_{VA} of 6.9 mm Hg/mL/ m^2 and the AV AT of 116 ms, this is likely to be true severe AS.

$$DI_{(Vmax)} = 0.6 \div 2.4 = 0.25 \qquad (3)$$

$$DI_{(VTI)} = 12 \div 56 = 0.21 \qquad (4)$$

$$Z_{VA} = (111 + 13) \div 18 = 6.9 \text{ mm Hg/mL/m}^2 \qquad (5)$$

22. **Answer: B.** There are two types of LF-LG severe AS (**Figure 19-20A**). One has normal left ventricular ejection fraction (LVEF; ≥50%), which is referred to as paradoxical LF-LG AS, and the other has abnormal LVEF (<50%), which is referred to as classical LF-LG AS. Both have low flow (indexed stroke volume ≤35 mL/m²) and low mean pressure gradient (≤40 mm Hg). In classical LF-LG AS, a stress (dobutamine or exercise) echocardiogram or computed tomography (CT) for calcium score is useful to differentiate true severe AS from pseudo-severe AS (**Figure 19-20B**). For patients with paradoxical LF-LG AS, other criteria can be considered to determine the likelihood of severe AS being present (**Figure 19-20C**).

KEY POINTS

▶ Use the step-by-step approach to assess AS by considering valve morphology, velocities and gradients, AVA, flow status, and the LVEF.

▶ LF-LG AS may be classical LF-LG AS with a depressed LVEF or paradoxical LF-LG AS with a normal LVEF.

▶ Classical LF-LG AS with a depressed LVEF may be true severe AS or pseudo-severe AS (differentiated by dobutamine stress echo and/or CT calcium score).

▶ Paradoxical LF-LG AS is recognized by identifying the cause of low flow; criteria that increase the likelihood of severe AS being present include clinical criteria, qualitative imaging data (e.g., LV hypertrophy), and quantitative imaging data (e.g., CT calcium score, AVA).

▶ An AV calcium score >1200 Agatston units (AU) (women) or >2000 AU (men) and an AV calcium density ≥300 AU/ cm² (women) or ≥500 AU/cm² (men) are used to identify hemodynamically severe AS.

23. **Answer: A.** A bicuspid aortic valve is best visualized in **Video 19-5A** and **Figure 19-6B** (systolic still frame). During systole, only two commissures are seen and a "raphe" is clearly identifiable. The valve is bicuspid with fusion of the right and noncoronary cusps. Observe that during diastole (see **Figure 19-6A**), the valve appears trileaflet; therefore, a BAV is best diagnosed during systole.

24. **Answer: B.** The patient has severe AS and moderate AR. **Table 19-11** lists the AS criteria for this study and the criteria for severe AS. This patient has a congenital bicuspid aortic valve with degenerative changes due to calcium build up on the valve from years of renal disease. Therefore, there is both congenital and degenerative aortic valve (AV) disease.

Table 19-12 lists the qualitative and semiquantitative parameters for AR severity. The vena contracta width of the AR jet is 0.44, which falls in the moderate range and there was no holodiastolic reversal of flow seen in the descending aorta, indicating a reduced likelihood of severe AR.

Table 19-11.

	This Study	**Severe AS**
AV V_{max} (m/s)	4.2	≥4.0
AV mean gradient (mm Hg)	46	≥40
DI	0.23	<0.25

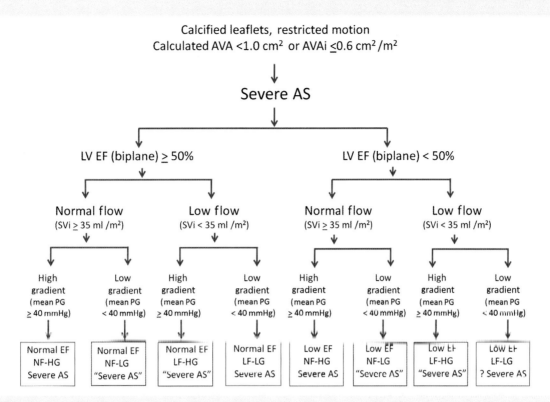

Figure 19-20A (From Piedmont Heart Institute.)

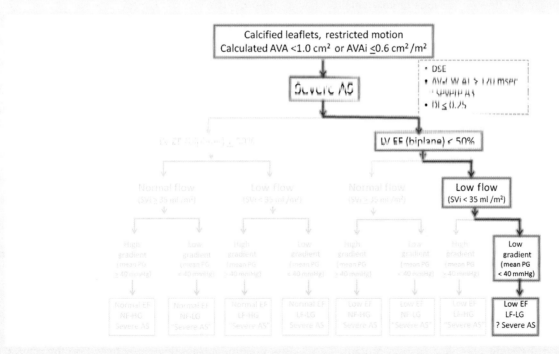

Figure 19-20B (From Piedmont Heart Institute.)

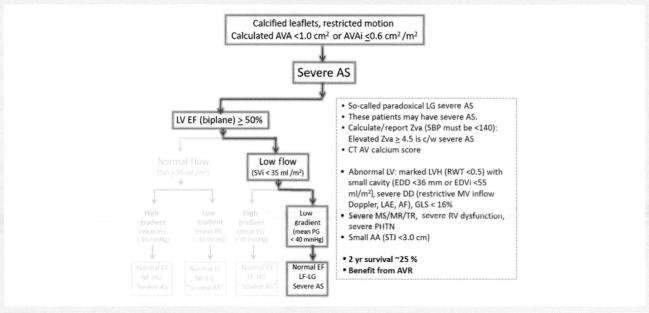

Figure 19-20C (From Piedmont Heart Institute.)

Table 19-12. Qualitative and Semiquantitative Parameters for Aortic Regurgitation Severity

| | Mild | Moderate | | Severe |
	Grade I	Grade II	Grade III	Grade IV
Jet width in LVOT, color flow	Small in central jets	Intermediate		
Flow convergence, color flow	None or very small	Intermediate		Large
Jet density, CWD	Incomplete or faint	Dense		Dense
PHT (ms)	>500	500-200		<200
Diastolic flow reversal in descending aorta, PWD	Brief, early diastolic reversal	Intermediate		Prominent holodiastolic reversal
VCW (cm)	<0.3	0.3 0.6		>0.6
Jet width/LVOT width, central jets (%)	<25	25-45	46-64	≥65
Jet CSA/LVOT CSA, central jets (%)	<5	5-20	21-59	≥60

CSA, cross-sectional area; CWD, continuous-wave Doppler; LVOT, left ventricular outflow tract; PHT, pressure half-time; PWD, pulsed-wave Doppler; VCW, vena contracta width.

Reprinted from Zoghbi WA, Adams D, Bonow RO, et al. Recommendations for noninvasive evaluation of native valvular regurgitation. A report from the American Society of Echocardiography developed in collaboration with the Society for Cardiovascular Magnetic Resonance. *J Am Soc Echocardiogr.* 2017;30(4):303-371. Copyright © 2017 by the American Society of Echocardiography. With permission.

25. **Answer: E.** The AR jet (color Doppler) looks moderate but is actually underestimated due to the eccentricity of the jet. The left ventricle (LV) is dilated in this case and the right coronary cusp is prolapsing into the LV. The AR is severe due to the malcoaptation of the noncoronary and right coronary cusps documented in this TEE. Answers A, B, and C are incorrect since there is no evidence of aortic cusp perforation (answer A), aortic cusp restriction (answer B), or aortic annulus dilatation and normal cusp motion (answer C).

26. **Answer: B.** A functional classification for AR has been proposed similar to the Carpentier classification for mitral regurgitation (**Figure 19-21**). For AR, the functional classification is based on the mechanisms of AR and the surgical repair techniques. In type I dysfunction, the aortic cusp motion is normal, and AR occurs due to dilatation of the aorta or due to cusp perforation. Type II dysfunction refers to leaflet prolapse as a result of excessive cusp tissue or commissural disruption. Type III refers to leaflet restriction, which may occur in bicuspid,

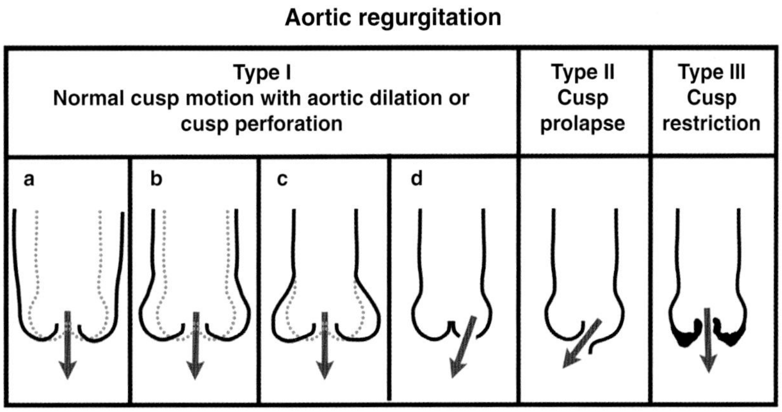

Aortic regurgitation

	Type I Normal cusp motion with aortic dilation or cusp perforation				Type II Cusp prolapse	Type III Cusp restriction
	a	b	c	d		

Figure 19-21 Functional classification of AR. Type Ia depicts sinotubular junction enlargement and dilatation of the ascending aorta. Type Ib depicts dilatation of the sinuses of Valsalva and sinotubular junction. Type Ic depicts dilatation of the ventriculoarterial junction (annulus). Type Id denotes aortic cusp perforation. Type II dysfunction refers to leaflet prolapse. Type III refers to leaflet restriction. (Reprinted from Zoghbi WA, Adams D, Bonow RO, et al. Recommendations for noninvasive evaluation of native valvular regurgitation. A report from the American Society of Echocardiography developed in collaboration with the Society for Cardiovascular Magnetic Resonance. *J Am Soc Echocardiogr.* 2017;30(4):303-371. Copyright © 2017 by the American Society of Echocardiography. With permission.)

degenerative, or rheumatic valvular disease and as a result of calcification, thickening, and fibrosis of the aortic leaflets. There is no type IV classification.

In this patient, there is AR secondary to cusp prolapse; therefore, this is type II dysfunction and answer B is correct.

27. **Answer: C.** The EROA in this case was calculated as 0.22 cm², which places the severity of aortic regurgitation (AR) in the moderate range. However, this is a case of severe AR with an eccentric AR jet. Although EROA is advantageous for the quantitative assessment of AR severity, it can be less accurate in eccentric jets. In addition, small errors in the radius measurement can lead to substantial errors in EROA due to squaring of the error.

Answer A is incorrect since the reduced compliance of the aorta, especially in elderly patients, can result in holodiastolic flow reversal in the aorta in the absence of severe AR; the aortic compliance does not affect the EROA calculation. Answer B is incorrect since the left ventricular (LV) compliance affects the AR pressure half-time (PHT), not the EROA calculation. For example, in patients with chronic severe AR with a compliant left ventricle, the AR PHT may be prolonged as the LV is able to accommodate an increase in volume without a significant increase in the LV diastolic pressure. In contrast, mild AR in patients with severe diastolic dysfunction may have a short PHT because the diastolic pressure in the noncompliant LV increases significantly with only a small increase in LV volume.

28. **Answer: A.** Myxomas are generally located in the left atrium; thus, answer B is incorrect. Papillary fibroelastomas are often located on the cardiac valves but are smaller (<1 cm); thus, answer C is

incorrect. Thrombi on native valves are extremely rare; thus, answer F is unlikely. A paraganglioma could be located in the aortic root but generally occurs in young adults and is relatively immobile; thus, answer D is incorrect. A rhabdomyoma could be located in the left ventricular outflow tract and/or at the level of the aortic valve; however, it occurs most often in children younger than 4 years. Thus, answer E is incorrect. Therefore, the most probable etiology of the mass is endocarditis; thus, the correct answer is A.

29. **Answer: B.** The AR as seen in the apical-5 chamber view (**Video 19-7E**) shows a central jet caused by the infective endocarditis (**Figure 19-7F**). On the continuous-wave Doppler tracing (**Figure 19-8**), the AR jet is dense, and the deceleration slope is steep. The pressure half time measured was 136 ms indicating severe AR (see **Table 19-12**).

30. **Answer: D.** The AR is a mild eccentric jet. The VCW was <0.3 cm (it was 0.22 cm) and the pressure half-time was >500 ms (it was 606 ms). These values confirm mild AR (see **Table 19-12**).

31. **Answer: C.** The AR was a mild eccentric jet confirmed by the vena contracta width <0.3 cm (2.2 cm) and the pressure half-time >500 ms (606 ms). The eccentric jet was directed posteriorly toward the mitral valve and basal inferolateral wall. This is an indirect sign of AR similar to high frequency fluttering and "reverse doming" of the anterior mitral valve leaflet. Answer A is incorrect as the AR severity is only mild. Answer B is incorrect since AR occurs in diastole and systolic anterior motion (SAM) of the mitral valve occurs in systole. Answer D is incorrect since the eccentric jet was not directed anteriorly toward the interventricular septum.

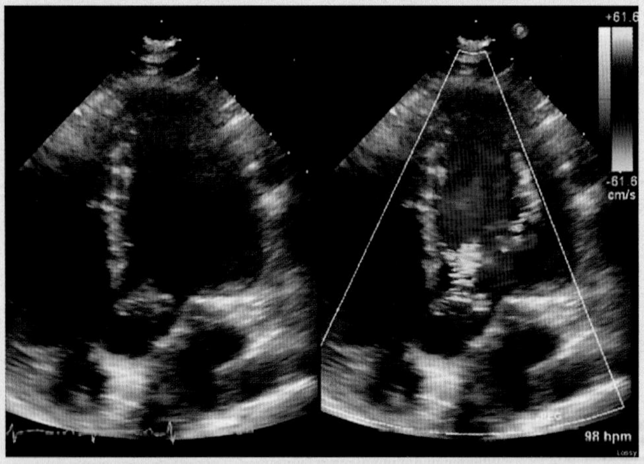

Figure 19-22

32. **Answer: A.** The vena contracta is defined as the narrowest part of the jet downstream from the narrowed (or regurgitant) orifice. Measurement of the VCW provides an estimate of the regurgitant orifice size. The VCW is measured perpendicular to the long axis of the AR jet. The VCW is best measured from the parasternal long-axis view with a zoomed and narrow sector. This allows optimal temporal and spatial resolution.

Answer B is incorrect since the standard technique for color Doppler imaging is to use a Nyquist limit of 50 to 70 cm/s as well as a high color gain that just eliminates random color speckle from nonmoving regions. The cutoff values listed in **Table 19-12** for the VCW and various grades of AR are based on measurements performed when the color Nyquist limit is set between 50 and 70 cm/s. Answer C is incorrect. Although the VCW may be used as a surrogate for the regurgitant orifice size, it is not the same as the effective regurgitant orifice area. Answer D is incorrect since the AR jet width or height is measured about 0.5 to 1.0 cm proximal to the aortic valve, in the left ventricular outflow tract, while the VCW is measured at the narrowest width of the jet, yielding a smaller value.

Table 19-13. Recommendations for Intervention in Patients With Severe AS (ESC/EACTS Guidelines 2017)

Symptomatic severe AS (surgical AVR or TAVI)	Class[a]	Level[b]
Indicated in severe high gradient AS (AV V$_{max}$ >4 m/s or mean gradient >40 mm Hg).	I	B
Indicated in patients with low-flow low-gradient severe AS with reduced ejection fraction and evidence of contractile reserve excluding pseudo-severe AS.	I	C
Should be considered in patients with low-flow low-gradient severe AS with preserved ejection fraction after careful confirmation of severe AS.	IIa	C
Should be considered in patients with low-flow low-gradient severe AS with reduced ejection fraction without evidence of contractile reserve, especially where CT calcium scoring confirms severe AS.	IIa	C
Should NOT be performed in patients with severe comorbidities where the intervention is unlikely to improve quality of life or survival.	III	C
Asymptomatic severe AS (surgical AVR only)		
Indicated in patients with severe AS and left ventricular systolic dysfunction (LVEF <50%) not due to another cause.	I	C
Indicated in patients with abnormal exercise test showing symptoms on exercise clearly related to AS.	I	C
Should be considered in patients with abnormal exercise test showing a decrease in blood pressure below baseline.	IIa	C
Should be considered if the surgical risk is low and one of the following abnormalities is present: • Very severe AS (AV V$_{max}$ >5.5 m/s). • Severe valve calcification with a rate of progression ≥0.3 m/s per year. • Markedly elevated BNP (>3-fold above age-corrected and sex-corrected normal range) confirmed by repeated measurements without other explanations. • Severe pulmonary hypertension (systolic pulmonary artery pressure >60 mm Hg at rest confirmed by invasive measurement) without other explanation.	IIa	C

AS, aortic stenosis; AV, aortic valve; BNP, B-type natriuretic peptide; LVEF, left ventricular ejection fraction; TAVI, transcatheter aortic valve implantation.

[a]Class of recommendation.
[b]Level of evidence. From Baumgartner H, Falk V, Bax JJ, et al. 2017 ESC/EACTS guidelines for the management of valvular heart disease. *Eur Heart J*. 2017;38(36):2739-2791. Copyright © 2017 European Society of Cardiology. Reproduced by permission of Oxford University Press.

33. **Answer: A.** The patient has severe AS and moderate AR. The AV peak velocity is 4.3 m/s (>4.0 m/s), mean gradient is 46 mmHg (>40 mm Hg), AVA is 0.8 cm² (<1 cm²), and DI is 0.22 (<0.25); all of these parameters are consistent with severe AS (values in the parentheses are the cutoff values for severe AS; see **Table 19-9**). For the AR, in this patient the VCW is 0.52 cm (0.3-0.5 cm), PHT is 432 ms (200-500 ms), and R$_{Vol}$ is 43 mL (30-59 mL); all of these parameters are consistent with moderate AR (values in the parentheses are the cutoff values for moderate AR; see **Tables 19-11** and **19-13**).

34. **Answer: C.** This patient has severe AS and moderate AR based on the values mentioned previously (see answer outline for Question 33). The patient's symptoms are likely related to severe AS. This patient has a class I indication for an aortic valve replacement (AVR); therefore, this patient should undergo a surgical AVR (SAVR) or a transcatheter AVR (TAVR) procedure (**Table 19-13**).

35. **Answer: E.** An aortic regurgitant volume of 50 mL is not a specific criterion for severe AR; this is moderate AR (see **Table 19-10**). An RVol >60 mL indicates severe AR. The remaining values and signs in answers A, B, C, and D are specific signs of chronic severe AR. The presence of four or more of these criteria indicates severe chronic AR. Importantly, no single measurement or Doppler parameter is precise enough to quantify AR in individual patients, and therefore, an integration of multiple parameters is required to determine the severity of AR.

Acknowledgments: The authors thank and acknowledge Mani Vannan, MBBS, Shizhen Liu, MD, PhD, for their assistance with this chapter. The authors also acknowledge the contributions from Marie-Annick Clavel, DVM, PhD, Sorin V. Pislaru, MD, PhD, Maurice Enriquez-Sarano, MD, and Philippe Pibarot, DMV, PhD (Chapter 16, Aortic Valve Disease) in *Clinical Echocardiography Review. A Self Assessment Tool, 2nd Edition,* edited by Allan L. Klein, Craig R. Asher, 2017.

SUGGESTED READINGS

Baumgartner H, Hung J, Bermejo J, et al. Recommendations on the echocardiographic assessment of aortic valve stenosis: a focused update from the European Association of Cardiovascular Imaging and the American Society of Echocardiography. *J Am Soc Echocardiogr.* 2017;30(4):372-392.

Clavel M-A, Magne J, Pibarot P. Low-gradient aortic stenosis. *Eur Heart J.* 2016;37(34):2645-2657.

Everett RJ, Clavel MA, Pibarot P, Dweck MR. Timing of intervention in aortic stenosis: a review of current and future strategies. *Heart.* 2018;104(24):2067-2076.

Harris P, Kuppurao L. Quantitative Doppler echocardiography. *BJA Educ.* 2015;16(2):46-52.

Zoghbi WA, Adams D, Bonow RO, et al. Recommendations for noninvasive evaluation of native valvular regurgitation: a report from the American Society of Echocardiography developed in collaboration with the Society for Cardiovascular Magnetic Resonance. *J Am Soc Echocardiogr.* 2017;30(4):303-371.

CHAPTER 20

Mitral Valve Disease

Contributors: Karen G. Zimmerman, BS, ACS, RDCS (AE/PE), RVT and Jennifer Mercandetti, BS, ACS, RDCS (AE/PE)

✪ Question 1

Which pressure half-time (PHT) measurement of the mitral valve inflow signal shown in **Figure 20-1** is correct?

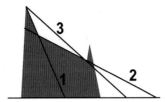

Figure 20-1

- **A.** Trace 1
- **B.** Trace 2
- **C.** Trace 3

✪✪✪ Question 2

Which of the following statements is true regarding the echocardiographic evaluation of mitral stenosis (MS)?

- **A.** The concept behind the pressure half-time (PHT) method is that the rate in which the transmitral pressure gradient decreases is directly proportional to the mitral valve area (MVA).
- **B.** The proximal isovelocity surface area (PISA) method for calculating the MVA is not accurate in the presence of significant mitral regurgitation (MR).
- **C.** The continuity equation for the calculation of the MVA is not dependent on the heart rate.

- **D.** The mitral valve resistance (resistance to flow caused by MS) has a high prognostic value and provides additional value for assessing MS severity.
- **E.** All of the above are true.

✪ Question 3

Which of the following statements is true regarding two-dimensional (2D) or three-dimensional (3D) planimetry of the mitral valve area (MVA)?

- **A.** Planimetry is an indirect measurement of MVA.
- **B.** When performing planimetry of the MVA, the measurement should be performed at end-diastole.
- **C.** MVA by planimetry is the reference measurement for stenosis severity in degenerative valve disease.
- **D.** When performing planimetry of the MVA, care should be taken to ensure the measurement is performed at the leaflet tips.

✪ Question 4

Which method in **Figure 20-2** demonstrates the correct measurement of the mean transmitral pressure gradient in mitral stenosis (MS)?

- **A.** Method a
- **B.** Method b
- **C.** Method c
- **D.** Method d
- **E.** All the above are correct

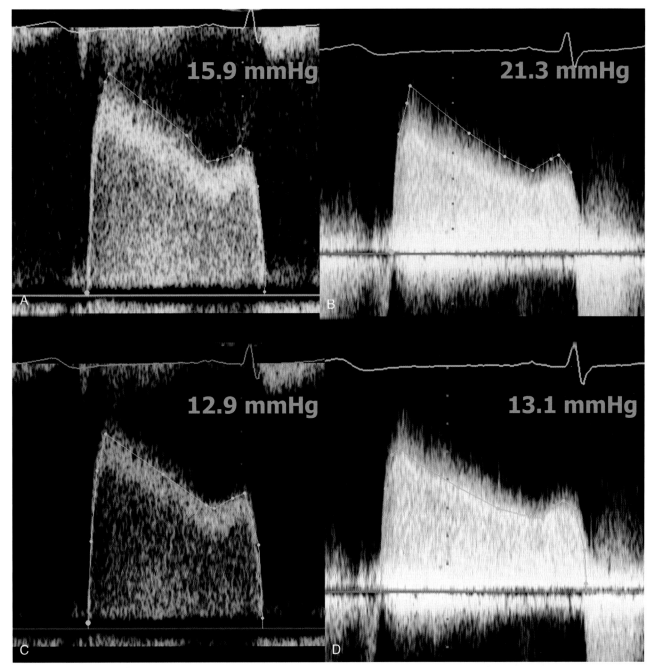

Figure 20-2

Question 5

Which of the following disease states is the most likely cause of the echocardiographic findings demonstrated in **Figure 20-3** and **Videos 20-1A** to **20-1D**, acquired in a 54-year-old woman?

   A. Rheumatic fever

   B. Chronic kidney disease

   C. Carcinoid heart disease

   D. Systemic bacterial endocarditis

Question 6

Which of the following mechanisms, demonstrated by 3D imaging of the mitral valve in **Figure 20-4**, is responsible for the increase in mitral valve area (MVA) following successful balloon valvuloplasty utilizing the Inoue technique?

   A. Tearing of the mitral valve leaflet(s)

   B. Separation of the fused and retracted chordae

   C. Splitting the commissures

   D. None of the above

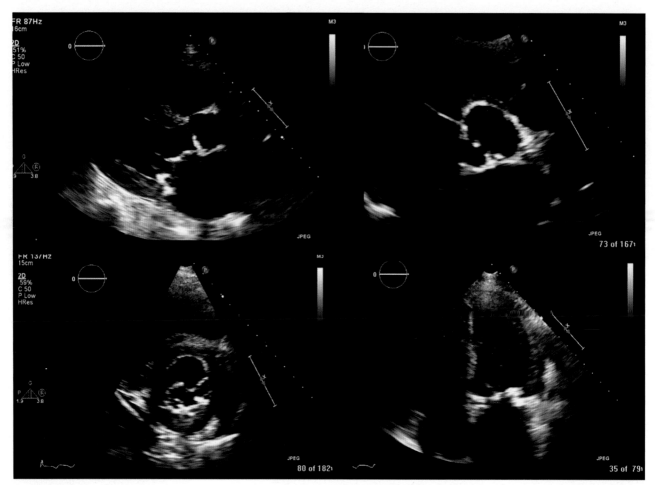

Figure 20-3

Question 7

Which of the following is not an echocardiographic scoring system that is used to assess the mitral valve anatomy prior to a percutaneous balloon mitral valvuloplasty (PBMV)?

- **A.** Cormier score
- **B.** McConnell score
- **C.** Padial score
- **D.** Wilkins score

✪✪ Question 8

Which of the following echocardiographic imaging planes is recommended for the evaluation of the mitral subvalvular apparatus in mitral stenosis (MS)?

- **A.** Transesophageal midesophageal long axis
- **B.** Transesophageal transgastric short axis
- **C.** Transthoracic parasternal short axis
- **D.** Transesophageal transgastric 2 chamber
- **E.** All of the above

✪✪ Question 9

In a patient with rheumatic mitral stenosis (MS), post percutaneous balloon mitral valvotomy (PBMV), what is the recommended method for assessing the degree of residual stenosis?

- **A.** Mean transmitral pressure gradient
- **B.** Deceleration time
- **C.** Direct planimetry of the mitral valve area (MVA)
- **D.** MVA via the proximal isovelocity surface area (PISA) method

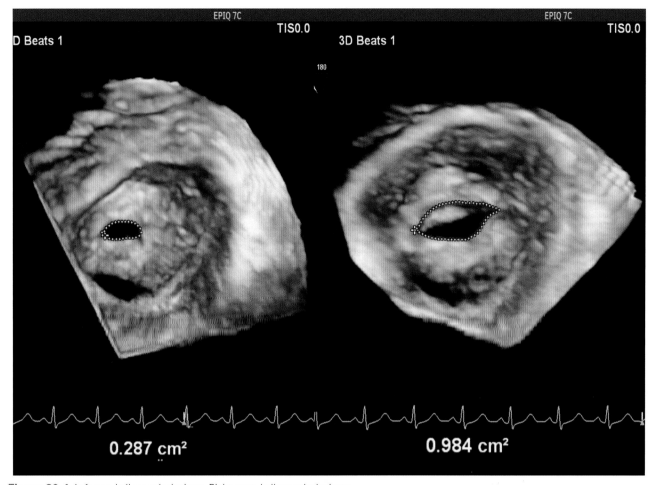

Figure 20-4 Left, pre–balloon valvuloplasty. Right, post–balloon valvuloplasty.

✪✪○ Question 10

The transesophageal echocardiographic (TEE) images in **Figure 20-5** and **Videos 20-2A** to **20-2C** were obtained in the cardiac catheterization laboratory to evaluate the mitral valve prior to percutaneous balloon valvuloplasty (PBMV). Based on the findings, which of the following statements is true?

A. The degree of mitral stenosis (MS) is only mild and does not warrant intervention.

B. There is moderate MS and moderate mitral regurgitation (MR), which is not suitable for PBMV.

C. There is severe MS with favorable anatomy that is suitable for PBMV.

D. The patient is at risk for systemic embolization and the intervention should be delayed at this time.

✪✪✪ Question 11

A 20-year-old woman is referred for an echocardiogram after noticing shortness of breath while training for an upcoming marathon. The echocardiogram demonstrates restriction of the anterior mitral leaflet with a "hockey stick" appearance, fusion of the lateral commissure, and trace mitral regurgitation (MR). The patient has a resting heart rate of 50 bpm. Her left atrial volume index (LAVI) is 35 mL/m², basal right ventricular (RV) dimension is 41 mm, peak tricuspid regurgitant (TR) velocity is 2.2 m/s, and the inferior vena cava is a normal size with normal inspiratory collapse. No other abnormalities are noted on the examination. What will be the most likely result of her mitral valve assessment?

A. Mitral valve area (MVA) of 2.0 cm² by direct planimetry

B. Mean transmitral pressure gradient of 11 mm Hg

C. MVA of 1.4 cm² by pressure half-time

D. MVA of 4.5 cm² by direct planimetry

E. There is insufficient information to comment on the mitral valve assessment

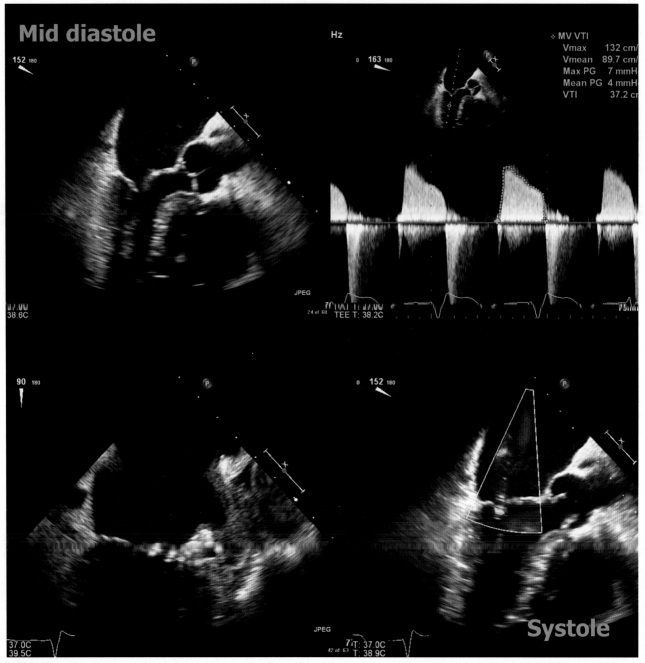

Figure 20-5

✪✪✪ Question 12

Which of the following patients is the best candidate for percutaneous balloon mitral valvuloplasty (PBMV)?

A. 93-year-old woman with a Wilkins score of 7, pressure half-time (PHT) of 240 ms, a mean transmitral gradient of 6 mm Hg at a heart rate of 55 bpm, mild mitral regurgitation (MR), and an estimated right ventricular systolic pressure (RVSP) of 49 mm Hg.

B. 54-year-old man with a history of lymphoma, Cormier group 3, a mean transmitral gradient of 12 mm Hg, moderate MR, and an estimated RVSP of 65 mm Hg.

C. 32-year-old man with end-stage renal disease, Padial score of 10 with extensive annular calcification and asymmetric heterogeneous fibrosis of the anterior leaflet, and a mean transmitral gradient of 8 mm Hg.

D. 18-year-old woman with a parachute mitral valve, a mean gradient of 10 mm Hg, and an estimated RVSP of 35 mm Hg.

✪ Question 13

▶ Which is the correct order of etiology of mitral valve disease demonstrated in **Figure 20-6** and **Videos 20-3A** to **20-3D**?
- **A.** a. Rheumatic, b. Degenerative, c. Congenital, d. Posterior reduction annuloplasty
- **B.** a. Degenerative, b. Congenital, c. Posterior reduction annuloplasty, d. Rheumatic
- **C.** a. Congenital, b. Posterior reduction annuloplasty, c. Rheumatic, d. Degenerative
- **D.** a. Posterior reduction annuloplasty, b. Degenerative, c. Rheumatic, d. Congenital

✪✪ Question 14

A transthoracic echocardiogram revealed the following: an effective regurgitant orifice area (EROA) of 40 cm^2, regurgitant volume (R$_{Vol}$) of 60 mL, an estimated left ventricular end-diastolic volume (LVEDV) of 170 mL, and a reduced left ventricular ejection fraction (LVEF) of 40%. Which grade of mitral regurgitation (MR) most likely applies to this scenario?
- **A.** Mild
- **B.** Moderate
- **C.** Severe
- **D.** Indeterminant

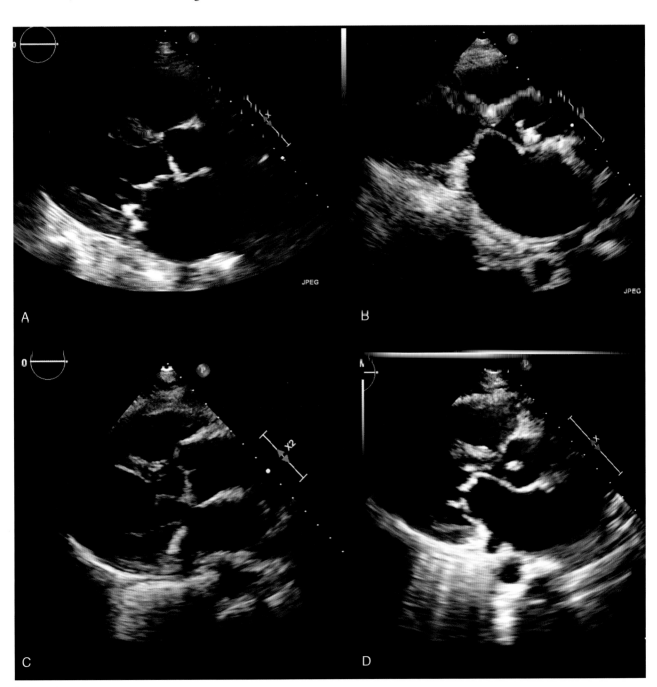

Figure 20-6

✪ Question 15

Mitral regurgitation (MR) resulting from degenerative disease, endocarditis, or rheumatic disease, where the valve itself is directly involved in the disease process, is identified as:

    A. Primary MR.
    B. Secondary MR.
    C. Functional MR.
    D. Carpentier MR.

✪ Question 16

Papillary muscle displacement and decreased interpapillary shortening is a result of:

    A. Primary mitral regurgitation (MR).
    B. Secondary MR.
    C. Fibroelastic deficiency (FED).
    D. Rheumatic mitral valve disease.

✪✪ Question 17

Mitral regurgitation (MR) in a young asymptomatic patient with bileaflet mitral valve prolapse (MVP) is likely due to:

    A. Rheumatic mitral valve disease.
    B. Fibroelastic deficiency (FED).
    C. Hypertrophic cardiomyopathy (HCM).
    D. Barlow disease.

✪ Question 18

The Carpentier classification for mitral leaflet dysfunction is based on leaflet motion in relation to the plane of the annulus. Which type of leaflet dysfunction is identified when the leaflets don't open in diastole?

    A. Type I
    B. Type II
    C. Type IIIa
    D. Type IIIb

✪✪ Question 19

During which phase of the cardiac cycle is the mitral annulus measured to obtain information needed for intervention planning?

    A. Systole
    B. Diastole
    C. Isovolumic relaxation
    D. Diastasis

✪ Question 20

▶ The 3D transesophageal en face view of the mitral valve shown in **Figure 20-7** and **Video 20-4** demonstrates ruptured chords involving:

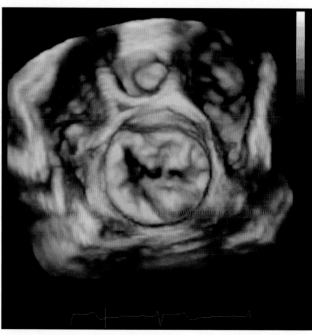

Figure 20-7

    A. The anterolateral aspect of A1.
    B. The anterolateral aspect of P3.
    C. The anterolateral aspect of P1.
    D. The posteromedial aspect of P2.

✪✪✪ Question 21

Which echocardiographic parameter is necessary for planning an intervention for patients with ischemic mitral regurgitation (IMR)?

    A. C-sept distance
    B. Leaflet length
    C. Left ventricular (LV) wall thickness
    D. Tenting area
    E. All of the above

✪✪ Question 22

Which type of myocardial infarction will cause asymmetric mitral leaflet tethering, which will be evident on the 2D and color Doppler echocardiographic examinations?

    A. Anterior
    B. Inferior
    C. Anterolateral
    D. Septal

✪ Question 23

In which direction would the mitral regurgitant (MR) jet most likely be directed with posterior mitral leaflet flail?

   A. Anteriorly
   B. Posteriorly
   C. Centrally
   D. Superiorly

✪✪ Question 24

In which direction would the mitral regurgitation (MR) jet most likely be directed with posterior leaflet tethering?

   A. Anteriorly
   B. Posteriorly
   C. Central
   D. Superiorly

✪✪ Question 25

Which of the settings described below would most often result in central mitral regurgitation (MR)?

   A. Annular dilation from fibroelastic deficiency (FED) and symmetric systolic restriction from a dilated cardiomyopathy
   B. Posterior myocardial infarction and isolated P3 flail from FED
   C. Anterior leaflet congenital cleft and posterior leaflet perforation from endocarditis
   D. Complex prolapse and flail from Barlow disease and posterior leaflet congenital cleft

✪ Question 26

In which direction would the mitral regurgitation (MR) jet most likely occur with bileaflet mitral valve prolapse?

   A. Anteriorly directed
   B. Posteriorly directed
   C. Centrally directed
   D. Possibly none of the above

✪ Question 27

Which of the following statements is false?

   A. Mitral valve prolapse (MVP) can be diagnosed from the parasternal long-axis view when one or more of the leaflet segments is seen billowing into the left atrium past the annular plane.

   B. MVP can be seen by M-mode echocardiography as late-systolic posterior motion of the leaflets.
   C. MVP can reliably be diagnosed from the 4-chamber view in most cases.
   D. Systolic flow reversals in the pulmonary veins are a sign of significant mitral regurgitation.

✪ Question 28

Which of the following parameters is most consistent with severe mitral regurgitation (MR)?

   A. Color jet area/left atrial area of 40%
   B. Regurgitant volume of 45 mL
   C. Vena contracta width of 0.75 cm
   D. Systolic dominance on the pulmonary venous trace
   E. All of the above

✪ Question 29

The PISA calculation is based on flow that:

   A. Accelerates distal to a regurgitant orifice.
   B. Accelerates proximal to a regurgitant orifice.
   C. Is perpendicular to a regurgitant orifice.
   D. Is turbulent downstream from a regurgitant orifice.

✪ Question 30

From the transthoracic apical views, in which direction is the color baseline shifted to find the aliasing velocity needed to calculate the mitral effective regurgitant orifice area (EROA) via the PISA method?

   A. Down
   B. Up
   C. Set the baseline to 15 cm/s
   D. Adjust the baseline to 100 cm/s

✪✪ Question 31

Which of these findings is not usually associated with significant mitral regurgitation (MR)?

   A. A dilated left atrium (LA)
   B. Atrial fibrillation
   C. An A-wave dominant transmitral inflow pattern
   D. Congestive heart failure

✪✪✪ Question 32

A V cut-off sign seen on the mitral regurgitant (MR) continuous-wave (CW) Doppler trace is consistent with:

A. High left atrial (LA) compliance.
B. A marked increase in LA pressure with systole.
C. A marked increase in left ventricular (LV) pressure with systole.
D. A and B.
E. A and C.

✪✪✪ Question 33

Which one of the statements regarding mitral regurgitation (MR) below is false?

A. The first sign of left ventricular (LV) systolic impairment in chronic MR is an increased end-systolic dimension.
B. The presence of pulmonary artery systolic pressure (PASP) >50 mm Hg at rest is an indication to proceed with surgery in asymptomatic patients with chronic secondary MR.
C. LV dilatation that occurs as a consequence of chronic MR tends to be spherical and global.
D. Acute severe MR is characterized by a large regurgitant orifice and LV dilatation.

✪✪ Question 34

Which of the following statements regarding the vena contracta width (VCW) is false?

A. VCW is valid when there are multiple jets.
B. VCW is less influenced by loading conditions than other color Doppler parameters.
C. VCW is reliable for both central and eccentric jets.
D. In patients with mitral regurgitation (MR) in which the jet is elliptical (as opposed to circular), the VCW width of the regurgitant jet may appear abnormally broad or as a double jet.

✪✪ Question 35

Which of the following statements regarding the benefits of cross-sectional 3D-derived vena contracta area (VCA) is false?

A. No assumptions are made regarding the shape of the regurgitant orifice.

B. VCA can be used with multiple jets.
C. Compared to the flow convergence method, VCA yields lower values for effective regurgitant orifice area (EROA).
D. VCA provides a measure of EROA.

✪✪ Question 36

Which of the following statements best describes the benefits of using color jet area and/or color jet length in assessing mitral regurgitation (MR)?

A. Color jet area is a useful screening tool for MR.
B. Color jet area is independent of loading conditions and a quick and reliable way to assess MR severity.
C. Color jet length is particularly helpful with assessment of eccentric MR.
D. MR wall-hugging jets, with a small jet area, are not usually severe.
E. All of the above.

✪✪ Question 37

Which statement regarding mitral regurgitation (MR) is true?

A. The elliptical shape of a mitral regurgitant orifice usually results in an overestimation of regurgitant flow using the proximal isovelocity surface area (PISA) method.
B. When flow convergence is nonhemispherical, decreasing the color aliasing velocity will make the flow convergence smaller and less prone to constraint.
C. The PISA for estimating the effective regurgitant orifice area (EROA) cannot be used for multiple jets.
D. Primary MR resulting from a flail leaflet generally has a more circular orifice, while the orifice resulting from secondary MR is usually more elliptical.

✪✪ Question 38

Which of the following statements regarding the proximal isovelocity surface area (PISA) method for mitral regurgitation (MR) is false?

A. PISA is most accurate for central MR.

B. PISA is taken from a single-frame image and will overestimate the MR severity if MR is not holosystolic.

C. Poor alignment of the MR jet will underestimate MR severity via the PISA method.

D. The simplified PISA method can be used for patients with very low blood pressures.

✪ Question 39

Which transesophageal view should be used to measure the vena contracta (VC) of mitral regurgitation (MR)?

A. Mid esophageal (ME) commissural view

B. ME long-axis view

C. ME 4-chamber view

D. Deep transgastric view

CASE 1

A 59-year-old woman was referred for evaluation of mitral stenosis and candidacy for percutaneous balloon mitral valvuloplasty (PBMV). She is clinically symptomatic, NYHA Class II to III with exertional dyspnea and exercise intolerance, and near syncope with bending and squatting. She has developed atrial fibrillation that required cardioversion. Her echocardiogram revealed a mitral valve with even thickening and restriction of leaflets, extending from tips to the midportion. There was evidence of fusion of both the lateral and medial commissures. There was a single area of calcification noted and trace mitral regurgitation along the lateral commissure. The chordae appeared thickened proximal to the leaflet tips. Heart rate at the time of the exam was 56 bpm in normal sinus rhythm. The mean transmitral gradient was 6.6 mm Hg, pressure half-time was 226.2 ms, and mitral valve area by 3D planimetry was 0.79 cm². There was no evidence of aortic stenosis, a trace of aortic insufficiency and mild tricuspid regurgitation.

✪✪ Question 40

Which of the following echocardiographic findings is not taken into consideration when predicting whether or not this patient is likely to develop severe mitral regurgitation (MR) after percutaneous balloon mitral valvuloplasty (PBMV)?

A. Fusion of both the lateral and medial commissures

B. Thickening and restriction of both leaflets

C. Single area of calcification along the lateral commissure

D. Chordae appeared thickened proximal to the leaflet tips

✪✪✪ Question 41

Which of the following statements is most accurate regarding the assessment of mitral valve anatomy in this patient?

A. The Wilkins score is 10, making this patient an ideal candidate for PBMV.

B. The patient is in group 2 based on the Cormier score, and should undergo PBMV.

C. The patient's Wilkins score is 7, and she is an ideal candidate for PBMV.

D. The patient is Cormier Group 1 and should receive a mitral valve replacement.

CASE 2

A 96-year-old woman presents for consultation for her valvular heart disease and consideration for percutaneous mitral balloon valvotomy (PBMV). She has a history of severe three-vessel coronary artery disease diagnosed following a non-Q wave apical myocardial infarction. She has had a permanent VVI pacemaker placed for sick sinus syndrome. She also has a history of atrial fibrillation and diabetes mellitus that have been well controlled. An echocardiogram performed at that time was notable for severe mitral stenosis with primarily anterolateral commissural fusion with calcification, a mean transmitral gradient of 10 mm Hg, and severe pulmonary hypertension (estimated right ventricular systolic pressure of 80 mm Hg). She was not considered an ideal operative candidate due to her age and a palliative PBMV was performed using the Inoue technique.

✪✪ Question 42

Which of the following complications can be seen in the transesophageal echocardiographic (TEE) image in **Figure 20-8**, following a single successful balloon dilation of the mitral valve?

A. Atrial septal defect (ASD)

B. Pericardial tamponade

C. Severe traumatic mitral regurgitation (MR)

D. Thromboembolic event

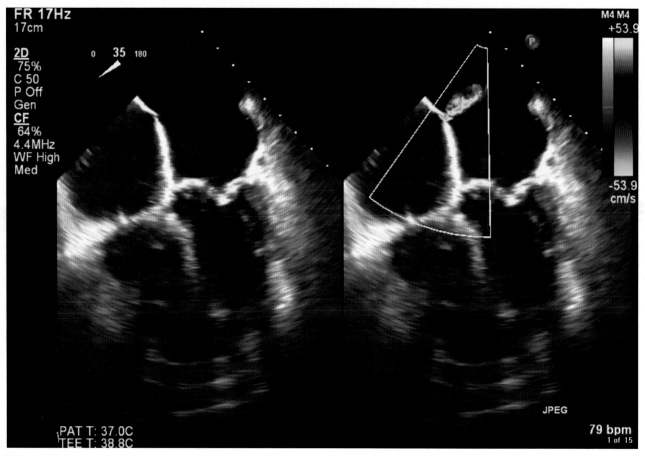

Figure 20-8

ANSWERS

1. **Answer: B. Figure 20-1** shows the various methods that can be used to measure PHT in nonlinear Doppler spectra. Trace 1 measures the PHT in early diastole by following the early diastolic slope. Trace 2 measures the PHT by measuring the slope from mid-diastole to end-diastolic velocity just prior to atrial contraction. Trace 3 measures the PHT by the "mean" slope method, which measures the slope from the peak early diastolic velocity to the peak end-diastolic velocity just prior to atrial contraction. The correct measurement technique is trace 2. Using trace 1 for measuring mitral valve PHT is a common mistake. The first part of the signal is reflective of both left atrial (LA) and left ventricular (LV) pressure, not only of mitral stenosis. In cases where the deceleration slope is nonlinear, the American Society of Echocardiography (ASE) recommends that the deceleration slope in mid-diastole rather than the early deceleration slope be measured.

2. **Answer: C.** The continuity equation for MS utilizes the concept of the conservation of mass; that is, what goes in equals what goes out. In the case of MS, the stroke volume passing through the mitral valve in diastole must be equal to the stroke volume exiting the aorta in systole. This is true regardless of heart rate; therefore, answer C is correct.

Answer A is incorrect. The PHT method for MVA is derived from the equation: MVA = 220 ÷ PHT. Therefore, the decrease in the PHT is inversely proportional to the MVA.

Answer B is incorrect as the PISA method for calculating the MVA can be used accurately in the presence of significant MR. This is because measurements are made during diastole. The accuracy of the PISA calculation is limited by errors in the measured radius of flow convergence, and the opening angle of the leaflets. Answer D is incorrect. The mitral valve resistance is defined as the ratio of mean mitral gradient to transmitral diastolic flow rate, which is calculated by dividing the stroke volume by the diastolic filling period. This parameter has been proposed as an alternative measurement of the severity of MS; however, it has not been shown to have an additional prognostic value, it has no additional value over

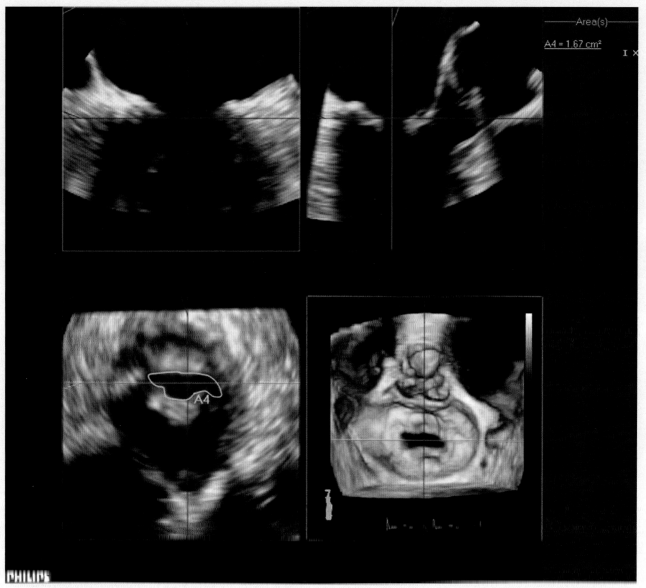

Figure 20-9 Measurement of mitral valve area (MVA) using multiplanar reconstruction. Axial 3D images of the mitral valve (MV) are shown. The frame with the largest diastolic opening of the MV has been chosen for analysis. The top left panel shows a commissural 2D slice; the top right image shows a long-axis 2D slice; the bottom left panel shows a short-axis slice at the level of the leaflet tips; the bottom right panel shows a volume-rendered 3D image in the surgical orientation from the left atrial aspect. In the commissural and long-axis quadrants, the red and green lines have been adjusted so they are positioned through the center of the mitral orifice, and the blue lines have been adjusted so they pass through the narrowest part of the mitral orifice. MVA has been measured with planimetry (bottom left panel). The measurement of 1.67 cm² indicates mild mitral stenosis. (Reproduced with permission of the Oxford Publishing Limited through PLSclear, from Sidebotham DA, Merry AF, Legget ME, et al, eds. *Practical Perioperative Transesophageal Echocardiography*. 3rd ed. Oxford, England: Oxford University Press; 2018:132.)

the MVA, and there is no clear threshold for MS severity. Therefore, this method is not recommended for clinical use.

3. **Answer: D.** When performing planimetry of the MVA, care should be taken to ensure the measurement is performed at the leaflet tips. Use of 3D, biplane, and/or careful 2D scanning from the apex to the base of the heart should be used to ensure that the measurement is obtained at the leaflet tips (**Figure 20-9**).

Answer A is incorrect as planimetry of the mitral orifice is a direct tracing of the anatomic MVA. It

is obtained from a parasternal short-axis view (or 3D dataset), with the scan plane perpendicular to the orifice. Answer B is incorrect since the mitral valve orifice should be identified and planimetered in mid-diastole. Answer C is incorrect as in degenerative mitral stenosis, the stenosis begins at the base and works its way to the leaflet tips and is more calcified in nature; this makes planimetry of the MVA less accurate.

4. **Answer: D.** Methods a and c are pulsed-wave (PW) Doppler traces as evidenced by the incomplete filling of the Doppler spectrum. PW Doppler is not

recommended for acquiring MS Doppler signals as the accuracy of measurements from these signals relies on the sample volume being placed at the narrowest region of flow. Therefore, methods a and c are incorrect for measuring the mean transmitral pressure gradient and answers A and C are incorrect. Continuous-wave (CW) Doppler is preferred to ensure maximal velocities are recorded. CW Doppler continuously "samples" along the entire length of the ultrasound beam; therefore, the maximal velocity will not be missed provided that the ultrasound beam is aligned parallel with flow. Method b overestimates the mean pressure gradient; therefore, answer B is incorrect. In Method d, the mean pressure gradient is traced along the densest edge of the signal; therefore, answer D is correct.

KEY POINTS

The mean transmitral pressure gradient in MS should be measured from a CW Doppler trace.

Optimization of gain settings, wall filters, beam orientation, and a good acoustic window are needed to obtain well-defined contours of the transmitral Doppler profile.

The mean gradient should be measured by tracing along the dense edge of the signal.

5. **Answer: B.** Valvular heart disease is common in patients with chronic kidney disease who are undergoing maintenance dialysis. Abnormalities include valvular and annular thickening and calcification of any of the heart valves, more commonly the aortic and mitral valves. The images provided show aortic and mitral valvular calcification. The anterior mitral leaflet and chordae appear normal in thickness and length and the valve orifice extends through to the commissures.

Answer A is incorrect as rheumatic heart disease results in thickening and calcification of the mitral leaflets, fusion of the commissures, and fibrosis and shortening of the chordae; these findings are not seen in the images provided. Answer C is incorrect as carcinoid heart disease causes thickening and dysfunction of the right-sided cardiac valves. Left-sided valves can be affected in the presence of an intracardiac shunt; however, both pulmonary and tricuspid valves appear normal in the parasternal short-axis view. Answer D is incorrect. Vegetations are the hallmark of infective endocarditis and are typically attached to the upstream side of the valve; that is, on the ventricular side for the semilunar valves and on the atrial side for atrioventricular valves. They typically present as an oscillating mass with a motion independent to that of the valve. Healed vegetations can calcify; however, this would be unlikely to result in echocardiographic findings shown in **Figure 20-3**.

6. **Answer: C.** The primary mechanism of stenosis in rheumatic mitral valve disease is fusion of the commissures. The goal of percutaneous balloon mitral valvotomy (PBMV) is to "crack" the commissures and increase the MVA. The 3D image of the MVA in **Figure 20-4** (viewed from the apex) demonstrates a threefold increase in valve area (0.3 cm^2 to almost 1.0 cm^2).

Answer A is incorrect as tears of the anterior or posterior leaflets during a PBMV result in moderate to severe mitral regurgitation and often require surgical intervention, making the procedure unsuccessful. Answer B is incorrect as separation of the fused and retracted chordae is achieved with open surgical commissurotomy.

7. **Answer: B.** Treatment of symptomatic mitral stenosis includes surgical mitral valve replacement or PBMV. The Cormier, Wilkins, and Padial scores are used to help determine the appropriate choice for the individual patient. The Cormier score (answer A) classifies patients into three groups, according to anterior leaflet mobility and extent of subvalvular disease, and their suitability for closed-heart commissurotomy, open-heart commissurotomy, or valve replacement (**Table 20-1**A). The Wilkins score is used to determine whether mitral valve morphology is suitable for PBMV (**Table 20-1**B). The criteria for scoring include an assessment of leaflet mobility, valve thickening, subvalvular fibrosis, and valve calcification. Each item is given a score of 1 to 4, with the total score being the sum of the four items (between 4 and 16). The lower the score, the more favorable the anatomy for PBMV. The Padial score is used to predict the development of severe mitral

Table 20-1A. Assessment of Mitral Valve Anatomy According to the Cormier Score

Echocardiographic Group	Mitral Valve Anatomy
Group 1	Pliable noncalcified anterior mitral leaflet and mild subvalvular disease (i.e., thin chordae >10 mm long)
Group 2	Pliable noncalcified anterior mitral leaflet and severe subvalvular disease (i.e., thickened chordae <10 mm long)
Group 3	Calcification of mitral valve of any extent, as assessed by fluoroscopy, whatever the state of subvalvular apparatus

From Iung B, Cormier B, Ducimetière P, et al. Immediate results of percutaneous mitral commissurotomy. A predictive model on a series of 1514 patients. *Circulation*. 1996;94(9):2124-2130.

Table 20-1B. Assessment of Mitral Valve Anatomy According to the Wilkins Score

Grade	Mobility	Subvalvular Thickening	Leaflet Thickening	Calcification
1	Highly mobile valve with only leaflet tips restricted	Minimal thickening just below the mitral leaflets	Leaflets near normal in thickness (4-5 mm)	A single area of increased echo brightness
2	Leaflet mid and basal portions have normal mobility	Thickening of chordal structures extending up to one-third of the chordal length	Mid-leaflets normal, considerable thickening of margins (5-8 mm)	Scattered areas of brightness confined to leaflet margins
3	Valve continues to move forward in diastole, mainly from the base	Thickening extending to the distal third of the chords	Thickening extending through the entire leaflet (5-8 mm)	Brightness extending into the midportion of the leaflets
4	No or minimal forward movement of the leaflets in diastole	Extensive thickening and shortening of all chordal structures extending down to the papillary muscles	Considerable thickening of all leaflet tissue (>8-10 mm)	Extensive brightness throughout much of the leaflet tissue

The total score is the sum of each of these echocardiographic features and ranges from 4-16.

From Wilkins GT, Weyman AE, Abascal VM, Block PC, Palacios IF. Percutaneous balloon dilatation of the mitral valve: an analysis of echocardiographic variables related to outcome and the mechanism of dilatation. Br Heart J. 1988;60(4):299-308.

regurgitation following PBMV (**Table 20-1C**). Scoring the mitral valve by the Padial criteria is based on the evaluation of subvalvular disease, commissural calcification, as well as the heterogeneity of fibrosis and calcification on each leaflet; each parameter is scored from 1 to 4, with the total score being between 4 and 16.

8. **Answer. D.** The goal of evaluating the subvalvular apparatus in MS is to determine the extent of thickening, fusion, and shortening of the chordae tendineae. Although the short-axis views (answers B and C) allow for visualization of chordal thickening,

and to some extent the amount of fusion, they do not demonstrate the full length of the chordae and therefore cannot be used to fully evaluate the extent of subvalvular involvement and overall reduction in chordal length and are therefore not the best choice. A long-axis view (answer A) is required for direct visualization of the chordal length. In the normal patient, the chordae are able to be viewed from transesophageal midesophageal views. However, with the ultrasound beam originating behind the left atrium, in the patient with MS, there is corresponding image dropout below the mitral valve; therefore,

Table 20-1C. Assessment of Mitral Valve Anatomy According to the Padial Score

Grade	Leaflet Thickening (Score Each Valve separately.)	Commissure Calcification	Subvalvular Disease
1	Leaflet near normal (4-5 mm) or with only a thick segment	Fibrosis and/or calcium in only one commissure	Minimal thickening of chordal structures just below the valve
2	Leaflet fibrotic and/or calcified evenly; no thin areas	Both commissures mildly affected	Thickening of chordae extending up to one-third of chordal length
3	Leaflet fibrotic and/or calcified with uneven distribution; thinner segments are mildly thickened (5-8 mm)	Calcium in both commissures; one markedly affected	Thickening of the distal third of the chordae
4	Leaflet fibrotic and/or calcified with uneven distribution; thinner segments are near normal (4-5 mm)	Calcium in both commissures; both markedly affected	Extensive thickening and shortening of all chordae extending down to the papillary muscle

The total score is the sum of each of these echocardiographic features and ranges from 4-16.

From Padial LR, Abascal VM, Moreno PR, Weyman AE, Levine RA, Palacios IF. Echocardiography can predict the development of severe mitral regurgitation after percutaneous mitral valvuloplasty by the Inoue technique. *Am J Cardiol.* 1999;83(8):1210-1213.

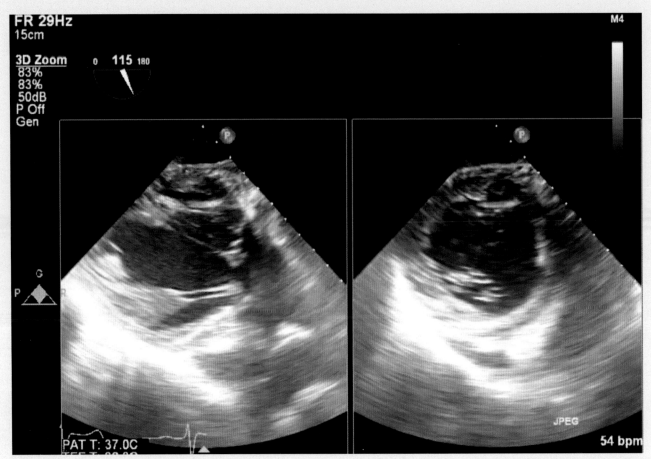

Figure 20-10 Transgastric biplane 2-chamber and short-axis views. Transesophageal transgastric 2-chamber view, shown on the left, clearly demonstrating the full extension of the chordae tendineae from the papillary muscles to the mitral valve leaflets. This view allows for the evaluation of the extent of chordal thickening, fusion, and subsequent reduction in chordal length that occurs with the rheumatic process. The cross-sectional view demonstrated by the biplane image on the right demonstrates the limitation in assessing chordae from the short-axis planes.

answer A is incorrect. The transgastric 2-chamber view avoids artifact at the valvular level and allows the best visualization of the subvalvular apparatus (**Figure 20-10**); therefore, answer D is correct.

9. **Answer: C.** The MVA is the specific parameter used to classify severity of MS. Direct measurement of the anatomic MVA is the reference measurement of choice, both pre- and post-PBMV, for determining the severity of MS. This is because unlike other methods, planimetry does not involve any hypothesis regarding flow conditions, cardiac chamber compliance, or associated valvular lesions.

    The mean transmitral gradient (answer A) is not a reliable marker for evaluation of severity since it is dependent on the MVA as well as a number of other factors that influence transmitral flow rate such as the heart rate, cardiac output, and associated mitral regurgitation (MR), which is common post-PBMV. Due to acute changes in cardiac hemodynamics post-PBMV, the pressure half-time method for calculating MVA (derived from the deceleration time) is inaccurate; therefore, answer B is incorrect. PISA calculation of the MVA (answer

D) can be used, even in the presence of MR; however, it is time consuming and technically demanding and is therefore not the recommended method of choice.

10. **Answer: D.** While the TEE images display favorable valve anatomy, and only mild MR, the lower left image in **Figure 20-5** and **Video 20-2B**, demonstrates thrombus within the left atrial appendage (LAA). This finding warrants delaying intervention until the patient is adequately anticoagulated and the LAA thrombus is resolved.

11. **Answer: A.** The four stages of mitral stenosis (MS) are defined by valve anatomy, valve hemodynamics, the consequences of valve obstruction on the left atrium (LA) and pulmonary circulation, and patient symptoms (**Table 20-2**). Based on the information provided, the patient exhibits features of progressive (Stage B) mitral valve disease: rheumatic valve changes with commissural fusion and diastolic doming of the mitral valve leaflets, mild LA enlargement (LAVI: 35 mL/m^2), and normal pulmonary artery systolic pressure (PASP) at rest (22 mm Hg calculated from the TR pressure gradient of

Table 20-2. Stages of Mitral Stenosis

Stage	Definition	Valve Anatomy	Valve Hemodynamics	Hemodynamic Consequences	Symptoms
A	At risk of MS	• Mild valve doming during diastole	• Normal transmitral flow velocity	• None	• None
B	Progressive MS	• Rheumatic valve changes with commissural fusion and diastolic doming of the mitral valve leaflets • Planimetered MVA >1.5 cm²	• Increased transmitral flow velocities • MVA >1.5 cm² • Diastolic pressure half-time <150 ms	• Mild-to-moderate LA enlargement • Normal pulmonary pressure at rest	• None
C	Asymptomatic severe MS	• Rheumatic valve changes with commissural fusion and diastolic doming of the mitral valve leaflets • Planimetered MVA ≤1.5 cm² • MVA ≤1.0 cm² with very severe MS	• MVA ≤1.5 cm² • (MVA ≤1.0 cm² with very severe MS) • Diastolic pressure half-time ≥150 ms • (Diastolic pressure half-time ≥220 ms with very severe MS)	• Severe LA enlargement • Elevated PASP >30 mm Hg	• None
D	Symptomatic severe MS	• Rheumatic valve changes with commissural fusion and diastolic doming of the mitral valve leaflets • Planimetered MVA ≤1.5 cm²	• MVA ≤1.5 cm² • (MVA ≤1.0 cm² with very severe MS) • Diastolic pressure half-time ≥150 ms • (Diastolic pressure half-time ≥220 ms with very severe MS	• Severe LA enlargement • Elevated PASP >30 mm Hg	• Decreased exercise tolerance • Exertional dyspnea

The transmitral mean pressure gradient should be obtained to further determine the hemodynamic effect of the MS and is usually >5-10 mm Hg in severe MS; however, due to the variability of the mean pressure gradient with heart rate and forward flow, it has not been included in the criteria for severity. LA, left atrial; LV, left ventricular; MS, mitral stenosis; MVA, mitral valve area; PASP, pulmonary artery systolic pressure.

From Nishimura RA, Otto CM, Bonow RO, et al. 2014 AHA/ACC guideline for the management of patients with valvular heart disease: a report of the American College of Cardiology/American Heart Association Task Force on Practice Guidelines. *Circulation*. 2014;129:2440-2492. With permissions from Lippincott Williams & Wilkins.

19 mm Hg + normal right atrial pressure of 3 mm Hg). In this stage, the planimetered MVA is greater than 1.5 cm²; therefore, answer A is correct.

Answer B is incorrect since a mean transmitral pressure gradient >10 mm Hg is consistent with severe MS and the hemodynamic consequences of severe MS include severe left atrial enlargement and an elevated pulmonary artery systolic pressure (PASP). Answer C is incorrect as an MVA ≤1.5 cm² is associated with elevated PASP and marked left atrial enlargement. Answer D is incorrect as a normal MVA is 4 to 5 cm² and this would not support her symptoms or echocardiographic findings.

12. **Answer: A.** As previously discussed, the Cormier, Wilkins and Padial scores are used to help determine the appropriate choice for the individual patient. A Cormier score of 3 (group 3) is considered unfavorable for a PBMV; therefore, answer B is incorrect. A Padial score of ≥10 identifies those patients likely to

develop severe MR following a mitral balloon valvuloplasty via the Inoue technique; therefore, answer C is incorrect. Mitral stenosis resulting from mantle radiation or chronic kidney disease is typically more calcified in nature and these patients should be referred for surgery when the time is right. Mitral stenosis resulting from abnormalities of the subvalvular apparatus (as in parachute mitral valve) is better treated by open commissurotomy or mitral valve replacement; therefore, answer D is incorrect. A Wilkins score of ≤8 recognizes patients who will have a good result post valvuloplasty; therefore, answer A is correct.

13. **Answer: B.** The main lesion in degenerative mitral stenosis (MS) is calcification of the mitral annulus. Due to the nature of the disease, it is frequently observed in the elderly. With calcific mitral stenosis, valve thickening or calcification mainly affects the base of the leaflets (demonstrated in **Figure 20-6A**,

Table 20-3. Quantitative Parameters for MR Severity

	Mild	Moderate		Severe
	Grade I	Grade II	Grade III	Grade IV
R_{Vol} (mL)	<30	30-44	45-59	≥60
RF (%)	<30	30-39	40-49	≥50
EROA (cm²)	<0.2	0.2-0.29	0.30-0.39	≥0.4

EROA, effective orifice area; MR, mitral regurgitation; RF, regurgitant fraction, R_{Vol}, regurgitant volume.

From Zoghbi WA, Adams D, Bonow RO, et al. Recommendations for noninvasive evaluation of native valvular regurgitation: a report from the American Society of Echocardiography developed in Collaboration with the Society for Cardiovascular Magnetic Resonance. *J Am Soc Echocardiogr.* 2017;30(4):303-371.

panel a and **Video 20-3A**). Congenital MS is primarily due to an abnormality of the subvalvular apparatus as demonstrated with a parachute mitral valve as seen in this 28-year-old patient with Shone syndrome (**Figure 20-6B**, panel b and **Video 20-3B**). The valve is supported by a single papillary muscle resulting in tethering of the leaflets and a funnel-shaped orifice. **Figure 20-6C**, panel c and **Video 20-3C** demonstrate mitral valve repair via posterior reduction annuloplasty. The echogenic structure noted along the posterior leaflet is the annuloplasty ring. The primary mechanism of rheumatic MS is fusion of the commissures resulting from the inflammatory response initiated by rheumatic fever. This fusion is demonstrated in the long-axis view of the mitral valve by the diastolic "hockey stick" appearance of the mitral valve (**Figure 20-6D**, panel d and **Video 20-3D**).

14. **Answer: C.** Mitral regurgitation is graded as mild (Grade I), moderate (Grade II and III) and severe (Grade IV). There are several parameters that can be used for evaluation of MR severity; quantitative parameters include the effective orifice area (EROA), regurgitant volume (R_{Vol}), and the regurgitant fraction (RF) (**Table 20-3**). According to the 2017 American Society of Echocardiography guidelines for the non-invasive evaluation of native valvular regurgitation, severe MR is considered with an EROA ≥0.40 cm², regurgitant fraction (RF) ≥50% and R_{Vol} ≥60 mL.

15. **Answer: A.** The etiology of MR is broadly categorized as primary and secondary. Primary (organic) mitral valve disease involves lesions that directly alter the anatomy of the valve, such as degenerative and rheumatic disease. Examples of lesions include thin or weak leaflets, infected tissue, displaced or excessive leaflets, or scarred tissue. Secondary (functional) mitral valve disease results from lesions that distort left ventricular geometry, such as ischemia and cardiomyopathies. In secondary valve disease, the valve is essentially normal and dysfunction results from a ventricular problem that distorts the mitral valve. **Figure 20-11**

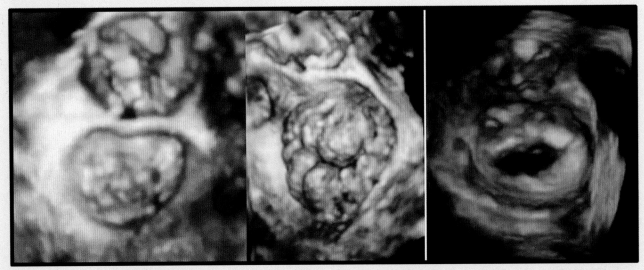

Figure 20-11 Examples of lesions in primary mitral valve disease that directly alter the anatomy of the valve itself. The left image displays thin or weak leaflets seen with fibroelastic deficiency or endocarditis. The middle image displays excessive leaflet tissue seen with Barlow disease. The right image shows scarred and thickened leaflet tissue seen with rheumatic disease.

shows various 3D echocardiographic examples of causes of MR.

16. **Answer: B.** As previously described, secondary valve disease is the result of a ventricular problem. Secondary MR is caused by left ventricular (LV) dilatation from coronary artery disease (regional or ischemic cardiomyopathies) and diffuse global or dilated cardiomyopathies. Dysfunction results from leaflet tethering during systole. The lesions that commonly result from myopathic disease are

displacement of the papillary muscles. Two patterns of lesions from cardiomyopathy are recognized: asymmetric and symmetric (**Figure 20-12**).

17. **Answer: D.** Barlow disease is a primary degenerative mitral valve disease identified by a dramatically enlarged mitral annulus with redundant leaflet tissue and/or chordal apparatus. The Barlow patient is typically younger and asymptomatic. This is a genetic disease and there is often tricuspid and aortic involvement. Lesions for

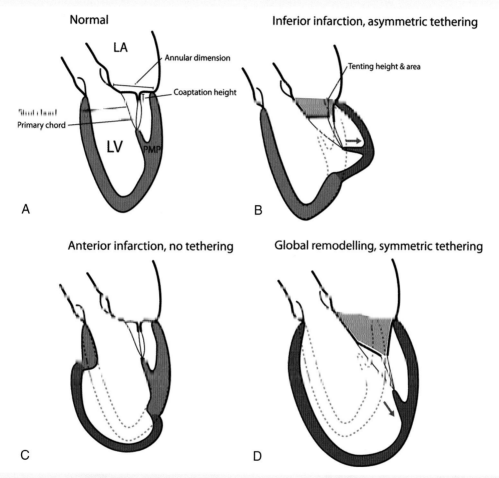

Figure 20-12 Leaflet tethering patterns and secondary (functional) MR. Panel A, Normal appearances of the mitral leaflets at end-systole. The plane of coaptation is at, or just below, the level of the annular plane, and there is significant leaflet overlap (coaptation height). Panel B, Asymmetric leaflet tethering following an inferior or posterior myocardial infarction. Localized remodeling (shaded blue) causes lateral displacement (indicated by the directional arrow) of the posteromedial papillary muscle (PMP), leading to bileaflet tethering, particularly of the posterior leaflet, and anterior leaflet override. Tension on the anterior leaflet from secondary chordae may cause bending of the midportion of the leaflet ("seagull sign"). If present, the jet of MR is posteriorly directed. The severity of leaflet tethering can be quantified by measuring tenting height and area. Tenting height is the distance from the coaptation point to the annular plane, and tenting area is the area bounded by leaflets and annular plane. Panel C, Effect of anterior myocardial infarction. Remodeling (shaded blue) after anterior infarction typically involves more myocardium than inferior infarction but causes less leaflet tethering. See text for details. Panel D, Symmetric leaflet tethering due to global LV remodeling. There is apical and lateral displacement (indicated by the red directional arrow) of both papillary muscles with bileaflet tethering. The coaptation point is displaced well into the left ventricle (LV), resulting in a marked increase in tenting height. There may be a central jet of MR. Symmetric tethering is associated with dilated cardiomyopathy and global remodeling after anterior myocardial infarction. If present, the jet of MR is typically central. LA = left atrium. (Reprinted from Sidebotham DA, Allen SJ, Gerber IL, et al. Intraoperative transesophageal echocardiography for surgical repair of mitral regurgitation. *J Am Soc Echocardiogr.* 2014;27(4):345-366. Copyright © 2014 American Society of Echocardiography. With permission.)

Barlow disease include excessive tissue, dramatic annular enlargement and chordal elongation (**Figure 20-13**). Regurgitation primarily results from leaflet prolapse due to chordal elongation and/or rupture.

Answer A is incorrect as MVP is not seen with rheumatic mitral valve disease. Answer B is incorrect since FED, which is characterized by thin delicate leaflet tissue, is typically seen in patients in their sixth decade. MR in these cases may occur as central regurgitation as a result of a lack of coaptation due to a mild or moderately dilated annulus or may occur when there is subsegmental prolapse. Furthermore, in FED there is usually a single, prolapsing segment (most commonly the middle scallop of the posterior leaflet) and bileaflet prolapse is uncommon. Answer D is incorrect since MR in patients with HCM is due to systolic anterior motion of the anterior mitral valve leaflet, not MVP.

18. **Answer: C.** The Carpentier classification of leaflet dysfunction is shown in **Figure 20-14**. Leaflet dysfunction where leaflet restriction occurs predominantly in diastole is type IIIa. Examples include rheumatic disease, radiation-induced valvulopathy, and dystrophic calcification. The lesions include thickened fibrotic tissue resulting in restricted leaflet motion during diastole.

19. **Answer: A.** Both percutaneous and surgical repair for mitral regurgitation attempt to restore normal systolic function. It is important to determine the anteroposterior axis and commissural axis annular dimensions to ensure the proper disease classification, for procedural planning, and to minimize the risk of postoperative systolic anterior motion (SAM). Remodeling annuloplasty is one of the most important principals of mitral repair. Reductive annuloplasty is important for many types of repair, but care must be taken to avoid mitral stenosis and SAM. Risk factors for SAM are shown in **Figure 20-15**

20. **Answer: D.** This 3D en face image of the mitral valve shows a partial flail of the posteromedial aspect of the P2 segment (**Figure 20-16**).

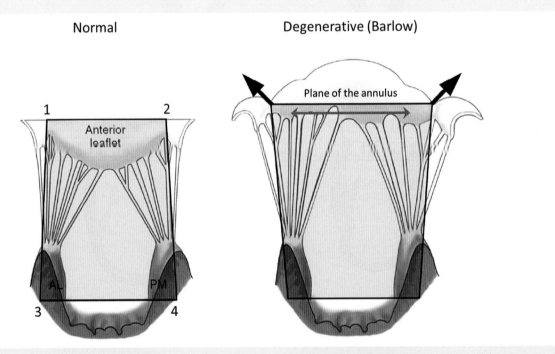

Figure 20-13 Left: The normal mitral trapezoid is defined by four points in a single plane: (1) the anterolateral commissure, (2) the posteromedial commissure, (3) the base of the anterolateral papillary muscle, and (4) the base of the posteromedial papillary muscle. The vertical sides of the trapezoid extend from the base of the papillary muscles to the commissures. Superiorly, the horizontal side of the trapezoid is defined as a line that that traverses the annulus between the two commissures (the mid-commissural annular width). Inferiorly, the horizontal line of the trapezoid extends between the bases of the papillary muscles (the interpapillary distance). Right: Degenerative disease (Barlow-type) results in annular enlargement, and elongation of the subvalvular apparatus. The interpapillary distance (inferior horizontal line) is usually normal; however, the mid-commissural width (superior horizontal line, plane of the annulus) is typically markedly increased and leaflets lie above the plane of the annulus. (Adapted from Drake DH, Zimmerman KG, Sidebotham DA. Transesophageal echocardiography for surgical repair of mitral regurgitation. In: Otto CM, ed. *Practice of Clinical Echocardiography*. 5th ed. Philadelphia, PA: Elsevier; 2017:346, chap 19. Reproduced with permission from David Sidebotham and Daniel Drake.)

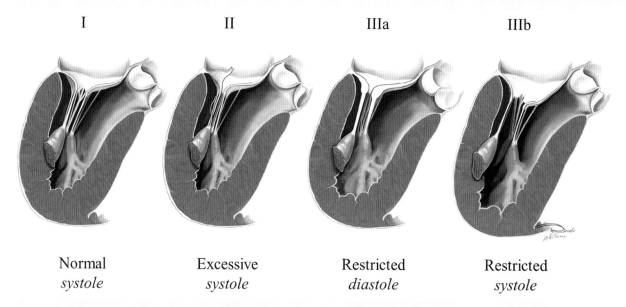

I	II	IIIa	IIIb
Normal *systole*	Excessive *systole*	Restricted *diastole*	Restricted *systole*

Figure 20-14 Carpentier classification for leaflet dysfunction. Type I dysfunction is defined as mitral regurgitation in the presence of normal leaflet motion; Examples include annular dilation, leaflet perforation, and leaflet cleft. Type I dysfunction can also result from the combination of degenerative and secondary disease. Type II dysfunction refers to excessive leaflet motion. Examples include leaflet prolapse and flail due to degenerative disease. Type III dysfunction refers to restricted leaflet motion. Type IIIa is leaflet restriction that occurs predominantly in diastole. Examples include rheumatic disease, radiation-induced valvulopathy, and dystrophic calcification. Type IIIb is leaflet restriction that occurs predominantly in systole. Type IIIb may be symmetric or asymmetric. Examples include dilated cardiomyopathy (symmetric) and myocardial infarction (asymmetric). (Adapted from Drake DH, Zimmerman KG, Sidebotham DA. Transesophageal echocardiography for surgical repair of mitral regurgitation. In: Otto CM, ed. *Practice of Clinical Echocardiography*. 5th ed. Philadelphia, PA: Elsevier; 2017:345, chap 19. Reproduced with permission from David Sidebotham and Daniel Drake.)

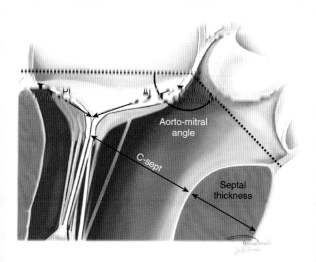

Figure 20-15 Echocardiographic measurements that can be performed in the prerepair echocardiogram include posterior leaflet length (PL), anterior leaflet length (AL), shortest distance between the coaptation point and the anterior septal wall (C-sept distance), aorto-mitral angle, septal thickness, and left ventricular (LV) end-diastolic diameter (not shown). Other than LV end-diastolic diameter, all measurements should be obtained in late systole in the mid-esophageal long-axis view. (From Drake DH, Zimmerman KG, Sidebotham DA. Transesophageal echocardiography for surgical repair of mitral regurgitation. In: Otto CM, ed. *Practice of Clinical Echocardiography*. 5th ed. Philadelphia, PA: Elsevier; 2017:359, chap 19. Reproduced with permission from David Sidebotham and Daniel Drake.)

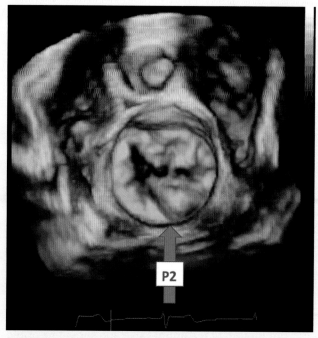

Figure 20-16 P2 leaflet located at the blue arrow is flail.

TEACHING POINT

Leaflet segments are named using the Carpentier nomenclature (**Figure 20-17**). With the mitral valve positioned in the surgeon's view, the aortic valve is above the mitral valve and the left atrial appendage is on the left. There are two minor indentations (sometimes called "clefts") in the posterior leaflet. These indentations divide the posterior leaflet into three segments. Using the Carpentier nomenclature, from left to right, these are termed P1, P2, and P3. The anterior leaflet has no indentations; however, the corresponding segments of the anterior leaflet are termed according to the opposing posterior leaflet segments as A1, A2, and A3.

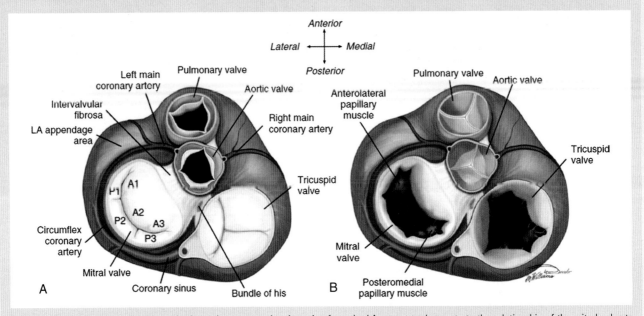

Figure 20-17 The base of the heart is shown in an anatomic orientation from the LA aspect to demonstrate the relationship of the mitral valve to adjacent cardiac structures. A is systole and B is diastole. The posterior leaflet of the mitral valve normally has two indentations (sometimes called "clefts"). These indentations divide the posterior leaflet into three segments that, using the Carpentier nomenclature, are termed P1, P2, and P3. Although there are no indentations in the anterior leaflet, the corresponding segments of the anterior leaflet are termed A1, A2, and A3. For purposes of echocardiographic orientation, it is useful to note that P1 is adjacent to the left atrial (LA) appendage and that P3 is adjacent to the tricuspid valve. (From Drake DH, Zimmerman KG, Sidebotham DA. Transesophageal echocardiography for surgical repair of mitral regurgitation. In: Otto CM, ed. *Practice of Clinical Echocardiography*. 5th ed. Philadelphia, PA: Elsevier; 2017:344, chap19. Reproduced with permission from David Sidebotham and Daniel Drake.)

21. **Answer: D.** There are multiple echocardiographic parameters used for guiding both percutaneous and surgical mitral repair or valve replacement; some of these have been mentioned already (see the answer outline for Question 19). For IMR, echocardiographic parameters considered for planning intervention include A2 and P2 closing angles, height of coaptation (or tenting height), tenting area, A2 bending angle, and interpapillary distance and shortening (**Figure 20-18**). Therefore, answer D is correct. Again, it is essential that the proper images are obtained to include all of this information.

C-sept distance (answer A), leaflet length (answer B), and LV wall thickness (answer C) are measurements that can be used to identify those at risk of developing postoperative systolic anterior motion of the mitral valve and should be noted on every mitral study. However, they are generally not used to quantitate the anatomy of IMR or plan intervention.

TEACHING POINT

For percutaneous mitral repair, the COAPT trial supports percutaneous IMR repair when the tenting height is 1.0 cm or less. For surgical repair, tenting areas of 1.0 cm² or less and a tenting height of <1.0 cm are associated with near uniform success with simple reductive ring annuloplasty. Note that tenting distance, tenting height, and height of coaptation are terms that are used interchangeably.

22. **Answer: B.** An inferior myocardial infarction is commonly the result of right coronary artery (RCA) occlusion. The RCA is frequently the only vessel supplying blood to the posteromedial papillary muscle. The posteromedial muscle inserts into the mid-inferior or inferolateral segment of the left ventricle. A posterior/inferior infarct may result in lateral displacement of the posteromedial papillary muscle, leading to bileaflet tethering, although

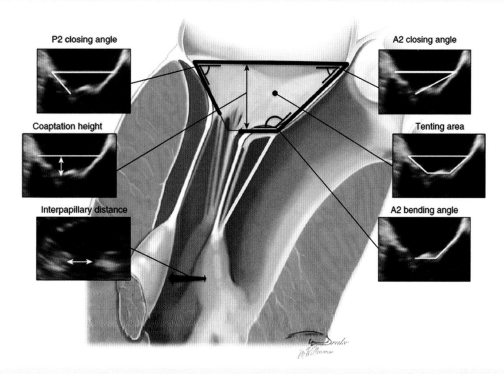

P2 closing angle

A2 closing angle

Coaptation height

Tenting area

Interpapillary distance

A2 bending angle

Figure 20-18 Indices of leaflet distortion with secondary mitral regurgitation. (From Drake DH, Zimmerman KG, Sidebotham DA. Transesophageal echocardiography for surgical repair of mitral regurgitation. In: Otto CM, ed. *Practice of Clinical Echocardiography*. 5th ed. Philadelphia, PA: Elsevier; 2017:361, chap 19. Reproduced with permission from David Sidebotham and Daniel Drake.)

more so of the posterior leaflet, with overriding of the anterior leaflet (see **Figure 20-19**). On the 2D echocardiographic examination, asymmetric tethering may cause bending of the midportion of the anterior mitral leaflet; this is known as the "seagull sign." On the color Doppler examination, the jet of MR is posteriorly directed.

23. **Answer: A.** The MR jet will usually be directed away from the affected area. Therefore, a flail posterior leaflet will usually result in an anteriorly directed MR jet (**Figure 20-19**).

24. **Answer: B.** With leaflet restriction the MR jet is usually directly toward the affected segment. Therefore, restriction of the posterior leaflet will usually result in a posteriorly directed MR jet. Restriction of the anterior leaflet will result in an anteriorly directed MR jet.

25. **Answer: A.** FED resulting in annular dilation without a flail segment typically produces a central MR jet. Similarly, a symmetric global cardiomyopathy can result in a central MR jet. Most other lesions are less predictable and tend to produce anterior, posterior, oblique, or complex jets.

26. **Answer: D.** The mere presence of bileaflet mitral valve prolapse (MVP) does not mean there is always significant MR. Bileaflet MVP is usually associated with redundant myxomatous leaflet tissue as seen from Barlow disease. These bulky leaflets may in fact prevent regurgitation. When MR is present with

these types of valves, it is usually the result of a dramatically dilated annulus, redundant leaflet tissue, and elongated and/or ruptured chordae tendineae. The resultant MR is complex and typically directed away from the segments with the most severe prolapse or flail segments.

27. **Answer: C.** The diagnosis of MVP via 2D echocardiography should not be made from the 4-chamber view. This is because the mitral annulus at end systole is saddle-shaped; as a result, the 4-chamber view slices the mitral valve obliquely (**Figure 20-20**). Therefore, from the 4-chamber view, the mitral valve may appear to prolapse simply due to the manner in which the valve is transected through the saddle-shaped annulus; hence, this view cannot be used to diagnose MVP.

28. **Answer: C.** The vena contracta (VC) is the narrowest portion of an MR jet that occurs at or just downstream from the regurgitant orifice (**Figure 20-21**). The VC width (VCW) measured perpendicular to the flow direction at the narrowest diameter or neck of the flow convergence, between the proximal isovelocity surface area and flow expansion into the left atrium (LA). The VCW reflects the diameter of the regurgitant orifice and is therefore considered a surrogate for the regurgitant orifice size. The advantage of this measurement is that it is independent of flow rate and driving pressure, it is less affected by instrument settings, and there is good

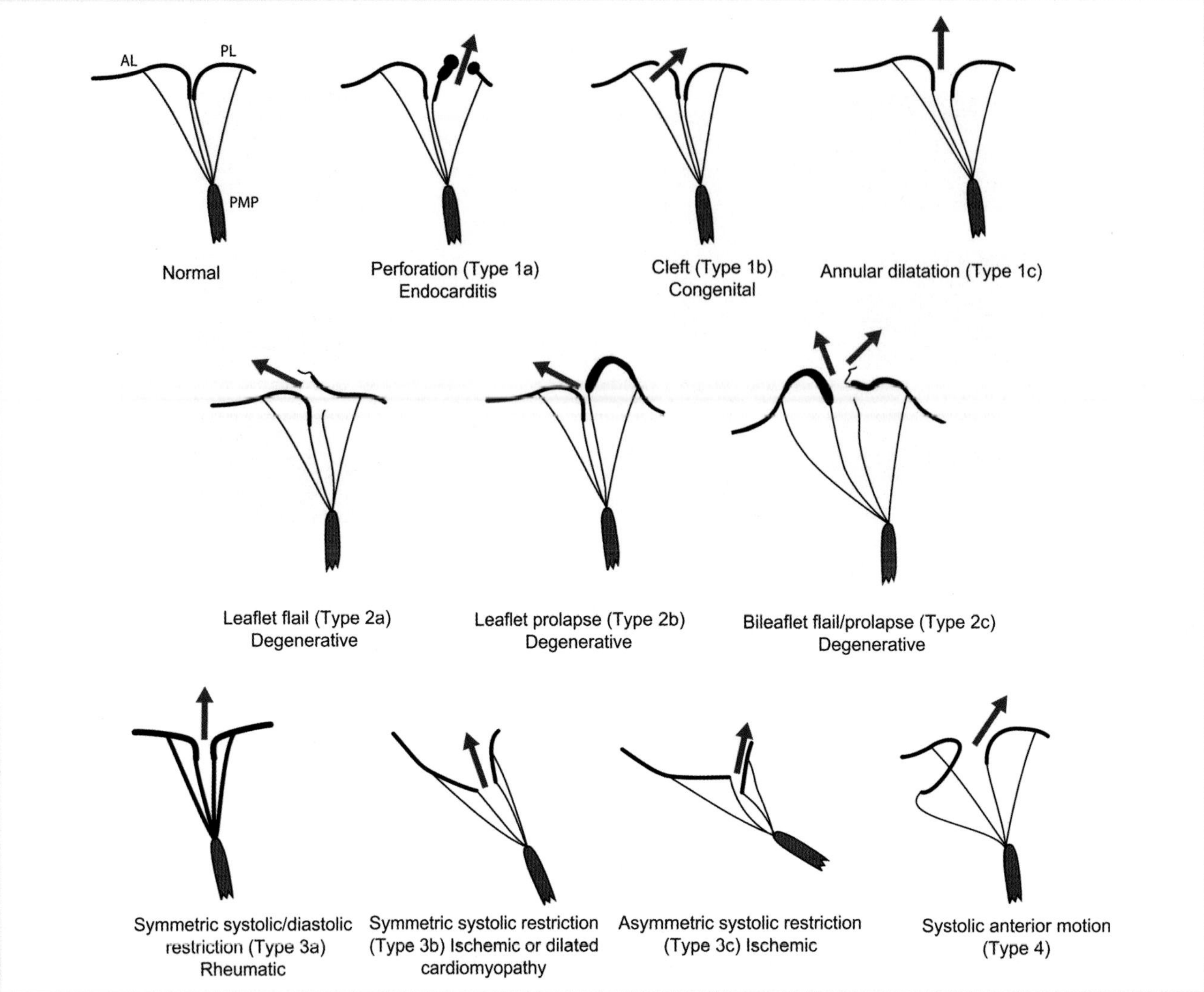

Figure 20-19 Echocardiographic classification of mitral valve pathology on the basis of leaflet motion. Arrows indicate the direction of the MR jet. (Reprinted from Sidebotham DA, Allen SJ, Gerber IL, et al. Intraoperative transesophageal echocardiography for surgical repair of mitral regurgitation. *J Am Soc Echocardiogr*. 2014;27(4):345-366. Copyright © 2014 American Society of Echocardiography. With permission.)

separation between mild MR (<0.3 cm) and severe MR (≥0.7 cm). A VCW of 0.75 cm is consistent with severe MR; therefore, answer C is correct.

Answer A is incorrect. Severe MR is described as having a color jet area >50% of the LA. Furthermore, the color jet area is no longer considered a reliable method for evaluating regurgitation due to numerous factors that increase or reduce the color Doppler jet area. Answer B is incorrect as a regurgitant volume of 45 mL is considered moderate to moderately severe; a regurgitant volume ≥60 mL indicates severe MR. Answer D is incorrect. Moderate and severe MR alter the pulmonary venous pulsed-wave Doppler waveform. Moderate regurgitation is associated with systolic blunting (S wave < D wave) and severe MR is associated with systolic flow reversal. Elevated LA pressure from mitral stenosis or left ventricular dysfunction also causes S-wave blunting. Systolic blunting or reversal may affect the pulmonary veins unequally, particularly for eccentric jets. Therefore, both left- and right-sided pulmonary veins should be evaluated.

29. **Answer: B.** As flow accelerates toward a narrowed orifice, the flow convergence zone proximal to the narrowing comprises a series of isovelocity hemispheric shells of increasing velocity and decreasing surface area; this is the basis of the proximal isovelocity surface area (PISA) principle. Because the heart is a closed system, the blood flow at a point of color aliasing proximal to the valve is equal to the blood flow through the regurgitant orifice. Color Doppler aliasing velocity is used to calculate the instantaneous regurgitant flow rate (RFR):

$$RFR = 2\pi r^2 \times V_N \qquad (1)$$

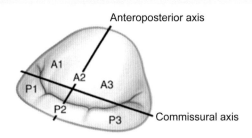

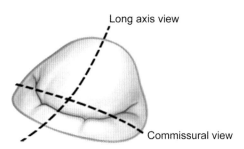

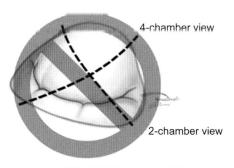

Figure 20-20 The image planes of the mid-esophageal long-axis, commissural, four-chamber, and two-chamber views are indicated. Observe that the four-chamber view is oblique to the axes of the valve. (Adapted from Drake DH, Zimmerman KG, Sidebotham DA. Transesophageal echocardiography for surgical repair of mitral regurgitation. In: Otto CM, ed. *Practice of Clinical Echocardiography*. 5th ed. Philadelphia, PA. Elsevier, 2017:361, chap 19. Reproduced with permission from David Sidebotham and Daniel Drake.)

where r is the PISA radius, $2\pi r^2$ is the surface area of a hemisphere and V_N is the aliasing velocity (or Nyquist limit).

The blood velocity increases as it approaches the narrow regurgitant orifice during systole. The Nyquist limit should be set to around 40 cm/s to optimize the PISA dome and to increase the accuracy of the PISA radius measurement.

The effective regurgitant orifice area (EROA) is then estimated by dividing the regurgitant flow rate (RFR) by the maximum velocity of the regurgitant jet (V_{max}):

$$EROA = RFR \div Vmax \qquad (2)$$

The regurgitant volume (R_{Vol}) is then calculated by multiplying the EROA by the velocity time integral (VTI) of the regurgitant jet (VTI_{RegJet}):

$$RVol = EROA \times VTI_{RegJet} \qquad (3)$$

It is important to note that when doing this calculation, all measurements are in cm or cm/s.

Flow convergence is more accurate for central jets than eccentric jets and assumes a circular regurgitant orifice.

30. **Answer: A.** The color baseline is shifted in the direction of flow to increase the size of the proximal isovelocity surface area (PISA) radius, which will improve measurement accuracy. To perform a PISA radius measurement, the image should be zoomed, and the sector narrowed, then the baseline is shifted in the direction of the mitral regurgitation (MR) jet. From the transthoracic apical views, the MR jet is directed away from the transducer, therefore, the color baseline is shifted downward. From

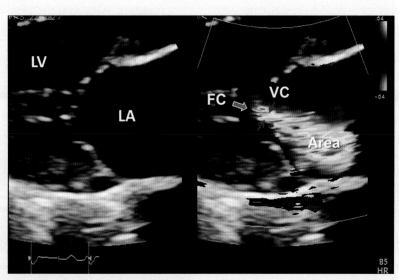

Figure 20-21 Three components of a color mitral regurgitant jet: flow convergence (FC), vena contracta (VC), and jet area. (Reprinted from Zoghbi WA, Adams D, Bonow RO, et al. Recommendations for noninvasive evaluation of native valvular regurgitation. A report from the American Society of Echocardiography developed in Collaboration with the Society for Cardiovascular Magnetic Resonance. *J Am Soc Echocardiogr.* 2017;30(4):303-371. Copyright © 2017 by the American Society of Echocardiography. With permission.)

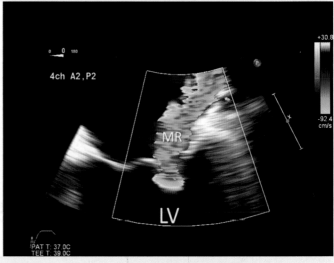

Figure 20-22 Mushroom-shaped PISA domes seen on a transthoracic echocardiographic (TTE) study (left) and a transesophageal echocardiographic (TEE) study (right) from two different patients. The color baseline is shifted in the direction of the MR jet. Therefore, on the TTE image, acquired from a zoomed apical 4-chamber view, the color baseline is shifted down to a color Nyquist limit of 37 cm/s. On the TEE image, acquired from the zoom 4-chamber view, the color baseline is shifted up to a color Nyquist limit of 31 cm/s.

the mid-esophagus transesophageal position, the baseline should be shifted upward. The ideal aliasing velocity is when a clean "mushroom-shaped" PISA dome can be visualized (**Figure 20-22**). The color Doppler Nyquist limit used in the PISA calculation of the EROA is the smaller of the two numbers shown at either end of the color velocity scale. PISA can be used for the calculation of other orifice areas besides that of MR. The key point to remember is to move the baseline in the direction of the regurgitant flow.

21. **Answer: C.** A dilated LA and left ventricle, atrial fibrillation, and congestive heart failure are signs commonly associated with severe MR. A dominant E wave transmitral inflow pattern ($E > 1.2$ m/s) is also associated with severe MR. In patients with significant MR, the flow across the mitral valve is the combination of the mitral regurgitant volume and the normal stroke volume returning from the lungs. Therefore, in patients with significant MR, the transmitral flow is often increased. This may be evidenced by an increased peak E velocity. In particular, an A-dominant (E to A ratio <1) pattern essentially excludes the presence of severe MR.

The rise in LA pressure in MR is related to the extra volume from the regurgitation and to the size and elasticity of the LA. This results in dilatation of the LA, which may in turn lead to atrial fibrillation. There is also a decrease in cardiac output due to the amount of blood not being ejected into the systemic circulation, but instead being "ejected" back into the LA; this leads to congestive heart failure.

32. **Answer: B.** The V cut-off sign may be seen when there is a marked increase in LA pressure with systole as in the case of acute severe MR. In this situation,

the LA pressure toward the end of systole increases significantly due to the increase in LA volume caused by severe MR. This increase in the v-wave pressure on the LA pressure trace results in a decrease in the LV-to-LA pressure gradient toward the end of systole. This results in an MR velocity spectrum that has a V-shaped appearance (**Figure 20-23**).

While the V cut-off sign is an indicator of a marked increase in the LA v-wave pressure, this is dependent on LA compliance. For example, this sign may be absent when there is severe MR and LA compliance is high, that is, the LA is able to accept a large volume of blood without a significant increase in LA pressure. Therefore, answers A and D are incorrect.

Answer C is incorrect. A marked increase in LV pressure with systole would simply increase the peak MR velocity. Remember that the peak MR velocity reflects the pressure difference between the LV and LA during systole. Hence, the higher the LV systolic pressure, the higher the peak MR velocity.

33. **Answer: D.** Acute severe MR has a large regurgitant orifice with minimal LV cavity dilatation. Acute severe MR may be brief with low regurgitant

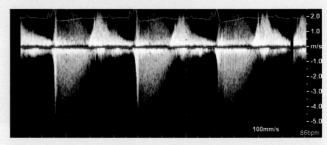

Figure 20-23 V cut-off sign on the MR CW Doppler signal due to a high LA v-wave pressure.

volume and little LV cavity dilatation due to rapid equalization of pressure that occurs with a low driving force for regurgitation. Cavity dilatation occurs when chronic MR imposes a volume load on the LV but also provides a low impedance pathway for systolic ejection. This combined effect leads to an increased LV end-diastolic dimension and, at least initially, a reduced LV end-systolic dimension with a supranormal LV ejection fraction (LVEF).

Answer A is a true statement as one of the first signs of systolic impairment is an increase in the LV end-systolic dimension and wall thickness creating what appears to be a "normal LVEF". While the LVEF remains within the so-called "normal range, this LVEF does not truly reflect the underlying reduction in LV contractile function. In decompensated chronic MR, LV systolic dysfunction develops due to prolonged LV volume overload which essentially stretches the LV to its limit and therefore reduces contractile function. As a result, a weakened LV can no longer adequately contract and LV end-systolic

volume increases. Answer B is a true statement as a PASP >50 mm Hg at rest is an indication to proceed with surgery in asymptomatic patients with chronic secondary MR (**Figure 20-24**). Answer C is a true statement as LV dilatation that occurs as a consequence of primary MR tends to be spherical and global. Conversely, LV dilatation that causes MR (secondary) may be regional (i.e., asymmetric tethering—see **Figure 20-12**).

34. **Answer: A.** VCW is a semi-quantitative measure of MR severity that assesses the regurgitant orifice in a linear dimension and is not accurate for multiple jets. VCW is a quick method for semi-quantifying MR. As previously discussed, the VCW is measured perpendicular to the flow direction at the narrowest diameter of the MR jet. One of the advantages of this measurement is that it is less influenced by loading conditions and is reliable for both central and eccentric jets. The main limitation of the VCW is the assumption that the regurgitation orifice is circular, which may not be the case. Therefore, the

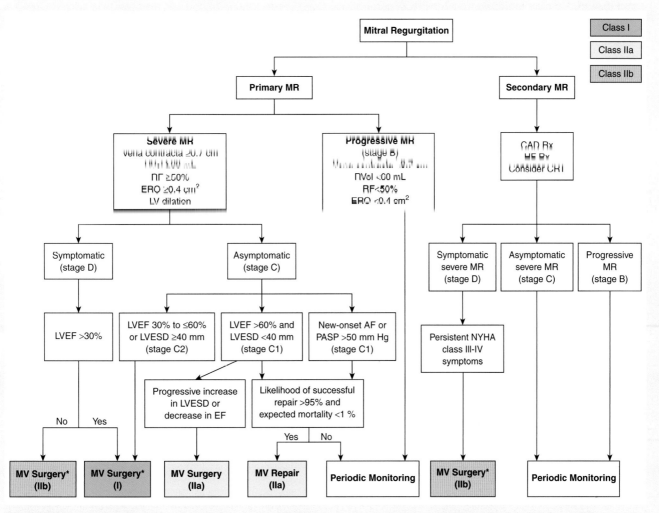

Figure 20-24 Indications for Surgery for chronic secondary MR. (Reprinted with permission from Nishimura RA, Otto CM, Bonow RO, et al. AHA/ACC guideline: 2017 AHA/ACC focused update of the 2014 AHA/ACC guideline for the management of patients with valvular heart disease. *Circulation*. 2017;135(25):e1159-e1195. Copyright © 2017 American Heart Association, Inc.)

VCW may overestimate MR severity if there is a markedly elliptical (noncircular) orifice shape, as often seen in secondary MR. For example, a 2-chamber view, which is oriented parallel to the line of leaflet coaptation, may show a wide vena contracta even in mild MR.

35. **Answer: C.** The VCA is a cross-sectional 3D direct measurement of the narrowest portion of regurgitant flow that occurs at or immediately downstream from the regurgitant orifice (**Figure 20-25**) and is slightly smaller than the anatomical regurgitant orifice. VCA is measured via 3D echocardiography using axial multiplanar reconstruction (MPR) analysis and provides a reliable measure of EROA; therefore, answer D is true. The advantage of being able to manipulate a 3D dataset for proper image alignment and analysis eliminates assumptions regarding the shape (often noncircular) of the regurgitant orifice; therefore, answer A is true. The VCA can also be used when there are multiple jets and the VCA can be measured for each jet; therefore, answer B is true. Multiple VCAs can be used to identify severe functional mitral regurgitation, which is often underestimated by PISA. VCA yields higher values for EROA compared

to the flow convergence method; therefore, answer C is false and the correct answer selection.

36. **Answer: A.** Jet area is a useful parameter for screening for MR. The color jet area is excellent for excluding MR but is not reliable for assessing MR severity. The color jet area and length are dependent on momentum and driving pressure and, therefore, are affected by loading conditions, ventricular function, atrial size and compliance, and color Doppler gain settings. The jet area will underestimate the severity of eccentric jets due to a loss of jet momentum. The color jet length is more reflective of the driving pressure than the severity of regurgitation. As a general rule, all wall-hugging jets should be considered severe. Therefore, MR severity should not be determined by "eyeballing" the MR color jet area and/or color jet length alone. Consideration of the origin of the jet (vena contracta) and its flow convergence will aid in the grading of MR. For example, a small jet area (<20% of the LA area) with a narrow vena contracta and no visible flow convergence region usually indicates mild MR, while a large jet area (>50% of the LA area) with a wide VC and a

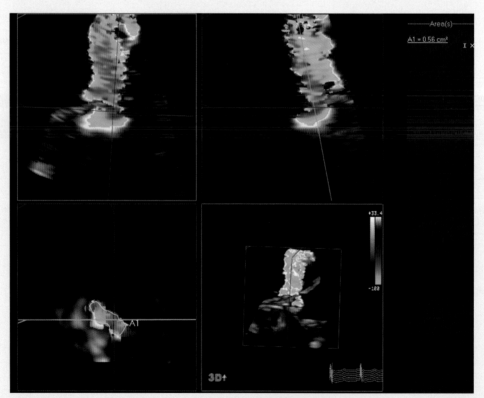

Figure 20-25 Measurement of vena contracta area by multiplanar reconstruction. Axial 3D images of the mitral valve with color Doppler imaging are shown. A late-systolic frame has been chosen for analysis. The top left panel shows a commissural 2D slice; the top right image shows a long-axis 2D slice; the bottom left panel shows a short-axis image at the level of the vena contracta; the bottom right panel shows a volume-rendered color 3D image in the surgical orientation from the left atrial aspect. In the commissural and long-axis quadrants, the red and green lines have been adjusted so they are positioned through the center of the jet, and the blue lines have been adjusted so they pass through the narrowest part of the jet (i.e., the vena contracta). The vena contracta area has then been measured with planimetry (bottom left panel). The value of 0.33 cm² indicates mild to moderate regurgitation. (Reproduced with permission of the Oxford Publishing Limited through PLSclear, from Sidebotham DA, Merry AF, Legget ME, et al, eds. *Practical Perioperative Transesophageal Echocardiography.* 3rd ed. Oxford, England: Oxford University Press; 2018:127.)

large flow convergence region usually indicates severe MR.

37. **Answer: D.** The shape of the regurgitant orifice in primary MR or organic disease as a result of a flail leaflet is generally more circular. In secondary or functional MR, the orifice resembles an elliptical or crescent-like shape.

Answer A is false as an elliptical MR regurgitant orifice, as seen with secondary MR, will lead to underestimation of the regurgitant flow by the PISA method. Answer B is false if the flow convergence is hemispherical due to constraint; increasing the color aliasing velocity may be attempted to make the flow convergence smaller and less prone to constraint. Angle correction may also be attempted. Answer C is false as PISA can be used for more than one orifice area with jets greater than mild. In this instance, the PISA method can be applied to each orifice and flows and EROA can be added together.

38. **Answer: D.** The simplified PISA method can be used to quickly estimate the effective regurgitant orifice area (EROA). Via this method, the PISA radius is measured at a color Nyquist limit (V_N) set to 40 cm/s and it is assumed that the peak MR velocity (V_{max}) is 5 m/s (or 500 cm/s), which yields a 100 mm Hg pressure difference between the left ventricle and left atrium in systole:

$$EROA = \left(2\pi r^2 \times V_N\right) \div Vmax$$

$$= \left(6.28 \times r^2 \times 40\right) \div 500$$

$$\left(r^2 \times r^2\right) = 500$$

$$= r^2 \cdot \left(500 \cdot 251\right)$$

$$\approx r^2/2$$

The vast majority of MR jet peak velocities are between 4 and 6 m/s; therefore, this can be a reasonable way to estimate the EROA (see **Table 20-3** for significance of the EROA for each MR grade). However, this simplified equation cannot be used with extremes in blood pressure (BP). For example, in patients with very low BP, the MR velocity will be much lower than 5 m/s.

Answer A is true since PISA is more accurate for central regurgitant jets than eccentric jets (circular versus noncircular orifices). Regurgitant orifices that are crescent-shaped, as in secondary MR, will result in underestimation of the EROA via PISA, which assumes a circular geometry.

Answer B is true as PISA calculated from a single frame will overestimate MR severity if not holosystolic. This is especially a problem with mitral valve prolapse where MR characteristically occurs during mid-to-late systole. Therefore, determining the

severity of MR based only on the EROA may overestimate the MR severity. In these cases, the regurgitant volume should be calculated.

Answer C is true as poor alignment of the continuous-wave Doppler cursor with an eccentric jet will lead to underestimation of the MR velocity and overestimation of the EROA.

39. **Answer: B.** Vena contracta width should be measured perpendicular to the coaptation line in the ME long-axis view. The Nyquist limit should be set to 40 to 70 cm/s and the narrowest part of the widest jet should be chosen for analysis (**Figure 20-26**, top). Because the commissural view (answer A) scans along the curved coaptation line, in patients with MR in which the jet is elliptical (as opposed to circular) the regurgitant jet may appear abnormally broad or as a double jet (**Figure 20-26**, bottom). Therefore, this view should not be used to measure the vena contracta. As discussed earlier, the 4-chamber view

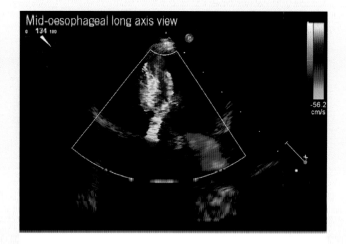

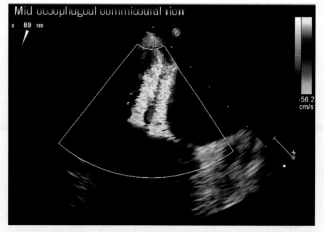

Figure 20-26 Mitral regurgitation demonstrated in the mid-esophageal long-axis and commissural views in the same patient. In the long-axis view, the image plane is perpendicular to the coaptation line, and a single jet of regurgitation is seen. In the commissural view, the image plane is parallel to the curved coaptation line, cutting it twice, and a double jet of mitral regurgitation is seen. (Reproduced with permission of the Oxford Publishing Limited through PLSclear, from Sidebotham DA, Merry AF, Legget ME, et al, eds. *Practical Perioperative Transesophageal Echocardiography.* 3rd ed. Oxford, England: Oxford University Press; 2018:114.)

(answer C) cuts through the valve obliquely; therefore, this view is not accurate for the VC measurement. The deep transgastric view (answer D) may be similar to a 4- or 5-chamber view, where it is not possible to know exactly where you are lined up with the valve segments; therefore, this view is not accurate for the VC measurement.

40. **Answer: A.** The score proposed by Padial and colleagues is used to predict which patients are more likely to develop severe MR with PBMV (see **Table 20-1C**). The echocardiographic features that are evaluated included in the score are location, thickness, and distribution of fibrosis/calcification of both anterior and posterior leaflets; the degree of calcification in one or both commissures; the extent of subvalvular disease. The score does not consider commissural fusion.

41. **Answer: C.** The Wilkins score is used to determine whether mitral valve morphology is suitable for PBMV (see **Table 20-1B**). A low Wilkins score (≤8) is indicative of a mobile valve with limited thickening, and this patient is an ideal candidate for PBMV;

therefore, answer C is correct. A Wilkins score >8 indicates unfavorable anatomy for PBMV (answer A is incorrect). Cormier Group 2 is defined by severe subvalvular disease and a pliable, noncalcified anterior leaflet; these patients are typically recommended for surgical commissurotomy (answer B is incorrect). Cormier Group 1 displays mild subvalvular disease and pliable anterior leaflet and closed-heart commissurotomy is recommended (answer D is incorrect).

42. **Answer: A.** The TEE demonstrates a right-to-left interatrial shunt through the iatrogenic ASD, resulting from the transseptal puncture. Most procedural ASDs will close in time; however, this finding was accompanied by a decrease in oxygen saturation (88%). The defect was subsequently closed with an Amplatzer septal occluder.

Acknowledgments: The authors thank and acknowledge Sorin V. Pislaru, MD, PhD, and Maurice Enriquez-Sarano, MD, for their inspiration based on Chapter 17, Mitral Valvular Disease in *Clinical Echocardiography Review: A Self-Assessment Tool, 2nd Edition*, edited by Allan L. Klein, Craig R. Asher, 2017.

SUGGESTED READINGS

Baumgartner H, Hung J, Bermejo J, et al. Echocardiographic assessment of valve stenosis: EAE/ASE recommendations for clinical practice. *J Am Soc Echocardiogr.* 2009;22(1):1-23.

Drake DH, Zimmerman KG, Hepner AM, Nichols CD. Echo-guided mitral repair. *Circ Cardiovasc Imaging.* 2014;7(1):132-141.

Drake DH, Zimmerman KG, Sidebotham DA. Transesophageal echocardiography for surgical repair of mitral regurgitation. In: Otto CM, ed. *The Practice of Clinical Echocardiography.* 5th ed. Philadelphia, Pennsylvania: Elsevier Saunders; 2017:chap 19

El-Tallawi KC, Messika-Zeitoun D, Zoghbi WA. Assessment of the severity of native mitral valve regurgitation. *Prog Cardiovasc Dis.* 2017;60(3):322-333.

Levine RA, Triulzi MO, Harrigan P, Weyman AE. The relationship of mitral annular shape to the diagnosis of mitral valve prolapse. *Circulation.* 1987;75(4):756-767.

Iung B, Cormier B, Ducimetière P, et al. Immediate results of percutaneous mitral commissurotomy. A predictive model on a series of 1514 patients. *Circulation.* 1996;94(9):2124-2130.

Padial LR, Abascal VM, Moreno PR, Weyman AE, Levine RA, Palacios IF. Echocardiography can predict the development of severe mitral regurgitation after percutaneous mitral valvuloplasty by the Inoue technique. *Am J Cardiol.* 1999;83(8):1210-1213.

Sidebotham DA, Drake DH, Zimmerman KG. Surgical repair of mitral valve disease. In: Sidebotham DA, Merry AF, Legget ME, Wright IG, eds. *Practical Perioperative Transesophageal Echocardiography.* 3rd ed. Oxford, England: Oxford University Press; 2018.

Wilkins GT, Weyman AE, Abascal VM, Block PC, Palacios IF. Percutaneous balloon dilatation of the mitral valve: an analysis of echocardiographic variables related to outcome and the mechanism of dilatation. *Br Heart J.* 1988;60(4):299-308.

Zoghbi WA, Adams D, Bonow RO, et al. Recommendations for noninvasive evaluation of native valvular regurgitation: a report from the American Society of Echocardiography developed in Collaboration with the Society for Cardiovascular Magnetic Resonance. *J Am Soc Echocardiogr.* 2017;30(4):303-371.

CHAPTER 21

Tricuspid and Pulmonary Valve Disease

Contributors: Margaret M. Park, BS, ACS, RDCS, RVT and Amy Kanta, RDCS

✪✪ Question 1

A 27-year-old is seen in the emergency room due to shortness of breath and a heart murmur. He has a previous history of heart surgery as a child. An echocardiogram shows a communication between the left ventricle (LV) and right atrium (RA) encompassing the tricuspid valve leaflets. This abnormality may be termed a(n):

- **A.** Atrial septal defect.
- **B.** Atrioventricular septal defect.
- **C.** Endocardial cushion defect.
- **D.** Gerbode defect.

✪ Question 2

The most common cause of pulmonic stenosis is:

- **A.** Congenital heart disease.
- **B.** Carcinoid heart disease.
- **C.** Rheumatic heart disease.
- **D.** Functional stenosis due to compression of the right ventricular outflow tract (RVOT).
- **E.** None of the above.

✪ Question 3

The most likely cause of pulmonic regurgitation (PR) is:

- **A.** Abnormal pulmonic valve leaflets due to congenital heart disease.
- **B.** Increased pulmonary artery pressures.
- **C.** Post balloon pulmonary valvuloplasty.
- **D.** Rheumatic heart disease.

✪✪ Question 4

Which of the following statements is not true with respect to echocardiographic imaging of rheumatic tricuspid stenosis (TS)?

- **A.** Imaging shows partial commissural fusion and leaflet tip fibrosis.
- **B.** There is systolic bowing and shortened tricuspid leaflets.
- **C.** There is thickening of the leaflets and chordae tendineae.
- **D.** Tricuspid leaflets are best visualized with 3D transesophageal echocardiography (TEE).

✪ Question 5

The most common cause of significant tricuspid regurgitation (TR) is:

- **A.** Infective endocarditis.
- **B.** Implantable device leads.
- **C.** Rheumatic heart disease.
- **D.** Tricuspid valve prolapse.
- **E.** Left heart disease resulting in pulmonary hypertension.

✪ Question 6

All of the following statements are true regarding physiological regurgitation except:

- **A.** Detection increases in individuals older than 50 years.
- **B.** Regurgitant jets are central and near the point of leaflet coaptation.
- **C.** Regurgitation may be detected in 75% of healthy individuals.
- **D.** Regurgitation is most frequently detected in the left-sided valves.
- **E.** Most individuals with physiological regurgitation have normal electrocardiograms.

✪✪✪ Question 7

All of the following are supportive 2D echocardiographic findings for significant, chronic tricuspid regurgitation (TR) except:

A. A dilated inferior vena cava (IVC).
B. A D-shaped left ventricle (LV).
C. An end-systolic right ventricular (RV) eccentricity index <2.
D. Leaflet tethering with a coaptation distance >8 mm.
E. Right ventricular enlargement.

✪✪ Question 8

▶ Based on the images provided (**Video 21-1** and **Figure 21-1**), the severity of pulmonic regurgitation (PR) is:

A. Trace.
B. Mild.
C. Moderate.
D. Severe.
E. Indeterminate.

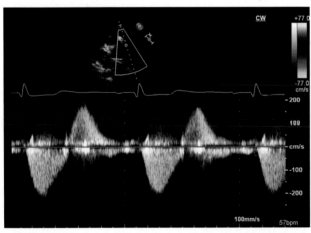

Figure 21-1

✪✪ Question 9

Which of the following echocardiographic findings is indirectly associated with significant tricuspid regurgitation (TR)?

A. Dominant hepatic vein systolic waves
B. Increased tricuspid inflow velocity >1.0 m/s
C. Increased tricuspid regurgitation velocity >3.0 m/s
D. Inferior vena cava (IVC) collapse upon inspiration
E. Pulmonary vein systolic flow reversal

✪✪ Question 10

A young man with mild pulmonary valve stenosis (PS) presents for an echocardiogram. He has a peak gradient across the pulmonary valve (PV) of 20 mm Hg. His peak tricuspid regurgitant (TR) velocity is 3 m/s and his right atrial (RA) size is normal. His IVC is not enlarged and decreases further upon sniffing. Which of the following is true?

A. His pulmonary artery systolic pressure (PASP) is normal.
B. His PASP is moderately elevated.
C. His PASP cannot be estimated when pulmonary stenosis is present.
D. He has severe pulmonary arterial hypertension.
E. None of the above.

✪✪ Question 11

Determining the grade of tricuspid regurgitation (TR) based on the color Doppler jet appearance, jet area, vena contracta, or the flow convergence radius or zone alone can be unreliable due to the:

A. Influence of hemodynamic factors.
B. Three or more papillary muscles associated with the tricuspid valve.
C. Assumption that the tricuspid annulus is saddle-shaped.
D. Multiple commissures and several scallops of the tricuspid valve.

✪✪ Question 12

Which of the following findings is consistent with severe pulmonic stenosis (PS)?

A. Normal right ventricular systolic pressure (RVSP)
B. Normal size of the pulmonary artery
C. Peak velocity >4 m/s across the pulmonic valve
D. Peak gradient <64 mm Hg
E. Right ventricular (RV) wall thickness of 0.3 cm

✪✪✪ Question 13

Which rare congenital cardiac abnormality of the tricuspid valve displayed in **Figure 21-2** is frequently seen with right ventricular hypoplasia, an atrial septal defect (ASD), and a ventricular septal defect (VSD)?

A. Ebstein anomaly
B. Tricuspid atresia
C. Noonan syndrome
D. Tetralogy of Fallot

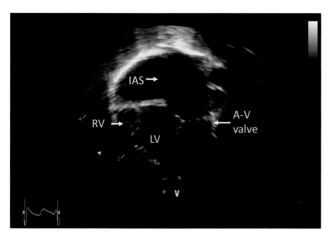

Figure 21-2

✪✪✪ Question 14

Which of the following semiquantitative color Doppler methods best correlates with the severity of pulmonic regurgitation (PR)?

A. PR effective orifice area (EROA)
B. PR jet area
C. PR jet length
D. PR jet width
E. All of the above

✪✪ Question 15

Which of the following is a functional cause of tricuspid regurgitation (TR)?

A. Carcinoid disease
B. Rheumatic heart disease
C. Pulmonary embolism
D. Endocarditis
E. Pacemaker lead insertion

✪✪ Question 16

Which of the following pressures can be estimated from a pulmonic regurgitation (PR) spectral Doppler signal?

A. Mean pulmonary artery pressure (mPAP)
B. Pulmonary artery systolic pressure (PASP)
C. Right ventricular end-diastolic pressure (RVEDP)
D. Right atrial pressure (RAP)
E. All of the above

✪✪ Question 17

When performing 2D/3D Doppler echocardiography in the operating room, which effect does general anesthesia have on the evaluation of tricuspid regurgitation (TR) severity?

A. TR will appear more severe during anesthesia.
B. TR will appear less severe during anesthesia.
C. No effect is seen on TR grade during anesthesia.

✪✪✪ Question 18

A 45-year-old woman with pulmonary hypertension has an echocardiogram. The echo reveals normal left and right ventricular size and function, mild right atrial dilation, mild pulmonary regurgitation (PR), and an IVC that is 1.99 cm and collapses <50%. The estimated mean pulmonary artery pressure (mPAP) based on the information provided and the continuous-wave Doppler trace of the PR jet (**Figure 21-3**) is:

A. 14 mm Hg.
B. 15 mm Hg.
C. 18 mm Hg.
D. 25 mm Hg.
E. None of the above.

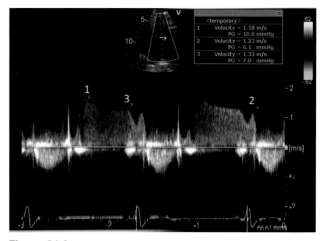

Figure 21-3

✪✪✪ Question 19

Using the information in the previous question, the estimated pulmonary artery end-diastolic pressure (PAEDP) is:

A. 14 mm Hg.
B. 15 mm Hg.
C. 18 mm Hg.
D. 25 mm Hg.
E. None of the above.

✪✪ Question 20

A patient with known tricuspid regurgitation (TR) undergoes an annual echocardiogram. The TR vena contracta measures 0.5 cm, the effective regurgitant orifice area (EROA) is calculated as 0.37 cm², and the regurgitant volume is 44 mL. Based on these measurements and calculations, the severity of TR is graded as:

 A. Mild.
 B. Moderate.
 C. Severe.
 D. Not enough information to grade.

✪✪✪ Question 21

Guidelines for imaging the tricuspid valve (TV) using 3D transesophageal echocardiography (TEE) recommend the image be displayed as an en face view, viewing the TV from either the right ventricle (RV) or right atrium (RA), with the septal TV leaflet positioned at:

 A. 9 o'clock (medial).
 B. 11 o'clock (superior position).
 C. 6 o'clock (inferior position).
 D. 3 o'clock (lateral).

✪✪ Question 22

The tricuspid valve (TV) consists of the following leaflets:

 A. Anterior, lateral, medial.
 B. Anterior, posterior, septal.
 C. Left, right, posterior.
 D. Moderator, anterior, posterior.
 E. Moderator, posterior, septal.

✪✪ Question 23

The relationship between the tricuspid valve (TV) annular diameter and the volume of tricuspid regurgitation (TR) is best described as:

 A. Linear.
 B. Inverse.
 C. Negatively correlated.
 D. Not correlated.

✪✪✪ Question 24

A patient with prior rheumatic heart disease presents for a transthoracic echocardiogram (TTE). Which of the following is true regarding the echocardiographic assessment of tricuspid stenosis (TS) in this condition?

 A. Doming and thickening of the tricuspid valve (TV) in systole are seen.
 B. Planimetry of the tricuspid valve area is readily obtained.
 C. The mean pressure gradient is at least 10 mm Hg in severe TS.

 D. The tricuspid valve area may be estimated by dividing 190 by the pressure half-time.
 E. TS is clinically significant in 25% of patients with coexistent rheumatic mitral stenosis.

✪✪✪ Question 25

Which of the following transthoracic echocardiographic (TTE) and transesophageal echocardiographic (TEE) views can show both the septal and posterior tricuspid leaflets in the same imaging plane?

 A. Parasternal short-axis (TTE) and midesophageal 90° (TEE) views
 B. Right ventricular inflow (TTE) and transgastric 0° (TEE) views
 C. Parasternal short-axis (TTE) and distal esophageal 0° (TEE) views
 D. Apical 4-chamber (TTE) and midesophageal 0° (TEE) views
 E. Right ventricular inflow (TTE) and deep gastric 90° (TEE) views

✪✪ Question 26

▶ A 55-year-old woman presents with signs of right heart failure, accompanied by facial flushing and stomach cramps. Based on the images provided (**Figure 21-4** and **Video 21-2**), the diagnosis is:

 A. Carcinoid heart disease.
 B. Ebstein anomaly.
 C. Endocarditis.
 D. Pheochromocytoma.
 E. Rheumatic heart disease.

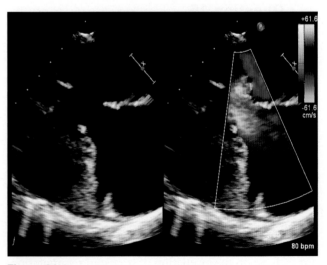

Figure 21-4

✪ Question 27

Based on the information provided in **Table 21-1** and assuming there is no significant tricuspid or aortic regurgitation, the estimated tricuspid valve area (TVA) is:

- **A.** 0.57 cm^2.
- **B.** 0.99 cm^2.
- **C.** 1.27 cm^2.
- **D.** 2.92 cm^2.
- **E.** Not enough information to calculate the TVA.

Table 21-1.

Left ventricular outflow tract (LVOT) diameter	2.2 cm
LVOT peak velocity	0.9 m/s
LVOT velocity-time integral (VTI)	17 cm
Right ventricular outflow tract (RVOT) diameter	2.5 cm
Tricuspid annular diameter	3.8 cm
Tricuspid peak E velocity	1.5 m/s
Tricuspid inflow VTI	65 cm

✪ Question 28

Based on the information provided in the previous question, the degree of tricuspid stenosis (TS) is considered to be:

- **A.** None.
- **B.** Mild.
- **C.** Moderate.
- **D.** Severe.

✪✪✪ Question 29

Based on the information provided in **Figure 21-5**, what is the pulmonic regurgitant volume and regurgitant fraction?

- **A.** 72 mL, 52%
- **B.** 45 mL, 62%
- **C.** 52 mL, 72%
- **D.** 62 mL, 45%

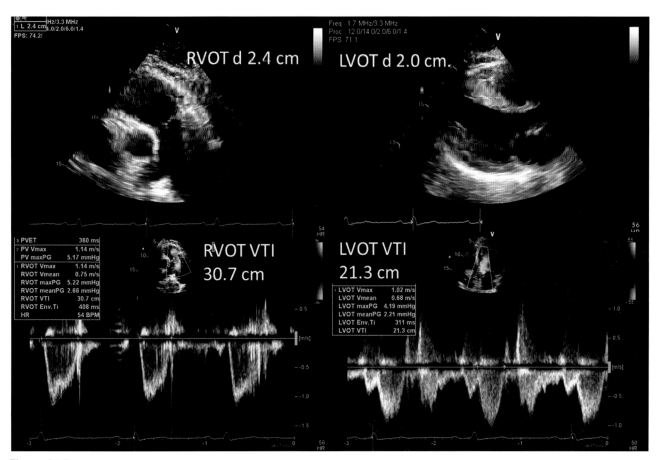

Figure 21-5

✪✪ Question 30

A pulmonic regurgitant fraction is calculated in the range of 25% to 30%. This value would suggest what degree of pulmonary regurgitation (PR) severity?

A. Trivial
B. Mild
C. Moderate
D. Severe

✪✪ Question 31

All of the following statements are true about the pulmonary valve except:

A. Pulmonary cusps are thinner than those of the tricuspid valve.
B. Branch pulmonary stenosis may cause pathologic pulmonary regurgitation (PR).
C. Pulmonary regurgitant pressure half-time is a specific sign of pressure equalization.
D. Right ventricular (RV) dilatation is a specific sign of severe PR.

✪✪ Question 32

▶ A 51-year-old man presented to the emergency room with acute pulmonary embolism. The transthoracic echocardiogram revealed a small mass on the tricuspid valve (TV). The patient had a prior history of intravenous drug use and TV infective endocarditis (15 years ago) but has been healthy and asymptomatic ever since. Based on the images provided (**Figure 21-6A to C** and **Video 21-3A** and **21-3B**), what is the diagnosis?

A. Lambl excrescence
B. Myxoma
C. Papillary fibroelastoma
D. Reoccurrence of a TV vegetation

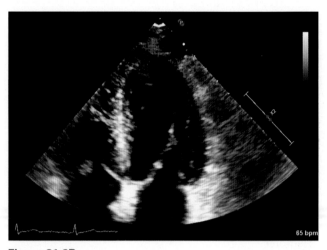

Figure 21-6B

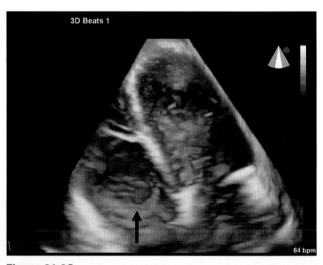

Figure 21-6C

✪✪✪ Question 33

From the schematic pulmonary valve M-mode patterns shown in **Figure 21-7**, which trace suggests infundibular stenosis?

A. A
B. B
C. C
D. D
E. E

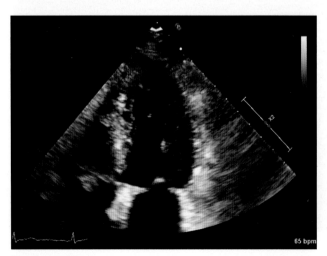

Figure 21-6A

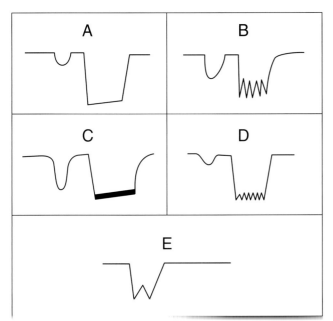

Figure 21-7 (Reprinted with permission from Armstrong WF, Ryan T, eds. Feigenbaum's Echocardiography. 8th ed. Philadelphia, PA: Wolters Kluwer; 2018.)

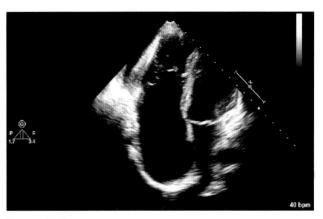

Figure 21-8

✪✪✪ Question 34

Which of the following statements about infundibular stenosis is correct?

A. Infundibular stenosis is part of a congenital syndrome.

B. The site of stenosis will be supravalular.

C. Doppler estimation of the pressure gradient across the infundibular stenosis is inaccurate except when valvular pulmonic stenosis coexists.

D. Infundibular stenosis is most accurately assessed from the apical imaging window.

E. Infundibular stenosis may cause a high velocity jet that impinges on the pulmonary valve, causing pulmonary regurgitation.

✪✪✪ Question 35

▶ A 30-year-old woman presents with right-sided heart failure. She has had a murmur since childhood but has only recently complained of fatigue and ankle edema. On admission, she developed a wide complex tachycardia at a fast rate and required immediate cardioversion. An apical 4-chamber view of her heart is shown in **Video 21-4** and **Figure 21-8**. What is the most likely cause of her heart failure?

A. Tachycardia-mediated cardiomyopathy

B. Severe tricuspid regurgitation (TR)

C. Severe pulmonary hypertension

D. Recent endocarditis

E. Right-to-left shunt at the atrial level

✪✪ Question 36

A young man with prior open-heart surgery has a transthoracic echocardiogram (TTE). He has significant **right** ventricular (RV) dilatation and some RV dysfunction. He has no prior TTE available and he is unaware of what surgery was performed as a child. Based on the parasternal short-axis image of the pulmonary valve (**Figure 21-9**), which of the following statements is most likely to be correct?

A. Mild pulmonary regurgitation is present.

B. There is an atrial septal defect with high flow through the pulmonary circuit.

C. There is severe pulmonary regurgitation (PR).

D. There is a patent ductus arteriosus.

E. A mechanical valve should be used if replacement of the pulmonic valve is required.

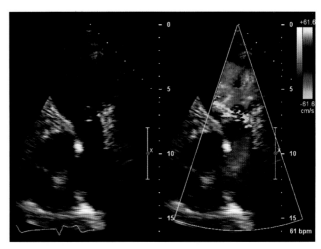

Figure 21-9

ANSWERS

1. ▶ **Answer: D.** A Gerbode-type defect is a communication between the LV and the RA; it is basically a ventricular septal defect (VSD). This defect is located within the atrioventricular (AV) septum and is almost always congenital in nature but can be acquired as a complication of endocarditis, or may result from trauma, acute myocardial infarction, or an aortic valve replacement. The true communication may be difficult to see on echocardiography, and the LV-to-RA jet, which is created from the high systolic pressure gradient between the LV and the RA, is often mistaken for tricuspid regurgitation (TR). As a result, pulmonary hypertension is misdiagnosed. Imaging off-axis with angulation of the transducer and a careful eye can reveal the true communication point (**Video 21-5**).

   An atrial septal defect (answer A) results in shunting between the left atrium (LA) and RA.

   An atrioventricular septal defect (answer B), sometimes called an endocardial cushion defect (answer C) or atrioventricular canal defect, generally consists of a spectrum of lesions characterized by the presence of a common AV junction, as opposed to separate right and left AV junctions, and abnormalities of the AV valve leaflets.

2. **Answer: A.** The etiology of pulmonary stenosis (PS) is almost always congenital; the valve may be trileaflet, bicuspid, unicuspid, or dysplastic. Dysplastic PS presents as thickened leaflets with usually poor mobility, characterized by disorganized myxomatous tissue. Acquired PS is uncommon with the most common cause of acquired PS being carcinoid heart disease. Rheumatic PS is also an acquired cause of PS but is very rare. Functional PS may occur due to compression of the RVOT from a tumor or mass but is not commonly encountered.

3. **Answer: B.** PR may be described as primary or secondary regurgitation. Secondary (or functional) PR is the most common cause. The pulmonary valve is morphologically normal, and regurgitation occurs due to dilatation of the pulmonary annulus. Secondary causes of PR include increased pulmonary artery pressures of any cause, RV volume overload, and connective tissue disorders. Primary (or organic) PR is caused by leaflet abnormalities. The most common primary causes for PR include iatrogenic (surgical valvotomy/valvectomy or balloon pulmonary valvuloplasty), infectious (infective endocarditis), immune-mediated (rheumatic heart disease), systemic disease (carcinoid disease), and congenital malformations. Like tricuspid regurgitation (TR), it is common to see trace to mild PR in the normal population (in up to 90% of individuals).

4. **Answer: B.** In rheumatic TS (and mitral stenosis), the leaflets may display bowing during opening in

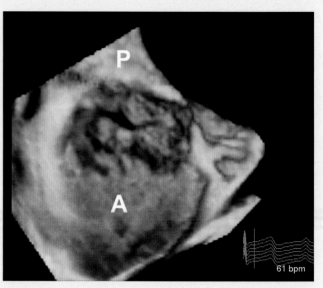

Figure 21-10A 3D TEE image of a rheumatic tricuspid valve (full-volume en face view from the right atrial perspective). The leaflets are thickened, and the leaflet edges are fibrosed with partial commissural fusion creating a bicuspidization of the TV. The ability of 2D echocardiography to detect these subtle changes in TV morphology is limited. A = anterior side of the patient, P = posterior side of the patient. (Reprinted with permission from Lambert S, Hynes MS. Tricuspid valve. In: Lang RM, Shernan SK, Shirali GS, et al. *Comprehensive Atlas of 3D Echocardiography*. 1st ed. Philadelphia, PA: Wolters Kluwer Health/Lippincott Williams & Wilkins; 2013:215, chap 10)

diastole but not during systole. In rheumatic TS, the leaflets may appear shortened, thickened and display *diastolic* bowing. With the aid of 3D TEE imaging, partial commissural fusion, leaflet tip fibrosis, and chordal thickening, which are also common findings in rheumatic TS, can be identified (**Figures 21-10A and 21-10B**).

5. **Answer: E.** As for pulmonic regurgitation (PR), the etiology of TR may be described as primary or secondary regurgitation. Primary (or organic) TR is caused by abnormalities of the tricuspid leaflets and/or subvalvular apparatus; while in secondary (or functional) TR, the tricuspid valve (TV) and subvalvular apparatus are morphologically normal and TR occurs due to annular dilatation and/or leaflet tethering. The most common cause of TR is functional regurgitation resulting from tricuspid annular dilation secondary to right atrial (RA) and/or right ventricular (RV) enlargement. RA and/or RV dilation may occur in a setting of RV dysfunction, RV pressure overload (e.g., pulmonary arterial hypertension, pulmonary hypertension due to left heart disease), and/or RV volume overload (e.g., significant PR or atrial septal defects).

   Infective endocarditis, implantable device leads, rheumatic heart disease, and tricuspid valve prolapse are all less common (primary) causes of TR.

6. **Answer: D.** Physiological regurgitation is most frequently detected in the right-sided valves, followed by the mitral valve. Physiological aortic

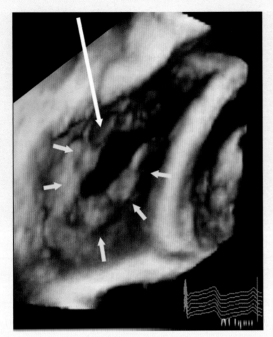

Figure 21-10B 3D TEE image full volume en face view of a rheumatic TV from the RV perspective. Yellow arrows point to thickened TV leaflets and the white arrow points to thickened chordae tendinae (brown spots). (Reprinted with permission from Lambert S, Hynes MS. Tricuspid Valve. In: Lang RM, Shernan SK, Shirali GS, et al. *Comprehensive Atlas of 3D Echocardiography*. 1st ed. Philadelphia, PA: Wolters Kluwer Health/Lippincott Williams & Wilkins; 2013:215.)

physiologic PR

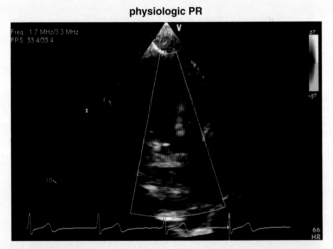

Figure 21-11A

physiologic TR

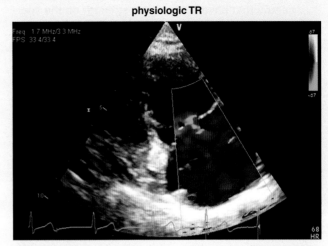

Figure 21-11B

physiologic MR

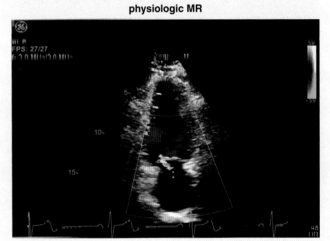

Figure 21-11C

physiologic AI

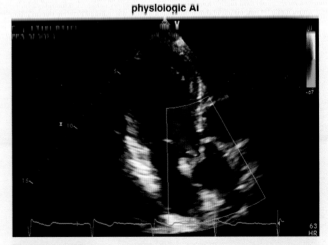

Figure 21-11D

regurgitation is less common in clinically normal individuals (especially in individuals younger than 50 years). **Figures 21-11A to 21-11D** were acquired from a 76-year-old woman with no previous cardiac history, and a normal physical examination free of murmurs. An echocardiogram was part of a preoperative examination. Physiological regurgitation of all four valves was noted.

Answers A, B, C, and E are all true features of physiological regurgitation. In the normal population, trace-mild regurgitation is detected in one, two, or three heart valves by color Doppler imaging about 60% to 75% of the time, partially due to increased sensitivity of the current ultrasound systems. When present, physiological regurgitation is localized to a small region near the point of leaflet coaptation and regurgitation jets are generally central that have a low signal strength on the spectral Doppler examination. Physiologic degrees of TR are associated with normal right ventricular (RV) and right atrial size and low systolic velocities, indicating a normal RV systolic pressure. Physiological regurgitation usually has no clinical significance and is generally considered a normal finding.

7. **Answer: C.** Significant, chronic TR leads to a right heart volume overload state. The end-systolic RV eccentricity index (RVEI), measured from the parasternal short-axis view at the LV papillary muscle level, is a simple quantification of RV geometry and the degree of RV dilatation (**Figure 21-12A**). An end-systolic RVEI >2 supports significant TR. Therefore, answer C is the correct answer as an RVEI <2 is not a 2D echocardiographic findings for significant, chronic TR.

Answer A is incorrect since the IVC is dilated when there is significant TR due to increased right atrial (RA) volume and backflow of the TR jet into the RA and IVC.

Answer B is incorrect as diastolic flattening of the interventricular septum (IVS) resulting in a D-shaped LV may be seen with right heart volume overload due to significant TR. If there is coexistent pulmonary hypertension, septal flattening with a D-shaped LV may be seen throughout the cardiac cycle.

Answer D is incorrect. Dilation of the right heart can lead to tricuspid valve annular dilation and leaflet tethering. This tethering can prevent complete tricuspid leaflet coaptation during systole. The coaptation distance or height is a measure of the degree of tethering. This distance is measured from the apical 4-chamber view in mid-systole as the distance between the tricuspid annular plane and the coaptation point between the anterior and septal tricuspid leaflets (**Figure 21-12B**). A coaptation

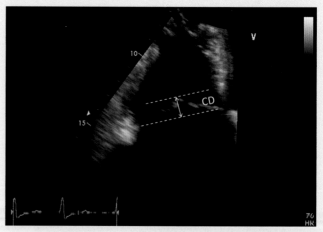

Figure 21-12B The coaptation distance (CD) is measured from a zoomed apical 4-chamber view in mid-systole as the distance between the tricuspid annular plane and the coaptation point between the anterior and septal tricuspid leaflets.

distance >8 mm represents significant tethering and is a sign of significant, chronic TR.

Answer E is not correct. As previously stated, in cases of significant TR, RV dilatation occurs due to RV volume overload.

8. **Answer: D.** The features of severe PR on the images provided include (1) a wide PR color jet filling the right ventricular outflow tract in diastole, (2) flow reversal in the main pulmonary artery (PA) and PA branches (**Video 21-1B**), (3) a dense PR signal on the continuous-wave (CW) Doppler trace, (4) a rapid PR deceleration slope, and (5) early termination of the PR signal.

Observe that the PR duration on the color Doppler image is short, which is often the reason why severe PR is missed with color Doppler imaging alone. The still-frame diastolic image from **Video 21-1B** is shown in **Figure 21-13A**. This image shows flow reversal in the pulmonary artery during diastole (red color). The spectral density of the CW Doppler trace is proportional to the number of red

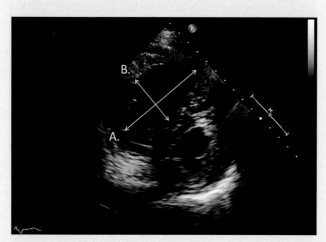

Figure 21-12A The RVEI, measured from the parasternal short-axis view at end-systole, is derived as a ratio between **Line A** and **Line B**. **Line B** is first measured as the line connecting the IVS and the RV free wall at the midpoint of the IVS and **Line A** is then measured as the RV longest lateral distance perpendicular to the **Line B**.

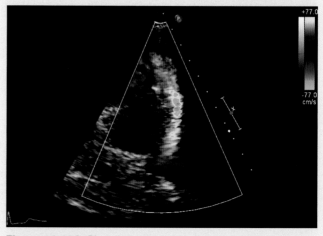

Figure 21-13A Diastolic flow reversal in the main PA and PA branches on color Doppler imaging.

blood cells (RBCs) creating Doppler shifts; the stronger the signal, the more RBCs and the more severe the regurgitation. Note, however, that an overlap between moderate and severe regurgitation exists with regard to the density. The PR deceleration slope is rapid, with a pressure half-time <100 ms, and early termination of the PR signal before onset of the QRS on the electrocardiogram (**Figure 12-13B**). This occurs as a result of early equalization of the PA and right ventricular (RV) pressures during diastole. The presence of diastolic flow reversal in the main pulmonary artery (PA) +/– the PA branches is supportive of severe PR (**Figure 21-13C**). Anticipate the RV to be dilated in cases of severe PR.

9. **Answer: B.** Significant TR can lead to an increased tricuspid inflow velocity due to the increase in flow through the valve as a result of the volume overload. This is because the total forward diastolic flow across the tricuspid valve (TV) is a combination of the usual forward stroke volume across the

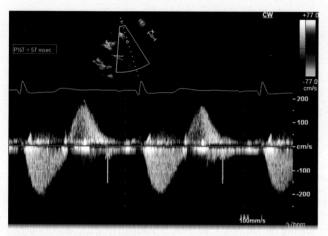

Figure 21-13B A short PR pressure half-time (P1/2T) < 100 ms and early termination of the PR signal (arrows).

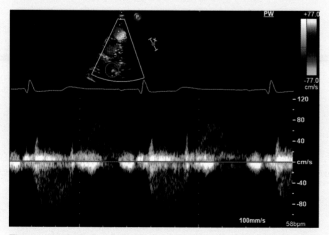

Figure 21-13C Diastolic flow reversal in the right PA branch on pulsed-wave Doppler appears above the zero-velocity baseline. The red circle indicates the position of the sample volume within the right PA branch.

valve plus the regurgitant volume (RVol) that leaked through the TV during systole.

Answer A is not correct. The normal hepatic venous flow profile demonstrates predominant forward flow during systole and diastole (seen below the zero-velocity baseline) and small antegrade velocities occurring with atrial and ventricular contraction (seen above the zero baseline). With increasing degrees of TR, the hepatic venous systolic velocity becomes blunted or reduced; with severe TR, systolic flow reversal may be seen as flow above the zero baseline in systole due to the backflow of blood into the right atrium (RA) and up into the hepatic veins.

Answer C is not correct. The TR velocity does not correlate with TR severity. In fact, severe TR may be associated with a low velocity with near equalization of right ventricular and RA systolic pressures.

Answer D is not correct since the IVC may not collapse with significant TR due to the increase in the RA pressure. Answer E is not correct. The pulmonary vein systolic flow reversal is associated with significant mitral regurgitation (MR), not significant TR.

10. **Answer: A.** Right ventricular systolic pressure (RVSP) can be estimated from the peak TR velocity (V_{TR}) and the RA pressure (RAP):

$$RVSP = 4V_{TR}^2 + RAP \qquad (1)$$

The peak TR velocity is 3 m/s and the RAP can be assumed to be normal (3 mm Hg) given the normal RA and IVC sizes. Therefore, the RVSP is:

$$RVSP = 4(3^2) + 3 = 36 + 3 = 39 \text{ mm Hg} \qquad (2)$$

The peak systolic pressure gradient across the pulmonary valve (ΔP_{PS}) is 20 mm Hg. Therefore, the PASP is approximately:

$$PASP = RVSP - \Delta P_{PS} = 39 - 20 = 19 \text{ mm Hg} \qquad (3)$$

As the PASP is < 40 mm Hg, this value is normal.

KEY POINTS

In patients with PS, the RVSP is greater than the PASP. The PASP can be estimated if the pressure gradient across the pulmonary valve is known.

11. **Answer: A.** Assessment of TR severity requires integration of multiple observations rather than an emphasis on a single measurement due to a number of hemodynamic factors that can influence the color jet characteristics. The color jet area is dependent on the driving pressure and jet direction. The shape of the jet may underestimate (eccentric) or

overestimate (central entrainment) the severity of TR. The vena contracta can be problematic with multiple jets, and flow convergence proximal to the TR jet needs to be clearly visualized for the assessment of the vena contracta. The proximal flow convergence radius or zone may be nonhemispheric in shape and is also unreliable with multiple jets.

12. **Answer: C.** Quantitative assessment of PS is based mainly on the transpulmonary peak pressure gradient (**Table 21-2**). Severe pulmonic stenosis is defined by Doppler echocardiography as a peak velocity across the valve >4 m/s and a peak gradient >64 mm Hg. Normal RV systolic pressure (answer A) should not occur with severe PS as the RVSP must exceed the pulmonary artery systolic pressure (PASP) as blood flows from a higher- to a lower-pressure chamber. A normal size of the pulmonary artery (answer B) is not characteristic of severe PS, where poststenotic dilatation is more common. An RV wall thickness of 0.3 cm (answer E) is normal. In patients with significant PS, RV hypertrophy (RVH) is expected. RVH is defined as an RV wall thickness >0.5 cm.

Of note: the PASP is usually normal in the setting of severe pulmonic stenosis.

Table 21-2. Grading of Pulmonary Stenosis

	Mild	Moderate	Severe
Peak velocity (m/s)	<3	3-4	>4
Peak pressure gradient (mm Hg)	<36	36-64	>64

From Baumgartner H, Hung J, Bermejo J, et al. Echocardiographic assessment of valve stenosis: EAE/ASE recommendations for clinical practice. J Am Soc Echocardiogr. 2009;22(1):1-23. Copyright © 2009 European Society of Cardiology. With permission.

13. Answer: B. Tricuspid atresia is the third most common form of cyanotic congenital heart disease and is characterized by the absence of a direct communication between the right ventricle (RV) and right atrium. The tricuspid valve (TV) leaflets themselves are not visible, and either they have failed to form or the formed leaflets have fused. There is a functionally single ventricle with the ventricle having a left ventricular morphology (**Video 21-6**). An opening in the interatrial septum (IAS) is necessary for survival and usually consists of a secundum-type ASD. Those with normal great artery anatomy (ventriculoarterial concordance) have a high incidence of subvalvular or valvular pulmonic stenosis. The majority will also have some form of rudimentary RV and a VSD.

Ebstein anomaly (answer A) is a congenital abnormality involving the TV. The TV leaflets are displaced toward the RV apex and a significant portion of the RV becomes "atrialized." Noonan syndrome

(answer C) is a genetic disorder associated with short stature and congenital heart disease. The most common cardiac defect is pulmonary stenosis, with or without a dysplastic pulmonary valve; ASDs are also common, and hypertrophic cardiomyopathy is present in about 20% of patients. Tetralogy of Fallot (answer D) is a combination of four cardiac defects: an overriding aorta, a malalignment VSD, infundibular or pulmonary stenosis, and RV hypertrophy.

14. **Answer: D.** The proximal PR jet width is the most widely used semiquantitative method to assess PR severity. A value >0.7 for the ratio of the PR jet width to the pulmonary annular diameter is associated with severe PR.

The effective orifice area by the proximal isovelocity surface area (PISA) method (answer A) can be performed; however, no studies have examined the accuracy of this method in quantifying PR severity. The PR jet area (answer B) can be used to assess PR severity but lacks reproducibility. PR jet length (answer C) can provide an indirect clue of nonsignificant PR; a PR jet length <10 mm represents insignificant PR. However, as with aortic regurgitation (AR), the color jet length does not correlate with severity and is more related to the driving pressure. It is also important to note that significant PR is often associated with laminar rather than turbulent flow because of a low-pressure gradient between the right ventricle and pulmonary artery during diastole.

15. **Answer: C.** As previously stated, in functional (or secondary) TR, the tricuspid valve (TV) and subvalvular apparatus are morphologically normal and TR occurs due to annular dilatation and/or leaflet tethering. As a result, TR occurs due to malcoaptation of the TV leaflets. Functional causes account for approximately 75% of TR cases. Causes include pulmonary hypertension, any cause of right ventricular (RV) myocardial disease, RV ischemia and infarction, and right atrial enlargement from atrial fibrillation. Therefore, answer C is correct. Pulmonary embolism causes acute RV dysfunction and dilation with an underlying increase in RV pressures and a structurally normal TV. The TR is a result of the acute RV volume overload (dilated RV) and increase in RV pressures.

Answers A, B, D, and E are incorrect as these are organic (or primary) causes of TR. Primary TR refers to abnormalities of the TV leaflets and/or subvalvular apparatus. TR due to pacemaker lead insertion is considered an iatrogenic cause.

16. **Answer: A.** The mean pulmonary artery pressure and the pulmonary artery end-diastolic pressure (PAEDP) can be estimated from the PR spectral Doppler signal:

$$mPAP = 4V_{PR-EaD}^2 + RAP \qquad (1)$$

$$PAEDP = 4V_{PR-ED}^2 + RAP \qquad (2)$$

where V_{PR-EaD} is the peak PR velocity in early diastole, V_{PR-ED} is the peak PR velocity at end-diastole and RAP is the right atrial pressure estimated from the IVC size and collapsibility (**Table 21-3**).

In the absence of pulmonic stenosis or right ventricular outflow tract obstruction, PASP (answer B) will equal right ventricular systolic pressure (RVSP), which is derived as:

$$RVSP = 4V_{TR}^2 + RAP \qquad (3)$$

where V_{TR} is the peak TR velocity and RAP is the right atrial pressure estimated from the IVC size and collapsibility (**Table 21-3**).

In the absence of tricuspid stenosis, the RVEDP (answer C) can be assumed to be the same as the estimated RAP.

17. **Answer: B.** General anesthesia will change the appearance of TR, making it seem less severe when compared to preanesthesia due to decreased volume of blood in the vascular system and consequent change in loading.

Table 21-3. IVC Size and Collapsibility for the Estimation of RAP

Range	IVC Diameter (cm)	IVC Collapsibility With Sniff (%)	Estimated RAP (mm Hg)
Normal	≤2.1	>50	3
High	>2.1	<50	15
Intermediate[a]	≤2.1	<50	8
	>2.1	>50	8

[a]When there are no secondary signs of increased RAP, the RAP can be downgraded to 3 mm Hg; when the IVC collapses <35% and there are secondary signs of increased RAP, then the RAP can be upgraded to 15 mm Hg. Secondary signs of elevated RAP include a restrictive tricuspid inflow filling profile, a tricuspid E/e' ratio >6, or a hepatic venous systolic filling fraction >55%.

18. **Answer: C.** Mean pulmonary artery pressure can be calculated as:

$$mPAP = 4V_{PR-EaD}^2 + RAP \qquad (1)$$

where V_{PR-EaD} is the peak PR velocity in early diastole and RAP is the right atrial pressure estimated from the IVC size and collapsibility (see **Table 21-3**).

In this case, the PR V_{max} in early diastole is 1.58 m/s and the IVC is normal in size but collapses less than 50%, so the RAP is estimated at 8 mm Hg. Therefore, the estimated mPAP is:

$$mPAP = 4(1.58^2) + 8 = 10 + 8 = 18 \text{ mm Hg} \qquad (2)$$

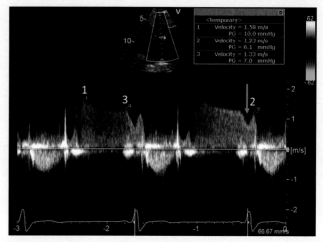
Figure 21-14

19. **Answer: A.** The PAEDP can be estimated as:

$$PAEDP = 4V_{PR-ED}^2 + RAP \qquad (1)$$

where V_{PR-ED} is the peak PR velocity at end-diastole and RAP is the right atrial pressure estimated from the IVC size and collapsibility (see **Table 21-2**).

From the PR trace in **Figure 21-3**, there are two measurements toward the end of diastole: 2 and 3. Measurement 3 is just prior to atrial contraction and measurement 2 is after atrial contraction. Atrial contraction is reflected by the "dip" in the trace (**Figure 21-14**, orange arrow). This dip reflects a transient increase in the right ventricular diastolic pressure and therefore a transient drop in the pressure gradient between the pulmonary artery and right ventricle at this instant in time. As end-diastole is defined as the closure of the tricuspid valve (following atrial contraction), the true end-diastolic velocity is measurement number 2. This variable is 1.23 m/s; the IVC is normal in size but collapses less than 50%, so the RAP is estimated at 8 mm Hg. Therefore, the estimated PAEDP is:

$$PAEDP = 4(1.23)^2 + 8 = 6 + 8 = 14 \text{ mm Hg} \qquad (2)$$

20. **Answer: B.** Based on the data in **Table 21-4**, a TR vena contracta of 0.5 cm, an effective regurgitant orifice area (EROA) of 0.37 cm², and a regurgitant volume of 44 mL is consistent with moderate TR.

Table 21-4. Features of TR Severity

	Mild	Moderate	Severe
Vena contracta (cm)	<0.3	0.3-0.69	≥0.7
EROA (cm²)	<0.2	0.2-0.4	>0.4
Regurgitant volume (mL)	<30	30-44	≥45

Reprinted from Zoghbi WA, Adams D, Bonow RO, et al. Recommendations for noninvasive evaluation of native valvular regurgitation. A report from the American Society of Echocardiography Developed in Collaboration with the Society for Cardiovascular Magnetic Resonance. *J Am Soc Echocardiogr*. 2017;30(4):303-371. Copyright © 2017 by the American Society of Echocardiography. With permission.

21. **Answer: C.** The en face view, viewing the TV from either the RV or RA, with the septal leaflet and the interatrial septum (IAS) positioned at 6 o'clock (or inferior position) is the recommended view for imaging the TV leaflets, as all three leaflets and the annulus can be seen in one view (**Figure 21-15**). The en face views are particularly helpful in localizing leaflet disease such as TV prolapse, perforation or vegetations, or for performing valve planimetry to assess the severity of tricuspid stenosis. A full-volume image displays a pyramidal volume of data that can be rotated or cropped in any direction in order to answer a relevant structural question. A full volume with color Doppler added enables analysis of the tricuspid regurgitation (TR) mechanism and location of the TR jet origin.

22. **Answer: B.** The tricuspid valve consists of three leaflets: anterior, septal, and posterior. There is some variation as to which TV leaflets are seen from the various transthoracic echocardiographic (TTE) views. From the parasternal long-axis right ventricular (RV) inflow view, the anterior leaflet is imaged superiorly and to the right, adjacent to the RV free wall and either the septal or posterior TV leaflet is imaged inferiorly and to the left. When the interventricular septum (IVS) is seen, this is the septal leaflet and when the IVS is not seen, this could be either the septal or posterior TV leaflet.

In the parasternal short-axis view (at the level of the aortic valve), the TV leaflet combination is again variable. The TV leaflet closest to the aorta is the anterior or septal leaflet, while the TV leaflet near the RV free wall is either the posterior or anterior leaflet.

From the apical 4-chamber view, the septal TV leaflet is seen closest to the IVS, while the TV leaflet against the RV free wall is usually the posterior TV leaflet; the anterior TV leaflet may be seen when this imaging plane is tilted anteriorly to the apical 5-chamber view. From the subcostal 4-chamber view,

the anterior leaflet is usually seen adjacent to the RV free wall and the septal leaflet adjacent to the IVS.

23. **Answer: A.** Typically, as the diameter of the TV annulus increases, so does the degree of TR, exemplifying a linear response or relationship. A linear relationship is one where increasing or decreasing one variable (n) times will cause a corresponding increase or decrease of (n) times in the other variable. In simpler words, if you double one variable, the other will double as well. An inverse response or relationship (answer B) would indicate the TR became less significant with a larger annulus, as an inverse relationship between two values is one whereby an increase in one value results in a decrease in the other value, and vice versa. A negative correlation (answer C) is essentially the same as an inverse relationship; that is, a negative correlation is a relationship between two variables in which one variable increases as the other decreases, and vice versa.

24. **Answer: D.** The constant used to estimate the tricuspid valve area (TVA) in TS by the pressure half-time method is 190 (it is 220 in mitral stenosis). Therefore, the TVA is calculated as:

$$\mathrm{TVA}\left(\mathrm{cm}\right)^{2} = 190 \div \mathrm{PHT} \tag{1}$$

where PHT is the pressure half-time measured in ms.

Answer A is not correct since doming of the TV in TS is seen in diastole, not systole.

Planimetry of the TVA (answer B) in a TTE is difficult in TS as it is difficult to get a true short-axis view of the valve. 3D TTE with good image quality may be useful for planimetry. However, with 3D TTE it is usually difficult to image the leaflets clearly for planimetry in most patients due to the distance of the probe from the valve leaflets, which causes some blurring of the image. Answer C is not

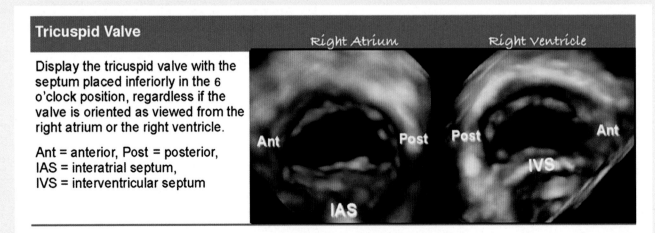

Tricuspid Valve

Display the tricuspid valve with the septum placed inferiorly in the 6 o'clock position, regardless if the valve is oriented as viewed from the right atrium or the right ventricle.

Ant = anterior, Post = posterior, IAS = interatrial septum, IVS = interventricular septum

Figure 21-15 (Reprinted from Lang RM, Badano LP, Tsang W, et al. EAE/ASE recommendations for image acquisition and display using three-dimensional echocardiography. *J Am Soc Echocardiogr.* 2012;25(1):3-46. Copyright © 2012 Elsevier. With permission.)

correct as the mean gradient in severe TS is ≥ 5 mm Hg. Answer E is not correct. Although rheumatic involvement of the TV occurs with some frequency, hemodynamically significant stenosis is relatively uncommon and is reported in about 5% of patients with rheumatic involvement of the mitral valve.

25. **Answer: D.** While there is some variability in the display of tricuspid valve (TV) leaflets, the apical 4-chamber (TTE) and midesophageal 0° (TEE) views display the septal and posterior tricuspid leaflet combination (**Figures 21-16A** and **21-16B**). Also, the TEE distal esophageal 90° view and the TTE parasternal short-axis (PSAX) view may demonstrate the septal and posterior TV leaflet combination. The deep transgastric 0°, transgastric 90°, and PSAX views may display all three tricuspid valve leaflets.

> **TEACHING POINT**
>
> A recent study compared 2D and 3D multiplanar reconstruction to determine which tricuspid leaflet combination is commonly seen on the TTE 2D examination (Addetia et al., 2016). Based on the results from this study, the tricuspid leaflet combination may include anterior and septal, anterior and posterior, anterior alone, posterior and septal, or posterior, anterior and septal. The frequency of leaflet combinations seen in the 2D TTE images is summarized in **Figure 21-16C**.

26. **Answer: A.** Carcinoid heart disease is a complication of a rare malignancy (carcinoid tumor). Usually only carcinoid tumors that invade the liver result in changes to the heart. Carcinoid tumors that are invasive and/or metastasize produce the carcinoid syndrome that is characterized by facial flushing, diarrhea, and bronchoconstriction. Carcinoid heart disease mainly affects the right heart (90% of the time) resulting in thickened, immobile, or "fixed" tricuspid and pulmonary valves. This is a result of exposure to serotonin, a common product of a carcinoid tumor. Left-sided valve disease occurs in 10% of patients. When seen on the left side, it occurs primarily in patients who have an intracardiac shunt, which allows serotonin-rich blood to bypass the filter of the lungs. In contrast, rheumatic heart disease (answer E) leads to a doming appearance of the leaflets when open, with decreased leaflet separation. Endocarditis (answer C) typically presents with a vegetation. Pheochromocytoma (answer D) is a tumor that grows on the adrenal glands and is associated with periods of systemic hypertension, tachycardia/palpitations, excessive sweating, and severe headaches. Ebstein anomaly (answer B) is a complex congenital lesion that primarily involves the tricuspid valve and atrialization of the RV.

27. **Answer: D.** In the absence of significant tricuspid and aortic regurgitation, it can be assumed that the stroke volume (SV) across both valves is the same; that is, the same SV ejected into the LVOT ultimately passes across the TV. This is the continuity principle.

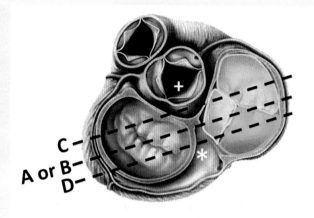

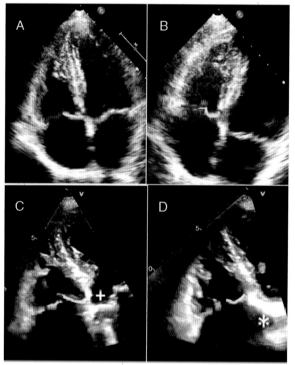

Figure 21-16A From the 4-chamber views of the right ventricle (A and B), the septal leaflet can be clearly identified; however, the opposing leaflet can be the anterior or the posterior leaflet (red line). Tilting the transducer anteriorly, so that a portion of the aorta (+) is imaged (C), will image the septal and anterior leaflets. Angling the transducer posterior so that a portion of the coronary sinus (*) is imaged (D) will image the septal and posterior leaflets. (Reprinted with permission from Hahn RT. State-of-the-art review of echocardiographic imaging in the evaluation and treatment of functional tricuspid regurgitation. *Circ Cardiovasc Imaging*. 2016;9(12):e005332.)

The SV is derived from the cross-sectional area (CSA) × VTI; therefore,

$$TVA \times TV_{TVI} = \left(0.785 \times LVOT_d^2\right) \times LVOT_{VTI} \tag{1}$$

where $(0.785 \times LVOT_d^2)$ is the CSA of the LVOT, TVA is the tricuspid valve area and TV_{VTI} is the VTI across the TV. Rearranging this equation, the TVA is calculated as:

$$TVA = \left[\left(0.785 \times LVOT_d^2\right) \times LVOT_{VTI}\right] \div TV_{TVI} \tag{2}$$

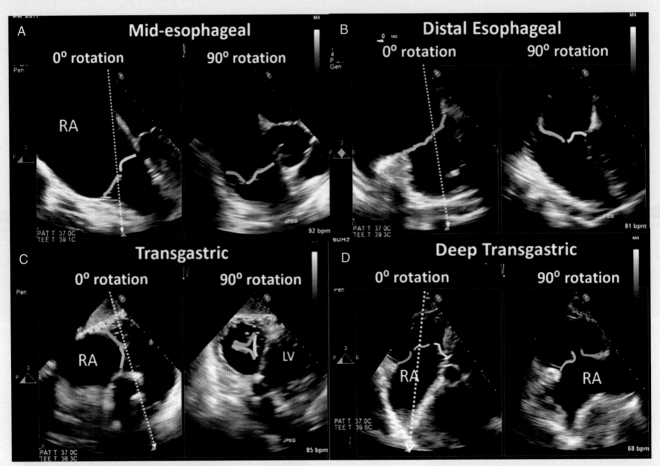

Figure 21-16B Multilevel imaging of the tricuspid valve (TV). A, Example of simultaneous multiplane imaging at the midesophageal depth. The 4-chamber view permits the visualization of the septal and typically the anterior leaflet; simultaneous biplane imaging may help clarify which leaflet is imaged because the anterior leaflet is typically seen adjacent to the aorta. Low esophageal views (B) at the level of the coronary sinus (*) typically image the posterior and anterior leaflets. Advancing the TEE probe into the stomach and rotating approximately 20° to 60° produces the transgastric basal short-axis view (C), which is the only 2D view that usually provides simultaneous visualization of all three TV leaflets. Using the simultaneous multiplane imaging mode, all the leaflet coaptation points can be imaged. Advancing the TEE probe along with rightward anterior flexion and returning the multiplane angle to 0° to 40° produces a deep transgastric view of the TV (D). (Reprinted with permission from Hahn RT. State of the art review of echocardiographic imaging in the evaluation and treatment of functional tricuspid regurgitation. *Circ Cardiovasc Imaging.* 2016;9(12):e005332.)

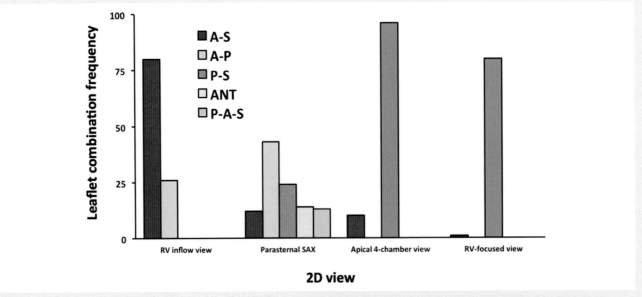

Figure 21-16C The frequency of tricuspid leaflet combinations seen on the 2D TTE. ANT (anterior alone), A-S (anterior-septal combination), A-P (anterior posterior combination), P-S (posterior-septal combination), P-A-S (posterior, anterior, and septal combination). (Reprinted from Addetia K, Yamat M, Mediratta A, et al. Comprehensive two-dimensional interrogation of the tricuspid valve using knowledge derived from three-dimensional echocardiography. *J Am Soc Echocardiogr.* 2016;29(1):74-82. Copyright © 2016 American Society of Echocardiography. With permission.)

Substituting the values in **Table 21-1**, the TVA is estimated as:

$$TVA = \left[\left(0.785 \times 2.2^2\right) \times 17\right] \div 65$$

$$= 64.59 \div 65 = 0.99 \, cm^2 \qquad (3)$$

The TVA can also be calculated from the SV derived from the RVOT by substituting the RVOT diameter and VTI measurements for the LVOT diameter and VTI measurements:

$$TVA = \left[\left(0.785 \times RVOT_d^2\right) \times RVOT_{VTI}\right] \div TV_{TVI} \qquad (1)$$

The main limitations of this continuity equation method for estimating the TVA is the accurate measurement of the tricuspid inflow VTI and the absence of any significant tricuspid regurgitation (TR) and/or aortic regurgitation (AR). When there is significant TR or AR, the continuity assumptions are violated as the SV across both areas is no longer the same. When there is significant TR, the tricuspid inflow VTI is increased and therefore the TVA will be underestimated. When there is significant AR, the LVOT stroke volume is overestimated and therefore the TVA will be overestimated.

28. **Answer: D.** The goal of echocardiographic assessment of TS is to recognize patients with significant TS, in which intervention may be necessary to relieve symptoms. **Table 21-5** indicates echocardiographic findings consistent with significant TS. In this patient from Question 27, the TVA was 0.99 cm² and the tricuspid inflow VTI was 65 cm; based on these parameters, severe TS is present.

Table 21-5. Findings Indicative of Hemodynamically Significant Tricuspid Stenosis (TS)

	Significant TS
Mean pressure gradient (mm Hg)	≥5
Inflow velocity-time integral (VTI) (cm)	>60
Pressure half-time (ms)	≥190
Valve area (cm²)	≤1

From Baumgartner H, Hung J, Bermejo J, et al. Echocardiographic assessment of valve stenosis: EAE/ASE recommendations for clinical practice. *J Am Soc Echocardiogr.* 2009;22(1):1-23. Copyright © 2009 European Society of Cardiology. With permission.

29. **Answer: A.** Pulmonic valve (PV) regurgitant volume (RVol) is calculated as the stroke volume (SV) of the right ventricular outflow tract (RVOT) minus the SV of the left ventricular outflow tract (LVOT) in units of mL:

$$RVol = SV \, RVOT - SV \, LVOT \qquad (1)$$

The regurgitant fraction (RF) is the ratio of regurgitant volume (RVol) and total flow across the regurgitant PV (SV RVOT):

$$RF = \left(RVol \div SV \, RVOT\right) \times 100 \qquad (2)$$

Using the respective outflow tract diameters and velocity-time integral (VTI) of both right and left valves, the SV across the LVOT and RVOT can be calculated. As previously described, the SV is derived from the cross-sectional area (CSA) × VTI; therefore, the SV LVOT is:

$$SV \, LVOT = \left(0.785 \times LVOT_d^2\right) \times LVOT_{VTI} \qquad (3)$$

Using the information provided in **Figure 21-5**:

$$SV \, LVOT = \left(0.785 \times 2.0^2\right) \times 21.3 = 67 \, mL \qquad (4)$$

Repeating the same process using the RVOT diameter and VTI for the SV RVOT:

$$SV \, RVOT = \left(0.785 \times 2.4^2\right) \times 30.7 = 139 \, mL \qquad (5)$$

Therefore, the pulmonary RVol using Equation 1 is:

$$RVol = 139 - 67 = 72 \, ml \qquad (6)$$

And the pulmonary RF using Equation 2 is:

$$RF = \left(72 \div 139\right) \times 100 = 52\% \qquad (7)$$

Note that this calculation assumes that there is no significant aortic regurgitation (AR). In cases of significant AR, the LVOT measurements can be substituted with the mitral annular measurements. These quantitative calculations can be used with multiple jets and eccentric jets. While these calculations can provide a quantitative estimation of pulmonic regurgitation (PR) severity, they are not usually performed routinely due to lack of experience, difficulty in measuring the RVOT diameter, and a lack of validation data for quantifying PR severity by these methods.

30. **Answer: C.** While the pulmonary regurgitant fraction (RF) can be estimated by echocardiography, RF data are primarily derived from cardiac magnetic resonance (CMR) for the grading of PR severity. Applying these CMR cutoff values to echocardiographic values in this case, the PR severity is graded as moderate (**Table 21-6**).

Table 21-6. RF for PR Severity

	Mild	Moderate	Severe
Regurgitant fraction (%)	<20	20-40	>40

Reprinted from Zoghbi WA, Adams D, Bonow RO, et al. Recommendations for noninvasive evaluation of native valvular regurgitation. A report from the American Society of Echocardiography Developed in Collaboration with the Society for Cardiovascular Magnetic Resonance. *J Am Soc Echocardiogr.* 2017;30(4):303-371. Copyright © 2017 by the American Society of Echocardiography. With permission.

31. **Answer: D.** Although significant PR can lead to enlargement of the RV, RV dilatation by itself is not a specific sign of significant PR since it can result from several other conditions. However, it is important to correlate the severity of RV enlargement with the degree of PR. Dilatation with significant PR may be localized to the right ventricular outflow tract in patients post tetralogy of Fallot repair. In functional PR, the degree of RV dysfunction, RV dilatation, and abnormal interventricular septal motion are related to the severity of the underlying disease process, such as pulmonary arterial hypertension, rather than to the degree of PR. Answer A is true; the pulmonic valve cusps are thinner than those of the tricuspid valve. Answer B is true; branch pulmonary stenosis may create more than physiologic PR due to elevated pulmonary artery pressure (PAP). Likewise, other conditions that lead to elevated PAP such as left ventricular dysfunction, acquired bronchopulmonary disease, or pulmonary vascular disease can have the same exacerbated effect on PR. It is important to note that the relief of branch pulmonary stenosis reduces PR in the swine model (*J Thorac Cardiovasc Surg.* 2009;138(2):382-389). Answer C is true; severe pulmonary regurgitation eventually causes pressure equalization between the RV and pulmonary artery in mid-diastole.

32. **Answer: C.** A papillary fibroelastoma (PFE) is a benign tumor of the heart valves; it is the most common primary valve tumor. The etiology of PFE is unknown, but a possible explanation may be previous mechanical damage to the endothelium. Although the echocardiographic appearance is similar to that of a vegetation, the patient did not present with symptoms associated with infective endocarditis, such as fever and chills. Also, PFEs tend to appear on the downstream side of the valve while vegetations tend to appear on the upstream side. Lambl excrescences are small fronds that occur at sites of valve closure. They originate as tiny thrombi on the endocardial surfaces at sites of minor endothelial damage (due to wear and tear). A myxoma is a benign tumor that arises primarily from the left atrial side of the interatrial septum.

33. **Answer: B.** The pulmonic M-mode tracing (B) in infundibular pulmonary obstruction demonstrates an exaggerated "a dip" as similarly seen in pulmonic stenosis plus erratic flutter waves throughout systole due to the turbulent flow proximal to the valve. Trace A displays a normal pulmonic valve M-mode tracing. Trace C shows a thickened leaflet and a very exaggerated a-wave of > 6 mm; these findings are characteristic of pulmonic stenosis. Note that the exaggerated "a dip" can only be identified when sinus rhythm is present and may be dependent upon the presence of RV hypertrophy. Trace D shows fine systolic flutter waves which may be seen with idiopathic dilatation of the pulmonary artery. Trace E shows mid-systolic notching, otherwise termed as "flying W" sign, which is associated with and is commonly seen in chronic pulmonary hypertension.

TEACHING TIP

M-mode pattern recognition alone is not diagnostic of any of the abnormalities shown in **Figure 21-7**. A comprehensive 2D/3D echocardiographic examination including color and spectral Doppler is required in all cases.

34. **Answer: E.** Right ventricular outflow tract (RVOT) obstruction may be valvular, subvalvular (infundibular), or supravalvular. Infundibular stenosis may give rise to a high-velocity jet that causes damage to the pulmonary valve leaflets leading to pulmonary regurgitation.

    Answer A is not correct as infundibular stenosis may be either congenital or acquired. It occurs not only in congenital heart diseases such as tetralogy of Fallot but also in hypertrophic cardiomyopathy, in tumors of the RVOT, or in infiltrative disorders. It may be discrete or consist of a more extensive region of fibromuscular thickening. Answer B is not correct since the site of infundibular stenosis is subvalvular, not supravalular. Answer C is not correct. Pressure gradients measured by Doppler across the infundibular stenosis are reasonably accurate. When concomitant pulmonic valvular stenosis is present, it is usually impossible to isolate the precise contribution of the pulmonic valve and infundibulum to the total gradient measured by continuous-wave Doppler across the RVOT. Answer D is not correct as infundibular stenosis is often best imaged and evaluated from a parasternal short-axis view or from the subcostal window.

35. **Answer: B.** This is a case of Ebstein anomaly. The usual cause of right-sided heart failure, at least with a later presentation, is TR. Answer A is not correct. Although tachycardia may occur in Ebstein anomaly (due to associated accessory pathways such as in Wolff-Parkinson-White syndrome), there is no evidence of cardiomyopathy on the images provided. Answer C is not correct as severe pulmonary hypertension is relatively rare. Answer D is not correct as there is no evidence of endocarditis. Answer E is not correct. While an atrial septal defect (ASD) occurs

in many patients with Ebstein anomaly, the patient would have been expected to present somewhat earlier if the ASD was associated with significant right-to-left shunting.

36. **Answer: C.** This is a case of severe PR with evidence of proximal flow convergence on the pulmonary artery (PA) side of the valve and a flail leaflet (note that **Figure 21-9** is acquired in diastole). It is consistent with RV dilation and RV dysfunction. The most common cause of severe PR is prior surgery for congenital heart disease involving the pulmonary valve or right ventricular outflow tract.

Answers A and B are not correct based on the above statement regarding the display of proximal flow convergence on the PA side of the valve and a flail leaflet. Answer D is not correct as a patent duc-

tus arteriosus will give rise to continuous flow into the PA above, not below, the valve. Answer E is not correct since a homograft or allograft is usually the valve replacement of choice at the pulmonic position. Mechanical valves are associated with higher rates of thrombosis at right-sided valve positions because of the lesser pressure gradient across them and are usually avoided. Transcatheter pulmonic valve replacement is a growing field, and a potential option in selected patients.

Acknowledgments: The authors thank and acknowledge the contributions from Roger Byrne and Brian P. Griffin (Chapter 18, Pulmonic and Tricuspid Valve Disease) in *Clinical Echocardiography Review: A Self-Assessment Tool*, 2nd edition, edited by Allan L. Klein, Craig R. Asher, 2017.

SUGGESTED READINGS

Addetia K, Yamat M, Mediratta A, et al. Comprehensive two-dimensional interrogation of the tricuspid valve using knowledge derived from three-dimensional echocardiography. *J Am Soc Echocardiogr.* 2016;29(1):74-82.

Armstrong WF, Ryan T. *Chapter 12 Tricuspid and Pulmonary Disease.* In: *Feigenbaum's Echocardiography.* 8th ed. Philadelphia: Wolters Kluwer Health/Lippincott Williams & Wilkins; 2019.

Arsalan M, Walther T, Smith RL II, Grayburn PA. Tricuspid regurgitation diagnosis and treatment. *Eur Heart J.* 2017;38(9):634-638.

Baumgartner H, Hung J, Bermejo J, et al. Echocardiographic assessment of valve stenosis: EAE/ASE recommendations for clinical practice. *J Am Soc Echocardiogr.* 2009;22(1):1-23.

Bouzas B, Milner PJ, Gatzoulis MA. Pulmonary regurgitation: not a benign lesion. *Eur Heart J.* 2005;26(5):433-439.

Hahn RT. State-of-the-Art Review of echocardiographic imaging in the evaluation and treatment of functional tricuspid regurgitation. *Circ Cardiovasc Imaging* 2016;9(12):pii: e005332.

Lancellotti P, Moura L, Pierard LA, et al. European Association of Echocardiography recommendations for the assessment of valvular regurgitation. Part 2: mitral and tricuspid regurgitation (native valve disease). *Eur J Echocardiogr.* 2010;11(4):307-332.

Lang RM, Badano LP, Tsang W, et al. EAE/ASE recommendations for image acquisition and display using three-dimensional echocardiography. *J Am Soc Echocardiogr.* 2012;25(1):3-46.

Lang RM, Shernan SK, Shirali GS, Mor-Avi V. Chapter 10, tricuspid valve. In: *Comprehensive Atlas of 3D Echocardiography.* Philadelphia: Wolters Kluwer Health/Lippincott Williams & Wilkins; 2013.

Petit CJ, Rome JJ. Relief of branch pulmonary artery stenosis reduces pulmonary valve insufficiency in a swine model. *J Thorac Cardiovasc Surg.* 2009;138(2):382-389.

Zoghbi WA, Adams D, Bonow RO, et al. Recommendations for non-invasive evaluation of native valvular regurgitation: a report from the American Society of Echocardiography Developed in Collaboration with the Society for Cardiovascular Magnetic Resonance. *J Am Soc Echocardiogr.* 2017;30(4):303-371.

Prosthetic Valves

Contributors: Thomas Van Houten, MPH, ACS, RDCS and Michael Rampoldi, ACS, RDCS, RVT

✪ Question 1

A 55-year-old man with prior aortic valve replacement presents with dyspnea on exertion that has been present since his surgery. Prosthesis-patient mismatch (PPM) is suspected. An indexed effective orifice area (EOA) ≤ _____ is used to define this syndrome.

- **A.** 0.55 cm²/m²
- **B.** 0.65 cm²/m²
- **C.** 0.75 cm²/m²
- **D.** 0.85 cm²/m²
- **E.** 0.95 cm²/m²

✪ Question 2

A 55-year-old man with a recent aortic valve replacement (AVR) undergoes postoperative echocardiography to establish baseline values for the valve. A peak AVR velocity of 2.5 m/s is recorded. This value:

- **A.** Is abnormally high, suggesting prosthesis-patient mismatch (PPM).
- **B.** Is abnormally high, suggesting AVR stenosis.
- **C.** May be normal depending on the size and type of the AVR.
- **D.** Is low, suggesting that the AVR is an allograft valve.
- **E.** Is abnormally low, suggesting that the patient has a reduced cardiac output.

✪ Question 3

A 72-year-old woman with a bioprosthetic mitral valve replacement (MVR) undergoes echocardiographic evaluation. Which of the following statements is true regarding the effective orifice area (EOA) and the pressure half-time (PHT)?

- **A.** EOA calculated as 220/PHT provides the best single measurement of the functional valve area.
- **B.** EOA calculated as 270/PHT provides the best single measurement of the functional valve area.
- **C.** EOA calculated as 1.5 × (220/PHT) provides the best single measurement of the functional valve area.
- **D.** EOA calculated as 150/PHT provides the best single measurement of the functional valve area.
- **E.** EOA calculated by the PHT method is inaccurate in patients with mitral prostheses.

✪✪ Question 4

A 63-year-old patient with prior aortic valve replacement (AVR) undergoes echocardiographic evaluation for new symptoms of dyspnea. In addition to recording the peak and mean pressure gradients, the Doppler velocity index (DVI) is also calculated as:

- **A.** Stroke volume ÷ AVR velocity-time integral (VTI).
- **B.** (Stroke volume × heart rate) ÷ peak AVR velocity.
- **C.** Left ventricular outflow tract (LVOT) VTI ÷ AVR VTI.
- **D.** (LVOT VTI × stroke volume) ÷ AVR VTI.
- **E.** Calculated EOA ÷ factory-specified normal EOA.

✪ Question 5

A 72-year-old woman with prior mitral valve replacement (MVR) is noted to have a new systolic murmur. An echocardiogram is performed. Based on **Figure 22-1**, what is the diagnosis?

   A. Bioprosthesis with paravalvular mitral regurgitation (MR)

   B. Bileaflet prosthesis with paravalvular MR

   C. Bioprosthesis with valvular MR

   D. Bileaflet prosthesis with normal closure jets

   E. Bileaflet prosthesis with valvular MR

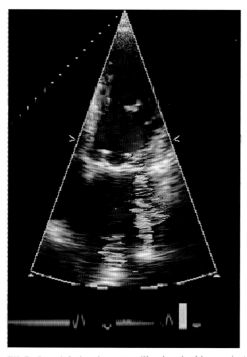

Figure 22-1 Apical 4-chamber view. (Reprinted with permission from Klein AL, Asher CR. *Clinical Echocardiography Review: A Self-Assessment Tool.* 2nd ed. Philadelphia, PA: Wolters Kluwer; 2017.)

✪✪ Question 6

A 75-year-old man with prior aortic valve replacement (AVR) undergoes echocardiographic evaluation because of dyspnea on exertion (**Figure 22-2**). The pulsed-wave Doppler spectrum recorded in the left ventricular outflow tract (LVOT) yields a velocity-time integral (VTI) of 10 cm. Continuous-wave Doppler recorded across the AVR yields a VTI of 67 cm. The LVOT diameter is 2.0 cm. What is the calculated Doppler velocity index (DVI)?

   A. 3.0

   B. 1.05

   C. 0.75

   D. 0.5

   E. 0.15

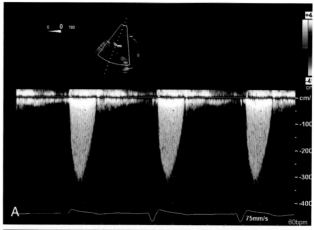

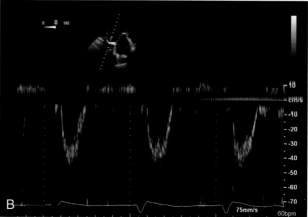

Figure 22-2 A, Continuous-wave (CW) Doppler, aortic position. B, Pulsed-wave (PW) Doppler, left ventricular outflow tract. (Reprinted with permission from Klein AL, Asher CR. *Clinical Echocardiography Review: A Self-Assessment Tool.* 2nd ed. Philadelphia, PA: Wolters Kluwer; 2017.)

✪✪ Question 7

▶ An 88-year-old woman with prior MVR is referred for echocardiographic evaluation following a transient ischemic attack (**Figure 22-3**, **Video 22-1A** and **B**). What type of prosthesis has been implanted?

   A. Bovine pericardial bioprosthesis

   B. Medtronic-Hall

   C. Porcine bioprosthesis

   D. St. Jude

   E. Starr-Edwards

✪✪✪ Question 8

▶ A 77-year-woman is referred for echocardiographic evaluation. Based on the images in **Figure 22-4** and **Video 22-2A-E**, what is shown?

   A. A tilting disc mitral valve replacement

   B. A mitral Alfieri stitch repair with ring

   C. An isolated mitral ring annuloplasty

   D. A bioprosthetic mitral valve replacement

   E. A bileaflet mitral valve replacement

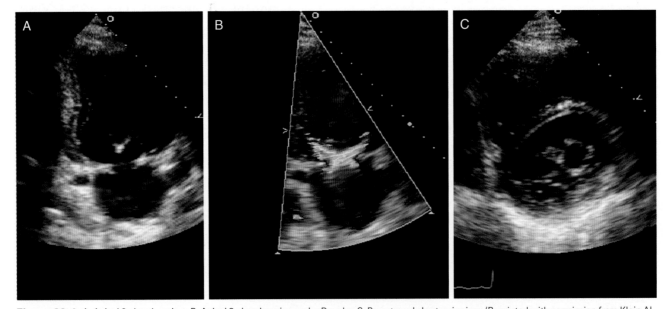

Figure 22-3 A, Apical 4-chamber view, diastole. B, Apical 4-chamber view, systole. C, Apical 4-chamber view, color Doppler. (Reprinted with permission from Klein AL, Asher CR. *Clinical Echocardiography Review: A Self Assessment Tool.* 2nd ed. Philadelphia, PA: Wolters Kluwer; 2017.)

✪✪ Question 9

A 63-year-old patient with prior bioprosthetic mitral valve replacement undergoes echocardiographic evaluation. The mean transvalvular pressure gradient is 10 mm Hg. To interpret this result, it is most important to know the patient's:

- **A.** Blood pressure.
- **B.** Heart rate.
- **C.** Height.
- **D.** Sex.
- **E.** Weight.

✪✪ Question 10

A 71-year-old patient with a bileaflet mitral valve prosthesis undergoes transthoracic echocardiographic evaluation with harmonic imaging. In the apical views, spontaneous microbubbles are seen in the left ventricle. This finding is most consistent with:

- **A.** A patent foramen ovale.
- **B.** Hemolysis.
- **C.** An imaging artifact.
- **D.** Normal prosthetic function.
- **E.** Paravalvular regurgitation.

Figure 22-4 A, Apical 2-chamber view. B, Apical 2-chamber view, color Doppler. C, Parasternal short-axis view. (Reprinted with permission from Klein AL, Asher CR. *Clinical Echocardiography Review: A Self-Assessment Tool.* 2nd ed. Philadelphia, PA: Wolters Kluwer; 2017.)

⭐ Question 11

An 81-year-old woman with prior bioprosthetic mitral valve replacement is noted to have a new systolic murmur and evidence of congestive heart failure. Transthoracic echocardiography (TTE) evaluation reveals only trace central mitral regurgitation (MR). Which of the following statements is correct?

A. Transesophageal echocardiography (TEE) is essential to evaluate the patient for paravalvular regurgitation.

B. A peak transmitral velocity of 2 m/s argues against undetected paravalvular regurgitation.

C. A mean transmitral pressure gradient of 10 mm Hg argues against undetected paravalvular regurgitation.

D. Normal (S-dominant) pulmonary venous flow excludes the possibility of paravalvular regurgitation.

E. Paravalvular regurgitation is best detected in the apical long-axis view.

⭐⭐ Question 12

A 22-year-old man presents for an echocardiographic follow-up 10 years after a Ross procedure. A 3/6 murmur is heard. Which complication is the echocardiogram most likely to demonstrate?

A. Aortic allograft stenosis

B. Aortic autograft stenosis

C. Aortic autograft regurgitation

D. Aortic allograft regurgitation

E. Pulmonary autograft regurgitation

⭐⭐⭐ Question 13

A 65-year-old woman underwent tricuspid valve replacement (TVR) for a traumatic flail tricuspid valve caused by deceleration injury in a car accident; 2 years later she presents with peripheral edema. Transthoracic echocardiography was performed. The images in **Figure 22-5** were recorded at a heart rate of 55 bpm and a blood pressure of 120/75 mm Hg. Which of the following diagnoses is most consistent with these findings?

A. Normal tricuspid prosthetic function with high output state

B. Normal tricuspid prosthetic function with rapid pressure recovery

C. Mild tricuspid prosthetic stenosis

D. Moderate tricuspid prosthetic stenosis

E. Severe tricuspid prosthetic stenosis

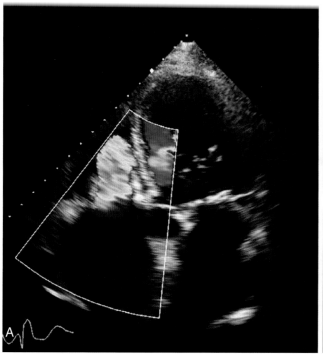
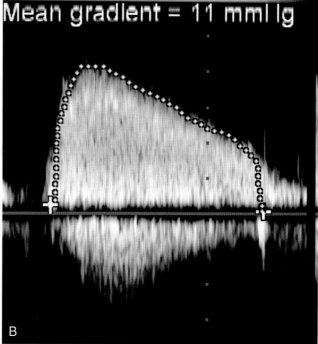

Figure 22-5 A, Apical 5-chamber view with color Doppler. B, Tricuspid valve continuous-wave (CW) Doppler. (Reprinted with permission from Klein AL, Asher CR. *Clinical Echocardiography Review: A Self-Assessment Tool.* 2nd ed. Philadelphia, PA: Wolters Kluwer; 2017.)

✪ Question 14

A 52-year-old man with prior mitral valve surgery undergoes three-dimensional (3D) transesophageal echocardiography (TEE) following a suspected neuroembolic event (**Figure 22-6**). What type of procedure has the patient undergone?

A. Mitral ring annuloplasty
B. Alfieri stitch valvuloplasty
C. Tilting disk mitral valve replacement
D. Bileaflet mitral valve replacement
E. Mitral allograft replacement

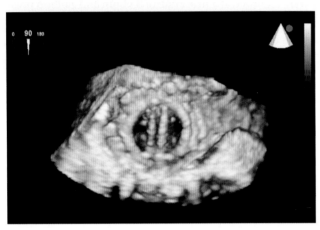

Figure 22-6 3D TEE of the mitral valve (Left atrial perspective). (Reprinted with permission from Klein AL, Asher CR. *Clinical Echocardiography Review: A Self-Assessment Tool.* 2nd ed. Philadelphia, PA: Wolters Kluwer; 2017.)

✪✪✪ Question 15

A 21-year-old man with recent allograft aortic valve replacement experiences a headache preceded by visual field deficits and undergoes a transesophageal echocardiogram (TEE) to rule out a cardiac source of embolism. He has been afebrile and Doppler evaluation reveals only trace aortic regurgitation. Based on the echocardiographic image in **Figure 22-7**, which would be an appropriate next step in management?

A. Urgent reoperation
B. Refer for coronary angiography
C. Initiate broad-spectrum antibiotics
D. Refer for cardiothoracic surgery evaluation
E. Provide reassurance that the appearance of the valve is normal

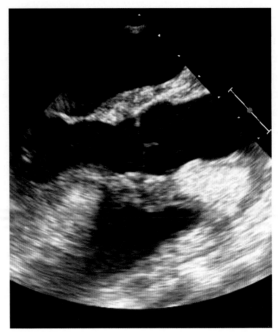

Figure 22-7 TEE image from the midesophageal long-axis view. (Reprinted with permission from Klein AL, Asher CR. *Clinical Echocardiography Review: A Self-Assessment Tool.* 2nd ed. Philadelphia, PA: Wolters Kluwer; 2017.)

✪✪ Question 16

A 62-year-woman undergoes mitral valve surgery. What type of prosthesis is shown in the perioperative transesophageal echocardiogram (TEE) in **Figure 22-8**?

A. Trileaflet disk
B. Tilting disk
C. Disk and cage
D. Bileaflet disk
E. Ball and cage

✪✪ Question 17

A 42-year-old man with a prior history of a mitral valve replacement presents with fever and dyspnea. Blood cultures are positive for methicillin-sensitive *Staphylococcus aureus*. A transesophageal echocardiogram is performed. Based on the findings shown in the images in **Figure 22-9A, B** and **Video 22-3A, B**, which is the most likely basis for the patient's dyspnea?

A. Left ventricular (LV) systolic dysfunction
B. LV diastolic dysfunction
C. Multiple septic pulmonary emboli
D. Severe prosthetic mitral regurgitation (MR)
E. Severe prosthetic mitral stenosis

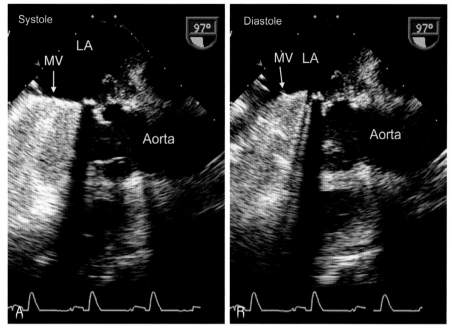

Figure 22-8 A. TEE, midesophageal long-axis view, systole. B. TEE, midesophageal long-axis view, diastole. (Reprinted with permission from Klein AL, Asher CR. *Clinical Echocardiography Review: A Self-Assessment Tool.* 2nd ed. Philadelphia, PA: Wolters Kluwer; 2017.)

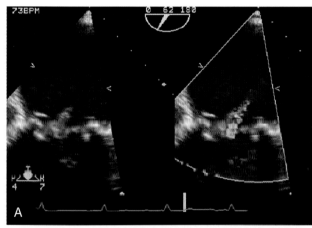

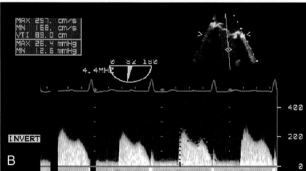

Figure 22-9 A, TEE, Midesophageal commissural view. B, TEE, Midesophageal commissural view, continuous-wave (CW) Doppler (inverted). (Reprinted with permission from Klein AL, Asher CR. *Clinical Echocardiography Review: A Self-Assessment Tool.* 2nd ed. Philadelphia, PA: Wolters Kluwer; 2017.)

✪ Question 18

A 46-year-old man undergoes a routine transthoracic echocardiogram to evaluate his mechanical aortic valve replacement (AVR). During the examination, there is too much shadowing to accurately measure the left ventricular outflow tract (LVOT) diameter. What is the best method for the aortic evaluation of the AVR function in this situation?

  A. Rely on AVR pressure gradients alone.
  B. Use the labeled prosthesis size as a substitute for the LVOT diameter.
  C. Use the LVOT diameter measurement from the previous echocardiogram.
  D. Consider the Doppler velocity index (DVI).

✪✪✪ Question 19

A 62-year-old woman with a bioprosthetic aortic valve replacement (AVR) presents with worsening dyspnea on exertion. A transthoracic echocardiogram revealed normal AVR hemodynamics. Which test should be performed next?

  A. Treadmill stress echocardiogram
  B. Dobutamine stress echocardiogram
  C. Cardiac catheterization
  D. Computed tomography (CT) scan
  E. Cinefluoroscopy of the valve

✪✪ Question 20

Which of the following is a complication of transcatheter aortic valve replacement (TAVR) that can be identified by transthoracic echocardiography (TTE)?

A. Aortic rupture or dissection
B. Pericardial effusion
C. Severe mitral regurgitation
D. Left ventricular dysfunction
E. All of the above

✪✪ Question 21

To accurately measure the left ventricular outflow tract (LVOT) stroke volume in a patient following the normal deployment of a balloon-expandable transcatheter aortic valve replacement (TAVR), the pulsed-wave (PW) Doppler sample volume is placed at which location in **Figure 22-10**?

A. 1
B. 2
C. 3
D. 4

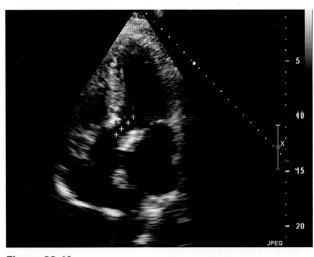

Figure 22-10

✪✪ Question 22

All of the following are examples of mechanical prosthetic heart valves, except the:

A. Starr-Edwards valve.
B. St. Jude valve.
C. Lillehei-Kaster valve.
D. Carpentier-Edwards valve.
E. Bjork-Shiley valve.

✪✪✪ Question 23

A 27-year-old-man with a mechanical aortic valve replacement (AVR) undergoes a routine transthoracic echocardiogram. The findings show a peak aortic velocity of 3.13 m/s, a Doppler velocity index (DVI) of 0.22, and an acceleration time (AT) of 120 ms. What is the most likely explanation for these findings?

A. Improper left ventricular outflow tract velocity measurement
B. Normal AVR function
C. AVR stenosis or obstruction
D. Underestimated AVR peak velocity

✪✪✪ Question 24

According to the appropriate use criteria for patients with prosthetic valves, what is the appropriate time frame for routine surveillance transthoracic echocardiography (TTE)?

A. ≥1 year
B. <1 year
C. ≥3 years
D. <3 years

✪✪✪ Question 25

In differentiating between pannus and thrombus formation, which of the following statements is false?

A. Prosthetic valve thrombosis is more common in mechanical than bioprosthetic valves.
B. Pannus is more common in bioprosthetic valves than in mechanical valves.
C. Differentiation between pannus and thrombus is important if thrombolytic therapy is a consideration.
D. Thrombi are larger and have an appearance or echo density similar to myocardium while pannus is smaller and more echo-dense.
E. Pannus formation typically occurs later after surgery compared with thrombosis.

✪ Question 26

What is the most common site of attachment for a vegetation on a prosthetic valve?

A. Valve stents
B. Bioprosthetic leaflets
C. Sewing ring of the valve
D. Mechanical occluder

Question 27

The following are spectral Doppler parameters suggestive of severe aortic prosthesis stenosis or obstruction, except:

A. A jet contour that is triangular and early peaking.
B. A Doppler velocity index of 0.24.
C. A mean pressure gradient of 36 mm Hg.
D. A peak velocity of 3.2 m/s.

Question 28

A 45-year-old woman presents 4 months following a mechanical mitral valve replacement (MVR) for rheumatic heart disease. She complains of worsening dyspnea and associated orthopnea for 1 week. She has an international normalized ratio (INR) of 1.30, a blood pressure of 100/90 mm Hg, and a heart rate of 95 bpm. Her echocardiogram demonstrates a significantly elevated mean pressure gradient across the MVR and a small echogenic mass that appears to be attached to the ventricular side of the MVR ring. Which is the most likely diagnosis?

A. Artifact
B. Pannus formation
C. Dehiscence of the sewing ring
D. Thrombus

Question 29

While evaluating a postoperative transcatheter aortic valve replacement (TAVR) patient, the echocardiographer identifies a paravalvular leak (PVL), which occupies 40% of the circumference of the valve in the parasternal short axis view with a pressure half-time (PHT) measurement of 190 ms. This best represents which of the following?

A. Trace PVL
B. Mild central PVL
C. Moderate PVL
D. Severe PVL

Question 30

In a patient with a transcatheter aortic valve replacement (TAVR), a smaller than expected effective orifice area (EOA) in relation to the patient's body surface area causing significantly elevated transvalvular pressure gradients is called:

A. Severe functional stenosis.
B. Underdeployed TAVR.

C. Bioprosthetic dysfunction.
D. Prosthesis-patient mismatch (PPM).

Question 31

Which of the following does not represent a limitation for evaluating mitral regurgitation (MR) in a mechanical mitral valve replacement (MVR) via transthoracic echocardiography (TTE)?

A. Different regurgitant flow patterns between all valve types
B. Differentiation between physiologic or "normal" washing MR jets and pathologic MR
C. Reverberation/shadowing from the prosthetic material, making the direct visualization of MR impossible
D. Complete visualization of the left atrium is obscured by artifacts from the prosthetic valve

Question 32

A 59-year-old woman undergoes a routine follow up transthoracic echocardiogram to evaluate her mechanical mitral valve replacement (MVR). She is found to have a peak MVR E velocity of 2.5 m/s, an MVR velocity-time integral (VTI) of 46 cm, a mean pressure gradient of 8 mm Hg, and a left ventricular outflow tract VTI of 17 cm. What is the mitral valve Doppler velocity index (DVI) and is it normal?

A. 0.15, abnormal
B. 0.17, normal
C. 2.40, normal
D. 2.70, abnormal

Question 33

A 56-year-old man with a 3-year-old mechanical mitral valve replacement (MVR) for rheumatic mitral stenosis was admitted for worsening shortness of breath and dyspnea on exertion 2 to 3 days prior to admission. On admission, the international normalized ratio was 1 and blood cultures were negative. The patient has a history of medication noncompliance. What is demonstrated in **Video 22-4**?

A. Pannus formation
B. Thrombus
C. Vegetation
D. Both A and B

Question 34

The insertion of an undersized transcatheter aortic valve replacement (TAVR) may result in which of the following complications?

A. Device migration
B. Aortic root conformation
C. Significant mitral regurgitation
D. Significant paravalvular aortic regurgitation
E. Both A and D

Question 35

The prosthetic valve in the mitral position as seen in **Video 22-5** is what type?

A. Mechanical mitral valve prosthesis
B. Bioprosthetic mitral valve
C. Transcatheter valve-in-valve
D. None of the above

Question 36

The image shown in **Video 22-6** is consistent with which of the following?

A. Posteriorly directed paravalvular leak in a transcatheter aortic valve replacement (TAVR)
B. Central paravalvular leak in a TAVR
C. Normal color Doppler in a mechanical aortic valve replacement
D. Paravalvular leak caused by an underdeployed TAVR

Question 37

The bileaflet mechanical valve in **Video 22-7** shows "washing jets." Which of the following statements is false regarding these jets?

A. These are built-in jets designed to prevent blood stasis and thrombus.
B. These jets tend to be of low velocity and are nonturbulent.
C. These jets are commonly seen in all types of prosthetic valves.
D. These jets are also referred to as leakage volumes.

Question 38

Which of the examples listed below are limitations in the assessment of infective endocarditis in prosthetic valves?

A. Distinguishing small vegetations from prosthetic material or suture structure
B. Reflectance of the prosthetic material
C. Vegetations can be similar in appearance to pannus or loose suture material
D. All of the above

Question 39

Other than true prosthetic valve stenosis or prosthetic valve obstruction, which of the following could result in increased pressure gradients across a prosthetic valve?

A. Prosthesis-patient mismatch (PPM)
B. Significant regurgitation
C. Increased heart rate
D. All of the above
E. Both A and C only

Question 40

A 68-year-old woman with a porcine aortic valve replacement (AVR) that was replaced 3 years prior presents with worsening dyspnea on exertion. A transthoracic echocardiogram is performed. Left ventricular (LV) function is normal and the mean bioprosthetic aortic valve gradient is found to be 16 mm Hg, which is a normal finding for this valve. A supine bicycle stress echocardiogram is ordered; the results show normal LV wall motion and an increase in the mean pressure gradient. Which mean pressure gradient at peak exercise would indicate a significant abnormal finding of prosthesis-patient mismatch (PPM) or obstruction?

A. 21 mm Hg
B. 26 mm Hg
C. 35 mm Hg
D. B and C
E. None of the above

ANSWERS

1. **Answer: D.** PPM occurs when the EOA of a normally functioning prosthetic valve is too small in relation to the patient's body size, leading to abnormally high transprosthetic pressure gradients compared with the normal range for the valve subtype and size. The parameter used to characterize PPM is the indexed EOA; that is, the EOA of the prosthesis divided by the patient's body surface area. For prostheses in the aortic position, the cutoff for PPM is defined as an indexed EOA ≤ 0.85 cm^2/m^2; this is

based on the observation that at smaller areas there is a rapid increase in transvalvular pressure gradients. An indexed EOA ≤0.65 cm²/m² is considered severe PPM. The major adverse outcomes associated with PPM are reduced short-term and long-term survival, particularly if associated with left ventricular dysfunction.

2. **Answer: C.** The best answer is C since there is significant variability in the normal values reported for AVRs, which are dependent upon the valve size and type.

   Answer A is incorrect since the diagnosis of PPM requires further information such as the effective orifice area (EOA) and the patient size. Answer B is incorrect as peak velocities less than 3 m/s are generally considered to be normal. In general, velocities >3.0 m/s prompt concern about pathological elevation due to a variety of causes, including PPM and intrinsic valve pathology (**Figure 22-11**). Note, however, that velocities >3.0 m/s may be normal for some AVRs. Answer E is incorrect since a peak velocity of 2.5 m/s may be within the normal range for many AVRs. Additionally, answer E is incorrect as the peak velocity does not provide direct information regarding the cardiac output; the cardiac output is derived from the stroke volume, which is derived from the left ventricular outflow tract cross-sectional area and velocity-time integral.

3. **Answer: E.** The pressure half-time may be used to estimate the mitral valve area (MVA) in native mitral stenosis (MS) using the equation: MVA = 220 ÷ PHT (where 220 is a constant). However, the PHT cannot be used to calculate the EOA in patients with an MVR. In these patients, the PHT method tends to grossly overestimate the EOA. However, while the PHT cannot be used to estimate the EOA, it still provides important information regarding the normality of MVR hemodynamics. For example, the PHT measurement may be used on serial studies to monitor for development of MVR stenosis or obstruction. Significant increases in PHT may be associated with MVR stenosis or obstruction.

KEY POINT

The PHT cannot be used to calculate the EOA in prosthetic mitral valves. The PHT, however, can be used to determine if the MVR is functioning normally or if there is evidence of MVR dysfunction.

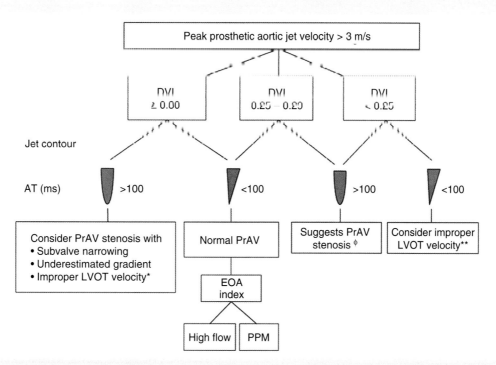

Figure 22-11 Algorithm for evaluation of elevated peak prosthetic aortic jet velocity. Algorithm for evaluation of elevated peak prosthetic aortic jet velocity incorporating Doppler velocity index (DVI), jet contour, and acceleration time (AT). *PW Doppler sample volume too close to the valve (particularly when jet velocity by CW Doppler is ≥4 m/s). **PW Doppler sample volume too far (apical) from the valve (particularly when jet velocity is 3-3.9 m/s). φ Stenosis further substantiated by effective orifice area (EOA) derivation compared with reference values if valve type and size are known. Fluoroscopy and TEE are helpful for further assessment, particularly in bileaflet valves. LVOT = left ventricular outflow tract; PPM = prosthesis-patient mismatch; PrAV = prosthetic aortic valve. (Reprinted from Zoghbi WA, Chambers JB, Dumesnil JG, et al. Recommendations for evaluation of prosthetic valves with echocardiography and Doppler ultrasound: a report from the American Society of Echocardiography's Guidelines and Standards Committee and the task force on prosthetic valves. *J Am Soc Echocardiogr.* 2009;22(9):975-1014. Copyright © 2009 American Society of Echocardiography. With permission.)

4. **Answer: C.** The DVI is defined as the ratio of LVOT VTI (or peak velocity) to the AVR VTI (or peak velocity):

$$DVI = V_{LVOT} \div V_{AV} \qquad (1)$$

$$DVI = VTI_{LVOT} \div VTI_{AV} \qquad (2)$$

where V_{AV} is the peak AVR velocity, VTI_{AV} is the AVR velocity-time integral, V_{LVOT} is the peak LVOT velocity, and VTI_{LVOT} is the LVOT velocity-time integral.

This ratio is particularly useful when image quality precludes accurate measurement of the LVOT diameter, as is needed to calculate EOA, and in the differentiation between prosthesis-patient mismatch (PPM) and AVR stenosis or obstruction (see **Figure 22-11**). A DVI <0.25 is suggestive of AVR stenosis or obstruction.

5. **Answer: A.** The MVR is identifiable as a stented bioprosthesis by the presence of clearly demarcated stents. There is an MR jet that clearly originates outside the sewing ring and extends back to the left atrium: this is paravalvular regurgitation. Although the image has not been optimized for proximal isovelocity surface area (PISA)-based quantitation, there is a significant PISA shell demarcated on the left ventricular side of the MVR. While spontaneous valve dehiscence may occur, hemodynamically significant new paravalvular jets raise the possibility of endocarditis as the cause.

6. **Answer: E.** As previously described, the DVI is defined as the ratio of LVOT velocity-time integral (VTI) or peak velocity to the AVR VTI or peak velocity. Using the VTI across the LVOT and AVR, the DVI is:

$$DVI = 10 \div 67 = 0.15$$

The DVI is easily calculated and may be used as an alternative to effective orifice area when the LVOT diameter is difficult to measure. Velocity measurements may also be used in place of VTI to calculate the DVI.

7. **Answer: E.** This appearance is typical for a Starr-Edwards ball and cage valve. Note that the ball appears larger than its actual size due to slower transmission of sound through the ball as opposed to tissue. With ball-cage valves, there is noncentral flow dynamics with lateral flow diverging around the ball occluder as seen in the color Doppler images (**Figure 22-3C** and **Video 22-1B**). Spontaneous microbubbles secondary to a degassing phenomenon are frequently seen as is evident in this case (see **Video 22-1A**).

8. **Answer: B.** These images demonstrate the double orifice that is typical of an Alfieri stitch mitral repair. **Figure 22-4C** is pathognomonic for this form of repair in which the A2 and P2 scallops are stitched together to create a double orifice valve that mimics congenitally double orifice mitral valve. Transcatheter mitral valve repair with the MitraClip is patterned on this type of repair.

9. **Answer: B.** Pressure gradients across mitral and tricuspid prostheses are heart rate dependent. Although a mean pressure gradient of 10 mm Hg at a heart rate of 60 beats per minute (bpm) would be abnormal, the same pressure gradient at a heart rate of 120 bpm would be "normal" for most mitral prostheses. While height and weight (answer C and E) and the calculated body surface area are important in evaluating patients for prosthesis-patient mismatch (indexed effective orifice area [EOA] <1.2 cm^2/m^2 for mitral prostheses), this assessment requires the calculation of EOA, which is not possible with mean pressure gradient only. It is important to record blood pressure (answer A) at the time of echocardiography for patients with mitral disease; however, its major impact is on regurgitation rather than stenosis. Sex (answer D) has no direct impact on valve pressure gradients.

10. **Answer: D.** With harmonic imaging, microbubbles are frequently seen with normally functioning mechanical valves. These microbubbles appear as very small, echogenic bubbles downstream from the valve that last for several seconds; this appearance is especially prominent with harmonic imaging and is thought to occur due to carbon dioxide degassing.

In the absence of intravenously injected micro bubbles, a patent foramen ovale (answer A) and associated right-to-left shunt will not result in left-sided microbubbles. These microbubbles are not imaging artifacts (answer C). In the era of fundamental imaging, microbubbles were reported as markers of hemolysis (answer B), which may be a feature of paravalvular regurgitation (answer E).

11. **Answer: A.** Due to acoustic shadowing and the eccentricity of paravalvular jets, TTE is relatively insensitive for detection of paravalvular regurgitation. Thus, TEE is indicated whenever paravalvular regurgitation is suspected. Elevated mitral pressure gradients (answers B and C) favor MR. Normal (S-dominant) flow (answer D) may be preserved in pulmonary veins remote from the jet when jets are eccentric. All apical views, including the apical long-axis view (answer E), should be used to assess for paravalvular regurgitation, but no single view is ideal.

12. **Answer: C.** The Ross procedure consists of moving the patient's pulmonary valve to the aortic position (aortic autograft) and placing an allograft (cadaveric) valve in the pulmonic position (pulmo-

nary allograft). Of the possible correct answers, aortic autograft regurgitation or aortic regurgitation is the most common due to progressive dilatation of the autograft root.

13. **Answer: E.** Although there are no large series of published normal values for TVR pressure gradients, the existing literature supports the diagnosis of prosthetic tricuspid stenosis whenever the mean pressure gradient exceeds 6 mm Hg. The mean pressure gradient of 11 mm Hg at a slow heart rate is consistent with severe prosthetic stenosis. Note that the pressure half-time method has not been validated for prosthetic tricuspid valves and should not be used as a means of determining the effective orifice area.

Answer A is unlikely with a heart rate of 55 bpm and even a significantly elevated stroke volume would typically not be associated with pressure gradient elevation of this degree at a slow heart rate. Answer B is incorrect since rapid pressure recovery does not occur with large bioprosthetic valves in the tricuspid position.

14. **Answer: D.** This is the typical three-dimensional (3D) view of a bileaflet mechanical mitral prosthesis as seen from the atrial perspective. Two orifices are identified in this diastolic frame with the occluders in the open position. For 3D images of other prostheses, readers are referred to the articles by Tsang et al. and Sugeng et al. as cited in the Suggested Readings section.

15. **Answer: E.** Aortic allografts are treated cadaveric aortic roots and valves, as well as portions of the tubular segment of the ascending aorta into which the native coronary arteries are reimplanted. The native aorta may be used to wrap the allograft aorta (the inclusion technique) or be resected. Particularly when the inclusion technique is used, the aortic root normally appears postoperatively as variably thickened, perhaps due in part to a hematoma. Over time, this resorbs, and the appearance of the valve resembles that of the native aortic valve. In a clinical scenario suggestive of endocarditis, it may be impossible to differentiate a normal allograft from an abscess. Comparison with the postimplantation perioperative TEE can be very helpful in resolving this dilemma. In the absence of clinical features of infection, the appearance shown here can be interpreted as normal.

16. **Answer: B.** This is a typical appearance for a tilting disk mechanical mitral prosthesis. The disk pivots from an eccentric pivot point and closure is associated with a prominent central jet. This valve should not be confused with bileaflet or ball and cage valves (**Figure 22-12**). There are no trileaflet mechanical valves.

17. **Answer: E.** At a heart rate of 73 bpm, a mean pressure gradient of 12.6 mm Hg is severely elevated and consistent with severe prosthetic mitral valve stenosis attributable to obstruction of the prosthesis by vegetations (**Table 22-1**).

Answer A is incorrect as no images of the left ventricle are provided; therefore, it is not possible to attribute the patient's dyspnea to LV systolic dysfunction. Answer B is incorrect as in the presence of an abnormal mitral prosthesis, it is impossible to assess LV diastolic function on the basis of an isolated mitral inflow spectrum. Answer C is incorrect as septic pulmonary emboli are not a complication in the absence of concomitant right-sided endocarditis. Answer D is incorrect since the color flow Doppler shows only trace MR.

18. **Answer: D.** The DVI is a useful flow-independent parameter that does not require the measurement of the LVOT diameter. This measurement can be used in the serial evaluation of an AVR.

Answer A is incorrect since pressure gradients are flow-dependent and therefore these pressure gradients may vary from study to study depending on the volumetric flow and heart rate. Answer B is incorrect as there is significant variation in the way prosthetic valve sizes are labeled and measured, so the AVR size should not be used as a substitute for a direct LVOT diameter measurement. Assuming a previous LVOT diameter measurement (answer C) is not recommended unless the accuracy of this measurement can be confirmed.

KEY POINT
The DVI is a useful flow-independent parameter that does not require the measurement of the LVOT diameter. In an individual patient, a baseline DVI value obtained in the early postoperative period can serve as the control value or "valve fingerprint" for future examinations. Provided prosthetic valve function remains normal, the DVI will remain constant even with changes in stroke volume.

19. **Answer: B.** At rest, the AVR hemodynamics are normal. As the patient reports worsening dyspnea on exertion, the next test would be a stress echocardiogram. Dobutamine and supine bicycle exercise are most commonly used as both of these tests enable the acquisition of AVR hemodynamics during stress and while the heart rate remains high. Therefore, answer B is correct.

Treadmill stress echocardiography (answer A) provides additional information about exercise capacity but is less frequently used because the AVR hemodynamics are taken in the recovery period and the hemodynamics may have rapidly returned to baseline. Cardiac catheterization (answer C) to assess prosthetic valves can provide additional correlative data but is not commonly performed. CT scans (answer D) and cinefluoroscopy (answer E) are valuable in the assessment of mechanical

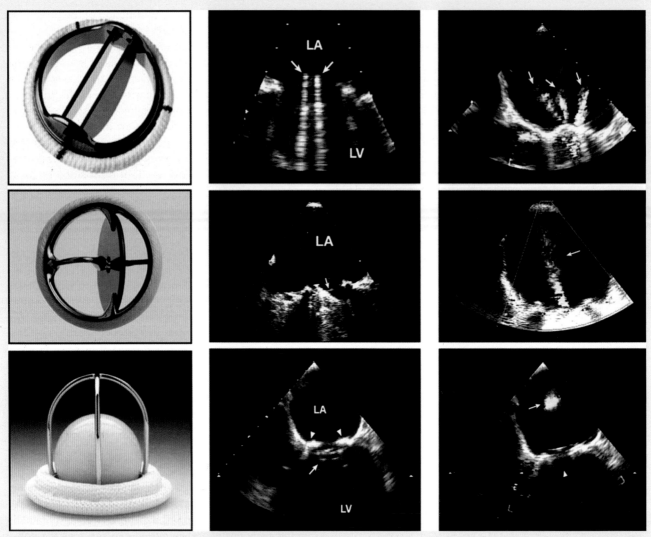

Figure 22-12 Mechanical valves. Examples of bileaflet, single-leaflet, and ball-cage mechanical valves and their transesophageal echocardiographic characteristics taken in the mitral position in diastole (middle) and in systole (right). The arrows in diastole point to the occluder mechanism of the valve and in systole to the characteristic physiologic regurgitation observed with each valve. (Reprinted with permission from Klein AL, Asher CR. *Clinical Echocardiography Review: A Self-Assessment Tool.* 2nd ed. Philadelphia, PA: Wolters Kluwer; 2017; and Modified from Zoghbi WA, Chambers JB, Dumesnil JG, et al. Recommendations for evaluation of prosthetic valves with echocardiography and Doppler ultrasound: a report from the American Society of Echocardiography's Guidelines and Standards Committee and the Task Force on Prosthetic Valves. *J Am Soc Echocardiogr.* 2009;22(9):975-1014; quiz 1082-1084. Copyright © 2009 The American Society of Echocardiography. With permission.)

prosthetic valves to assess disk motion and opening/closing angles when AVR pressure gradients are abnormally high. CT may also allow imaging of the cusps of bioprosthetic valves to identify leaflet thickening, calcification, or thrombus.

20. **Answer: E.** All of the complications listed may occur following TAVR and can be identified by TTE. Aortic dissection and/or rupture can occur during or after deployment of the valve. Pericardial effusion may result from chamber perforation or aortic dissection during deployment. Mitral regurgitation can result from perforation, ruptured chordae, or tethering of the leaflets. If coronary ostia are compromised by the valve placement, left ventricular regional wall motion abnormalities are visualized.

21. **Answer: B.** For TAVR, LVOT measurements should be performed immediately proximal to the stent (prestent region) rather than at the base of the pros-

thetic valve leaflets (in-stent precusp region). Therefore, the LVOT PW Doppler sample volume should be placed apical to the proximal edge of the stent (prestent region) due to the flow acceleration that occurs once inside the stent cage (in-stent precusp region).

22. **Answer: D.** The Carpentier-Edwards valve is an example of a porcine or bovine xenograft. These stented valves may be an entire valve from a single pig or a composite from two or three individual pigs with the leaflet mounted on a flexible frame. Xenograft means from one species to another.

The Starr-Edwards valve (answer A) is an example of a ball-cage valve that consists of a silastic ball (poppet) housed within a stellite alloy cage composed of three or four U-shaped, monocast struts joining at the apex.

The St. Jude valve (answer B) is an example of a bileaflet tilting disk. These valves consist of two

Table 22-1. Doppler Parameters of Prosthetic Mitral Valve Function

	Normal[a]	Possible Stenosis[b]	Suggests Significant Stenosis[a,b]
Peak velocity (m/s)[c,d]	<1.9	1.9-2.5	≥2.5
Mean pressure gradient (mm Hg)[c,d]	≤5	6-10	>10
VTI_{MVR}/VTI_{LVOT}[c,d]	<2.2	2.2-2.5	>2.5
EOA (cm²)	≥2.0	1-2	<1
PHT (ms)	<130	130-200	>200

EOA, effective orifice area; MVR, mitral valve replacement; PHT, pressure half-time; VTI_{LVOT}, velocity-time integral of LVOT; VTI_{MVR}, velocity-time integral of the MVR.

[a]Best specificity for normality or abnormality is seen if the majority of the parameters listed are normal or abnormal, respectively.
[b]Values of the parameters should prompt a closer evaluation of valve function and/or other considerations such as increased flow, increased heart rate, or prosthesis-patient mismatch.
[c]Slightly higher cutoff values than shown may be seen in some bioprosthetic valves.
[d]These parameters are also abnormal in the presence of significant prosthetic MR.

Modified from Zoghbi WA, Chambers JB, Dumesnil JG, et al. Recommendations for evaluation of prosthetic valves with echocardiography and Doppler ultrasound: a report from the American Society of Echocardiography's Guidelines and Standards Committee and the task force on prosthetic valves. *J Am Soc Echocardiogr.* 2009;22(9):975-1014. Copyright © 2009 American Society of Echocardiography. With permission.

equal-sized semicircular disks attached to a central hinge. The open valve consists of three orifices: one small, slit-like central orifice between open disks and two larger semicircular lateral orifices. There are several types of bileaflet tilting disk valves with the design differing in the composition and purity of pyrolytic carbon, the shape and opening angle of the leaflets, the design of the pivots, the size and shape of the housing, and the design of the sewing ring.

The Lillehei-Kaster (answer C) and the Bjork-Shiley valve (answer E) are examples of single tilting disk valves. These valves consist of a single hinged circular disk within a rigid annulus. The open valve consists of two distinct orifices of different sizes. There are several types of single tilting disk valves with the designs differing based on the opening angles.

23. Answer: C. When evaluating an AVR, one must rely on several factors when determining if the valve is functioning normally or if there is a pathological process. Some normally functioning mechanical AVRs have velocities of close to or over 3 m/s, which is higher than a native valve, but that does not necessarily indicate stenosis. Therefore, the peak velocity should be examined in conjunction with DVI (normal being ≥0.30) and the AT (normal being <80 ms). A peak velocity >3 m/s, a DVI <0.25, and an AT >100 ms are suggestive of AVR stenosis or obstruction (Table 22-2 and see Figure 22-11, answer outline for Question 2). Therefore, with the patient in question these three metrics indicate probable AVR stenosis or obstruction.

Table 22-2. Doppler Parameters of Prosthetic Aortic Valve Function[a]

	Normal	Possible Stenosis	Suggests Significant Stenosis
Peak velocity (m/s)[b]	<3	3-4	>4
Mean pressure gradient (mm Hg)[b]	<20	20-35	>35
DVI	≥30	0.29-0.25	<0.25
EOA (cm²)	>1.2	1.2-0.8	<0.8
Contour of AVR jet[c]	Triangular, early peaking	Triangular to intermediate	Rounded, symmetrical
Acceleration time (ms)[c]	<80	80-100	>100

AVR, aortic valve replacement; DVI, Doppler velocity index; EOA, effective orifice area.

[a]In conditions of normal or near-normal stroke volume (50-70 mL) through the aortic valve.
[b]These parameters are more affected by flow, including low cardiac output and concomitant prosthetic valve regurgitation.
[c]These parameters are highly influenced by left ventricular chronotropy and function.

Modified from Zoghbi WA, Chambers JB, Dumesnil JG, et al. Recommendations for evaluation of prosthetic valves with echocardiography and Doppler ultrasound: a report from the American Society of Echocardiography's Guidelines and Standards Committee and the Task Force on Prosthetic Valves. *J Am Soc Echocardiogr.* 2009;22(9):975-1014, with permission from Elsevier.

24. **Answer: C.** With no new symptoms and no known or suspected valve dysfunction the recommended time frame for routine surveillance TTE is ≥3 years after valve implantation. TTE is also considered appropriate for the initial postoperative evaluation of prosthetic valves for establishment of baseline function, for the evaluation of prosthetic valves with suspected dysfunction or a change in clinical status and/or cardiac examination, and for the reevaluation of known prosthetic valve dysfunction when it would change management or guide therapy. TTE is considered rarely appropriate for the routine surveillance (<3 years after valve implantation) of a prosthetic valve if no known or suspected valve dysfunction exists.

25. **Answer: B.** Prosthetic valve thrombosis refers to the formation of a blood clot around the prosthetic valve while pannus refers to a slow ingrowth of fibrous tissue over the prosthetic valve sewing ring. While pannus formation has been observed in both mechanical and bioprosthetic valves, pannus is more commonly encountered with mechanical valves; therefore, answer B is the false statement.

    Answer A is a true statement. Prosthetic valve thrombosis may occur in both mechanical and bioprosthetic valves but is more commonly seen in mechanical valves where there is inadequate antithrombotic therapy. Answer C is a true statement as prosthetic valve thrombosis may be treatable with thrombolytic therapy while thrombolysis is ineffective in pannus. Answer D is a true statement as thrombi are larger and have an appearance or echo density similar to myocardium while pannus is smaller and has an echo-dense appearance. Answer E is a true statement. Pannus forms as part of the healing response whereby excessive scarring or keloid formation occurs; therefore, pannus formation occurs later following surgery. Thrombosis may occur at any time; however, if this occurs later, it is usually associated with pannus.

26. **Answer: C.** The sewing ring of the leaflets is the most common location for infective endocarditis on a prosthetic valve; vegetations may spread to the leaflet of the prosthetic valve, stent, or occluder and impair the opening and closing of the valve. Vegetations are usually irregularly shaped and can be recognized on echocardiography as independently mobile structures of relatively low echogenicity.

27. **Answer: A.** In a normally functioning aortic valve replacement (AVR), the jet contour is similar to that seen with mild native aortic valve stenosis with a triangular shape that peaks in early systole. With increasing stenosis or obstruction, there is a longer ejection duration and a more delayed peaking of the AVR velocity. When there is severe stenosis or obstruction, the jet contour becomes rounded with a symmetrical contour that peaks in mid-systole. Therefore, the acceleration time as well as the ejection time is prolonged. This occurs because it takes more time for the left ventricle to eject blood flow through a stenotic valve, causing a delay in valve closure compared to a normal prosthetic valve. Refer to **Figure 22-11** in the answer outline for Question 2 and **Table 22-2** in the answer outline for Question 23.

28. **Answer: D.** A few key elements identified thrombus versus all other answers, including a postoperative period of less than 6 months, subtherapeutic INR (≤2.5), and acuteness of symptoms. Pannus formation (answer A) usually occurs at least 6 months or more after surgery and without acute symptoms. Dehiscence of the sewing ring (answer C) would not cause an increased MVR mean pressure gradient. Artifact (answer D) is common in mechanical valves, but this cannot account for the increased pressure gradients.

TEACHING POINT

The international normalized ratio (INR) is a measure of how long it takes blood to form a clot. For normal patients who are not on anticoagulation, the INR is usually 1.0. For patients with mitral prosthetic valves and on anticoagulant therapy, a target INR of 3.0 (range 2.5-3.5) is recommended. For mechanical aortic valves, a target INR of 2.5 (range 2.0-3.0) is recommended.

29. **Answer: D.** The circumferential extent of the regurgitant jet in relation to the total circumference of the prosthetic valve ring is a useful parameter for assessing the severity of paravalvular regurgitation following a TAVR. A continuous circumferential extent of aortic regurgitation (AR) greater than 30% is indicative of severe AR. Since the number of jets also reflects severity, an extensive search for all jets should be performed from all imaging windows, including off-axis imaging planes. When there are multiple jets, these are summed and then divided by the total circumference of the prosthetic valve ring. A PHT of less than 200 ms is also consistent with severe regurgitation, including paravalvular leak (PVL). However, it should be remembered that the AR PHT is influenced by left ventricular compliance and other factors.

KEY POINT

The circumferential extent of paravalvular regurgitation (PVR) in a TAVR is used to determine the severity. When there are multiple jets, the circumferential extent is measured as the sum of the circumferential lengths of each regurgitant jet vena contracta (not including the nonregurgitant space between the separate jets) divided by the circumference of the outer edge of the valve. Mild PVR is <10%, moderate PVR is 10% to 29%, and severe PVR is ≥30%. It is important to note that the circumferential extent of PVR should not be used alone, but in combination with other qualitative and quantitative Doppler parameters.

30. **Answer: D.** PPM was first described in 1978 as a problem associated with valve replacement where inappropriate valve sizing could cause obstruction to the inflow and/or outflow. Severe functional stenosis (answer A) may be a result of PPM. An under-deployed TAVR (answer B) will result in paravalvular leak, not stenosis. Bioprosthetic dysfunction (answer C) is a general term used to describe any number of problems related to a dysfunctional prosthetic valve, such as leaflet tearing, degradation, thrombosis/pannus formation, PPM, prosthetic valve stenosis or obstruction, prosthetic valve regurgitation, prosthetic valve dehiscence, and prosthetic valve endocarditis.

31. **Answer: B.** Washing jets and pathologic MR are somewhat easy to differentiate due to the location, timing, and direction. Each mechanical valve has distinguishing washing jets located between the sewing ring or disk. During the closing phase, there is a period of regurgitant flow caused by a small gap, which in some cases is meant to "clean" the valve from thrombi. Answers C and D are limitations for assessing MR in a mechanical MVR via TTE as visualization of regurgitation into the left atrium is virtually impossible due to shadowing/reverberation artifacts which also preclude the accurate calculation of left atrial volumes. Answer A is a limitation for assessing MR in a mechanical MVR since regurgitant flow patterns can differ greatly between different types of prosthetic valves, especially mechanical valves in the mitral position, making it difficult to accurately assess the extent of mitral regurgitation.

32. **Answer: D.** The equation for the DVI in an MVR is:

$$DVI = VTI_{MVR} \div VTI_{LVOT} \qquad (1)$$

where VTI_{LVOT} is the LVOT velocity-time integral and VTI_{MVR} is the MVR velocity-time integral.

Note that this index is the opposite of the DVI for prosthetic aortic valves where the LVOT VTI is divided by the VTI of the AVR.

In this case, the mitral DVI is calculated as:

$$DVI = 46 \div 17 = 2.7 \qquad (2)$$

A ratio of <2.2 is considered normal for prosthetic valves. A mitral DVI >2.2 plus elevated pressure gradients is indicative of MVR dysfunction, either regurgitation or obstruction. If the pressure half-time (PHT) is prolonged (>130 ms), this suggests obstruction; if the PHT is <130 ms, this suggests hemodynamically significant regurgitation.

33. **Answer: B.** Just from this image, thrombus is the most obvious answer due to a patient history of medication noncompliance and a subtherapeutic international normalized ratio (≤2.5) with a mechanical MVR. Negative blood cultures exclude vegetations. It is possible that this patient also has pannus, but this cannot be specifically ascertained from this video.

34. **Answer: E.** Inappropriate fitting of an undersized TAVR may leave a circumferential orifice between the valve and aortic root, causing significant paravalvular aortic leak or complete dislodging of the valve resulting in device migration. Answer B is incorrect; the aortic root will not shrink in size to conform to a valve. Answer D is incorrect, as significant mitral regurgitation is not a direct result of undersizing.

35. **Answer: B. Video 22-5** shows a bioprosthetic valve that is identified by the large struts and hypoechoic middle space. A mechanical valve (answer A) would create imaging artifacts, which would be seen moving with the opening and closing of the valve. A transcatheter valve-in-valve (answer C) would have a somewhat similar appearance as a bioprosthetic valve but with lower-profile struts.

36. **Answer: A.** The valve appearance is typical of a CoreValve (a self-expandable stent within a nitinol frame). The color Doppler jet is crossing the valve in a posterior fashion. Answer B is incorrect as centrally located regurgitation cannot be paravalvular; however, a central jet that is eccentric may give the appearance of a paravalvular leak. Answer C is incorrect as a mechanical valve will demonstrate significant reverberation and shadowing artifacts through the left atrium. Answer D is incorrect since there does not appear to be a gap between the TAVR and the aortic root.

37. **Answer: C.** While physiological regurgitation is detected in all types of prosthetic valves, washing jets are unique to mechanical valves. These "built-in" washing jets are described by their evenly distributed and directional trace of regurgitant flow, which aids in preventing blood stasis and thrombus formation due to the consistent active movement of blood in and out of the valve. As these are generated by the closing velocity of the leaflet and not the pressure gradient across the valve, these jets tend to be of low velocity and are nonturbulent. Washing jets are also referred to as normal leakage volumes; these jets appear at the hinge points of the occluder.

38. **Answer: D.** Each of these examples are limitations in imaging and identifying infective endocarditis in a prosthetic valve. Differentiation between vegetations and other echogenic masses, such as pannus, thrombus, sutures, torn cusps, or residual chordal tissue, is very difficult. However, consideration of the clinical presentation as well as comparison of the current study with the baseline study is very useful in determining the nature of these masses.

39. **Answer: D.** Elevated pressure gradients across prosthetic valves are not only caused by prosthetic valve stenosis or obstruction. Elevated gradients

may also occur secondary to PPM (as previously discussed), high flow conditions (high output states including increased heart rates), prosthetic valve regurgitation, or rapid pressure recovery (RPR). RPR is a complex phenomenon particular to small-sized bileaflet mechanical valves whereby the velocity at the smaller central orifice is higher than the velocities at the larger lateral orifices.

40. **Answer: C.** Stress echocardiography may be useful to identify PPM or pathologic obstruction when the resting hemodynamics of the AVR are normal. While there is no established cutoff for an AVR, an increase pointing toward significant obstruction would be similar to those of native valves. Therefore, an increase in the mean pressure gradient of 15 mm Hg or greater would be considered significant.

Acknowledgments: The authors thank and acknowledge Allan Klein, MD, and Craig Asher, MD, along with the contributions from Linda D. Gillam, MD, MPH, Konstantinos P. Koulogiannis, MD, and Leo Marcoff, MD (Chapter 19 Prosthetic Valves) in *Clinical Echocardiography Review: A Self-Assessment Tool*, 2nd Edition, edited by Allan L. Klein, Craig R. Asher, 2017.

SUGGESTED READINGS

Anderson B. Chapter 10 prosthetic valves. In: *A Sonographer's Guide to the Assessment of Heart Disease.* Brisbane, Australia: MGA Graphics; 2014.

Douglas PS, Garcia MJ, Haines DE, et al. ACCF/ASE/AHA/ASNC/HFSA/HRS/SCAI/SCCM/SCCT/SCMR 2011 Appropriate use criteria for echocardiography. A report of the American College of Cardiology Foundation appropriate use criteria task force, American Society of Echocardiography, American Heart Association, American Society of Nuclear Cardiology, Heart Failure Society of America, Heart Rhythm Society, Society for Cardiovascular angiography and Interventions, Society of Critical Care Medicine, Society of Cardiovascular Computed Tomography, Society for Cardiovascular Magnetic Resonance American College of Chest Physicians. *J Am Soc Echocardiogr.* 2011;24(3):229-267.

Hillier SD, Burstow DJ. Mitral prosthetic valves. In: Lang RM, Goldstein SA, Kronzon I, Khandheria BK, Mor-Avi V, eds. *ASE's Comprehensive Echocardiography.* 2nd ed. Philadelphia, PA: Elsevier Saunders; 2016:chap 129.

Lancellotti P, Pibarot P, Chambers J, et al. Recommendations for the imaging assessment of prosthetic heart valves: a report from the European Association of Cardiovascular Imaging endorsed by the Chinese Society of Echocardiography, the Inter-American Society of Echocardiography, and the Brazilian Department of Cardiovascular Imaging. *Eur Heart J Cardiovasc Imaging.* 2016;17(6): 589-590.

Roper D, Burstow DJ. Chapter 128: aortic prosthetic valves. In: Lang RM, Goldstein SA, Kronzon I, Khandheria BK, Mor-Avi V, eds. *ASE's Comprehensive Echocardiography.* 2nd ed. Philadelphia, PA: Elsevier Saunders; 2016.

Sugeng L, Shernan SK, Weinert L, et al. Real-time three-dimensional transesophageal echocardiography in valve disease: comparison with surgical findings and evaluation of prosthetic valves. *J Am Soc Echocardiogr.* 2008;21:1347-1354.

Tsang W, Weinert L, Kronzon I, Lang RM. Three-dimensional echocardiography in the assessment of prosthetic valves. *Rev Esp Cardiol.* 2011;64(1):1-7.

Zoghbi WA, Chambers JB, Dumesnil JG, et al. Recommendations for evaluation of prosthetic valves with echocardiography and Doppler ultrasound: a report from the American Society of Echocardiography's Guidelines and Standards Committee and the task force on prosthetic valves. *J Am Soc Echocardiogr.* 2009;22(9):975-1014; quiz 1082-1084.

Zoghbi WA, Asch FM, Bruce C, et al. Guidelines for the evaluation of valvular regurgitation after percutaneous valve repair or replacement: a report from the American Society of Echocardiography developed in collaboration with the Society for Cardiovascular Angiography and Interventions, Japanese Society of Echocardiography, and Society for Cardiovascular Magnetic Resonance. *J Am Soc Echocardiogr.* 2019;32(4):431-475.

CHAPTER 23

Infective Endocarditis

Contributors: Bonnie J. Kane, BS, RDCS and Kate A. Marriott, BSc App (HMS), M Cardiac Ultrasound

⊕ Question 1

Echocardiography plays a central role in evaluating patients with a clinical suspicion of infective endocarditis (IE). In patients with native valve endocarditis, which is the smallest left-sided vegetation that can be detected by two-dimensional (2D) transthoracic echocardiography (TTE)?

A. 1 mm
B. 3 mm
C. 5 mm
D. 7 mm
E. 9 mm

⊕⊕ Question 2

Which of the following is associated with a higher risk for an embolic event in a patient with infective endocarditis?

A. Sessile vegetation
B. *Staphylococcus* species
C. Vegetation 8 mm in size
D. Positive response to antibiotic therapy (<4 days)

⊕ Question 3

Which of the following best describes the 2D echocardiographic appearance of a typical vegetation during the acute phase of infective endocarditis (IE)?

A. A discrete echolucent mass adherent to native valves or intracardiac prosthetic devices with high-frequency motion independent of the underlying cardiac structure. The mass cannot be imaged in multiple views throughout the cardiac cycle.

B. A discrete echogenic dense mass adherent to native valves or intracardiac prosthetic devices with high-frequency motion independent of the underlying cardiac structure. The mass cannot be imaged in multiple views throughout the cardiac cycle.

C. A discrete echogenic calcified mass adherent to native valves or intracardiac prosthetic devices with high-frequency motion independent of the underlying cardiac structure. The mass can be imaged in multiple views throughout the cardiac cycle.

D. A discrete echogenic mass adherent to native valves or intracardiac prosthetic devices with high-frequency motion independent of the underlying cardiac structure. The mass can be imaged in multiple views throughout the cardiac cycle.

⊕ Question 4

According to the modified Duke criteria, which of the following is not a major clinical criterion for infective endocarditis (IE)?

A. New partial dehiscence of prosthetic valve
B. New valvular regurgitation
C. Predisposing heart condition or history of intravenous (IV) drug use
D. Two positive blood cultures for infective endocarditis

✪ Question 5

Peripheral clinical signs are considered minor criteria in the Duke criteria for diagnosis of infective endocarditis. Which of these conditions presents as a retinal hemorrhage as opposed to a cutaneous lesion?

A. Janeway lesions
B. Osler nodes
C. Petechiae
D. Roth spots
E. Splinter hemorrhages

✪✪ Question 6

A patient with a membranous ventricular septal defect (VSD) presents with a high likelihood of infective endocarditis. Where would a vegetation arising from the jet lesion most likely be located?

A. Anterior leaflet of the mitral valve
B. Aortic valve
C. Left ventricular outflow tract
D. Pulmonic valve
E. Septal leaflet of the tricuspid valve

✪✪✪ Question 7

▶ A 25-year-old man who is an intravenous (IV) drug abuser presents with fever and shortness of breath. Two sets of blood cultures are growing gram-positive cocci in clusters. A transthoracic echocardiogram is performed and shows a vegetation of 2.5 cm × 3.5 cm on the tricuspid valve (**Figure 23-1** and **Video 23-1**). Which leaflet of the tricuspid valve is the vegetation attached to?

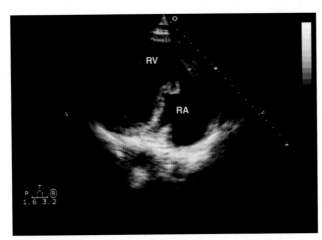

Figure 23-1 RA, right atrium; RV, right ventricle.

A. Anterior leaflet
B. Septal leaflet
C. Posterior leaflet
D. A or B
E. B or C

✪ Question 8

What is the most frequent location of an abscess in patients presenting with infective endocarditis (IE)?

A. Aortic root
B. Mitral valve annulus
C. Myocardium
D. Pericardial space
E. Tricuspid valve annulus

✪✪ Question 9

Which of the following is most likely to be confused with a mitral annular abscess on TTE?

A. A dilated coronary sinus
B. Caseous calcification of the mitral annulus
C. Epicardial fat
D. The descending thoracic aorta

✪✪ Question 10

Which of the following statements about nonbacterial thrombotic endocarditis (NBTE) is incorrect?

A. NBTE can be described as Libman-Sacks endocarditis or verrucous or marantic vegetations.
B. NBTE is often associated with conditions such as malignancies and autoimmune disorders such as systemic lupus erythematosus (SLE).
C. NBTE usually appears as a heterogeneous echo density with high reflectance in central regions consistent with connective tissue or calcific changes.
D. There is often gross and microscopic evidence of leaflet destruction in NBTE.

✪✪ Question 11

Which condition is most likely to be confused with a mitral valve aneurysm?

A. Mitral valve prolapse
B. Mitral valve blood cyst
C. Mitral valve flail segment
D. Mitral valve repair with Alfieri stitch

⊛ Question 12

A pulsatile, perivalvular echo-free space, in which flow is detected via color Doppler imaging, best describes which of the following echocardiographic findings of infective endocarditis?

A. Abscess
B. Fistula
C. Perforation
D. Pseudoaneurysm

⊛ Question 13

In a patient with infective endocarditis of a native mitral valve, the most typical location for a vegetation would be:

A. On the atrial side of the leaflet near the coaptation point.
B. On the atrial side of the leaflet near the medial annulus.
C. On the ventricular side of the leaflet near the coaptation point.
D. On the ventricular side of the leaflet near the medial annulus.

⊛⊛ Question 14

Abscess formation adjacent to which aortic cusps (leaflets) is most commonly associated with heart block rhythm disturbances?

A. Left and right coronary cusps
B. Noncoronary and right coronary cusps
C. Noncoronary, right, and left coronary cusps
D. Noncoronary and left coronary cusps

⊛⊛⊛ Question 15

Patients who are at high risk of endocarditis are expected to have prophylactic antibiotics prior to having dental procedures that disrupt the gingiva. Which of these microorganisms is most likely to cause endocarditis from oral bacteria?

A. Enterococcus
B. Fungi
C. *Staphylococcus aureus*
D. *Streptococcus viridans*

⊛⊛ Question 16

Considering the current guidelines for antibiotic prophylaxis, should a patient with an indwelling catheter have antibiotics prior to having a dental procedure?

A. Yes, for all dental procedures
B. Yes, but only if the dental procedure is deemed high-risk
C. No, does not meet current guidelines
D. No, there is no risk of infective endocarditis (IE) to this patient

CASE 1

▶ A 28-year-old man with a history of congenital kidney disease and a kidney transplant with subsequent graft failure and removal presents for an echocardiogram. He is currently on hemodialysis and has developed a fever. Blood was drawn for blood culture. **Video 23-2** is a low parasternal short-axis view showing a hemodialysis catheter in the right atrium (RA).

⊛⊛ Question 17

Upon review of **Video 23-2** and taking the patient's clinical history into account, the most likely location of vegetations is:

A. On the right atrial wall.
B. On the tricuspid valve (TV).
C. On the hemodialysis catheter.
D. B and C.
E. Any of the above.

CASE 2

▶ A 65-year-old woman presents with progressive shortness of breath. Four weeks ago, she was diagnosed with endocarditis and is being treated with antibiotics. **Videos 23-3A** and **23-3B** represent transthoracic echocardiography (TTE) parasternal long-axis views of the mitral valve and the same view with color Doppler imaging, respectively. **Video 23-3C** illustrates a TTE parasternal short-axis view of the mitral valve with color Doppler imaging.

⊛ Question 18

Which of the following statements is true about the mitral valve?

A. A vegetation is present on the mitral valve with associated mitral regurgitation (MR).
B. There is an anterior mitral leaflet perforation associated with MR.
C. There is mitral valve prolapse with MR.
D. There is a cleft of the anterior mitral leaflet with MR.

✪✪ Question 19

Where is the origin of the mitral regurgitant (MR) jet?
- **A.** The MR jet is located at A1.
- **B.** The MR jet is located at A2.
- **C.** The MR jet is located at P1.
- **D.** The MR jet is located at the junction of P2 and P1.
- **E.** The MR jet is centrally located between A2 and P2.

CASE 3

▶ A 24-year-old man patient presents to the hospital with fever and malaise. Three months prior to this admission, the patient underwent a mitral valve repair with false chords and an annuloplasty ring. **Video 23-4** is a zoomed parasternal long-axis view acquired in this patient.

✪✪ Question 20

Based on the image provided, there is:
- **A.** A vegetation on the anterior mitral leaflet.
- **B.** A vegetation on the posterior mitral leaflet.
- **C.** A vegetation on the prosthetic ring.
- **D.** No vegetation present.
- **E.** A, B, and C.

CASE 4

▶ A 33-year-old man presents with increasing fatigue, night sweats, and dyspnea on exertion. The patient is diagnosed with pneumonia and treated with oral antibiotics. Two weeks later he presents with pulmonary edema, ischemic hepatitis, and renal failure. Loud systolic and diastolic murmurs are heard on cardiac auscultation. A transthoracic echocardiogram is performed and obvious vegetations on the aortic and tricuspid valves are visualized. **Videos 23-5A**, **23-5B**, and **23-5C** were acquired from a parasternal short-axis view and the apical window.

✪✪✪ Question 21

Other than the obvious vegetations noted, which additional echocardiographic finding is shown?
- **A.** An aorta to right atrium fistula
- **B.** An atrial septal defect (ASD) with right-to-left shunting
- **C.** A membranous ventricular septal defect (VSD)
- **D.** A ruptured sinus of Valsalva aneurysm
- **E.** Severe tricuspid regurgitation

✪✪ Question 22

What is the likely morphology of the aortic valve?
- **A.** Unicuspid aortic valve
- **B.** Bicuspid aortic valve
- **C.** Trileaflet aortic valve
- **D.** Indeterminate aortic valve morphology

CASE 5

▶ A 43-year-old man presents to the hospital with multiple-foci cryptogenic stroke, with a C-reactive protein (CRP) of 2 mg/L. He denies any recent viral illness or fevers. The images from the transthoracic echocardiogram are shown in **Videos 23-6A** to **23-6D**.

✪✪✪ Question 23

Considering the clinical history and the appearance of the mitral valve shown in the images provided, which is the least likely differential for this abnormal mitral valve?
- **A.** Acute vegetation (active infective endocarditis)
- **B.** Papillary fibroelastoma
- **C.** Myxoma
- **D.** Nonbacterial thrombotic (NBTE) or marantic endocarditis

CASE 6

▶ A 45-year-old man presents with end-stage renal failure on hemodialysis via permcath. He is referred for a transthoracic echocardiogram and a transesophageal echocardiogram (TEE). He has a diagnosis of enterococcus bacteremia and endocarditis treated with vancomycin. The images from the TEE are shown in **Videos 23-7A** to **23-7D**.

✪✪✪ Question 24

Based on the images provided, all of the following are present except:
- **A.** A "kissing lesion" on the noncoronary cusp.
- **B.** Destruction and prolapse of the tip of the right coronary cusp.
- **C.** A large pedunculated vegetation on the right coronary cusp.
- **D.** Perivalvular extension and root abscess.
- **E.** Severe aortic regurgitation.

ANSWERS

1. **Answer: C.** Studies comparing transthoracic echocardiography (TTE) with transesophageal echocardiography (TEE) for the detection of vegetations with TEE as the gold standard have shown that the sensitivity of TTE is dependent on vegetation size. Sensitivity varies from 0% to 25% for vegetations <5 mm and 84% to 100% for vegetations of >10 mm. Therefore, vegetations of <5 mm can easily be missed by TTE even with the application of harmonic imaging. The sensitivity of TTE to detect vegetations is also affected by image quality.

2. **Answer: B.** *Staphylococcus* endocarditis increases the risk of an embolic event due to the aggressive nature of the bacteria. Nonmobile or sessile vegetations do not increase the risk of embolism. Vegetations smaller than 10 mm in size do not confer an increased risk of an embolic event. A patient responding to antibiotic therapy within 1 days indicates that the infective endocarditis is not creating a high risk of embolism. Large mobile vegetations (>10 mm), vegetations located on the mitral valve, increasing size of the vegetation while on antibiotic therapy, and multivalvular infection also identify patients at high risk for embolic events.

3. **Answer: D.** An active vegetation is an echogenic mass with an irregular shape. It is usually located at or near the lines of valve closure at the low-pressure end of the regurgitant jet lesion with high-frequency motion independent of the underlying cardiac structure. The mass can be associated with valve dysfunction. Chronic healed vegetations become echo dense masses due to fibrin, collagen, and calcium deposition. The echocardiographic identification of vegetation or abscess is considered a major criterion for IE in the widely used modified Duke criteria (**Table 23-1**). A definite diagnosis of IE requires the presence of two major criteria, or one major criterion and three minor criteria, or five minor criteria. According to the modified Duke criteria, a vegetation is defined as "an oscillating intracardiac mass on valves or supporting structures, or in the path of regurgitant jets, or on implanted material, in the absence of an alternative anatomical explanation." Compared with infective vegetations, noninfective vegetations from marantic or Libman-Sacks endocarditis have similar morphologic features and can only be differentiated from infective vegetations on the basis of the clinical findings.

4. **Answer: C.** A patient with a predisposing heart condition or history of IV drug use is considered a minor criterion for IE in the Duke criteria (see **Table 23-1**). Positive blood cultures for IE and the presence of new complications of IE such as dehiscence of a prosthetic valve or new valvular regurgitation would all be considered major criteria.

5. **Answer: D.** Roth spots are hemorrhages that form in the retina and can be seen by an ophthalmologic examination. Osler nodes have been attributed to an autoimmune-mediated phenomenon, but some suspect that they are embolic in nature as are the Janeway lesions, splinter hemorrhages, and

Table 23-1. Summary of the Modified Duke Criteria for the Diagnosis of Infective Endocarditis (IE)

Major Criteria

- Positive blood culture for infective endocarditis
  - Two positive blood cultures with a typical organism in the absence of a known source, or persistently positive blood cultures, or single positive blood culture or positive serology for *Coxiella burnetii*
- Evidence of endocardial involvement
  - Positive echocardiographic findings of vegetation, abscess or new dehiscence of prosthetic valve, or new valvular regurgitation

Minor Criteria

- Predisposing heart condition or intravenous drug use
- Fever (>38°C or >100.4°F)
- Vascular phenomena
- Immunologic phenomena
- Positive blood culture but not meeting major criterion, or serologic evidence of active infection with organism consistent with infective endocarditis

Interpretation

Definite Infective Endocarditis
- Pathologic criteria
  - Microorganisms: demonstrated by culture or histology in a vegetation, or in a vegetation that has embolized, or in an intracardiac abscess, or
  - Pathologic lesions: vegetation or intracardiac abscess confirmed by histology examination showing active endocarditis
- Clinical criteria
  - Two major criteria, or
  - One major and three minor criteria, or
  - Five minor criteria

Possible Infective Endocarditis
- One major criterion and one minor criterion; or
- Three minor criteria

Rejected
- Firm alternate diagnosis explaining evidence of endocarditis; or
- Resolution of IE syndrome with antibiotic therapy for 4 days or less; or
- No pathologic evidence of IE at surgery or autopsy, after antibiotic therapy for 4 days or less

From Li JS, Sexton DJ, Mick N, et al. Proposed modifications to the Duke criteria for the diagnosis of infective endocarditis. *Clin Infect Dis.* 2000;30(4):633-638. Copyright © 2000 by the Infectious Diseases Society of America. Adapted by permission of Oxford University Press.

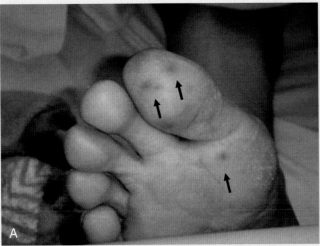
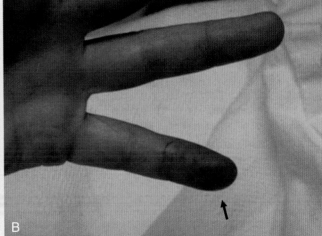

Figure 23-2 (Images courtesy of J. Flaherty MD.)

petechiae. Osler nodes have a painful component, whereas the other cutaneous lesions are generally not painful. **Figure 23-2** shows examples of Janeway lesions of the toes and Osler nodes on a finger.

6. **Answer: E.** The septal leaflet of the tricuspid valve is usually affected due to its close proximity to the VSD. However, right ventricular outflow tract and subpulmonic vegetations have also been described in patients with a VSD presenting with infective endocarditis.

7. **Answer: B.** The images shown were acquired from the right ventricular (RV) inflow view. From this view, the anterior leaflet (anterior on the screen) and septal leaflet (posterior on the screen) of the tricuspid valve are typically seen, although the posterior leaflet can also be imaged from this view (posterior on the screen). Since the interventricular septum (IVS) is seen in the images provided, the tricuspid leaflet is in fact the septal leaflet (not the posterior leaflet).

KEY POINT
In the RV inflow view, the tricuspid valve leaflet seen to the right of the 2D image is always the anterior leaflet. When the 2D plane intersects the IVS, the tricuspid valve leaflets are the anterior and septal leaflets. When the IVS is not seen in the 2D plane, the tricuspid leaflet combination imaged could be anterior and septal or anterior and posterior.

8. ▶ **Answer: A.** An abscess is a complication of IE where there is extension and penetration of the infection to surrounding tissue. Abscesses form cavities that contain purulent material (pus or phlegmon) and do not communicate with the circulation. They are most commonly associated with prosthetic valve and aortic valve IE. In aortic valve IE, abscesses are predominantly located at the aortic root and mitral aortic intervalvular fibrosa. On the echocardiographic examination, an abscess may appear as

a localized abnormal nonhomogeneous perivalvular thickening or as an echolucent space within the perivalvular tissue; they are nonpulsatile and they do not communicate with the surrounding cardiac chambers (**Figure 23-3** and **Video 23-8**). Myocardial abscesses are associated with very high mortality. The development of heart block in this setting is an indication of abscess formation involving the interventricular septum. A pericardial abscess usually represents a fistula formation between an annular abscess and the pericardial space.

9. **Answer: B.** Caseous calcification of the mitral annulus can present as an echolucent space within the calcification of the mitral annulus, simulating a mitral valve annulus abscess. To differentiate from an abscess, other echocardiographic features need to be sought, such as a vegetation, perforation of the leaflet, or valve dysfunction.

A dilated coronary sinus, epicardial fat, and the descending thoracic aorta can be easily distinguished from an abscess in the presence of normal mitral valve anatomy and function.

10. **Answer: D.** Nonbacterial thrombotic endocarditis is a noninfectious process that results in thrombotic deposits on the cardiac valves, most commonly on the left heart valves. NBTE is also known as marantic or verrucous vegetations or Libman-Sacks endocarditis and is a condition often associated with advanced malignancies such as adenocarcinomas, hypercoagulable states, and autoimmune disorders such as systemic lupus erythematosus and antiphospholipid syndrome. It can be difficult to differentiate between NBTE and infective endocarditis (IE) vegetations purely on the echocardiographic appearance of the mass itself. The presence of leaflet destruction and associated abnormalities such as abscess formation and perforation would all be indicators of IE rather than NBTE. The clinical context of the patient also needs to be considered in the differentiation

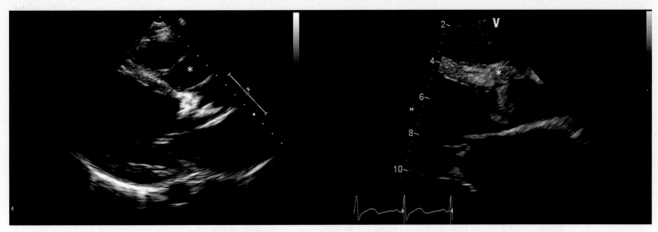

Figure 23-3 These two parasternal long-axis images, acquired from two different patients, show an anterior aortic root abscess (*). In the left image the abscess cavity is echolucent; in the right image, the abscess cavity is echo-dense. Both cases also show grossly abnormal aortic valve leaflets. On real-time imaging, the abscess cavity is nonpulsatile (see **Video 23-8**).

between NBTE and IE. While systemic embolization and vasculitic phenomena can be seen in both conditions, the presence of fever and positive blood cultures are hallmark features of IE.

11. **Answer: A.** Mitral valve prolapse (MVP) can sometimes mimic a mitral valve aneurysm because of the systolic bulging of the mitral valve leaflet toward the left atrium (LA). However, the absence of vegetation and valve disruption favor the diagnosis of MVP. A mitral valve (MV) blood cyst (answer B) is a very rare condition that can present as an immobile echogenic mass on the MV leaflet. A flail MV leaflet (answer C) is usually associated with ruptured chordae that can be identified by the typical "snake-tongue" appearance of the corresponding mitral leaflet protruding into the LA during systole. Mitral valve repair with an Alfieri stitch (answer D) presents as a double-orifice MV on the parasternal short axis view. On the parasternal long-axis view, the MV leaflets appear thickened and restricted.

12. ▶ **Answer: D.** A pseudoaneurysm is a further complication of an abscess where the perivalvular cavity (abscess) now communicates with the circulation (**Videos 23-9A** and **23-9B** and **Figure 23-4**). As previously described, an abscess (answer A) may appear as localized nonhomogeneous thickening (echo-dense) or as an echolucent space; it is nonpulsatile and does not communicate with the surrounding cardiac chambers. A perforation (answer C) is the interruption of endocardial tissue continuity and typically occurs as a complication of a valve aneurysm. On the color Doppler examination, a valve perforation is suspected when the regurgitant jet is located away from the site of leaflet coaptation. A fistula (answer B) is an abnormal communication between cardiac chambers or a cardiac chamber and great vessel and occurs due to weakening of infected tissue. On the color Doppler examination, the fistulous communication between two neighboring cavities through a perforation will be seen.

KEY POINTS

An abscess is a perivalvular cavity with necrosis and purulent material that does not communicate with the circulation. On the echocardiographic examination, this appears as a thickened, nonhomogeneous perivalvular area with an echo-dense or echolucent appearance.

A pseudoaneurysm is a perivalvular (abscess) cavity that communicates with the circulation. On the echocardiographic examination, a pseudoaneurysm appears as a pulsatile perivalvular echo-free space, with intracavity flow detected on the color Doppler examination.

A perforation is an interruption of endocardial tissue continuity. On the echocardiographic examination, a perforation is identified as discontinuity of the endocardial tissue with flow detected across the perforation on the color Doppler examination.

A fistula is a communication between two neighboring cavities through a perforation. On the echocardiographic examination, the perforation is identified as above, and the color Doppler examination confirms the communication between neighboring cavities via a perforation.

13. ▶ **Answer: A.** The lesions typically form on the upstream side of the valve and in a native valve, often near the coaptation point of the leaflets. Therefore, for the mitral valve (MV), it is common to see an infective vegetation on the left atrial side of the leaflets, generally closer to the coaptation point. The lesion will prolapse into the left ventricle in diastole and buckle back into the left atrium in systole (**Video 23-10**).

14. **Answer: B. Figure 23-5** shows the relationship between the conduction system (atrioventricular node and branches) and the three cusps of the aortic valve. This close association between the noncoronary and right coronary cusps and the conduction pathway explains why abscess development can disrupt the conduction system, leading to rhythm abnormalities such as heart block.

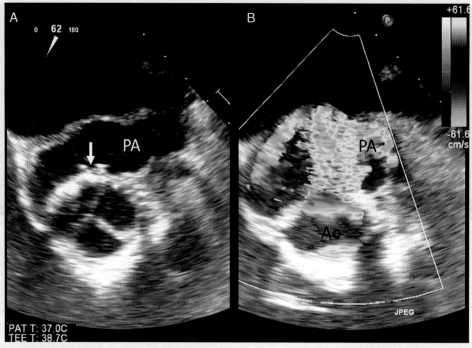

Figure 23-4 Ao, aorta; PA, pulmonary artery.

15. **Answer: D.** The viridans group streptococci (VGS) are a heterogeneous group of organisms and are known oral inhabitants. When the gingival tissue is disrupted with procedures such as teeth cleaning, bacteremia with Strep viridans group can occur and potentially lead to endocarditis in susceptible individuals. Staph species and fungi more often arise from the skin, and enterococcus organisms arise from the gut.

16. **Answer: C.** Although this patient has an indwelling catheter that may predispose him to a greater risk of endocarditis, current American Heart Association

(AHA)/American College of Cardiology (ACC) and European Society of Cardiology (ESC) guidelines do not recommend antibiotic prophylaxis for indwelling catheters.

Antibiotic prophylaxis is recommended for high-risk dental procedures and high-risk patients. High-risk dental procedures involve manipulation of the gingiva (gums) or periapical region of the teeth or perforation of the oral mucosa. High-risk patients include those with prosthetic valves, or where prosthetic material has been used to repair a valve, patients with previous IE, and patients with congenital heart disease that is unrepaired, in the first 6 months after repair with prosthetic material, or with residual valvular or shunt defects. The AHA/ACC also recommends antibiotic prophylaxis in cardiac transplants with valve regurgitation due to a structurally abnormal valve; however, the ESC does not recommend antibiotic prophylaxis for heart transplants with structural heart abnormalities.

17. **Answer: E.** This patient has a primary vegetation on the hemodialysis catheter and satellite vegetations on his tricuspid valve (TV) and the free wall of the right atrium (RA). On the real-time image (**Video 23-2**), a small vegetation is seen on the septal leaflet of the TV, and larger vegetations are seen in the RA attached to the hemodialysis catheter and RA free wall. **Figure 23-6** shows the indwelling catheter.

Staphylococcus capitis was isolated from the blood culture. Prosthetic material in the heart predisposes patients to a higher risk of infective

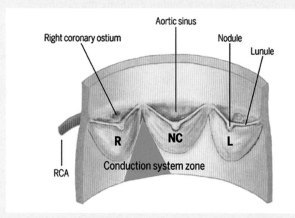

Figure 23-5 Spatial relationship between the three cusps of the aortic valve and the zone where the left bundle branch emerges beneath the membranous septum. L, left cusp; NC, noncoronary cusp; R, right cusp; RCA, right coronary artery. (From Mangieri A, Montalto C, Pagnesi M, et al. TAVI and post procedural cardiac conduction abnormalities. *Front Cardiovasc Med.* 2018;5:85. https://creativecommons.org/licenses/by/4.0/. Copyright © 2018 Mangieri, Montalto, Pagnesi, Lanzillo, Demir, Testa, Colombo and Latib.)

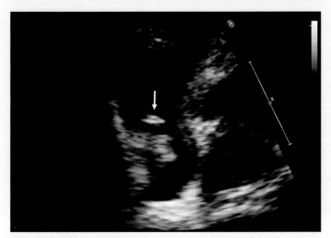

Figure 23-6 The arrow indicates the hemodialysis catheter.

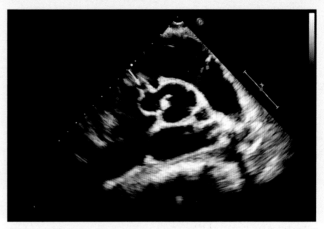

Figure 23-7 This still frame image acquired from the parasternal short-axis view shows an aortic root abscess cavity with a fistulous communication to the right atrium (arrow).

endocarditis (IE). Sonographers should interrogate all of the valves and chambers from different views and angles when IE is suspected.

18. **Answer: B.** The MV leaflets appear normal with no prolapse, but color Doppler imaging shows a perforation of the anterior leaflet. The regurgitant jet does not originate from the coaptation site but rather from the body of the leaflet suggesting leaflet perforation. The perforation is not well seen on 2D imaging. No mitral valve cleft is present.

19. **Answer: A.** The MR jet is located at the A1 segment of the mitral leaflet. The parasternal short-axis view with color Doppler imaging clearly demonstrates that the jet is located laterally at the A1 scallop and is directed posteriorly.

20. **Answer: B.** There is an independently mobile mass attached to the left atrial side of the anterior prosthetic ring. In this clinical setting, the appearance is consistent with a vegetation. There are no obvious vegetations associated with the mitral valve leaflets. Prosthetic material in the heart allows for a greater incidence for a circulating microorganism to seed endocardial tissue and form a vegetation. The vegetations consist of platelets, fibrin, anti-inflammatory cells, and causative microorganisms. Once the infection starts, it can then spread to the surrounding valve leaflets. Three-dimensional (3D) transesophageal echocardiography would be beneficial in identifying the location and extent of the vegetative lesion in this patient.

21. **Answer: A.** This patient has vegetations on the aortic and tricuspid valves. Often when the infection is this expansive, other complications such as an aortic abscess form, leading to even further tissue destruction, resulting in a pseudoaneurysm or a fistula. In this case, the patient has an aortic root abscess that has ruptured, resulting in a fistulous communication between the aorta and right atrium, shown by the arrow in **Figure 23-7**. There is no ASD

or VSD in this patient. While there may be tricuspid regurgitation present, the primary abnormality is the aorta to right atrium fistula.

22. **Answer: B.** A bicuspid aortic valve (BAV) can be identified from the parasternal short-axis view during systole by identifying just two commissural attachments to the aortic root. In this patient, there appears to be a raphe between the right and left coronary cusps with only two commissures opening out to the aortic root at the 9- and 3-o'clock positions (**Figure 23-8**).

Patients with a BAV are at markedly increased risk of infective endocarditis and aortic root abscess relative to patients with a trileaflet aortic valve.

23. **Answer: A.** The CRP test checks for infection or inflammation. A normal CRP is below 2 mg/L. A CRP between 100 and 500 mg/L is considered highly predictive of inflammation due to bacterial infection, and CRP concentrations between 2 and 10 mg/L are considered as metabolic inflammation. Therefore, a CRP of 2 mg/L in this patient is

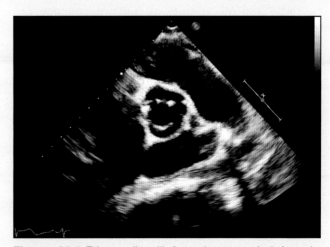

Figure 23-8 This systolic still frame image acquired from the parasternal short-axis view shows a BAV with two commissures opening out to the aortic root.

Table 23-2. Echo Appearance and Clinical Findings of Differentials for an Abnormal Mitral Valve

Differentials	Echo Appearance and Clinical Findings
Acute vegetation—infective endocarditis	• Homogeneous soft-tissue density • Independently mobile • Commonly associated with leaflet destruction and associated complications such as abscess formation, perforation, and new regurgitation
Papillary fibroelastoma	• Most common tumor of cardiac valves • Small, homogeneous masses often attached to the valve by a stalk • Not associated with destruction of valve leaflets
Myxoma	• Circumscribed and often speckled appearance • Most commonly located within left atrium attached to the atrial septum • Not associated with destruction of valve leaflets
NBTE or marantic endocarditis	• Can be difficult to differentiate from echocardiographic appearance of IE • Systemic embolization and vasculitic phenomena can be seen in NBTE • Not associated with destruction of leaflets

IE, infective endocarditis; NBTE, nonbacterial thrombotic endocarditis.

not indicative of infection. Therefore, the echocardiographic densities seen on the mitral valve (MV) and the absence of leaflet destruction are not likely to represent infective endocarditis (IE) in this patient. While the appearance of the mitral valve could also represent a "healed" vegetation, this was not one of the offered answers. **Table 23-2** provides a summary of the echocardiographic appearances and clinical findings that may be helpful in differentiating among IE vegetations, papillary fibroelastomas, myxomas, and NBTE or marantic endocarditis.

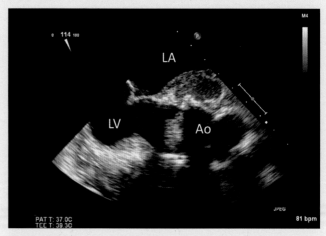

Figure 23-9 Observe the large, thickened nonhomogeneous appearance of the aortic root abscess located in the aorto-mitral curtain in this TEE image. Ao, aorta; LA, left atrium; LV, left ventricle.

24. ▶ **Answer: D.** The images provided display all of the aforementioned options except for perivalvular extension and root abscess. While abscess formation in the aortic root is a common complication of infective endocarditis (IE), in this case, the aortic root appears unremarkable.

An example of perivalvular extension and aortic root abscess is shown in **Figure 23-9** and **Video 23-11**.

KEY POINTS

▶ Leaflet perforation should be considered when the regurgitant jet is located away from the coaptation point of the leaflets.

▶ According to the current guidelines, patients should undergo early surgery when there is IE with valve dysfunction associated with heart failure.

▶ The presence of leaflet destruction and the patient's clinical condition (i.e., fever) are key determinants in diagnosing IE as opposed to NBTE.

▶ Abscess formation near the noncoronary and right coronary cusps of the aortic valve can lead to disruption in the conduction system and ultimately cause abnormalities such as heart block.

▶ Prosthetic material in the heart allows for a greater incidence for a circulating microorganism to seed endocardial tissue and form a vegetation.

Acknowledgments: The authors thank and acknowledge Ying Tung Sia, MD, MSc, Guillaume Marquis Gravel, MD, MSc and Kwan Leung Chan, MD (Chapter 20, Endocarditis) in Clinical Echocardiography Review: A Self-Assessment Tool, 2nd Edition, edited by Allan L. Klein, Craig R. Asher, 2017.

SUGGESTED READINGS

Anderson B. Infective endocarditis and cardiac masses. In: *A Sonographer's Guide to the Assessment of Heart Disease*. Brisbane, Australia: Echotext Pty Ltd; 2014:chap 13.

Armstrong WF, Ryan T. Infectious endocarditis. In: *Feigenbaum's Echocardiography*. 8th ed. Philadelphia, PA: Lippincott Williams and Wilkins; 2018:chap 13.

Baddour LM, Wilson WR, Bayer AS, et al. Infective endocarditis in adults: diagnosis, antimicrobial therapy, and management of complications. A scientific statement for healthcare professionals from the American Heart Association. *Circulation*. 2015;132(15):1435-1486.

Freeman WK. Infectious endocarditis. In: Oh JK, Kane GC, eds. *The Echo Manual*. 4th ed. Philadelphia, PA and Rochester, MN: Wolters Kluwer and Mayo Foundation for Medical Education and Research; 2019:chap 15.

Habib G, Lancellotti P, Antunes MJ, et al. 2015 ESC guidelines for the management of infective endocarditis: the task force for the management of infective endocarditis of the European Society of Cardiology (ESC). *Eur Heart J*. 2015;36(44):3075-3128.

Murdoch DR, Corey GR, Hoen B, et al. Clinical presentation, etiology, and outcome of infective endocarditis in the 21st century: the International Collaboration on Endocarditis-Prospective Cohort Study. *Arch Intern Med*. 2009;169(5):463-473.

Otto CM. Endocarditis. In: *Textbook of Clinical Echocardiography*. 6th ed. Philadelphia, PA: Elsevier; 2018:chap 14.

Saric M, Armour A, Arnaout MS, et al. Guidelines for the use of echocardiography in the evaluation of a cardiac source of embolism. *J Am Soc Echocardiogr*. 2016;29(1):1-42.

Sedgwick JF, Burstow DJ. Update on echocardiography in the management of infective endocarditis. *Curr Infect Dis Rep*. 2012;14(4): 373-380.

CHAPTER 24

Tumors, Masses, and Sources of Emboli

Contributors: Margaret M. Park, BS, ACS, RDCS, RVT and Sarah H. Park, RDCS

✪✪ Question 1

A paradoxical embolism is best described as:
- **A.** A thromboembolism that straddles the branch pulmonary artery after surgery.
- **B.** Septic emboli occurring as a result of infective endocarditis.
- **C.** A venous embolism that becomes a systemic embolism through an intracardiac shunt.
- **D.** An identified deep vein thrombosis (DVT) in a pregnant woman.

✪✪✪ Question 2

Which are the best views to image the left atrial appendage (LAA) to exclude thrombus formation?
- **A.** Transesophageal echocardiography (TEE) midesophageal 2-chamber and midesophageal aortic valve short-axis views
- **B.** Transthoracic echocardiography (TTE) apical 4-chamber, apical 2-chamber, and parasternal right ventricle (RV) inflow views
- **C.** TEE deep transgastric short-axis and modified long-axis views
- **D.** TTE apical 4-chamber, apical 2-chamber, and subcostal views

✪✪ Question 3

The three factors that form Virchow's triad include:
- **A.** Low arterial blood pressure, distended neck veins, and muffled heart sounds.
- **B.** Blood stasis, vessel wall injury, and hypercoagulability.
- **C.** Tachycardia, tachypnea, and tender hepatomegaly.
- **D.** Chest pain, heart failure, and syncope.

✪ Question 4

The most common chamber for thrombus formation following a large anterior wall myocardial infarction (MI) is the:
- **A.** Left atrium (LA).
- **B.** Right atrium (RA).
- **C.** Right ventricle (RV).
- **D.** Left ventricle (LV).

✪✪ Question 5

With respect to the distinction between benign and malignant tumors, which of the following statements is false?
- **A.** Benign tumors are well-differentiated while malignant tumors are poorly differentiated.
- **B.** Benign tumors are slower growing and may regress while malignant tumors are usually rapid growing.
- **C.** Benign tumors are fixed to adjacent structures while malignant tumors are freely mobile in relation to adjacent structures.
- **D.** Benign tumors do not metastasize while malignant tumors frequently metastasize.

✪✪ Question 6

Which is the most common primary benign cardiac tumor in adults and in children?
- **A.** Lipoma in adults and myxoma in children
- **B.** Myxoma in adults and rhabdomyoma in children
- **C.** Myxoma in both adults and children
- **D.** Papillary fibroelastoma in adults and rhabdomyoma in children
- **E.** Rhabdomyoma in adults and myxoma in children

✪✪ Question 7

Which is the most common primary malignant cardiac tumor in adults and in children?

A. Angiosarcoma in adults and rhabdomyosarcoma in children

B. Angiosarcoma in both adults and children

C. Leiomyosarcoma in adults and rhabdomyosarcoma in children

D. Rhabdomyosarcoma in adults and leiomyosarcoma in children

E. Synovial sarcoma in adults and angiosarcoma in children

✪ Question 8

Which of the following statements regarding the use of ultrasound enhancing agents (UEAs) in the differentiation of thrombus from vascularized tumors is true?

A. A thrombus will be highly vascularized while a tumor will show only mild vascularity if any.

B. A thrombus will have a high uptake of contrast, and a tumor will have no uptake.

C. A thrombus will have no uptake of contrast while many tumors are highly perfused.

D. UEAs have little value in differentiating a tumor from a thrombus.

✪✪ Question 9

Which of the following types of cancer metastasize to the heart?

A. Breast, lung, and melanoma

B. Colon, rectal, and esophageal

C. Liver, renal, and thyroid

D. Thyroid, brain, and leukemia

✪ Question 10

▶ An echocardiogram is ordered for a patient with shortness of breath. Based on the images provided in **Video 24-1**, which type of tumor is most likely?

A. Leiomyosarcoma

B. Papillary fibroelastoma

C. Renal cell carcinoma

D. Myxoma

✪ Question 11

Identify the structure (arrow) in the right ventricle (**Figures 24-1A** and **24-1B**) that is often mistaken for a thrombus.

A. Device lead

B. Moderator band

C. Chiari network

D. Ventricular septal defect (VSD) repair patch

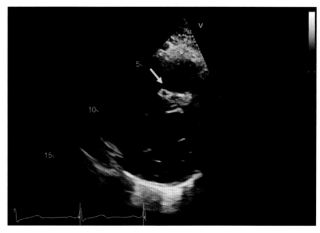

Figure 24-1A

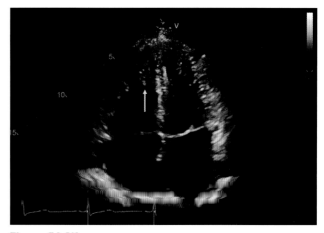

Figure 24-1B

✪ Question 12

A patient presents with a stroke, and an echocardiogram is performed. A large, mobile, heterogeneous mass with an apparent attachment to the fossa ovalis via a stalk is visualized in the left atrium and is assumed to be the source of emboli until further testing can be done. The mass is most likely a(n):

A. Angiosarcoma.

B. Myxoma.

C. Papillary fibroelastoma.

D. Renal cell carcinoma.

✪ Question 13

A middle-aged man complains of swelling, redness, and pain in his calf several days after a long plane flight. His doctor orders a duplex ultrasound examination of his leg and an echocardiogram due to a soft murmur heard on physical examination. The echocardiogram shows a large, highly mobile, snake-like structure in the right atrium (RA), appearing to enter from the inferior vena cava (IVC). Which is the likely diagnosis?

A. Leiomyosarcoma
B. Myxoma
C. Renal cell carcinoma
D. Thrombus

✪✪ Question 14

Which of the following signs is not associated with acute pulmonary embolism?

A. Flattening and paradoxical motion of the interventricular septum
B. Midsystolic notching on the right ventricular outflow tract (RVOT) Doppler trace
C. A right ventricular (RV) acceleration time <60 ms and right ventricular systolic pressure (RVSP)>60 mm Hg
D. RV free wall akinesis with preserved apical function

✪✪ Question 15

The following statements are true with respect to left ventricular (LV) thrombus except:

A. An ultrasound enhancing agent (UEA) can be a valuable tool in identification of LV thrombus.
B. Laminated thrombus is very easily detected by echocardiography.
C. LV thrombus is a common complication of myocardial infarction.
D. LV thrombus is more likely to develop in the presence of low cardiac output.
E. "Smoke" is a precursor to development of thrombus.

✪✪ Question 16

▶ Based on the images provided (**Videos 24-2A** and **24-2B**), the risk for thrombus embolization is:

A. Low.
B. Moderate.
C. High.
D. Zero.

✪✪ Question 17

A 21-year-old college student in good health seeks medical clearance to travel abroad. She has no family history of heart disease and no symptoms. She has no history of rheumatic fever, night sweats, or chills and has had all childhood and youth vaccinations. On examination, palpitations are noted, and an echocardiogram is ordered. The left ventricular (LV) chamber size is normal and the ejection fraction (EF) is low normal. A large echo density is noted on the parasternal long- and short-axis LV images (**Figures 24-2A** and **24-2B**). This abnormality is most likely a(n):

A. Large pericardial mass.
B. Large LV cavity tumor.
C. LV aneurysm filled with thrombus.
D. Mass embedded within the LV walls.

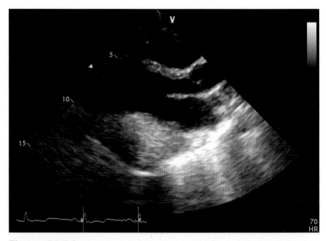

Figure 24-2A

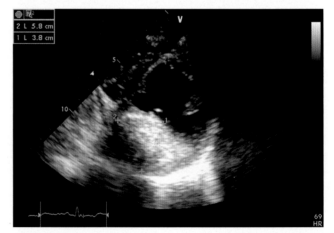

Figure 24-2B

✪✪✪ Question 18

A 65-year-old female with a heart murmur since childhood has complaints of worsening shortness of breath and lightheadedness when bending over or squatting. She is referred to the cardiology clinic for evaluation of hypertrophic obstructive cardiomyopathy (HOCM). From the apical 4-chamber view (**Video 24-3**), which is the likely abnormality?

A. Fatty infiltration

B. Giant tricuspid valve papillary fibroelastoma

C. Marked tricuspid annular calcification

D. Right atrial myxoma

✪✪ Question 19

Which echocardiographic feature is not a criterion for defining a vegetation?

A. Amorphous, irregular shape

B. Attached to downstream side of valve

C. Soft tissue density

D. Mobile and oscillating

✪✪✪ Question 20

A 44-year-old male executive is experiencing mild chest pain at rest and with exercise. His physical examination is unremarkable, and a 1/6 systolic murmur is heard at the lower left sternal border on auscultation. A stress echocardiogram is ordered to further evaluate his chest pain and murmur. Based on the images provided (**Videos 24-4A to 24-4D**), which best describes the abnormality shown?

A. A blood-filled cyst

B. A homogeneous thrombus

C. Schistosomiasis invasion

D. Unusual presentation of lipoma

✪✪✪ Question 21

A 72-year-old woman with symptomatic aortic stenosis has a cardiac catheterization and is approved for percutaneous transvalvular aortic valve replacement (TAVR). Based on the images from her discharge echocardiogram (**Videos 24-5A to 24-5D**), which finding is present?

A. Thickened nodules of Arantius

B. Moderate mitral annular calcification

C. Lambl's excrescences

D. Caseous calcification of the mitral annulus

E. An abscess involving the anterior mitral valve leaflet

✪✪ Question 22

A 69-year-old woman is 2 weeks post total knee replacement and presents in the emergency room (ER) with confusion and marked shortness of breath. A bedside echocardiogram performed in the ER was technically difficult due to the patient's body habitus, position, and irritability. The sonographer sees movement in the right atrium (RA) only from the parasternal long-axis view of right ventricular inflow (**Figure 24-3**). The reading physician recommends a stat transesophageal echocardiogram (**Videos 24-6A** and **24-6B**). Based on the images provided, the echocardiographic findings are consistent with the mass being:

A. Adipose tissue.

B. A Chiari network.

C. A eustachian valve.

D. A thrombus

E. A vegetation.

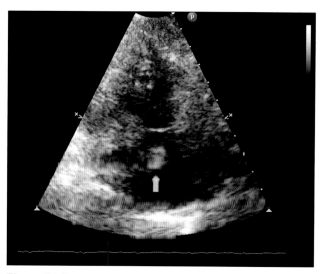

Figure 24-3

✪✪ Question 23

Technical tips for increasing visualization of left ventricular (LV) apical thrombus include all the following except:

A. Moving the focal zone to the apex in zoom mode.

B. Using a lower transducer frequency.

C. Using nonstandardized views and off-axis imaging.

D. Imaging at a shallow depth setting.

E. Use of an ultrasound enhancing agent (UEA).

✪✪ Question 24

All the following are associated with Libman-Sacks endocarditis except:

    A. Verrucous endocarditis.
    B. Autoimmune disease.
    C. Systemic lupus erythematosus.
    D. Nonbacterial thrombotic endocarditis.
    E. Positive blood cultures.

✪ Question 25

▶ A 34-year-old female athlete is experiencing recent episodes of chest pain. She has a family history of premature coronary artery disease. A cardiac stress test reveals no abnormalities at maximum effort with the patient reaching 95% maximum heart rate. An echocardiogram is performed. From the images provided (**Videos 24-7A** and **24-7B**), the most likely diagnosis is:

    A. Renal cell carcinoma.
    B. Right atrial (RA) myxoma.
    C. RA thrombus.
    D. Tricuspid valve papillary fibroelastoma (PFE).

✪ Question 26

▶ Regarding the mass in the previous question (Question 25, **Videos 24-7A** and **24-7B**), the mass can be accurately be described as:

    A. Pedunculated.
    B. Laminated.
    C. Protruding.
    D. Calcified.
    E. Homogeneous.

✪✪ Question 27

▶ A 75-year-old woman with a history of diabetes, hypertension, and a transit ischemic attack (TIA) has a transthoracic echocardiogram (TTE) followed by a transesophageal echocardiogram (TEE). Based on the videos provided (**Videos 24-8A** and **24-8B**), which is the likely diagnosis of her tricuspid valve abnormality?

    A. Nodules of Arantius
    B. Lambl's excrescences
    C. Bacterial endocarditis
    D. Papillary fibroelastoma

✪✪✪ Question 28

▶ A 25-year-old woman with a history of cardiomyopathy and an implantable cardioverter defibrilla-

tor (ICD) is admitted with increasing shortness of breath and general weakness. A previous transthoracic echocardiogram (TTE) revealed depressed left ventricular (LV) function (ejection fraction of 25%), right ventricular (RV) dysfunction, and mild tricuspid regurgitation. She has a repeat TTE to evaluate her LV function. With this limited clinical information and based on the images provided (**Figure 24-4** and **Videos 24-9A** and **24-9B**), which statement best describes the echocardiographic findings of this study?

    A. There is a right atrial (RA) thrombus on an indwelling central line.
    B. There is a thrombus attached to the pacemaker wire.
    C. A venous thrombus has traveled through the inferior vena cava (IVC) and has embolized to the right-sided chambers becoming entangled in the tricuspid valve apparatus.
    D. There is a large vegetation attached to the pacemaker wire.
    E. Any of the above options may be correct.

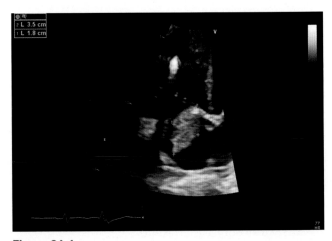

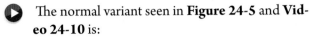

Figure 24-4

✪✪ Question 29

▶ The normal variant seen in **Figure 24-5** and **Video 24-10** is:

    A. A Chiari network.
    B. The crista terminalis.
    C. A cor triatriatum dexter.
    D. A pectinate muscle.
    E. A eustachian valve.

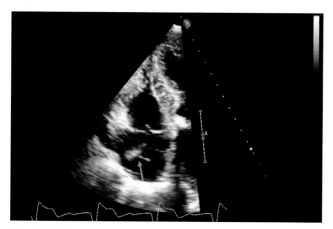

Figure 24-5

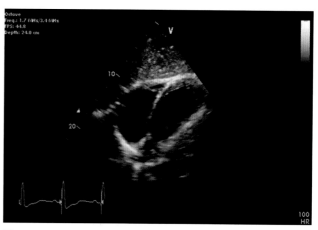

Figure 24-6B

✪✪ Question 30

A 52-year-old male with no significant past medical history develops a persistent cough. After 3 months, he develops lower extremity swelling, fatigue, and increased shortness of breath with exercise. He has no murmur and a normal blood pressure with a heart rate of 88 bpm. From the parasternal short-axis image at the level of the great vessels (**Figure 24-6A**) and subcostal 4-chamber view (**Figure 24-6B**), a large mediastinal mass with compression of underlying cardiac structures is seen. There was no significant gradient across the pulmonary valve, and the right ventricular systolic pressure (RVSP) was estimated at 35 mm Hg. There was no definitive infiltration of the cardiac chambers or pericardium. Which is the imaging modality of choice in the further evaluation of mediastinal lesions exterior to the heart?

    A. Conventional radiology (chest X-ray)
    B. Computed tomography (CT)
    C. Chest ultrasonography
    D. Magnetic resonance imaging (MRI)

✪✪✪ Question 31

In reference to the patient in Question 30 above, the mediastinal mass was diagnosed by CT scan as a germ cell tumor. Of the following statements, which is false regarding germ cell tumors?

    A. These tumors occur most frequently in the gonad.
    B. These tumors may be benign or malignant.
    C. Teratomas are a type of germ cell tumor.
    D. One-third of patients with these tumors will be symptomatic.
    E. 95% of these tumors arise in the posterior mediastinum.

✪✪✪ Question 32

Transesophageal echocardiography (TEE) is important in the assessment of the left atrial appendage (LAA). The primary indications for TEE assessment include to rule out the presence of LAA thrombus and to assess LAA function via pulsed-wave Doppler (PWD). Based on the TEE image in **Figure 24-7**, which peak (late diastolic) emptying velocity (PEV) would be expected on PWD of this LAA?

    A. PEV of 40 to 45 cm/s
    B. PEV of 30 to 35 cm/s
    C. PEV of 15 to 20 cm/s
    D. PEV of 0 cm/s

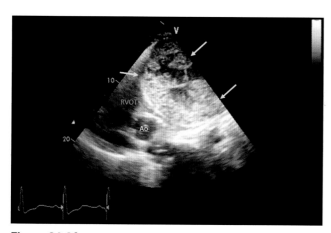

Figure 24-6A

✪✪ Question 33

▶ A 52-year-old woman has a transthoracic echocardiogram with agitated saline ordered to evaluate a possible cardiac shunt. The sonographer performs two saline bubble injections, one with and one without a Valsalva maneuver. Later in the study, an ultrasound enhancing agent (UEA) is used to improve image quality. Based on the images provided in **Videos 24-11A** to **24-11C**, there is a:

A. Laminated left ventricular (LV) mass with perfusion and a negative bubble study.

B. Laminated LV mass with no perfusion and a negative bubble study.

C. Mobile protruding LV mass with no perfusion and a negative bubble study.

D. Mobile protruding LV mass with perfusion and a negative bubble study.

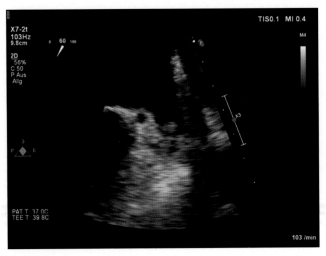

Figure 24-7

ANSWERS

1. ▶ **Answer: C.** A paradoxical embolism is an embolism that starts on the systemic venous side of the circulatory system and crosses through an intracardiac defect such as a patent foramen ovale (PFO) to the systemic arterial side of the circulation. The definitive diagnosis of paradoxical embolism requires detection of thrombus lodged within the PFO (**Video 24-12**). However, when an actual thrombus crossing a PFO or other intracardiac defect is not seen, the diagnosis of paradoxical embolism may be suspected when there is (1) a systemic embolism without an apparent source in the left heart or proximal arterial tree, (2) evidence of venous thrombus or pulmonary embolus as an embolic source, and (3) evidence of a PFO with right-to-left shunting.

   A bubble study (agitated saline) is warranted for a patient with stroke-like symptoms to rule out an intracardiac shunt. The early appearance of saline bubbles in the left heart (within 3 beats) is most consistent with intracardiac shunting and the late appearance of saline bubbles (after 5-7 beats) is most suggestive of pulmonary arteriovenous shunting.

2. ▶ **Answer: A.** The best way to image the LAA to exclude or confirm thrombus formation is on a TEE in the midesophageal 2-chamber view and the midesophageal aortic valve short-axis view (**Figure 24-8A**).

   Occasionally, the LAA can be seen on the TTE exam in the apical 4-chamber (**Figure 24-8B**), (**Video 24-13A**) apical 2-chamber, and parasternal short-axis (**Figure 24-8C**) (**Video 24-13B**) views; however,

TEE imaging is superior due to the closer proximity to the heart and increased sensitivity and specificity. Commercial echo contrast enhancement can help to better delineate the LAA and identify thrombus activity with certainty during TEE.

3. **Answer: B.** Virchow's triad refers to the three primary risk factors or predisposing conditions that influence the formation of thrombus. This includes blood stasis, vessel wall injury, and hypercoagulability. These three factors are thought to contribute to venous thrombus formation. Stasis includes long periods of immobility (for example, long duration car or plane trips or being bed bound), varicose veins, or any change in blood flow. Vessel wall injury includes trauma, hypertension, and inflammation. Lastly, hypercoagulability can be genetic or due to other risk factors such as trauma, obesity, cancer, pregnancy, advanced age, race, smoking, and oral contraceptives.

4. **Answer: D.** The most common site for thrombus formation following a large anterior wall MI (or any large MI) is the LV due to akinesis or dyskinesis of the LV segments and pooling of blood. A globally depressed ejection fraction from congestive heart failure can also cause LV thrombus. It is very important to interrogate the LV, especially the apex, for thrombus in these settings. An ultrasound enhancing agent (UEA) should be utilized whenever the apex is not well visualized or in the setting of a low ejection fraction, significant wall motion abnormalities, and/or aneurysms. In particular, the use of UEAs facilitates LV thrombus detection by providing opacification within the cardiac chambers to demonstrate the "filling defect" appearance of an intracardiac thrombus.

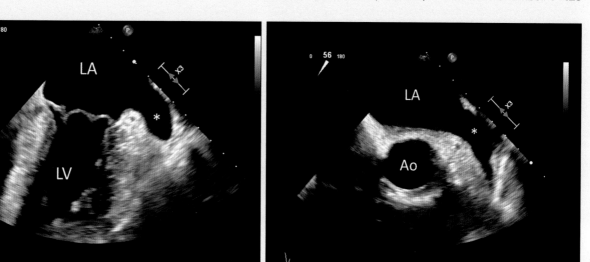

Figure 24-8A The TEE midesophageal 2-chamber view (left) and the midesophageal aortic valve (AV) short-axis view (right) show the LAA (*). LA, left atrium; LAA, left atrial appendage; LV, left ventricle; RA, right atrium; TEE, transesophageal echocardiography.

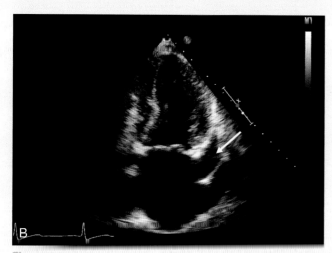

Figure 24-8B The arrow points to the LAA.

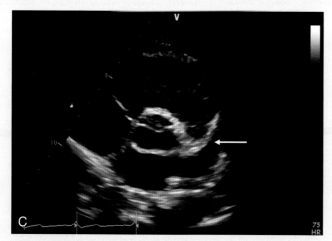

Figure 24-8C The arrow points to the LAA.

5. Answer: C. Benign tumors are freely mobile in relation to adjacent structures while malignant tumors are fixed to adjacent structures. Furthermore, benign tumors are well-circumscribed or encapsulated and do not invade or infiltrate sur-

rounding normal tissue. Malignant tumors, on the other hand, are poorly circumscribed and have an indistinct irregular shape, they are not encapsulated, and they tend to be locally invasive, infiltrating surrounding tissue.

Answer A is a true statement since benign tumors are well-differentiated while malignant tumors are poorly differentiated. This means that benign tumors may be composed of cells resembling the mature normal cells of the tissue of origin of the neoplasm while the cells of malignant tumors are primitive-appearing, unspecialized cells. Answer B is a true statement as benign tumors are slower growing and may regress while malignant tumors tend to be rapid growing. However, malignant tumors may also be slow growing. Answer D is a true statement as benign tumors do not metastasize although they can reoccur after being surgically resected. Malignant tumors frequently metastasize. The spread of malignant tumors occurs via (1) direct seeding of body cavities or surfaces, (2) lymphatic spread, or (3) hematogenous spread.

Both types of tumors can cause a host of signs/symptoms including dyspnea, embolism, fever, chills, chest pain, weight loss, arrhythmias, left ventricular outflow tract obstruction, valvular leaks/stenosis, and heart failure. Resection and biopsy (if possible) are a vital part of diagnosis and treatment.

6. Answer: B. The differential diagnoses for primary cardiac tumors can be aided by the age of the patient. The most common benign cardiac tumor in the adult population is a myxoma. These are typically located in the left atrium (75%) but can also be found in the right atrium and rarely in the left or right ventricle. Myxomas are usually connected to the fossa ovalis by a narrow stalk. Rhabdomyomas are the most common benign cardiac tumor in children, particularly in those with tuberous sclerosis (a rare multisystem genetic disease that causes non-cancerous tumors to grow in the brain and other vital organs such as the kidneys, heart, liver, eyes, lungs, and skin). Rhabdomyomas are often multiple and located in the right ventricle (RV) or RV outflow tract, although they can occur in either ventricle. These tumors may regress spontaneously. Papillary fibroelastomas are the most common tumors of the cardiac valves and the second most common primary cardiac tumors in adults. While these tumors most frequently occur on aortic and mitral valves, they can also be found on the tricuspid and pulmonary valves, papillary muscles, chordae, or the left or right atrium. Lipomas can be found in any part of the heart. Most of these tumors arise in the subendocardium, but they can also occur in the pericardium and on the cardiac valves.

KEY POINT

In the adult, the most common primary benign cardiac tumor is the myxoma, which is usually seen in the left atrium. In children, the most common primary benign cardiac tumor is the rhabdomyoma, which is most commonly seen in the RV or RV outflow tract.

7. **Answer: A.** As previously discussed, the differential diagnoses for primary cardiac tumors can be aided by the age of the patient. The most common primary malignant cardiac tumor in adults is the angiosarcoma. Cardiac angiosarcomas are generally located in the right atrium and are very aggressive; by the time of diagnosis there is usually metastasis. Rhabdomyosarcomas are the most common primary malignant cardiac tumor in children. These tumors arise from the ventricular and atrial walls and are very aggressive. Leiomyosarcomas are made of smooth muscle cells and are most often found in the left atrium, especially near the pulmonary veins. Synovial sarcomas rarely occur in the heart, almost always on the right side. The most common site for synovial sarcoma is a lower limb.

KEY POINT

In adults, the most common primary malignant tumor is the angiosarcoma, which is most commonly seen in the right atrium. In children, the most common primary malignant tumor is the rhabdomyosarcoma, which can arise from any cardiac structure.

8. **Answer: C.** The purpose of administering a UEA (or contrast agent) while evaluating a mass is to demonstrate vascularity. A tumor that is vascularized will be highly enhanced with the UEA (**Video 24-14A**). Thrombus is avascular and therefore will have no uptake of contrast (**Video 24-14B**). Echocardiographic perfusion imaging has also been demonstrated to characterize vascularity of cardiac masses and assist with the differentiation of malig-

nant, highly vascular tumors from benign tumors or thrombi. Importantly, not all cardiac tumors are highly vascular. Myxomas have a poor blood supply and therefore have low uptake and appear partially enhanced. Papillary fibroelastomas are avascular and therefore show no enhancement.

9. **Answer: A.** Common types of cancer known to spread to the heart include breast cancers, lung cancers, and melanoma as well as renal cell carcinoma, esophageal cancers, leukemia, lymphoma, and carcinoid. Breast cancer, lung cancer, melanoma, esophageal cancer, leukemia, and lymphoma are often carried to the heart through blood or the lymphatic system. Renal cell carcinoma enters into the right heart directly through the inferior vena cava (IVC). Carcinoid tumors are neuroendocrine tumors that usually arise from the gastrointestinal tract and, rarely, from other sites such as the bronchus, biliary tract, pancreas, ovaries, or testes. The secretion of substances from metastatic carcinoid tumors results in the deposition of fibrous plaques on right-sided cardiac valves, leading to thickening, shortening, and retraction of tricuspid and pulmonic valves. Malignant pericardial effusions are also caused by lung cancer, breast cancer, melanoma, lymphoma, and leukemia. These effusions may result in cardiac tamponade.

10. **Answer: C.** A mass in the right atrium (RA) appears to arise from the inferior vena cava (IVC) and therefore most likely represents a renal cell carcinoma. Leiomyosarcomas (answer A) tend to be in the left atrium (LA), and papillary fibroelastomas (answer B) are usually attached to valves. Myxomas (answer D) are most commonly found in the LA but can occur in other locations such as the RA, right ventricle, left ventricle, and attached to atrioventricular valves. Typically, myxomas are attached by a stalk and would not originate from the IVC.

TEACHING POINT

Echocardiography is a fast and inexpensive way to evaluate tumors and monitor changes in tumor size. Computed tomography (CT) and/or cardiac magnetic resonance imaging (MRI) with contrast may be needed to better characterize a cardiac tumor in terms of size, morphology, composition, attachment site, and extension.

11. **Answer: B.** The moderator band in the right ventricle (RV), when prominent, can sometimes be mistaken for a thrombus or other mass due to its location and size. There are numerous normal cardiac structures that can be confused for intracardiac masses or tumors. This includes normal structures in the left ventricle such as false tendons and hypertrophied papillary muscles and structures in the RV such as device leads and trabeculations. Suture lines and mitral annular calcification seen in the left atrium may be confused for intracardiac masses or

tumors. Normal structures confused with thrombus or an intracardiac mass in the right atrium include the Chiari network, crista terminalis, and Eustachian valve. Prominent lipomatous hypertrophy of the interatrial septum may also be mistaken for an intracardiac mass or tumor. All of these structures have characteristic echocardiographic features, and a thorough echocardiographic examination should be able to distinguish each from an intracardiac mass or tumor.

12. **Answer: B.** A large, mobile, heterogeneous mass in the left atrium with a stalk attachment to the fossa ovalis is most likely a myxoma. Myxomas can be smooth or rough and can have thrombi attached to them leading to fragments breaking off and embolizing. The differential diagnosis would be a left atrial thrombus, so further imaging is needed. Angiosarcomas (answer A) are also heterogeneous and may have an area of hemorrhage but are not attached by a stalk and may also have pericardial involvement. Papillary fibroelastomas (answer C) tend to be small, mobile, and homogeneous in appearance and are usually attached to left-sided cardiac valves by a small stalk, but these benign tumors can be seen elsewhere in the heart. Renal cell carcinomas (answer D) enter the heart through the inferior vena cava and are solid masses.

13. **Answer: D.** The "structure" most likely represents a dislodged deep venous thrombus (DVT). When a DVT embolizes, it travels directly into the heart via the IVC. When it becomes entangled within the tricuspid valve apparatus, it may be seen on the echocardiogram. This migratory thrombus appears very mobile. The patient's recent travel history along with symptoms of possible lower extremity DVT are very strong indicators that this is a thrombus.

Leiomyosarcomas (answer A) are rarely seen in the RA and are not typically highly mobile. Myxomas (answer B) are usually attached to the fossa

ovalis and are more round or oval shaped. Renal cell carcinomas (answer C) also originate from the IVC, but given the patient's presentation, a thrombus is more likely.

14. **Answer: C.** Following acute pulmonary embolism (APE), the RV is unable to generate pressures more than 40 to 50 mm Hg. In addition, there is a marked shortening of the RV acceleration time (RVAT) due to the sudden increase in afterload caused by an APE. Therefore, an RVAT ≤60 ms in addition to a tricuspid regurgitant (TR) pressure gradient ≤60 mm Hg is referred to as the "60/60 sign" (**Figure 24-9**). This sign is specific but not sensitive for an APE. Note that it is the TR pressure gradient, not the right ventricular systolic pressure (RVSP), that is considered for the "60/60" sign.

Answer A is a true statement since flattening and paradoxical motion of the interventricular septum (IVS) is seen in patients with an APE due to severe dilatation of the RV and underfilling of the LV (Video 24-15A). Answer B is a true statement. An APE causes an acute increase in RV afterload, and this results in midsystolic notching on the RVOT Doppler signal (see **Figure 24-9**, left). Answer D is a true statement. RV free wall akinesis with preserved apical function, also known as the McConnell sign, has been described in patients with APE (**Video 24-15B**). In particular, the presence of both the "60/60 sign" and McConnell sign are reliable but not sensitive signs of APE.

15. **Answer: B.** Laminated thrombus can be very difficult to detect on some echocardiograms even with the use of a UEA. The laminated thrombus can be difficult to distinguish from the true myocardium and may not be well seen due to the field of view or may be mistaken for normal myocardial wall tissue in an otherwise thinned and akinetic myocardium. Laminated thrombus is best ruled out using a UEA with multiple off-axis imaging views in addition to

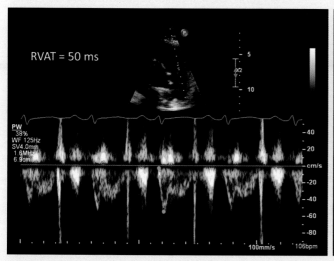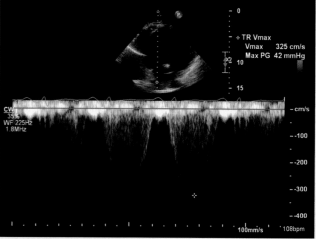

Figure 24-9 The "60/60" sign in a case of acute pulmonary embolism. The RV acceleration time (RVAT) is ≤60 ms and the TR pressure gradient (TR maxPG) is ≤60 mm Hg. Midsystolic notching is also seen on the right ventricular outflow tract (RVOT) trace (left).

the normal apical views. Decreasing the depth or utilizing the zoom feature is also helpful. Increasing the transducer frequency, changing the B-mode color hues, and moving the focal zone to the apex are necessary adjustments that can help tease out a laminated apical thrombus.

16. **Answer: C.** Left ventricular (LV) thrombi may be laminated, pedunculated, or mobile. This LV thrombus appears pedunculated in that it appears to hang by a thread to the LV apex. Although small in comparison to the LV, as this thrombus is protruding into the cavity, is very mobile, and has only a thin string-like attachment to the LV apex, there is a very high risk of embolization. Potential for embolization depends on the size, degree of protrusion, and mobility of the thrombus. For example, the likelihood of embolization is greater for thrombi that are either pedunculated or mobile and is highest when the thrombus is both pedunculated and mobile as in this case.

17. **Answer: D.** This mass appears to be embedded within the LV intramural layers of the inferolateral and inferior LV walls. This mass is possibly an intramural tumor such as a fibroma or rhabdomyoma. On the echocardiogram, a fibroma usually appears as a distinct, well-demarcated, noncontractile and solid, highly echogenic mass within the myocardium. The most common locations for fibromas are the LV lateral wall and right ventricular free wall or the interventricular septum. A rhabdomyoma can occur within a cavity as a pedunculated mass or may be embedded within the myocardium. These tumors usually involve the LV free wall and are associated with ventricular arrhythmias. On echocardiography, rhabdomyomas appear as well circumscribed, homogeneous masses with acoustic properties similar to the myocardium. The distinction between fibromas and rhabdomyomas can be made via computed tomography and/or cardiac magnetic resonance imaging.

Answer A is not correct since the mass clearly appears to be located within the LV myocardium and not outside the heart. Answer B is not correct as this mass does not protrude into the LV cavity. Answer C is unlikely as there is no history of previous cardiac disease and the LV size and function are normal.

18. **Answer: A.** Anatomic normal variants are frequently confused with pathological structures. Frequently fatty infiltration in the atrioventricular groove around the tricuspid valve (TV) is often mistaken for tumor. On echocardiography, fatty filtration appears echo-bright as in this example. This patient was sent for cardiac magnetic resonance imaging to better evaluate the structure. The results reported a benign condition of right ventricular (RV) free wall invagination with prominent, overlying epicardial fat, which resulted in a reduction of the TV annulus size. It was thought to be related to the patient's pectus deformity. The patient's symptoms were related to her HOCM with a significant left ventricular outflow tract obstruction due to systolic anterior motion of the mitral valve.

Answer B is not correct as a TV papillary fibroelastoma (PFE) is almost always found on the right atrial side of the tricuspid valve. Typically, PFEs are small and usually circular in shape; however, giant PFEs have been reported. On the echocardiographic examination, PFEs characteristically appear as small, round, homogeneous masses attached to the valve. Most commonly, PFEs are attached to the valve via a stalk, and therefore, they display highly mobile and independent motion.

Answer C is not correct. While tricuspid annular calcification is possible, there is an absence of acoustic shadowing distal to the mass, making calcification unlikely.

Answer D is not correct. A myxoma is usually connected to the interatrial septum by a short stalk and most commonly these tumors are found in the left atrium. On echocardiography, myxomas typically appear globular and finely speckled, not echobright as in this case.

19. **Answer: B.** It is essential to search for evidence of ongoing infection whenever a vegetation is suspected. Endocarditis can manifest as an abscess and/or a fistula, but the most common and direct evidence of endocarditis is the finding of a vegetation on a valve or valve apparatus. An echocardiographic characteristic of a vegetation is an attachment to the *upstream* side of the heart valves; that is, the ventricular side for the semilunar valves and the atrial side for the atrioventricular valves. Other characteristic features include an amorphous, irregular shape (answer A), a density similar to that of soft tissue (answer B), and high mobility (answer D). Vegetations come in all sizes and can have separate mobile attachments. Vegetations can be sessile or pedunculated but almost always have a motion pattern independent of the valve itself. The absence of mobility may indicate a healed vegetation. Fungal vegetations tend to be much larger than bacterial vegetations. Vegetations can also grow on indwelling catheters, pacemaker wires, and prosthetic valve sewing rings as well as on chamber walls or chordae attachments.

20. **Answer: A.** This mass measuring 1.6 cm × 1.8 cm is circular in shape and appears to have an echolucent center. The echolucency and thin border suggest a blood-filled cyst. The mass is attached to the tip of the anterior mitral valve leaflet and appears to "ping pong" back and forth with each cardiac cycle, an obvious risk for embolization. Transesophageal echocardiography and cardiac magnetic resonance imaging (MRI) were also performed to help delin-

eate this mass. The cardiac MRI reported "a benign-appearing intracavitary mass attached to the tip of the anterolateral papillary muscle as it gives rise to the chordae of the anterior mitral valve. Pedunculated and gelatinous appearing, malleable but solid, highly mobile, with no evidence of malignancy, including neovascularity or pericardial effusion. There was no evidence of fibrosis to suggest a myxoma on cardiac MRI."

Small blood-filled cysts of the heart valves have been observed postmortem on infant exams, but a large cyst found in an adult is extremely rare. This cyst was removed surgically, and a mitral valve repair was performed.

Thrombus (answer B) would be an unusual finding in a nonsymptomatic healthy individual with normal left ventricular (LV) ejection fraction. Schistosomiasis (answer C) is a disease caused by parasitic worms in freshwater snails that affect the bladder and other organs in humans; the primary cardiopulmonary manifestation of this disease is pulmonary arterial hypertension. Lipoma (answer D) is a rare benign cardiac primary tumor typically found in the right atrium and LV; these tumors originate in the subendocardium 50% of the time and can be identified by an increased T1 signal on cardiac MRI.

21. **Answer: D.** Mitral annular calcification (MAC) is commonly seen in the elderly and considered part of normal cardiac aging; it is also one of the most common findings found on autopsy. MAC, more common in females than males, can be seen in younger adults with advanced renal disease and other metabolic disorders that result in abnormal calcium metabolism. Sonographically, MAC is easily recognizable as increased accumulation of calcium, primarily involving the posterior aspect of the annulus. Caseous calcification of the mitral annulus (CCMA) or mitral annular liquification is a rare and benign variant of MAC. As MAC progresses to CCMA, the MAC becomes rounded in shape with smooth edges and appears to have an echolucent or liquid center on echocardiography. The contents of the cavity have been described as "toothpaste-like" or a "putty-like" mixture of fatty acids, cholesterol, and calcium. Studies have shown that some patients with CCMA recalcify. CCMA is seen rarely on echocardiography and, when identified, is perhaps best appreciated by transesophageal echocardiography. Sonographers should have the knowledge to recognize and identify CCMA. CCMA may be differentiated from MAC (answer B) based on central areas of echolucency.

The nodules of Arantius (answer A) are small nodules usually found on the free margin of the aortic and pulmonic valves. Lambl's excrescences (answer C) are thin, mobile, string-like echo densities most commonly seen on the mitral (atrial surface) and aortic (ventricular surface) valves. CCMA may mimic a paravalvular abscess (answer E), but usually the clinical presentation of an abscess would include signs associated with infection.

22. **Answer: D.** Considering the clinical setting, location, and appearance, this is a thrombus in transit and the source of cardiac emboli. Clinically, this is also the most likely diagnosis in a patient 2 weeks post total knee replacement. As previously discussed, thrombus formation is most likely to occur during conditions of blood stasis, vessel wall injury, and hypercoagulability.

Adipose tissue or fat (answer A) is usually seen near the tricuspid valve in the atrioventricular groove and may accumulate in the left and right atrial walls or in the interatrial septum (IAS) in cases of lipomatous hypertrophy.

A Chiari network (answer B) and the eustachian valve (answer C) are normal variants commonly mistaken for a mass, vegetation, or thrombus. These structures are found in the RA near the inferior vena cava (IVC). On the echocardiographic examination, the eustachian valve appears as a mobile linear structure stretching from the orifice of the IVC to the IAS. The Chiari network displays a more erratic motion during the cardiac cycle. This "network" appears as small moving targets with fast chaotic motion within the RA.

A vegetation (answer E) is a possible correct answer but there is no clinical suggestion that bacterial endocarditis should be considered in this situation. Keep in mind that clinical data often supply needed information about the identity of a cardiac mass discovered on imaging.

23. **Answer: D.** To improve visualization at the LV apex, the highest transducer frequency that still allows for adequate penetration should be employed (for example, frequencies between 5-7 MHz).

Moving the focal zone to the apex in zoom mode (answer A) and imaging at a shallow depth setting (answer D) will improve the spatial resolution at the apex. Off-axis imaging (answer C) can bring into view a small thrombus that is not visible in the standard apical views. A recently formed fresh thrombus may not be echogenic under normal circumstances and could be missed if a UEA is not used. Therefore, in the setting of poor LV contractility, a recent anterior ST segment elevation myocardial infarction (STEMI), or other clinical predictors for apical thrombus, it is recommended that a commercially available UEA be administered even when good endocardial border visualization is present (answer E).

24. **Answer: E.** Libman-Sacks endocarditis (LSE) is a nonbacterial thrombotic endocarditis (NBTE), and therefore, blood cultures will be negative (answer E is correct).

Answer A is a true statement as LSE is often referred to as verrucous (wart-like) endocarditis (or marantic or NBTE). Answers B and C are true statements as LSE may occur in patients with auto-immune diseases such as systemic lupus erythematosus and antiphospholipid syndrome with positive antiphospholipid antibodies.

TEACHING POINT

NBTE typically affects only the left-sided heart valves and can cause valvular dysfunction and may embolize. Most of the lesions are found on the mitral valve either at the base, middle, or tip of the leaflets. On the aortic valve, lesions are particular to the aortic side of the valve. These vegetations are rarely found on the right-sided valves. A distinguishing feature of these vegetations is valvular thickening and regurgitation, rarely stenosis. NBTE vegetations do not move as erratically as vegetations associated with infective endocarditis (IE) and the clinical presentation is different from in patients with IE. Patients with NBTE are typically asymptomatic until embolization occurs. The vegetations in NBTE consist of thrombi interwoven with strands of fibrin and thrombotic deposits on the valves, which can lead to valvular fibrosis and scarring.

25. **Answer: B.** Taking into consideration the location, size, features, and clinical history, this mass is most likely a RA myxoma, a benign primary cardiac tumor. In this example, the myxoma appears attached to or near the septal tricuspid valve leaflet. The motion of the mass is very dramatic as it prolapses through the open tricuspid valve into the right ventricle (RV) during diastole and pops back into the RA during systole. Doppler examination across the tricuspid valve will yield waveforms that mimic tricuspid stenosis. On auscultation, a tumor plop may be appreciated. Symptoms may include fever, malaise, symptoms of embolic events such dyspnea and chest pain, and symptoms of valve obstruction such as abdominal discomfort and a fluttering discomfort in the neck (caused by tall "a" waves in the jugular venous pulse).

A renal cell carcinoma (answer A) would present with a different clinical scenario, and the mass would be seen entering from the inferior vena cava into the RA. This mass would not be considered typical for an RA thrombus (answer C), as normal RA function exists, plus there is no history of atrial fibrillation or a previous pulmonary vein antral ablation procedure. Papillary fibroelastoma (answer D) is a potential differential diagnosis. PFEs are usually seen on the RA side of the tricuspid valve as in this example. While PFEs range in size from 8 to 40 mm, they are usually not this large. Furthermore, in this example, the mass appears multilobular which fits with an RA myxoma rather than a PFE.

TEACHING POINTS

Myxomas arise from the area of the fossa ovalis by a short stalk in the LA 75% of the time, 18% in the RA, 4% in the RV, and 4% in the LV. On echocardiography, myxomas often appear as gelatinous-appearing masses that can be globular, ovoid, or multilobular and they often have an echolucent center, and sometimes areas of calcification are seen. Myxomas generally have smooth well-defined edges and present as a singular mass. Multiple small myxomas forming a cluster have been described as having protruding fronds or a "cluster of grapes" appearance. A myxoma can be an incidental finding on an echocardiogram ordered for a different clinical indication.

26. ▶ **Answer: A.** Pedunculated is the best answer choice. A mass such as this is said to be pedunculated if it is supported by a peduncle, which is a narrow stalk of tissue. This tumor shows a pedunculated motion very descriptive for myxomas and the cause of the "tumor plop" heard on auscultation. The mass prolapses in diastole through the open tricuspid valve and then swings back into the right atrium during systole. There is a slight pause after the tricuspid valve opens before the tumor is "sucked up" through the valve in diastole. This motion can be recorded on M-mode trace and may help in displaying the motion of the myxoma (**Figures 24-10A** and **24-10B**). An example of a large left atrial myxoma prolapsing through the mitral valve is shown in **Video 24-16**.

27. **Answer: D.** The patient was being evaluated due to a possible TIA and hypertension. There is a mobile mass attached to the right atrial side of the tricuspid valve; this appearance is most consistent with a papillary fibroelastoma (PFE). Papillary fibroelastomas are typically small, highly mobile spherical masses attached to valves. PFE can occur on any valve but tends to favor the aortic and mitral valves. PFE can also occur attached to the atria walls, chordae, and/

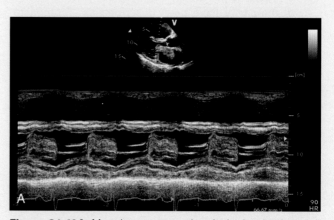

Figure 24-10A M-mode trace across the mitral valve showing a left atrial myxoma prolapsing through the mitral valve during diastole.

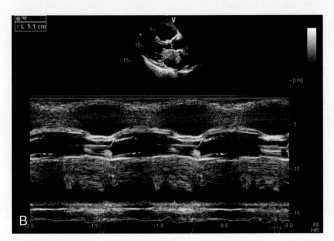

Figure 24-10B M-mode trace through the aorta and left atrium (LA) showing an LA myxoma within the LA cavity.

or papillary muscles and may be supported by a short stalk. PFE usually presents as a single mass, but there have been reports of multiple PFEs documented. If clinical symptoms of embolization are present, the PFE may be surgically removed. Yearly follow-up serial echocardiograms in this patient have documented no change in the PFE size or further accounts of TIA. The patient remains otherwise asymptomatic.

Answers A and B are not correct. Nodules of Arantius are small nodules found at the central coaptation area on semilunar valves. Lambl's excrescences are very small, thin, mobile linear echoes seen on the downstream side of a valve, most commonly the aortic valve.

Answer C is not correct. While the appearance of a PFE may be like a vegetation, the clinical scenario will not be the same. Furthermore, unlike vegetations, PFE have rounded edges. They are usually very mobile and may appear to "oscillate." This patient had no symptoms or clinical indication of infection, fever, or chills; therefore, a valvular vegetation due to bacterial endocarditis is not likely.

28. **Answer: B.** The images provided show an echogenic, independently mobile mass measuring 3.5 cm × 1.8 cm that appears to be attached to the pacemaker lead. It is serpentine in appearance and extends to the IVC. Although statements B, C, and D may be possible, the best answer in this clinical scenario is B. There is no mention of fever or infection or indications of endocarditis. The mass attached to the pacemaker wire is likely a thrombus, especially considering the underlying dilated cardiomyopathy and reduced RV contractility. Clinically, there is no mention of deep vein thrombosis (DVT) or a known reason to suspect a venous embolization. Answer A is not correct. Although thrombus can be seen on an indwelling central line due to RA wall injury, there is no mention of this patient having a central line in situ.

29. **Answer: A.** Based on the location of this structure in the right atrium (RA) near the RA-inferior vena cava (IVC) junction and the web-like appearance and hypermobility of this structure on the real-time image, it is most likely a Chiari network. Chiari network is thought to be a variant of the eustachian valve. The eustachian valve (answer E) is a remnant of the embryologic valve responsible for directing IVC blood across the foramen ovale in the interatrial septum to the left atrium. Lack of normal regression can result in a persistent eustachian valve. The Chiari network and eustachian valve can be differentiated echocardiographically by the "web-like" appearance and characteristic chaotic, random motion of the former. Both the Chiari network and eustachian valve are normal variants and should not be confused with tricuspid vegetations, flail leaflets, tumor, or thrombus. The crista terminalis (answer B) is a C-shaped fibromuscular ridge that divides the trabeculated RA appendage from the smooth-walled RA cavity. When prominent, this structure can protrude into the RA cavity and may resemble an intracardiac mass. Pectinate muscles (answer D) are prominent parallel ridges of atrial muscle that originate from the crista terminalis and are located within the atrial appendages. RA pectinate muscles are not normally seen on the transthoracic echocardiogram. Cor triatriatum dexter (answer C) is not a variant of normal anatomy but rather a rare congenital heart anomaly where the RA is divided into two chambers by a membrane.

KEY POINT

There are a number of normal RA variants that may be mistaken for pathologic masses, tumors, vegetations, or thrombus. Knowledge of the location and typical echocardiographic appearance of each normal RA variant will aid in the distinction of these masses from each other and from pathology.

30. **Answer: B.** Computed tomography is the imaging modality of choice in the evaluation of mediastinal lesions. CT has the capability to determine the exact location of the mediastinal tumor/mass, as well as its relationship to adjacent structures. CT is useful in differentiating masses that originate in the mediastinum from those that encroach upon the mediastinum from the lung or other structures. CT scans are highly accurate in differentiating fluid, fat, calcification, and cysts from solid tumors. CT may be used to assess the degree of vascularity of mediastinal tumors and in differentiating various tissue attenuations. Ultrasound (answer C) is being used more frequently in the pediatric population as it is highly sensitive in determining a cystic mass from a solid mediastinal mass and avoids radiation exposure. MRI (answer D) is mostly used as an adjunct to CT for evaluation of mediastinal tumors/masses.

MRI may provide additional information about the nature, location, and extent of disease. MRI has been found to be accurate for evaluation of superior vena cava syndrome and/or mediastinal and thoracic-inlet venous obstruction caused by mediastinal tumors. Conventional chest X-rays (answer A), often obtained for other reasons, frequently discover mediastinal masses as an incidental finding. The lateral view can often identify in which compartment of the mediastinum the mass lies (anterior compartment in this case) and may provide clues to pathology.

31. **Answer: E.** Approximately 95% of teratomas and other germ cell tumors arise in the anterior, not posterior, mediastinum. The anterior mediastinum or anterior compartment extends from the posterior surface of the sternum to the anterior surface of the pericardium and great vessels. It normally contains the thymus gland, adipose tissue, and lymph nodes. Germ cell tumors may be found incidentally in otherwise asymptomatic patients; those with seminomatous involvement are usually symptomatic (about 1/3 of patients). Teratomas are a type of germ cell tumor, and germ cell tumors may be malignant or benign depending on origin.

32. **Answer: C.** The TEE image provided shows an LAA thrombus (**Figure 24-11A**, arrow). Specific PWD flow patterns, reflecting LAA function, have been characterized for normal sinus rhythm and various abnormal cardiac rhythms. When performed correctly, these PWD patterns of the LAA can identify when a high risk of thrombus formation is likely. The positive reflection immediately after the P wave on the electrocardiogram (or just prior to the QRS complex when the patient is in atrial fibrillation or atrial flutter) reflects the late diastolic emptying velocity, which is believed to result from LAA contraction and is thus a marker of LAA contractile function **Figure 24-11B**). Normal values are >50 cm/s; a value <20 cm/s is

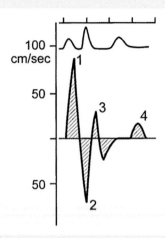

Figure 24-11B Diagram of left atrial appendage (LAA) flow in sinus rhythm. 1, LAA contraction (LAA emptying velocity); 2, LAA filling; 3, systolic reflection waves (positive and negative); 4, early diastolic LAA outflow. (Reprinted from Agmon Y, Khandheria BK, Gentile F, et al. Echocardiographic assessment of the left atrial appendage. *J Am Coll Cardiol.* 1999;34(7):1867-1877. Copyright © 1999 American College of Cardiology. With permission.)

considered abnormal and at risk for thrombus formation. In this patient, as there is LAA thrombus, the PEV will be decreased; therefore, answer C is correct.

TECHNICAL POINTS

As previously discussed, the TEE midesophageal 2-chamber view and the midesophageal aortic valve short-axis view are best for imaging the LAA (see the answer outline for Question 2). For the PWD examination of the LAA, the sample volume (SV) should be placed within the proximal one-third of the LAA, toward the left atrium, with care taken to avoid artifact from the LAA wall (**Figure 24-11C**). The signals are optimized by keeping the Doppler gains low and SV parallel to flow; the LAA PEV is identified just after the P wave on the electrocardiogram or just prior to the QRS complex when the patient is in atrial fibrillation or atrial flutter (**Figure 24-11D**, arrows).

KEY POINTS

The LAA is a common source of cardiac thrombus formation associated with systemic embolism. TEE allows a detailed evaluation of the structure and function of the LAA by 2D imaging and spectral Doppler interrogation of appendage flow. Specific flow patterns, reflecting LAA function, have been characterized for normal sinus rhythm and various abnormal cardiac rhythms. LAA dysfunction has been associated with LAA spontaneous echocardiographic contrast, thrombus formation, and thromboembolism. These associations have been studied extensively in patients with atrial fibrillation or atrial flutter, in patients undergoing cardioversion of atrial arrhythmias, and in patients with mitral valve disease.

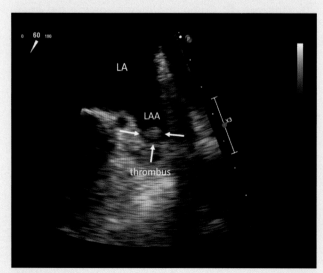

Figure 24-11A

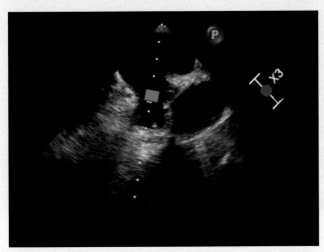

Figure 24-11C Placement for pulsed-wave Doppler sample position in LAA for flow assessment of thrombus risk.

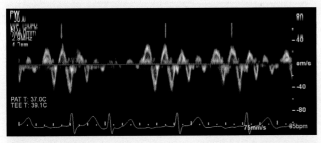

Figure 24-11D

33. Answer: D. A mobile protruding LV mass with perfusion and a negative bubble study is the best description of the series of images displayed. During the bubble study (**Video 24-11B**),

no bubbles cross into the left heart, indicating no shunt is detected on echo. On the image with the UEA (**Video 24-11C**), contrast is seen surrounding the mass and at times seen between the mass and the LV myocardium, indicating that the mass is not totally attached to the LV wall. It is easy to see movement of the mass as it protrudes further into the LV cavity during each cardiac cycle. The mass appears nonhomogeneous prior to contrast administration (**Video 24-11A**), with minimal contrast uptake predominantly in the section of the mass from 9 to 11 o'clock (**Video 24-11C**). The mass uptake is minimal in comparison to the amount of perfusion (uptake) occurring in the myocardium of the septum. Imaging with very low mechanical index (VLMI) software using flash (to clear the myocardium and mass from the UEA) would give a better evaluation of the true uptake. VLMI imaging with flash software was not available on the system at the time of this study. This mass was thought to be a thrombus, as the LV was dilated with significantly depressed LV ejection fraction (25%) and moderately decreased right ventricular systolic function.

TEACHING POINT

A laminated mass is often difficult to detect on standard echocardiography as it may just appear as increased wall thickness. A UEA can be used to bring out the difference in the wall layers and thrombus. Other LV thrombus and masses can be described as protruding, laminar (layered), globular (cluster of grapes), pedunculated (back and forth), and embedded.

SUGGESTED READINGS

Agmon Y, Khandheria BK, Gentile F, Seward JB. Echocardiographic assessment of the left atrial appendage. *J Am Coll Cardiol.* 1999;34(7):1867-1877.

Anderson B. Infective endocarditis and cardiac masses. In: *A Sonographer's Guide to the Assessment of Heart Disease.* Brisbane: MGA Graphics; 2014:chap 13.

Bruce CJ. Cardiac tumours: diagnosis and management. *Heart.* 2011;97(2):151-160.

Mankad R, Herrmann J. Cardiac tumors: echo assessment. *Echo Res Pract.* 2016;3(4):R65-R77.

Klarich KW, Oh JK, Maleszewski JJ. Cardiac tumors and masses. In: Oh JK, Kane GC, eds. *The Echo Manual.* 4th ed. Philadelphia, PA and Rochester, MN: Wolters Kluwer and Mayo Foundation for Medical Education and Research; 2019:chap 19.

Porter TR, Mulvagh SL, Abdelmoneim SS, et al. Clinical applications of ultrasonic enhancing agents in echocardiography: 2018 American Society of Echocardiography Guidelines Update. *J Am Soc Echocardiogr.* 2018;31(3):241-274.

Saric M, Armour AC, Arnaout MS, et al. Guidelines for the use of echocardiography in the evaluation of a cardiac source of embolism. *J Am Soc Echocardiogr.* 2016;29(1):1-42.

Silvestry FE, Cohen MS, Armsby LB, et al. Guidelines for the echocardiograpic assessment of atrial septal defect and patent foramne ovale: from the American Society of Echocardiography and Society for Cardiac Angiography and Interventions. *J Am Soc Echocardiogr.* 2015;28(8):910-958.

CHAPTER 25

Pericardial Disease

Contributors: Merri L. Bremer, EdD, RN, ACS, RDCS and Amy Dillenbeck, MS, ACS, RDCS

✪ Question 1

The pericardium is a membranous sac that consists of multiple layers. Which of the following layers of the pericardium is also known as the epicardium?

A. Visceral
B. Fibrous
C. Serous
D. Parietal

✪ Question 2

Under normal conditions, the pericardial space may contain up to which of the following amounts of fluid?

A. 25 mL
B. 50 mL
C. 100 mL
D. 150 mL

✪✪ Question 3

The serous pericardium is invaginated by the heart and great vessels. Reflections of the serous pericardium form sinuses and recesses. Which pericardial sinus/recess is indicated by the arrow in this transesophageal echocardiographic (TEE) image (**Figure 25-1**)?

A. Postcaval
B. Oblique
C. Superior
D. Transverse

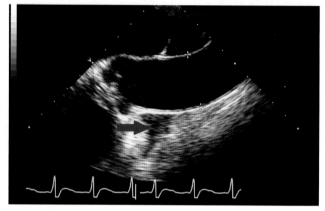

Figure 25-1

✪✪ Question 4

In **Figure 25-2**, which pericardial sinus/recess is indicated by the asterisk (*)?

A. Postcaval
B. Oblique
C. Superior
D. Transverse

✪✪ Question 5

Of the following, which is the most common cause of acute pericarditis in the "Western" world?

A. Autoimmune
B. Traumatic
C. Idiopathic
D. Neoplastic

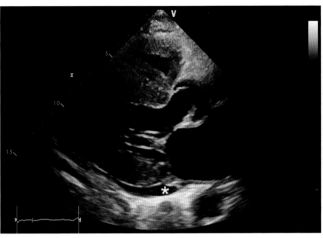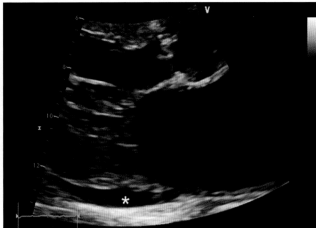

Figure 25-2

✪ Question 6

Which of the following is the echocardiographic finding that most supports the diagnosis of acute pericarditis?

A. Thickened pericardium
B. Patchy left ventricular (LV) dysfunction
C. Pericardial effusion
D. Decrease in LV ejection fraction

✪ Question 7

Which of the following is an echocardiographic feature of a pericardial cyst?

A. It is commonly located behind the atrium.
B. It is usually located at the cardiophrenic angle.
C. It is usually located near the left or right atria apex.
D. It is usually located near the transverse sinus.

✪✪✪ Question 8

▶ A 35-year-old male patient presents with intermittent nonexertional chest pain. During his transthoracic echocardiogram (TTE), the following apical view (**Video 25-1**) was obtained. Which of the following is the most likely diagnosis?

A. Normal echocardiogram
B. Acute pericarditis
C. Absent pericardium
D. Pectus excavatum

✪✪✪ Question 9

Which of the following is most common in patients with congenital absence of the pericardium?

A. Absence of entire pericardium
B. Absence of right hemipericardium
C. Absence of left hemipericardium
D. Absence of lateral hemipericardium

✪✪ Question 10

▶ How is the labeled portion (white arrow) of this parasternal long-axis image in **Video 25-2** best described?

A. Epicardial fat pad
B. Small anterior transudative pericardial effusion
C. Small anterior exudative pericardial effusion
D. No pericardial effusion, no epicardial fat pad

✪✪✪ Question 11

▶ A 53-year-old woman presents to the emergency department (ED) with chest pain and shortness of breath. She has a history of metastatic adenocarcinoma of the lung. A transthoracic echocardiogram was performed (**Videos 25-3A to 25-3D**). Which of the following best describes the findings?

A. Loculated hemorrhagic pericardial effusion
B. Circumferential hemorrhagic pericardial effusion
C. Large transudative pericardial effusion
D. Bilateral pleural effusions

✪✪ Question 12

There can be significant variability of pericardial fluid in location and linear dimension throughout the cardiac cycle. According to the 2013 ASE Guidelines on Multimodality Imaging of Pericardial Disease, a moderate pericardial effusion will measure _____ at _____.

A. 15 to 20 mm; end-diastole
B. 10 to 20 mm; end-systole
C. >20 mm; end-systole
D. 10 to 20 mm; end-diastole

✪✪ Question 13

The labeled portion (white arrow) of the two-dimensional echocardiographic image in **Figure 25-3** is consistent with:

- **A.** Pleural effusion.
- **B.** Pericardial effusion.
- **C.** Pericardial cyst.
- **D.** Mediastinal cyst.

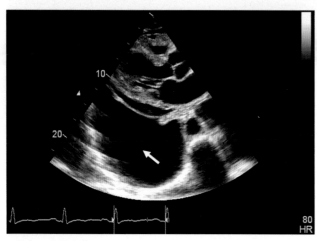

Figure 25-3

✪✪ Question 14

▶ A 35-year-old woman presented with shortness of breath for 1 week. Chest X-ray showed cardiomegaly (cardiac-thoracic ratio of 65%) and a left-sided pleural effusion. Her echocardiogram revealed a large pericardial effusion. She underwent an echo-guided pericardiocentesis. Part of the procedure is shown in **Video 25-4**. The echocardiogram is consistent with:

- **A.** Blood coagulum in the pericardial cavity.
- **B.** Spontaneous echo contrast in the pericardial cavity.
- **C.** Identification of a pericardial-pleural fistula.
- **D.** Injection of agitated saline contrast.

✪✪✪ Question 15

In which of the following clinical scenarios does the presence of pericardial effusion **most** imply a poor prognosis?

- **A.** Chronic renal failure
- **B.** Acute heart failure
- **C.** Pulmonary arterial hypertension
- **D.** Constrictive pericarditis

✪✪ Question 16

Cardiac tamponade occurs when:

- **A.** Intrapericardial pressure increases and causes impaired ventricular filling.
- **B.** Intrapericardial pressure decreases and causes impaired ventricular filling.
- **C.** Intracardiac pressure increases and causes impaired ventricular filling.
- **D.** Intracardiac pressure decreases and causes impaired ventricular filling.

✪✪✪ Question 17

Tachycardia and elevated jugular venous pressure (JVP) are frequently noted with cardiac tamponade. With which of the following are these clinical signs **most consistent**?

- **A.** Compensatory response to increased cardiac filling
- **B.** Excessive stimulation of the sympathetic nervous system
- **C.** Excessive stimulation of the parasympathetic nervous system
- **D.** Compensatory response to decreased cardiac filling

✪✪ Question 18

With normal physiology, right heart filling typically increases during inspiration and decreases during expiration, while left heart filling shows minimal variation. Cardiac tamponade causes an exaggeration of this normal variation in filling and may be manifested clinically as which of the following?

- **A.** Pulsus alternans
- **B.** Pulsus paradoxus
- **C.** Pulsus bisferiens
- **D.** Pulsus parvus et tardus

✪✪ Question 19

Which of the following clinical scenarios is most likely to present with signs and symptoms of **acute** cardiac tamponade?

- **A.** 50-year-old internal medicine patient with untreated hypothyroidism
- **B.** 40-year-old patient with renal failure being seen in the emergency department
- **C.** 60-year-old transplant patient status/post right ventricular biopsy
- **D.** 25-year-old hematology patient with a mediastinal mass

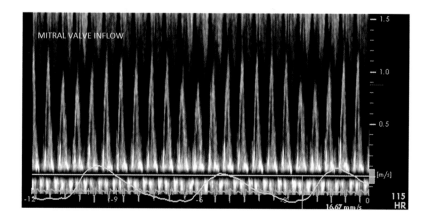

Figure 25-4

⊕⊕ Question 20

Which of the following is the single most useful parameter to exclude a hemodynamically significant pericardial effusion?
- **A.** Right atrial (RA) collapse
- **B.** Right ventricular (RV) free wall inversion
- **C.** Transmitral flow pulsed-wave (PW) Doppler respiratory variation
- **D.** Inferior vena cava (IVC) size

⊕ Question 21

The M-mode echocardiographic features shown in Figure 25-4 are suggestive of:
- **A.** A pleural effusion.
- **B.** Constrictive pericarditis.
- **C.** A large pericardial effusion.
- **D.** Cardiac tamponade.

⊕ Question 22

Transmitral and transtricuspid flow profiles shown in **Figure 25-5A, B** in a patient with a large pericardial effusion are suggestive of:
- **A.** Cardiac tamponade.
- **B.** Constrictive pericarditis.
- **C.** Normal respiratory variation.
- **D.** Accompanying pulmonary hypertension.

⊕⊕ Question 23

Which of the following may prevent right ventricular (RV) free wall diastolic collapse in a patient with a pericardial effusion?
- **A.** Rapid collection of the pericardial fluid
- **B.** A highly compliant pericardial sac
- **C.** Pulmonary hypertension in cor pulmonale
- **D.** Congenital partial absence of the pericardium

Figure 25-5A

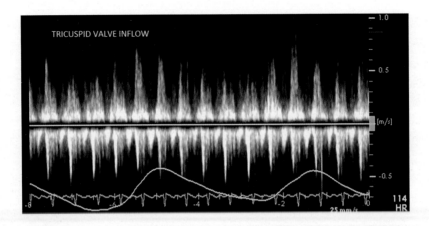

Figure 25-5B

✪✪✪ Question 24

What effect does mechanical ventilation have on spectral Doppler findings in cardiac tamponade?

  A. During positive-pressure ventilation, the respiratory variation on the spectral Doppler examination is opposite to the usual findings in cardiac tamponade.
  B. Positive-pressure ventilation has no effect on the spectral Doppler examination findings of a patient in cardiac tamponade.
  C. During positive-pressure ventilation, there is increased transmitral inflow respiratory variation.
  D. During positive-pressure ventilation, spectral Doppler analysis of the left ventricular outflow tract demonstrates an increase of inspiratory-to-expiratory variation of >25%.

✪✪✪ Question 25

A 63-year-old female with a history of end-stage renal disease and recent hemodialysis presents to the emergency department with fatigue and shortness of breath. The transthoracic echocardiogram reveals a moderate-sized, echo-free space adjacent to the right ventricle (RV) with diastolic RV chamber collapse, significant respiratory variation in the transmitral E wave velocity and isovolumic relaxation time, and a small inferior vena cava (IVC) that collapses >50% with inspiration. These echocardiographic findings are most consistent with:

  A. A pericardial cyst.
  B. Low-pressure cardiac tamponade.
  C. Classic cardiac tamponade.
  D. Effusive-constrictive pericarditis.

✪✪ Question 26

Cardiac tamponade is unique in patients with pulmonary hypertension. In this scenario, which of the following feature(s) is most commonly absent?

  A. Dilated IVC and hepatic veins
  B. Hypotension
  C. Pulsus paradoxus
  D. Right atrial (RA) and right ventricular (RV) chamber collapse

✪ Question 27

Currently, what is the most common etiology for constrictive pericarditis (CP) in developed countries?

  A. Radiation to the chest
  B. Previous pericarditis
  C. Neoplasm (primary or metastatic)
  D. Previous cardiac surgery

✪ Question 28

Which of the following auscultation findings is commonly associated with constrictive pericarditis?

  A. Pericardial rub
  B. Pericardial knock
  C. Pericardial honk
  D. Pleuropericardial rub

✪✪ Question 29

Enhanced respiratory variation of ventricular filling represents which pathophysiologic feature of constrictive pericarditis?

  A. Elevated ventricular filling pressure
  B. Enhanced ventricular interdependence
  C. Equalization of intrathoracic and extrathoracic pressures
  D. Intrathoracic and extrathoracic dissociation

✪ Question 30

Demonstration of which of the following is essential for the diagnosis of constrictive pericarditis (CP)?

A. Abnormal hemodynamics
B. Pericardial thickening/calcification
C. Pulmonary hypertension
D. Severe biatrial enlargement

✪✪ Question 31

Which of the following echocardiographic findings is common in both cardiac tamponade and constrictive pericarditis (CP)?

A. Diastolic right atrial compression
B. Diastolic right ventricular compression
C. Mitral annulus reversus (medial e' > lateral e')
D. Respiratory variation of interventricular septal (IVS) position and transmitral inflow profile

✪✪ Question 32

What is the suggested cutoff value of longitudinal early diastolic annular velocities for differentiating constrictive pericarditis (CP) from restrictive cardiomyopathy?

A. 4 cm/s
B. 8 cm/s
C. 15 cm/s
D. 12 cm/s

✪✪ Question 33

The M-mode echocardiogram shown in **Figure 25-6** (arrows 1 and 2) refers to the early diastolic motion of the interventricular septum and left ventricular posterior wall. This unique motion pattern is seen in which of the following pericardial diseases?

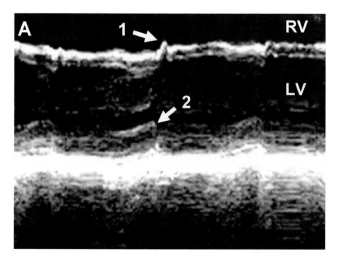

Figure 25-6

A. Absent pericardium
B. Cardiac tamponade
C. Chronic constrictive pericarditis
D. Chronic pericardial effusion

✪✪ Question 34

Figure 25-7 shows a pulsed-wave Doppler trace acquired from the hepatic vein. The features present on this trace are consistent with:

A. Expiratory diastolic flow reversals seen in acute pericarditis.
B. Expiratory diastolic flow reversals seen in chronic constrictive pericarditis (CP).
C. Inspiratory systolic flow augmentation seen in acute pericarditis.
D. Inspiratory systolic flow augmentation seen in chronic CP.

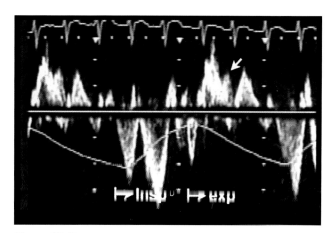

Figure 25-7

✪✪ Question 35

Which of the following is the Doppler finding that most reliably differentiates between chronic obstructive pulmonary disease (COPD) and constrictive pericarditis (CP)?

A. Hepatic vein flow
B. Mitral inflow velocity
C. Superior vena cava (SVC) flow
D. Tricuspid inflow velocity

✪✪✪ Question 36

A 75-year-old woman 6 months status post coronary artery bypass grafts presents with dyspnea, lower extremity edema, and jugular venous pressure elevation. On echocardiography, which of the following echocardiographic findings are most likely to be seen?

A. Flattened interventricular septum (IVS), E/A ratio = 0.9, medial e′ = 10 cm/s, lateral e′ = 12 cm/s, hepatic vein systolic flow reversal, dilated inferior vena cava (IVC).

B. Respirophasic ventricular septal motion, E/A ratio = 0.9 (variable velocity), medial e′ = 10 cm/s, lateral e′ = 12 cm/s, hepatic vein expiratory diastolic flow reversal, small IVC, exaggerated respiratory variation of superior vena cava (SVC) forward systolic flow.

C. Flattened IVS, E/A = 1.5, medial e′ = 3 cm/s, lateral e′ = 5 cm/s, hepatic vein inspiratory diastolic flow reversal, dilated IVC.

D. Respirophasic ventricular septal motion, E/A = 1.5 (variable velocity), medial e′ = 12 cm/s, lateral e′ = 10 cm/s, hepatic vein expiratory diastolic flow reversal, dilated IVC, minimal respiratory variation of SVC systolic forward flow.

CASE EXAMPLE

▶ A 22-year-old woman presented with shortness of breath and chest pain. Vital signs included blood pressure (BP) of 139/88 mm Hg, pulse rate of 130 bpm, respiratory rate of 40/min, and peripheral capillary oxygen saturation (SpO$_2$) of 100%. Her past medical history was remarkable for systemic lupus erythematosus and interstitial lung disease with pulmonary fibrosis. Her echocardiogram revealed a moderately large pericardial effusion around the right ventricle with evidence of cardiac tamponade physiology. She underwent successful pericardiocentesis and was sent home on Colchicine and Indocin. She returned 2 weeks later with recurrent symptoms and the echocardiogram was repeated (**Videos 25-5A** to **25-5D** and **Figures 25-14A to 25-14D**).

✪✪✪ Question 37

The echocardiogram is suggestive of:
A. Effusive-constrictive pericarditis.
B. Constrictive pericarditis.
C. A pericardial mass.
D. A pericardial effusion with hemodynamic compromise.

✪✪ Question 38

This case exhibits annulus paradoxus. To what does this term refer?
A. The relationship between the septal and lateral mitral annular velocities is reversed in patients with constrictive pericarditis (CP)
B. The reversal of the strong positive linear relationship between the pulmonary capillary wedge pressure (PCWP) and mitral E/e′ ratio in patients with CP
C. The reversal of the relationship between the transmitral inflow velocities and the transtricuspid inflow velocities with either CP or cardiac tamponade
D. The large decrease in stroke volume and systolic blood pressure during inspiration in patients with cardiac tamponade

✪✪ Question 39

During the imaging workup for differentiation between constrictive pericarditis (CP) and restrictive cardiomyopathy (RCM), the term annulus reversus on a tissue Doppler imaging (TDI) study reflects the:
A. Relationship between the septal and lateral mitral annular velocities, which are reversed in patients with CP.
B. Reversed relationship between E/e′ and left atrial (LA) pressure in patients with CP
C. Opposite of what happens in RCM whereby mitral annular velocities are increased in patients with CP.
D. Opposite of normal whereby mitral annular velocities change significantly in relation to respiration in patients with RCM.

✪✪✪ Question 40

Which of the following figures shows the characteristic strain pattern of constrictive pericarditis (CP)?
A. Figure 25-8A
B. Figure 25-8B
C. Figure 25-8C
D. Figure 25-8D

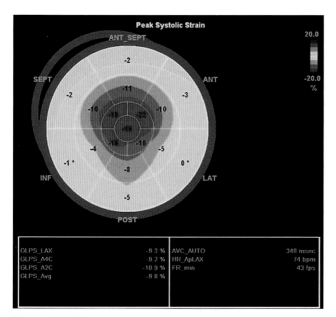

Figure 25-8A

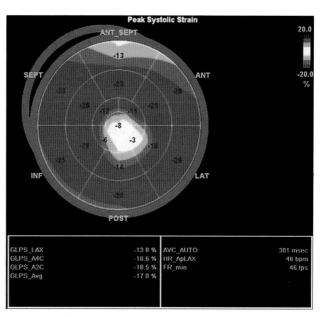

Figure 25-8B

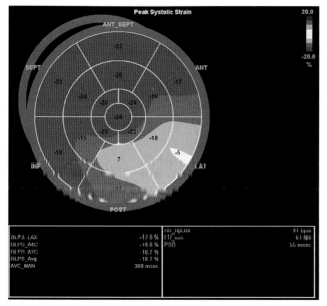

Figure 25-8C

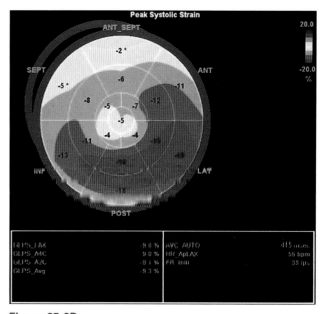

Figure 25-8D

ANSWERS

1. **Answer: A.** The normal pericardial sac consists of a thin outer fibrous layer and an inner serous layer that lines the pericardial cavity (**Figure 25-9**). The serous pericardium consists of two layers: the visceral pericardium (also known as the epicardium) and the parietal pericardium.

2. **Answer: B.** Typically, up to 50 mL of fluid is present in the pericardial space. Physiologic pericardial fluid acts as a lubricant to decrease friction between the parietal and visceral layers of the pericardium as the heart contracts.

3. **Answer: D.** The transverse sinus is tunnel-like. It is located posterior to the ascending aorta and main pulmonary trunk and anterior to the left atrium (LA); this is where the aorta and pulmonary artery leave the heart. On the TEE image, the transverse sinus is seen between the LA and the aorta (**Figure 25-10A**). The transverse sinus may also be seen on the transthoracic echocardiogram (TTE) (**Figure 25-10B**).

   The postcaval recess (answer A) is one of several pericardial recesses (or pockets) extending from or toward the transverse pericardial sinus; these

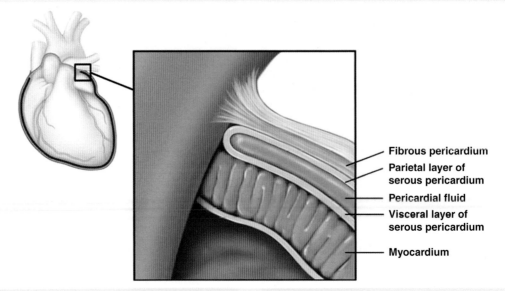

Fibrous pericardium

Parietal layer of
serous pericardium

Pericardial fluid

Visceral layer of
serous pericardium

Myocardium

Figure 25-9 (Reproduced with permission of the Cleveland Clinic Center for Continuing Education. Phelan D, Collier P, Grimm RA. Pericardial Disease. Disease management project. http://www.clevelandclinicmeded.com/medicalpubs/diseasemanagement/cardiology/pericardial-disease/. © 2000-2018 The Cleveland Clinic Foundation. All rights reserved.)

recesses are formed by reflections of the pericardium. The postcaval recess lies behind and on the right lateral aspect of the superior vena cava (SVC). It is separated from the transverse sinus by the reflection of the serous pericardium that covers the SVC across the right pulmonary artery and right superior pulmonary vein.

The oblique sinus (answer B) is the posterior extension of the pericardium and lies posterior to the LA and anterior to the esophagus; this is where the pulmonary veins and the inferior and superior venae cavae enter the heart. The superior sinus or superior aortic recess (answer C) is a pericardial recess that arises from the superior margin of the transverse pericardial sinus and lies between the SVC and the aorta. This recess surrounds the root of the ascending aorta and is indicated by the arrow in **Figure 25-10A.**

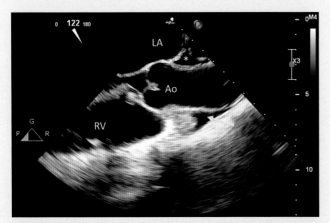

Figure 25-10A The transverse sinus is indicated by the *; the superior sinus or superior aortic recess is indicated by the arrow. Ao, aorta; LA, left atrium; RV, right ventricle.

KEY POINT
Several pericardial sinuses and recesses are formed by reflections of the serous pericardium (**Figure 25-11**). The identification of each is based on the anatomic location relative to the aorta, right and left pulmonary arteries, inferior and superior venae cavae, and the pulmonary veins. On the TTE, only the transverse and oblique sinuses are usually seen. On TEE, the transverse and oblique sinuses as well as the superior aortic recess may be seen.

4. **Answer: B.** As previously discussed, the oblique sinus is the posterior extension of the pericardium and lies posterior to the left atrium (LA) and anterior to the esophagus; this is where the pulmonary veins and the inferior and superior venae cavae enter the heart. Therefore, from the parasternal long-axis (PLAX) view, the oblique pericardial sinus is seen posterior to the LA and the atrioventricular groove. In this example, there is a small pericardial effusion present that highlights the oblique pericardial sinus.

   Answers A and C are not correct as these recesses will not be seen from the PLAX view. Answer D is not correct. From this PLAX view, the transverse sinus would be seen posterior to the aorta and anterior to the LA (see **Figure 25-10B**).

5. **Answer: C.** Acute pericarditis is characterized by inflammation of the pericardial sac. Most cases of pericarditis in Western Europe and North America are thought to be of viral etiology and are typically referred to as "idiopathic." Other causes of acute pericarditis include acute myocardial infarction, infections, malignancy, trauma, autoimmune disorders (such as rheumatoid arthritis, systemic lupus erythematosus, and systemic sclerosis), and inflammatory disorders (such as amyloidosis and sarcoidosis).

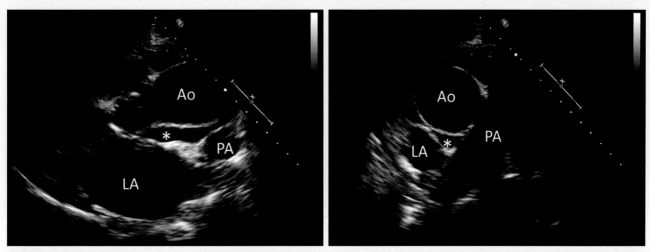

Figure 25-10B On TTE, the transverse sinus may be seen in the parasternal long-axis view (left) and the parasternal short-axis view (right). From these views, the transverse sinus is seen posterior to the aortic root (Ao) and anterior to the left atrium (LA). PA, pulmonary artery.

6   **Answer: C.** Most patients with acute pericarditis have unremarkable echocardiographic findings, although the presence of a thickened pericardium and pericardial effusion support the diagnosis. It is sometimes difficult to identify mild thickening of the pericardium with echocardiography, but the

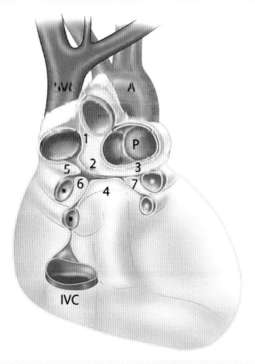

Figure 25-11 Drawing of interior of the serosal pericardial sac after resection of large vessels. A, aorta; P, pulmonary trunk; SVC, superior vena cava; IVC, inferior vena cava; *, pulmonary vein; 1, superior aortic recess of transverse sinus; 2, right pulmonic recess of transverse sinus; 3, left pulmonic recess of transverse sinus; 4, oblique sinus; 5, postcaval recess; 6, right pulmonary venous recess; 7, left pulmonary venous recess. (Reproduced from Shroff GS, Boonsirikamchai P, Viswanathan C, et al. Differentiating pericardial recesses from mediastinal adenopathy: potential pitfalls in oncological imaging. *Clin Radiol.* 2014;69(3):307-314. Copyright © 2013 The Royal College of Radiologists. With permission.)

presence of pericardial effusion is easily noted and is most helpful in this clinical setting.

7. **Answer: B.** The most common location of a pericardial cyst is in the right cardiophrenic angle; thus, these cysts are usually seen adjacent to the right atrium. On two-dimensional (2D) echocardiography, a pericardial cyst appears as an echo-free structure adjacent to the cardiac border. Pericardial cysts are typically 2 to 4 cm in diameter, although some may be larger (**Video 25-6**).

8. **Answer: C.** This image (**Video 25-1**) is consistent with typical echocardiographic findings in congenital absence of the pericardium. Patients with this rare disorder are typically asymptomatic, and the diagnosis is often made incidentally during cardiac imaging. Absence of the pericardium may be complete or partial. The most common echocardiographic findings may include an extremely lateral transducer position for the parasternal and apical windows, abnormal ventricular septal motion, exaggerated mobility of the heart due to loss of pericardial restraint, and the appearance of right-sided chamber enlargement due to levoposition of the heart. Elongation of the atria with widened, bulbous ventricles creates an inverted "tear-drop" shape of the heart.

9. **Answer: C.** Absence of the pericardium may be complete or partial, with left-sided absence being most common. Absence of the right hemopericardium and complete absence of the pericardium are uncommon. Congenital absence of the pericardium often occurs in isolation but can be associated with other congenital defects including atrial septal defect, bicuspid aortic valve, and bronchogenic cysts.

10. **Answer: A.** Spaces anterior to the heart are a common finding on transthoracic echocardiographic studies. Epicardial fat is typically more echogenic

than the myocardium, has a speckled or granular appearance, and tends to move with the heart.

11. **Answer: B.** 2D echocardiography differentiates whether a pericardial effusion is loculated (localized pocket) or circumferential (as in this case). Echocardiography can also differentiate some characteristics of pericardial fluid: transudative (consisting of watery fluid), exudative (made up of protein-rich fluid), and hemorrhagic (bloody pericardial effusion, fibrin strands, and clots). The images in this case reveal echogenic structures attached to the outer surface of both the left and right ventricles that are suggestive of thrombus. This finding and the clinical context support characterization of this effusion as hemorrhagic and possibly metastatic in nature. A transudative pericardial effusion (answer C) would more typically appear as an echo-free space because of its watery fluid appearance and lack of echogenic structures in the pericardial space. Exudative pericardial effusions most commonly occur secondary to infection, and on 2D echocardiography these effusions do not appear echo-free; these effusions may also show stranding, adhesions, or an uneven distribution. Pleural effusions (answer D) may mimic pericardial effusions. In this case, bilateral pleural effusions can be excluded as the effusion (pericardial) is seen anterior and posterior to the heart from the subcostal view (**Video 25-3D**).

12. **Answer: D.** By 2D echocardiography, a pericardial effusion is semiquantitatively described on the basis of the size of the echo-free space seen between the parietal and visceral layers of the pericardium at end-diastole: trivial (seen only in systole), small (<10 mm), moderate (10-20 mm), large (>20 mm), or very large (>25 mm).

13. **Answer: A.** Left pleural effusions can present as large echo-free spaces that resemble pericardial effusions. These can be recognized because they appear as very large posterior spaces without any anterior component. Generally, in the parasternal long-axis view, pleural effusions are located posterior to the descending thoracic aorta, whereas pericardial effusions are located anterior to the descending thoracic aorta. In **Figure 25-3**, a small pericardial effusion is also present posterior to the left ventricle and anterior to the descending thoracic aorta and the left pleural effusion.

14. **Answer: D.** A cross-sectional contrast echocardiogram showing the pericardial space containing a cloud of echogenic bubbles is seen. Although pericardiocentesis is a relatively safe procedure, there are hazards particularly suspected when hemorrhagic fluid is aspirated. Having the opportunity to outline the space from which the fluid is withdrawn is of particular interest in this situation. A current technique of echocardiography with contrast enhancement involves injection of a few milliliters of agitated saline solution. In the pericardium, contrast movement is slow and swirling and has a longer half-life. Performing this procedure helps in ensuring that the catheter is within the pericardial cavity and not within the cardiac chambers.

KEY POINT

Contrast echocardiography is a simple, effective technique that aids in localization of catheter position during pericardiocentesis.

15. **Answer: C.** The presence of even small pericardial effusions in patients with pulmonary arterial hypertension (PAH) is independently associated with poor survival. It is not well understood why pericardial effusion develops in some patients with PAH, although the mechanism is thought to be related to impaired fluid reabsorption by way of venous or lymphatic channels.

16. **Answer: A.** When sufficient pericardial fluid has accumulated so that intrapericardial pressure (IPP) exceeds diastolic intracardiac pressure, normal diastolic filling of the heart is impeded.

TEACHING POINT

In the normal situation, the intracardiac pressure (ICP) is usually positive and the IPP is negative (approximately the same as the intrathoracic pressure). Therefore, the transmural filling pressure (TMFP), which is the difference between the ICP and the IPP, is positive. This positive TMFP maintains the shape of the cardiac chambers and prevents them from collapsing at end-diastole when the ICP falls to zero.

In cardiac tamponade, the IPP is increased. As the IPP rises, the ICP also rises to maintain a positive TMFP and an adequate cardiac output. With further increases in the IPP there is a fall in the TMFP which results in impeded diastolic filling of the heart and a subsequent reduction in cardiac output. When the TMFP becomes negative, that is, when the IPP exceeds the ICP, there is collapse (compression) of the cardiac chambers.

17. **Answer: D.** In cardiac tamponade, central venous pressure (CVP) rises to maintain transmural filling pressure (TMFP) and to improve cardiac filling. Tachycardia is a compensatory measure to maintain or increase cardiac output in the setting of decreased cardiac filling resulting from cardiac tamponade.

KEY POINT

Cardiac tamponade is initially a diastolic problem, with limitation of ventricular filling due to increased pericardial fluid and pressure. Subsequently, impaired diastolic filling leads to limitation of cardiac output with characteristic clinical signs and symptoms and the typical echocardiographic findings in cardiac tamponade.

18. **Answer: B.** Pulsus paradoxus is defined as an abnormally large decrease in systolic blood pressure (>10 mm Hg) on inspiration and is a direct result of enhanced ventricular interdependence. With cardiac tamponade, exaggerated right ventricular (RV) filling occurs during inspiration, but left ventricular (LV) filling is compromised because the heart occupies a fixed space within the pericardial effusion. Thus, LV stroke volume decreases during inspiration, as demonstrated on the LV outflow tract pulsed-wave Doppler tracing in **Figure 25-12**.

   Answer A is not correct since pulsus alternans refers to an alternating force of the arterial pulse from beat to beat; this pulse is commonly associated with LV failure. Answer C is not correct as pulsus bisferiens refers to the appearance of two systolic peaks per cardiac cycle; this pulse is associated with significant aortic regurgitation. Answer D is not correct as pulsus parvus et tardus refers to a weak (parvus) and delayed (tardus) carotid upstroke; this pulse is associated with severe aortic stenosis.

19. **Answer: C.** Intrapericardial pressure is influenced by both the volume of fluid and the rate at which it accumulates. The pericardium is relatively distensible over a long period of time; thus, slow accumulation of a large amount of pericardial fluid may occur without causing frank cardiac tamponade physiology. Conversely, rapid accumulation of relatively small amounts of fluid in the pericardial space, as may occur with complications during or after invasive cardiac procedures, may cause acute cardiac tamponade within minutes.

20. **Answer: D.** A plethoric IVC is a specific marker of raised central venous pressure. Plethora of the IVC reflects impaired systemic venous return to the right atrium caused by RA pressure elevation and/or RA compression that occurs secondary to increased intrapericardial pressure. Although this sign may not manifest if the patient has undergone brisk diuresis or is severely dehydrated, its absence

usually makes the diagnosis of advanced or hemodynamically significant pericardial disease unlikely.

21. **Answer: D. Figure 25-4** shows M-mode features of early diastolic collapse of the right ventricular (RV) free wall in cardiac tamponade. The yellow arrows point to RV diastolic collapse. The * denotes the pericardial effusion. RV collapse occurs when the intrapericardial pressure exceeds the RV pressure; this usually occurs during early to mid-diastole when the RV pressure is at its lowest point. The pericardium has some degree of distensibility; but once this limit is reached, the ventricles must compete with each other for the fixed volume determined by the increased intrapericardial pressure. Therefore, RV collapse is exaggerated during expiration when right heart filling is reduced.

22. **Answer: A.** The respiratory variation of transmitral and transtricuspid flow velocities in cardiac tamponade is greatly increased and out of phase, reflecting the increased ventricular interdependence in which the hemodynamics of the left and right heart chambers are directly influenced by each other to a greater degree than normal. The pathophysiology of cardiac tamponade relates to the effect of the excessive pericardial fluid limiting cardiac filling as the cardiac chambers compete with the pericardial fluid in the "fixed" and noncompliant space. Ventricular diastolic filling is reduced because of reduced inflow pressure gradients. Inspiration increases venous return to the right heart, with a simultaneous decrease in left heart filling, while expiration increases left heart filling with a decrease in right heart filling. This explains the opposite respiratory variation of transmitral and transtricuspid inflow by pulsed-wave Doppler echocardiography. For the peak transmitral E inflow velocity, the maximal drop occurs with the first beat of inspiration and the first beat of expiration and usually exceeds >30% respiratory variation. For peak transtricuspid E inflow velocity, the maximal drop is on the first

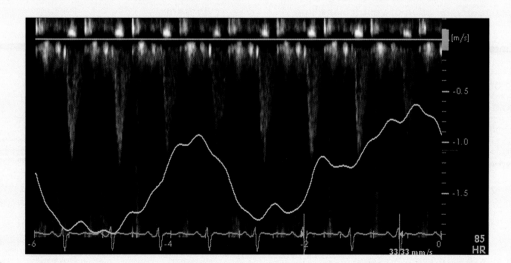

Figure 25-12

beat in expiration at the same time as the hepatic vein atrial reversal and usually exceeds >60% respiratory variation. Significant respiratory variation of the transmitral and transtricuspid inflows should not be used as a stand-alone criterion for cardiac tamponade without the presence of other features suggestive of cardiac tamponade such as chamber collapse. This is because in constrictive pericarditis (CP), the pattern of transmitral and transtricuspid flow variation with respiration is similar to that observed in cardiac tamponade. However, in CP the respiratory variation is usually less; for example, the transtricuspid peak E velocity increases >40% and the transmitral peak E velocity is considered abnormal with a drop of >25%. Other differences between cardiac tamponade and CP are listed in **Table 25-1**.

23. **Answer: C.** One of the 2D echocardiographic features of a hemodynamically significant pericardial effusion is RV diastolic collapse and/or right atrial (RA) collapse lasting more than 1/3 of the cardiac cycle. As previously discussed, these findings reflect the changes in the intrapericardial pressure (IPP) and the transmural filling pressure (TMFP). That is, when the IPP exceeds the intracardiac pressure, the TMFP becomes negative and there is collapse (compression) of the cardiac chambers. This effect is mostly seen in the cardiac chambers with the lowest pressures and will be reflected as indentation or collapse of the right-sided chambers during diastole. However, when right-sided pressures are abnormally high, as in severe pulmonary hypertension, pressures of the right ventricle and right atrium might increase to a pressure equal to or even higher than that of the pericardial pressure, thus preventing right-sided diastolic collapse.

24. **Answer: A.** The echocardiographic criteria to diagnose tamponade on the basis of transmitral inflow patterns are different during positive-pressure ventilation as opposed to spontaneous breathing. Positive-pressure ventilation causes an increase in intrathoracic pressure instead of the usual decrease; therefore, the spectral Doppler findings are opposite to those seen in the spontaneous breathing patient; that is, there is an increase in transmitral E velocity and decrease in transtricuspid E velocity on the first beat of inspiration.

25. **Answer: B.** Low-pressure cardiac tamponade is caused by a compressive pericardial effusion when the intravascular blood volume is considerably depleted. Low-pressure cardiac tamponade resulting from hypovolemia may mask the clinical findings of cardiac tamponade, complicating the diagnosis. In these cases, the central venous pressure is normal or often low; thus, the jugular venous distension normally seen in classic cardiac tamponade is absent. Therefore, the IVC may demonstrate respiratory variation and may not be dilated. Diastolic right atrial and RV chamber indentation or collapse on 2D echocardiography is particularly important in the diagnosis of low-pressure cardiac tamponade, when IVC dilation is minimal or absent. Exaggerated respiratory changes in the spectral Doppler profiles, as seen in classic cardiac tamponade, are also seen in low-pressure cardiac tamponade. Potential causes of low-pressure cardiac tamponade due to severe hypovolemia include traumatic hemorrhage, hemodialysis or ultrafiltration, or over-diuresis.

Table 25-1. Similarities and Differences Between Constrictive Pericarditis and Cardiac Tamponade

	Cardiac Tamponade	Constrictive Pericarditis
Fixed cardiac volume limiting cardiac filling	Present	Present
Increased respiratory variation of ventricular filling	Present	Present
Ventricular interdependence (septal shift)	Present	Present
Dissociation of intracardiac and intrathoracic pressures	Present	Present
Equal left- and right-sided diastolic pressures	Present	Present
Dilated noncollapsing inferior vena cava	Present	Present
Exaggerated (>10 mm Hg) fall in systolic blood pressure with inspiration (Paradoxical pulse)	Common	Uncommon
Systemic venous wave morphology	Absent Y descent	Prominent Y descent (M or W shaped)
Inspiratory change in systemic venous pressure	Decrease (normal)	Increase or no change (Kussmaul sign)
Square root sign in ventricular pressure	Absent	Present

KEY POINT

Low-pressure cardiac tamponade occurs due to intravascular fluid depletion which occurs as a result of severe hypovolemia, hemorrhage, or advanced malignancy. The hemodynamic significance of low-pressure cardiac tamponade is based on right heart chamber collapse and typical respiratory variations in the spectral Doppler examination. The IVC size and respiratory variation is usually normal in these cases.

26. **Answer: D.** The lack of right-sided diastolic chamber collapse may be seen when right-sided pressures are increased due to pulmonary hypertension. Chamber collapse is typically only seen when the intra-pericardial pressure is higher than the RA and RV diastolic pressures.

TEACHING POINT

The absence of any right heart chamber collapse has a very high negative predictive value for cardiac tamponade. However, right heart collapse may be absent when there is significant RV hypertrophy (RVH) or severe pulmonary hypertension. Recall that chamber collapse occurs when the intrapericardial pressure (IPP) exceeds the intracardiac pressure. Hence, when the right heart pressures are significantly elevated, chamber collapse may not occur despite the presence of cardiac tamponade. Likewise, when there is significant RVH, the thick, noncompliant RV wall is not compressed despite elevation in IPP.

27. **Answer: B.** CP is a condition in which an inflamed, thickened, scarred, or calcified pericardium becomes noncompliant, thus limiting diastolic filling of the ventricles. Worldwide, the most common cause of CP is tuberculosis. The most common cause of CP in developed countries is pericardial injury due to previous cardiac surgery. This is followed by pericarditis, previous pericardial effusion, and radiotherapy. Less common etiologies include radiation, neoplasms, infection, idiopathic CP, connective tissue disorders, and uremia.

28. **Answer: B.** The pericardial knock is a loud third heart sound occurring when the ventricular filling abruptly stops at the end of the early rapid filling phase of the ventricles. It is classically associated with severe constrictive pericarditis. The pericardial knock is relatively high in pitch and increases in intensity with inspiration.

Answer A is not correct as a pericardial (friction) rub is generated by the friction of two inflamed layers of the pericardium and occurs during the maximal movement of the heart within its pericardial sac. This heart sound is used in the diagnosis of pericarditis.

Answer C is not correct. A pericardial honk is a fictitious heart sound. A "precordial" honk is a short musical systolic murmur that is often preceded by a click and occurring in mid- or late systole. This murmur is most commonly associated with mitral valve prolapse.

Answer D is not correct. A pleuropericardial rub results from the friction between the inflamed pleura and the parietal pericardium. This heart sound indicates primary inflammatory, neoplastic, or traumatic pleural disease or inflammation secondary to infection or neoplasm.

29. **Answer: B.** In patients with constrictive pericarditis, the pulmonary capillary wedge pressure (PCWP) is influenced by the inspiratory fall in thoracic pressure, whereas the left ventricular (LV) pressure is shielded from respiratory pressure variations by the constrictive pericardial shell. Thus, with inspiration there is a fall in the PCWP and left atrial pressure, but not LV diastolic pressure, which decreases the pressure gradient for LV filling. This less favorable LV filling pressure gradient during inspiration explains the decline in LV filling velocity, which is reflected as a decline in the transmitral E velocity with inspiration. Reciprocal changes occur in right ventricular (RV) filling; that is, with inspiration RV filling is accentuated and this is reflected as an increase in the transtricuspid E velocity with inspiration. These changes are mediated by the interventricular septum (IVS), not by increased systemic venous return and represent features of exaggerated or enhanced ventricular interdependence.

TEACHING POINT

The ventricles share a common IVS and are confined within the pericardium. Therefore, any changes to the size, shape, pressure, and volume of one ventricle affects the size, shape, pressure, and volume of the other ventricle. This is referred to as ventricular interdependence. Normally, ventricular interaction is minimal. With inspiration, the IVS shifts slightly toward the left, resulting in a slight increase in RV filling and a minimal decrease in LV filling. However, when there is dissociation between intrathoracic pressure (ITP) and intracardiac pressure (ICP), ventricular interdependence is exaggerated or enhanced. Therefore, with inspiration there is a greater increase in RV filling, which occurs at the expense of LV filling. With expiration, the IVS shifts toward the right leading to an increase in LV filling, which occurs at the expense of RV filling. These changes are reflected on the transmitral and transtricuspid inflow profiles. With inspiration, there is an increase in transtricuspid inflow velocities and a decrease in transmitral inflow velocities. With expiration, the opposite occurs so there is a decrease in transtricuspid inflow velocities and an increase in transmitral inflow velocities.

30. **Answer: A.** Demonstration of constrictive physiology and elevated filling pressure are key requisites for the diagnosis of CP and can occur in the absence of a thickened pericardium. Significant pulmonary hypertension and severe atrial enlargement are not typical features of CP. Severe atrial enlargement is more characteristic of a restrictive cardiomyopathy.

31. **Answer: D.** Respiratory variation of IVS motion and the transmitral inflow profile is seen in both CP and cardiac tamponade. In both cases, this effect is due to dissociation between intrathoracic pressure (ITP) and intracardiac pressure (ICP) resulting in exaggerated or enhanced ventricular interdependence (see Teaching Tip in the answer outline for Question 29). In cardiac tamponade, the effect is caused by increased intrapericardial pressure (IPP); with constriction, a thickened, fibrotic pericardium prevents full transmission of ITP changes. The first two answers are typically seen in cardiac tamponade, but not in CP, while answer C is seen in CP and not in cardiac tamponade.

32. **Answer: B.** An e′ >8 cm/s has approximately 95% sensitivity and 96% specificity for the diagnosis of CP (Ha et al., 2004). In normal subjects, mitral lateral e′ velocity is higher than the medial e′ velocity. The presence of relatively normal lateral and/or septal mitral annular velocities suggests the presence of CP. However, the lateral e′ velocity is usually lower than the medial e′ velocity, resulting in annulus reversus. This finding is likely due to the tethering of the adjacent fibrotic and scarred pericardium, which influences the lateral mitral annulus of patients with CP.

33. **Answer: C.** In constrictive pericarditis, when intracardiac volume is less due to the stiff pericardium, diastolic filling is unimpeded, and early diastolic filling occurs abnormally rapidly because venous pressure is elevated. The rapid early diastolic filling, which is halted abruptly when intracardiac volume reaches the limit set by the noncompliant pericardium, is reflected by the abrupt displacement of the interventricular septum into the left ventricle during early diastole (i.e., the septal bounce, indicated by Arrow 1). Arrow 2 points out rapid early relaxation of the posterior wall. During the remainder of diastole, little posterior wall motion occurs because of continued impairment of diastolic filling.

34. **Answer: B.** Hepatic vein diastolic flow reversal with expiration suggests CP, even when the transmitral flow velocity pattern may not be diagnostic. The absence of typical respiratory flow velocity changes in transmitral flow should not exclude the diagnosis, because up to one-half of patients with CP may not meet these criteria. In such a situation, hepatic vein diastolic flow reversal that increases with expiration may still be seen and reflect the enhanced ventricular interaction and dissociation between the intracardiac and intrathoracic pressures. The white arrow in **Figure 25-7** refers to hepatic vein diastolic flow reversal.

35. **Answer: C.** In COPD, SVC systolic and diastolic forward flow is markedly increased with inspiration due to exaggerated inspiratory effort and a resultant exaggerated decrease in intrathoracic pressure (**Figure 25-13A**). This finding may also be noted in patients with obesity. In contrast, SVC systolic flow velocities show minimal changes in inspiratory forward flow in patients with CP (**Figure 25-13B**).

36. **Answer: D.** These echocardiographic findings are all consistent with a diagnosis of constrictive pericarditis. Findings that do not fit with the diagnosis include a flattened IVS, lateral e′ > medial e′, a transmitral inflow abnormal relaxation pattern (E/A < 1), the absence of hepatic vein expiratory diastolic flow reversals, exaggerated respiratory SVC forward flow, and presence of a normal or small IVC.

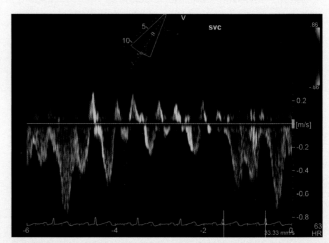

Figure 25-13A SVC pulsed-wave Doppler profile in a patient with COPD.

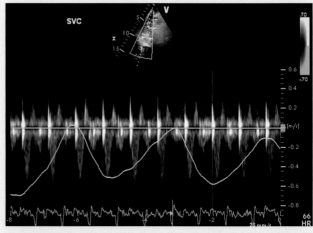

Figure 25-13B SVC pulsed-wave Doppler profile in a patient with CP.

37. Answer: A. The images provided for this echocardiogram show evidence of effusive-constrictive pericarditis. In this case, there is residual loculated anterior pericardial effusion with right ventricular compression (**Videos 25-5C** and **25-5D**). Respiratory variation of the pulsed-wave Doppler transmitral and hepatic venous profiles (**Figures 25-14A** and **25-14B**), prominent septal bounce (**Videos 25-5A** to **25-D**), pericardial thickening (**Videos 25-5A** and **25-5B**), and annulus paradoxus (**Figures 25-14C** and **25-14D**) are also present. Effusive-constrictive pericarditis is a clinical syndrome that may be seen in post-pericardiocentesis patients. In this scenario, pericardial constriction due to inflammation is present, as well as residual pericardial fluid and increased intrapericardial pressure leading to constrictive physiology. Echocardiographic spectral Doppler assessment may be useful to assess residual hemodynamic findings of constrictive physiology following pericardiocentesis.

00. Answer: D. Paradoxical to the positive correlation between mitral E/e' and PCWP in patients with abnormal diastolic function, an inverse relationship is typically found in patients with CP; that is, in patients with CP and an elevated PCWP, the E/e' is normal to low. This is reversed to that which is usually seen whereby the E/e' is high when the PCWP is elevated. This inverse relationship in CP is termed "annulus paradoxus" and occurs because mitral annular velocities are relatively normal or even increased in patients with CP due to the increased longitudinal motion of the heart, which compensates for the reduced ventricular filling from constricted radial expansion of the heart.

KEY POINT

Annulus paradoxus refers a low or normal E/e' ratio despite elevated LV filling pressures in CP. This phenomenon is primarily due to an increase in the e' velocity, particularly medially, that occurs when there is an increase in longitudinal motion. This increase in longitudinal motion compensates for reduced ventricular filling caused by the constricting pericardium which limits the radial expansion of the heart.

38. Answer: A. In normal subjects, the TDI e' velocity is higher at the lateral annulus compared to the medial (septal) annulus. In patients with CP, septal e' usually exceeds lateral mitral annulus e' (see **Figures 25-14C** and **25-14D**). This reversed relationship

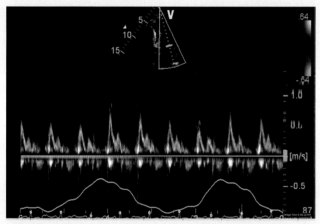

Figure 25-14A Transmitral inflow pulsed-wave (PW) Doppler.

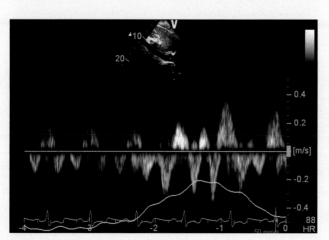

Figure 25-14B Hepatic vein PW Doppler.

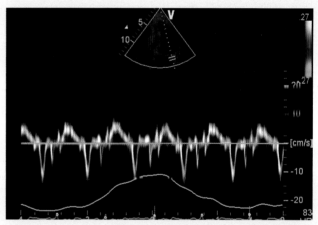

Figure 25-14C Lateral mitral annular tissue Doppler imaging (TDI).

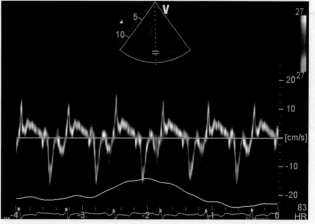

Figure 25-14D Medial mitral annular TDI.

between the lateral and medial e' velocity is referred to as "annulus reversus." This phenomenon is attributed to the tethering of the left ventricular lateral free wall to the adjacent pericardium.

A reversed relation between E/e' and LA pressure (answer B) is called "annulus paradoxus," which occurs because, in contrast to what happens in RCM, mitral annular velocities are normal or increased in patients with CP (see the answer outline for Question 38).

Answer C is not correct. While mitral annular velocities are increased in patients with CP compared with patients with RCM, this is not "annulus reversus."

Answer D is not correct as mitral annular velocities do not change significantly in relation to respiration in patients with CP or RCM.

40. **Answer: C.** In CP, the free wall of the left ventricle is tethered to the pericardium. Therefore, the lateral wall strain values are typically less negative than septal strain values. **Figure 25-8A** is the typical apical sparing pattern seen in cardiac amyloidosis. **Figure 25-8B** is consistent with apical hypertrophic cardiomyopathy, and **Figure 25-8D** is a patient with ischemic cardiomyopathy.

Acknowledgments: The authors thank and acknowledge the contributions from Alaa Mabrouk Omar, MD, PhD, and Partho P. Sengupta, MD, DM (Chapter 25 Pericardial Disease) in *Clinical Echocardiography Review: A Self-Assessment Tool*, 2nd edition, edited by Allan L. Klein, Craig R. Asher, 2017.

SUGGESTED READINGS

Anderson B. Pericardial disease. In: *A Sonographer's Guide to the Assessment of Heart Disease*. Australia: MGA Graphics; 2014:343-371.

Armstrong WF, Ryan T, Feigenbaum H. Pericardial disease. In: *Feigenbaum's Echocardiography*. 7th ed. Philadelphia: Wolters Kluwer Health/Lippincott Williams & Wilkins; 2010:241-262.

Ha JW, Ommen SR, Tajik AJ. Differentiation of constrictive pericarditis from restrictive cardiomyopathy using mitral annular velocity by tissue Doppler echocardiography. *Am J Cardiol*. 2004;94(3):316-319.

Hayes SN, Freeman WK, Gersh BJ. Low pressure cardiac tamponade: diagnosis facilitated by Doppler echocardiography. *Br Heart J*. 1990;63(2):136-140.

Klein AL, Abbara S, Agler DA, et al. American Society of Echocardiography clinical recommendations for multimodality cardiovascular imaging of patients with pericardial disease. *J Am Soc Echocardiogr*. 2013;26(9):982-983.

Kronzon I, Giovannone S, Donnino R, et al. Pericardial disease. In: Lang RM, Goldstein SA, Kronzon I, Khandheria BK, Mor-Avi V, eds. *ASE's Comprehensive Echocardiography*. 2nd ed. Philadelphia, PA: Saunders, an Imprint of Elsevier Inc.; 2016.

Oh J. Pericardial diseases. In: *The Echo Manual*. 4th ed: Wolters Kluwer; 2019:273-305.

Otto CM. Pericardial disease. In: *Textbook of Clinical Echocardiography*. 6th ed. Philadelphia, PA: Elsevier Inc.; 2018.

Otto CM. Pericardial disease. In: *Practice of Clinical Echocardiography*. 5th ed. Philadelphia, PA: Elsevier Inc.; 2017.

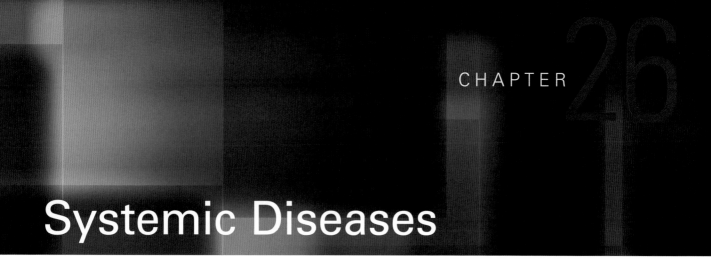

CHAPTER 26

Systemic Diseases

Contributors: Rebecca Perry, PhD, DMU (Cardiac), BSc and Ashwin Venkateshvaran, PhD, RCS, RDCS

✪✪ Question 1

Cardiac involvement in hereditary hemochromatosis typically manifests as:

A. Left ventricular (LV) dilatation and systolic dysfunction.
B. Increased LV wall thickness.
C. Regional wall motion abnormalities.
D. Pulmonary hypertension.
E. Pericardial effusion.

✪✪ Question 2

A 15-year-old boy with severe ataxia is referred for an echocardiogram. Which of the following constellation of echocardiographic findings is most characteristic of Friedreich ataxia?

A. Dilated cardiomyopathy
B. Severe left ventricular (LV) hypertrophy mimicking hypertrophic cardiomyopathy
C. Normal LV dimensions, preserved systolic function with isolated severe diastolic dysfunction
D. Regional wall motion abnormalities (RWMA) in a noncoronary distribution

✪✪ Question 3

A 66-year-old woman who appears younger than her stated age presents with complaints of dyspnea, arthralgias, and swelling of her hands and feet. A transthoracic echocardiogram is performed, and a short-axis view is provided in **Figure 26-1**. What is the most likely diagnosis?

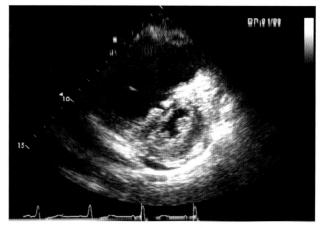

Figure 26-1

A. Cardiac amyloidosis
B. Scleroderma
C. Hemochromatosis
D. Rheumatoid arthritis

✪✪ Question 4

Which of the findings listed is considered a classical finding on the transthoracic examination in patients with cardiac amyloidosis?

A. Normal LV wall thickness
B. Uniformly reduced segmental global longitudinal myocardial strain
C. Short mitral deceleration time associated with worsening prognosis
D. Increased systolic and early diastolic velocities of the mitral annulus on tissue Doppler imaging
E. Interventricular septal "bounce"

✪ Question 5

In patients with more advanced stages of cardiac amyloidosis, a combined relaxation abnormality and a mild increase in left atrial pressure (LAP) will result in which of the following?

   A. Grade I diastolic dysfunction (impaired relaxation)
   B. Grade II diastolic dysfunction (pseudonormalized)
   C. Decreasing pulmonary venous atrial reversal velocity
   D. Decreasing left ventricular (LV) end-diastolic pressure

✪ Question 6

The 2D, color Doppler, and spectral Doppler images shown in **Figures 26-2A** to **26-2C** were acquired of the right ventricular outflow tract in a patient with metastatic carcinoid disease. In addition, she has features of severe tricuspid regurgitation (TR) and right heart failure. What specific lesion do these images suggest is present?

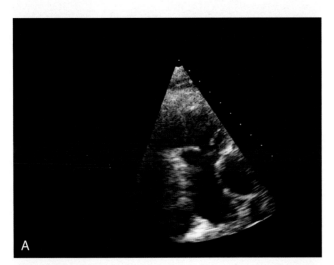

Figure 26-2A

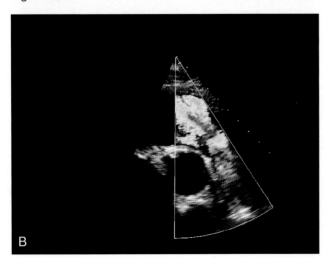

Figure 26-2B

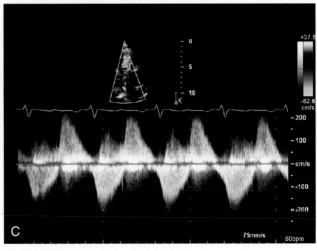

Figure 26-2C

   A. Severe pulmonary regurgitation
   B. Severe pulmonary stenosis
   C. Severe pulmonary hypertension
   D. Patent ductus arteriosus

✪✪✪ Question 7

Which of the following findings best describe the most typical echocardiographic appearance of hereditary hemochromatosis?

   A. Nondilated left ventricular (LV) cavity with severely increased wall thickness
   B. Restrictive diastolic filling pattern with normal LV wall thickness
   C. Mildly dilated LV cavity with global dysfunction and normal or mildly increased wall thickness
   D. Severely dilated LV cavity with regional dysfunction and severely increased wall thickness

✪✪✪ Question 8

A transesophageal echocardiogram (TEE) is obtained in a 29-year-old woman who presents with symptoms of arthralgias, low-grade fever, chest pain, skin rash, and photosensitivity. There is no history of illicit drug use. Chest X-ray demonstrates small bilateral pleural effusions. Initial laboratory tests demonstrate a mildly elevated white blood cell count, elevated creatinine level of 1.5 mg/dL, and an elevated erythrocyte sedimentation rate of 45 mm/h. Based on the TEE image (120°) shown in **Figure 26-3**, the most likely diagnosis is:

   A. Ergot-alkaloid use.
   B. Infective endocarditis.
   C. Libman–Sacks endocarditis.
   D. Rheumatic mitral valve disease.

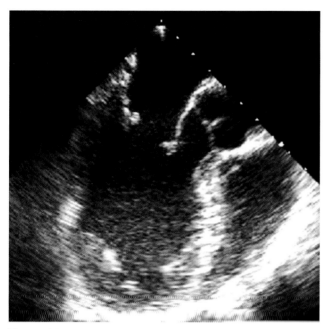

Figure 26-3

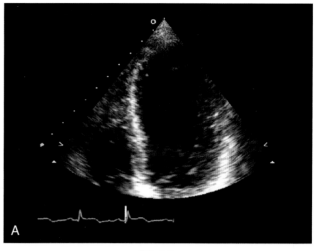

Diastole

Figure 26-4A

✪✪ Question 9

What is the most common cardiovascular abnormality seen in patients with a human immunodeficiency virus (HIV) infection?

- **A.** Dilated cardiomyopathy
- **B.** Pericardial effusion
- **C.** Kaposi sarcoma of the heart
- **D.** Primary pulmonary hypertension

✪✪ Question 10

A 67-year-old woman with no prior history of cardiac disease presented with severe chest pain and dyspnea over the past 24 hours. The initial electrocardiogram demonstrated ST elevation in the anterior precordial leads, and she was taken emergently to the cardiac catheterization laboratory. Coronary angiography demonstrated only mild epicardial coronary artery disease. A transthoracic echocardiogram was performed, and representative end-diastolic and end-systolic apical 4-chamber images are shown in **Figures 26-4A** and **26-4B**. Which of the following may be present in this patient?

- **A.** Persistent left ventricular (LV) systolic dysfunction at 1 year
- **B.** Dynamic left ventricular outflow tract (LVOT) obstruction
- **C.** Markedly increased cardiac biomarkers
- **D.** Hypertrophic cardiomyopathy

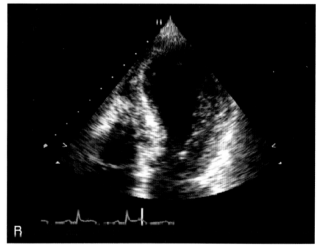

Systole

Figure 26-4B

✪ Question 11

A 23-year-old man is sent for an echocardiogram because of a widened mediastinum appreciated on chest X-ray performed during a routine preemployment physical examination. He has a history of lens dislocation as a child. His grandfather died suddenly of unknown cause. The pertinent echocardiographic images are shown in **Figure 26-5**. Which of the following is not likely in this patient?

- **A.** Marfan syndrome
- **B.** Aortic regurgitation
- **C.** Aortic coarctation
- **D.** Mitral regurgitation

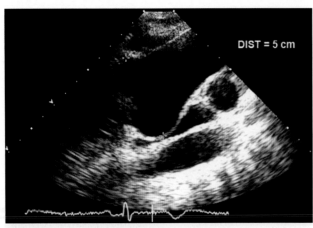

DIST = 5 cm

High parasternal long axis view

Figure 26-5

✪✪ Question 12

A 35-year-old man from Latin America with a low-risk cardiovascular profile presents to the echocardiography laboratory with nonspecific symptoms and general weakness. His electrocardiogram (ECG) demonstrates a right bundle branch block (RBBB) associated with left anterior hemiblock (LAHB). The transthoracic echocardiogram demonstrates mild left ventricular (LV) dilatation with mildly depressed function and an apical aneurysm. The patient had impaired diastolic relaxation with no signs of elevated filling pressures. Which of the following is the patient likely to have?

   A. Ischemic cardiomyopathy
   B. Chagas cardiomyopathy
   C. Restrictive cardiomyopathy
   D. Infiltrative cardiomyopathy

✪✪ Question 13

In the echocardiographic assessment of suspected Kawasaki disease, which one of the following settings is least likely to enhance visualization of the coronary arteries:

   A. Using the highest possible transducer frequency.
   B. Reducing depth and sector width.
   C. Magnifying the area of interest.
   D. Enhancing compression.

✪✪✪ Question 14

Which of the following echocardiographic features is least likely to suggest cardiac sarcoidosis?

   A. Dilated left ventricle
   B. Thinning or thickening of the interventricular septum
   C. Wall motion abnormalities in noncoronary distribution
   D. Significant aortic regurgitation

✪✪ Question 15

In a patient with rheumatoid arthritis, the most frequent cardiac complication is:

   A. Pericardial effusion.
   B. Cardiac tamponade.
   C. Constrictive pericarditis.
   D. Pericardial masses.

✪✪✪ Question 16

A 65-year-old male farmer is referred to the clinic for the evaluation of dyspnea. He presents with New York Heart Association functional class III symptoms; he is diabetic and has documented hepatic dysfunction. His skin appears noticeably bronzed. The physical exam reveals a blood pressure of 110/70 mm Hg, heart rate of 70 bpm, and an S3 gallop on auscultation. His echocardiogram reveals a significantly depressed left ventricular (LV) function with bi-atrial enlargement and severe mitral regurgitation. Which of the following diagnoses is most in agreement with the presented clinical picture?

   A. Cardiac hemochromatosis
   B. Cardiac amyloidosis
   C. Cardiac sarcoidosis
   D. Fabry disease

✪✪ Question 17

▶ **Figure 26-6A** and **Video 26-1** demonstrate an apical 4-chamber view in a patient who was referred for weakness and fatigue. **Figure 26-6B** demonstrates the pulsed-wave (PW) Doppler transmitral inflow waveform and **Figure 26-6C** shows the septal mitral annular tissue Doppler imaging (TDI) waveform. These findings are most consistent with:

   A. Cardiac sarcoid.
   B. Carcinoid heart disease.
   C. Hypertrophic cardiomyopathy.
   D. Infiltrative cardiomyopathy.

✪✪ Question 18

A 49-year-old man with an adrenal pheochromocytoma and uncontrollable hypertension presents for an echocardiogram. The most common echocardiographic feature of pheochromocytoma is:

   A. Left ventricular (LV) wall motion abnormalities.
   B. LV hypertrophy.
   C. Right ventricular (RV) wall motion abnormalities.
   D. RV hypertrophy.

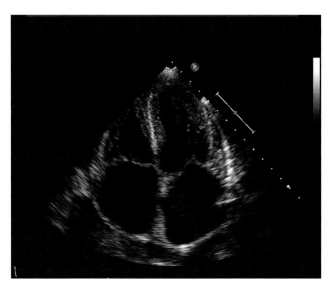

Figure 26-6A

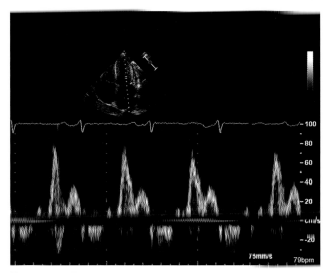

Figure 26-6B

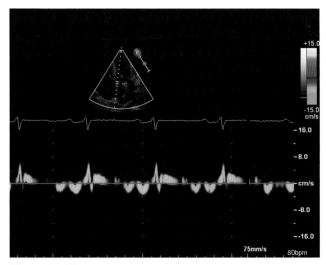

Figure 26-6C

⭐ Question 19

▶ A patient with acute chest pain presents to the hospital emergency room where an urgent echo-cardiogram is ordered. **Video 26-2** and **Figure 26-7** (systolic frame) demonstrate the apical long-axis view. The most likely systemic cause for this echocardio-graphic appearance is:

   A. Type 2 diabetes mellitus.
   B. Carcinoid heart disease.
   C. Hypereosinophilic syndrome.
   D. Duchenne muscular dystrophy.

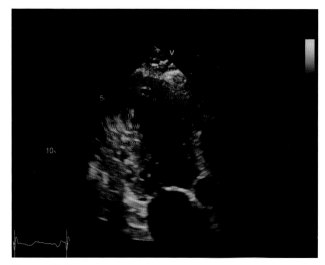

Figure 26-7

✰✰ Question 20

Figure 26-8 shows a parasternal long axis view in a young patient with a diastolic murmur. The most likely systemic disorder responsible for this appearance is:

   A. Rheumatoid arthritis.
   B. Ankylosing spondylitis.
   C. Systemic lupus erythematosus.
   D. Amyloidosis.

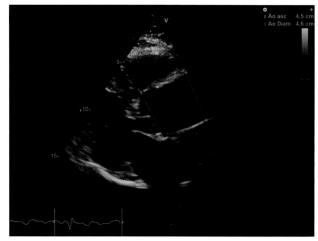

Figure 26-8

✪ Question 21

The most common echocardiographic feature seen in Duchenne muscular dystrophy is:

A. Left ventricular wall thickening.
B. Valvular regurgitation.
C. Pulmonary hypertension.
D. Dilated cardiomyopathy.

✪ Question 22

Figure 26-9 is a regional longitudinal strain (LS) map that demonstrates:

A. Reduced global LS consistent with a global process.
B. Reduced regional LS in the apical regions consistent with takotsubo cardiomyopathy.
C. Reduced regional LS in the basal and middle regions with apical sparing consistent with cardiac amyloidosis.
D. Reduced LS in the anteroseptal and apical regions consistent with left anterior descending coronary artery disease.

✪ Question 23

A patient with a history of scleroderma and shortness of breath presents for an echocardiogram. The most likely finding will be:

A. Restrictive cardiomyopathy.
B. Ventricular septal defect.
C. Atrial septal defect.
D. Elevated right ventricular systolic pressure.

✪ Question 24

▶ A 79-year-old man presents with right heart failure. The electrocardiogram (ECG) is shown in **Figure 26-10A**. The parasternal long-axis view is shown in **Figure 26-10B** and **Video 26-3**. The most likely diagnosis is:

A. Hypertrophic cardiomyopathy.
B. Fabry disease.
C. Cardiac amyloidosis.
D. Hypertension.

✪✪ Question 25

The most common type of amyloidosis seen with cardiac manifestations is:

A. Acquired immunoglobulin light chain (AL, or primary) amyloidosis.
B. Acquired serum amyloid A (AA, or secondary) amyloidosis.
C. Acquired transthyretin (ATTR, or senile type) amyloidosis.
D. Hereditary ATTR (or familial) amyloidosis.

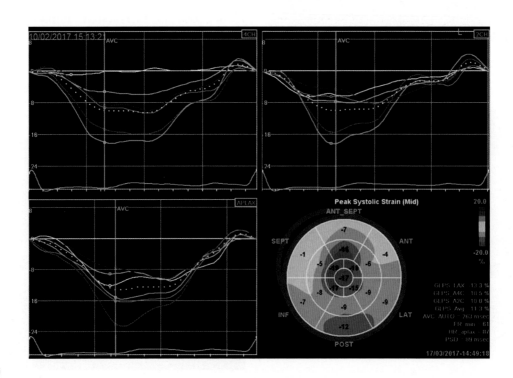

Figure 26-9

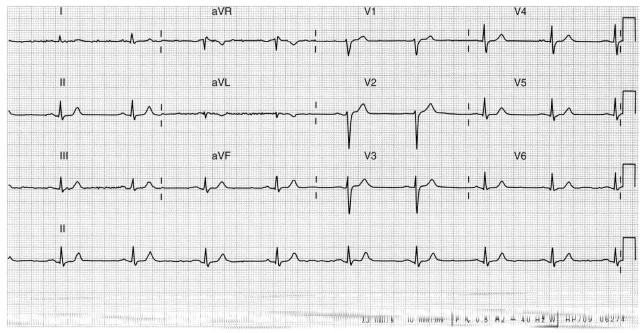

Figure 26-10A

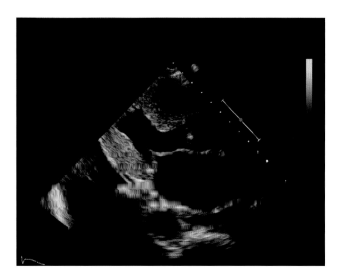

Figure 26-10B

⊗ Question 26

The atria are generally dilated in amyloid heart disease due to:
- **A.** Persistent atrial fibrillation.
- **B.** Restrictive filling of the ventricles.
- **C.** Significant valvular regurgitation.
- **D.** Significant valvular stenosis.

⊗⊗⊗ Question 27

▶ A 52-year-old woman presents with atypical chest pain and syncope. An echocardiogram is ordered to assess left ventricular (LV) function. **Video 26-4** and **Figure 26-11** (systolic frame) demonstrate the parasternal long-axis view. What is the most likely diagnosis?

- **A.** Left anterior descending myocardial infarction
- **B.** Takotsubo cardiomyopathy
- **C.** Dilated cardiomyopathy
- **D.** Cardiac sarcoidosis

⊗⊗⊗ Question 28

Sarcoidosis presents in the following sequential stages:
- **A.** Edema, granuloma formation, and fibrosis.
- **B.** Fibrosis, granuloma formation, and cell death.
- **C.** Granuloma formation, edema, and fibrosis.
- **D.** Edema, fibrosis, and granuloma formation.

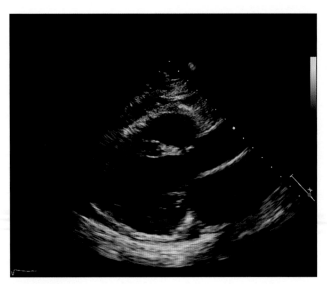

Figure 26-11

✪✪✪ Question 29

Patients with cardiac sarcoidosis often present with arrhythmias. An arrhythmia seen in sarcoidosis is:

A. Complete heart block.
B. Ventricular tachycardia.
C. Ventricular fibrillation.
D. All of the above.

✪ Question 30

A 72-year-old man with recent surgery to remove a tumor of the small intestine presents with right heart failure. **Figure 26-12** demonstrates a continuous-wave (CW) Doppler signal from the tricuspid valve. This image demonstrates:

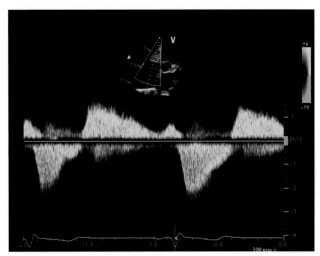

Figure 26-12

A. Severe tricuspid regurgitation.
B. Severe tricuspid stenosis.
C. Pulmonary hypertension.
D. Mixed tricuspid valve disease.

✪✪ Question 31

▶ The apical 4-chamber images displayed in **Figures 26-13A** and **26-13B** and **Videos 26-5A** and **26-5B** were acquired from the same patient as presented in **Question 30**. Based on these images, the most likely diagnosis is:

A. Ebstein anomaly.
B. Arrhythmogenic right ventricular dysplasia.
C. Carcinoid heart disease.
D. Tricuspid valve endocarditis.

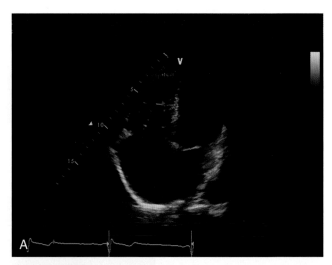

Figure 26-13A

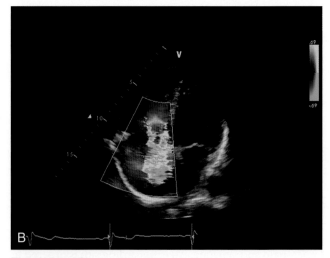

Figure 26-13B

⊛ Question 32

A patient with a carcinoid tumor demonstrates retracted and thickened mitral valve leaflets with free-flowing mitral regurgitation. What additional pathology is likely present in this situation?

   A. Pericardial effusion
   B. A right-to-left intracardiac shunt
   C. A left-to-right intracardiac shunt
   D. LV hypertrophy

⊛⊛⊛ Question 33

Hypereosinophilic syndrome (HES) occurs in three stages. On the echocardiogram, those three stages would appear as:

   A. Unexplained wall thickening followed by apical thrombus and then restrictive cardiomyopathy.
   B. Apical thrombus followed by unexplained wall thickening and then restrictive cardiomyopathy.
   C. Restrictive cardiomyopathy, unexplained wall thickening and then apical thrombus.
   D. Unexplained wall thickening followed by restrictive cardiomyopathy and then apical thrombus.

⊛⊛ Question 34

▶ An echocardiogram is ordered in a 49-year-old man with persistently elevated eosinophil count to rule out cardiac manifestations. An apical 4-chamber view is shown in **Figure 26-14** and **Video 26-6A**, with the corresponding contrast image shown in **Video 26-6B**. What is another name for this type of appearance?

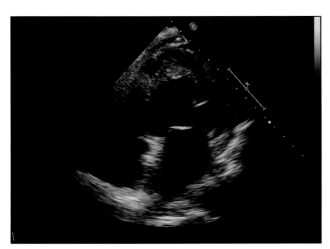

Figure 26-14

   A. Libman-Sacks endocarditis
   B. Apical akinesis
   C. Loeffler endocarditis
   D. Apical hypertrophic cardiomyopathy

⊛⊛ Question 35

Symptom status usually correlates with the stage of hypereosinophilic syndrome (HES). The second stage is most likely linked to which clinical sequela?

   A. Cerebral vascular accident
   B. Heart failure
   C. Mitral regurgitation
   D. Myocardial infarction

⊛⊛⊛ Question 36

A patient presents with endomyocardial fibrosis (EMF) on cardiovascular magnetic resonance imaging. EMF due to hypereosinophilic syndrome (HES) can be differentiated from tropical EMF based on:

   A. The pattern of ventricular involvement as tropical EMF mainly affects the right ventricle (RV), whereas HES can affect either ventricle.
   B. The degree of left ventricular (LV) hypertrophy as tropical EMF leads to asymmetric septal hypertrophy, whereas HES leads to concentric LV hypertrophy.
   C. valvular regurgitation as tropical EMF leads to right-sided valvular regurgitation, whereas HES leads to left-sided valvular regurgitation.
   D. Valvular stenosis as tropical EMF leads to right-sided valvular stenosis, whereas HES leads to left-sided valvular stenosis.

⊛⊛⊛ Question 37

A family in which the grandfather is positive for a cardiac-specific mutation of Fabry disease presents to determine which family members may also have this disease. The most likely early cardiac manifestation of Fabry disease on the echocardiogram will be:

   A. Systolic left ventricular (LV) dysfunction with globally reduced longitudinal strain.
   B. Mild concentric LV wall thickening with reduced longitudinal strain.
   C. Concentric LV wall thickening without reduction in longitudinal strain.
   D. Restrictive cardiomyopathy.

✪✪✪ Question 38

In a patient with advanced Fabry cardiomyopathy, myocardial longitudinal strain is normally reduced:

A. At the apex.

B. In the right ventricular free wall.

C. In the basal inferolateral region.

D. In the mid anteroseptal region.

✪✪✪ Question 39

Fabry disease is an X-linked recessive disorder. Which of the following statements best describes the mode of inheritance for this disease?

A. When one parent has the defective gene, there is a 50% chance that the child will inherit the faulty gene and will therefore be affected by or be predisposed to developing the disease.

B. When the father has the defective gene and the mother is a carrier of the defective gene, there is a 50% chance that each son will inherit the faulty gene and will therefore be affected by the disease.

C. When both parents carry the defective gene, there is a 25% chance for the child to inherit both defective genes and therefore be affected by the disease.

D. When both parents carry the defective gene, there is a 75% chance for the child to inherit the defective gene and therefore be affected by or predisposed to developing the disease.

✪✪ Question 40

Which of the following statements regarding Loeys-Dietz syndrome (LDS) is an incorrect statement?

A. LDS is an inherited autosomal recessive connective tissue disorder.

B. The cardiovascular manifestations of LDS are very similar to Marfan syndrome.

C. Congenital heart lesions such as a bicuspid aortic valve are more common in those with LDS than in the normal population.

D. An important complication of LDS is aortic dissection, which can occur without marked aortic dilatation.

ANSWERS

1. **Answer: A.** Hereditary hemochromatosis is an autosomal recessive iron-storage disease seen almost entirely in people of northern European descent. There is accumulation of iron in the heart, liver, pancreas, skin, and gonads. When cardiac involvement is present, the disease is usually in the advanced stage with multiorgan involvement (diabetes, cirrhosis, arthritis, and impotence). The severity of myocardial dysfunction is proportional to the extent of myocardial iron deposition. Cardiac manifestations include congestive heart failure, arrhythmias, and conduction abnormalities.

   Echocardiographic findings usually consist of mild LV dilatation, systolic dysfunction, normal or mildly increased wall thickness, relatively normal cardiac valves, and bi-atrial enlargement (see **Table 26-1**). The LV diastolic filling pattern is usually restrictive and morphologic 2D echocardiographic features are essentially those of dilated cardiomyopathy. Therefore, answer A (dilated left ventricle and systolic dysfunction) is correct. While LV wall thickness may be mildly increased, it is frequently normal. Regional wall motion abnormalities are not typically present. Although secondary pulmonary hypertension may be present due to restrictive LV physiology, this is not a prominent finding. Pericardial effusion is not typical.

2. **Answer: B.** Friedreich ataxia, an autosomal recessive degenerative disorder, is the most common hereditary ataxia and is manifested clinically by neurologic dysfunction, cardiomyopathy, and diabetes mellitus. Echocardiographic abnormalities are common, reported in 86% of patients, and are useful in confirming a diagnosis of Friedreich ataxia since cardiac involvement is not present in other ataxic disorders. The most common echocardiographic abnormality is concentrically increased wall thickness occasionally mimicking hypertrophic cardiomyopathy (see **Table 26-1**). Therefore, answer B is correct. Asymmetric septal thickening and dilated cardiomyopathy are uncommon. Other findings include globally decreased LV function and decreased LV end-diastolic diameter. RWMA in a noncoronary distribution are typically seen in infiltrative disorders, such as granulomatosis with polyangiitis and sarcoidosis.

3. **Answer: B.** The 2D echocardiographic findings of a pericardial effusion and an enlarged right ventricle with a D-shaped left ventricular cavity due to pulmonary hypertension should alert the operator to the differential diagnosis of scleroderma. The clinical

presentation of a patient who appears younger than her stated age, likely due to taut facial skin, dyspnea, arthralgias, and swelling of the hands and feet is also consistent with a diagnosis of scleroderma.

The most common primary cardiac abnormality associated with scleroderma is a pericardial effusion, often small (see **Table 26-1**). The myocardium may be involved by fibrosis or sclerosis and systolic and diastolic dysfunction may be present. Both systemic and pulmonary hypertension are prominent secondary complications of scleroderma.

Cardiac amyloidosis (answer A) is an infiltrative cardiomyopathy that results in a restrictive disease and is characterized by increased biventricular wall thickness. Hemochromatosis (answer C) can lead to a dilated cardiomyopathy due to excess deposition of iron within the myocardium. Finally, cardiac manifestations of rheumatoid arthritis (answer D) include pericarditis and less commonly, dilated cardiomyopathy with congestive heart failure.

4. **Answer: C.** A mitral deceleration time ≤150 ms in patients with biopsy-proven cardiac amyloidosis has been shown to correlate with a significantly worse

Table 26-1. Systemic Diseases, Disease Type, and Common Echocardiographic Findings

Systemic Disease	Disease Type	Common Echocardiographic Findings
Amyloidosis	Infiltrative	• Increased LV wall thickness • Diastolic dysfunction (restrictive in later stages) • Pericardial effusion • Valvular thickening
Ankylosing spondylitis	Connective tissue	• Aortic root dilatation • Aortic regurgitation • Mitral regurgitation
Carcinoid syndrome	Endocrine	• Thickened and retracted tricuspid and/or pulmonary valve • Tricuspid/pulmonary regurgitation • Left-sided valvular disease in the presence of an intracardiac shunt
Chagas disease	Parasitic	• Pericardial effusion • RWMA • LV dilatation • Apical aneurysm
Diabetes mellitus	Endocrine	• RWMA (from coronary artery disease) • LV hypertrophy (from systemic hypertension) • Diastolic dysfunction
Duchenne muscular dystrophy	Neuromuscular	• Dilated cardiomyopathy
Ehlers-Danlos syndrome (Type IV)	Connective tissue	• Aortic root dilatation ± aortic regurgitation • Aortic valve prolapse • Mitral valve prolapse ± mitral regurgitation • Aortic aneurysm at the sinuses of Valsalva • Type A aortic dissection
Fabry disease	Storage	• Hypertrophic cardiomyopathy • Diastolic dysfunction • Valvular disease
Friedreich ataxia	Neuromuscular	• Hypertrophic cardiomyopathy • Diastolic dysfunction
Hemochromatosis	Storage	• Dilated cardiomyopathy • Bi-atrial enlargement • Diastolic dysfunction
Hypereosinophilic syndrome	Endomyocardial	• Mural apical thrombus • Endocardial fibrosis • Posterior mitral leaflet tethering
Human immunodeficiency virus (HIV)	Immune/infectious	• Pericardial effusion • Dilated cardiomyopathy • Pulmonary hypertension

Table 26-1. Systemic Diseases, Disease Type, and Common Echocardiographic Findings (Continued)

Systemic Disease	Disease Type	Common Echocardiographic Findings
Kawasaki disease	Inflammatory	• Coronary artery dilatation/aneurysm • RWMA
Marfan syndrome	Connective tissue	• Aortic root dilatation • Aortic regurgitation • Aortic dissection • Mitral valve prolapse
Loeys-Dietz syndrome	Connective tissue	• Aortic root dilatation and aortic aneurysms +/- aortic regurgitation • Aortic valve prolapse • Mitral valve prolapse ± mitral regurgitation • Type A aortic dissection
Pheochromocytoma	Endocrine	• LV hypertrophy (from systemic hypertension)
Rheumatoid arthritis	Connective tissue	• Pericarditis/pericardial effusion • Valvular disease
Sarcoidosis	Infiltrative	• Dilated cardiomyopathy • Thinning of basal interventricular septum • RWMA inconsistent with coronary artery distribution
Scleroderma	Connective tissue	• Pulmonary hypertension • Pericardial disease
Systemic lupus erythematosus (SLE)	Connective tissue	• Pericarditis/pericardial effusion • Libman-Sacks endocarditis
Takotsubo cardiomyopathy	Endocrine (catecholamine mediated)	• LV RWMA inconsistent with coronary artery distribution • Most common LV regional wall motion pattern is apical akinesis/ballooning with normal/hyperdynamic basal regions

LV, left ventricular; RWMA, regional wall motion abnormalities.

prognosis and risk of cardiac death over an 18-month period, with a relative risk for cardiac death nearly five times greater than those patients with a deceleration time >150 ms. Therefore, answer C is correct. Similarly, 1-year cardiac survival of patients with an increased mitral E/A ratio (≥2.1) was less than that of patients with normal or decreased mitral E/A ratio (<2.1).

5. **Answer: B.** In most, if not all cardiac disease, as with cardiac amyloidosis, the initial diastolic dysfunction stage is impaired relaxation (Grade I diastolic dysfunction). In Grade I diastolic dysfunction, LAP is normal. With disease progression, continued impaired relaxation ultimately results in mild to moderate increases in LAP that can cause the mitral inflow velocity pattern to appear similar to a normal filling pattern; this is Grade II diastolic dysfunction or a pseudonormal profile. Therefore, answer B is correct.

In the pseudonormal profile, the E/A ratio is typically 1 to 1.5 and the E-wave deceleration time is usually between 160 and 220 ms. The best way to identify a pseudonormal filling profile or Grade II

diastolic dysfunction is by an average E/e′ >14, tricuspid regurgitant (TR) velocity >2.8 m/s, and a left atrial volume index (LAVi) >34 mL/m² (in the setting of normal LV systolic function) as per 2016 American Society of Echocardiography diastology guidelines. In patients with known systolic dysfunction or abnormally increased wall thickness, a normal E/A ratio suggests that increased LAP is masking abnormal relaxation. By decreasing preload (that is, via the Valsalva maneuver), one may unmask the underlying impaired LV relaxation by causing the E/A ratio to decrease by 0.5 or more, thus reversing the E/A ratio. In addition, color M-mode of the mitral inflow can determine rate of flow propagation into the left ventricle, and with worsening diastolic function, myocardial relaxation is always impaired and flow propagation is slow even when LAP and mitral E-wave velocity are increased.

6. **Answer: A.** The echocardiographic images are suggestive of severe pulmonary regurgitation, which is seen in about two-thirds of patients with carcinoid heart disease. The 2D image demonstrates significant thickening and retraction of the pulmonary

cusps (**Figure 26-2A**). Color flow demonstrates a broad-based regurgitation jet secondary to possible non-coaptation in diastole (**Figure 26-2B**). The continuous-wave Doppler signal is dense and demonstrates rapid equalization of pressures (**Figure 26-2C**). Severe pulmonary stenosis (answer B) is characterized by doming of the cusps in systole and a high systolic antegrade flow velocity across the pulmonary valve. While the velocity across the pulmonary valve is slightly accentuated owing to significant regurgitation, a velocity of less than 2 m/s is not suggestive of significant stenosis. Given the low pulmonary end-diastolic velocities of the pulmonary regurgitant jet, significant pulmonary hypertension (answer C) is unlikely. A shunt through a patent ductus arteriosus (answer D) is generally seen as a communication between the main pulmonary artery and the descending thoracic aorta with persistent flow throughout the cardiac cycle.

7. **Answer: C.** Hemochromatosis is a form of iron storage disease with deposition in various organs including the myocardial cells of the heart. It may be hereditary (primary) or acquired. By the American Heart Association classification of cardiomyopathies, it is characterized as a secondary cardiomyopathy since it is part of a systemic disease. Since hemochromatosis is not an infiltrative disorder, wall thickness is generally not significantly increased. The atria, ventricles, and atrioventricular conduction system may be involved. Supraventricular arrhythmias are common. Cardiac involvement in hereditary hemochromatosis evolves through a progression of structural and functional abnormalities. In the early stages, diastolic dysfunction, including tissue Doppler imaging abnormalities, may be the first manifestation, despite normal LV size, wall thickness, and systolic function. As the disease progresses, there is a decrease in LV systolic function and dilatation of the left ventricle and both atria. LV wall thickness is usually normal or mildly increased even in the later stages. Therefore, answer C (mildly dilated LV cavity with global dysfunction and normal or mildly increased wall thickness) is correct. A restrictive filling pattern is a late manifestation of the condition when there is LV dysfunction (see **Table 26-1**). Identification of cardiac hemochromatosis is important since treatment with chelating agents or phlebotomy may improve cardiac function.

8. **Answer: C.** The TEE image demonstrates small verrucous valvular lesions on the tips of the mitral valve leaflets. In the clinical setting of a young woman with arthralgias, low-grade fever, skin rash, photosensitivity, elevated white blood cell count, pleural effusion, and no history of illicit drug use, the most likely diagnosis is systemic lupus erythematosus (SLE) with Libman–Sacks endocarditis. Libman–Sacks endocarditis (also known as nonbacterial

thrombotic endocarditis or marantic endocarditis) refers to a characteristic verrucous valvular lesion that usually affects the mitral valve in patients with systemic lupus erythematosus (see **Table 26-1**). The lesion is typically present on the ventricular aspect of the mitral leaflets and may extend to the chordal and papillary structures.

Ergot-alkaloid use (answer A) is associated with valvulopathy and valvular regurgitation usually affecting the aortic and mitral valves. Echocardiographic features of infective endocarditis (answer B) are an oscillating intracardiac mass on a valve or other cardiac structure, abscesses, and dehiscence of a prosthetic valve. The vegetations are typically on the "upstream" surface of the regurgitant jet of the affected valve, that is, on the atrial aspect of atrioventricular valves and on the ventricular aspect of the aortic valve. Rheumatic mitral valve disease (answer D) is associated with thickened and calcified mitral leaflets and subvalvular apparatus, "hockey-stick" deformity of the anterior leaflet and relative immobility of the posterior leaflet, and associated stenosis or regurgitation.

9. **Answer: B.** A variety of cardiac abnormalities have been associated with HIV infection, including pericardial effusion, dilated cardiomyopathy, primary pulmonary hypertension, and Kaposi sarcoma of the heart (see **Table 26-1**). Of these, pericardial effusion is most common.

The cardiac manifestations of HIV disease have been greatly altered by the introduction of highly active antiretroviral therapy (ART). As overall survival has improved, and HIV has become a chronic infection, coronary artery disease has become the most important cardiovascular complication and attention has focused on aggressive risk factor modification.

The most common clinical manifestation of HIV disease in the pre-ART era was pericardial effusion, seen in approximately 20% to 40% of patients. This remains the case in the developing world and in resource-limited settings where access to ART is limited. Pericardial effusion is typically asymptomatic but serves as a marker of advanced disease and worse prognosis. It is much less common in the ART era.

Dilated cardiomyopathy (answer A) has been described in 8% to 16% of patients with HIV, but these data are from the pre-ART era. The prevalence is considerably lower in the ART-treated patients. Kaposi sarcoma (answer C) involving the heart is very rare and usually diagnosed as an incidental finding at autopsy. When present, it is typically found in subepicardial adipose tissue. Primary pulmonary hypertension (answer D) has been reported but is a rare finding seen in less than 0.5% of AIDS patients.

10. **Answer: B.** The echocardiogram demonstrates significant apical and mid-ventricular akinesis. The patient is a postmenopausal woman with a presentation that simulates acute myocardial infarction. These features are all consistent with apical ballooning syndrome.

Transient LV apical ballooning syndrome (also known as takotsubo cardiomyopathy or stress-induced cardiomyopathy) is a reversible cardiomyopathy triggered by profound psychological or physical stress and has a clinical presentation that is similar to acute myocardial infarction. Most patients are postmenopausal women. Proposed criteria for the diagnosis of apical ballooning require all four of the following characteristics: (1) electrocardiographic abnormalities (usually ST elevations followed by T wave inversion), (2) transient apical and mid-ventricular wall motion abnormalities, (3) absence of obstructive coronary artery disease or acute plaque rupture, and (4) absence of other conditions, such as significant head trauma, intracranial hemorrhage, pheochromocytoma, or another etiology of myocardial dysfunction. Catecholamine-induced microvascular dysfunction is currently postulated as a likely mechanism. According to recent reports, right ventricular (RV) apical dysfunction may be present in 30% to 40% of cases. Dynamic LVOT obstruction, which is due to basal hyperkinesis, is a well-described complication of apical ballooning syndrome and may result in hypotension; therefore, answer B is correct. Persistent LV systolic dysfunction (answer A) is not an expected complication in stress-induced cardiomyopathy. Although cardiac biomarkers are always elevated (answer C), the elevation is usually mild and disproportionate to the degree of cardiac compromise. Although the walls appear thickened, it is not the typical appearance of hypertrophic cardiomyopathy (answer D).

It is important to remember that apical ballooning syndrome is a diagnosis of exclusion and can only be diagnosed once obstructive coronary disease and acute plaque rupture have been excluded. Similar wall motion abnormalities can also result from myocardial infarction due to occlusion of a large wraparound left anterior descending (LAD) coronary artery. Hence, coronary angiography is required for the diagnosis even in the setting of typical regional wall motion abnormalities.

11. **Answer: C.** This young man has Marfan syndrome. The characteristic pear-shaped dilatation of the aortic root (aortic sinuses) is characteristic and a major diagnostic criterion of this autosomal dominant inherited condition, usually resulting from a fibrillin 1 gene mutation. The aortic root dilatation causes incomplete coaptation of the aortic valve leaflets giving rise to aortic regurgitation. Mitral regurgitation is also common in Marfan syndrome due to coexisting mitral valve prolapse (see **Table 26-1**). Aortic coarctation is not an association with Marfan syndrome; therefore, answer C is correct. Patients with Marfan syndrome have an increased risk of aortic dissection or rupture when the aortic caliber reaches a dimension of 50 mm with elective aortic root replacement indicated as first-line therapy. This patient should preferentially undergo aortic surgery in the near future due to the size of the aorta and family history of sudden death, presumed to be related to aortic dissection.

12. **Answer: B.** The presence of an apical aneurysm in a young Latin American should alert the sonographer to the possible presence of Chagas disease, a parasitic disease caused by *Trypanosoma cruzi* and transmitted by the reduviid bug endemic to Central America. The most common ECG findings include atrial fibrillation, RBBB, and variable degrees of atrioventricular block. Echocardiography generally reveals segmental hypokinesis, LV dilatation with systolic dysfunction, and apical aneurysms (see **Table 26-1**). Advanced Chagas cardiomyopathy often presents with atrial and ventricular dilation, diffuse biventricular hypokinesis, and ventricular aneurysms. Ischemic cardiomyopathy (answer A) is unlikely in a young male with no cardiovascular risk factors. Subjects with restrictive cardiomyopathy (answer C) generally demonstrate significant diastolic dysfunction. Infiltrative cardiomyopathy (answer D) rarely presents with myocardial thinning or dyskinesis.

13. **Answer: D.** Imaging the coronary arteries constitutes a standard component of the echocardiographic examination in pediatric subjects. In the setting of Kawasaki disease, both an initial focused coronary assessment and serial examinations may be required to study disease progression. Employing the highest possible frequency transducer (answer A) in keeping with the subject's size and build provides for superior gray scale resolution of the coronary arteries. Reducing the depth and sector width (answer B) enhances frame rate, which may be of value while imaging small, superficial structures in children with relatively faster heart rates. Magnifying the area of interest (answer C) may be helpful, particularly when images are adequately optimized. Enhancing compression (answer D), on the other hand, may obscure the vessel lumen by filtering out low-level sound waves, and hence is least likely to improve visualization.

14. **Answer: D.** Sarcoidosis is a rare inflammatory disorder characterized by the accumulation of white blood cell clusters, termed granulomas, in various parts of the body, which includes heart valve tissue and the myocardium. Given that granulomatous deposition can be localized to small areas of the myocardium, the sensitivity of an echocardiogram

to diagnose this disorder is low. However, certain signs can alert the sonographer to cardiac sarcoidosis as a potential differential diagnosis, particularly when accompanied by arrhythmias or a clinical history. Left ventricular (LV) morphological and structural alterations, which include dilatation (answer A), local aneurysms, septal thickening or thinning (answer B), and wall motion abnormalities (answer C), may be seen. While the presence of valvular irregularities may not be common, these may be limited to the mitral valve secondary to geometric changes in the left ventricle, or the tricuspid valve secondary to pulmonary hypertension. It is unlikely that aortic regurgitation (answer D) is coexistent in the setting of sarcoidosis.

15. **Answer: A.** Rheumatoid arthritis (RA) is commonly characterized by chronic inflammation of the joints, but extra-articular features are also known to develop. Pericardial disease is regarded as the most common cardiac manifestation of RA, affecting up to a third of patients (see **Table 26-1**). It has been found that the risk of developing pericardial effusion was 10-fold higher in patients with rheumatoid arthritis compared to patients without. Patients often present with small or moderate amounts of pericardial effusion as an expression of higher systemic inflammation. However, rarely does this pose a significant hemodynamic consequence. Both cardiac tamponade (answer B) and constrictive pericarditis (answer C) are rare in this setting. Pericardial masses (answer D) are not especially associated with RA.

16. **Answer: A.** A dilated cardiomyopathy like image in the setting of hepatic dysfunction and diabetes is suggestive of cardiac hemochromatosis. This systemic disorder is characterized by excessive deposition of iron in the myocytes, leading to reduced ventricular compliance and subsequent heart failure. Doppler echocardiography demonstrates abnormal LV filling during initial phases, and subsequent ventricular dilation and systolic dysfunction. Diagnosis is critical, as treatment by iron depletion or excretion by chemical chelation effectively restores the ventricle to health. There are two main types of iron overload cardiomyopathy (IOC), a familial idiopathic IOC and secondary haemochromatosis from iron overload. This results in excessive iron in various organs, including the heart, liver, and pancreas, leading to damage and impairment. While cardiovascular magnetic resonance imaging is the gold standard for noninvasive imaging in patients with or suspected to have IOC due to its ability to determine myocardial iron content, echocardiography is a valuable tool for screening and follow-up of these patients. Patients may present with different phenotypes depending on the degree of iron overload and may include diastolic dysfunction, increased LV wall

thickness, dilated cardiomyopathy, and/or restrictive cardiomyopathy.

17. **Answer: D.** The images demonstrate increased left ventricular (LV) mass with "ground glass" appearance, bi-atrial dilatation, and increased LV filling; this is in keeping with an infiltrative cardiomyopathy; the most common of which is cardiac amyloid. Diastolic dysfunction is a key feature of infiltrative cardiomyopathies due to the stiffening of the LV walls due to the infiltrate. Bi-atrial dilatation occurs due to the increased LV filling pressures. While diastolic dysfunction can occur in cardiac sarcoid, carcinoid heart disease, and hypertrophic cardiomyopathy, the 2D echocardiographic features on the apical 4-chamber view differ. Cardiac sarcoid (answer A) can show increased LV wall thickness due to granulomatous expansion, but the wall thickness does not usually become severe due to fibrosis after the granulomas heal. Carcinoid heart disease (answer B) commonly demonstrates right atrial dilatation due to severe tricuspid regurgitation from an abnormal tricuspid valve with thickened and retracted leaflets that remain in a fixed semiopen position throughout the cardiac cycle. Hypertrophic cardiomyopathy (answer C) generally presents with regional hypertrophy (usually asymmetrical septal hypertrophy but may also be concentric or apical).

18. **Answer: B.** A pheochromocytoma is a neuroendocrine tumor of the adrenal glands (originating in the chromaffin cells), or extra-adrenal chromaffin tissue that failed to involute after birth, that secretes high amounts of catecholamines. Pheochromocytoma is diagnosed based on the detection of increased levels of catecholamines in the blood and urine. Most patients with pheochromocytoma have systemic hypertension resulting in LV hypertrophy, this is the most common cardiac manifestation (see **Table 26-1**). Very rarely a cardiac pheochromocytoma may be detected in the myocardium. While LV wall motion abnormalities (answer A) may occur during hypertensive crisis, this is rare and results in a transient takotsubo type cardiomyopathy. RV wall motion abnormalities and RV hypertrophy (answers C and D) are not characteristic features of pheochromocytoma.

19. **Answer: A.** The images demonstrate regional wall motion abnormalities consistent with left anterior descending coronary artery disease. Type 2 diabetes mellitus (T2DM) is a risk factor for myocardial infarction (see **Table 26-1**). T2DM is due to a combination of decreased insulin secretion and insulin resistance. The diagnosis of T2DM is based on fasting plasma glucose. Coronary artery disease is the leading cause of morbidity and mortality in T2DM.

Carcinoid heart disease (answer B) results in right heart disease with tricuspid and/or pulmonary valve retraction and resultant regurgitation.

Hypereosinophilic syndrome (answer C) results in LV thrombus formation without related wall motion abnormalities. Duchenne muscular dystrophy (Answer D) most commonly results in a dilated cardiomyopathy.

20. **Answer: B.** Ankylosing spondylitis is a connective tissue inflammatory disorder that involves the vertebral and sacroiliac joints causing inflammatory back pain. It can result in aortitis, resulting in fusiform dilatation of the aortic root (see **Table 26-1**). It may also cause thickening of the aortomitral junction creating a "subaortic bump." The aortic root dilatation can result in aortic regurgitation. The most common presentation of rheumatoid arthritis (answer A) is pericardial effusion. Systemic lupus erythematosus (answer C) results in Libman-Sacks vegetations and pericardial effusions. Cardiac involvement with amyloidosis (answer D) results in increased ventricular wall thickness, valvular thickening, and small pericardial effusions.

21. **Answer: D.** Duchenne and Becker muscular dystrophy includes a group of X-linked muscular diseases responsible for over 80% of all cases of muscular dystrophy. Cardiac disease in Duchenne muscular dystrophy is progressive and leads to ventricular dysfunction, usually accompanied by ventricular dilation (see **Table 26-1**). By the third decade, most patients with Duchenne muscular dystrophy have dilated cardiomyopathy, which is the leading cause of death in these patients.

22. **Answer: C.** This regional strain map demonstrates reduced LS in the basal and middle regions with apical sparing, which is consistent with cardiac amyloidosis. Strain and strain rate are sensitive in assessing early left ventricular (LV) systolic dysfunction in amyloid heart disease. It is now well recognized that there is a specific strain "pattern" demonstrated in cardiac amyloidosis, with a severe impairment of basal LS along with preserved strain in the apical regions. This relative apical sparing pattern observed along with the apical-to-base gradient in LS parallels the larger extent of amyloid infiltration at basal level compared to the apex. The characteristic bulls-eye graph appearance has been described as "a cherry on top." Moreover, this apical sparing pattern is observed in both AL (light-chain) and ATTR (transthyretin) cardiac amyloid, and the basal-to-apical LS abnormalities are similar across both types, reflecting the amyloid burden. A loss of this apical sparing has been shown to predict major adverse cardiac events. Furthermore, it has been demonstrated that the pattern of relative apical sparing has a high accuracy to differentiate cardiac amyloidosis from other causes of LV hypertrophy. In fact, a relative apical LS (defined as average apical LS/[average basal LS + mid-LS]) of 1.0 was 93% sensitive and 82% specific in differentiating cardiac

amyloidosis from LV hypertrophy due to hypertrophic cardiomyopathy or aortic stenosis (Phelan et al., 2012).

23. **Answer: D.** Scleroderma with pulmonary involvement causes fibrosis in the pulmonary vasculature, resulting in pulmonary hypertension, which may elevate the right ventricular systolic pressure. A restrictive cardiomyopathy is rare. These patients have the same risk of septal defects as the general population.

24. **Answer: C.** The parasternal images (**Figure 26-10B** and **Video 26-3**) demonstrate concentric left ventricular (LV) wall thickening with a small LV cavity, right ventricular wall thickening, and small pericardial effusion. The ECG (**Figure 26-10A**) is not consistent with LV hypertrophy. Therefore, based on the echocardiographic features in the parasternal images and the ECG, the most likely diagnosis is cardiac amyloidosis.

Hypertrophic cardiomyopathy (answer A) generally presents with regional hypertrophy (usually asymmetrical septal hypertrophy but may also be concentric or apical). Fabry disease (answer B) and hypertension (answer D) usually present with concentric LV wall thickening; however, this is usually less prominent in these diseases compared with cardiac amyloidosis. It is important to note that cardiac amyloidosis is not LV hypertrophy; the increased LV mass is due to interstitial amyloid fibril deposition. As a result, the ECG voltages in cardiac amyloidosis are not consistent with LV hypertrophy. Certain clues may be seen on the ECG pointing to possible cardiac amyloidosis, including low QRS voltages in the limb leads and a pseudo-infarction pattern in the chest leads.

25. **Answer: A.** Cardiac amyloidosis is the involvement of the heart by amyloid deposition and may be cardiac specific or more commonly part of systemic amyloidosis. Light-chain or primary (AL), familial or senile (ATTR), and secondary (AA) amyloidosis are the three most common types of amyloidosis. These amyloid types differ in disease profile and long-term outcome. The most common form of cardiac amyloid disease is systemic AL (primary amyloidosis), where the protein deposited is a monoclonal immunoglobulin light chain. In the majority of cases, this occurs in the setting of multiple myeloma, with 15% to 30% of myeloma patients developing AL cardiac amyloidosis. Signs and symptoms of cardiac involvement occur in up to 50% of patients with AL amyloidosis compared to less than 5% of patients with AA amyloidosis. Unlike AL amyloidosis, systemic AA or secondary amyloidosis (answer B) rarely involves the heart. ATTR amyloidosis (answers C and D) is caused by the deposition of wild-type or mutated transthyretin (TTR, a protein that is produced in the liver). Cardiac involvement varies with the type of

mutation and there are over 100 different mutations that have been described in ATTR amyloidosis. Cardiac mutations of ATTR amyloidosis can be associated with significant increase in left ventricular wall thickness (especially senile systemic amyloidosis, SSA). Hemodynamic alterations are less common, and the disease runs a less aggressive course compared to AL amyloidosis.

26. **Answer: B.** Diastolic dysfunction is a key feature of cardiac amyloidosis due to the stiffening of the left ventricular (LV) walls due to the amyloid deposition. Bi-atrial dilatation occurs due to the increased LV filling pressures. While this can lead to atrial fibrillation and/or atrioventricular valvular regurgitation, this is usually not the cause of atrial dilatation.

KEY POINTS

▶ Cardiac amyloidosis is an infiltrative disease.

▶ The amyloid proteins preferentially invade the basal and middle regions of the ventricles rather than the apex.

▶ Amyloid infiltration results in thickened and rigid left and right ventricular walls.

▶ Diastolic dysfunction is always present.

27. **Answer: D.** The images demonstrate isolated basal septal thinning, which is not consistent with any coronary artery distribution. Cardiac sarcoidosis gives a regional pattern of dysfunction depending upon the extent of myocardial involvement. The presence of basal interventricular septal thinning is suggestive of cardiac sarcoidosis (see Table 26-1). The published diagnostic echocardiography criteria for cardiac sarcoidosis include basal thinning of the interventricular septum, LV dilatation, reduced LV ejection fraction <50%, and wall motion abnormalities with wall thickening or thinning outside of a coronary distribution pattern. Cardiac sarcoidosis is difficult to diagnose due to the focal nature or "patchiness" of the disease with endocardial biopsy findings only 20% to 30% sensitive for a positive diagnosis (Cooper et al., 2007).

A left anterior descending myocardial infarction (answer A) would result in reduced wall motion in the septum and apex, takotsubo cardiomyopathy (answer B) would result in akinesis and ballooning of the distal and apical regions of the left ventricle, and a dilated cardiomyopathy (answer C) would demonstrate globally reduced LV function.

28. **Answer: A.** Sarcoidosis is an idiopathic disease associated with collection and progression of inflammatory cells in the form of granulomas that affect several organs of the body, disrupting normal organ function. It results in noncaseating (nonnecrotizing) granulomatous infiltration (the histopathological hallmark of the disease). Although the cause of sarcoidosis is unknown, it is likely that it results from an immunological response to an unidentified antigen in genetically susceptible individuals. There are three sequential stages of the disease: edema, granuloma formation, and fibrosis leading to scar formation.

29. **Answer: D.** The myocardial edema, granulomas, and fibrosis in cardiac sarcoidosis interrupt the conduction system. This can occur near the atrioventricular node causing complete heart block. Myocardial fibrosis in either ventricle is a substrate for ventricular arrhythmias, often leading to sudden cardiac death if defibrillation is unavailable.

KEY POINTS

▶ Cardiac sarcoidosis causes myocardial edema, granulomas, and fibrosis.

▶ It is difficult to diagnose on echocardiography; however, a thinned basal septum in the presence of a dilated cardiomyopathy with or without complete heart block may assist with the diagnosis.

30. **Answer: D.** This CW Doppler signal demonstrates a dense and high-velocity tricuspid inflow waveform consistent with some degree of tricuspid stenosis and a dense tricuspid regurgitation (TR) waveform with a "v cutoff" sign, which is consistent with rapid equalization of pressures between the right atrium (RA) and right ventricle (RV). This "v cutoff" sign is seen in severe/free-flowing TR. Pulmonary hypertension (answer C) is likely but is not clearly demonstrated in this Doppler tracing as the velocity is low due to the rapid equalization of pressures between the RA and RV. The right atrial pressure is likely to be high in this case.

31. **Answer: C.** These images show thickening and malcoaptation of the tricuspid valve leaflets with severe/free flowing tricuspid regurgitation (TR). This is a typical appearance of carcinoid heart disease. The characteristic echocardiographic features of carcinoid heart disease include progressive thickening and reduced mobility of the tricuspid valve leaflets with a combination of tricuspid stenosis and regurgitation. Tricuspid stenosis is usually mild with the predominant lesion being severe TR. Pulmonary valve thickening and reduced mobility also occur in two-thirds of patients with carcinoid heart disease with the primary lesion being pulmonary regurgitation. Occasionally, pulmonary valve cusp thickening and annulus narrowing cause right ventricular outflow tract obstruction. Intramyocardial metastases also rarely occur.

Ebstein anomaly (answer A) is a congenital cardiac disorder that involves apical displacement of the septal and posterior tricuspid leaflets and variable tethering of the anterior leaflet. TR is a common finding in patients with Ebstein anomaly. Additional echocardiographic features include right atrial enlargement and atrial septal defect or patent foramen ovale. Arrhythmogenic right ventricular (RV) dysplasia (answer B) is characterized by ventricular arrhythmias and fatty replacement of the RV free wall. The fibrofatty replacement of the RV myocardium leads to RV thinning, aneurysmal dilatation, and regional or global RV systolic dysfunction.

Tricuspid valve endocarditis (answer D) appears as a highly mobile vegetation usually attached to the right atrial side of the tricuspid leaflets. Bacterial endocarditis of the tricuspid valve leaflets can result in severe TR; however, a vegetation is not seen in this case study.

32. **Answer: B.** Carcinoid heart disease occurs as a result of high circulating hormone levels, mainly serotonin. These substances form thick, pearly white plaque-like deposits on the right-sided valves causing them to become thickened, retracted, and rigid. Therefore, the valve becomes both stenotic and regurgitant; the tricuspid valve is most commonly affected. Because the humoral substances are inactivated by the lungs, cardiac lesions of the left side of the heart are rare. However, if there is a right-to-left shunt present across a patent foramen ovale, some of the serotonin-rich blood traverses into the left heart chambers without being filtered by the lungs. Left-sided carcinoid valve disease is characterized by thickening and reduced mobility of the mitral valve leaflets and/or aortic valve cusps. Left-sided valve disease is also found in patients with very active carcinoid syndrome and high levels of circulating serotonin.

KEY POINTS

▶ Carcinoid heart disease results from damage due to serotonin secretion from a metastatic carcinoid tumor (usually found in the gut).

▶ The serotonin is deactivated by the lungs; therefore, in the absence of an intracardiac shunt, the left heart valves are usually unaffected.

▶ The tricuspid and/or pulmonary valves become thickened, retracted, and rigid, resulting in regurgitation ± stenosis.

33. **Answer: A.** While the development may be unpredictable, and stages may overlap, HES typically occurs in three stages: an acute necrotic stage (eosinophilic infiltration of the endocardium and myocardium), thrombotic stage (thrombus formation due to damaged endocardium), and fibrotic stage (causing restrictive or dilated cardiomyopathy). Therefore, on the echocardiogram, these three stages would appear as unexplained wall thickening followed by apical thrombus then restrictive cardiomyopathy (answer A).

34. **Answer: C.** Videos **26-6A** and **26-6B** demonstrate a large apical thrombus in the setting of near-normal function of the apex. The apex in this patient is obliterated in systole due to the thrombus formation, which has been caused by eosinophilic infiltration damaging the endocardium, also known as Loeffler endocarditis. Loeffler endocarditis is a rare restrictive cardiomyopathy caused by abnormal endomyocardial infiltration of eosinophils, with subsequent tissue damage leading to thrombus formation and myocardial fibrosis. Libman-Sacks endocarditis (answer A) is associated with systemic lupus erythematosus and these lesions are seen on the mitral and/or aortic valves. Apical hypertrophic cardiomyopathy (answer D) is a form of hypertrophic cardiomyopathy that involves hypertrophy of the myocardium at the apex of the left ventricle. The contrast images clearly demonstrate that this is not part of the myocardium but is indeed thrombus formation. Apical akinesis (answer B) is not evident on the images provided.

35. **Answer: A.** The second stage of HES is the thrombotic stage where thrombus forms in both the left and right ventricular cavities due to damaged endocardium. Therefore, the most likely clinical sequela would be a cerebral vascular accident.

The fibrotic stage (third phase) affects both ventricles as well as the mitral valve leading to systolic dysfunction, mitral regurgitation, and restrictive cardiomyopathy where the symptoms of heart failure (answer B) and mitral regurgitation (answer C) are more apparent. There is no direct link between increased risk of myocardial infarction (answer D) and hypereosinophilic syndrome.

36. **Answer: A.** Tropical EMF usually affects the RV in isolation, whereas both ventricles can be involved in HES. Answer B is not correct. Stage 1 of HES can lead to a mild degree of LV hypertrophy; however, tropical EMF is not associated with hypertrophy.

Answer C is not correct since only HES is associated with mitral regurgitation due to posterior mitral leaflet tethering/adhesion to the LV wall.

Answer D is not correct since neither disease is associated with valvular stenosis.

KEY POINTS

▶ Cardiac involvement in hypereosinophilic syndrome involves three stages: an acute necrotic stage (eosinophilic infiltration of the endocardium and myocardium), thrombotic stage (thrombus formation due to damaged endocardium), and fibrotic stage (causing restrictive or dilated cardiomyopathy)

37. **Answer: B.** Fabry disease or Anderson-Fabry disease is a rare X-linked inherited metabolic disorder that results in a deficiency or absence of the enzyme alpha-galactosidase, leading to the accumulation of glycosphingolipids in various cells and organs, including the heart. Cardiac involvement is common and results in LV wall thickening, myocardial

inflammation, and regional fibrosis. Reduction in longitudinal strain has been shown in patients with Fabry disease both with and without increased LV wall thickening. This reduction in longitudinal strain is usually demonstrated in the basal regions of the left ventricle, in particular the basal inferolateral region. Despite the reduction in LV longitudinal strain, overt systolic dysfunction (answer A), as demonstrated by a reduction in ejection fraction, or restrictive cardiomyopathy (answer D) in Fabry disease is rare and only occurs late in the disease process. Concentric LV wall thickening without reduction in longitudinal strain (answer C) is not expected in Fabry disease.

38. **Answer: C.** Myocardial replacement fibrosis is a typical feature of an advanced Fabry cardiomyopathy. The gold standard for detection of myocardial replacement fibrosis is late gadolinium enhancement using cardiovascular magnetic resonance imaging, where the most typical area of replacement fibrosis in Fabry disease is the basal inferolateral region. However, speckle tracking strain demonstrates lower deformation values in these regions of replacement fibrosis and the degree of strain abnormality is proportional to the amount of replacement fibrosis. The abnormal longitudinal systolic strain is mainly found in the typical location for late gadolinium enhancement, the basal inferolateral region.

KEY POINTS

▶ Fabry disease is a rare X-linked disease, most commonly expressed in affected males, that often have cardiac manifestations.

▶ Fabry disease is inherited from an affected father and/or from a carrier mother.

▶ LV wall thickening and/or fibrosis may be present, particularly in the later stages of the disease.

39. **Answer: B.** As previously stated, Fabry disease is an X-linked recessive disorder. Therefore, the disease is inherited when the defective gene causing the disease is passed on by a female carrier and/or an affected father. Therefore, if the father has the defective gene and the mother is a carrier of the defective gene, there is a 50% chance that each

son will inherit the faulty gene and will therefore be affected by the disease. There is also a 50% probability that each daughter will either become a carrier of the disease or inherit the disease. This disease can also be passed on from an unaffected father and a carrier mother or from an affected father and an unaffected mother.

Answers A and D are not correct as these statements describe the mode of inheritance of autosomal dominant disorders. Answer C is not correct as this statement describes the mode of inheritance for autosomal recessive disorders.

40. **Answer: A.** LDS is an inherited, autosomal dominant (not recessive) connective tissue disorder. LDS is characterized by aortic aneurysms in children and has widespread systemic involvement.

Answer B is a true statement. The cardiovascular manifestations of LDS are very similar to Marfan syndrome and Ehlers-Danlos syndrome (EDS). A difference being that LDS is more aggressive and widespread than Marfan syndrome or EDS.

Answer C is a true statement. Congenital heart lesions such as a bicuspid aortic valve are more common in those with LDS than in the normal population. Other congenital heart lesions more commonly seen in LDS include atrial septal defects and patent ductus arteriosus.

Answer D is a true statement. An important complication of LDS is aortic dissection, which can occur without marked aortic dilatation. Furthermore, aortic dissection or rupture commonly occurs in childhood. Therefore, due to the aggressive nature of this syndrome, aortic imaging is required at frequent intervals, usually every 6 months, to monitor the status and growth of the ascending aorta.

Acknowledgments: The authors thank and acknowledge the following contributions from Imran Shafi Syed, MD, Charles James Bruce, MD and Heidi M. Connolly, MD (Chapter 24, Systemic Disease); Patrick Collier, MD, PhD, Andrew O. Zurick III, MD, David Verhaert, MD and Allan L. Klein, MD (Chapter 13, Diastology); Jorge Betancor, MD and Craig R. Asher, MD (Chapter 22, Cardiomyopathies) in *Clinical Echocardiography Review: A Self-Assessment Tool*, 2nd ed., edited by Allan L. Klein, Craig R. Asher, 2017.

SUGGESTED READINGS

Anderson B. Systemic diseases. In: *A Sonographer's Guide to the Assessment of Heart Disease*. Brisbane: Echotext Pty Ltd; 2014:chap 14.

Blankstein R, Waller AH. Evaluation of known or suspected cardiac sarcoidosis. *Circ Cardiovasc Imaging*. 2016;9(3):e000867.

Cooper LT, Baughman KL, Feldman AM, et al. The role of endomyocardial biopsy in the management of cardiovascular disease: a scientific statement from the American Heart Association, the American College of Cardiology, and the European Society of Cardiology Endorsed by the Heart Failure Society of America and the Heart Failure Association of the European Society of Cardiology. *J Am Coll Cardiol*. 2007;50(19):1914-1931.

Falk RH, Alexander KM, Liao R, Dorbala S. AL (light-chain) cardiac amyloidosis: a review of diagnosis and therapy. *J Am Coll Cardiol*. 2016;68(12):1323-1341.

Gulati V, Harikrishnan P, Palaniswamy C, Aronow WS, Jain D, Frishman WH. Cardiac involvement in hemochromatosis. *Cardiol Rev*. 2014;22(2):56-68.

Mankad R, Bonnichsen C, Mankad S. Hypereosinophilic syndrome: cardiac diagnosis and management. *Heart*. 2016;102(2):100-106.

Mankad R, Ball C, Myasoedova E, Matteson E. Non-atherosclerotic cardiac manifestations of rheumatoid arthritis. In: Semb AG, ed. *Handbook of Cardiovascular Disease Management in Rheumatoid Arthritis*. Switzerland: ADIS; 2017:chap 2.

Mavrogeni S, Markousis-Mavrogenis G, Papavasiliou A, Kolovou G. Cardiac involvement in Duchenne and Becker muscular dystrophy. *World J Cardiol.* 2015;7(7):410-414.

Nagueh SF, Smiseth OA, Appleton CP, et al. Recommendations for the evaluation of left ventricular diastolic function by echocardiography: an update from the American Society of Echocardiography and the European Association of Cardiovascular Imaging. *J Am Soc Echocardiogr.* 2016;29(4):277-314.

Perry R, Shah R, Saiedi M, et al. State of the art review: the role of cardiac imaging in the diagnosis and management of Anderson-Fabry disease. *JACC Cardiovasc Imaging.* 2019;12(7 Pt 1):1230-1242.

Perry R, Selvanayagam JB. Echocardiography in infiltrative cardiomyopathy. *Heart Lung Circ.* 2019;28(9):1365-1375.

Phelan D, Collier P, Thavendiranathan P, et al. Relative apical sparing of longitudinal strain using two-dimensional speckle-tracking echocardiography is both sensitive and specific for the diagnosis of cardiac amyloidosis. *Heart.* 2012;98(19):1442-1448.

CHAPTER 27

Noncyanotic Congenital Heart Disease

Contributors: Neha Soni-Patel, BS, RDCS (AE/PE), RCCS, Stephanie Nay, MBA, RCCS, and Melissa A. Wasserman, RDCS (AE/PE), RCCS

✪ Question 1

The flap of the foramen ovale is created by the:
- **A.** Septum primum.
- **B.** Septum secundum.
- **C.** Coronary sinus.
- **D.** Eustachian valve.

✪✪ Question 2

Atrial septal defects are classified according to their location relative to the:
- **A.** Bundle of His.
- **B.** Endocardial cushions
- **C.** Fossa ovalis.
- **D.** Truncal swellings.

✪✪✪ Question 3

▶ The type of defect verified by the saline bubble study in **Video 27-1** is a(n):
- **A.** Arteriovenous malformation (AVM).
- **B.** Patent foramen ovale (PFO).
- **C.** Persistent left superior vena cava (LSVC).
- **D.** Ventricular septal defect (VSD).

✪✪ Question 4

Which echocardiographic scan plane is optimal to define a secundum atrial septal defect?
- **A.** Apical 4-chamber view
- **B.** Parasternal long-axis view
- **C.** Parasternal short-axis view
- **D.** Subcostal 4-chamber view
- **E.** Suprasternal long-axis view

✪✪ Question 5

Ostium primum atrial septal defects are commonly associated with which other structural anomaly?
- **A.** Bicuspid aortic valve
- **B.** Cleft mitral valve
- **C.** Partial anomalous pulmonary venous return
- **D.** Total anomalous pulmonary venous return

✪✪ Question 6

The direction in which blood flows across an atrial septal defect (ASD) is primarily related to which of the following anatomic or hemodynamic factors?
- **A.** Pulmonary vascular resistance
- **B.** Relative atrial pressures
- **C.** Relative compliances of the ventricles
- **D.** Size and morphology of the ASD
- **E.** Systemic vascular resistance

✪✪ Question 7

The spectral Doppler waveform across an uncomplicated atrial septal defect (ASD) will:
- **A.** Appear predominantly biphasic.
- **B.** Appear similar to that across the semilunar valves.
- **C.** Be continuous, with similar velocities throughout systole and diastole.
- **D.** Display a sharp upstroke with diastolic runoff.

✪ Question 8

A long-standing atrial septal defect (ASD) will lead to:
- **A.** Left ventricular (LV) pressure overload.
- **B.** LV volume overload.
- **C.** Right ventricular (RV) pressure overload.
- **D.** RV volume overload.

✪ Question 9

What is the likelihood of spontaneous closure of a small muscular ventricular septal defect (VSD)?
- **A.** 5% to 10%
- **B.** 20% to 30%
- **C.** 40% to 50%
- **D.** 60% to 70%
- **E.** 80% to 90%

✪ Question 10

Which ventricular septal defect (VSD) is associated with tricuspid valve pouch tissue (VSD septal aneurysm)?
- **A.** Malalignment
- **B.** Outlet
- **C.** Perimembranous
- **D.** Trabecular

✪✪ Question 11

An anterior malalignment ventricular septal defect (VSD) can lead to:
- **A.** Aortic stenosis.
- **B.** Mitral stenosis.
- **C.** Pulmonary stenosis.
- **D.** Tricuspid stenosis.

✪✪ Question 12

A posterior malalignment ventricular septal defect (VSD) can lead to:
- **A.** Aortic stenosis.
- **B.** Mitral stenosis.
- **C.** Pulmonary stenosis.
- **D.** Tricuspid stenosis.

✪✪ Question 13

Which type of ventricular septal defect (VSD) occurs in the outlet portion of the ventricular septum and is defined as a partial or complete absence of muscle?
- **A.** Atrioventricular canal
- **B.** Conal septal
- **C.** Membranous
- **D.** Muscular

✪✪ Question 14

Which type of ventricular septal defect (VSD) is associated with an atrioventricular canal defect?
- **A.** Conal septal
- **B.** Inlet
- **C.** Muscular
- **D.** Perimembranous

✪✪✪ Question 15

Which of the following is the most commonly acquired lesion resulting from a subpulmonary ventricular septal defect (VSD)?
- **A.** Aortic insufficiency
- **B.** Aortic stenosis
- **C.** Left ventricular outflow tract (LVOT) obstruction
- **D.** Pulmonary stenosis
- **E.** Right ventricular outflow tract (RVOT) obstruction

✪✪ Question 16

▶ Which type of atrial septal defect (ASD) is seen in **Video 27-2**?
- **A.** Coronary sinus
- **B.** Inferior sinus venosus
- **C.** Patent foramen ovale
- **D.** Primum
- **E.** Secundum

✪ Question 17

An uncomplicated ventricular septal defect (VSD) will first lead to:
- **A.** Right ventricular (RV) volume overload.
- **B.** Left ventricular (LV) volume overload.
- **C.** RV pressure overload.
- **D.** LV pressure overload.

✪✪ Question 18

The best echocardiographic view for identifying an inlet ventricular septal defect (VSD) is the:
- **A.** Parasternal long axis.
- **B.** Parasternal short axis at the papillary muscle level.
- **C.** Apical 4 chamber.
- **D.** Apical 5 chamber.

✪ Question 19

Which of the following is the most common type of ventricular septal defect (VSD)?
  A. Anterior malalignment
  B. Apical muscular
  C. Inlet
  D. Perimembranous
  E. Subpulmonary

✪✪ Question 20

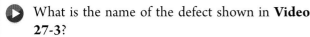

What is the name of the defect shown in **Video 27-3**?
  A. Gerbode defect
  B. Malalignment ventricular septal defect (VSD)
  C. Perimembranous VSD
  D. Supracristal VSD

✪ Question 21

Video 27-4, acquired from a parasternal short-axis view, depicts a:
  A. Patent ductus venosus.
  B. Patent ductus arteriosus.
  C. Patent foramen ovale.
  D. Vertebral artery.

✪✪ Question 22

With a large patent ductus arteriosus (PDA), pan-diastolic flow reversal can be seen in the:
  A. Pulmonary artery branches.
  B. Right upper pulmonary vein.
  C. Coronary arteries.
  D. Abdominal aorta.
  E. All of the above.

✪✪ Question 23

A patent ductus arteriosus (PDA) will result in:
  A. Left-sided pressure overload.
  B. Right-sided pressure overload.
  C. Left-sided volume overload.
  D. Right-sided volume overload.

✪ Question 24

If a newborn has persistent pulmonary hypertension, the patent ductus arteriosus (PDA) shunt will be:
  A. Bidirectional.
  B. Right-to-left.
  C. Left-to-right.

✪✪ Question 25

An example of an anatomic blockage of left ventricular output is:
  A. Ostium primum atrial septal defect.
  B. Large conoventricular septal defect.
  C. Large anterior malalignment ventricular septal defect.
  D. Subaortic membrane.

✪ Question 26

Which lesion is associated with Shone syndrome?
  A. Hypoplastic right ventricle
  B. Muscular ventricular septal defect
  C. Parachute mitral valve
  D. Right ventricular outflow tract obstruction
  E. All of the above

✪✪ Question 27

The physiology of an aortopulmonary window is similar to:
  A. Aortic stenosis.
  B. Atrial septal defect.
  C. Patent ductus arteriosus.
  D. Ventricular septal defect.

✪✪✪ Question 28

Which congenitally stenotic aortic valve morphology is not usually suitable for a balloon valvotomy?
  A. Unicuspid valve
  B. Bicuspid valve
  C. Trileaflet valve
  D. Quadricuspid valve

✪✪ Question 29

The type of pulmonary stenosis shown in **Video 27-5** is:
  A. Valvar.
  B. Branch pulmonary artery.
  C. Subvalvar.
  D. Supravalvar.

✪ Question 30

The most common site of right ventricular outflow obstruction is at which level?
  A. Subvalvar
  B. Valvar
  C. Supravalvar
  D. Peripheral branches

✪✪ Question 31

A child's branch pulmonary arteries are considered hypoplastic when:

    A. The z-score is greater than +2.

    B. The z-score is less than −2.

    C. The z-score is zero.

    D. Z-scores are not a marker to determine hypoplasia.

✪ Question 32

The most common associated finding in aortic coarctation is:

    A. A bicuspid aortic valve.

    B. A ventricular septal defect.

    C. Subvalvar aortic stenosis.

    D. Mitral stenosis.

✪✪ Question 33

When assessing a coarctation of the aorta, from which view should a spectral Doppler signal be obtained in addition to the suprasternal long-axis of the aortic arch?

    A. Apical 5 chamber

    B. Parasternal long axis

    C. Right sternal border

    D. Subcostal

✪✪ Question 34

A coarctation can be misdiagnosed due to:

    A. Poor axial resolution.

    B. Poor lateral resolution.

    C. Reverberation artifacts.

    D. Shadowing artifacts.

    E. All of the above.

✪✪ Question 35

▶ The patent ductus arteriosus (PDA) flow seen in **Video 27-6** can be described as:

    A. Bidirectional.

    B. Right-to-left.

    C. Left-to-right.

    D. Indeterminate.

    E. Both A and B.

✪✪ Question 36

In **Figure 27-1**, the structures labeled A to C are:

    A. A = left pulmonary artery; B = right pulmonary artery; C = patent ductus arteriosus.

    B. A = patent ductus arteriosus; B = right pulmonary artery; C = left pulmonary artery.

    C. A = right pulmonary artery; B = left pulmonary artery; C = patent ductus arteriosus.

    D. A = right pulmonary artery; B = patent ductus arteriosus; C = left pulmonary artery.

    E. A = left pulmonary artery; B = patent ductus arteriosus; B = right pulmonary artery.

✪✪✪ Question 37

The direction of the patent ductus arteriosus (PDA) flow seen in **Figure 27-1** (Question 36) can be described as:

    A. Right-to-left.

    B. Left-to-right.

    C. Bidirectional.

    D. Indeterminate.

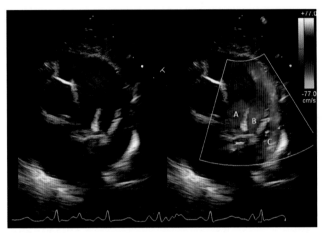

Figure 27-1

CASE 1

▶ A 13-year-old boy is referred for a murmur and right bundle branch block (RBBB) on his electrocardiogram. Representative images from this study are shown in **Figure 27-2A** to **27-2C** and **Video 27-7**.

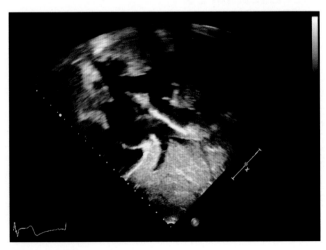

Figure 27-2A

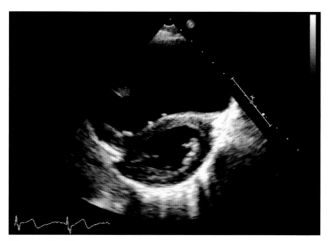

Figure 27-2B

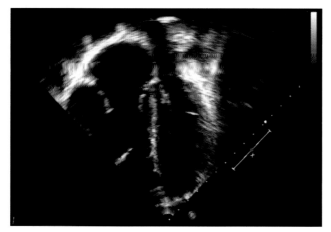

Figure 27-2C

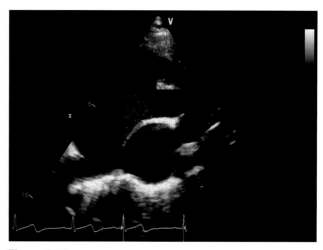

Figure 27-3

⊛⊛ Question 40

Which cardiac anomaly is most commonly associated with the defect seen in this case?
- **A.** Interrupted inferior vena cava
- **B.** Partial anomalous pulmonary venous return
- **C.** Persistent left superior vena cava
- **D.** Total anomalous pulmonary venous return

CASE 2

⏵ An 8-year-old boy is referred for an aortic valve murmur. Representative images from this study are shown in **Videos 27-8A** to **27-8B**.

⊛ Question 38

The type of cardiac defect displayed is a(n):
- **A.** Inferior vena cava-type sinus venosus atrial septal defect (ASD).
- **B.** Primum ASD.
- **C.** Secundum ASD.
- **D.** Superior vena cava–type sinus venosus ASD.

⊛ Question 39

Which echocardiographic view shown in **Figure 27-3** would also be useful in identifying the cardiac defect in this case?
- **A.** Parasternal long axis of left ventricle
- **B.** Parasternal short axis, level of aorta
- **C.** Right upper parasternal
- **D.** Suprasternal sagittal

⊛ Question 41

The congenital aortic valve anomaly demonstrated is:
- **A.** Bicuspid.
- **B.** Hypoplastic.
- **C.** Unicuspid.
- **D.** Quadricuspid.

⊛ Question 42

Aortic insufficiency seen in this case can lead to which secondary finding?
- **A.** Right ventricular dilatation
- **B.** Right atrial dilatation
- **C.** Left ventricular hypertrophy
- **D.** Left ventricular dilatation

✪✪ Question 43

Other parasternal long-axis view clues to the presence of the congenital aortic valve anomaly shown in this case may include:

A. A hypoplastic aortic root and dilated ascending aorta.

B. A central closure line of the aortic valve leaflets and dilatation of the sinotubular junction.

C. An eccentric closure line of the aortic valve leaflets and aortic root dilatation.

D. A hypoplastic aortic annulus and dilated aortic root.

ANSWERS

1. ▶ **Answer: A.** The septum primum appears on the posterosuperior wall of the primitive atrial chamber and grows toward the endocardial cushions. A large, temporary opening exists between the lower free edge of the septum primum and the endocardial cushions called the foramen primum. The flap of the foramen ovale is composed of the septum primum, which is more associated with the left atrium. The foramen ovale is a normal interatrial communication that is present throughout fetal life. Postnatally the pulmonic pressures decrease, and systemic pressures increase as fetal shunts begin to close. The closure of the foramen ovale occurs as pressure in the left atrium exceeds that in the right atrium. As a result, the valve of the fossa ovalis is pressed against the limbus and closes the opening. A permanent seal forms during the first year of life. Anatomic closure does not occur in 25% to 30% of people and is called a patent foramen ovale (**Figure 27-4** and **Video 27-9**).

2. **Answer: C.** An atrial septal defect (ASD) is a communication between the two atria. The foramen ovale should close soon after birth and is located centrally with the septum formed by the flaps of the septum primum and septum secundum. A sinus venosus ASD is located superiorly and is due to the failure of the interatrial septum to attach to the roof of the atria. A primum ASD is a failure of the interatrial septum to attach to the annulus at the level of the atrioventricular valves. Secundum ASDs occur centrally in the interatrial septum.

3. **Answer: A.** Arteriovenous malformations (AVMs) are abnormal connections between pulmonary arteries and pulmonary veins. AVMs can create direct shunting from the pulmonary arteries to the pulmonary veins without gas exchange in the lungs. Many patients will develop dyspnea and cyanosis later in life. A saline bubble study is an essential tool for screening and diagnosis. Five to 10 mL of agitated saline is injected and quickly will fill the right ventricle. In the presence of an atrial shunt such as a PFO (answer B), the bubbles will appear within 1 to 3 beats in the left atrium. If the microbubbles appear after 4 to 5 beats, then this confirms the presence of AVMs. This is because it takes time to travel through the pulmonary vasculature and therefore the microbubbles will appear later. In the presence of a persistent LSVC (answer C), the bubbles will appear first within the coronary sinus before entering the right atrium and right ventricle. This is best demonstrated in the apical 4-chamber view, oriented posteriorly to view the coronary sinus and by injecting into the left arm vein.

4. **Answer: D.** The subcostal imaging window is optimal for the interrogation of the interatrial septum (IAS) and to identify any associated atrial septal defects (ASDs) that may be present. To visualize the IAS without potential drop-out, the imaging plane should be perpendicular to the cardiac structure of interest. Therefore, the imaging plane that is nearly perpendicular to the IAS is utilized in the subcostal 4-chamber and sagittal (short-axis) views. ASDs can be demonstrated in other imaging windows including the parasternal short-axis, apical 4-chamber, and high right parasternal views, but care must be taken not to diagnose an ASD when the imaging plane is more parallel to the IAS, creating the potential for false drop-out in the two-dimensional image. The addition of color Doppler and spectral Doppler interrogation in these views may also facilitate the diagnosis of an ASD.

5. **Answer: B.** An ostium primum atrial septal defect (1° ASD) occurs between the inferior margin of the true interatrial septum (IAS) and the superior aspect

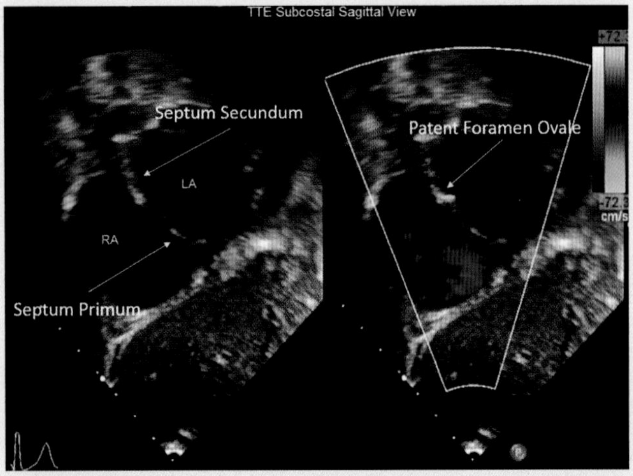

Figure 27-4

of the atrioventricular (AV) valves. These defects are also referred to as partial atrioventricular septal defects. Defects occur when the endocardial cushion, which also contributes to the formation of the AV valves, fails to fuse with the IAS in utero. This results in a 1° ASD and most commonly a cleft in the anterior leaflet of the mitral valve with associated mitral regurgitation (MR). The best echocardiographic view to image a 1° ASD is the apical 4-chamber view. From this view, the degree of MR arising from the cleft mitral valve can also be appreciated.

6. **Answer: C.** The direction of atrial level shunt is primarily related to the compliance of the ventricles. The right ventricle is typically more compliant than the left ventricle, which causes characteristic left-to-right shunting. These other factors noted in the question also contribute to the degree and direction of atrial level shunt, but ventricular compliance is most important.

7. **Answer: A.** An uncomplicated ASD is one that has no other associated defects. With the pulsed-wave Doppler sample volume in the right atrium adjacent to the ASD, a characteristic spectral Doppler pattern of left-to-right shunting will be seen. This will appear as low velocity (0.2-1.0 m/s) biphasic flow above the zero-velocity baseline that peaks in late ventricular systole and following atrial systole (**Figure 27-5**). Lack of phasic flow may be an indicator of a significant pressure gradient between the left and right atria due to a restrictive (small) defect. Continuous flow profiles with similar velocities throughout systole and diastole (answer C) are seen when there is a continuous pressure gradient of the same magnitude between chambers and/or vessels. Spectral Doppler patterns with a sharp upstroke and diastolic runoff (answer D) are used to describe obstructive defects such as coarctation of the aorta.

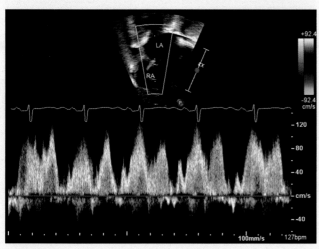

Figure 27-5

8. **Answer: D.** Because pulmonary pressures are normally lower than systemic pressures (and RV compliance is less than LV compliance), blood will shunt from left-to-right across an ASD. Due to the increased volume of flow on the right side of the heart, the right atrium (RA) and right ventricle (RV) respond by dilating (**Figure 27-6**). Dilatation of the tricuspid annulus will lead to tricuspid regurgitation. Another common finding in patients with a dilated right atrium and right ventricle is flow acceleration across the pulmonary valve. This does not mean that the patient has pulmonary stenosis. However, increased flow in the right heart leads to increased flow across the pulmonary valve.

9. **Answer: E.** Most (80%-90%) of muscular VSDs close spontaneously by late childhood. When small, the majority will close within the first few years of life, but spontaneous closure with these muscular defects can occur later in childhood and even in adulthood.

10. **Answer: C.** Perimembranous VSDs are the most common type of VSD and are known to close spontaneously. These defects occur in the upper section of the ventricular septum, near the tricuspid and aortic valves, and occur due to a deficiency of tissue in the region of the membranous septum or due to malalignment of the outlet septum with the muscular ventricular septum. Because of their location (adjacent to the tricuspid valve), these defects can lead to distortion of the tricuspid valve tissue. Accessory tissue from the tricuspid valve septal leaflet or the septal leaflet itself can partially or completely close the defect (**Video 27-10**).

11. **Answer: C.** Malalignment VSDs are characterized by malalignment of the outlet (conal or infundibular) septum to the muscular ventricular septum. The gap caused by malalignment of the outlet septum can be due to either anterior or posterior deviation of the outlet septum. Conal truncal malformations are commonly associated with malalignment defects; this includes transposition of the great arteries or double outlet ventricle. Tetralogy of Fallot occurs when the great arteries are normally related and there is anterior malalignment of the VSD, which impinges on the right ventricle and subpulmonary region, resulting in pulmonary stenosis (**Figure 27-7**).

12. **Answer: A.** Similar to the malalignment discussion in the previous question, if the great arteries are normally related, a posterior malalignment VSD will impinge on the left ventricle and subaortic region, resulting in aortic stenosis (**Figure 27-8**). Posterior and anterior malalignment VSDs never close spontaneously.

13. **Answer: B.** Conal septal defects, also known as outlet VSD, doubly committed VSD, or supracristal VSD, do not close spontaneously and often require a surgical approach for closure. From the parasternal

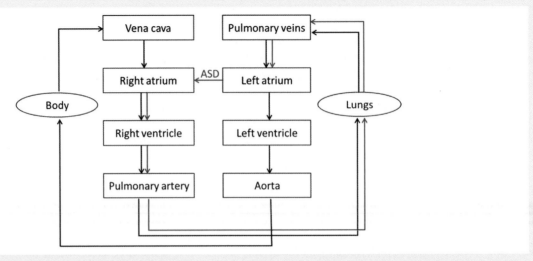

Figure 27-6 Left-to-right shunting across an ASD results in increased flow to the right atrium and right ventricle, leading to dilatation of these chambers.

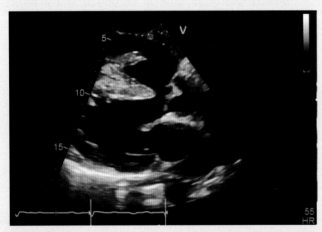

Figure 27-7

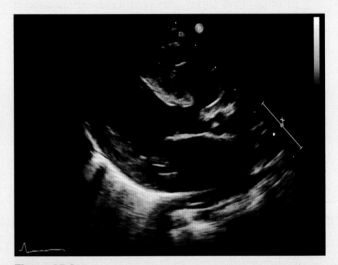

Figure 27-8

short-axis view, these defects appear between 12 and 3 o'clock (**Figure 27-9**). Due to the proximity of these defects to the right coronary cusp of the aortic valve, there is a propensity for aortic valve prolapse to occur into the VSD, resulting in partial or complete closure. Resulting severe aortic regurgitation is an indication for surgical repair.

14. **Answer: B.** An inlet-type VSD is associated with atrioventricular (AV) canal defect. These defects occur when there is abnormal embryologic development of the endocardial cushions. Inlet-type VSDs are located adjacent to the AV valves and can be associated with primum atrial septal defects, as well as AV valve abnormalities. An inlet-type VSD is best imaged in apical 4-chamber views to appreciate its proximity to the AV valves (**Figure 27-10**, arrow).

15. **Answer: A.** Aortic insufficiency (or regurgitation) is the most common associated abnormality because of prolapse of the aortic cusp into a subpulmonary VSD. While this associated prolapse of aortic tissue limits the size of the VSD and can lessen the left-to-right shunt, the progression of aortic insufficiency due to distortion of the aortic valve is well

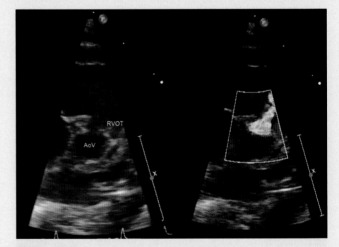

Figure 27-9

recognized. If this regurgitation is significant and progresses, surgical closure is indicated (and is not dependent upon the size of the left-to-right shunt).

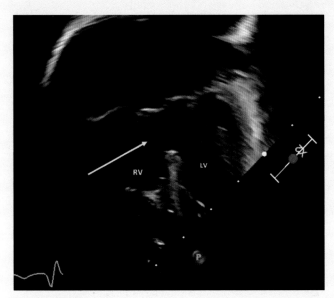

Figure 27-10

LVOT obstruction (answer C) is more characteristically present in patients with a septal defect while RVOT obstruction (answer E) is the hallmark of anterior malalignment VSDs in tetralogy of Fallot. Pulmonary stenosis (answer D) and aortic stenosis (answer B) are not characteristic findings in a patient with a subpulmonary VSD.

16. **Answer: A.** A coronary sinus ASD is a very rare type of anomaly that results from partial or complete unroofing of the tissue that separates the coronary sinus from the left atrium. As the coronary sinus runs in the posterior left atrioventricular groove, this lack of tissue will allow shunting of blood between the left and right atria, through the coronary sinus. It is important for the sonographer to rule out a persistent left superior vena caval connection to the coronary sinus.

17. **Answer: B.** With normal cardiac physiology, systemic pressures are higher than pulmonary pressures, leading to left-to-right shunting across the VSD. The blood shunting across the VSD will flow from the left ventricle to the right ventricle to the pulmonary arteries and then return to the left side of the heart via the pulmonary veins. This increase in volume, not pressure, leads to dilatation of the left heart chambers (**Figure 27-11**).

18. **Answer: C.** An inlet VSD is located posteriorly and immediately adjacent to both atrioventricular (AV) valves. The VSD will be seen best at the level of the AV valves in an apical 4-chamber view. An inlet VSD can be isolated but is most likely associated with the class of defects called atrioventricular septal defects. Atrioventricular septal defects can often be seen in patients with trisomy 21 but can also occur in isolation.

19. **Answer: D.** The most common type of VSD is a perimembranous defect (**Figure 27-12**). These defects account for approximately 80% of all VSDs and are located beneath the aortic valve bordering the septal tricuspid leaflet and inferior to the crista supraventricularis.

20. **Answer: A.** A Gerbode defect occurs within the atrioventricular septum, resulting in a communication between the right atrium (RA) and left ventricle (LV). A true Gerbode defect (in contrast to defects that result from adherence of the tricuspid valve commissure to the VSD rim) is extremely rare. It is important not to confuse the shunt through a Gerbode defect with tricuspid regurgitation to avoid overestimating right ventricular systolic pressure. The peak velocity of flow through the Gerbode defect reflects the pressure gradient between the LV and RA.

21. **Answer: B.** A patent ductus arteriosus (PDA) occurs when the ductus arteriosus from the fetal circulation fails to close. When evaluating a PDA, it is important

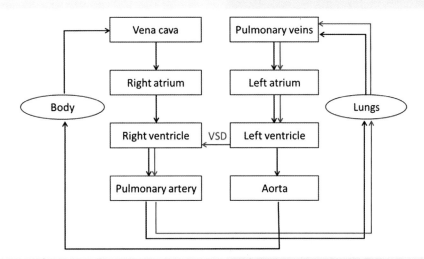

Figure 27-11 Left-to-right shunting across a VSD results in increased flow to the right ventricle, pulmonary artery, and lungs. This increases the pulmonary venous return leading to dilatation of left atrium and left ventricle.

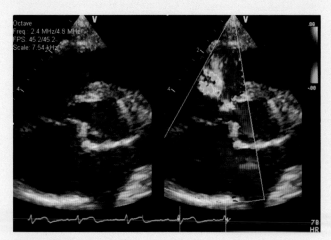

Figure 27-12

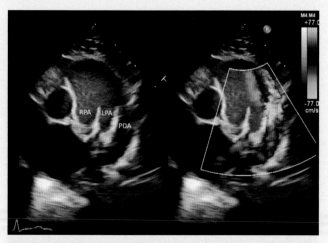

Figure 27-13C

to determine the diameter, length, and blood flow direction within the vessel, as well as the pressure gradient between the PDA and descending aorta. A PDA is best visualized in the upper left parasternal short-axis view, as well as in suprasternal views (**Figure 27-13A** to **27-13C**). In a patient with normal pulmonary pressures, blood will shunt from the

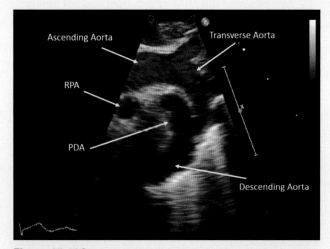

Figure 27-13A

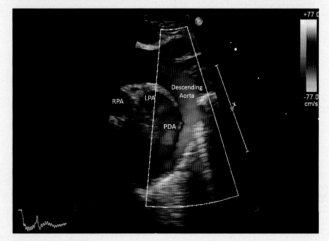

Figure 27-13B

aorta (left) to the pulmonary artery (right) because systemic (aortic) pressures are higher than pulmonary pressures.

22. **Answer: D.** Similar to severe aortic insufficiency, a large PDA displays pan-diastolic flow reversal in the abdominal aorta. Pan-diastolic flow reversal in the abdominal occurs when there is diastolic flow from the aorta into another lower-pressure chamber or vessel. In the case of a PDA, this occurs due to left-to-right shunting of blood from the aorta to the lower-pressure pulmonary artery. When grading the amount of left-to-right shunting across the PDA, it is important to use pulsed-wave Doppler to interrogate the abdominal aorta looking for flow below the zero-velocity baseline in diastole.

23. **Answer: C.** If the PDA is large, left-to-right shunting over time will cause left heart dilatation. This is because the extra volume of blood going into the branch pulmonary arteries from the PDA ultimately returns back to the left heart via the pulmonary veins (**Figure 27-14**). It is not uncommon to see torrential flow through the pulmonary veins, left atrial and left ventricular dilation, and mitral regurgitation in the prolonged presence of a moderate to large PDA.

In the setting of increased pulmonary pressures, blood will shunt bidirectionally across the PDA. In cases of severe pulmonary hypertension, blood will shunt completely right-to-left across the PDA, from the pulmonary artery to the aorta. These can be difficult to identify as there is also systolic flow seen in the branch pulmonary arteries and descending aorta all in the same region. Therefore, it is important to differentiate the PDA from the branch pulmonary arteries.

24. **Answer: B.** Newborns are born with increased pulmonary pressures. This is because they have received oxygen via the umbilical vein in utero and their lungs have never actually expanded. It is common to see equal pulmonary and systemic pressures in the first few hours of life. In a normal

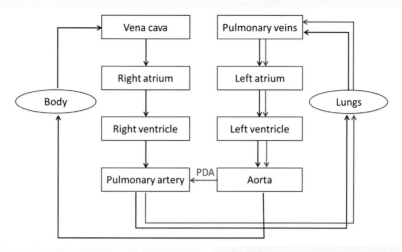

Figure 27-14 Left-to-right shunting across a PDA results in increased flow to the pulmonary artery and lungs. This increases the pulmonary venous return, leading to dilatation of left atrium and left ventricle.

newborn, this would result in bidirectional shunting across the PDA initially. As the baby breathes and the lungs expand, the pulmonary vascular resistance drops, leading to a decrease in pulmonary pressures, ultimately becoming less than systemic pressures. This is demonstrated by left-to-right shunting across the PDA. In the case of persistent pulmonary hypertension, the pressure in the lungs remains high. This is commonly seen in premature infants with primary lung disease. Because their lungs are underdeveloped and are not fully functioning, pulmonary pressures remain elevated and can even exceed systemic pressures. This is termed "supra-systemic" pulmonary pressures. In this case, blood will shunt from the pulmonary artery to the aorta (right-to-left) across the PDA. These patients also tend to have right ventricular hypertrophy and a flattened ventricular septum.

25. **Answer: D.** Congenital left ventricular outflow tract (LVOT) obstruction is defined as an anatomic blockage of left ventricular output. Obstruction may involve the subvalvar, valvar, or supravalvar portion of the aortic valve complex. A subaortic membrane is the most common type of subaortic stenosis. It is a discrete "shelf-like" membrane that grows below the aortic valve in the LVOT. It is more common in males and can be familial. The membrane can be seen with 2D echocardiography in any view when the LVOT is imaged; this includes the parasternal and apical long-axis views and the apical 5-chamber view (**Figure 27-15**). The best views for imaging of the subaortic membrane are the apical views where the ultrasound beam is perpendicular to the membrane. In the parasternal long-axis view, the ultrasound beam is parallel to a subaortic membrane and therefore this can be missed. The hemodynamics are similar to aortic stenosis in that the membrane makes the LVOT narrower, causing blood to flow faster across it. Therefore, continuous-wave Doppler

will most likely be used to display increased velocities across the LVOT. Color Doppler imaging is especially useful in identifying the level of obstruction (**Video 27-11**). It is not uncommon to see left ventricular hypertrophy in patients with a subaortic membrane. A discrete subaortic membrane can be surgically removed, but there is a possibility of regrowth of the tissue. Importantly, follow-up exams after resection should include a detailed evaluation with color flow and pulsed-wave Doppler to identify new membrane tissue growth.

26. **Answer: C.** The original description of Shone's syndrome included four left heart obstructive defects: supravalvular mitral ring, parachute mitral valve, subaortic stenosis, and coarctation of the aorta. Bicuspid aortic valve has also been included as a lesion associated with this syndrome. A parachute

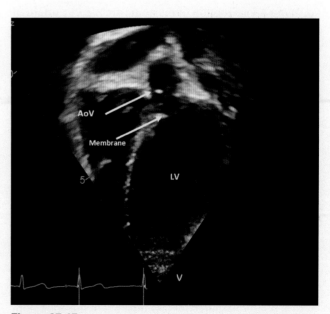

Figure 27-15

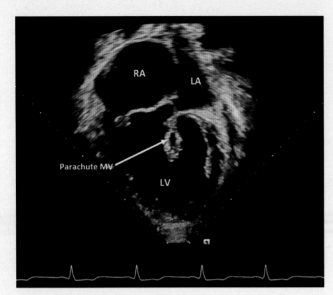

Figure 27-16

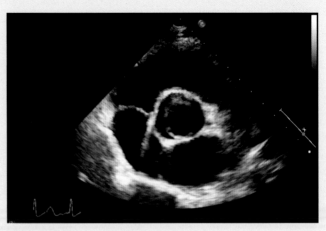

Figure 27-17

mitral valve is characterized by a single papillary muscle to which all the mitral chordae are attached. **Figure 27-16** and **Video 27-12** show an example of a parachute mitral valve.

27. **Answer: C.** An aortopulmonary (AP) window is a communication between the aorta and pulmonary artery above the semilunar valve. An AP window differs from a patent ductus arteriosus (PDA) because the AP window results from failure of complete septation of the truncus arteriosus embryologically, whereas a PDA occurs when the fetal ductal arteriosus fails to close after birth. In both cases, there is left-to-right shunting of blood from the aorta to the pulmonary artery, resulting in dilatation of the left heart chambers.

Approximately 50% of patients with an AP window have other associated anomalies. These include type A interruption of the aortic arch, aortic origin of the right pulmonary artery, anomalous origin of one or both coronary arteries from the pulmonary artery, tetralogy of Fallot, right aortic arch, ventricular septal defect, and transposition of the great arteries.

28. ▶ **Answer: A.** A unicuspid aortic valve (UAV) is a very rare lesion that occurs when there is fusion between two of the three developing aortic valve cusps or fusion of all three developing cusps resulting in an abnormal valve with a solitary opening. These valves are usually stenotic at birth. UAVs may be acommissural or unicommissural. In an acommissural UAV, there is a single membrane-like leaflet with a central orifice and no apparent commissural attachment to the aortic root. The unicommissural UAV, which is more common, has an eccentric orifice with one commissural attachment to the aorta (**Figure 27-17** and **Video 27-13**).

A UAV accounts for less than 5% of the adult population with aortic stenosis that requires surgery.

Adults with a UAV usually present in the third to fifth decade of life with severe aortic stenosis or regurgitation. Due to the lack of commissures and raphes in a UVA, surgery achieves better outcomes than balloon valvuloplasty.

29. **Answer: C.** There is discrete narrowing of the pulmonary artery in the supravalvular region (**Figure 27-18**). This is called supravalvar pulmonary stenosis (PS). There are four different levels for right ventricular outflow tract obstruction: subvalvar PS, when there is narrowing below the valve in the right ventricular outflow tract; valvar PS, with narrowing at the valve level; supravalvar PS, when the main pulmonary artery is narrowed just above the pulmonary valve; and stenosis in the pulmonary artery branches (also known as peripheral stenosis). With supravalvar PS, the pulmonary valve leaflets themselves could be normal; however, there will be flow acceleration through the narrowed pulmonary artery. It is important to frequently assess the gradient of all types of PS found in newborns, as the pulmonary vascular resistance (PVR) changes. As the PVR drops, the gradient across the narrowed pulmonary region will increase. PS is graded according

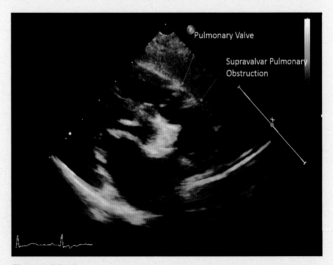

Figure 27-18

to peak gradient measurements: Mild PS is defined as a peak gradient between 30 and 40 mm Hg, moderate PS is defined as a peak gradient between 40 and 60 mm Hg, and severe PS is defined a peak gradient greater than 60 mm Hg. PS causes a pressure overload of the right ventricle, and this results in right ventricular hypertrophy.

30. **Answer: B.** With valvar pulmonary stenosis (PS), the pulmonary valve is typically thickened, with systolic doming. The valve is often bicuspid and poststenotic dilatation of the main pulmonary artery can often be noted. Valvular PS is associated with Noonan syndrome, with approximately 15% of patients with Noonan syndrome having PS. Pulmonary valve stenosis can also be associated with severe dysplasia of the pulmonary valve leaflets; this is most typically seen in association with Noonan syndrome.

31. **Answer: B.** A z-score represents the number of standard deviations (σ) a given value falls from the population mean value (**Figure 27-19**). A z-score of 0 will signify the normal population mean. In pediatrics, a z-score of +2 represents the upper limit of normal and −2 represents the lower limit of normal. Any score greater than +2 will start to qualify an enlarged structure as larger than normal. A score less than −2 will qualify a structure as hypoplastic. Z-scores are especially useful in pediatric cardiology as they provide method for charting serial measurements by considering age and growth of body size. For example, the normal heart size for an 8-year-old ballerina and a 12-year-old high school football player will not be the same; therefore, the z-score can be used to determine normal values based on the age and size of the child.

32. **Answer: A.** The bicuspid aortic valve, specifically the underdevelopment of the intercoronary commissure, is often associated with coarctation of the aorta. Fusion of the right and left coronary cusps is the most common form of intercoronary commissure fusion in patients with coarctation of the aorta. The ridge of tissue resulting from fusion of the intercoronary commissures is also known as a raphe.

33. **Answer: D.** Coarctation of the aorta represents a congenital narrowing of the aorta, most often occurring just distal to the left subclavian artery and adjacent to the site of insertion of the ductus arteriosus. As the ductus arteriosus closes and forms the ligamentum arteriosum, the intimal lining of the descending aorta is constricted, leading to a narrowing in the descending aorta. The suprasternal view is considered the best window for imaging a coarctation of the aorta. From this view, a coarctation is characterized by an echo-dense shelf of tissue narrowing the aortic lumen, and the color Doppler examination demonstrates an area of flow acceleration proximal to this narrowed aortic segment (**Video 27-14**). On the continuous-wave Doppler examination, the characteristic flow pattern displays a "sawtooth" appearance, with antegrade flow extending into diastole (**Figure 27-20A**). In addition to suprasternal notch imaging, the sonographer should also obtain a pulsed-wave Doppler tracing of the abdominal aortic flow. In the presence of a coarctation, the abdominal aortic flow will have a delayed arterial upstroke with slow diastolic runoff or blunted aortic flow depending upon the severity of the obstruction (**Figure 27-20B**).

34. **Answer: B.** Poor lateral resolution can create a false appearance of a coarctation shelf from the suprasternal notch window. Adjusting the transmit focus will help reduce the incidence of false-positive imaging. Decreasing the transducer frequency, allowing increased depth penetration, can help image the distal portion of the descending thoracic aorta.

35. **Answer: A.** When intracardiac pressures are normal, shunting across a PDA occurs from the higher-pressure aorta to the lower-pressure pulmonary artery (PA) and, therefore, shunting is left-to-right.

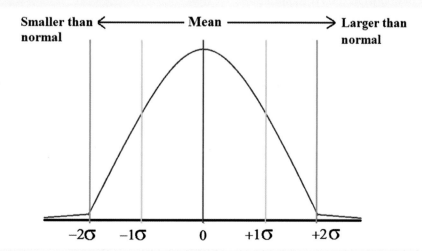

Smaller than normal ← Mean → Larger than normal

−2σ   −1σ   0   +1σ   +2σ

Figure 27-19

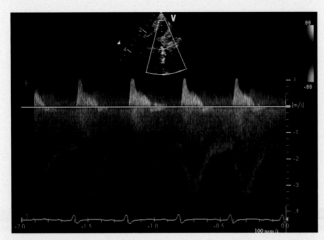

Figure 27-20A

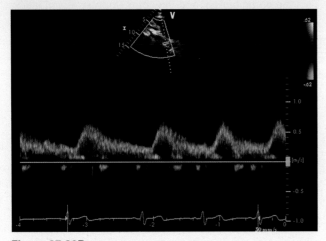

Figure 27-20B

Furthermore, as the pressure in the aorta is higher than the pressure in the PA in both systole and diastole, this shunting is continuous. On the color Doppler examination, PDA flow appears as red continuous flow toward the transducer. However, in the setting of increased pulmonary pressures, blood will shunt bidirectionally across the PDA as in this example. Bidirectional shunting is described as right-to-left shunting from the PA to the aorta in

systole and left-to-right shunting from the aorta to the PA in diastole. On the color Doppler examination, this appears as blue flow away from the transducer in systole and red flow toward the transducer in diastole (**Figure 27-21**).

36. **Answer: C.** This image shows the right pulmonary artery (A), left pulmonary artery (B), and a large patent ductus arteriosus (C).

37. **Answer: A.** True confirmation of the direction of the PDA shunt requires real-time imaging. However, as there is blue flow away from the transducer, this indicates that shunting is either bidirectional or right-to-left. As previously described, bidirectional shunting, which involves right-to-left shunting from the pulmonary artery (PA) to the aorta in systole and left-to-right shunting from the aorta to the PA in diastole, occurs when the pulmonary pressures are increased. On the color Doppler examination, this appears as blue flow away from the transducer in systole and red flow toward the transducer in diastole. In cases of severe pulmonary hypertension, shunting is completely right-to-left, from the PA to the aorta throughout the cardiac cycle. On the color Doppler examination, this appears as blue continuous flow away from the transducer. Right-to-left shunting across a PDA can be difficult to identify as there is also systolic flow seen in the branch pulmonary arteries and descending aorta all in the same region. Therefore, it is important to differentiate the PDA from the branch pulmonary arteries during the 2D exam.

Answer B is incorrect because left-to-right shunting will appear as red flow toward the transducer (see answer outline for Question 35).

38. **Answer: D.** ASDs account for approximately 15% of all congenital cardiac anomalies. They are named according to which part of the atrial septum is deficient. The ostium secundum ASD is most common, followed by ostium primum ASD and sinus venosus ASDs. Sinus venosus ASDs can be either superior, involving the superior vena cava (SVC), or inferior, involving the inferior vena cava. In this case, the

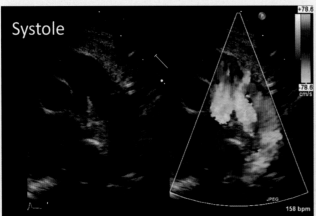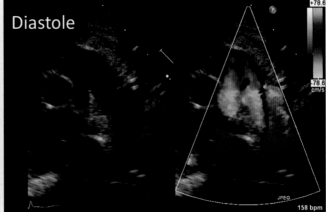

Figure 27-21

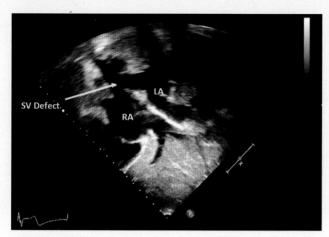

Figure 27-22

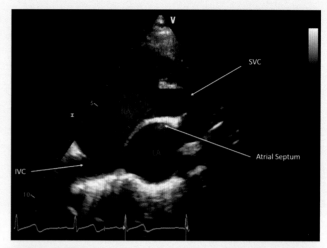

Figure 27-23A

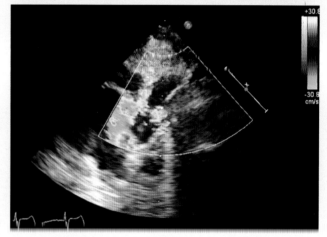

Figure 27-23B

SVC is seen draining into both the right atrium and left atrium and no superior atrial septum is seen (**Figure 27-22**, arrow). As the left atrial pressure is higher than right atrial pressure, blood shunts from left-to-right across the ASD. Large ASDs with left-to-right shunting lead to increased volume in the right atrium and right ventricle and subsequent dilatation of these chambers.

39. **Answer: C.** The right upper parasternal view is an excellent view for profiling the superior vena cava (SVC) and inferior vena cava (IVC) as they drain into the right atrium (RA) and for profiling the atrial septum between the left atrium (LA) and RA (**Figure 27-23A**). The blunt end of the secundum atrial septum, the lack of superior atrial septum, and the SVC draining into both the right and left atria can be seen in the case of an SVC-type sinus venosus atrial septal defect (**Figure 27-23B**).

40. **Answer: B.** Partial anomalous pulmonary venous return is the most commonly associated cardiac anomaly with superior vena cava (SVC)-type sinus venosus atrial septal defects. In utero, the pulmonary veins begin growing from the lungs, working their way to the left atrium where they normally attach. If there is no atrial septal wall near the SVC, the growing right upper pulmonary vein will find the SVC and attach itself to it, while the other three pulmonary veins all drain normally into the left atrium. This is also demonstrated in the right upper parasternal view.

41. **Answer: A.** Approximately 2% of the general population have a bicuspid aortic valve (BAV), and it is twice as common in males as in females. It is the most common congenital aortic valve anomaly. BAV occurs when two of the three aortic cusps fail to separate in utero. The most common type of BAV is fusion of the right and left coronary cusps. The echocardiographic diagnosis of a BAV is made from the parasternal short-axis view by observing only two, instead of three, commissural attachments to the aortic root.

42. **Answer: D.** Aortic insufficiency leads to volume overload of the left ventricle. Over time, the increased volume causes the left ventricle to dilate to accommodate the extra diastolic blood volume. In cases of long-standing moderate to severe aortic insufficiency, the mitral annulus will dilate with the left ventricle, leading to mitral regurgitation and left atrial dilatation. Therefore, it is not uncommon to see left heart dilatation with moderate to severe aortic insufficiency. It is also important to perform spectral Doppler interrogation of the descending aorta and the abdominal aorta to look for pan-diastolic flow reversal, which assists with grading the degree of aortic insufficiency.

43. **Answer: C.** While the best echocardiographic view to diagnose a bicuspid aortic valve (BAV) is the parasternal short-axis view, there are clues that can be seen in the parasternal long-axis view as well. Since the two aortic valve leaflets are often unequal in size and shape, when they close during diastole, the closure line is not perfectly in the middle of the aortic annulus. Instead, they have an abnormal closure, leading to eccentric closure lines. BAV is also

associated with aortic root and ascending aortic dilatation. These measurements should be made in the parasternal long-axis view. In addition, diastolic and/or systolic doming of the aortic valve are clues to the presence of a BAV.

Acknowledgments: The authors thank and acknowledge the contributions from Benjamin W. Eidem, MD (Chapter 30 Noncyanotic Congenital Heart Disease) in *Clinical Echocardiography Review: A Self-Assessment Tool*, 2nd Edition, edited by Allan L. Klein, Craig R. Asher, 2017.

SUGGESTED READINGS

Allen HD, Shaddy RE, Penny DJ, Feltes TF, Cetta F. *Moss & Adams' Heart Disease in Infants, Children, and Adolescents: Including the Fetus and Young Adult*. 9th ed. Philadelphia, PA: Wolters Kluwer; 2016.

Eidem B, O'Leary P, Cetta F. *Echocardiography in Pediatric and Adult Congenital Heart Disease*. 2nd ed. Philadelphia, PA: Wolters Kluwer Health; 2015.

Everett AD, Lim DS. *Illustrated Field Guide to Congenital Heart Disease and Repair*. 2nd ed. Charlottesville, VA: Scientific Software Solutions Inc; 2007.

Harry MJ. *Cardiac Doppler Hemodynamic Handbook: An Illustrative Guide*. Des Moines, IA: Iowa Heart Institute; 1994.

Harry MJ. *Essentials of Echocardiography and Cardiac Hemodynamics*. Forney, TX: Pegasus Lectures; 2007.

Heiden K. *Congenital Heart Defects, Simplified*. Milwaukee, WI: Midwest EchoSolutions; 2009.

Lai W, Mertens L, Cohen M, Geva T. *Echocardiography in Pediatric and Congenital Heart Disease - From Fetus to Adult*. 2nd ed. West Sussex, UK: John Wiley & Sons; 2016.

Lewin MB, Stout K. *Echocardiography in Congenital Heart Disease*. Philadelphia, PA: Elsevier Saunders; 2012.

Pansky B. *Review of Medical Embryology*. New Jersey: Macmillan; 1982.

Reynold T. *The Pediatric Echocardiographer's Pocket Reference*. 3rd ed. Phoenix, AZ: Arizona Heart Institute; 2002.

Shabana A. Bicuspid aortic valve: an article from the e-journal of the ESC Council for Cardiology Practice. *E-Journal of Cardiology Practice*. 2014;13(2). https://www.escardio.org/Journals/E-Journal of Cardiology Practice/Volume-13/Bicuspid-aortic-valve.

Singh S, Ghayal P, Mathur A, et al. Unicuspid unicommissural aortic valve: an extremely rare congenital anomaly. *Tex Heart Inst J*. 2015;42(3):273-276.

Cyanotic Congenital Heart Disease

Contributors: Heidi S. Borchers, BS, RDCS (AE, PE), Colleen D. Cailes, AS, RDCS, RCS, and Cathy West, DMU (Cardiac), EACVI CHD, MSc

✪ Question 1

What is the most common form of transposition of the great arteries (TGA)?

- **A.** Levo-transposition of the great arteries (l-TGA)
- **B.** Taussig-Bing transposition with double outlet right ventricle (DORV)
- **C.** Dextro-transposition of the great arteries (d-TGA)
- **D.** Congenitally corrected transposition of the great arteries (cc-TGA)

✪ Question 2

A 2-month-old baby girl presents to the pediatric cardiology clinic with the indication of failure to thrive and enlarged heart on X-ray. An echocardiogram is ordered to assess cardiac anatomy. Based on the image of the subcostal 4-chamber view (**Figure 28-1**), which is the most likely diagnosis?

- **A.** Total anomalous pulmonary venous return
- **B.** Truncus arteriosus
- **C.** Ebstein anomaly with pulmonary hypertension
- **D.** Small muscular ventricular septal defect

✪ Question 3

Which of the four options below correctly describes the four congenital heart abnormalities that form tetralogy of Fallot?

- **A.** Septal deviation, infundibular stenosis, RVH, VSD
- **B.** Subvalvular PS, ASD, overriding aorta, RVH
- **C.** VSD, dilated aortic root, pulmonary stenosis, RVH
- **D.** VSD, infundibular PS, RVH, overriding aorta

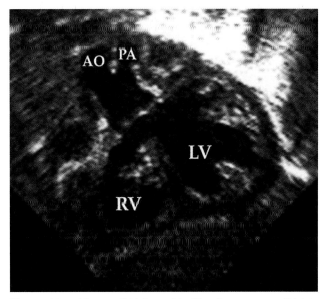

Figure 28-1 AO, aorta; LV, left ventricle; PA, pulmonary artery; RV, right ventricle. (Reprinted with permission from MacDonald MG, Seshia MM. *Avery's Neonatology.* 7th ed. Philadelphia, PA: Wolters Kluwer; 2015.)

ASD = atrial septal defect; PS = pulmonary stenosis; RVH = right ventricular hypertrophy; VSD = ventricular septal defect.

✪ Question 4

Which type of total anomalous pulmonary venous return (TAPVR) presents with a dilated innominate vein?

- **A.** Cardiac TAPVR directly to the right atrium (RA)
- **B.** Cardiac TAPVR with return via the coronary sinus
- **C.** Infracardiac TAPVR to the portal vein system
- **D.** Supracardiac TAPVR to the right superior vena cava (SVC)
- **E.** Supracardiac TAPVR via a left vertical vein

✪ Question 5

An echocardiogram is performed on a 10-year-old with Ebstein anomaly—**Figure 28-2** shows the apical 4-chamber view. Saturations have been normal in the past, but today it is reading lower than usual. In addition to the obvious abnormality of the tricuspid valve, what other defect must be present for the patient to have cyanosis?

A. A patent ductus arteriosus
B. A patent foramen ovale
C. Pulmonary hypertension
D. Severe pulmonary insufficiency
E. Severe tricuspid regurgitation

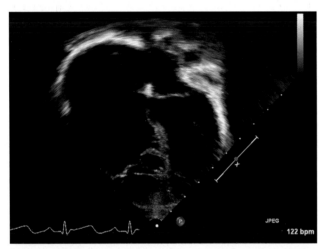

Figure 28-2

✪ Question 6

Which of the following statements specifically relates to Eisenmenger syndrome?

A. A left-to-right shunt which becomes bidirectional or right-to-left
B. Central cyanosis with blue lips and tongue
C. Right-to-left shunting causing hypoxia
D. Suprasystemic pulmonary pressures

✪ Question 7

In the initial pediatric echocardiographic examination, the pulmonary artery (PA) is identified by:

A. Its relationship to the aorta.
B. Its bifurcation pattern.
C. The length of the vessel.
D. The ventricle from which it originates.

✪✪ Question 8

Based on **Figure 28-3**, the most likely diagnosis is:

A. Tetralogy of Fallot (TOF).
B. Double outlet right ventricle (DORV).
C. Truncus arteriosus.
D. A or C.
E. Any of the above.

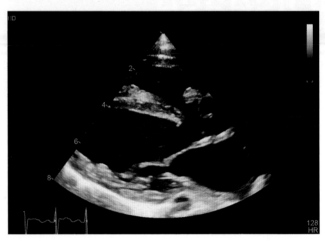

Figure 28-3

✪ Question 9

The degree of cyanosis observed in tetralogy of Fallot (TOF) is primarily determined by which of the following?

A. The size of the ventricular septal defect (VSD)
B. The size of the right ventricle (RV)
C. The degree of right ventricular outflow tract (RVOT) obstruction
D. The degree of aortic override

✪ Question 10

With which of the following syndromes is tetralogy of Fallot most commonly associated?

A. Williams syndrome
B. Noonan syndrome
C. Eisenmenger syndrome
D. Down syndrome

✪✪ Question 11

Which of the following pathologies hemodynamically mimics unobstructed total anomalous pulmonary venous return (TAPVR)?

A. Large atrial septal defect (ASD) with left-to-right shunting

B. Mitral valve prolapse (MVP) with moderate mitral regurgitation

C. Moderate patent ductus arteriosus (PDA) with left-to-right shunting

D. Moderate pulmonary valve stenosis with moderate pulmonary regurgitation

E. Moderate ventricular septal defect (VSD) with left-to-right shunting

✪✪ Question 12

What is the MOST common type of tricuspid atresia?

A. Normally related great arteries, intact ventricular septum, pulmonary atresia

B. Normally related great arteries, small ventricular septal defect (VSD), pulmonary stenosis

C. Transposed great arteries, large VSD, pulmonary atresia

D. Transposed great arteries, small VSD, aortic stenosis

E. Transposed great arteries, VSD, normal size great arteries

✪✪ Question 13

Which of the following statements regarding double outlet right ventricle (DORV) is incorrect?

A. DORV is commonly associated with Ebstein anomaly.

B. The aorta overrides the ventricular septal defect (VSD) by more than 50%.

C. The location of the VSD determines the surgical approach to repair.

D. There can be ventriculoarterial concordance or discordance.

✪✪ Question 14

What anatomy is critical to assess when presented with a cyanotic newborn that has Ebstein anomaly?

A. The pulmonary arteries

B. The pulmonary valve

C. The tricuspid valve

D. The interventricular septum

✪✪ Question 15

When a patient presents with atrioventricular (AV) concordance with ventriculoarterial (VA) discordance which of the following best describes the pathway of blood?

A. RA to RV to PA and LA to LV to AO

B. RA to LV to PA and LA to RV to AO

C. RA to RV to AO and LA to LV to PA

D. RA to LV to AO and LA to RV to PA

AO = aorta; LA = left atrium; LV = left ventricle; PA = pulmonary artery; RA = right atrium; RV = right ventricle.

✪✪ Question 16

As a baby with truncus arteriosus gets older, heart failure worsens. Which of the following changes is the most likely contributing factor?

A. The patent ductus arteriosus (PDA) closes.

B. The pulmonary arteries grow.

C. Systemic vascular resistance (SVR) decreases.

D. Pulmonary vascular resistance (PVR) decreases.

✪✪ Question 17

What is the embryological defect that causes the four lesions seen in tetralogy of Fallot (TOF)?

A. Right ventricular dysplasia

B. Anterocephalad deviation of the outlet septum

C. Excessive reabsorption of the ventricular septum

D. Anterocephalad deviation of the perimembranous septum

✪✪ Question 18

Which type of total anomalous pulmonary venous return (TAPVR) is not likely to present with obstruction?

A. Cardiac TAPVR with return via the coronary sinus to the right atrium

B. Infracardiac TAPVR with drainage in the liver

C. Supracardiac TAPVR through a right vertical vein to the superior vena cava (SVC)

D. Supracardiac TAPVR via left vertical vein to the innominate vein

✪✪ Question 19

Which of the following statements regarding truncus arteriosus is false?

A. The truncal valve can have between two and five leaflets.

B. Truncus patients can have a widened pulse pressure.

C. Truncus arteriosus is best imaged from the short-axis views.

D. Truncus arteriosus is an abnormal structure in embryonic development.

✪✪ Question 20

The most commonly associated conditions observed with tricuspid atresia include all of the following except:

A. Transposition of the great arteries.

B. Ventricular septal defect.

C. Pulmonary stenosis.

D. Subaortic stenosis.

E. Primum atrial septal defect.

✪✪ Question 21

In a patient with truncus arteriosus, which of the following findings would be most concerning?

A. A high-velocity ventricular septal defect (VSD) jet

B. A low-velocity VSD jet

C. A quadricuspid valve

D. A patent ductus arteriosus

✪✪ Question 22

Which of the following pathologies is not commonly associated with tetralogy of Fallot (TOF)?

A. A right aortic arch

B. A persistent left superior vena cava (SVC)

C. Coronary anomalies

D. Tricuspid valve dysplasia

✪✪ Question 23

A 3-month-old baby boy presents with symptoms of heart failure. Chest X-ray shows cardiomegaly, blood tests reveal hypocalcemia, and echocardiography reveals a diagnosis of truncus arteriosus. The baby has unusual facial features. The most likely syndrome for this patient is:

A. Turner syndrome.

B. Marfan syndrome.

C. DiGeorge syndrome.

D. Williams syndrome.

✪✪ Question 24

Which variant of tetralogy of Fallot (TOF) is ductal-dependent?

A. "Pink" TOF

B. TOF with pulmonary atresia

C. TOF with absent pulmonary valve syndrome

D. TOF with major aortopulmonary collateral arteries (MAPCAs)

✪✪✪ Question 25

A newborn in the neonatal intensive care unit presents with significant acute respiratory distress. The patient is tachypneic and has oxygen saturations in the low 80% range. Physical exam reveals a 2/6 systolic ejection murmur and normal femoral pulses. A chest X-ray shows increased pulmonary vascular markings and "ground glass" appearance to the lungs. The plan is to place the patient on extracorporeal membrane oxygenation (ECMO). An echocardiogram is ordered, and the following images are obtained (**Figures 28-4A to 28-4D**). Based on the images shown, should ECMO cannulation proceed?

A. Yes, proceed with ECMO cannulation.

B. No, further radiologic testing is needed.

C. No, surgery to correct the heart defect is needed.

D. No, place the patient on inhaled nitric oxide.

E. No, this patient needs an interventional cardiac catheterization procedure to correct the cardiac issue.

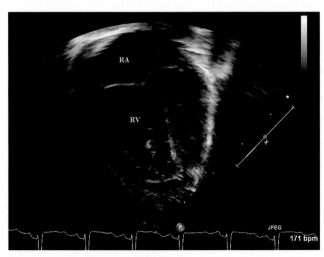

Figure 28-4A Apical 4-chamber view.

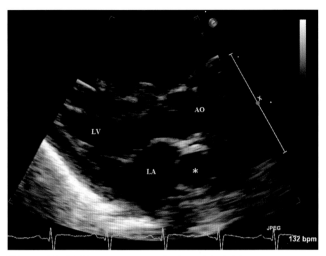

Figure 28-4B Parasternal long-axis view of the left heart structures.

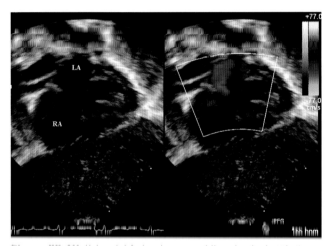

Figure 28-4C Subcostal 4 chamber view of the interatrial septum

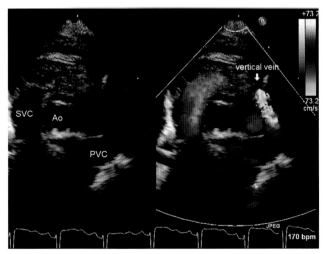

Figure 28-4D Parasternal short-axis view above the level of the left atrium.

✪✪✪ Question 26

A newborn is found to have tricuspid atresia with normally related great arteries, a small ventricular septal defect (VSD), and pulmonary stenosis. Oxygen satu-

ration readings are in the mid 80% range on room air and no elevation is seen in the central venous pressure (CVP) readings. The next step to stabilize this patient would be:

    A. A balloon atrial septostomy.

    B. A pulmonary balloon valvuloplasty.

    C. A Blalock-Taussig-Thomas (BTT) shunt.

    D. Pulmonary artery banding.

    E. No immediate intervention as the patient is stable.

✪✪✪ Question 27

In cases of pulmonary atresia and intact ventricular septum which of the following conditions is most commonly present?

    A. Cleft mitral valve

    B. Coronary artery sinusoids

    C. Partial anomalous pulmonary venous return

    D. Persistent left superior vena cava (SVC)

✪✪✪ Question 28

An initial echocardiogram demonstrates d-transposition of the great arteries (TGA) with a small atrial shunt, no ventricular septal defect, and a small, restrictive patent ductus arteriosus (PDA). The patient's oxygen saturations are rapidly decreasing and are now in the 60% range. What procedure would be performed to quickly stabilize the patient and increase saturations?

    A. Balloon atrial septostomy

    B. Immediate surgical repair

    C. Stenting open the interatrial septum

    D. Stenting open the patent ductus arteriosus

✪✪✪ Question 29

In the initial diagnosis of tetralogy of Fallot (TOF), it is important to establish the anatomy of the coronary arteries for which of the following reasons?

    A. Reduced coronary flow results from cyanosis.

    B. Coronary artery fistulae are well described in TOF patients.

    C. TOF patients are at increased risk of ischemic heart disease in early life.

    D. Anomalous coronary artery anatomy can interfere with the approach for corrective surgery.

✪✪✪ Question 30

An image of the abdominal aorta is obtained in a patient with total anomalous pulmonary venous return (TAPVR) (**Figure 28-5**). What vascular structure is located anterior to the aorta, denoted with a question mark?

    A. Azygous vein
    B. Hepatic vein
    C. Inferior vena cava
    D. Portal vein
    E. Vertical vein

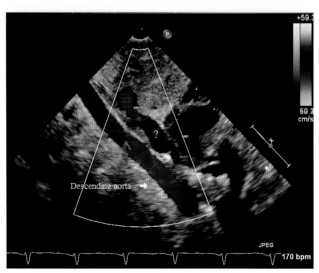

Figure 28-5

CASE STUDY 1

▶ A 2-day-old baby boy was transferred to a tertiary care center and was found to have a decreased oxygen saturation before discharge. His oxygen saturation was 80% and did not improve with 100% O_2. Echocardiography is as shown in **Video 28-1A** (parasternal long-axis view) and **Video 28-1B** (parasternal short-axis view).

✪✪✪ Question 31

Based on the images provided, what is the diagnosis?

    A. Double-outlet right ventricle
    B. Anomalous origin of coronary arteries
    C. Congenitally corrected transposition
    D. d-Transposition of great arteries (d-TGA)
    E. Truncus arteriosus

✪✪✪ Question 32

What is the most common associated anomaly with this condition?

    A. Left ventricular outflow tract (LVOT) obstruction
    B. Coarctation of the aorta

    C. Ventricular septal defect (VSD)
    D. Atrial septal defect (ASD)
    E. Coronary anomalies

✪✪✪ Question 33

In this condition, intracardiac mixing is:

    A. Primarily at the atrial level through a large ASD.
    B. Primarily at the ventricular level via a large VSD.
    C. Primarily at the great arterial level through a large PDA.
    D. More influenced by defect size than location.

CASE STUDY 2

An infant with mild cyanosis and cardiomegaly on chest X-ray is having an echocardiogram to examine the source of the cyanosis. There are four chambers and four valves with a normal relationship between the great arteries. Total anomalous pulmonary venous return (TAPVR) is suspected when the right heart is noted to be large and a right-to-left atrial shunt is seen.

✪✪✪ Question 34

▶ Which is the true statement about the type of TAPVR shown in this suprasternal view in **Video 28-2**?

    A. Obstruction is never present in this type of TAPVR.
    B. This type of TAPVR is almost always associated with pulmonary venous obstruction.
    C. This type of TAPVR is associated with an intact atrial septum.
    D. This is the most common form of TAPVR.
    E. This form of TAPVR produces profound cyanosis of the newborn.

✪✪✪ Question 35

Which of the following echocardiographic features describes this condition?

    A. The left atrium (LA) is usually normal in size.
    B. The pulmonary artery is often mildly hypoplastic.
    C. The right ventricle (RV) is dilated in all types of TAPVR.
    D. The atrial and ventricular septa bow into the right side of the heart.
    E. Doppler echocardiography is usually not helpful to establish the pulmonary venous connection.

✪✪✪ Question 36

With TAPVR, in order to identify the location of the pulmonary veins, the echocardiographer needs to examine:

A. The aorta.
B. The ductus arteriosus.
C. The left ventricle.
D. The right ventricle.
E. The systemic veins.

CASE STUDY 3

A 2-month-old infant arrives at the emergency department in acute respiratory failure and with oxygen saturations in the 90% range. There is generalized edema and tachypnea. An echocardiogram is ordered to assess cardiac anatomy and function.

✪✪✪ Question 37

▶ What is the primary diagnosis based on **Video 28-3A**?

A. Cor triatriatum with restricted atrial shunt
B. Hypoplastic left heart syndrome (HLHS)
C. Pulmonary atresia with intact ventricular septum
D. Tricuspid atresia with ventricular septal defect (VSD)

✪✪✪ Question 38

▶ Based on the information provided in **Videos 28-3B** and **28-3C**, what can be assumed regarding the estimated pulmonary artery pressure (PAP)?

A. PAP is normal.
B. PAP is mildly elevated.
C. PAP is near or equal to systemic pressure.
D. Cannot determine based on information provided.

✪✪✪ Question 39

Clinically this patient is in congestive heart failure. Which of the following echocardiographic findings would not support the diagnosis of congestive heart failure in this patient?

A. Pericardial effusion
B. Right heart enlargement
C. Unrestricted pulmonary blood flow
D. Left ventricular noncompaction (LVNC) with reduced LV function
E. Low-velocity bidirectional shunting at the ventricular level

CASE STUDY 4

An echocardiogram reveals significant mitral hypoplasia and aortic hypoplasia. A patent ductus arteriosus (PDA) is present with systolic right-to-left shunting.

✪✪✪ Question 40

▶ What cardiac defect is seen in **Video 28-4A**?

A. Hypoplastic right heart syndrome (HRHS)
B. Hypoplastic left heart syndrome (HLHS)
C. Double outlet right ventricle (DORV)
D. Double inlet left ventricle (DILV)

✪✪✪ Question 41

▶ In **Video 28-4B**, why is the systolic flow in the **proximal** descending aorta retrograde but antegrade in the **distal** aorta?

A. There is low output through the aortic valve.
B. There is an arteriovenous malformation in the head.
C. There is a large bidirectional patent ductus arteriosus.
D. There are aortopulmonary collaterals causing the reversal in flow.

✪✪✪ Question 42

The interrogation of which additional intracardiac structure is important in order to stabilize this patient?

A. Mitral valve
B. Tricuspid valve
C. Pulmonary valve
D. Interatrial septum
E. Interventricular septum

ANSWERS

1. **Answer: C.** Dextro-transposition of the great arteries is the most common form of TGA with an incidence of approximately 31 per 100,000 live births. In d-TGA, there is atrioventricular (AV) concordance and ventriculoarterial (VA) discordance (**Figures 28-6A to 28-6E**). That is, the atria and ventricles are connected normally (AV concordance), but the great arteries arise from the incorrect ventricles (VA discordance) with the aorta, which is anterior and to the right of the pulmonary artery, arising from the right ventricle (RV) and the pulmonary artery (PA) arising from the left ventricle (LV). Thus, systemic venous return to the heart is directed out of the aorta with no oxygenation taking place. Pulmonary venous return to the heart is directed through the PA and back to the lungs. As a result, there is no mixing of the circulation except at the atrial level (via a patent foramen ovale or atrial septal defect) and ductal level (via a patent ductus arteriosus). In answers A and D, the terms levo-transposition (l-TGA) and congenitally corrected transposition of the great arteries (cc-TGA) refer to the same

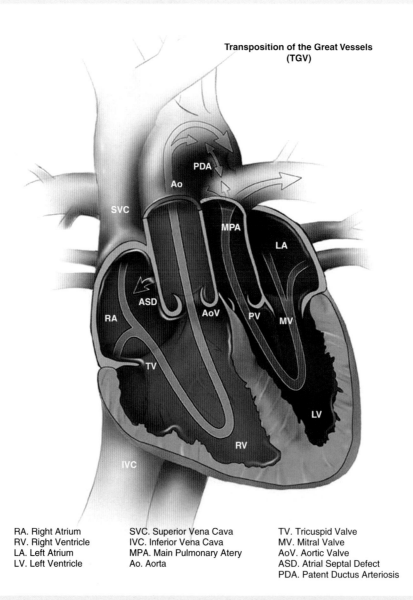

Transposition of the Great Vessels (TGV)

RA. Right Atrium	SVC. Superior Vena Cava	TV. Tricuspid Valve
RV. Right Ventricle	IVC. Inferior Vena Cava	MV. Mitral Valve
LA. Left Atrium	MPA. Main Pulmonary Atery	AoV. Aortic Valve
LV. Left Ventricle	Ao. Aorta	ASD. Atrial Septal Defect
		PDA. Patent Ductus Arteriosis

Figure 28-6A Diagram of d-TGA. The aorta arises from the right ventricle and the pulmonary artery from the left ventricle. The position of the aorta is to the right and anterior relative to the position of the pulmonary artery. Arrows designate the direction of blood flow. Mixing of blood is shown across an atrial septal defect (ASD) and a patent ductus arteriosus (PDA). (From https://www.cdc.gov/ncbddd/heartdefects/d-tga.html. Courtesy of Centers for Disease Control and Prevention, National Center on Birth Defects and Developmental Disabilities.)

condition. In cc-TGA or I-TGA, there is atrioventricular discordance and ventriculoarterial discordance. That is, systemic venous return to the right atrium (RA) courses through the morphological LV and then to the PA. Pulmonary venous return to the left atrium (LA) courses through the morphological RV and to the aorta, which is anterior and leftward of the PA (**Figures 28-6E** and **28-6F**). In essence, the circulation is correct but through an abnormal connection of chambers and valves. Taussig-Bing anomaly (answer B) is a form of double outlet RV with a subpulmonic ventricular septal defect (VSD). In this anomaly, the great arteries can be transposed, malpositioned, side by side, or normally related. The key is that the pulmonary artery arises over the VSD.

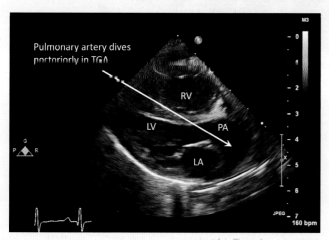

Figure 28-6B Parasternal long-axis view of d-TGA. The pulmonary artery dives posteriorly, where PA is pulmonary artery, RV is right ventricle, LV is left ventricle, and LA is left atrium. (Reprinted with permission from Franco KL, Thourani VH. *Cardiothoracic Surgery Review*. 1st ed. Philadelphia, PA: Wolters Kluwer Health/Lippincott Williams & Wilkins; 2011.)

TEACHING POINT

According to the currently used Van Praagh classification, d-TGA refers to ventriculoarterial connections and not spatial relationships. In most cases the aorta is anterior and rightward of the PA. Therefore, the aorta arises from the RV and the PA arises from the LV. Careful initial echocardiographic studies include establishing atrial and ventricular connections and determining atrial situs and following a segmental analysis protocol.

2. **Answer: B.** The subcostal 4-chamber image demonstrates truncus arteriosus (**Figure 28-7A**). Later imaging revealed truncus type I where the main pulmonary artery (PA) arises from the truncal root and then bifurcates into the right and left branch pulmonary arteries. There are three main types of truncus arteriosus: type I, as in the presented patient; type II, in which each PA arises separately from the posterior portion of the truncal root; and type III, in which the right and left PA branches originate from the sides of the truncal root (**Figure 28-7B**). Some descriptions classify a type IV with bronchial arteries arising from the descending aorta, but there are arguments that say it is a form of pulmonary atresia. The schematic in **Figure 28-7C** shows the circulatory pathway in truncus arteriosus.

3. **Answer: D.** The four congenital heart abnormalities that form tetralogy of Fallot (TOF) include (1) a malaligned VSD, (2) an aorta overriding the VSD, (3) right ventricular outflow tract (RVOT) obstruction (usually infundibular but can also be at the valvular level), and (4) right ventricular hypertrophy (RVH). These abnormalities are illustrated in **Figures 28-8A** and **28-8B**. Answer A is incorrect

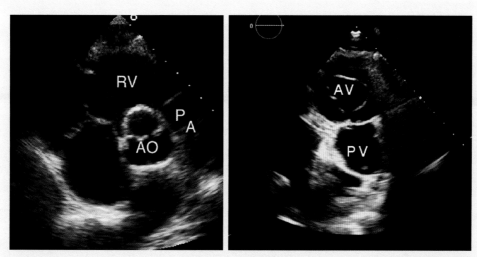

Figure 28-6C Parasternal short-axis view showing the normal great artery relationship (left) and the relationship in d-TGA (right). Normally, the aortic valve (AV) is posterior and the RV outflow tract (RV) and pulmonary artery (PA) appear to wrap around the aorta (AO). With d-TGA, the aorta is anterior, and the two great vessels arise in parallel. PV, pulmonary valve. (Reprinted with permission from Armstrong WF, Ryan T. *Feigenbaum's Echocardiography*. 8th ed. Philadelphia, PA: Wolters Kluwer; 2018.)

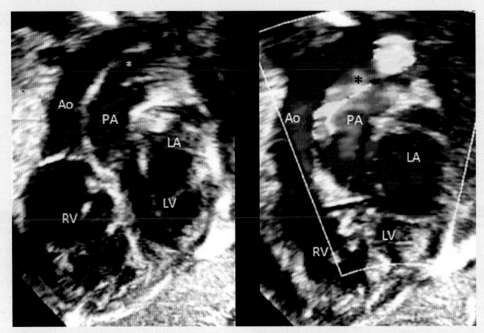

Figure 28-6D Sagittal images of d-TGA. These subcostal, sagittal plane images also demonstrate the discordant (abnormal) connection of the right and left ventricles to the great arteries. However, one can also appreciate the parallel ascending course taken by the aorta (Ao) and pulmonary artery (PA) in these patients. These images allow visualization of the patent ductus arteriosus (asterisk in both panels) connecting the two circulations and allowing for desaturated blood from the aorta to reach the PA (red color flow on the right, asterisk). LA, left atrium; LV, left ventricle; RV, right ventricle. (Reprinted with permission from Oh JK, Kane GC. *The Echo Manual.* 4th ed. Philadelphia, PA: Wolters Kluwer; 2018.)

because although there is septal deviation in TOF, it is not considered one of the four lesions; rather, septal deviation is the embryological malformation that leads to the development of the lesions. This includes an overriding aorta, which is omitted from this answer. Answer B is incorrect because atrial septal defects are not part of the TOF criteria.

However, ASDs are associated with TOF in about a third of patients and when they occur in combination with TOF, this is referred to as the "Pentalogy of Fallot." Answer C is incorrect as the overriding aorta is omitted. Dilated aortic roots are seen commonly in TOF patients, due to the increased flow from both ventricles.

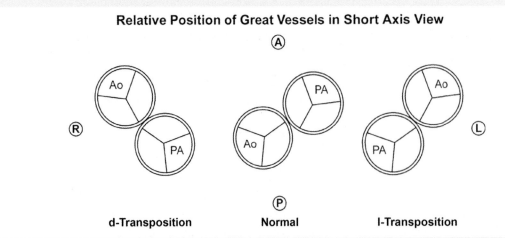

Figure 28-6E Relative position of great arteries in TGA. Normal position of great arteries (center): the aorta (Ao) is posterior and the pulmonary artery (PA) wraps anteriorly around the aorta. d-transposition (left): great arteries run parallel, with the aorta anterior and to the right of the PA. l-transposition (right): great arteries run parallel with the aorta anterior and to the left of the PA. A, anterior; L, left; P, posterior; R, right. (Reprinted with permission from Griffin BP, Kapadia SR, Rimmerman CM. *Cleveland Clinic Cardiology Board Review.* 2nd ed. Philadelphia, PA: Wolters Kluwer Health/Lippincott Williams & Wilkins; 2012.)

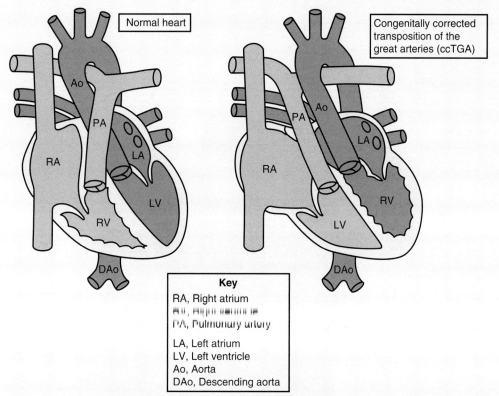

Key
RA, Right atrium
A̶o̶,̶ ̶R̶i̶g̶h̶t̶ ̶a̶t̶r̶i̶u̶m̶
P̶A̶,̶ ̶P̶u̶l̶m̶o̶n̶a̶r̶y̶ ̶a̶r̶t̶e̶r̶y̶

LA, Left atrium
LV, Left ventricle
Ao, Aorta
DAo, Descending aorta

Figure 28-6F l-TGA or cc-TGA is atrioventricular and ventriculoarterial discordance. This allows for blood to course through an abnormal sequence of chambers to reach the correct destination. Patients would not present with cyanosis in this condition. (Reprinted with permission from Franco KL, Thourani VH. *Cardiothoracic Surgery Review*. 1st ed. Philadelphia, PA: Wolters Kluwer Health/Lippincott Williams & Wilkins; 2011.)

TEACHING POINT

The severity of right ventricular outflow tract (RVOT) obstruction will determine the age presentation of patients with TOF. The more severe obstructions will result in more right-to-left shunting and more cyanosis; therefore, an earlier diagnosis is made, usually in the first weeks of life. However, in the setting of milder degrees of RVOT obstruction, good pulmonary blood flow is still maintained, and cyanosis will be less; together, these factors may delay the diagnosis. Commonly, patients are diagnosed within the first 12 months of life, but in cases with very mild RVOT obstruction, the diagnosis may not be made until adulthood. The usual presentation in a baby is failure to gain weight, onset of bluish skin tone during crying or feeding (also known as "Tet spells"), and shortness of breath.

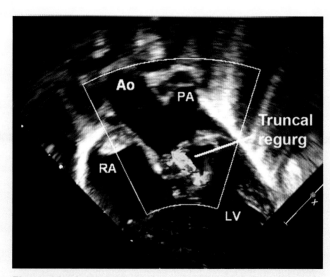

Figure 28-7A This is a subcostal left anterior oblique view of a patient with type I truncus arteriosus. The aorta (Ao) and pulmonary artery (PA) arise from the same trunk. The truncal valve in this patient is thickened and doming with truncal regurgitation seen (truncal regurg). LV, left ventricle; RA, right atrium. (Reprinted with permission from Kaiser L, Kron IL, Spray TL. *Mastery of Cardiothoracic Surgery*. 3rd ed. Philadelphia, PA: Wolters Kluwer Health/Lippincott Williams & Wilkins; 2013.)

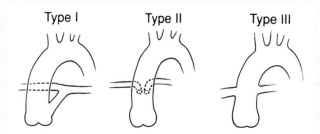

Figure 28-7B These diagrams illustrate the basic forms of the original Collett-Edwards classification of persistent truncus arteriosus. (Reprinted with permission from Brandt WE, Helms CA. *Brandt and Helms Solution*. 3rd ed. Philadelphia, PA: Wolters Kluwer Health/Lippincott Williams & Wilkins; 2006.)

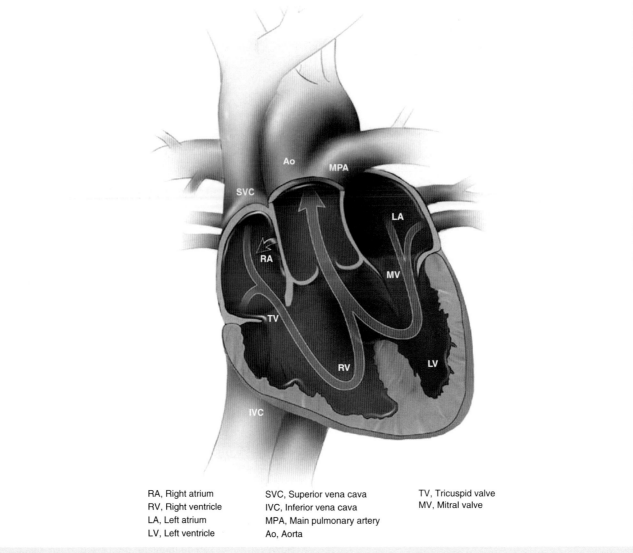

RA, Right atrium   SVC, Superior vena cava   TV, Tricuspid valve
RV, Right ventricle   IVC, Inferior vena cava   MV, Mitral valve
LA, Left atrium   MPA, Main pulmonary artery
LV, Left ventricle   Ao, Aorta

Figure 28-7C Diagram of truncus arteriosus. Arrows designate the direction of blood flow. An atrial septal defect (red arrow) is also shown. (From https://www.cdc.gov/ncbddd/heartdefects/d-tga.html. Courtesy of Centers for Disease Control and Prevention, National Center on Birth Defects and Developmental Disabilities.)

4. **Answer: E.** The left vertical vein allows decompression of the pulmonary venous confluence and directs flow superiorly to the left innominate vein, causing dilation of venous vasculature downstream until it reaches the atrium (**Figure 28-9**). Supracardiac TAPVR with return to the right SVC (answer D) would result in dilation from the entry into the right SVC to the RA. Cardiac TAPVR to the RA (answer A), cardiac TAPVR to the coronary sinus (answer B), or infracardiac TAVPR to the portal vein system (answer C) has no volume overload to the SVC or the above veins. Dilation of any systemic vasculature with no evident reason warrants further investigation.

TEACHING POINT

TAPVR, also known as total anomalous pulmonary venous connection (TAPVC), is classified based on the location of pulmonary venous drainage. In the supracardiac type, seen in 35% to 50% of cases, the pulmonary venous confluence (PVC) drains through a left vertical (ascending) vein into the left innominate (brachiocephalic) vein, or rarely to the SVC, a left SVC, or to the azygous system. In the infracardiac type, seen in approximately 20% of cases, the PVC drains by way of a descending vein, below the diaphragm, to the portal vein, hepatic vein, inferior vena cava (IVC), or ductus venosus. In the cardiac type, seen in approximately 20% of cases, the PVC drains directly to the coronary sinus or to the veins connecting to the RA. The mixed type of TAPVR, seen in approximately 10% of cases, is a combination of the other forms with the PVC drainage into at least two different locations, above or below the diaphragm.

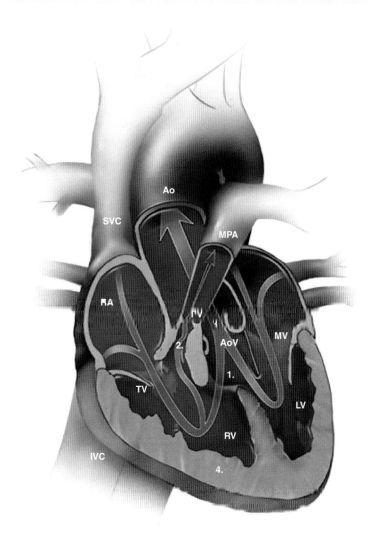

RA, Right atrium	SVC, Superior vena cava	TV, Tricuspid valve
RV, Right ventricle	IVC, Inferior vena cava	MV, Mitral valve
LA, Left atrium	MPA, Main pulmonary artery	PV, Pulmonary valve
LV, Left ventricle	Ao, Aorta	AoV, Aortic valve

Figure 28-8A Tetralogy of Fallot. The four elements are shown: 1. malaligned VSD, 2. infundibular stenosis, 3. overriding aorta, 4. RV hypertrophy. (From https://www.cdc.gov/ncbddd/heartdefects/d-tga.html. Courtesy of Centers for Disease Control and Prevention, National Center on Birth Defects and Developmental Disabilities.)

5. **Answer: B.** This figure shows features consistent with Ebstein anomaly based on significant inferior displacement of the septal tricuspid valve with atrialization of the right ventricle and tethering of the septal and posterior tricuspid leaflets to the interventricular septum (IVS) and free wall. Cyanosis in Ebstein anomaly occurs when a high right atrial pressure results in right-to-left shunting of deoxygenated blood across a patent foramen ovale (PFO) or across an atrial septal defect (ASD).

TEACHING POINT

The diagnosis of Ebstein anomaly is confirmed by the identification of apical displacement of the septal tricuspid valve leaflet. A displacement index corrected for the body surface area (BSA) has been described. This index is derived from the apical 4-chamber view as the distance from the septal mitral hinge point to the delaminated tricuspid septal leaflet hinge point, divided by the BSA. An index greater than 8 mm/m^2 is consistent with Ebstein anomaly. There is a spectrum of severity of the leaflet displacement. As the septal leaflet becomes more inferiorly displaced, tethering of the leaflets increases. This restricted motion results in increased tricuspid regurgitation, poor forward flow, and a greater potential for right-to-left shunting across a PFO or ASD.

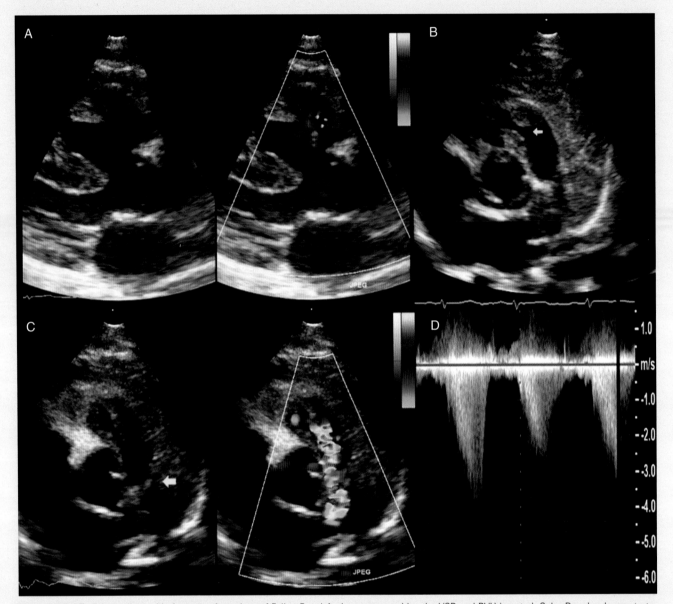

Figure 28-8B Echocardiographic features of tetralogy of Fallot. Panel A: the aorta overrides the VSD and RVH is noted. Color Doppler demonstrates laminar flow across the VSD, suggesting significantly elevated RV pressure. Panel B: the arrow points to discrete infundibular thickening. Panel C: the arrow indicates the pulmonary valve, and turbulent flow is seen well below the valve level. Panel D: late-peaking systolic Doppler is noted on the continuous-wave Doppler trace, indicating the dynamic nature of obstruction, causing elevated RV pressure.

6. **Answer: A.** Eisenmenger syndrome starts as a defect with a left-to-right shunt which, if left untreated, may go on to cause damage to the pulmonary vascular bed from the increased pulmonary blood flow. This in turn results in raised pulmonary pressures and eventually the shunt direction will change. Bidirectional or right-to-left shunting both allow for deoxygenated blood to mix with arterial blood, resulting in cyanosis. Answer B is incorrect, as central cyanosis is a manifestation of some noncardiac pathologies such as disorders of the blood, central nervous and respiratory systems. Answer C is incorrect as this could occur in pathologies with reduced pulmonary blood flow, for example, due to severe pulmonary obstruction as in TOF, without significant damage to the pulmonary bed. Answer D is incorrect because suprasystemic pulmonary pressures can result from various forms of pulmonary hypertension, even without cardiac shunts.

7. **Answer: B.** The pulmonary artery is identified by its branching into the right and left pulmonary arteries, which occurs approximately 4 to 5 cm from the level of the valve. The aorta is defined by its arching and by the origin of the head vessels and the coronary arteries.

   Answers A, C, and D are not correct. The anatomic relationship of the PA to the aorta as well as the ventricle from which it originates does not help identify the PA. The obvious example is I-transposition

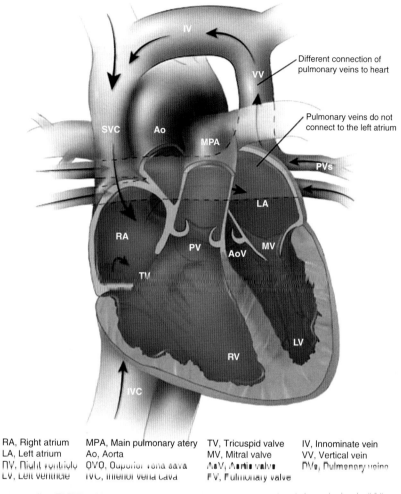

RA, Right atrium	MPA, Main pulmonary atery	TV, Tricuspid valve	IV, Innominate vein
LA, Left atrium	Ao, Aorta	MV, Mitral valve	VV, Vertical vein
RV, Right ventricle	SVC, Superior vena cava	AoV, Aortic valve	PVs, Pulmonary veins
LV, Left ventricle	IVC, Inferior vena cava	PV, Pulmonary valve	

Figure 28-9 Diagram of supracardiac TAPVR with pulmonary veins (PVs) returning through a left vertical vein (VV) to the innominate vein (IV) and eventual return to the right atrium (RA). Dilation of the right heart is present secondary to the volume overload state. (From https://www.cdc.gov/ncbddd/heartdefects/d-tga.html. Courtesy of Centers for Disease Control and Prevention, National Center on Birth Defects and Developmental Disabilities.)

of the great arteries (I-TGA). In I-TGA, the great arteries run parallel, with the aorta anterior and to the left of the pulmonary artery (PA). The PA arises from the morphologic left ventricle and the aorta arises from the morphologic right ventricle (see the answer outline for Question 1 for more information).

8. **Answer: D.** In this parasternal long axis-view, there is a large VSD and a great artery straddling the ventricular septal defect (VSD). This could be either truncus arteriosus or TOF. More information is required to differentiate between these two lesions with careful inspection of the origin of the pulmonary artery. DORV (answer B) is excluded because the VSD is aligned to the center of the vessel. DORV may be identified when the aorta overrides the ventricular septum more than 50%; that is, DORV is considered when at least half of the aorta arises from the right ventricle, which is not seen in this case. Furthermore, with a DORV there is an absence of fibrous continuity between the anterior mitral leaflet and the aorta.

9. **Answer: C.** The degree of obstruction is a major determinant for symptoms and cyanosis in TOF. In severe stenosis, there will be reduced blood flow to the lungs and increased right-to-left shunting across the VSD, which causes cyanosis, or bluish discoloration of the skin, particularly the lips and fingernail beds. Cyanosis is dangerous because it results in reduced oxygen levels in the coronary arteries, the brain, and major visceral organs.

Answers A, B, and D are incorrect because it is pressure that determines the volume of a shunt more so than the size of the VSD, the size of the RV, or the degree of aortic override. However, the size of the VSD is an important determinant for repair.

TEACHING POINT

Patients with TOF and mild RVOT obstruction can present later in life, even into adulthood. These are so-called "pink tets" as they can maintain sufficient pulmonary blood flow with physiology similar to a simple VSD.

10. **Answer: D.** Down syndrome or Trisomy 21 is strongly associated with congenital heart disease, which occurs in up to 50% of patients. The most common congenital heart lesions associated with this syndrome are atrial septal defect, ventricular septal defect, atrioventricular septal defects (most common), and TOF. Williams syndrome (answer A) is associated with supravalvular aortic stenosis or peripheral pulmonary stenosis. Noonan syndrome (answer B) is associated with pulmonary stenosis, hypertrophic cardiomyopathy, and atrial septal defects. Eisenmenger syndrome (answer C) can result from a range of shunt lesions that start at birth with a left-to-right shunt, but over time, as pulmonary pressures progress to systemic or suprasystemic levels, the shunt becomes bidirectional or reverses to right-to-left shunting.

11. **Answer: A.** TAPVR presents with right heart volume overload and mimics a large ASD. With an ASD, there is moderate left-to-right shunting that occurs at the atrial level. This will result in right heart enlargement and volume overload to the lungs (**Figure 28-10A**). In TAPVR, both pulmonary and systemic venous return is to the right atrium (RA). A portion of the mixed saturated blood must shunt right-to-left at the atrial level to maintain systemic flow. A moderate volume overload to the right heart and lungs remains (**Figure 28-10B**). The only difference between a large ASD and TAPVR is that there is cyanosis present in the latter.

Answers C and E are incorrect since both a VSD and a PDA result in left heart volume overload.

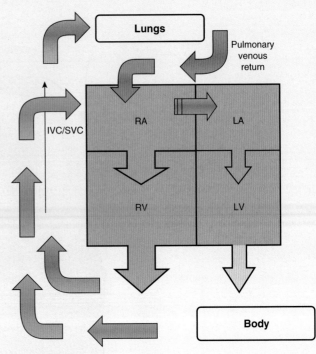

Figure 28-10B This is a box diagram showing circulation for TAPVR. Note that the pulmonary venous return to the right heart results in right heart dilatation. Unlike an isolated ASD as shown in **Figure 28-10A**, in TAPVR, there is cyanosis due to right-to-left shunting across an ASD.

MVP with moderate mitral regurgitation (answer B) results in left atrial enlargement and increased back pressure to the lungs. Moderate pulmonary stenosis with moderate pulmonary regurgitation (answer D) results in right heart pressure and volume overload and would result in primarily right ventricular dilatation and hypertrophy with a normal RA size.

KEY POINT

When mild right heart enlargement presents with no evident reason, always consider the possibility of partial anomalous pulmonary venous return (PAPVR). Unlike TAPVR, PAPVR can go undetected into adulthood. If a thorough interrogation of the interatrial septum reveals no defect, then consider PAPVR. Hemodynamically, an anomalous connection of a single pulmonary vein is equivalent to a small ASD.

12. **Answer: B.** Tricuspid atresia (TA) is characterized by absence of the tricuspid valve. There are three major variants based on the associated relationship of the great vessels and these three variants can be further subclassified based on the presence or absence of an accompanying VSD and pulmonary valve pathology (**Figure 28-11**). TA type I is characterized by normally related great arteries and this type has the highest prevalence, accounting for about two-thirds of all TA cases. Type Ib, pulmonary hypoplasia with subpulmonary stenosis, diminutive right ventricle (RV), and small VSD (**Figure 28-11, B**), is the most common type of TA. TA type II is characterized

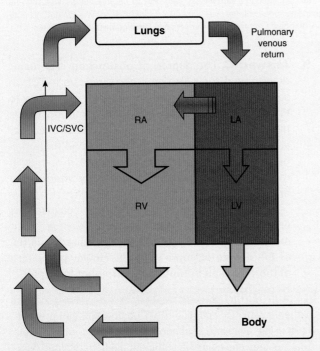

Figure 28-10A This is a box diagram showing circulation with a large ASD. Note that shunting of blood across the ASD results in right heart dilatation.

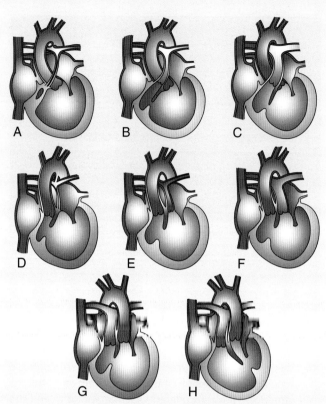

Figure 28-11 Type I tricuspid atresia without TGA includes type Ia, pulmonary atresia with virtual absence of the RV (A); type Ib, pulmonary hypoplasia with subpulmonary stenosis, diminutive RV, and small VSD (B); and type Ic, no pulmonary hypoplasia and a diminutive RV (C). Type II, tricuspid atresia with d-TGA includes type IIa, pulmonary atresia, aorta arises from the RV (D); type IIb, pulmonary or subpulmonary stenosis (E); and type IIc, normal or enlarged pulmonary artery (F). Type III tricuspid atresia with l-TGA includes type IIIa, pulmonary or subpulmonary stenosis (G), and type IIIb, subaortic stenosis (H). There is ventricular inversion. (Reprinted with permission from Hensley LA, Gravle GP, Martin DE, *Practical Approach to Cardiac Anesthesia*. 5th ed. Philadelphia, PA: Wolters Kluwer Health/ Lippincott Williams & Wilkins, 2012.)

by d-transposition of the great arteries (TGA); this type of TA accounts for approximately one-third of TA cases. TA type III is characterized by l-TGA; this type of TA is rare and accounts for a very small fraction of cases.

13. **Answer: A.** Ebstein anomaly is not commonly associated with DORV. As the name suggests, in DORV both great arteries arise from the RV. Often, one vessel is overriding the VSD by more than 50%, a criterion that is important to differentiate DORV from tetralogy of Fallot. The location of the VSD is important for the natural history and the surgical approach. VSDs are usually subaortic but can also be subpulmonary, both subaortic and subpulmonary, or muscular (also called remote, as they are distant from the great vessels). The VSD is the only outlet from the left ventricle and so forms part of the left ventricular outflow tract. For this reason, nonrestrictive VSDs provide better conditions for left ventricular outflow. The great vessels can be either concordant or normally related (DORV-tetralogy type), or discordant or abnormally related (DORV-transposition type).

14. **Answer: B.** Determining pulmonary valve patency is critical when assessing an infant with Ebstein anomaly. With a hypoplastic or atretic pulmonary valve, cyanosis is a result of right-to-left shunting at the atrial level because of poor or absent forward flow through the pulmonary valve. In this situation, pulmonary circulation is ductal-dependent. The degree of forward flow through the pulmonary valve is also based on the severity of tricuspid regurgitation and overall right ventricular volume. In this instance, there may be a normal-appearing pulmonary valve, but an insufficient pressure is generated to open the valve. In these cases, close monitoring of the pulmonary valve as the pulmonary vascular resistance decreases and maintaining ductal patency is the typical approach to early management. In the less severe form of Ebstein anomaly, no cyanosis is present, and this defect can go undiagnosed into adulthood.

TEACHING POINT
There is an association of left ventricular noncompaction (LVNC) with Ebstein anomaly. Therefore, close assessment of the LV anatomy and long-term function is important. **Figure 28-12** is an example of LVNC with Ebstein anomaly.

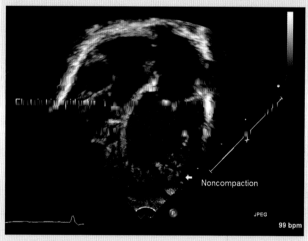

Figure 28-12 Apical 4-chamber view of Ebstein anomaly and LVNC.

15. **Answer: C.** In d-transposition of the great arteries (TGA), there is a normal relationship between the atria and the ventricles (AV concordance) and an abnormal relationship between the ventricles and the great arteries (VA discordance). Concordance refers to a normal relationship and discordance refers to an abnormal relationship. In answer A there is concordance between the atria, ventricles, and great arteries; therefore, anatomy is normal. Answer B describes discordance between the atria and ventricles (AV discordance) and between the ventricles and great arteries (VA discordance); this describes congenitally corrected transposition or l-TGA. Answer D, AV discordance and VA concordance,

is a rare form of complex congenital heart disease, an example of which is isolated ventricular inversion.

KEY POINTS

The terms concordance and discordance are used to describe the relationships between the atria, ventricles, and great arteries. Concordance refers to a normal relationship and discordance refers to an abnormal relationship. Therefore:

▶ AV concordance implies the normal connection between the atria and the ventricles; thus, the RA connects to the RV and the LA connects to the LV.

▶ AV discordance implies abnormal connection between the atria and the ventricles; thus, the RA connects to the LV and the LA connects to the RV.

▶ VA concordance implies the normal connection between the ventricles and the great arteries; thus, the RV connects to the PA and the LV connects to the aorta.

▶ VA discordance implies abnormal connection between the ventricles and the great arteries; thus, the RV connects to the aorta and the LV connects to the PA.

16. **Answer: D.** It is normal that the PVR decreases after birth as the baby starts to breathe and the pulmonary circulation develops. At birth, the PVR is not very different from the SVR and the circulation through both systems in truncus arteriosus is similar. As the PVR drops, the difference between the SVR and PVR becomes greater. In truncus arteriosus, this encourages more left-to-right shunting at the truncal level, which floods the lungs with increased pulmonary flow, leading to heart failure.

Answer A is incorrect. While the PDA does close, this is not significant because the aorta and pulmonary arteries remain connected via the common arterial trunk. Answer B is incorrect because growth of the pulmonary arteries occurs slowly over time and is not a significant contributing factor to heart failure. Answer C is incorrect because the SVR is low in utero, becomes high at birth, and remains high.

17. **Answer: B.** Antero (frontal) cephalad (superior) deviation of the outlet (ventricular) septum is the single anatomical lesion that causes TOF. The deviation of the outlet septum causes malalignment between the outlet and muscular septum creating the ventricular septal defect (VSD). This deviation also causes the aorta to override the VSD. Furthermore, the anterocephalad deviation of the outlet septum pushes it anteriorly toward the sternum and superiorly toward the head, which narrows the right ventricular outflow tract (RVOT), leading to infundibular stenosis and subsequent right ventricular hypertrophy (RVH) **(Figure 28-13)**.

18. **Answer: A.** Pulmonary venous return via the coronary sinus does not typically present with obstruction. This type of TAPVR can go undiagnosed beyond the

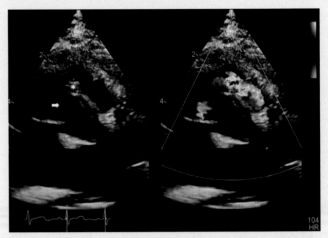

Figure 28-13 Anterocephalad outlet septal deviation creates the four lesions associated with TOF. A large malalignment VSD is noted (arrow) as a result of the malaligned septum. The outlet septum (asterisk) has deviated anteriorly and causes RVOT obstruction demonstrated by the turbulent flow seen with color Doppler imaging. The aorta overrides the VSD and subsequent RVH develops due to RVOT obstruction.

perinatal period if there is no restriction to shunting at the atrial level. In supracardiac TAPVR, obstruction is a result of compression of the vertical vein as it courses superiorly through dilated vascular anatomy and the left/right bronchus **(Figures 28-14A and 28-14B)**. Infracardiac TAPVR can present with obstruction at the level of the diaphragmatic hiatus. The descending vertical vein, along with the esophagus, courses through the hiatus of the diaphragm and becomes compressed with engorgement of the esophagus during feeding. Drainage into the hepatic venous system can restrict return with closure of the ductus venosus or because of the extensive course from the portal vein to the hepatic vein system **(Figure 28-14C)**.

19. **Answer: D.** Truncus arteriosus is a normal structure in embryonic development that, together with the bulbus cordis, represents the outflow of the ventricles. As development continues, the truncus arteriosus divides and separates into the ascending aorta and main pulmonary artery. Failure to septate results in a persistent truncus arteriosus, which in everyday practice, is commonly referred to as "truncus arteriosus." Answer A is a true statement as the truncal valve, which usually has three leaflets, can have anywhere between two and five leaflets. This valve is often dysplastic with regurgitation, but stenosis is also described. Answer B is a true statement. The pulse pressure is the difference between the systolic and diastolic blood pressures. A widened pulse pressure in truncus patients occurs because in diastole, blood in the common arterial trunk continues to flow into the pulmonary arteries, resulting in less blood volume in the aorta; therefore, the diastolic blood pressure is lower than normal. Answer C is a true statement since the short-axis views, either from the subcostal or parasternal window, are excellent for identifying the pulmonary artery anatomy and forming the basis for classification

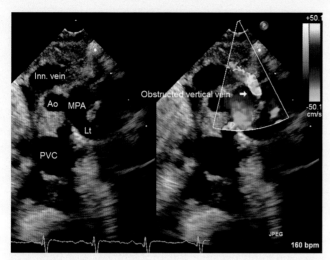

Figure 28-14A Parasternal short-axis view showing obstruction of the left vertical vein in a supracardiac TAPVR.

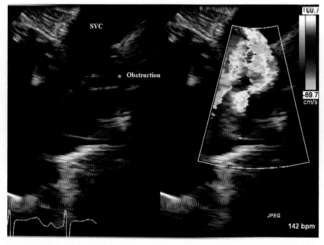

Figure 28-14B Right parasternal long axis view showing obstruction (*) of a right vertical vein entering into the right SVC in a supracardiac TAPVR.

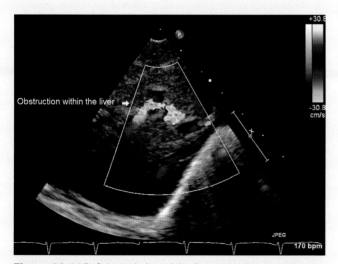

Figure 28-14C Subcostal view of the liver optimizing the obstruction of the flow from the pulmonary veins into the hepatic system in an infracardiac TAPVR case.

of the type of truncus arteriosus. While the parasternal long-axis view will display the aorta overriding a ventricular septal defect, further investigation is required to differentiate between truncus arteriosus and tetralogy of Fallot.

20. **Answer: E.** A secundum atrial septal defect (ASD) is the type of atrial shunt associated with this pathology, not a primum ASD. Answer A is not correct as tricuspid atresia can present with normally related or transposed great arteries. When the great arteries are transposed, this is usually d-transposition of the great arteries (TGA); l-TGA is also possible but is rare. Answer B is not correct as the interventricular septum can be intact or there may be a ventricular septal defect (VSD) present. The VSD, when present, can be of a varied size. A smaller VSD would result in restricted blood flow to the great artery arising from the hypoplastic right ventricle. Answers C and D are not correct as subpulmonary artery stenosis, valvular stenosis, hypoplastic pulmonary artery branches, and pulmonary atresia may be present in tricuspid atresia when the great arteries are normally related. In the instance of transposed great arteries, subaortic stenosis, valve stenosis, aortic atresia, hypoplastic aortic arch, and interruption of the arch are possible. This gives a broad spectrum of types of tricuspid atresia.

21. **Answer: A.** In truncus arteriosus, the VSD forms part of the ventricular outflow. A high-velocity jet, or restrictive VSD, would behave like an outflow obstruction, reducing the flow and pressure loading the ventricle. A low-velocity VSD jet or laminar flow (answer B) suggests low resistance to outflow and an easy passage of blood from the ventricles through the VSD to the common arterial trunk; therefore, this would be of no concern. Truncal valves can have between two and five leaflets, but usually have three or four leaflets. Therefore, a quadricuspid valve (answer C) is not unexpected and is not of concern. The ductus arteriosus is absent in about 50% of cases. When present, it does not usually remain patent unless associated with an interrupted aortic arch, which is associated with truncus arteriosus in ~30% of cases. Therefore, the presence of a patent ductus arteriosus (answer D) in truncus arteriosus is of no concern.

22. **Answer: D.** The tricuspid valve is not usually affected by TOF. Right aortic arch (~30%), persistent left SVC (~10%), and coronary anomalies (~10%) are well described common associations with TOF; with the prevalence for each noted in the brackets.

23. **Answer: C.** Up to 40% of patients with DiGeorge syndrome, also known as 22q11 deletion, have congenital heart defects, primarily associated with conotruncal abnormalities such as truncus arteriosus, tetralogy of Fallot, or pulmonary atresia. Hypocalcemia is common and causes convulsions. This syndrome is also associated with developmental delay and patients have a reduced immunity making them susceptible to recurrent infections. Answer A is incorrect.

Turner syndrome is caused by loss of all or part of an X chromosome in females and is associated with bicuspid aortic valve and coarctation. Answer B is not correct. Marfan syndrome is a connective tissue disorder with associated heart defects including aortic root dilatation or mitral valve prolapse. Answer D is not correct. Williams syndrome, which occurs due to a mutation in the elastin gene, is associated with arterial abnormalities such as supravalvular aortic or peripheral pulmonary artery stenosis.

24. **Answer: B.** As the name suggests, ductal-dependent congenital heart lesions are dependent upon the presence of a patent ductus arteriosus (PDA) to supply pulmonary or systemic blood flow, or to allow adequate mixing between parallel circulations. TOF with pulmonary atresia has no established connection between the right ventricle and the pulmonary arteries. Therefore, the only flow to the lungs is provided through the ductus arteriosus; hence, this is a ductal-dependent lesion.

    Pink TOF (answer A) has balanced flow with no undercirculation to the lungs, so additional flow from a ductus is not needed. TOF with absent pulmonary valve syndrome (answer C) is a rare type of TOF in which there is no identifiable pulmonary valve tissue and in its place is a linear fibrous shelf. As the pulmonary valve is absent, there is to-and-fro flow across the outflow, resulting in severe dilation of the main pulmonary artery and its branches. This is not a ductal-dependent lesion. TOF with MAPCAs (answer D) has continued blood supply to the lungs from major collaterals directly from the aorta; hence, this is not a ductal-dependent lesion.

KEY POINTS

Ductal-dependent congenital heart lesions are dependent upon a PDA to supply pulmonary or systemic blood flow, or to allow adequate mixing between parallel circulations. Examples of ductal-dependent congenital heart lesions include:
▶ Critical aortic valve stenosis
▶ Critical coarctation of the aorta
▶ Critical pulmonary stenosis
▶ d-Transposition of the great arteries (d-TGA)
▶ Ebstein anomaly—severe cases with extreme cyanosis
▶ Hypoplastic left heart syndrome (HLHS)
▶ Interrupted aortic arch
▶ Obstructed TAPVR
▶ Pulmonary atresia with intact IVS
▶ TOF with pulmonary atresia or critical right ventricular outflow tract (RVOT) obstruction
▶ Tricuspid atresia with severe RVOT obstruction

25. **Answer: C.** This patient has supracardiac TAPVR with return through a left vertical vein; therefore, surgery to correct a heart defect is needed. **Figure 28-4A**

shows right heart enlargement with a normally developed left ventricle. The right ventricle is apex-forming. **Figure 28-4B** shows the common pulmonary venous confluence superior to the left atrium (*). **Figure 28-4C** shows the right-to-left atrial shunting across the interatrial septum that is a classic finding in TAPVR. **Figure 28-4D** shows the pulmonary venous confluence (PVC) in a parasternal short-axis view with a left vertical vein coursing superiorly to the dilated innominate vein.

Answer A is not correct. A patient diagnosed with TAPVR would not be placed on ECMO because ECMO will not correct the anatomical abnormality that is present. A patient placed on ECMO may improve but will eventually return to the initial presentation because the problem has not been corrected. Answer B is not correct. Radiologic testing such as a computed tomography (CT) scan is not required, as the echocardiogram provided sufficient information for the diagnosis. Answer D is not correct. A pulmonary vasodilator such as inhaled nitric oxide will not help this patient since the problem is drainage of the pulmonary vascular bed. Answer E is not correct. An interventional cardiac catheterization cannot correct this problem. The only correction is cardiac surgery to reestablish pulmonary venous return to the left atrium. The typical surgical repair is to create a connection between the common pulmonary vein confluence and the left atrium.

KEY POINT
Echocardiography is often utilized to evaluate a patient prior to being placed on extracorporeal membrane oxygenation (ECMO). The echocardiogram is used as a screening tool to assess for any congenital heart defects that would be a contraindication to placing a patient on ECMO. With TAPVR, intracardiac anatomy appears relatively normal with the exception of pulmonary venous return. Right-to-left atrial shunting is the most important echocardiographic feature that should alert the sonographer to the possibility of TAPVR. Complete right-to-left shunting is unusual with a normal 4-chambered heart.

26. **Answer: E.** The most common form of tricuspid atresia is normally related great arteries, a small VSD, and pulmonary stenosis (see the answer outline for Question 12). Oxygenated and deoxygenated blood mix at the atrial level, leaving the systemic output saturation readings decreased until the left and right heart circulations can be separated surgically. Saturation readings in the mid 80% range are an acceptable reading indicating that there is no over-circulation or undercirculation to the lungs. There is currently no need to increase pulmonary blood flow with either a balloon valvuloplasty (answer B) or BTT shunt (answer C). A normal CVP reading indicates normal right atrial pressure and no obstruction to shunting at the atrial level. An atrial balloon

septostomy (answer A) is not indicated. A small VSD will restrict the amount of blood flow to the pulmonary vascular bed, limiting overcirculation, so a pulmonary artery band (answer D) would be not be indicated. When the shunting allows for a balance in the flow (no overcirculation or undercirculation), the patient will present as clinically stable. Intervention should not be considered at this time, but close monitoring of the patient is essential to determine when and what intervention needs to take place.

27. **Answer: B.** Pulmonary atresia with intact ventricular septum is characterized by complete obstruction to right ventricular outflow with varying degrees of right ventricular and tricuspid valve hypoplasia (**Figure 28-15A**). Coronary artery sinusoids are commonly seen and are well visualized in cases of pulmonary atresia with intact ventricular septum. The severely hypertrophied right ventricle (RV) is under significantly high pressure and has no outlet. The two main escape routes for blood in the RV is through the sinusoids and as tricuspid regurgitation (TR). To decompress the RV, coronary

artery fistulas (sinusoids) form, allowing blood to return through the cardiac vein to the right atrium (RA) and eventually across the interatrial septum (right-to-left shunt to the LA). Typically, the tricuspid valve is hypoplastic and can be patent. The tricuspid valve may present with some TR as the blood flow is forced back to the RA without a forward pathway due to the atretic pulmonary valve. **Figure 28-15B** shows a RV angiogram from a left anterior oblique projection (LAO) of a hypoplastic RV with coronary artery sinusoids draining to the aorta. **Figure 28-15C** shows a parasternal long-axis view of the left ventricle demonstrating reversal of flow in the right coronary artery. **Figure 28-15D** is an apical 4-chamber view showing a hypoplastic tricuspid annulus in pulmonary atresia with intact ventricular septum.

Partial anomalous pulmonary venous return (answer C) is not a common finding with pulmonary atresia. Left SVC (answer D) and cleft mitral valve (answer A) are also not commonly associated with pulmonary atresia with intact ventricular septum.

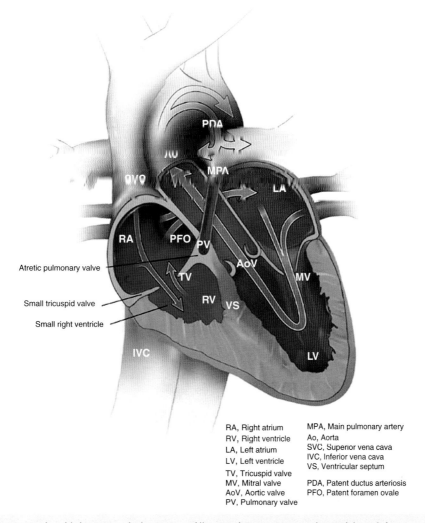

RA, Right atrium
RV, Right ventricle
LA, Left atrium
LV, Left ventricle
TV, Tricuspid valve
MV, Mitral valve
AoV, Aortic valve
PV, Pulmonary valve

MPA, Main pulmonary artery
Ao, Aorta
SVC, Superior vena cava
IVC, Inferior vena cava
VS, Ventricular septum

PDA, Patent ductus arteriosis
PFO, Patent foramen ovale

Figure 28-15A Pulmonary atresia with intact ventricular septum. All systemic venous return shunts right to left across the patent foramen ovale and pulmonary artery supply is through a left-to-right patent ductus arteriosus. (From https://www.cdc.gov/ncbddd/heartdefects/d-tga.html. Courtesy of Centers for Disease Control and Prevention, National Center on Birth Defects and Developmental Disabilities.)

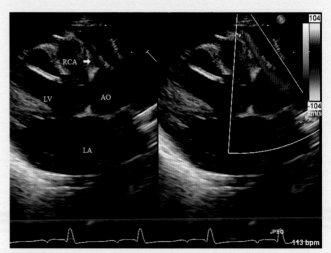

Figure 28-15C Parasternal long-axis view of the LV demonstrating reversal of flow in the right coronary artery.

Figure 28-15B RV angiogram from a left anterior oblique (LAO) projection of a hypoplastic RV with coronary artery sinusoids draining to the aorta.

28. Answer: A. Balloon atrial septostomy (Rashkind procedure) is performed during the perinatal period in cases of significant cyanosis to increase mixing of blood for improved oxygen saturations (**Figure 28-16A and 28-16B**). Bedside septostomy is common in emergent situations and is quick to set up. Echocardiography is used to confirm the correct position of the balloon catheter prior to performing the atrial septostomy (**Figure 28-16C**) as well as reducing the exposure to radiation from X-ray. Complications from poor positioning can result in damage to the mitral valve. Post procedure, echocardiography is used to confirm adequate atrial shunting. Balloon atrial septostomy may also be performed in the cardiac catherization laboratory depending on the interventionalist's preference and the urgency of the patient's situation.

Answer B is incorrect as the surgeon likes to wait until the patient has grown and stabilized in order to achieve the best surgical outcome for the patient. In very rare cases when the balloon septostomy is unsuccessful the patient may be taken to the operating room for a surgical atrial septectomy, but the complete repair would be performed when the patient is stable. Coronary stents are sometimes, but rarely placed in the interatrial septum and the patent ductus arteriosus to increase atrial shunting and ductal patency, so answers C and D are not preferred procedures in these circumstances.

TEACHING POINT

Atrial septostomy is also used in other cases of complex congenital heart disease to alleviate restriction of shunting at the atrial level and increase mixing of oxygenated and deoxygenated blood. Hypoplastic left heart syndrome (HLHS) is one of the complex cardiac pathologies where oxygenation is low, and patients will benefit from this procedure.

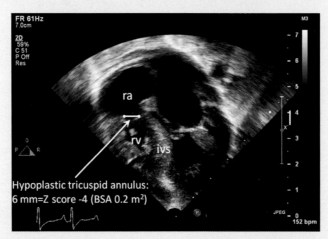

Figure 28-15D Hypoplastic tricuspid annulus in pulmonary atresia with intact ventricular septum (A4C). ivs, interventricular septum; ra, right atrium; rv, right ventricle. (Reprinted with permission from Franco KL, Thourani VH. *Cardiothoracic Surgery Review*. 1st ed. Philadelphia, PA: Wolters Kluwer Health/Lippincott Williams & Wilkins; 2011).

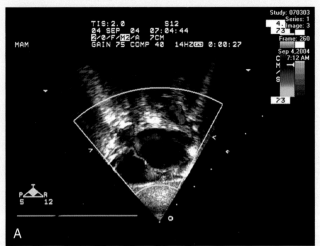

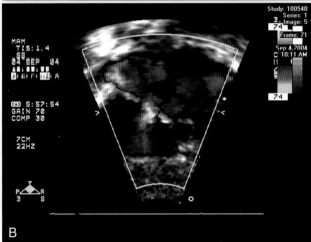

Figure 28-16A, B Restrictive atrial septum in a newborn with transposition of the great arteries. (A): Two-dimensional echocardiogram with color Doppler from the subcostal window demonstrating a tiny PFO with left-to-right flow across the atrial septum. (B): Following successful balloon atrial septostomy, a wide communication now exists between the left and right atria. LA, left atrium; PFO, patent foramen ovale; RA, right atrium. (Reprinted with permission from MacDonald MG, Seshia MM. *Avery's Neonatology.* 7th ed. Philadelphia, PA: Wolters Kluwer Health/Lippincott Williams & Wilkins; 2015.)

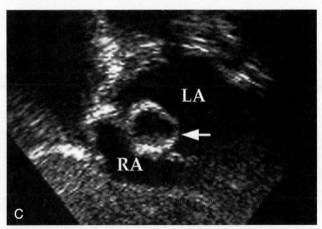

Figure 28-16C Echocardiographic subxiphoid view demonstrating a balloon septostomy catheter with the inflated balloon (arrow) being pulled from the left atrium (LA) to the right atrium (RA) through the foramen ovale. This septostomy technique is used in neonates with d-TGA to create an atrial septal defect to increase intracardiac mixing of fully and incompletely oxygenated blood, thereby improving systemic oxygenation. (Reprinted with permission from MacDonald MG, Seshia MM. *Avery's Neonatology.* 7th ed. Philadelphia, PA: Wolters Kluwer Health/Lippincott Williams & Wilkins; 2015.)

29. **Answer: D.** The anomalous origin of the left anterior descending (LAD) coronary artery arising from the right coronary artery (RCA) is a well-described coronary anomaly in TOF and has significant implications for repair. The anterior course of the LAD across the right ventricular outflow tract can interfere with the surgical approach for infundibular repair and may necessitate the insertion of an extra-cardiac right ventricle-to-pulmonary artery conduit in addition to the native outflow tract.

30. **Answer: E.** In this patient with TAPVR, there is a descending vertical vein decompressing the pulmonary venous confluence inferiorly. The vertical vein descends inferiorly through the diaphragm and typically empties into the liver. This vascular structure is anterior to the aorta and is usually venous in nature. The color Doppler signal is the same as the descending aorta, so the flow is coursing away from the thoracic cavity into the abdominal cavity. The inferior vena cava, hepatic veins, and the portal vein (Answers B, C, and D) are abdominal venous structures with a superior course; however, they do not enter the thoracic cavity. The azygous vein (answer A) is situated posterior to the aorta and along either side of the spine. It courses superiorly and eventually drains into the upper systemic venous system. This azygous vein would appear as a venous signal coursing in the opposite direction of the aorta.

KEY POINT

By definition, a vein is a vascular structure that courses toward the heart. The vertical vein in TAPVR is noted to be coursing away from the heart, whether superiorly or inferiorly. This vein would seem very out of place and close interrogation of the pulmonary venous return would be warranted in this instance.

31. **Answer: D.** The parasternal long-axis view shows two great artery side-by-side; the parasternal short-axis view displays the two semilunar valves in short axis. These features are consistent with d-TGA. In d-TGA, the aorta arises from the right ventricle, usually in a position that is anterior and rightward of the pulmonary valve. The two great arteries course parallel to one another; a distinctly different arrangement from the normal pulmonary artery crossing over the aortic root. Echocardiographically, the posterior great artery, which is the pulmonary artery, will be seen taking an immediate posterior course, typical of the pulmonary artery (see **Video 28-1A**).

32. **Answer: C.** VSD is common and present in about 40%–45% cases of d-TGA. There are basically two forms of transposition: (1) with intact ventricular septum and (2) with VSD (usually perimembranous) (**Figure 28-17**). Nearly half of the hearts with d-TGA have no other anomaly except a persistent patent foramen ovale or a patent ductus arteriosus (PDA). Answer A is not correct since LVOT obstruction

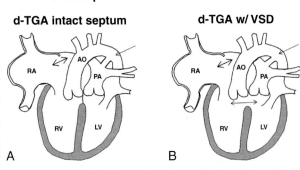

d-Transposition of the Great Arteries

d-TGA intact septum   d-TGA w/ VSD

A   B

Figure 28-17

is present in only 5% and 10% of cases of d-TGA with intact ventricular septum and d-TGA with VSD, respectively. Answer E is not correct as the coronary anatomy is normal in approximately two-thirds of cases of d-TGA. However, when present, common coronary abnormalities are a circumflex from the right coronary artery, single coronary artery, or inverted arrangement of coronary arteries (listed in decreasing frequency). Other associated defects include an ASD (answer D), coarctation of the aorta (answer B), pulmonary stenosis (subvalvular, valvular), and a PDA.

33. ▶ **Answer: A.** In d-TGA, desaturated blood returning to the right ventricle enters the aorta and returns to the systemic circulation ("parallel" circulation). This causes severe systemic desaturation (cyanosis). In a similar manner, fully saturated pulmonary venous blood returns to the left atrium, enters the left ventricle, and then the pulmonary artery. This oxygenated blood then returns to the lungs where further saturation with oxygen cannot occur. It is important to remember that desaturated blood needs to go from the systemic circulation into the pulmonary circulation in order to get oxygenated. At the same time, oxygenated blood needs to enter the systemic circulation in order to supply oxygen to the body. Without intracardiac mixing of systemic venous or pulmonary venous blood, this physiology results in fatal hypoxia. Survival in children with d-TGA depends on the presence of intracardiac (ASD, VSD) or extracardiac (PDA) shunts that allow mixing of systemic venous and pulmonary venous blood.

The level of arterial oxygen saturation is influenced primarily by the pulmonary-to-systemic blood flow ratio. This ratio, in turn, depends on adequate size of anatomic shunting sites, local pressure gradient, and vascular resistance in each of the circulations. In the presence of a large shunting site, atrial-level shunting is affected the least out of all three shunting sites by vascular resistance in systemic and pulmonary circulation. The pressure gradient between the two atria will be minimal, if any, whereas that is not true for VSD and PDA shunting sites. In summary, given the choices, the primary source of intracardiac mixing

is at the atrial level through a large ASD; therefore, answer A is the correct answer.

It is very important to evaluate the adequate size of any atrial septal communication. In the case of a restrictive atrial septal communication, the child may need emergency balloon atrial septostomy to establish an area of adequate mixing and therefore adequate saturation. **Video 28-5A** shows balloon septostomy done for a restricted atrial septal communication. After balloon septostomy, an adequate atrial septal defect is seen without any flow acceleration (**Video 28-5B**).

KEY POINTS FOR CASE 1

▶ d-TGA produces profound early cyanosis.

▶ The posterior great artery is the pulmonary artery and courses posteriorly from its origin.

▶ VSD is a common associated anomaly.

▶ Areas of potential mixing at atrial, ductal, and ventricular levels are important for survival preoperatively and need to be identified.

34. **Answer: D.** Echocardiography shows TAPVR of the supracardiac type. As previously discussed (see answer outline for Question 4), the supracardiac TAPVR is the most common form of TAPVR seen in 35%–50% of cases.

Answers A and B are not correct. In the supracardiac type, some form of obstruction is present in 50% of cases, but it is often mild. Obstruction of venous return is virtually always present when the pulmonary venous return is below the diaphragm, or infracardiac. Obstruction is rarely seen in the cardiac type of TAPVR. Answer C is not correct. In all forms of TAPVR, some form of atrial communication is almost always present. Answer E is not correct since profound cyanosis is unusual at any age. As a result, some forms of TAPVR may go undetected until later in life, although this is unusual.

35. **Answer: C.** TAPVR is a cyanotic congenital heart disease with right-sided volume overload. The right atrium (RA) will receive systemic as well as pulmonary venous return. This results in dilatation of the RA and RV as well as the pulmonary arteries. This is true for all types of TAPVR. In obstructed TAPVR, development of pulmonary hypertension can also lead to right ventricular hypertrophy.

Answer A is incorrect as the left-sided cardiac chambers are often smaller in size. Also remember that a part of the LA is formed by absorption of pulmonary veins which does not happen in TAPVR, resulting in a smaller LA. Answer B is incorrect. As stated above, the pulmonary arteries are dilated in TAPVR. Answer D is incorrect since the atrial and ventricular septa bow into the left side because of volume and/or pressure overload on the right side. Answer E is incorrect as Doppler echocardiography, particularly color flow Doppler, is very useful to establish the connection of pulmonary veins in normal hearts as well as in cases of TAPVR.

36. ▶ **Answer: E.** The scenario presented here is typical of a case of TAPVR. The first thing that needs to occur is an index of suspicion. In the case of small left heart or enlarged right heart or both, TAPVR should be suspected. When this is combined with right-to-left atrial shunting, a very strong suspicion for this entity should be present. The next phase of the echocardiographic evaluation involves a search of the systemic venous system for sources of abnormal flow. This includes the superior caval system and innominate vein, the coronary sinus, the liver and hepatic veins, and the RA. Color flow Doppler interrogation of the flows in these areas is essential to identifying the abnormal veins. Often the abnormal flow will produce very turbulent flow in some of these areas as well as unusually large venous structures. An example of infracardiac TAPVR is shown in Video 28-8 with an unusual, obstructed flow signal in the liver and hepatic veins that eventually drains into the IVC. Spectral Doppler interrogation is also important when obstruction is suspected from the color flow examination.

37. **Answer: D.** This video clip is an apical 4-chamber view with no formation of the tricuspid valve. There is a large VSD present.

Answer A is not correct as in cor triatriatum there is a membrane within the left atrium (LA) that divides the pulmonary venous return from the remainder of the LA and restricts flow from entering into the left ventricle; this is not seen in this video. Answer B is not correct as in HLHS there is poor development of the left heart structures and chambers; this is not present in this video. Answer C is not correct. While pulmonary atresia with intact ventricular septum can result in a hypoplastic right ventricle, a VSD and not an intact ventricular septum is seen in this video.

38. **Answer: C.** In the parasternal short-axis view, the VSD demonstrates low-velocity bidirectional shunting. In the subcostal view, there is no pulmonary outflow obstruction present. With no restriction to shunting at the ventricular level and no obstruction to flow at the pulmonary level, there is overcirculation to the lungs, resulting in an eventual increase in the pulmonary vascular resistance (PVR). This is the case with this patient, so the PAP is near or equal to systemic pressure.

39. **Answer: B.** There is no right heart enlargement because the patient has a hypoplastic right ventricle. Poor LV function is present as this patient also has LVNC, a form of cardiomyopathy. Prolonged unrestricted flow through the pulmonary outflow will result in increased PVR. Elevated pulmonary artery pressures will result and is demonstrated in the low-velocity bidirectional shunting at the VSD. A small to moderate degree of pericardial effusion is also present, suggesting third spacing in this fluid overload state.

These findings, in combination with the patient's clinical presentation, are all conclusive of congestive heart failure. In this single ventricular pathology, the presence of LVNC and significant left ventricular dysfunction leaves cardiac transplantation as the only option for this patient.

TEACHING POINT

The oxygen saturation reading in the 90% range would suggest overcirculation to the lungs. Normal oxygen saturation readings for a patient with tricuspid atresia with balanced flow would be in the mid 80% range. A larger volume of blood flow to the lungs would result in an increased volume of blood returning to the left atrium, thus giving a higher oxygen saturation reading. Undercirculation would be seen as oxygen saturation readings below the lower 70% range. With chronic overcirculation, the pulmonary vascular bed would increase resistance to try and protect the lungs from the extra volume.

40. ▶ **Answer: E.** Video 28-4A shows an underdeveloped left heart with a hypoplastic mitral valve; these features are consistent with HLHS. HLHS is a combination of hypoplasia or atresia of the mitral and aortic valves, underdevelopment of the LV, and hypoplasia of the aortic arch (**Figure 28-18**). The right ventricle will be dilated and apex-forming. In HLHS, the circulation through the left heart is not adequate to support systemic output. This is a ductal-dependent lesion until a stable systemic outflow is established and the patient can be removed from prostaglandin.

41. **Answer: A.** There is low output through the aortic valve because it is significantly hypoplastic. Ductal flow is right to left in order to supply blood systemically. The retrograde flow in the descending aorta above the level of the ductus is to provide perfusion to the head, neck, and coronary arteries since cardiac output through the aortic valve is insufficient. There is right-to-left systolic shunting through the ductus, but it is not the cause for the reversal of flow in this location. Aortopulmonary collaterals have continuous flow away from the aorta. An arteriovenous malformation in the head can cause reversal of flow in the proximal descending aorta, but this would be diastolic reversal and not systolic.

42. **Answer: D.** Unrestricted left-to-right flow through the interatrial septum is key in stabilizing a patient with the diagnosis of HLHS. If the atrial shunt is restricted, a balloon atrial septostomy needs to be performed. In addition, prostaglandin administration will be started to maintain ductal patency.

Acknowledgments: The authors thank and acknowledge the contributions from Richard A. Humes MD and James M. Galas MD (Chapter 31: Cyanotic Congenital Heart Disease) in *Clinical Echocardiography Review: A Self-Assessment Tool, 2nd Edition,* edited by Allan L. Klein, Craig R. Asher, 2017.

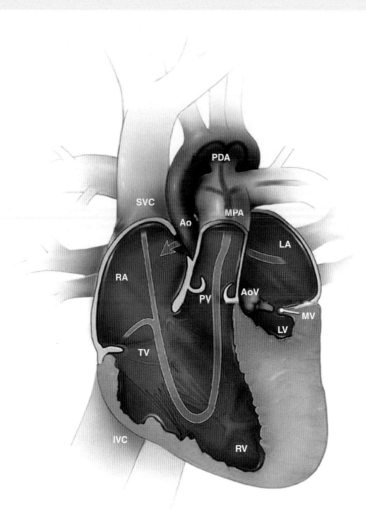

RA, Right atrium	SVC, Superior vena cava	TV, Tricuspid valve
RV, Right ventricle	IVC, Inferior vena cava	MV, Mitral valve
LA, Left atrium	MPA, Main pulmonary artery	PV, Pulmonary valve
LV, Left ventricle	Ao, Aorta	AoV, Aortic valve
	PDA, Patent ductus arteriosis	

Figure 28-18 Diagram of HLHS. Left heart structures are severely underdeveloped with little to no prograde flow present. Pulmonary venous return to the left atrium shunts left to right across an atrial septal defect and systemic blood supply is through the PDA. (From https://www.cdc.gov/ncbddd/heartdefects/d-tga.html. Courtesy of Centers for Disease Control and Prevention, National Center on Birth Defects and Developmental Disabilities.

SUGGESTED READINGS

Doty D, Doty J. *Cardiac Surgery.* 2nd ed. Philadelphia, PA: Elsevier Saunders; 2012.

Driscoll D. *Fundamentals of Pediatric Cardiology.* Philadelphia, PA: Wolters Kluwer Health; 2015.

Eidem B, O'Leary P, Cetta F. *Echocardiography in Pediatric and Adult Congenital Heart Disease.* 2nd ed. Philadelphia, PA: Wolters Kluwer Health; 2015.

Gatzoulis M, Webb G, Daubeney P. *Diagnosis and Management of Adult Congenital Heart Disease.* Philadelphia, PA: Elsevier Saunders; 2011.

Ho S, Rigby M, Anderson R. *Echocardiography in Congenital Heart Disease Made Simple.* London: Imperial College Press; 2005.

Johnson W, Moller J. *Pediatric Cardiology.* Chichester, West Sussex: John Wiley & Sons; 2014.

Lai W, Mertens L, Cohen M, Geva T. *Echocardiography in Pediatric and Congenital Heart Disease - From Fetus to Adult.* 2nd ed. John Wiley & Sons; 2016.

Park M. *Pediatric Cardiology for Practitioners.* Philadelphia, PA: Mosby/Elsevier; 2008.

Perloff J, Marelli A. *Perloff's Clinical Recognition of Congenital Heart Disease.* Philadelphia: Elsevier Saunders; 2012.

Reynolds T, Yan P, Dubovec P. *The Pediatric Echocardiographer's Pocket Reference.* 3rd ed. Phoenix: Arizona Heart Institute; 2002.

Silverman N. *Pediatric Echocardiography.* Baltimore: Williams & Wilkins; 1993.

Snider A, Serwer G, Ritter S. Echocardiography. In: *Pediatric Heart Disease.* St. Louis: Mosby; 1997.

CHAPTER 29

Adult Congenital Heart Disease

Contributors: G. Monet Strachan, ACS, RDCS (AE, PE) and Erik Echegaray, BS, ACS, RDCS (AE, PE, FE)

✪ Question 1

After a device closure of a secundum atrial septal defect (ASD), which potential complication(s) should be excluded by an echocardiogram?

A. Embolization or poorly seated device with a residual shunt
B. Device-caused erosion of cardiac structures
C. Pericardial effusion
D. Thrombus on device
E. All of the above

✪ Question 2

Which of the following is not a type of repair used for coarctation of the aorta (COA)?

A. Interposition graft
B. Modified Bentall
C. Subclavian flap
D. Angioplasty with or without a stent
E. Resection of COA with end-to-end anastomosis

✪✪ Question 3

Which of the following is not a long-term complication of ventricular septal defect (VSD) repair?

A. Aortic regurgitation
B. Left heart dilatation
C. Outflow tract obstruction
D. Residual ventricular septal defect (VSD)
E. Tricuspid regurgitation

✪ Question 4

An adult patient with a transannular patch post tetralogy of Fallot (TOF) repair is most likely to show which of the following on an echocardiogram?

A. Suprapulmonic stenosis
B. Normal right ventricular (RV) size
C. Pulmonic annulus stenosis secondary to obstruction from the patch
D. Diastolic flow reversal in the pulmonary artery (PA) and PA branches
E. Subpulmonic obstruction from the patch being passively pulled into the outflow tract during systole

✪✪ Question 5

Which selection is an uncommon complication following tetralogy of Fallot (TOF) repair involving a transannular patch?

A. Subpulmonic aneurysm
B. Severe pulmonic regurgitation (PR)
C. Thrombus formation on the patch
D. Subpulmonic obstruction secondary to endothelial growth on the patch
E. Subpulmonic obstruction secondary to transannular patch movement into the right ventricular outflow tract (RVOT)

✪✪✪ Question 6

The continuous-wave (CW) Doppler trace shown in **Figure 29-1** was obtained from an off-axis apical window in an adult patient with normal sinus rhythm, tetralogy of Fallot repair (Rastelli procedure), and no other interventions. This Doppler trace demonstrates:

A. A ventricular septal defect (VSD) baffle leak with bidirectional shunting.

B. Congenital mitral stenosis and regurgitation.

C. Congenital tricuspid stenosis and regurgitation with evidence of a significantly elevated right ventricular systolic pressure.

D. Pulmonic (conduit) stenosis and regurgitation.

E. No determinate finding.

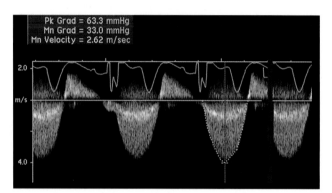

Figure 29-1

✪✪✪ Question 7

The continuous-wave Doppler trace in **Figure 29-2** was acquired from a high parasternal long-axis view angled leftward in a patient with tetralogy of Fallot repair who has been lost to follow up. The left arm blood pressure was 124/78 mm Hg and right ventricular systolic pressure (RVSP) estimated from the tricuspid regurgitant velocity was 50 mm Hg. Which of the following statements is correct?

A. Flow above the baseline represents a residual ventricular septal defect (VSD) with right ventricular (RV) pressures nearing systemic pressures.

B. Flow through the pulmonary valve is coming toward the probe and is around 2 m/s, suggesting mild pulmonary stenosis.

C. There is mild right ventricular outflow tract obstruction with a "dagger"-shaped signal, suggesting dynamic obstruction.

D. This pattern represents severe pulmonary regurgitation (PR).

E. This profile likely reflects mild or moderate PR.

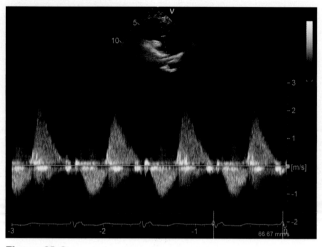

Figure 29-2

✪✪✪ Question 8

The images shown in **Figure 29-3A** to **C** are systolic frames acquired from the parasternal short-axis (PSAX) view in a 21-year-old man with tetralogy of Fallot repair and a 29 mm bovine pulmonary valve replacement. The left arm blood pressure was 139/80 mm Hg. Based on this information, which statement is correct?

A. There is a residual ventricular septal defect (VSD) at the posterior patch margin with low gradient reflecting significantly elevated right ventricular systolic pressure (RVSP).

B. There is a ruptured sinus of Valsalva aneurysm with an RVSP of 100 mm Hg.

C. There is eccentric aortic regurgitation with a color Doppler artifact in the right atrium.

D. There is eccentric mitral regurgitation through an anterior cleft in the mitral valve.

E. There is tricuspid regurgitation at the septal commissure with an RVSP of 39 mm Hg + right atrial pressure.

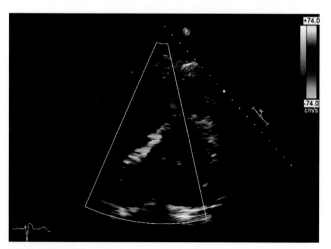

Figure 29-3A

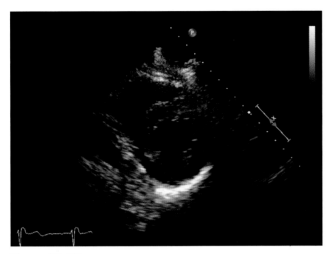

Figure 29-3B

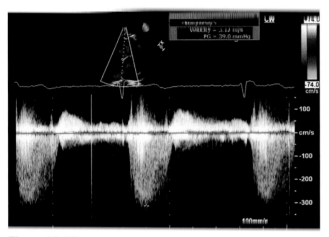

Figure 29-3C

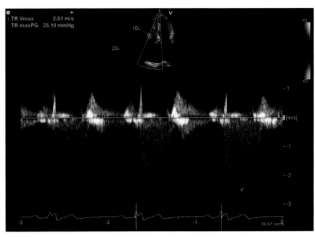

Figure 29-4

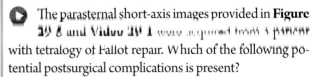

✪✪ Question 10

🔘 The parasternal short-axis images provided in **Figure 29-5 and Video 29-1** were acquired from a patient with tetralogy of Fallot repair. Which of the following potential postsurgical complications is present?

A. An aneurysm of the right ventricular outflow tract (RVOT)

B. Aortic dilatation

C. Prosthetic pulmonic valve dysfunction

D. Residual RVOT obstruction

E. Ventricular septal defect patch rupture

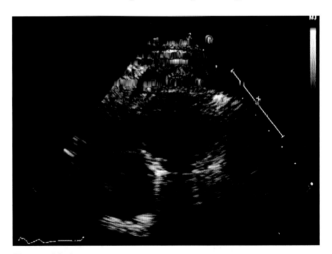

Figure 29-5

✪✪ Question 9

The tricuspid regurgitant (TR) Doppler waveform shown in **Figure 29-4** was obtained in a patient with tetralogy of Fallot repair. Mean right atrial pressure (RAP) was estimated as 5 mm Hg. The pulmonic gradient was not able to be obtained in this patient due to poor acoustic windows. Based on this information, which statement is correct?

A. A ventricular septal defect (VSD) is suspected.

B. An atrial septal defect (ASD) is suspected.

C. The peak pulmonic outflow gradient is likely less than 30 mm Hg.

D. The peak pulmonic outflow gradient is likely more than 30 mm Hg.

E. Nothing can be said regarding the peak pulmonic outflow gradient.

✪✪ Question 11

Which of the following is not a complication seen post–truncus arteriosus repair in the adult?

A. Arch repair restenosis

B. Patent ductus arteriosus (PDA)

C. Right ventricle-pulmonary artery (RV-PA) conduit stenosis/regurgitation

D. Severe truncal valve regurgitation/stenosis

E. Ventricular septal defect (VSD) patch leak

✪✪✪ Question 12

Which of the following statements regarding the surgical repair for dextro-transposition of the great arteries (d-TGA {S,D,D}) is false?

A. After an atrial switch operation, the right ventricle (RV) is connected to the aorta and the left ventricle (LV) is connected to the pulmonary artery (PA).

B. The LeCompte maneuver is usually performed during an arterial switch operation.

C. The presence of ventricular inversion dictates whether an atrial or arterial switch operation is performed.

D. The Rastelli, REV, and Nikaido procedures may be performed in some patients with d-TGA.

E. There are many potential variations of coronary artery origins and course, some of which may affect the arterial switch operation.

✪✪✪ Question 13

Which of the following correctly identifies the anatomy in this parasternal long-axis (PLAX) view (**Figure 29-6A** and **B**) acquired in a patient with a Senning repair for dextro-transposition of the great arteries (d-TGA)?

A. 1 = pulmonary artery (PA); 2 = aorta (Ao); 3 = pulmonary venous baffle (PVB); 4 = systemic venous baffle (SVB); 5 = descending aorta (DAo)

B. 1 = PA; 2 = Ao; 3 = SVB; 4 = PVB; 5 = DAo

C. 1 = Ao; 2 = PA; 3 = PVB; 4 = SVB; 5 = DAo

D. 1 = Ao; 2 = PA; 3 = SVB; 4 = PVB; 5 = DAo

E. 1 = Ao; 2 = PA; 3 = SVB; 4 = PVB; 5 = coronary sinus

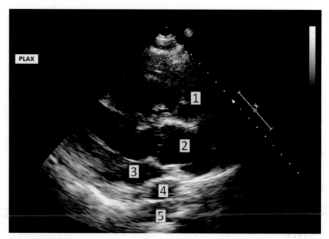

Figure 29-6B

✪✪ Question 14

Which statement regarding the atrial switch operation for dextro-transposition of the great arteries (d-TGA) is false?

A. Senning and Mustard procedures are both examples of an atrial switch operation.

B. The left ventricle (LV) becomes the systemic pumping chamber.

C. Pulmonic venous and systemic venous baffles are created whereby the pulmonary venous baffle (PVB) directs oxygenated blood to the right ventricle (RV) and the systemic venous baffle (SVB) directs deoxygenated blood to the left ventricle.

D. Baffle leaks can occur anywhere and more typically shunt from PVB to SVB, which causes significant LV volume overload if the shunt is large.

E. Baffle stenosis can occur anywhere but more often occurs in the superior limb of the SVB and at the superior end of the PVB.

✪✪✪ Question 15

Figure 29-7 shows a pulsed-wave Doppler trace recorded across the pulmonary venous baffle (PVB) in a patient with an atrial switch operation for dextro-transposition of the great arteries (d-TGA) and a junctional rhythm. This trace is consistent with:

A. Normal PVB flow.

B. Significant mitral regurgitation (MR).

C. Significant tricuspid regurgitation (TR).

D. A low junctional rhythm.

E. C and D.

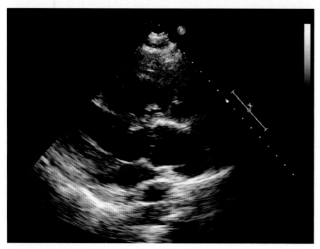

Figure 29-6A

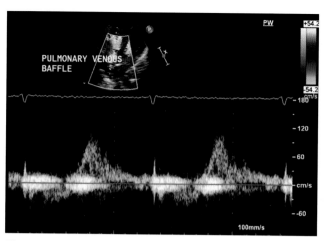

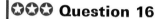

Figure 29-7

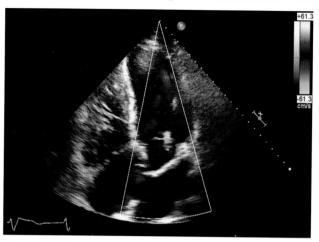

Figure 29-8A

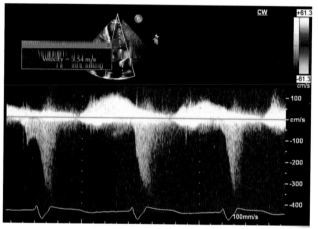

Figure 29-8B

✪✪✪ Question 16

The images shown in Figures 29-8A and B were acquired from a patient with an atrial switch operation for dextro-transposition of the great arteries (d-TGA). Assuming that there is no outflow tract obstruction, which of the following statements regarding the continuous-wave Doppler trace is correct?

A. This is mitral regurgitation (MR) and the pulmonary artery systolic pressure (PASP) is at least 50 mm Hg.
B. This is MR and the patient is significantly hypotensive.
C. This is tricuspid regurgitation (TR) and the PASP is at least 50 mm Hg.
D. This is TR and the patient is significantly hypotensive.
E. None of the above is true.

✪✪ Question 17

The images shown in **Figure 29-9** were acquired from a patient with dextro-transposition of the great arteries (d-TGA). Based on these images, what surgery was performed and what is the complication seen?

A. Arterial switch operation (ASO) with branch pulmonary artery (PA) stenosis
B. ASO with ascending aortic stenosis
C. Rastelli procedure with conduit stenosis
D. Rastelli procedure with a residual ventricular septal defect
E. Atrial switch with a baffle leak

✪✪ Question 18

▶ Based on the images provided (**Figure 29-10A** and **B** and **Video 29-2**), which surgical repair is likely to be performed in this patient with dextro-transposition of the great arteries (d-TGA)?

A. Atrial switch
B. Arterial switch operation
C. Rastelli procedure
D. Unrepairable

✪✪ Question 19

▶ Based on the images provided (**Figure 29-11A** and **B** and **Video 29-3A** and **B**) the likely repair in this patient with dextro-transposition of the great arteries (d-TGA) is:

A. An atrial switch.
B. An arterial switch.
C. A Rastelli procedure.
D. Indeterminate.

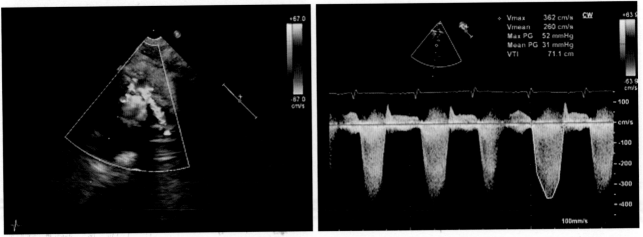

Figure 29-9 Left: Parasternal short-axis view showing the Doppler cursor position; Right: Continuous-wave Doppler trace from the left image.

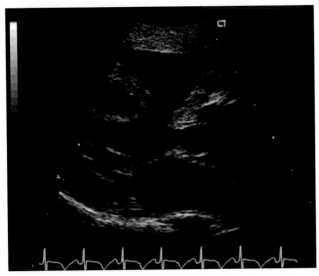

Figure 29-10A

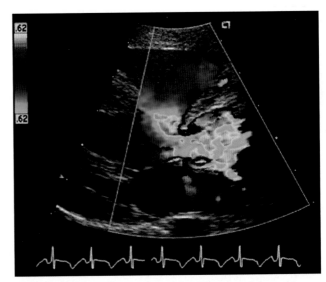

Figure 29-10B

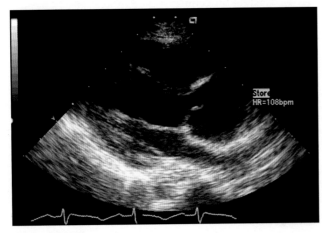

Figure 29-11A

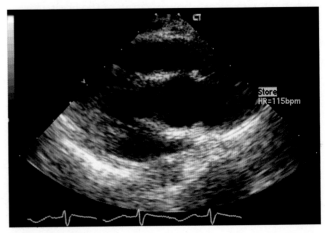

Figure 29-11B

✪✪✪ Question 20

▶ Based on the images provided (**Figure 29-12A** and **B** and **Video 29-4A** and **B**), the likely repair and complication in this patient with dextro-transposition of the great arteries (d-TGA) is:

A. An atrial switch with systemic venous baffle obstruction.

B. An arterial switch with pulmonary stenosis.

C. A Rastelli procedure with conduit stenosis.

D. A Rastelli procedure with a residual ventricular septal defect.

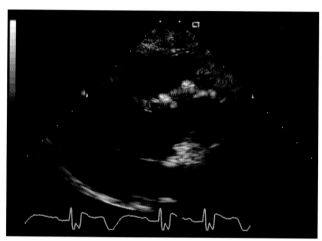

Figure 29-12A

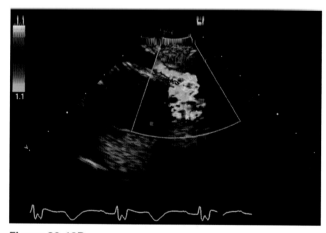

Figure 29-12B

✪✪ Question 21

Which of the following is not a typical feature of unrepaired congenitally corrected transposition of the great arteries (cc-TGA)?

A. The aortic valve usually lies anterior and to the left of the pulmonic valve.

B. The great arteries are in parallel arrangement.

C. The left ventricle gives rise to the pulmonary artery and the right ventricle gives rise to the aorta.

D. There is mitral-aortic fibrous continuity.

E. There is ventricular inversion.

✪✪ Question 22

The Fontan operation is:

A. Any operation that diverts the flow of pulmonary venous blood to the body without passing through a ventricle.

B. Any operation that diverts the systemic venous return to the pulmonary artery without passing through a ventricle.

C. A connection between the right atrial appendage and the pulmonary artery.

D. A direct anastomosis between the aorta and the pulmonary trunk.

E. A procedure that normalizes the circulation in patients with a single ventricular morphology.

✪✪ Question 23

A fenestrated Fontan operation includes:

A. A creation of a small defect between the Fontan and the left atrium.

B. A creation of a small defect between the Fontan and the right atrium.

C. A creation of a small defect between the Fontan and the single ventricle.

D. A repair of a fenestration between the right and left atria.

E. A repair of a fenestration in the atrioventricular valve.

✪✪✪ Question 24

This suprasternal notch image **Figure 29-13** was recorded in a 23-year-old man with a history of hypoplastic left heart syndrome with a Norwood procedure, bidirectional Glenn shunt, and a lateral Fontan. The distance between the yellow arrows measured 7.4 mm. Which of the following statements is correct?

A. The superior vena cava (SVC) flow may be abnormal.

B. The left pulmonary artery (LPA) is narrow.

C. This is a retro-aortic innominate vein.

D. The Fontan baffle is narrowing.

E. A and B.

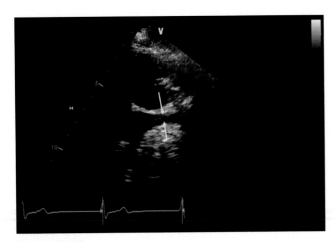

Figure 29-13

✪✪✪ Question 25

Which of the following echocardiographic findings is not a cause for increased pulmonary vascular resistance (PVR) in a patient with hypoplastic right heart syndrome (HRHS) and a Fontan circuit?

A. Fontan baffle obstruction and cavopulmonary anastomosis site narrowing
B. Narrow interatrial communication
C. Narrow pulmonary arteries
D. Pulmonary vein stenosis
E. Severe systemic atrioventricular (AV) valve regurgitation

✪✪ Question 26

In this patient with tricuspid atresia, the dilated (5.7 cm) structure marked by the yellow arrow in **Figure 29-14** is the:

A. Aorta.
B. Coronary sinus.
C. Fontan baffle.
D. Pulmonary venous channel.
E. Systemic venous channel.

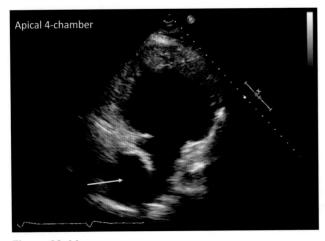

Apical 4-chamber

Figure 29-14

✪✪✪ Question 27

This zoomed apical 4-chamber view of the atria (**Figure 29-15**) was acquired from a 31-year-old man with complex congenital heart disease and a lateral Fontan. What is the color Doppler flow that measures 5 mm in width and what is the likely sequela?

A. Fontan fenestration: lower arterial oxygen saturation
B. Pulmonary vein stenosis secondary to encroachment from the Fontan: pulmonary venous hypertension
C. Atrioventricular (AV) valve regurgitation: pulmonary hypertension
D. AV valve stenosis: systemic venous hypertension

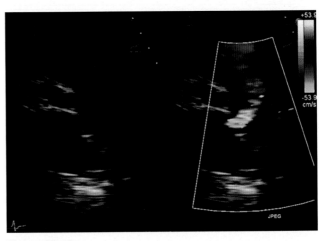

Figure 29-15

CASE 1

A 58-year-old man with a history of tetralogy of Fallot repair and a 27 mm pericardial tissue pulmonary valve replacement and right ventricular outflow tract reconstruction using a bovine pericardial patch presents for routine follow-up. On the current echocardiogram, there is marked left and right ventricular dysfunction and tricuspid regurgitation.

⭐ Question 28

▶ **Figure 29-16** and **Video 29-5**, taken with the transducer at the right sternal border (RSB), show which of the following complications?
A. Aortic dilatation
B. Prosthetic pulmonic valve dysfunction
C. Residual right ventricular outflow tract (RVOT) obstruction
D. RVOT aneurysm
E. Ventricular septal defect (VSD) patch rupture

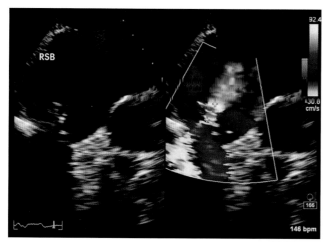

Figure 29-16

⚙⚙⚙ Question 29

▶ On a 3-month follow-up echocardiogram, **Figure 29-17A** and **B** and **Video 29-6** were acquired from a parasternal long-axis (PLAX) view with the transducer tilted leftward. Which of the following complications is shown?

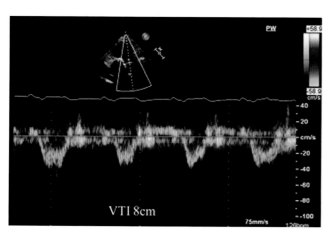

Figure 29-17A

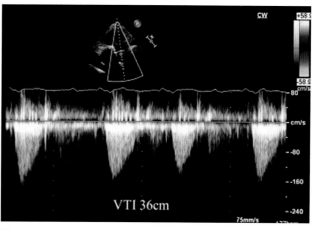

Figure 29-17B

A. Right ventricular outflow tract (RVOT) aneurysm
B. Residual RVOT obstruction
C. Prosthetic pulmonic valve dysfunction
D. Ventricular septal defect (VSD) patch rupture
E. None of the above

CASE 2

A 31-year-old woman with a congenital heart defect presented for an echocardiogram.

⚙⚙⚙ Question 30

▶ Based on the images provided (**Video 29-7A** and **B**), what is the most likely diagnosis?
A. Complete atrioventricular canal defect
B. Congenitally corrected transposition of the great arteries
C. Ebstein anomaly
D. Hypoplastic left heart syndrome
E. Pulmonary atresia with an intact ventricular septum

⚙⚙⚙ Question 31

This patient went on to have a "one-and-a-half" ventricle repair which for her means:
A. A Fontan circuit was completed.
B. A modified Blalock-Taussig (BT) shunt was the end-repair.
C. The right ventricle (RV) was surgically reconstructed.
D. A superior cavopulmonary anastomosis was the end-repair.

CASE 3

A 30-year-old woman who was lost to follow up with medical records not yet available presents for an echocardiogram.

✪✪✪ Question 32

▶ Based on the images provided (**Figure 29-18A and B** and **Video 29-8**), there is:

A. A single ventricle with a Fontan circuit and an atrial stent.

B. Dextro-transposition of the great arteries (d-TGA) with atrial switch and a stent in the superior venous baffle (SVB).

C. d-TGA with Rastelli repair and conduit narrowing

D. Congenitally corrected transposition of the great arteries (cc-TGA) with double switch and a pulmonary venous baffle (PVB) stent.

E. cc-TGA with double switch and a pulmonary conduit.

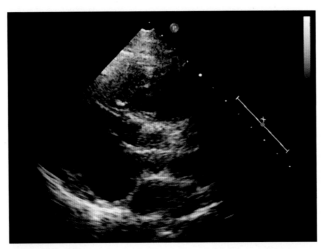

Figure 29-18A

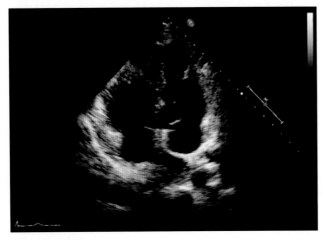

Figure 29-18B

✪✪✪ Question 33

Figure 29-19 is a high parasternal long-axis view of the great arteries. This image shows:

A. A coarctation of the aorta.

B. A patent ductus arteriosus.

C. A pulmonary artery (PA) band.

D. Left PA stenosis.

E. Right PA stenosis.

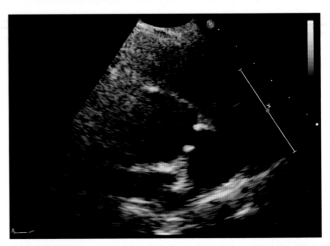

Figure 29-19

CASE 4

▶ A 44-year-old man with a Mustard repair and ventricular septal defect (VSD) closure for dextro-transposition of the great arteries presents for an echocardiogram. The left arm blood pressure (BP) was 110/66 mm Hg. A residual VSD was noted and there was negligible pulmonic valvular stenosis and no obstruction of the right ventricular outflow tract, aortic valve, descending aorta, or left subclavian artery. Representative images from the parasternal long-axis (PLAX) (**Figure 29-20A and B** and **Video 29-9A**) and parasternal short-axis (PSAX) views of the left ventricular outflow tract and pulmonary valve (**Figures 29-20C to E** and **Video 29-9B and C**) are provided.

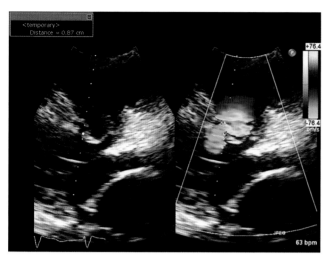

Figure 29-20A

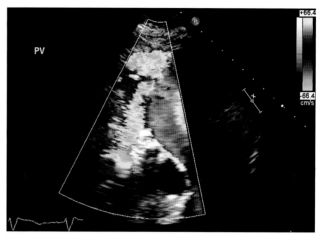

Figure 29-20D

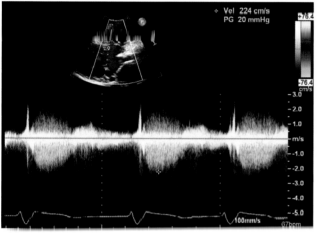

Figure 29 20D

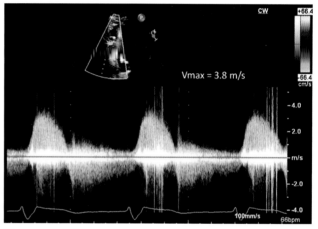

Figure 29-20E

A. There is a left ventricle (LV)-to-right ventricle (RV) shunt with an estimated right ventricular systolic pressure (RVSP) of 20 mm Hg.

B. There is an LV-to-RV shunt with an estimated RVSP of 90 mm Hg.

C. There is an RV-to-LV shunt with an estimated left ventricular systolic pressure (LVSP) of 20 mm Hg.

D. There is an RV-to-LV shunt with an estimated LVSP of 90 mm Hg.

E. The shunt direction or systolic pressure in either ventricle cannot be determined with the data given.

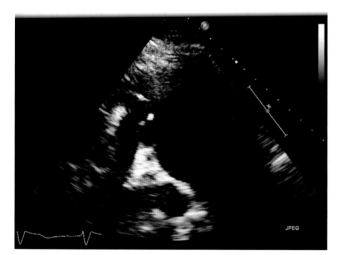

Figure 29-20C

✪✪✪ Question 34

Based on the information and images provided for this case, which of the following statements regarding the ventricular septal defect (VSD) is most correct?

✪✪✪ Question 35

Based on the information and images provided and using prior data determined in this case, the estimated pulmonary artery systolic pressure (PASP) is:

A. 33 mm Hg.

B. 53 mm Hg.

C. 57 mm Hg.

D. 90 mm Hg.

E. Indeterminate.

CASE 5

A 38-year-old active man with a Mustard repair for dextro-transposition of the great arteries presents with a chief complaint of dyspnea on exertion (DOE) when walking up hills. Results from a cardiopulmonary exercise test were unremarkable. Findings on his echocardiogram include a right ventricular fractional area change (RVFAC) of 35%, tricuspid annular systolic plane excursion (TAPSE) of 0.9 cm, and a tricuspid annular s' velocity of 6 cm/s.

✪✪✪ Question 36

▶ Based on the images provided (**Video 29-10A** to **C**), what is a likely cause of his DOE?

A. Pulmonary venous baffle (PVB) stenosis and subsequent pulmonary venous hypertension

B. Large secundum atrial septal defect (ASD) with subsequent pulmonary overcirculation

C. Pulmonary hypertension as evidenced by a flattened interventricular septum (IVS)

D. Severely enlarged right ventricle (RV) with severe systolic dysfunction

E. None of the above

✪✪ Question 37

What is this structure (identified by yellow arrow in **Figure 29-21**) and what transducer maneuver can be done to better visualize it from this parasternal long-axis (PLAX) view?

A. Dilated coronary sinus; tilt transducer rightward and rotate to open up

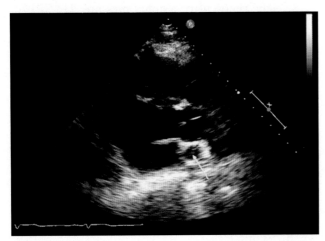

Figure 29-21

B. Systemic venous baffle; tilt transducer rightward and rotate to open up

C. Pulmonary venous baffle; tilt transducer rightward and rotate to open up

D. Left pulmonary artery branch; tilt transducer leftward and rotate to open up

E. Right pulmonary artery branch; tilt transducer rightward and rotate to open up

✪✪✪ Question 38

▶ Based on **Video 29-11** and **Figure 29-22**, what abnormality is shown and what is the sequela that could arise?

A. Unroofed coronary sinus; left-to-right shunt

B. Systemic venous baffle (SVB) leak; left-to-right shunt

C. SVB stenosis; upper systemic venous congestion

D. Pulmonary venous baffle (PVB) leak; left-to-right shunt

E. PVB stenosis; pulmonary venous hypertension

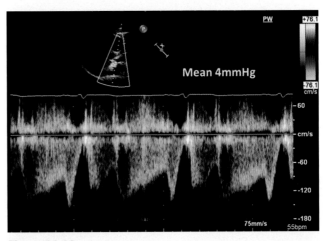

Figure 29-22

✪✪✪ Question 39

▶ Additional findings in this case study are shown in **Figure 29-23A** and **B** and **Video 29-12**. What is the color flow seen (yellow arrow in **Figure 29-23A**)?

A. Baffle leak with predominant left (pulmonary venous baffle [PVB])-to-right (systemic venous baffle [SVB]) shunt

B. Baffle leak with predominant left (SVB)-to-right (PVB) shunt

C. Baffle leak with predominant right (PVB)-to-left (SVB) shunt

D. Baffle leak with predominant right (SVB)-to-left (PVB) shunt

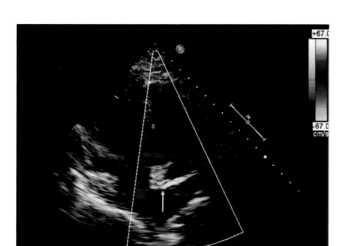

Figure 29-23A

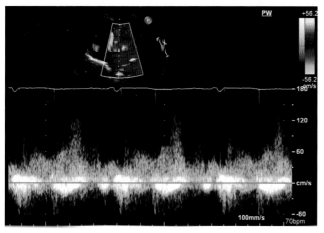

Figure 29-23B

D. Pulmonary venous confluence and stent to the left atrium

E. Pericardial effusion from an atrial septal defect device–induced erosion of the atrial wall

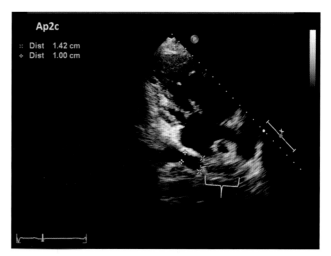

Figure 29-24A

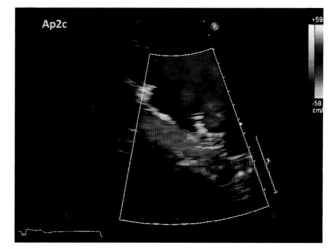

Figure 29-24B

CASE 6

This is a study of an 18-year-old man with complex congenital heart disease (right ventricular dominant unbalanced atrioventricular canal defect, double outlet right ventricle, and pulmonary stenosis). Prior cardiac surgeries included a bidirectional Glenn shunt and an external fenestrated Fontan. Three years prior to this echocardiogram, the patient had a cardiac arrest and was successfully resuscitated.

✪✪✪ Question 40

The images shown in **Figure 29-24A** to **C** were acquired from an apical 2-chamber (Ap2c) view. What is the structure being measured and what is the yellow bracket pointing to in **Figure 29-24A**?

A. Glenn shunt and stent

B. Left superior vena cava and stent

C. Fontan conduit and stent

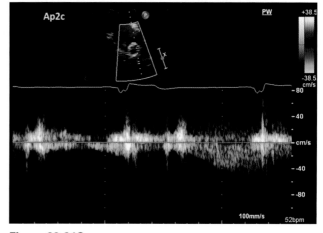

Figure 29-24C

✪✪✪ Question 41

After his cardiac arrest, the patient also developed thrombus in the left superior vena cava (LSVC) for which a stent was placed. **Figure 29-25A** to C shows the 2D, color Doppler and spectral Doppler interrogation of the stent from the left supraclavicular win-

dow (the stent is marked by the yellow bracket in **Figure 29-25A** and **B**). The LSVC stent is:

A. Mildly narrowed.
B. Moderately narrowed.
C. Severely narrowed.
D. Widely patent.

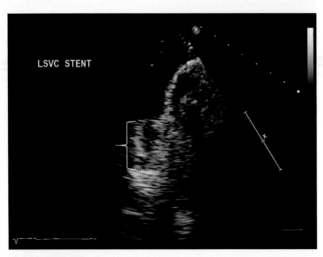

Figure 29-25A

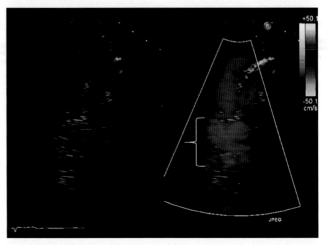

Figure 29-25B

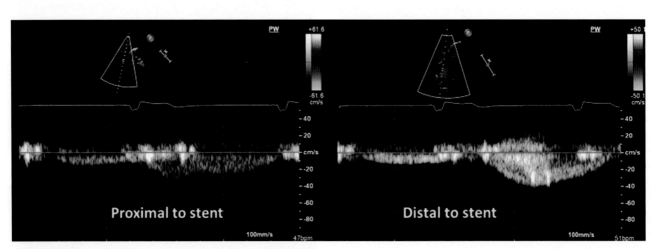

Figure 29-25C

✪✪✪ Question 42

Based on the images provided (**Figure 29-26A** and **B**) and assuming a mean Fontan pressure of 10 mm Hg, which of the following is true?

A. Mean atrial pressure is 3 mm Hg
B. Mean atrial pressure is 17 mm Hg
C. Transpulmonary mean gradient is 3 mm Hg
D. Transpulmonary mean gradient is 17 mm Hg

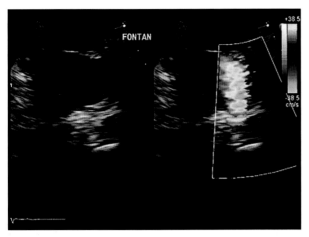

Figure 29-26A

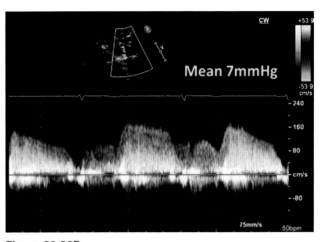

Figure 29-26B

ANSWERS

1. **Answer: E.** Secundum ASDs are the third most common congenital heart defect, many of which are amenable to transcatheter device closure. Complications following the procedure are uncommon. A large ASD with a diminutive or absent posterior/inferior rim is at a higher risk for poor device positioning or embolization of the device. Therefore, the preprocedure assessment for adequate rims for device capture is of paramount importance. Larger devices have been implicated in erosion of cardiac structures such as the mitral valve, aortic root, and atrial wall. Pericardial effusion can be a sequela of the procedure or erosion. Thrombus on the device disk has been reported even with full heparinization at the time of implantation.

2. **Answer: B.** The Bentall procedure is a surgical repair of an ascending aortic or aortic root aneurysm in combination with aortic valve disease.

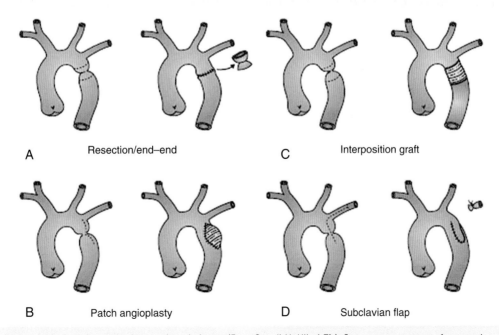

Figure 29-27 Major surgical aortic coarctation repair techniques. (From Suradi H, Hijazi ZM. Current management of coarctation of the aorta. *Glob Cardiol Sci Pract.* 2015;2015(4):44. https://creativecommons.org/licenses/by/4.0/. Copyright © 2015 Suradi, Hijazi, licensee Bloomsbury Qatar Foundation Journals.)

Less commonly, it is used to repair aortic dissection affecting the aortic root and valve.

Major surgical COA repair techniques are illustrated in **Figure 29-27**. Interposition grafts (answer A) can be used in the adult with recurrent COA or newly discovered COA. Since the graft will not grow, this is not widely used in infants. The subclavian flap procedure (answer C) has the advantage of using the patient's own native tissue (subclavian artery) and COA recurrence rate is low, but the subclavian artery is sacrificed. A bypass graft from the carotid or innominate artery to the ongoing subclavian artery can be performed for arm ischemia. Angioplasty/stent for COA (answer D) has been in use since the mid-1990s and has the advantage of being delivered transcutaneously with minimal recovery time and if COA recurs, angioplasty can be repeated and/or a stent can be expanded. Ideally a stent will be expandable from 12 to 22 mm. For the end-to-end repair (answer E), the area of COA is first resected, and then the two aortic ends brought together and sutured. Recurrence of COA can occur at the anastomosis site.

Other COA repairs include bypass grafts and jump grafts. Bypass grafts use a conduit from the transverse aorta or subclavian artery to the descending aorta and jump grafts (**Figure 29-28** and **Video 29-13**) use a conduit from the ascending aorta to the descending aorta. These grafts are used for complex, long-segment, or recurrent COA.

3. **Answer: B.** Left heart dilatation with a VSD results from volume overload but resolves over time after the VSD is closed, and therefore is not a long-term complication. Aortic regurgitation (answer A) can be a result of aortic valve damage from prolapse caused by the Venturi effect whereby the cusp (usually the right coronary) gets sucked into the VSD,

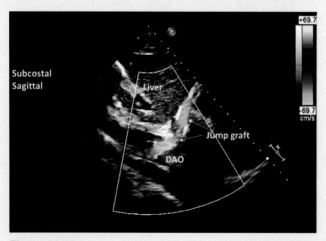

Figure 29-28

mostly seen with supracristal-type VSD. If there is damage to the aortic valve and a repair was done, the valve can degenerate over time and precipitate aortic regurgitation. Outflow tract obstruction (answer C) can be a direct consequence of the patch protruding into the outflow tract (usually pulmonic outflow). If the VSD closure was a baffle patch closure, such as seen with complex congenital heart defects and a Rastelli operation, then the VSD acts as a part of the outflow as it channels blood from the left ventricle through the VSD and to the aorta. In this case, systemic outflow tract obstruction occurs by the growth of the ventricular septum into the VSD. Residual VSDs (answer D) as a result of patch failure can occur and have been shown to increase in prevalence with a larger, more extensive patch such as seen with large VSDs or with baffle patches. Baffle patches have a longer distance to traverse. Tricuspid regurgitation (answer E) is a complication caused by leaflet trauma or valve apparatus entrapment during placement of a patch or a transcatheter device. It should be noted that if a ventriculotomy was performed, then damage to the myocardium or coronary artery can result in long-term complications such as ventricular dysfunction and aneurysm. Arrhythmias are also seen whether due to the ventriculotomy, or by a patch, or by device-caused damage to the atrioventricular node and conduction system. Ventricular tachycardia and heart block rhythms may necessitate a pacemaker or an implantable cardioverter defibrillator.

4. **Answer: D.** In TOF repair, the ventricular septal defect (VSD) is closed and the anteriorly deviated conus and hypertrophied muscle bundles are resected and a patch that spans the pulmonic annulus (transannular patch) is placed to enlarge the hypoplastic RV outflow tract. It is highly unlikely for a transannular patch to cause stenosis at any level. RV enlargement is the norm and is likely to be more than mild from severe long-standing pulmonic regurgitation. The pulmonic valve is severely compromised leading to significant regurgitation. A significantly incompetent pulmonic valve can no longer protect the PA and PA branches from the effects of RV diastolic expansion and annulus descent, which creates a suction of blood backward through the pulmonary arteries, causing diastolic flow reversal.

5. **Answer: A.** As previously described, a transannular patch that spans the pulmonic annulus is placed to enlarge the hypoplastic RVOT in patients with TOF. Although transatrial and transpulmonary approaches for TOF repair can be done, avoidance of a right ventriculotomy may not be possible. A right ventriculotomy damages myocardium and leaves a

scar that can cause thinning of the myocardium and surrounding area. This can be exacerbated if a coronary artery was inadvertently cut. Therefore, a right ventriculotomy, with or without an RVOT patch or transannular patch, can cause RVOT aneurysms. RVOT aneurysms are less common and can be seen in as many as 25% of patients who have TOF repair. RVOT aneurysms may lead to right ventricular (RV) dysfunction and, rarely, thrombus formation. RVOT aneurysms are more likely to occur in the presence of residual subpulmonic obstruction (which causes higher upstream RV pressures), residual VSD shunts (which cause higher RV volume load), and larger transannular patches (weaker and can bulge out under pressure).

Severe PR (answer B) is a common complication from TOF/transannular patch surgery and is expected. Pericardial patches are used for their low thrombogenicity and it is exceedingly rare to see thrombus on a patch and therefore answer C is not the best answer. Subpulmonic obstruction is due to a residual RVOT muscle bundle or a previously overlooked hypertrophied muscle bundle and not due to secondary endothelial growth on the patch (answer D) or transannular patch movement (answer E).

6. **Answer: D.** A Rastelli procedure involves closure of the VSD and the placement of an external conduit from the right ventricular outflow tract to the pulmonary artery. A clue to identifying this CW Doppler trace is the presence of presystolic flow below the zero-velocity baseline that occurs following atrial contraction (white arrow **Figure 29-29**). Answer A can be excluded, as a VSD with bidirectional shunting would demonstrate a lower systolic velocity. Answers B and C can be excluded, as there is no forward flow with atrial

contraction; that is, there is no A wave. Therefore, this trace is most consistent with pulmonic stenosis and regurgitation. The presystolic flow below the zero-velocity baseline represents a high right ventricular end-diastolic pressure (RVEDP) following atrial contraction. When the RVEDP exceeds the pulmonary artery end-diastolic pressure, there is presystolic forward flow across the pulmonary valve. Presystolic flow reversal can also be seen in the setting of first-degree or higher atrioventricular heart block; however, in this example (**Figure 29-1**), the PR interval is clearly less than 200 ms. There is also a bright signal at about 1 m/s that is in keeping with the right ventricular outflow tract waveform, making answer D the best answer.

7. ▶ **Answer: D.** This pattern is typical of severe PR. Note that the diastolic waveform above the baseline represents PR, while the trace below the baseline represents forward flow across the pulmonary valve during systole. The PR signal is steep (pressure half-time <100 ms) and falls all the way down to the baseline before the end of diastole, which means the diastolic pulmonary artery and right ventricular (RV) pressures equalize and do so early. This is in keeping with severe PR and not mild or moderate PR. **Video 29-14** shows color Doppler imaging from this study. Observe that on the color Doppler image, the PR signal does not look impressively severe; however, the holodiastolic flow reversal in the main pulmonary artery and branches can be clearly seen and should alert the sonographer to significant PR.

Answer A is incorrect since it is stated that the RVSP is 50 mm Hg, which is less than half of the systolic blood pressure. While a residual VSD may be bidirectional, this would occur when the RVSP reaches systemic pressures. Answer B is incorrect since the flow above the baseline occurs during diastole and therefore cannot represent forward flow through a stenotic pulmonic valve. Answer C is incorrect as there is no "dagger" shaped, late-systolic peak in this Doppler signal.

8. **Answer: E.** It is not uncommon to see tricuspid regurgitation (TR) originate from the septal/VSD patch intersection as seen in this case. A surgical stitch from the VSD patch may have captured a tricuspid valve chord or a small part of the septal leaflet. The peak TR velocity is 3.12 m/s, yielding a right ventricular to right atrial systolic pressure gradient of 39 mm Hg; therefore, the estimated RVSP is 39 mm Hg + right atrial pressure.

Answer A is incorrect because although residual VSD patch leaks can certainly occur in this area, the absence of systolic septal flattening rules out a

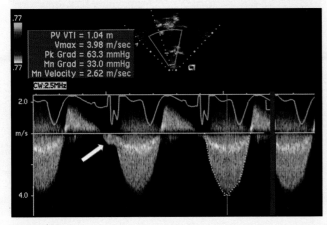

Figure 29-29

VSD with elevated RVSP. Care should be taken to obtain an accurate jet velocity as this can help differentiate TR from VSD when the RVSP is normal or mildly elevated. However, it may be impossible to differentiate a 4 to 5 m/s TR jet from a VSD jet of similar velocity when they occur in this location. A careful investigation from multiple views will be the best chance at differentiating the origin of this jet; TR originates from the RV, while a VSD originates from the LV. Answer B is incorrect since this jet clearly originates below the aortic valve and, therefore, is not a ruptured sinus of Valsalva. Also, the PSAX view shows the interventricular septum to be in a normal systolic position, i.e., no septal flattening, which suggests that RVSP is not 100 mm Hg. Answer C is incorrect as this is a systolic event and therefore cannot be aortic regurgitation. Answer D is incorrect as the jet clearly does not originate at the mitral valve and there is no color artifact present.

9. **Answer: C.** Based on the information provided, the RVSP is 30 mm Hg:

$$RVSP = 4V_{TR^2} + RAP$$
$$= 25 + 5 = 30 \, mm \, Hg$$

There is always a pressure drop downstream from a stenotic area. Therefore, the pulmonic pressure gradient must be less than 30 mm Hg. This underlies the importance of a good TR signal.

There is no way to say anything regarding the presence or absence of a VSD or ASD from this limited datum.

10. **Answer: A.** The arrows in **Figure 29-30** point to an RVOT aneurysm. As many as 25% of patients who have tetralogy of Fallot repair can have RVOT aneurysms. See the answer outline for question 5 for further information about this complication.

11. **Answer: B.** The most common truncus arteriosus types do not have a PDA. However, truncus with interrupted aortic arch (IAA) and truncus with a remotely located pulmonary artery (PA) branch do have a PDA (the PDA is connected to the remotely located PA branch). In these instances, the PDA will be closed at the time of repair and poses no real risk of postoperative complications in the adult; therefore, answer B is correct.

Patients with truncus arteriosus and a coarctation of the aorta or truncus arteriosus with an IAA may require further intervention for arch restenosis (answer A) or aortic aneurysm. Aneurysms typically occur after the stenotic area as shown in this patient with transverse aortic arch hypoplasia (**Figure 29-31**). RV-PA conduits can be placed with or without a valve and either type is prone to RV-PA conduit regurgitation and stenosis (answer C). Most truncal valves have three cusps but are dysplastic making truncal valve regurgitation and/ or stenosis (answer D) the most common complication. VSD patch leaks (answer E) are uncommon but do occur.

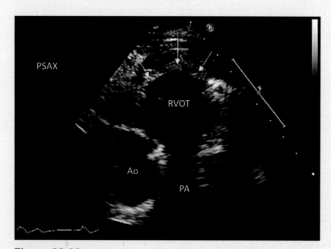

Figure 29-30

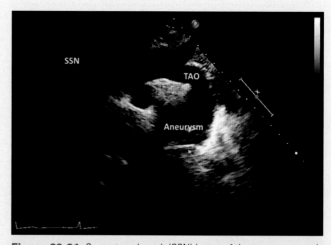

Figure 29-31 Suprasternal notch (SSN) image of the transverse aortic arch (TAO) with an aneurysm.

12. Answer: C. In d-TGA {S,D,D}, ventricular inversion is not present, therefore this is not a surgical consideration and Answer C is incorrect. In d-TGA, there is normal rightward ventricular looping (d-looping) and the ventricles are normally positioned. Ventricular inversion refers to the positioning of the ventricles whereby the anatomic RV has left-sided chirality and is on the left.

Answers A and B are true statements. In unrepaired d-TGA there is atrioventricular (AV) concordance (the right atrium connects to the RV and the left atrium connects to the LV) and ventriculoarterial (VA) discordance (the RV connects to the aorta and the LV connects to the PA). The two main operations for the repair of "simple" d-TGA include the atrial and arterial switch operations (**Figure 29-32**). The atrial switch procedures (Senning or Mustard procedures) use baffles to redirect the systemic and pulmonary venous blood flow. The pulmonary venous baffle directs oxygenated blood to the RV, which then ejects the blood into the aorta. The systemic venous baffle directs deoxygenated blood to the LV, from which the blood is pumped to the PA. A patient with d-TGA born before the late 1980s to early 1990s is more likely to have an atrial switch procedure. The arterial switch operation (ASO) has now replaced the atrial switch procedure. The ASO switches the aorta and PA such that there are concordant VA connections (LV to aorta and RV to PA). Note that while the arteries switch, the semilunar valves remain in their original positions; hence a thorough presurgery evaluation of size and morphology of the pulmonic valve is needed as it will become the systemic semilunar valve. Postsurgical regurgitation of this valve is not uncommon. A Lecompte maneuver is almost always performed as part of the ASO whereby the PA is brought anterior to the aorta and the PA branches straddle the ascending aorta. Answer D is a true statement. The Rastelli, REV (Réparation à l'Etage Ventriculaire), and Nikaido procedures may be performed in patients with d-TGA, a ventricular septal defect, and a left or right ventricular outflow tract obstruction. The most common of these is the Rastelli procedure, in which the VSD is used to baffle blood from the LV to the aorta, the PA is ligated, and an RV-PA conduit is placed. In cases where there is subvalvular outflow obstruction, a Konno procedure may also be done in conjunction with the ASO.

Answer E is a true statement. Coronary artery anatomy is varied and complex in d-TGA but must be elucidated since in the ASO the aorta and PA will be transected and repositioned as will be the coronary artery "button(s)."

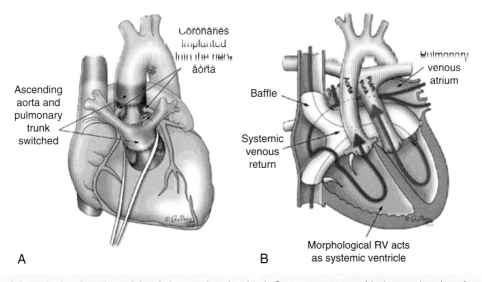

Figure 29-32 A, Schematic drawing of arterial switch operation showing LeCompte maneuver with the translocation of aortic and pulmonary arteries. B, Schematic drawing of an atrial switch (Mustard/Senning) for transposition of the great arteries. Systemic (blue) blood is directed from the superior caval vein and inferior caval vein into the left atrium, then via the mitral valve to the left ventricle and then to the pulmonary artery. Pulmonary (red blood) is directed from the pulmonary veins to the right atrium, then via the tricuspid valve to the right ventricle and then the aorta. (Images produced with permission from Gemma Price. From Zuluaga MA, Burgos N, Mendelson AF, Taylor AM, Ourselin S. Voxelwise atlas rating for computer assisted diagnosis: Application to congenital heart diseases of the great arteries. *Med Image Anal.* 2015;26(1):185-194. doi:10.1016/j.media.2015.09.001.)

TEACHING POINT

The Van Praagh classification provides a systematic method for describing congenital heart defects. This is based on a segmental notation using braces { } to describe a three-letter subset. The first member of the set represents visceroatrial situs, the second, ventricular looping, and the third, great artery situs. The visceroatrial notation can be S for situs solitus, I for inversus, or A for ambiguous. Ventricular loop notation can be D for D loop or L for L loop. The great artery notation can be S for solitus normal or I for inversus if the pulmonary artery arises above the right ventricle and aorta normally above the left ventricle, or D for the aortic valve to the right, L for aortic valve to the left, or A for the aortic valve directly anterior to the pulmonary valve. In cases where the information is insufficient to determine the particular segment, that notation may be represented by the letter X. In a normal heart, the segmental notation is {S,D,S}.

In d-TGA, the segmental notation is {S,D,D} where "S" = "solitus" meaning the organs are in their correct locations and therefore the inferior vena cava and abdominal aorta are right and left, respectively, of the spine; "D" = D-looped ventricles (which is the normal looping) and so the anatomic LV is on the left and the anatomic RV is on the right (**Figure 29-33**); "D" = "dextro" meaning the aortic valve is located anterior and rightward to the pulmonic valve. It is also possible to have other d-TGA variations such as {S,D,A} where the aortic valve is directly anterior (hence the "A"), and {S,D,L} where the aortic valve is anterior and leftward of the pulmonary valve. The position of the aorta has ramifications for the ASO surgery.

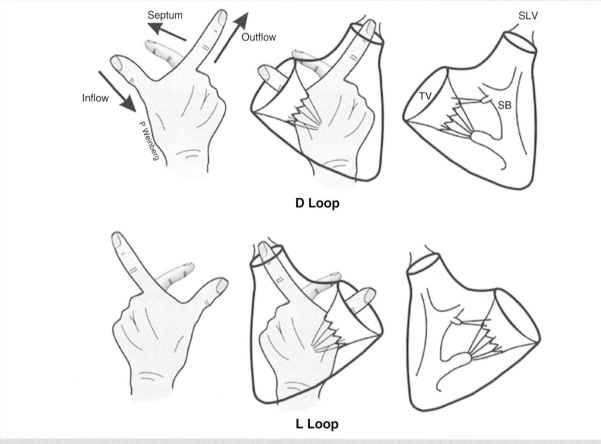

Figure 29-33 Ventricular loop and handedness. Ventricular loop or situs is determined by the internal organization of the ventricles. Right ventricular organization shown schematically at the right is compared with the right hand; thumb, index finger, and middle finger held mutually orthogonally and representing ventricular inflow, outflow, and septum, respectively. In D loop, placing the right hand on the RV side of the septum, the thumb would be in the inflow and the index finger would point to the outflow. In L loop, placing the left hand on the RV side of the septum, the thumb would be in the inflow and the index finger would point to the outflow. SB, septal band; SLV, semilunar valve; TV, tricuspid valve. (Reprinted with permission from Weinberg PM. Anatomy and classification of congenital heart disease. In: Kaiser L, Kron IL, Spray TL, eds. *Mastery of Cardiothoracic Surgery.* 3rd ed. Philadelphia, PA: Wolters Kluwer Health/Lippincott Williams & Wilkins; 2013:chap 71.)

13. **Answer: D.** An atrial switch procedure, such as the Senning or Mustard procedure, does not alter the great artery relationship, therefore 1 is the aorta and 2 is the PA. The left ventricle (LV) is still the posterior and leftward ventricle, therefore 3 is the SVB bringing deoxygenated blood to the LV and out the PA, and 4 is the PVB bringing oxygenated blood to the RV and out the aorta. Number 5 is the descending aorta with the coronary sinus barely seen and in its usual location.

14. **Answer: B.** Answers A and C are true statements. The Senning procedures uses the patient's own atrial septum to create the pulmonary and systemic baffles while the Mustard procedure uses a pericardial or Dacron patch to create the pulmonary and systemic baffles. Therefore, the circulatory pathway is correct in that the PVB directs oxygenated blood to the RV and out the aorta and the SVB directs deoxygenated blood to the LV and out the PA (Figure 29-34). However, the LV remains the subpulmonic systemic ventricle and therefore, answer B is the false statement.

Answer D is a true statement. The PVB (analogous to the left atrium [LA]) is usually higher pressure than the SVB (analogous to the right atrium [RA]). Therefore, with a baffle leak the shunt is from the PVB to the SVB (analogous to a LA-to-RA shunt in a normal heart). As the SVB directs blood to the LV, a significant PVB-to-SVB shunt will result in LV dilatation.

Answer E is a true statement since baffle stenosis more often occurs in the superior limb of the SVB and at the superior end of the PVB. The superior limb (or superior vena caval limb) of the SVB must make a turn to the left and run posterior to the pulmonary artery to baffle blood to the LV and can

kink/stenose. Likewise, the PVB makes a turn to the right and inferiorly to baffle blood to the RV and can kink/stenose.

TEACHING POINT

Baffle leaks from the SVB to the PVB may also occur when the SVB pressure is higher than the PVB pressure; examples include severe mitral regurgitation or a baffle leak on the upstream side of an SVB stenosis. A saline contrast injection ("bubble study") can be instrumental in baffle leak detection, especially if the leak is in the outlying, hard to image areas of the baffle.

15. **Answer: C.** In **Figure 29-7**, late-systolic flow reversal below the baseline is present. With an atrial switch operation for d-TGA, the PVB directs blood to the right ventricle (RV), which is the systemic ventricle. The atrioventricular valve connected to the RV is always the tricuspid valve. Therefore, significant TR that causes systolic flow reversal in the PVB much like severe MR causes pulmonary venous flow reversal in a normally arranged heart.

Answer A is incorrect since normal PVB flow is antegrade in systole and diastole and therefore, flow should appear above the zero-velocity baseline during systole and diastole (**Figure 29-35**). Answer B is incorrect as the mitral valve is connected to the left ventricle, which does not connect with the PVB and therefore, this systolic flow reversal cannot be due to MR. Answer D is incorrect. With a low junctional rhythm, the P waves are seen in or after the QRS which essentially means that atrial and ventricular contraction occur simultaneously. Atrial contraction against a closed tricuspid valve causes flow to reverse, however, this will be a brief phenomenon and does not last throughout systole as seen here.

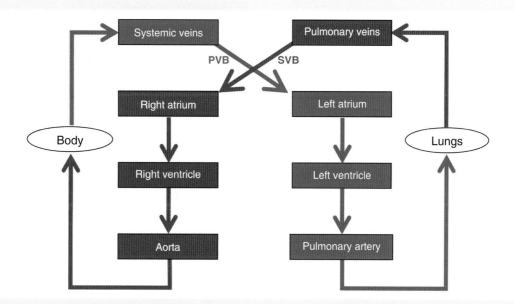

Figure 29-34

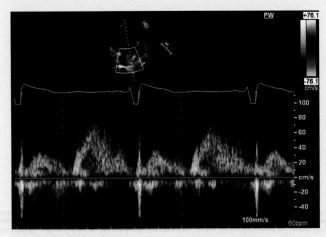

Figure 29-35 Normal PVB flow.

16. **Answer: A.** These images show MR. In d-TGA with an atrial switch, the systemic veins (inferior and super vena cava) return deoxygenated blood to the systemic venous baffle, then to the left ventricle (LV) and out the pulmonary artery (see **Figure 29-34**, answer outline for Question 14). Therefore, in the absence of left ventricular outflow tract obstruction or pulmonic stenosis, the MR velocity reflects PASP:

$$PASP = 4V_{MR}^2 + CVP$$

where CVP = central venous pressure.

Therefore, in this example, the PASP is 50 mm Hg + CVP.

The pulmonary veins return oxygenated blood to the pulmonary venous baffle, then to the right ventricle (RV) and out the aorta (see **Figure 29-34**, answer outline for Question 14). Therefore, in the absence of right ventricular outflow tract obstruction or aortic stenosis, the TR velocity reflects aortic systolic pressure (AoSP):

$$AoSP = 4V_{TR}^2 + PVP$$

where PVP is the pulmonary venous pressure.

KEY POINT

In d-TGA with an atrial switch, the LV remains the pulmonic ventricle (pumps blood to the lungs) and therefore it is the MR (not TR) that reflects PASP in the absence of left ventricular outflow tract or pulmonary stenosis. In order to avoid confusion, MR may be referred to as pulmonic atrioventricular valve regurgitation (pulmonic AVVR).

17. ▶ **Answer: A.** In this high parasternal short-axis (PSAX) view, the anterior great artery bifurcates, therefore must be the PA. Its branches are seen straddling the posteriorly located aorta (**Figure 29-36A**). This is the new location of the pulmonary arteries after the ASO with Lecompte maneuver. The peak pressure gradient across the right PA branch is 52 mm Hg. It is not uncommon to see mild or even moderate branch PA (BPA) stenosis as well as see BPA with stents. Care should be taken to interrogate the BPAs from every window. The peak gradient from the PSAX view was falsely low. When interrogated from the right parasternal bicaval view, a peak gradient of 78 mm Hg was recorded, consistent with severe right PA stenosis (**Figure 29-36B** and **Video 29-15**).

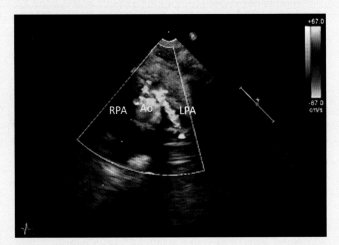

Figure 29-36A

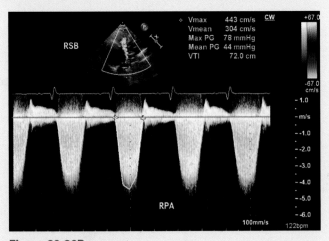

Figure 29-36B

The LeCompte maneuver is a surgical technique whereby the PA is brought anteriorly with the PA branches straddling the ascending aorta; it is almost always performed in an ASO. Branch PA obstruction is a well-recognized complication of this maneuver and is likely precipitated by the "stretched" and possibly kinked course of the PA branches. However, if the great arteries are side-by-side, the PA is brought rightward instead of anterior, and so the PA branches may not have to straddle the aorta. Likewise, in the rare cases where the aorta is leftward, the ASO may not necessitate that the PA branches straddle the aorta. There are exceptions, however, and the decision to straddle or not is made by assessing the best path for the PA branches that will cause the least stretching, kinking, and stenosis for the given anatomy. **Figure 29-37** illustrates the great artery relationships in d-TGA and their possible PA branch locations before (left) and after (right) an arterial switch operation (ASO).

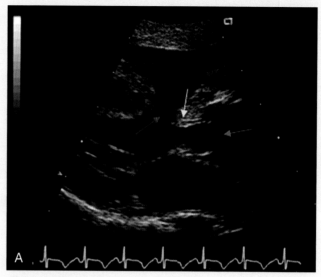

Figure 29-38A Yellow arrow = marked posterior deviation of the conal septum into the LV; red arrow = large VSD; blue arrow = dysmorphic and domed, stenotic pulmonic valve.

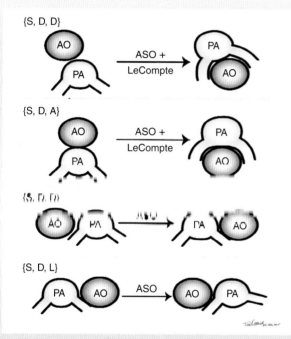

Figure 29-37 {S,D,D} = d-TGA with situs solitus, D-looped ventricles and aortic valve located anterior and rightward to the pulmonic valve. {S,D,A} = d-TGA with situs solitus, D-looped ventricles and ambiguous aortic valve. {S,D,L} = d-TGA with situs solitus, D-looped ventricles and aortic valve located anterior and leftward to the pulmonic valve (see Teaching Point in the answer outline for Question 12 regarding the { } segmental notation). Illustration by Teri Dittrich.

18. **Answer: C.** In addition to d-TGA, there is a large ventricular septal defect (VSD), marked posterior deviation of the conal septum into the left ventricular outflow tract, and a dysmorphic and domed, stenotic pulmonic valve (see **Figure 29-38A**). These findings make the Rastelli operation the likely choice.

The Rastelli operation is used when there is significant left ventricular/pulmonic outflow obstruction. This operation utilizes the existing large VSD and a single patch is employed to baffle oxygenated blood from the left ventricle to the aorta; the VSD is not closed and becomes part of the outflow and the left ventricle is the systemic ventricle. In addition, the Rastelli operation utilizes a right ventricle-to-pulmonary artery (RV-PA) conduit to establish pulmonary flow while the native PA is ligated/divided and the valve often over sown. **Figure 29-38B** illustrates the circulatory pathway following a Rastelli operation.

19. **Answer: B.** The left atrium shows no evidence of a baffle; therefore, this is not an atrial switch (answer A). No ventricular septal defect baffle to the anterior great artery is present; therefore, this is not a Rastelli procedure (answer C). There are notable echodensities seen in the posterior great artery (**Figure 29-39**, arrows) which are in keeping with the suture/scars from transected great arteries such as is done with an arterial switch; therefore, answer B is correct.

The neo-aortic root in **Figure 29-11A** and **B** is dilated. To clarify the term "neo-aortic root" it should be known that although the great arteries are switched at the time of an arterial switch operation (ASO), the semilunar valves are not switched; therefore, the posterior semilunar valve remains the native pulmonic valve and the anterior semilunar valve remains the native aortic valve. To avoid confusion, the native pulmonic valve and the switched aorta are referred to as "neo-aortic valve" and "neo-aortic root," respectively, while the native aortic valve and switched pulmonary artery are referred to as the "neo-pulmonary valve" and "neo-pulmonary artery."

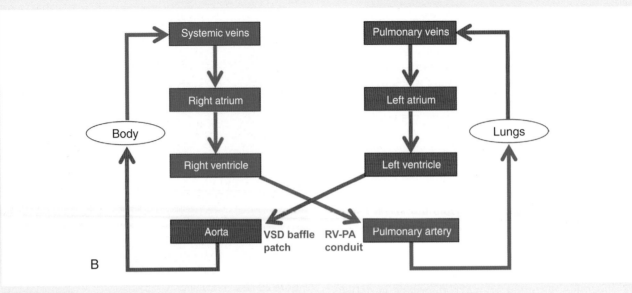

Figure 29-38B

20. **Answer: C.** There are notable bright and irregular echoes seen from the crest of the ventricular septum to the anterior part of the aorta; these are consistent with a ventricular septal defect (VSD) baffle patch. **Figure 29-12A** and **Video 29-4A** show the subaortic conus separating the mitral and aortic valves (see * in **Figure 29-40**), whereas with an arterial switch operation (ASO) the mitral and pulmonic (neo-aortic) valves are in fibrous continuity (see **Figure 29-11A**); therefore, answer B is excluded. **Figure 29-12B** and **Video 29-4B** show the right ventricle-to-pulmonary artery (RV-PA) conduit with turbulent flow during systole. Therefore, these images are consistent with a Rastelli repair with conduit stenosis. As the turbulent flow originates above the aortic valve level, this flow cannot be a residual VSD, so Answer D is excluded. Answer A (an atrial switch with systemic venous baffle obstruction) is excluded as no atrial baffles are seen.

21. **Answer: D.** There is no mitral-aortic fibrous continuity in cc-TGA.

In cc-TGA, also known as levo-TGA or l-TGA, there is atrioventricular (AV) and ventriculoarterial (VA) discordance. The great arteries are transposed and are parallel to each other; therefore, the aorta arises from the right ventricle (RV) and the pulmonary artery arises from the left ventricle (LV). The aortic valve is usually located anterior and leftward

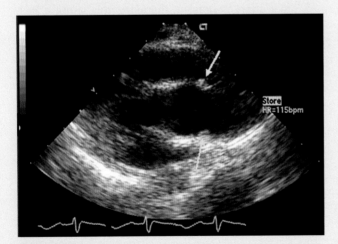

Figure 29-39

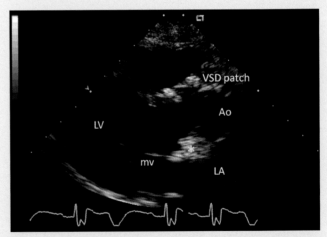

Figure 29-40 Rastelli repair showing a ventricular septal defect (VSD) baffle patch. Ao = aorta; LA = left atrium; LV = left ventricle; mv = mitral valve; * = subaortic conus.

of the pulmonic valve; however, other locations are also possible. There is ventricular inversion (L-looped ventricles) and the LV is on the right while the RV is on the left such that if you placed the palm of your left hand on the RV side of the septum, your thumb would be in the inflow and your finger in the outflow (see **Figure 29-33** in the answer outline for Question 12).

cc-TGA and d-TGA are similar in that the great arteries run parallel and are transposed with the aorta arising from the right ventricle and the pulmonary artery arising from the left ventricle. This VA discordance associated with both anomalies also means that the normal mitral-aortic fibrous continuity is lost. Unlike d-TGA, where there is normal ventricular looping (D-looping), in cc-TGA ventricular looping is inverted (L-looped ventricles) so that the LV is on the right while the RV is on the left. Also, unlike d-TGA, patients with cc-TGA are not cyanotic. In d-TGA, AV concordance and VA discordance results in parallel pulmonary and systemic circulations (**Figure 29-41**, left). In cc-TGA, despite AV discordance and VA discordance, the pulmonary circulation is connected in series with the systemic circulation (**Figure 29-41**, right).

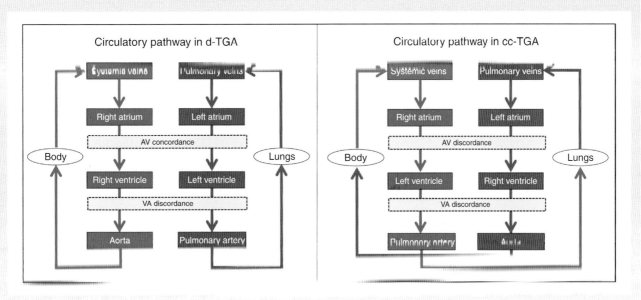

Figure 29-41

22. Answer: B. The Fontan operation is a palliative surgical procedure performed in patients with a functional or anatomic single ventricle. This operation effectively diverts systemic venous return to the lungs without a ventricular pump. This operation is usually performed in three stages (**Figure 29-42**). Stage 1 is performed in the newborn and usually involves a modified Blalock-Taussig shunt between the subclavian artery and the pulmonary artery that increases pulmonary blood flow. Stage 2 is a superior cavopulmonary anastomosis or Glenn shunt (a surgical anastomosis between the superior vena cava and the pulmonary circulation) which is typically performed between 4 and 6 months of life. Stage 3 is the completion of the Fontan circulation whereby the inferior vena cava is connected to the pulmonary arteries; this is usually performed between 2 and 4 years of life. The Fontan circulation can be completed by way of: (1) a classic atriopulmonary (AP) connection where the right atrial appendage is connected to the pulmonary artery; (2) an intra-atrial baffle (also known as a lateral tunnel [LT]), which is an amalgam of right atrial (RA) wall, atrial septum, and a synthetic (e.g., Gore-Tex) patch fashioned into a tube; (3) an extracardiac (EC) synthetic conduit that sits entirely outside of the right atrium; or (4) a Bjork-modified (RA-right ventricle) Fontan. The Bjork-Fontan procedure was used in patients with tricuspid atresia, a ventricular septal defect, and normally related great vessels who are deemed to have adequate right ventricular size and function and an adequate pulmonary artery to support pulmonary circulation.

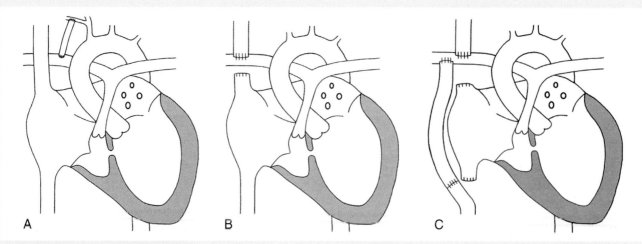

Figure 29-42 The three different stages of Fontan palliation in tricuspid atresia. A, First stage: artificial shunt placed between right subclavian artery and right pulmonary artery. B, Second stage: anastomosis between right pulmonary artery and superior vena cava. C, Third stage: completion of the Fontan circulation (extracardiac conduit allowing total cavopulmonary connection shown). (From Nayak S, Booker PD. The Fontan circulation. *Contin Educ Anesthes Crit Care Pain.* 2008;8(1):26-30. Copyright © 2008 The Board of Management and Trustees of the British Journal of Anaesthesia. Reproduced by permission of Oxford University Press.)

TEACHING POINT

Numerous modifications to the Fontan operation have been made over the years and include the AP Fontan, LT Fontan, EC Fontan, and Bjork-modified Fontan. Importantly, the completed Fontan circulation can be done in many ways depending on the anatomy and surgeon's preference. Examples include (1) right superior vena cava (RSVC) to right pulmonary artery (RPA) anastomosis and an inferior vena cava (IVC) to RPA connection, (2) a left superior vena cava (LSVC) to left pulmonary artery (LPA) anastomosis and IVC to RPA connection, (3) an RSVC to RPA anastomosis and an RA to RPA connection, and (4) LSVC to LPA anastomosis and RA to RPA connection.

In the modern era, the Fontan operation (inferior cavopulmonary anastomosis) involves using either an extracardiac conduit or an intra-atrial tunnel that directs blood flow from the IVC to the RPA. A superior cavopulmonary anastomosis connecting the SVC to the RPA (Glenn or Hemi-Fontan) is typically done prior to the completion of the inferior cavopulmonary anastomosis, although, less commonly, may be done at the same time. The superior cavopulmonary anastomosis may be end-to-end or end-to-side and is typically bidirectional allowing for flow to either the RPA or LPA. The Glenn operation is an end-to-side anastomosis of the SVC to the branch pulmonary artery (PA). In this operation, the cardiac end of the SVC is divided and sutured closed. The Hemi-Fontan operation uses an anterior homograft patch to augment the RA/SVC and branch PA junction. The branch PA is extensively augmented with this homograft patch as well. As opposed to the Glenn, the Hemi-Fontan leaves the SVC intact with the RA but closes the orifice to the RA with a posterior homograft patch ("dam"). The "dam" can easily be excised when the lateral tunnel Fontan baffle connection is completed at a later date.

23. **Answer: B.** A fenestrated Fontan operation is where a small defect between the Fontan and the right atrium (RA) is created. This functions as a "pop-off valve" allowing right-to-left shunting between the Fontan and the RA that can relieve elevated Fontan pressures, increase ventricular preload to the systemic ventricle, and increase cardiac output. In later years, fenestrations may be closed to reduce cyanosis associated with the right-to-left shunting.

TEACHING POINT

In the Fontan circuit, flow is as follows: Fontan → pulmonary artery (PA) → lungs → pulmonary veins → atria. Therefore, in the absence of PA stenosis, the pressure in the Fontan pathway is equal to the PA pressure. The difference between the PA and pulmonary venous pressures is called the transpulmonary pressure gradient (TPG). When there is a Fontan fenestration, the fenestration flow is directed into the functional left atrium (LA) and in the absence of pulmonary venous stenosis, the LA pressure is equal to the pulmonary venous pressure. As the Fontan pressure is equal to the PA pressure, the pressure drop across the fenestration is the same as the pressure difference between the PA and pulmonary veins. Thus, the mean fenestration gradient equals the TPG.

24. ▶ **Answer: E.** In Fontan patients, maintaining a low pulmonary vascular resistance (PVR) is key to providing adequate Fontan-circuit flow through the lungs and for providing the best possible ventricular preload to the systemic ventricle and, therefore a good cardiac output. Stenosis

anywhere along the line from the Fontan circuit to the ventricle increases the PVR and is very detrimental to cardiac output. The arrows show a narrow LPA. **Video 29-16** shows the presence of a stent at this location and the presence of spontaneous echo contrast, which indicates slow flow. As the LPA was perpendicular to the imaging plane, an accurate Doppler signal could not be obtained. Therefore, accurate 2D measurement of the LPA was key to finding this stenosis. Upstream flow, such as in the SVC, also provided additional clues to the presence of downstream stenosis. Normal Fontan flow is respiratory phasic with greater flow seen during inspiration. This is due to a drop in thoracic pressure and increase in venous return. Also, normal Fontan Doppler flow tends to drop to the baseline or even transiently reverse. A downstream obstruction can cause even higher systemic venous pressures that are no longer susceptible to thoracic pressure changes. The pulsed-wave Doppler waveform obtained from his SVC (**Figure 29-43**) showed loss of respiratory changes. The patient was in a junctional rhythm and a tiny reversal wave is noted (arrow in **Figure 29-43**).

25. **Answer: B.** Any impediment to flow from the Fontan through the lungs and into the systemic ventricle can increase PVR. This includes Fontan baffle obstruction and cavopulmonary anastomosis site narrowing (answer A), narrow pulmonary arteries (answer C), and pulmonary vein stenosis (answer D). Severe systemic AV valve regurgitation (answer E) will also increase pulmonary venous pressure and therefore PVR. In this patient with underlying HRHS, the pulmonary venous flow returning to the left atrium (LA) does not need to cross the atrial septum and a narrow interatrial communication would not cause increased pulmonary venous pressure or PVR. Therefore, answer B is correct. In this case, only flow from the coronary sinus needs to return through the atrial communication. However, in hypoplastic left heart syndrome with a Fontan circuit, the pulmonary venous flow returning to the LA must then pass through an atrial septectomy (or atrial septal defect) on its way to the right atrium and right ventricle. In this case, narrowing through the interatrial communication can cause pulmonary venous hypertension and increased PVR.

26. **Answer: C.** In this apical 4-chamber view there is no tricuspid valve or right ventricle (RV) seen, which is consistent with tricuspid atresia and a severely hypoplastic RV. The structure seen is a Fontan baffle that lies within the heart (note its location relative to the pericardium) making this a lateral tunnel Fontan baffle. The lateral Fontan is partly composed of the right atrial sinus venarum (the smooth-walled section of the right atrium located posteriorly). After prolonged exposure to elevated systemic venous pressure, the Fontan baffle can become quite dilated, which commonly precipitates atrial arrhythmias. It is important to visualize the Fontan baffle from the inferior vena cava all the way to the pulmonary artery. In this case, a counterclockwise rotation and rightward tilt of the transducer was able to open up the length of the Fontan baffle (**Figure 29-44**) from the inferior margin toward the superior margin; this view would aid in the visualization of complications such as baffle narrowing, thrombus, or leaks.

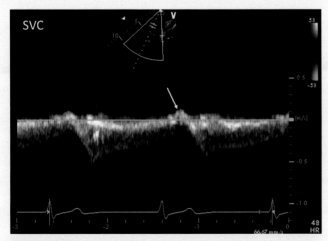

Figure 29-43

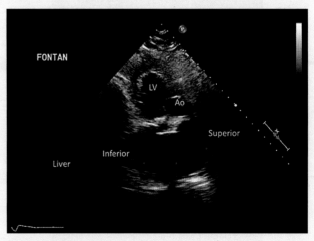

Figure 29-44

TEACHING POINT

It should be noted that the Fontan baffle may not always be on the patient's right. The left image in **Figure 29-45** shows an unbalanced atrioventricular canal defect (AVCD) with the Fontan baffle on the patient's right (yellow arrow), whereas the image on the left shows an unbalanced AVCD with the Fontan on the patient's left (red arrow).

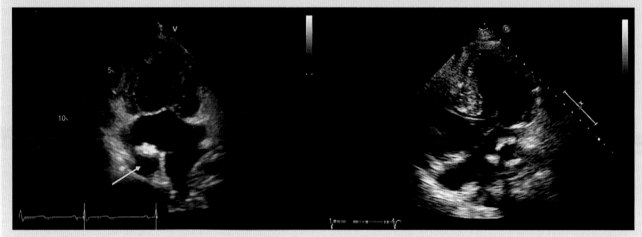

Figure 29-45

27. **Answer: A.** The structure outlined with arrows in **Figure 29-46** is the Fontan baffle and the color Doppler jet shows flow from the baffle into the atria. Anywhere from 1 to 3 fenestrations are made at the time of surgery and typically range in size from 3 to 5 mm. This 5-mm communication is within the range of a fenestration or a baffle leak. The purpose of a fenestration is twofold. One, it decreases systemic venous pressure and two, increases ventricular preload to the systemic ventricle and therefore increases cardiac output. It does these two things at the expense of arterial desaturation. Pulse oximetry showed the arterial oxygen saturation to be in the low 80% range.

28. **Answer: A.** From this RSB image, the aortic root and valve are well seen. There is aortic root dilatation with severe aortic regurgitation (AR). It is important to utilize all available windows, including this right parasternal window, for a comprehensive evaluation. This window provided the best image quality as well as a parallel line for spectral Doppler interrogation and was best for quantitative assessment of the AR (see **Figure 29-47A** and **B**). The RSB images are typically best when acquired with the patient lying in a right lateral decubitus position.

Figure 29-46

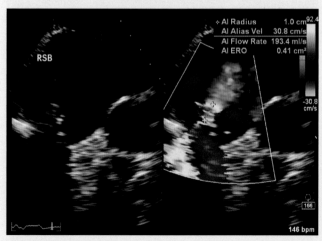

Figure 29-47A

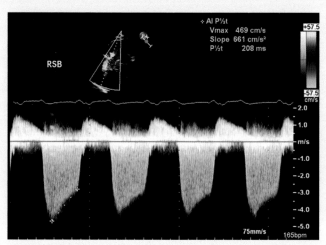

Figure 29-47B

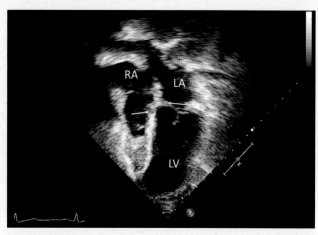

Figure 29-48 Arrows identify offset insertion of the atrioventricular (AV) valves.

29. **Answer: C. Video 29-6** shows the 27 mm pulmonary valve replacement (PVR). A leftward tilt of the transducer from the standard PLAX view will image the pulmonic valve and at times will allow for clearer imaging of the pulmonic valve than the parasternal short-axis view since the transducer can sit in between the ribs rather than across them; however, both views should be used. **Figure 29-17A** shows the pulsed-wave Doppler sample volume below the PVR in the RVOT, while **Figure 29-17B** shows the continuous-wave (CW) Doppler trace obtained through the PVR. Even though the CW Doppler velocity is just below 1.6 m/s and would be considered normal for this PVR, the RVOT velocity is only 40 cm/s which is in keeping with severe right ventricular (RV) dysfunction and/or tricuspid regurgitation and should alert the sonographer to a potential "low-flow, low-gradient" scenario. An over fourfold increase in the velocity-time integral (VTI) is seen across the PVR (VTI$_{PVR}$) compared with the VTI across the RVOT (VTI$_{RVOT}$), yielding a dimensionless index (DI) of 0.22, which is suggestive of PVR stenosis:

$$DI = VTI_{RVOT} \div VTI_{PVR}$$
$$= 8 \div 36 = 0.22$$

30. **Answer: E.** The images provided show a hypoplastic right heart, which is the norm for pulmonary atresia with an intact ventricular septum (PA/IVS). The right ventricle (RV) can be described as a triangle with inlet, apical, and outlet sections representing the three sides. This apical section is completely undeveloped. Coronary sinusoids (right ventricle [RV] to coronary communications) are also commonly seen in PA/IVS but are not shown here. The most common form of PA/IVS is valvular atresia with a well-developed pulmonary artery.

There is an offset insertion of the atrioventricular (AV) valves (arrows in **Figure 29-48**), which rules out an AV canal defect (answer A). The left ventricle (LV) is on the left, and RV on the right with the more apically inserted AV valve revealing the tricuspid valve and therefore the RV. Ventricular inversion is not present and therefore this is not cc-LTGA (answer B). Ebstein anomaly (answer C) cannot be the diagnosis due to insufficient apical displacement of the septal tricuspid valve (TV) leaflet as well as absence of an elongated and tethered anterior TV leaflet. Also, there is an absence of the right atrial (RA) enlargement that is seen with Ebstein anomaly. The left heart is well-developed; therefore this cannot be a hypoplastic left heart syndrome (answer D).

31. **Answer: D.** A one-and-a-half ventricle repair consists of a superior cavopulmonary anastomosis (Glenn procedure) while leaving the RV in the pulmonary circulation. It is used when the RV is hypoplastic and unable to handle pulmonary circulation needs by itself but is considered able to contribute in some significant capacity and therefore is left in the pulmonary circulation pathway. The Glenn connection offloads the small RV and aids with pulmonary circulation. The Fontan circulation is not completed in this case and blood from the inferior vena cava continues to return to the right atrium, RV, and out the pulmonary artery. Although a modified BT shunt (answer B) was done in infancy as a palliation, it was not the end-repair. Answer C is incorrect as the RV cannot be surgically reconstructed.

32. ▶ **Answer: B.** Two ventricles are clearly seen and in their normal locations so this cannot be a single ventricle (answer A), nor can it be cc-TGA (answers D or E). There is no ventricular septal defect or baffle patch to the aorta present so this cannot be a Rastelli procedure (answer C). d-TGA with atrial switch can develop baffle stenosis and the superior limb of the SVB is a common site. Observe on the real-time image acquired from the parasternal long-axis view, the SVB with a stent is

seen posterior to the great arteries. The superior vena cava (SVC) and inferior vena cava (IVC) limbs of the SVB join in the atria and advance as one to the pulmonic ventricle giving the SVB the appearance of a "Y" when viewed from the suprasternal short-axis view (**Figure 29-49A** and **Video 29-17**). The superior limb can be difficult to image, and all windows should be used to interrogate this area. The Doppler waveform taken from the SVC limb stent

showed normal venous flow (**Figure 29-49B**). The PVB has the appearance of a "C" when viewed from the apical 4-chamber view (**Figure 29-49C**).

33. ▶ **Answer: C.** Patients with an atrial switch for dextro-transposition of the great arteries do not have their great arteries switched; therefore the anterior artery is the aorta (Ao) and the posterior great artery is the PA. The PA is seen to be "pinched" (yellow arrows in **Figure 29-50A**). A PA band (PAB) has been surgically implanted around the main PA and tightened to intentionally create stenosis. This was done to "train" the pulmonic left ventricle (LV) to adapt to higher pressures, maintaining adequate LV size, mass, and function so it could be converted into a systemic ventricle if the systemic right ventricle (RV) were to fail in the future. These bands can be quite restrictive as the idea is to subject the LV to near systemic pressures as seen in the spectral Doppler trace showing a 71 mm Hg gradient across the PAB (**Figure 29-50B**).

34. **Answer: D.** The RV is connected to the aorta; therefore in the absence of outflow stenosis between the RV and the blood pressure cuff (i.e., no obstruction to the right ventricular outflow tract, aortic valve,

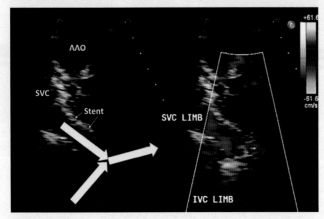

Figure 29-49A

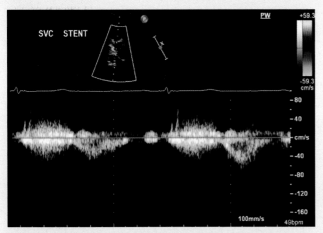

Figure 29-49B

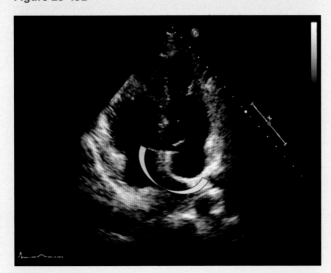

Figure 29-49C

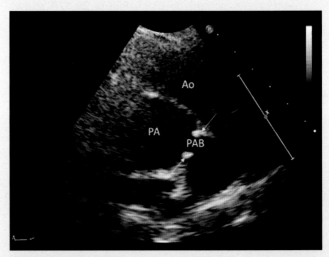

Figure 29-50A

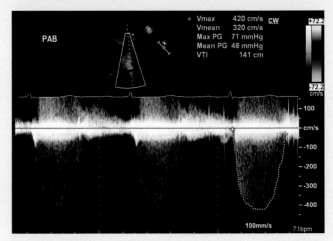

Figure 29-50B

descending aorta, or left subclavian artery), the RVSP is assumed to be the same as the cuff systolic BP (SBP) of 110 mm Hg. The VSD shunt is from the RV to LV; therefore:

$$4V_{VSD}^2 = RVSP - LVSP$$

According to the continuous-wave Doppler signal, the VSD velocity is 2.24 m/s, yielding a 20 mm Hg pressure drop from the RV to the LV using $4V^2$. Therefore, the LVSP is 90 mm Hg:

$$LVSP = SBP - 4V_{VSD}^2$$
$$= 110 - 20 = 90 \, mm \, Hg$$

35. **Answer: A.** Even if assuming negligible pulmonic valvular stenosis, there is still substantial subvalvular left ventricular outflow obstruction (LVOTO) caused by the bowing of the ventricular septal defect (VSD) patch and subpulmonic conus (yellow and red arrows, respectively **Figure 29-51**). The previously estimated left ventricular systolic pressure (LVSP) was 90 mm Hg (see answer outline for Question 34). Since there is a peak velocity of 3.77 m/s across the LVOTO (**Figure 29-20E**), the PASP is estimated as:

$$PASP = LVSP - 4V_{LVOTO}^2$$
$$= 90 - 4(3.77)^2$$
$$= 90 - 57$$
$$= 33 \, mm \, Hg$$

KEY POINT

Although the pulmonic ventricle has near-systemic pressures of 90 mm Hg, the LVOTO "protects" the lungs from this high pressure.

36. ▶ **Answer: E.** The PVB is widely patent, which gives the appearance of a large secundum ASD seen in **Video 29-10A**; however this is a normal finding in the atrial switch. A flattened IVS, as seen in **Video 29-10C**, is expected since the RV is functioning as the systemic ventricle and is not an indication of pulmonary hypertension; if the IVS was *not* flattened, pulmonary hypertension would be suspected. The RV, as seen in **Video 29-10B**, appears mildly enlarged and the systolic function appears to be borderline low with RVFAC of 35%. The TAPSE and RV s′ were low as is expected postpericardiotomy.

TEACHING POINTS

The systemic RV is known to develop dysfunction and cause heart failure at earlier ages. However, the echocardiographic assessment of RV function is difficult with no clear best parameter that has emerged. Therefore, for the assessment of RV systolic function, multiple parameters are best and may serve as the patient's own internal standard for serial echocardiographic comparisons. This includes parameters such as the RVFAC, TAPSE, tricuspid annular s′ velocity, dP/dt, and the RV myocardial performance index. Global longitudinal RV free wall strain, 3D RV ejection fraction, and the isovolumic acceleration can also be performed.

37. **Answer: B.** This is the inferior end of the superior vena caval limb of the systematic venous baffle (SVB) which was located posterior to and rightward of the pulmonary artery. Tilting the transducer rightward and rotating opens up the SVB as shown in **Figure 29-52**; clear communication of this structure to the systemic venous atria is now seen. This demonstrates the importance of careful transducer movement to better delineate structures.

38. ▶ **Answer: C.** The parasternal long-axis view in **Video 29-11** was obtained by moving the transducer up an intercostal space to generate a better

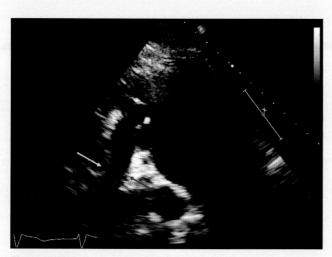

Figure 29-51

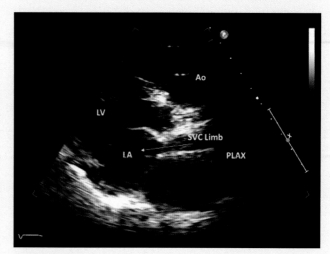

Figure 29-52

Doppler angle of the superior vena caval (SVC) limb. The Doppler signal shows a mean pressure gradient of 4 mm Hg, which is elevated for SVC flow; however, the signal nearly drops back down to the baseline, suggesting only mild stenosis. The concern with SVC limb stenosis would be for upper systemic venous congestion (SVC syndrome), although the patient had none of the symptoms. A second concern would be for further narrowing of this area if a transcutaneous pacemaker lead were implanted. A stent would be placed in the SVC limb prior to pacemaker lead implant.

39. **Answer: A.** Images show a small (5.2 mm) baffle leak with predominant left (PVB)-to-right (SVB) shunt as evidenced by spectral Doppler flow above the zero-velocity baseline. An agitated saline bubble study without the Valsalva maneuver revealed >25 bubbles crossing right to left (yellow arrows in **Figure 29-53**) and this may be an indication for device closure of this baffle leak.

40. **Answer: C.** The bracket outlines a stent placed in the Fontan conduit. The Fontan conduit is extracardiac and small. Shortly after his cardiac arrest, the patient was found to have organized thrombus in the Fontan conduit with conduit stenosis and a mean pressure of 20 mm Hg at cardiac catheterization. Therefore, a stent was placed in the Fontan conduit. Now, normal Fontan flow appears restored with low-velocity respiratory phasic flow seen in **Figure 29-24C**.

41. **Answer: D.** There is no evidence for stenosis of any degree. The color Doppler image (**Figure 29-25B**) shows blue laminar flow in the LSVC stent. The spectral Doppler traces (**Figure 29-25C**) show good

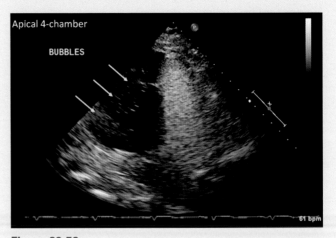

Figure 29-53

respiratory phasic flow proximally and at the distal end of the stent.

42. **Answer: A.** The Fontan fenestration mean pressure gradient represents the pressure gradient between the Fontan "chamber" and the atrial "chamber." Therefore, if the Fontan mean pressure is 10 mm Hg and dropped 7 mm Hg across the fenestration, then the atrial mean pressure must be 3 mm Hg. The Fontan fenestration mean pressure gradient is equal to the transpulmonary pressure gradient (see Teaching Point in the answer outline for Question 23). Fontan circulations that are functioning well are associated with mean fenestration (transpulmonary) gradients of 5 to 8 mm Hg. An elevated mean fenestration (transpulmonary) gradient may reflect an elevated pulmonary vascular resistance (PVR). A low PVR is a key determinant of positive outcomes in patients with Fontan circulations.

SUGGESTED READINGS

Backer CL, Mavroudis C. The Rastelli operation. *Oper Tech Thorac Cardiovasc Surg.* 2003;8(3):121-130.

DiLorenzo MP, Bhatt SM, Mercer-Rosa L. How best to assess right ventricular function by echocardiography. *Cardiol Young.* 2015;25(8):1473-1481.

Eidem BW, O'Leary PW, Cetta F, eds. *Echocardiography in Pediatric and Adult Congenital Heart Disease.* 2nd ed. Philadelphia, PA: Wolters Kluwer/Lippincott Williams & Wilkins; 2015.

Gewillig M, Brown SC. The Fontan circulation after 45 years: update in physiology. *Heart.* 2016;102(14):1081-1086.

Iriart X, Roubertie F, Jalal Z, Thambo JB. Quantification of systemic right ventricle by echocardiography. *Arch Cardiovasc Dis.* 2016;109(2):120-127.

Khairy P, Clair M, Fernandes SM, et al. Cardiovascular outcomes after the arterial switch operation for D-transposition of the great arteries. *Circulation.* 2013;127(3):331-339.

Konstantinov IE, Alexi-Meskishvili VV, Williams WG, Freedom RM, Van Praagh R. Atrial switch operation: past, present, and future. *Ann Thorac Surg.* 2004;77(6):2250-2258.

Lai WW, Mertens LL, Cohen MS, Geva T, eds. *Echocardiography in Pediatric and Congenital Heart Disease from Fetus to Adult.* 2nd ed. West Sussex, UK: Wiley Blackwell; 2015.

Nayak S, Booker PD. The Fontan circulation. *Contin Educ Anesthes Crit Care Pain.* 2008;8(1):26-30.

Rios R, Ginde S, Saudek D, Loomba RS, Stelter J, Frommelt P. Quantitative echocardiographic measures in the assessment of single ventricle function post-Fontan: incorporation into routine clinical practice. *Echocardiography.* 2017;34(1):108-115.

Seybold-Epting W, Chiariello L, Hallman GL, Cooley DA. Aneurysm of pericardial right ventricular outflow tract patches. *Ann Thorac Surg.* 1977;24(3):237-240.

CHAPTER 30

Three-Dimensional Echocardiography

Contributors: Natalie F. A. Edwards, M Cardiac Ultrasound, B Ex Sci, ACS, Keith A. Collins, MS, RDCS, and Megan Yamat, RDCS, RCS, ACS

✪✪ Question 1

Which statement is correct about modern three-dimensional (3D) ultrasound transducers?

A. The fully sampled matrix array typically contains about 128 elements.

B. The fully sampled phased array typically contains about 3000 piezoelectric elements.

C. The fully sampled matrix array typically contains about 3000 piezoelectric elements.

D. The fully sampled phased array typically contains about 128 piezoelectric elements.

✪ Question 2

To achieve a higher volume rate (volumes per second), the operator should make the following adjustment on the ultrasound system:

A. Choose a single-beat/live acquisition.

B. Increase magnification.

C. Choose a multibeat acquisition.

D. All of the above.

✪✪ Question 3

Obtaining useful and high-quality 3D echocardiography (3DE) images to answer the clinical question is a balance between spatial and temporal resolution. The relationship between temporal resolution (volume rate), and spatial resolution can be described by which of the following statements?

A. Decreasing the volume size reduces temporal resolution.

B. Improvements in spatial resolution can be achieved by decreasing the scan-line density.

C. Temporal resolution can be increased by increasing the volume depth and width of the image sector.

D. There is an inverse relationship between temporal and spatial resolution.

✪ Question 4

Following acquisition of a 3D data set, the ultrasound software allows visualization of images using three main categories. Match the following images (**Figure 30-1**; panels 1 to 3) to the different types of postacquisition display.

A. (1) Multibeat acquisition; (2) volume analysis; (3) 2D tomographic slices

B. (1) Surface rendering; (2) volume rendering; (3) 2D tomographic slices

C. (1) Volume rendering; (2) volume analysis; (3) 2D tomographic slices

D. (1) Volume rendering; (2) surface rendering; (3) 2D tomographic slices

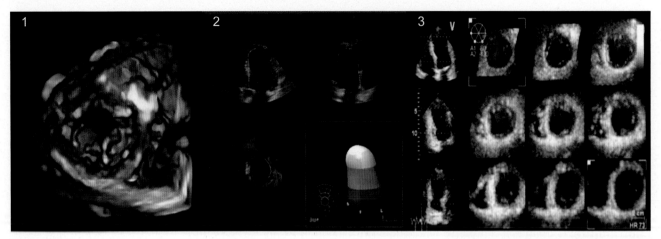

Figure 30-1

✪✪ Question 5

▶ With reference to **Figure 30-2** and **Video 30-1**, which 3D echocardiographic imaging modality was used to acquire the image of the mitral valve?

   A. Multibeat acquisition

   B. Real-time narrow sector acquisition

   C. Real-time zoom acquisition

   D. Single-beat acquisition

   A. The frame rate (volume rate) is too low.

   B. The image is not obtained en face.

   C. The image is undergained causing tissue dropout.

   D. There is a stitch artifact present.

   E. Nothing. The image is fine for analysis.

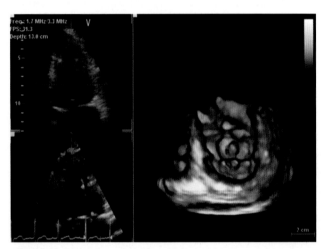

Figure 30-2

✪✪ Question 6

▶ A 68-year-old female patient with a history of syncope and dizziness was referred for a transthoracic echocardiogram with an agitated-saline study. The echo showed a moderately enlarged right ventricle with preserved function. A markedly positive saline study revealed a large atrial septal defect. A transesophageal echocardiogram was ordered to evaluate the defect for closure. A zoomed 3D volume was obtained to size the defect (**Figures 30-3**, **Video 30-2**). What is the major problem with the image?

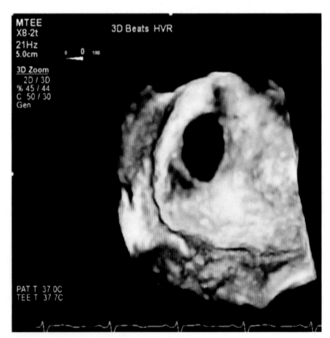

Figure 30-3

✪✪ Question 7

▶ A patient with chronic aortic regurgitation is being serially evaluated. Left ventricular (LV) volumes are monitored for dilatation. The 3D full volume of the left ventricle was acquired for analysis (**Video 30-3**). What is the problem with the volume acquisition and how could it be corrected in another acquisition?

A. There is a motion artifact that may be corrected with a breath hold with a multibeat acquisition.

B. There is a near-field artifact that might be eliminated by reducing the near-field gains and changing the apical position.

C. There is a stitch artifact that may be avoided by reducing the number of beats in the acquisition and with a breath hold.

D. There is chord artifact that may be avoided by tilting the probe or by changing the apical position to avoid the chordal structure.

E. There is interference from a calcified mass in the apex causing ring-down artifact in all angles and the image is unlikely to be improved from another acquisition.

✪✪ Question 8

A 79-year-old female patient with a history of moderate coronary artery disease is brought in by ambulance to the emergency department with chest pain and shortness of breath following the recent death of her spouse. A transthoracic echocardiogram (TTE) revealed normal left ventricular (LV) size with mildly impaired systolic function. The ejection fraction (EF) was calculated to be 51%. From the 3D LV volume analysis (**Figure 30-4**), which of the following statements is the most correct and how has 3D echocardiography (3DE) aided in this diagnosis?

A. There is a left anterior descending infarct or stress-induced cardiomyopathy (takotsubo cardiomyopathy); 3DE has enabled a more accurate assessment of LV function.

B. There is a left anterior descending infarct; 3DE has not added any significant benefit over conventional 2D imaging.

C. There is a left anterior descending infarct; 3DE has enabled a more accurate assessment of LV function.

D. There is a stress-induced cardiomyopathy (takotsubo cardiomyopathy); 3DE has enabled a more accurate assessment of LV function.

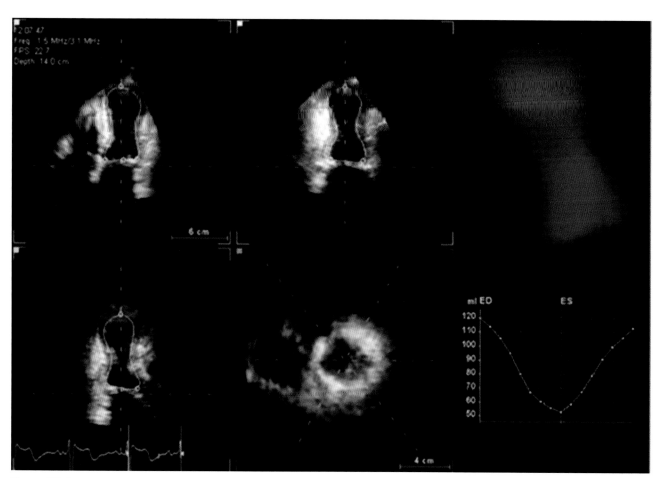

Figure 30-4

✪ Question 9

Which statement pertaining to assessment of the right ventricle by 3D echocardiography (3DE) is most correct?

- **A.** Quantitation of right ventricular (RV) function by 3DE is an online program using the method of disks.
- **B.** Quantification of RV volumes is accurate and reproducible using the method of disks.
- **C.** Quantification of RV volumes is a widespread application since it is accurate and reproducible.
- **D.** Quantification of RV volumes involves geometric modeling and mathematical equations easily performed off-line.
- **E.** Quantification of RV volumes is similar to LV assessment using a bullet-shaped geometric model.

✪ Question 10

Which modality is most accurate and reliable for measuring or calculating the mitral valve area (MVA) after balloon mitral valvuloplasty for mitral stenosis?

- **A.** 2D planimetry
- **B.** 3D planimetry
- **C.** Continuity equation
- **D.** Flow convergence method
- **E.** Pressure half-time method

✪ Question 11

A 41-year-old female patient from Xian, China, had a history of rheumatic fever as a child with balloon valvuloplasty performed on the mitral valve in her early 20s. The patient now complains of shortness of breath upon exertion. Transthoracic and transesophageal echocardiograms were performed. From the corresponding continuous-wave Doppler trace (**Figure 30-5A**) and 3D image (**Figure 30-5B**), what is the most likely diagnosis for this patient?

- **A.** Flail P2 prolapse with severe eccentric mitral regurgitation
- **B.** Normal mitral valve opening consistent with successful balloon valvuloplasty
- **C.** Restricted mitral valve opening due to restenosis
- **D.** Severe mitral stenosis with severely reduced cardiac output

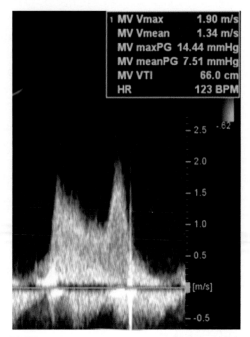

1 MV Vmax	1.90 m/s
MV Vmean	1.34 m/s
MV maxPG	14.44 mmHg
MV meanPG	7.51 mmHg
MV VTI	66.0 cm
HR	123 BPM

Figure 30-5A

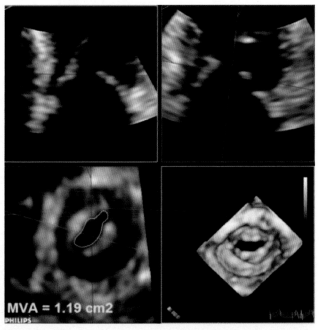

MVA = 1.19 cm2

Figure 30-5B

✪✪ Question 12

From the patient presented in question 11, mitral valve area obtained by 2D planimetry of the mitral valve orifice was significantly smaller than that derived from 3D echocardiography (**Figure 30-5B**). What is the likely reasoning for the mismatch in these measurements?

A. Cropping of a 3D volume of the mitral valve allows an en-face measurement of the effective orifice area
B. 2D measures are more limited by artifact caused by the calcified mitral valve leaflets
C. 2D images cannot account for the saddle shape of the mitral valve, but 3D volumes can
D. A and B
E. A and C

✪✪ Question 13

A 51-year-old man is referred to a cardiologist for a systolic murmur, new onset of atrial fibrillation, and dyspnea on exertion. A transthoracic echocardiogram showed low normal left ventricular systolic function, mild central mitral regurgitation, and calcified mitral chordae. Due to poor image quality, a transesophageal echocardiogram (TEE) was performed with the following 3D volume data set obtained (**Figure 30-6**, **Video 30-4**). The patient appears to have:

A. Bileaflet, multisegmental prolapse with billowing.
B. Mild A2, A3, P2, P3 prolapse.
C. Posterior leaflet prolapse and redundant chordae.
D. Posterior leaflet prolapse with flail P3.
E. Severe P2 and P3 prolapse with mild A3 prolapse.

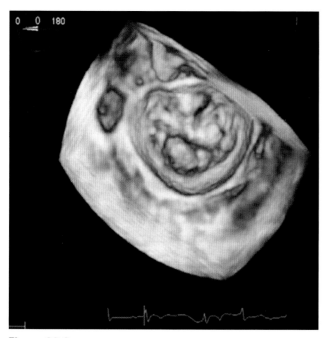

Figure 30-6

✪✪ Question 14

A 73-year-old male patient was referred for an echocardiogram by his primary care physician for a loud systolic murmur. The transthoracic echocardiogram revealed a normal EF of 62% with severe mitral regurgitation (MR), based on the calculated effective regurgitant orifice area of 0.4 cm². A transesophageal echocardiogram was performed to ascertain the mechanism of the regurgitation. The corresponding 3D volume depicted from the left atrial perspective (**Figure 30-7**, **Video 30-5**) was obtained. What is the mechanism of the MR?

A. Flail P2
B. Flail P3
C. Prolapse and flail P3
D. Prolapse P2 and P3
E. More images are necessary to diagnose the etiology

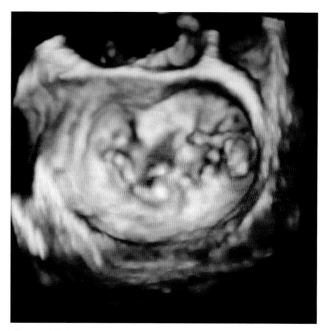

Figure 30-7

✪✪✪ Question 15

A 61-year-old male patient was admitted to the hospital following an inferior myocardial infarction. During cardiac angiography, the patient received three stents, in the right, left anterior descending, and left circumflex coronary arteries. The patient experienced cardiogenic shock toward the end of the procedure and was placed on intra-aortic balloon pump therapy. Subsequently, a loud systolic murmur was heard on auscultation. The transthoracic echocardiogram showed normal left ventricular size and low normal systolic function with extensive regional wall motion abnormalities. The right ventricle (RV) was mildly dilated with severely impaired systolic function. From the 3D color Doppler transesophageal echocardiographic (TEE) image shown in **Video 30-6**, what is the likely cause of the systolic murmur?

A. Severe mitral regurgitation secondary to tethering of the leaflets following myocardial infarction

B. Ventricular rupture post myocardial infarction

C. Ruptured anterolateral papillary muscles resulting in severe mitral regurgitation

D. Serpentine, postinfarct ventricular septal defect (VSD) with predominantly left to right shunting

✪✪✪ Question 16

3D color Doppler imaging was performed to grade mitral regurgitation severity in a patient where two of the four pulmonary veins showed systolic flow reversal and the other two showed systolic blunting. What approach should be used to display the 3D color Doppler data?

A. Only one view should be used to determine the regurgitant jet severity.

B. At least two different views should be used to understand the orientation of the jet.

C. Cropping of a 3D color Doppler data set should be performed only at the vena contracta.

D. The vena contracta should be measured with the color baseline shifted in the direction of flow.

E. All of the above.

✪✪ Question 17

3D transthoracic echocardiographic zoom acquisition of the aortic valve is displayed from the aortic perspective in **Figure 30-8** and **Video 30-7**. Which of the following labelings of the aortic valve leaflets is correct?

A. 1 = right coronary cusp; 2 = left coronary cusp; 3 = noncoronary cusp

B. 1 = left coronary cusp; 2 = noncoronary cusp; 3 = right coronary cusp

C. 1 = left coronary cusp; 2 = right coronary cusp; 3 = noncoronary cusp

D. 1 = noncoronary cusp; 2 = right coronary cusp; 3 = left coronary cusp

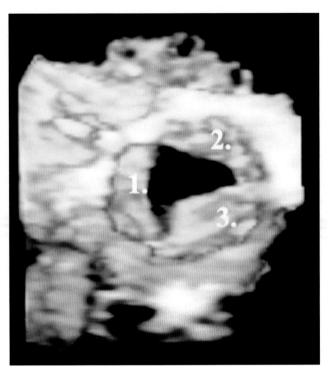

Figure 30-8

✪✪✪ Question 18

A 44-year-old man presents to the emergency department in respiratory distress and is febrile. His prior medical history includes poor medical compliance for hypertension and congestive heart failure (CHF), resulting in septic emboli and a *cerebrovascular accident* (CVA). His prior EF was 26%. He initially refuses treatment but consents to a transthoracic echocardiogram (TTE), not a transesophageal echocardiogram. A comprehensive TTE was performed with 3D echocardiography (**Figure 30-9**, **Videos 30-8A** and **30-8B**). What interpretations may be made of the aortic valve pathology?

A. There are multiple mobile vegetations with at least moderate eccentric regurgitation.

B. There are either flail portions of the noncoronary or left coronary cusp, or vegetations with mild-to-moderate aortic regurgitation.

C. There is a large mass attached to the right coronary cusp, which may be flail or likely a calcified vegetation. Perforation is likely and severe aortic regurgitation is present.

D. Calcified Lambl excrescences and hypertension are likely causes of moderate aortic regurgitation.

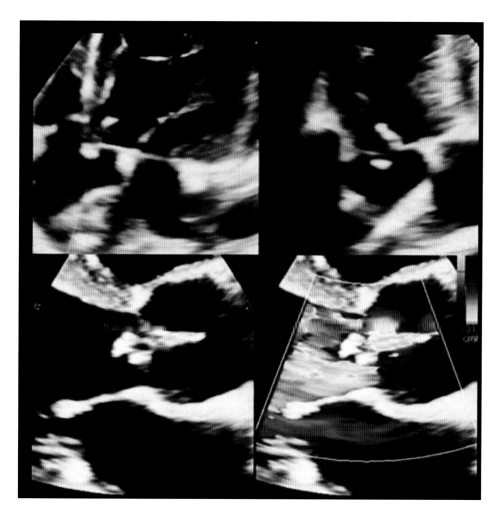

Figure 30-9

⭐ Question 19

▶ 3D zoom acquisition of the tricuspid valve is displayed from the right ventricular (RV) perspective in **Figure 30-10** and **Video 30-9**. Which of the following labelings of the tricuspid valve leaflets is correct?

A. 1 = posterior leaflet; 2 = anterior leaflet; 3 = septal leaflet

B. 1 = anterior leaflet; 2 = posterior leaflet; 3 = septal leaflet

C. 1 = septal leaflet; 2 = anterior leaflet; 3 = posterior leaflet

D. 1 = posterior leaflet; 2 = septal leaflet; 3 = anterior leaflet

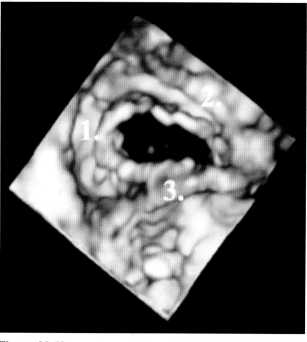

Figure 30-10

✪✪ Question 20

A 34-year-old man has a family history of sudden cardiac death, globally reduced left ventricular function, and an implantable cardioverter defibrillator (ICD). Recently, he complained of recurrent fevers but had negative blood cultures. On transthoracic echocardiography, the pulmonary artery pressure was 28 mm Hg. Based on the 3D volumes provided (**Video 30-10A** showing the right ventricular view of the tricuspid valve and **Video 30-10B** showing the views from the right ventricle [left] and right atrium [right]), which statement is correct?

A. There are multiple vegetations on the pacing lead.

B. There is perforation of the septal tricuspid valve leaflet and the pacing lead is without vegetations.

C. There is a coaptation defect of the tricuspid valve due to an abnormal pacing lead position.

D. There is normal pacing lead placement and the pacing lead is without vegetations.

E. There is septal leaflet impingement by the pacing lead without vegetations.

✪✪✪ Question 21

This is a 62-year-old female patient with a history of multiple myocardial infarctions and an ischemic cardiomyopathy requiring orthotopic cardiac transplantation. Subsequently she underwent serial endomyocardial biopsies (EMBs) and now has developed a left parasternal cardiac murmur, which augmented with inspiration. Based on the images provided (**Figure 30-11A** and **30-11B**), what is the likely cause for the murmur?

A. A flail tricuspid valve leaflet

B. A Gerbode defect

C. A ventricular septal defect

D. Tricuspid valve leaflet prolapse

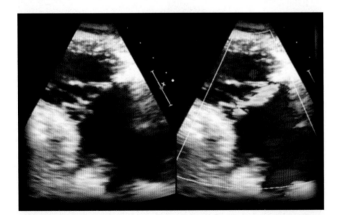

Figure 30-11A

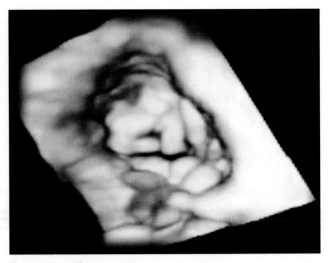

Figure 30-11B

✪✪✪ Question 22

A 69-year-old male patient with a history of a 31 mm ATS mitral valve replacement (MVR) and a 25 mm ATS aortic valve replacement (AVR) is referred for a transesophageal echocardiogram due to bacteremia. From the corresponding images of the MVR (**Figure 30-12** and **Video 30-11A**) and AVR (**Video 30-11B**), which of the following statements best describes the findings?

A. There is a dehisced MVR with a large mobile echodensity attached to the anterior aspect of the MVR and a number of smaller echodensities around the valve rim, and a mobile echodensity attached to the anterior aspect of the AVR.

B. There is a large echodensity attached to the posterior aspect of the MVR rim with numerous smaller echodensities around the valve rim, and a mobile echodensity attached to the anterior aspect of AVR on the aortic root side.

C. There is a large echodensity attached to the posterior aspect of the MVR rim with numerous smaller echodensities around the valve rim, and fixed AVR occluders with a large echodensity attached to the disk.

D. There is restriction of the MVR occluders with a large echodensity attached to the posterior aspect of the MVR rim; numerous smaller echodensities around the valve rim, and a mobile echodensity attached to anterior aspect of the AVR on the aortic root side.

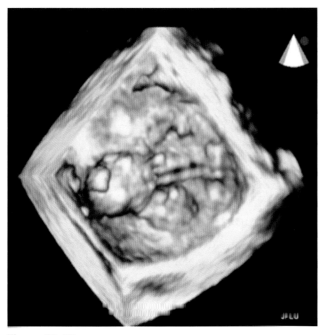

Figure 30-12

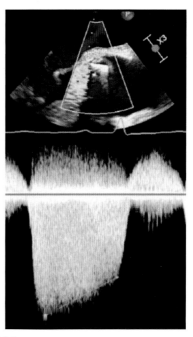

Figure 30-13A

✪✪ Question 23

▶ A 69-year-old man with a prior history of coronary artery disease and status post aortic valve replacement (AVR) for aortic stenosis presents with extreme dyspnea on exertion and reduced functional capacity. Immediate postoperative echocardiographic assessments showed a normally functioning AVR with minimal gradient. Two months postoperative, a new diastolic murmur is heard. He prefers to avoid repeat valve surgery. A 3D transesophageal echocardiogram is performed in the cardiac catheterization laboratory. What interpretation of the 3D and 2D echo data may be made from the provided images (**Figure 30-13A** and **30-13B** and **Video 30-12**)?

A. There is an associated ventricular septal defect (VSD).

B. There is embolization and dehiscence of the bioprosthetic AVR.

C. There is mild-to-moderate paravalvular aortic regurgitation following a percutaneous transcatheter AVR (valve-in-valve AVR).

D. There is moderate-to-severe paravalvular aortic regurgitation, resulting from an abscess surrounding the bioprosthetic AVR.

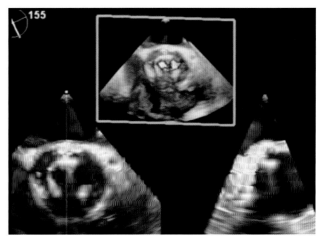

Figure 30-13B

✪✪ Question 24

A 48-year-old female patient with a history of trisomy 21 (Down syndrome) was referred for a follow-up transthoracic echocardiogram. The study showed normal left ventricular size and systolic function, a small primum atrial septal defect, an aneurysmal ventricular septal defect with a trivial left to right shunt, and moderate mitral and tricuspid regurgitation. The patient has not had a prior surgical procedure. From the corresponding image (**Figure 30-14**), what is the most likely cause of mitral regurgitation (MR)?

A. Cleft anterior mitral leaflet

B. Mitral annular dilatation

C. Posterior mitral leaflet prolapse

D. Anterior mitral leaflet prolapse

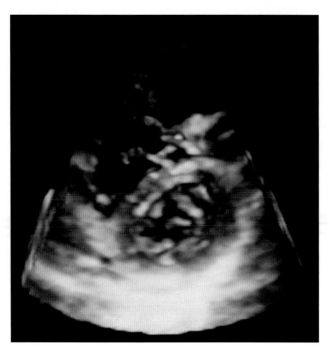

Figure 30-14

✪✪ Question 25

▶ A 61-year-old female patient with a history of hypertension and paroxysmal atrial fibrillation has undergone a procedure. A 3D transthoracic echocardiogram was performed post intervention. Based on the 3D echocardiographic images provided (**Videos 30-13A** and **30-13B**) from a zoom acquisition displayed from the right atrial (RA) perspective, what was the procedure and what is the postprocedural complication?

A. The patient underwent a surgical stitch closure for an atrial septal defect and there is no postprocedural complication.

B. The patient underwent a surgical patch closure for an atrial septal defect and there is a residual left-to-right shunt noted.

C. The patient had an Amplatzer device placed to close an atrial septal defect and there is a residual left-to-right shunt noted.

D. The patient has had a Watchman device closure of the left atrial appendage and there is slight dislodgement of this device.

✪ Question 26

▶ A 71-year-old female patient with a history of ischemic cardiomyopathy presented for a transthoracic echocardiogram. The left ventricle was severely dilated (end-diastolic volume = 94 mL/m²) with severe regional systolic dysfunction and an ejection fraction of 19%. There was mild mitral annular dilatation with mild thickening of the mitral leaflets

resulting in severe (grade 4/4) mitral regurgitation (MR) arising from the P2/P3 junction. The following day the patient underwent an interventional procedure. From the corresponding 3D transesophageal echocardiographic (TEE) videos (**Videos 30-14A** to **30-14C**), what procedure has been performed?

A. Amplatzer atrial septal defect device occlusion

B. MitraClip

C. Reduced left atrial pressure device

D. Transcatheter aortic valve replacement

✪✪✪ Question 27

▶ A 75-year-old male patient with a history of transluminal alcohol septal ablation (TASH) for septal hypertrophy undergoes a transthoracic echocardiogram that shows normal left ventricular (LV) size and systolic function with moderately increased LV wall thickness (16 mm). There is mild chordal systolic anterior motion and no dynamic outflow tract obstruction. There is diffuse thickening of the aortic valve with a resultant valve area of 0.9 cm² using the right ventricular outflow tract stroke volume. From the corresponding 3D transesophageal echocardiographic (TEE) images (**Videos 30-15A** and **30-15B**), what is the likely procedure and the resultant outcome of this procedure?

A. MitraClip with mild residual mitral regurgitation

B. Amplatzer atrial septal defect (ASD) device occlusion with mild residual shunting detected on color Doppler

C. Repeat TASH with mild residual gradients

D. Transcatheter aortic valve replacement (TAVR) with moderate paravalvular aortic regurgitation (AR)

✪✪ Question 28

A patient with chronic atrial fibrillation is referred for left atrial appendage (LAA) closure with a Watchman device. 3D transesophageal echocardiography (TEE) is requested to guide the procedure. Why is 3D echo useful in Watchman LAA closure assessment?

A. In difficult 2D imaging, 3D volumes may provide and/or confirm the necessary preprocedural measurements at difficult angles.

B. Color Doppler imaging may clarify the severity and extent of flow around the device.

C. A measured vena contracta around the Watchman device of less than 5 mm indicates acceptable positioning of the device.

D. A and B only.

E. All of the above.

ANSWERS

1. **Answer: C.** 3D transducers are fully sampled matrix array transducers that are typically composed of about 3000 individually connected piezoelectric elements with operating frequencies ranging from 2 to 4 MHz for transthoracic 3D transducers and 5 to 7 MHz for transesophageal transducers. The piezoelectric elements are arranged in a matrix configuration (rectangular grid) with phasic firing generating a scan line that propagates radially or axially (y-axis) and can be steered in the lateral or azimuthal (x-axis) and elevational (z-axis) planes to acquire the 3D pyramidal volume of data (**Figure 30-15A**).

   Conventional two-dimensional (2D) transducers are phased array transducers and are composed of 128 piezoelectric elements. Each are electrically isolated and arranged in a single row with each ultrasound pulse generated by firing individual elements in a specific sequence with a delay phase with respect to the transmit initiation time. 2D transducers use only the x and y dimensions (**Figure 30-15B**); thus, the information displayed is "triangular" and "flat" rather than pyramidal and 3D.

2. **Answer: C.** Compared to single-beat, three-dimensional (3D) acquisition, multibeat enables the capture of specific intracardiac structures or the entire heart at a much higher temporal resolution or volume rate while still maintaining a high spatial resolution. Single-beat, live 3D is where the ultrasound system scans in real time; that is, if the transducer is removed from the patient's chest, the image disappears. Single-beat, live 3D images are acquired from multiple pyramidal data sets per second in a single heart beat (**Figure 30-16A**). The limitation of this technique is poor temporal and spatial resolution; thus, answer A is incorrect. A multibeat acquisition uses the electrocardiogram to acquire multiple beats of narrow data and then stitches the subvolumes together to create a single, full-volume data set (**Figure 30-16B**). Thus, pyramidal volume size is maintained and temporal resolution (volume rate) is improved. The major limitation of a multibeat acquisition is the stitch artifact. If the position of the structure of interest changes from beat-to-beat during the acquisition due to either translation of the heart, respiration, transducer movement, or arrhythmias, the cross section of the sector will not match when stitched together, causing a stitch artifact.

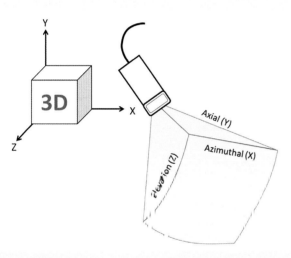

Figure 30-15A

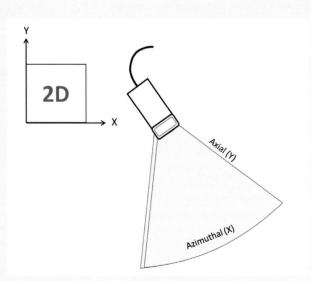

Figure 30-15B

Single-beat acquisition

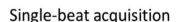
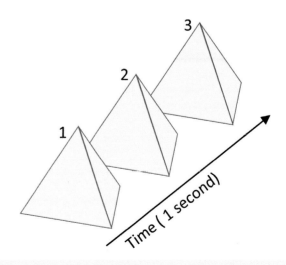

Figure 30-16A

Multibeat acquisition

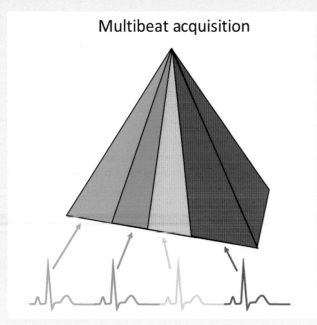

Figure 30-16B

Increased magnification (answer B) does not change spatial or temporal resolution. However, decreasing the imaging depth, decreasing sector width (elevation and lateral), and using a zoom mode of imaging will also increase the volume rate.

3. **Answer: D.** There is an inverse relationship between temporal and spatial resolution. The laws of physics still apply to 3DE. 3DE images are limited by (1) spatial resolution; (2) temporal resolution (volume rate); and (3) the sector or volume size. Increasing any two of the above will sacrifice the third. Increasing the temporal resolution (by transmitting fewer scan lines that are wider apart) will cause the spatial resolution to be compromised. Increasing the spatial resolution (by increasing the density of scan lines) will cause the temporal resolution to decrease. Increasing the volume size (by sending scan lines that are farther apart) will cause the spatial resolution to be compromised. Therefore, temporal and spatial resolution can be adjusted to the specific needs of the type of scan by either changing the volume width or depth. Small volumes of data with high temporal resolution are required for displaying intracardiac structures such as valves. Larger volumes with slightly lower temporal resolution are satisfactory for left ventricular volume analysis.

Answer A is not correct as decreasing the volume size increases temporal resolution. Answer B is not correct since spatial resolution can be achieved by increasing, not decreasing, the scan-line density. Answer C is not correct as temporal resolution is decreased, not increased, when the volume depth and width of the image sector are increased.

4. **Answer: D. Figure 30-1** (panel 1) shows volume-rendered 3D data sets. Volume rendering is used to enable visualization of cardiac structures from any desired view and in relation to surrounding intracardiac structures by electronically segmenting and sectioning by cropping, slicing, and rotating the image. When using the volume rendering modality, color maps are applied to convey depth perception of the 3D image on a 2D monitor to the user. Commonly, lighter shades are used for structures closer to the observer and darker shades are placed in the background for deeper structures.

Figure 30-1 (panel 2) shows surface rendering. Surface rendering displays the 3D surface of cardiac structures, such as the left ventricular (LV) or right ventricular (RV) volume. This provides the "beutel" of the left ventricle, which can be appreciated contracting and relaxing throughout the cardiac cycle for assessment of size and function. This is achieved by using semiautomated or more recently, fully automated border detection algorithms by the ultrasound software to trace and track the endocardium from a series of 2D cross-sectional images generated by the 3D full-volume acquisition. Wireframe rendering is an alternative to the surface rendering technique and is achieved by the ultrasound software by identifying equidistant points on the surface of the 3D volume and connecting these using lines to create a mesh-like appearance.

Figure 30-1 (panel 3) shows 2D tomographic slices. From the 3D full-volume data set, multiple simultaneous 2D views can be visualized in a cine loop format. **Figure 30-1C** shows nine transverse slices of the left ventricle from the mitral valve to the apex. The position of the lowest and highest transverse planes as well as the thickness of the slices can be adjusted by the operator. Using this modality, the limitations of 2D imaging can be overcome as acquisition of unique cut planes can be obtained in virtually any acoustic window.

5. **Answer: A.** There is a stitch artifact present within this image, which is consistent with multibeat acquisition. As previously described, multibeat 3D acquisition provides higher temporal resolution compared to single-beat acquisition methods. The ultrasound system achieves this by acquiring multiple acquisitions of narrow volumes of data over two to six cardiac cycles, which are then stitched together to create a single volumetric data set. This is advantageous since larger pyramidal volumes of data can be acquired while maintaining the temporal resolution (volume rate). If there is interference such as transducer movement, cardiac translation during respiration or cardiac motion, or an irregular cardiac rhythm during the acquisition, a "stitch" artifact will occur. A stitch artifact results from misalignment of adjacent subvolumes of data.

Answer B is not correct as real-time narrow sector acquisition produces a display of a 300 × 600 pyramidal volume. The size of the sector is insufficient to visualize the entirety of a single structure in any one imaging place. Answer C is not correct as real-time zoom acquisition is an imaging modality within single-beat acquisition and is therefore not limited by the stitching artifact. Real-time zoom permits a focused, wide sector of cardiac structures. Answer D is not correct as the stitch artifact present is not a phenomenon associated with single-beat acquisition. Single-beat acquisition acquires multiple pyramidal data sets per second in a single heartbeat. It overcomes the limitations associated with irregular rhythms and movement caused by the transducer or respiration, however, is limited by lower temporal and spatial resolution.

6. **Answer: C.** The image was obtained in a 3D zoom high volume rate (HVR) mode, with a narrow sector to obtain acceptable frame (volume) rates for a relatively nonmobile structure. In HVR mode, the volume is reconstructed in real time, so stitch artifacts are negligible. The defect may be visualized by cropping and reorienting the 3D volume data set. However, reduced gains give the appearance of multiple fenestrations, rather than a discrete singular defect. Dropout in the atrial wall as well as the interatrial septum suggests undergaining. Dropout artifacts appear as false holes in the rendered 3D volume surfaces where no real holes are present (**Figure 30-17**). The cause of dropout artifacts is when a structure such as the interatrial septum, aortic valve cusps, or tricuspid valve leaflets are too thin to reflect enough echo signal intensity and appear as a loss In the 3D surface. Too little gain also causes a dropout artifact.

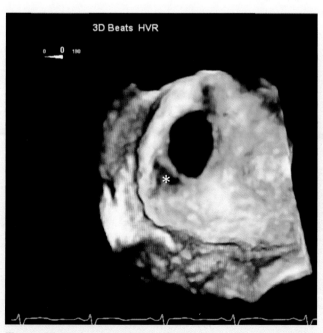

Figure 30-17 A dropout artifact of the atrial wall (*) has occurred due to undergaining of the 3D image.

7. **Answer: B.** Near-field artifact and chord artifact appear similar in many acquisitions. Chord brightness may generate a ring-down effect into the atria. This may compromise the endocardial border definition in diastole and in particular, systole, when the cavity is smaller. However, this is not the main problem with this image; therefore, answer D is not correct.

Answer A is not correct. There is no evidence of motion artifact within the left ventricle. Answer C is not correct. There is no evidence of stitch artifact within the left ventricle during the six-beat acquisition with a breath hold. Answer E is incorrect. While difficult to interpret LV mass or thrombus, a large calcified mass is unlikely in this position, adjacent to the anteroseptum and anterior wall, but not in the apex. Dropout of the ultrasound signal, or striping, adjacent to the brightness in the apical 2-chamber view suggests a rib artifact. However, the apex appears free of this mass in the biplane apical 2-chamber view.

Correction of the artifact by reducing near-field gains and changing the apical position leads to better border detection and reliable analysis, as seen in the accompanying video (**Video 30-16**).

8. **Answer: A.** There is either a left anterior descending infarct or stress-induced cardiomyopathy (takotsubo cardiomyopathy) and 3DE has enabled a more accurate assessment of LV function. Since the patient has a history of preexisting coronary artery disease as well as a significant emotional stressful event, a cardiac angiogram needs to be performed to determine the likely cause of regional wall motion abnormalities. In this case, the angiogram showed that although there was extensive diffuse coronary artery disease, there was no significant obstruction or flow impairment. The left ventriculogram revealed findings that were consistent with takotsubo cardiomyopathy (**Figure 30-18**). Takotsubo cardiomyopathy (stress-induced cardiomyopathy) is a nonischemic cardiomyopathy where there is a sudden and temporary weakening of the heart muscle, particularly within the apical region, triggered by emotional stressors.

3DE is beneficial in this case as it requires no geometric assumptions, even in patients with regional wall motion abnormalities. Measurement of LV volume by 3DE has been shown to be superior to 2D echocardiography when compared to cardiac magnetic resonance imaging as a gold standard. 3D LV volumes show less intra- and interobserver variability and eliminate foreshortening errors.

9. **Answer: B.** The right ventricle has been described as a crescent-shaped ventricle not easily conforming to any geometric shape. Therefore, its quantitative assessment is very difficult. RV imaging has previously required a reconstructive 3D method using

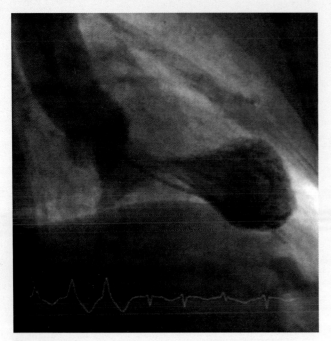

Figure 30-18

either rotation or a freehand approach, but currently real-time 3DE is the method of choice. Most efforts in quantitation of the right ventricle have utilized the method of disks. This method results in accurate and reproducible assessment. Off-line assessment using a rotation approach and automated border detection has also been proven to be accurate but does not have widespread use.

10. **Answer: B.** Following percutaneous balloon mitral valvuloplasty (PBMV), 3D echocardiographic measurements of the MVA are more accurate and reliable compared with the pressure half-time method (answer E) and 2D planimetry (answer A). The pressure half-time (P½t) is not only inversely related to the MVA but is also directly proportional to other factors such as the peak transmitral gradient and chamber compliance. In particular, acute changes in left atrial compliance immediately following PBMV alters the relationship between the P½t and the MVA, reducing accuracy of the pressure half-time method.

The continuity equation (answer C) cannot be used in the setting of coexisting aortic regurgitation (AR) or mitral regurgitation (MR), the latter being a frequent complication of valvuloplasty. Calculation of the MVA via the continuity equation assumes that stroke volume across the mitral valve is the same as the stroke volume across the left ventricular outflow tract (LVOT). However, when there is coexistent AR and/or MR, this assumption is no longer valid and the MVA cannot be accurately calculated. Furthermore, this method estimates the effective orifice area (EOA) rather than the anatomic orifice area and the EOA tends to be slightly smaller than the

anatomic orifice area. While the flow convergence method (answer D) can be used to estimate the MVA, this technique is not as accurate or as reliable as 3D echocardiography and provides an estimation of the EOA rather than the anatomic mitral orifice area.

11. **Answer: C.** Restricted mitral valve opening due to restenosis. The 3D data set is a zoomed view of the mitral valve from the left ventricle perspective. The 3D image from the short-axis view shows leaflet thickening and anterior mitral leaflet doming ("hockey-stick" appearances) with medial and lateral commissural fusion. Answer A is not correct since there is no evidence of a flail P2 segment on the 2D and 3D images. Answer B is not correct since the anterior and posterior leaflets are calcified and demonstrate restricted opening with an elevated mean gradient. Answer D is not correct since severe mitral stenosis is indicated when the mean pressure gradient is >10 mm Hg and the mitral valve area is <1.0 cm². In this case the mean pressure gradient is 7.5 mm Hg, which may be due to reduced cardiac output; however, the maximal gradient suggests a relatively normal cardiac output.

12. **Answer: A.** Using multiplanar reconstruction, a 2D cut plane can be placed at the tips of the mitral leaflets en face to the valve opening. Following mitral balloon valvuloplasty, 3D measurement of the mitral orifice is the most accurate and reliable method compared to pressure half-time and 2D planimetry. Since mitral regurgitation is a common complication of valvuloplasty, the continuity equation cannot be used for estimation of valve area.

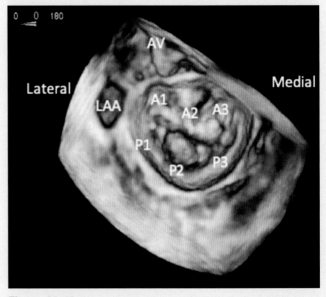

Figure 30-19

13. **Answer: A.** The corresponding 3D TEE image and video assess the mitral valve from the left atrium (LA) and demonstrate bileaflet, multisegmental prolapse with billowing. **Figure 30-19** shows the labeled segments of the mitral valve and it can be appreciated that there is prolapse of all anterior segments and a flail P2. The leaflet thickening, large redundant leaflets, chordal elongation, and annular dilatation are all characteristic features of Barlow disease, which is represented in this example. Barlow disease is a degenerative process and is often multisegmental, affecting both leaflets in up to 40% of patients.

14. **Answer: B.** While further 2D and 3D images may be helpful, the diagnosis may be made with the images provided. **Figure 30-7** and **Video 30-5** were acquired from the left atrial perspective ("en-face" view) of the mitral valve. The labeled scallops of the mitral valve can be appreciated in **Figure 30-20**. The uniform coaptation of the anterior and posterior leaflets excludes prolapse; however, the P3 segment (labeled as an *) appears to "bulge" into the left atrium, although with a thin, echogenic structure most likely consistent with a ruptured chord.

15. ▶ **Answer: D.** Video 30-6 and **Figure 30-21** (*represents the VSD) demonstrates a serpiginous, postinfarct VSD with predominantly left to right shunting. Post–myocardial infarction VSD is an increasing, rare complication of myocardial infarction and most commonly develops within a few days following a transmural infarct involving the septum. 3D (Video 30-17A) and color (Video 30-17B) biplane TEE also nicely demonstrate the serpiginous nature and extent of the VSD. Although

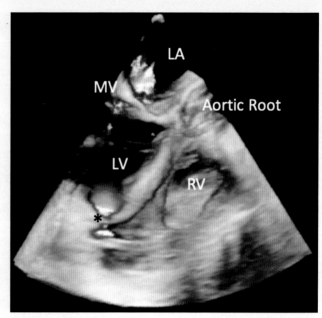

Figure 30-21 * indicates the ventricular septal defect with color noted across the septum.

the mitral valve leaflets are mildly thickened and tethered, answer A is not correct as there is only mild to moderate regurgitation present in **Video 30-6**. Answer B is not correct since the color flow is directed into the right ventricle, which is confirmed on biplane TEE. Answer C is not correct as there is no evidence of papillary muscle rupture which would result in severe mitral regurgitation. Papillary muscle rupture is associated with a linear echo density attached to the mitral valve and can be seen prolapsing through the mitral valve into the left atrium.

16. **Answer: B.** 3D color Doppler data are best displayed in two long-axis views, along the narrowest and widest portions of the jet using multiplanar cut planes. These views limit the inherent "bleed" of color Doppler data, allowing for greater precision of the color Doppler measurements. 3D color Doppler data may also be displayed using a volume-rendered image in addition to the multiplanar views, as was performed with this case (**Figure 30-22**).

17. **Answer: C.** The aortic valve is displayed from the aortic perspective on this 3D zoom acquisition. The leaflet labeled 1 is the left coronary cusp, the leaflet labeled 2 is the right coronary cusp, and the leaflet labeled 3 is the noncoronary cusp. When performing 3D echocardiography, it is extremely important to know from which perspective the image is being viewed so the cusps can be correctly identified (**Figure 30-23**).

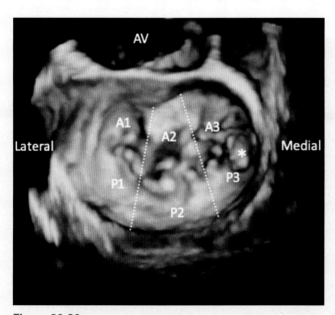

Figure 30-20

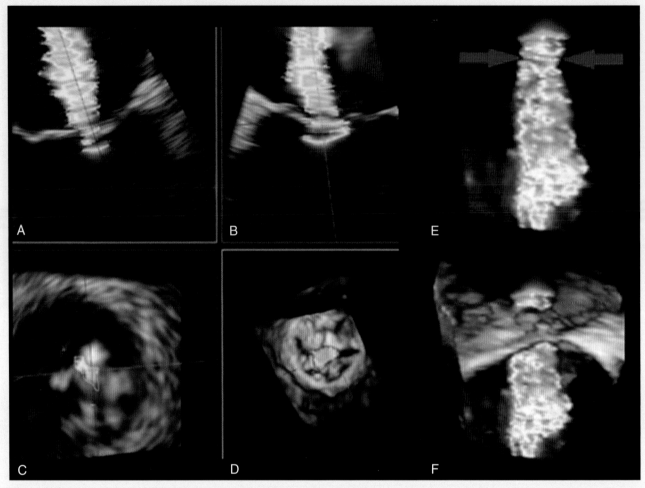

Figure 30-22 From three multiplanar views (panel A-C), a volume-rendered 3D color-flow Doppler image of the mitral valve is obtainable. The vena contracta of the mitral regurgitant jet is able to be planimetered from the short-axis view (panels C and D) and appreciated from the long-axis view (panel E—red arrows). The volume-rendered 3D color-flow Doppler image of the regurgitant jet is appreciated in panel F.

TEACHING TIP

When visualizing the aortic valve on 3D echocardiography from the aortic perspective, the leaflets are right-left inverted compared with the transthoracic echocardiographic parasternal short-axis view (**Figure 30-23**).

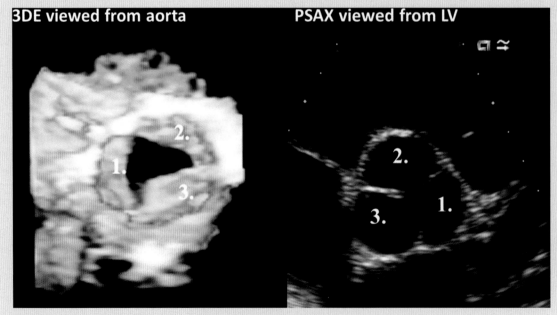

Figure 30-23 1 = left coronary cusp; 2 = right coronary cusp; 3 = noncoronary cusp.

18. ▶ **Answer: C.** The 2D and 3D imaging shows significant degeneration of the aortic valve (**Figure 30-9** and **Videos 30-8A** and **30-8B**). There are multiple bright, likely calcified attachments to the right coronary cusp, with one long filamentous mass on the ventricular side and another on the ascending aortic side. Color Doppler shows two aortic regurgitant (AR) jets with different origins, one traversing the body of the right cusp, suggesting perforation (**Figure 30-9**, bottom right). Biplane imaging (another form of 3D imaging) was also used in multiple views to determine the attachment of mobile structures to the leaflets. The 3D-zoom view of the aortic valve obtained from the parasternal long-axis view was cropped into the coaptation line of the right and noncoronary cusps and is angled to display a perforation in the leaflet (**Video 30-18**).

Spectral Doppler interrogation of the eccentric AR jet is shown in **Figure 30-24**, left. Pan-diastolic flow reversal in the descending aorta was also noted (**Figure 30-24**, right). Multibeat acquisition and a narrow sector allowed a sufficient frame rate for Doppler analysis.

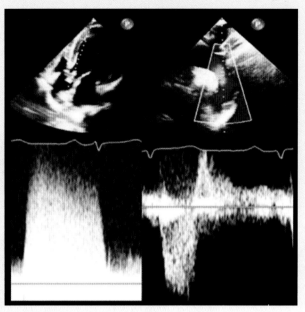

Figure 30-24

KEY POINT

In challenging examinations, biplane and 3D data sets may provide valuable supporting or novel information, perhaps avoiding the need for another imaging test.

19. ▶ **Answer: A.** These 3D zoom images of the tricuspid valve are displayed from the RV perspective. On the real-time clip (**Video 30-9**), the mitral valve can be seen "below" the tricuspid valve; thus, leaflet 3 is the septal tricuspid leaflet. The anterior tricuspid leaflet is largest; therefore, this is leaflet 2 and leaflet 1 is the posterior leaflet.

KEY POINT

When performing 3D echocardiography, it is extremely important to know the perspective from which the image is being viewed so the cusps can be correctly identified. By inverting this image, the tricuspid valve would then be viewed "en face" from the atrial perspective; this is also referred to as the "surgeon's view."

20. **Answer: D.** The most common implantation of a pacemaker lead is between the septal and posterior tricuspid valve leaflets as seen in this case. The pacemaker lead appears bright without any mobile echo densities suggestive of vegetations associated with it.

TEACHING POINT

▶ As the right ventricle dilates with increased volume and/or pressure, a coaptation defect of the leaflets may be seen (**Figure 30-25A** and **Video 30-19A**). This may result in migration of the pacing lead. The septal leaflet appears pliable and coapts to the other leaflets in systole, so no impingement is present.

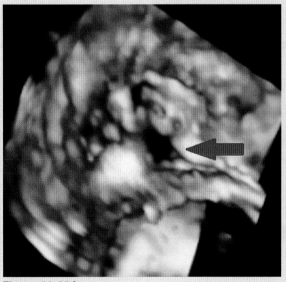

Figure 30-25A

Recall that the proper orientation for 3D echocardiographic display of the tricuspid valve, according to the joint EAE/ASE recommendations for image acquisition and display using three-dimensional echocardiography, is with the interventricular septum (IVS) displayed on the bottom and the septal leaflet positioned at 6 o'clock. Rotating clockwise from the IVS, the posterior and anterior leaflets are displayed on top (**Figure 30-25B**). Compare the normal leaflet coaptation to the pacemaker lead position between the leaflets (**Video 30-19B**) with the coaptation defect in a patient with severely dilated RV, and migration of the pacemaker lead toward the center of the leaflet opening (**Video 30-19A**).

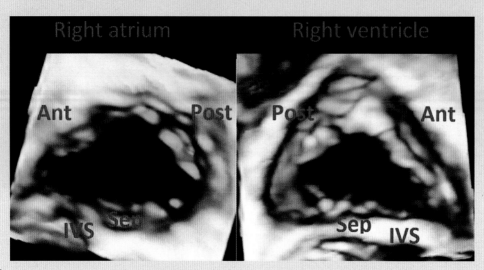

Figure 30-25B

21. **Answer: A.** The clue to the answer for this question is the new murmur and the history of serial endomyocardial biopsies. **Figure 30-11B** is a 3D zoom acquisition of the tricuspid valve displayed from the right atrial perspective. This image shows a flail component of the tricuspid valve on the septal leaflet (**Figure 30-26**). The color Doppler image (**Figure 30-11A**) demonstrates an eccentric tricuspid regurgitant jet that appears to be almost horizontal to the valve plane. In this case the 3D acquisition confirmed the mechanism of the EMB-induced tricuspid regurgitation.

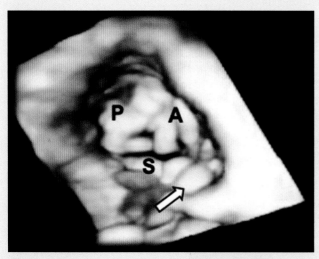

Figure 30-26 The arrow indicates the flail component of the septal tricuspid valve leaflet. A, anterior; P, posterior; S, septal.

22. **Answer: B.** The MVR appears well seated and the occluders appear to open without significant restriction. There is a large irregular echodensity attached to the posterior aspect of the mitral valve rim at the hinge point of the occluders. There are numerous other smaller mobile echodensities around the valve rim, including at the posteromedial and anterior hinge points. The AVR appears well seated with no restriction of the occluders. There is a mobile echodensity attached to the anterior aspect of the valve rim on the aortic root side. Given the clinical setting of bacteremia, these findings are most consistent with prosthetic valve vegetations.

23. **Answer: D.** Using the limited data provided, there is at least moderate paravalvular aortic regurgitation (AR). The vena contracta of the color jet and density of the continuous-wave (CW) Doppler waveform suggest moderate-to-severe AR. The regurgitant jet is shown to arise from an echo-free space or abscess cavity surrounding the prosthesis. A VSD (answer A) is excluded as the AR jet enters the left ventricle and the CW Doppler signal occurs during diastole. Answer B is excluded as the valve has not embolized or dehisced based on the stable appearance of the AVR. Answer C is excluded as the 3D appearance of the AVR is not consistent with a valve-in-valve procedure having been performed.

TEACHING POINT

To repair this defect, interventionalists along with echocardiographers used 3D echocardiographic guidance to lead a guide wire into the abscess and then deployed an Amplatzer occluder device. **Figure 30-27** displays the guide wire insertion (left and middle panels) and the resultant closure device well seated without significant paravalvular regurgitation in the abscess (right panel).

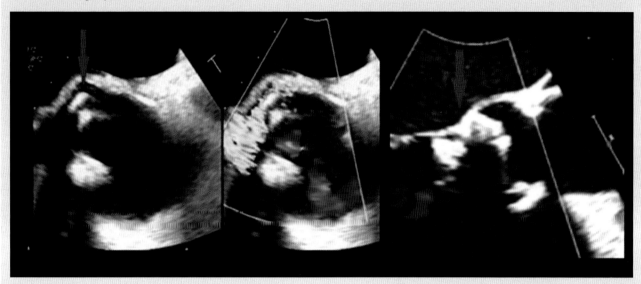

Figure 30-27

24. **Answer: A.** The figure provided for this question (**Figure 30-15**) is a 3D transthoracic echocardiographic image of the short axis of the mitral valve taken from the left ventricular perspective. There is a "gap" within the A1/A2 portion of the anterior mitral valve leaflet represented by the red arrow in **Figure 30-20**.

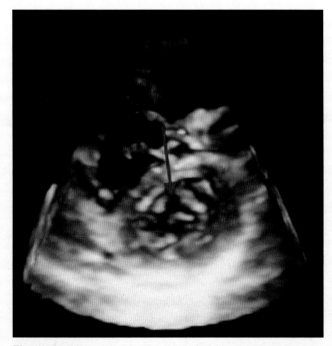

Figure 30-28

TEACHING POINTS

Color Doppler imaging would also be useful in confirming the cleft as this is where the MR jet would originate. 3D echocardiography is useful to show the 3D anatomical structure, spatial orientation, and extent of the cleft.

25. **Answer: C.** The images provided show 3D full-volume acquisition of an Amplatzer device. The clue to this case is the Amplatzer device itself, which resembles a "figure-of-8" on the 3D echocardiographic images. After reviewing the color Doppler image, a red "en-face" jet is visualized from the RA perspective demonstrating a residual left-to-right shunt. The 3D color full volume acquisition is helpful in identifying the exact location of the residual shunt.

26. ▶ **Answer: B.** The images from this 3D TEE study show the various stages of insertion of a Mitra-Clip device. This procedure is performed in patients with severe MR who are not suitable for open heart surgery. One or more clips are clamped across the mitral valve leaflets via a transcatheter approach. Ideally, the MR severity is reduced by two grades. **Video 30-14A** shows a wire crossing the interatrial septum into the left atrium. Once the catheter travels across to the left side of the heart, toward the mitral valve, the MitraClip device is used to catch the mitral valve leaflet tissue that is causing the valve to leak (**Video 30-14B**). Once the MitraClip is tested to ensure the leak is reduced, the catheter is removed, and the result is a double orifice (**Video 30-14C**).

A similar procedure, the Alfieri stitch, can be performed surgically. Unlike the MitraClip procedure, the Alfieri repair shows no clips or "stem." Both procedures result in a double orifice with two distinct regurgitant jet orifices. **Figure 30-29A** and **Video 30-20A** are 3D echocardiographic en-face images of an Alfieri stich and **Figure 30-29B** and **Video 30-20B** are 3D echocardiographic en-face images of a MitraClip. Observe that the MitraClip device has a brighter echo appearance and displays a "stem."

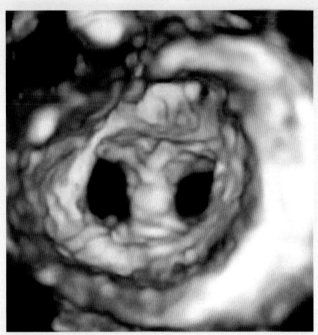

Figure 30-29A

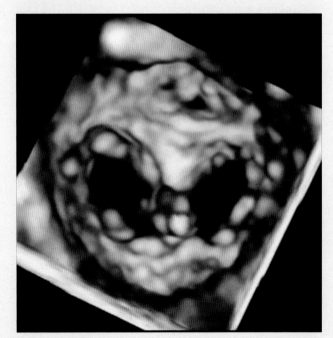

Figure 30-29B

TEACHING POINT

3D echocardiographic intraprocedural guidance for the MitraClip procedure is necessary to ensure that there is significant capture of the mitral leaflets, in addition to the assessment of MR severity reduction.

27. ▶ **Answer: D.** The corresponding **Videos 30-15A** and **30-15B** is taken immediately post deployment of a TAVR for severe aortic stenosis. From **Video 30-15A** the wire frame of the stent can be appreciated along with the thin leaflets of the valve within the center of the device. Therefore this device could not be a MitraClip or Amplatzer ASD device and answers A and B are not correct. Answer C is not correct since the patient did not require an additional TASH as there was no dynamic or significant outflow tract gradient prior to this procedure. **Figure 30-30** is a still frame taken from **Video 30-15B** with an arrow pointing the origin of the jet. **Video 30-21** is a 3D biplane TEE view interrogating the severity of the jet immediately following deployment. 3D TEE is useful immediately following TAVR particularly when a rapid assessment is required to determine the position and function of the valve. This includes identification and severity of aortic regurgitation.

28. **Answer: E.** 3D TEE is important in the preplanning for Watchman LAA closure, to verify the morphology and suitability of the LAA, for device sizing, and to certify that no LAA clot exists. Measurement of the LAA ostial dimensions using 3D flexi-slice is shown in **Figure 30-31A**. The LAA orifice is able to be cropped and displayed through its short axis instead of single-plane measurements via 2D TEE. These additional measurements help to confirm the accuracy of 2D

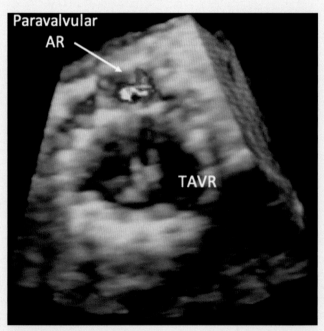

Figure 30-30

TEE measurements. The 3D volume data set may be cropped at appropriate angles (0°, 45°, 90°, 135°) to ensure that the correct size of the device can be implanted and be well seated. 3D color TEE is more effective for visualization of residual leaks and their severity compared to conventional 2D TEE (**Figure 30-31B**). From **Figure 30-31B**, a small, residual shunt can be visualized on color 3D echocardiography.

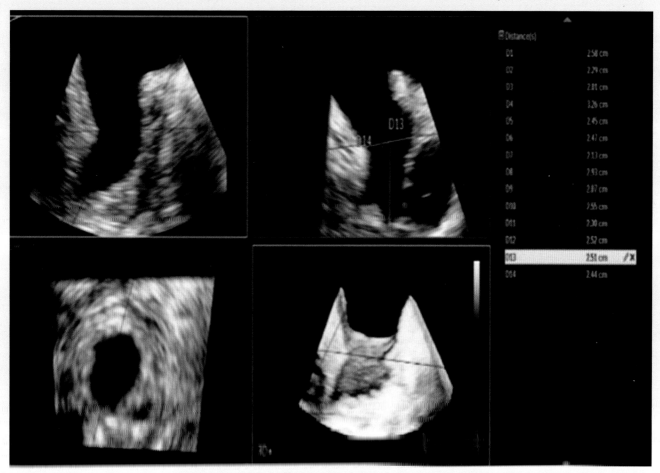

Figure 30-31A

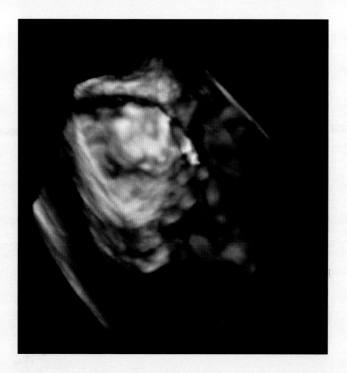

Figure 30-31B

Acknowledgments: The authors thank and acknowledge the contributions from Ben A. Lin, MD, PhD, and Lissa Suseng, MD, MPH (Chapter 5, Three-Dimensional Echocardiography) in *Clinical Echocardiography Review: A Self-Assessment Tool*, 2nd Edition, edited by Allan L. Klein, Craig R. Asher, 2017.

SUGGESTED READINGS

Addetia K, More-Avi V, Weinert L, et al. A new definition for an old entity: improved definition of mitral valve prolapse using three-dimensional echocardiography and color-coded parametric models. *J Am Soc Echocardiogr.* 2014;27(1):8-16.

Baumgartber H, Hung J, Bermejo J, et al. Echocardiographic assessment of valve stenosis: EAE/ASE recommendations for clinical practice. *J Am Soc Echocardiogr.* 2009;22(1):1-23.

Lang RM, Badano LP, Mor-Avi V, et al. Recommendations for cardiac chamber quantification by echocardiography in adults: an update from the American Society of Echocardiography and the European Association of Cardiovascular Imaging. *J Am Soc Echocardiogr.* 2015;28(1):1-39.

Lang RM, Badano LP, Tasang W, et al. EAE/ASE recommendations for image acquisition and display using three-dimensional echocardiography. *J Am Soc Echocardiogr.* 2012;25(1):3-46.

CHAPTER 31

Myocardial Mechanics and Strain Imaging

Contributors: Jeffrey C. Hill, BS, ACS, Daniel P. Bourque, MS, RCS, and Bryan Doldt, BS, RDCS

✪✪ Question 1

In which direction does the left ventricular apex rotate during systole?

A. Clockwise
B. Counterclockwise
C. Counterclockwise and clockwise
D. None of the above

✪ Question 2

At which point on the electrocardiogram (ECG) do normal peak myocardial strains occur?

A. Onset of the P wave
B. On the R wave
C. On the S wave
D. End of the T wave

✪✪✪ Question 3

A 69-year-old man with a history of hypertension and coronary artery disease presents with borderline tachycardia and ST-segment-elevation myocardial infarction (STEMI) involving the proximal left anterior descending coronary artery (LAD). Based on **Figure 31-1**, which answer best reflects the patient's myocardial mechanics?

A. Abnormal rotation
B. Abnormal radial strain
C. Abnormal longitudinal strain
D. Abnormal circumferential strain

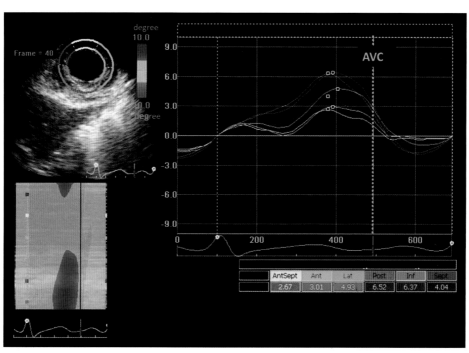

Figure 31-1

✪ Question 4

Which type of left ventricular strain was measured in **Figure 31-2A to 31-2D**?

    A. End-systolic longitudinal strain

    B. Peak systolic longitudinal strain

    C. Postsystolic longitudinal strain

    D. Peak longitudinal strain

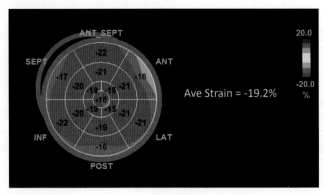

Figure 31-2D

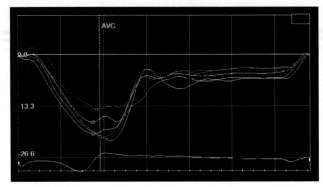

Figure 31-2A

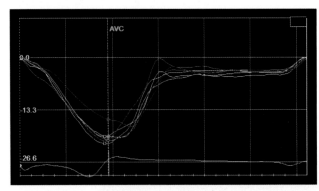

Figure 31-2B

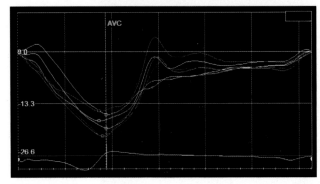

Figure 31-2C

✪✪✪ Question 5

If two-dimensional strain imaging is used to evaluate pathologic processes involving the subendocardium, the preferred measure should be:

    A. Rotation.

    B. Radial strain.

    C. Longitudinal strain.

    D. Circumferential strain.

✪ Question 6

The calculation of strain or the amount of deformation along an axis is defined as a:

    A. Change in length divided by the original length.

    B. Change in length minus the original length.

    C. Change in length multiplied by the original length.

    D. Change in length plus the original length.

✪✪ Question 7

Which type of left ventricular strain is measured in **Figure 31-3**?

    A. Circumferential strain

    B. Radial strain

    C. Circumferential strain rate

    D. Longitudinal strain

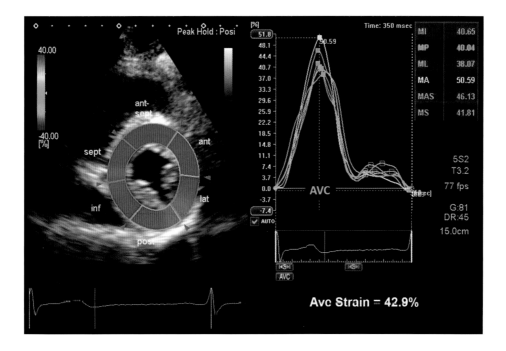

Figure 31-3

✪✪ Question 8

When reporting global longitudinal strain (GLS), it is important to consider the impact of:

    A. Vendor.

    B. Gender.

    C. Age.

    D. All of the above.

✪ Question 9

The two-dimensional (2D) views required to complete a bull's-eye plot for the calculation of global longitudinal strain (GLS) include the:

    A. Apical 4-chamber, apical long-axis, and apical 2-chamber views.

    B. Parasternal short-axis, apical long-axis, and parasternal long-axis views.

    C. Apical 4-chamber, parasternal long-axis, and apical 2-chamber views.

    D. Parasternal long-axis, apical 2-chamber, and apical long-axis views.

✪ Question 10

Normal mean global longitudinal strain (GLS) of the left ventricle (LV) is:

    A. −23.3%.

    B. 47.3%.

    C. −19.7%.

    D. 10.5%.

✪✪✪ Question 11

Based on the expert consensus for multimodality imaging of the adult patient during and after cancer therapy, subclinical left ventricular (LV) dysfunction is defined as a:

    A. 10% reduction in global longitudinal strain (GLS) when compared to baseline value.

    B. 12% reduction in GLS when compared to baseline value.

    C. 15% reduction in GLS when compared to baseline value.

    D. 25% reduction in GLS when compared to baseline value.

✪ Question 12

A source of two-dimensional (2D) imaging artifact resulting in an underestimation of the true myocardial deformation includes all of the following except:

    A. Acoustic shadowing.

    B. Reverberation.

    C. Side lobe.

    D. Wall filter saturation.

✪✪ Question 13

Optimal frames per second (fps) for acquisition of two-dimensional (2D) speckle tracking is:

    A. 40 to 60.

    B. 10 to 30.

    C. 0 to 20.

    D. 20 to 40.

✪✪✪ Question 14

In patients with acute heart failure, which of the following is a powerful predictor of cardiac events and appears to be a better parameter than left ventricular ejection fraction (LVEF)?

A. Global longitudinal strain
B. Global longitudinal strain rate
C. Global radial strain
D. Global circumferential strain

✪✪ Question 15

Which two-dimensional (2D) strain modality is most commonly used for the assessment of right ventricular (RV) myocardial mechanics?

A. Circumferential strain
B. Longitudinal strain
C. Radial strain
D. Transverse strain

✪ Question 16

When obtaining two-dimensional (2D) imaging for speckle tracking strain analysis, the sonographer should instruct the patient to:

A. Breathe in during acquisition of the 2D image.
B. Breathe in and out during acquisition of the 2D image.
C. Breathe out during acquisition of the 2D image.
D. Cease breathing during acquisition of the 2D image.

✪✪✪ Question 17

When interpreting strain imaging, which of the following variables may influence the results of the strain values being reported?

A. Blood pressure
B. Height
C. Weight
D. Transducer frequency
E. All of the above

✪ Question 18

Longitudinal and circumferential strain measure which component of heart deformation?

A. Peak lengthening during diastole
B. Peak shortening during systole
C. Peak thickening during systole
D. Peak thinning during diastole

✪✪ Question 19

Which type of left ventricular strain is measured in this bull's-eye plot in **Figure 31-4**?

A. End-systolic longitudinal strain
B. End-diastolic radial strain
C. End-systolic circumferential strain
D. End-diastolic longitudinal strain

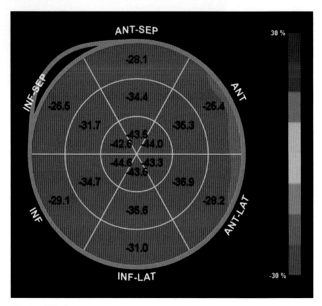

Figure 31-4

✪ Question 20

Normal mean global circumferential strain (GCS) for the left ventricle (LV) is:

A. −19.7%.
B. 47.3%.
C. −23.3%.
D. 62.5%.

✪✪✪ Question 21

Which type of strain is measured in **Figure 31-5**?

A. Three-dimensional (3D) radial strain
B. Two-dimensional (2D) circumferential strain rate
C. 3D longitudinal strain
D. 2D circumferential strain

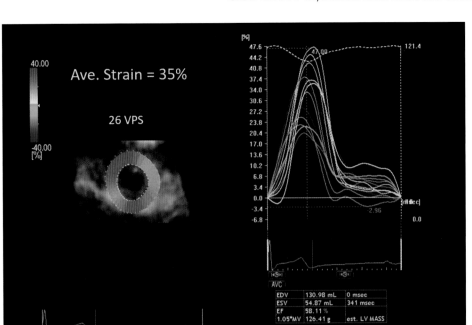

Figure 31-5

✪ Question 22

Which myocardial imaging modality was used to study the parasternal short-axis image in **Figure 31-6**?

  A. Longitudinal strain rate imaging
  B. Radial strain imaging
  C. Circumferential strain rate imaging
  D. Longitudinal strain imaging

✪✪✪ Question 23

The 2019 publication from the World Alliance Societies of Echocardiography (WASE) reported normal echocardiography values from around the world. Which country would the values shown in **Figures 31-7A** and **31-7B** be considered the lowest limits of normal for global longitudinal strain (GLS) in a male patient?

  A. Australia
  B. India
  C. Korea
  D. United States of America

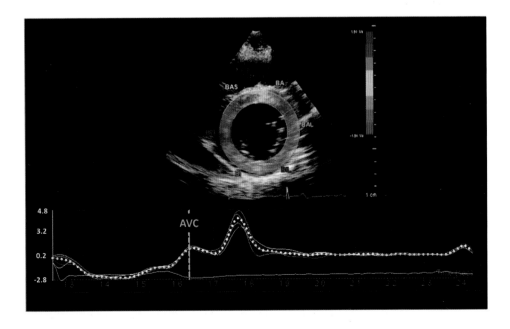

Figure 31-6

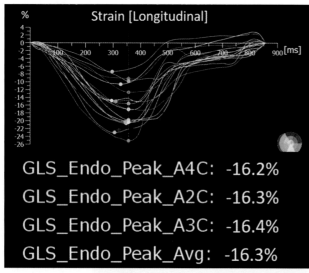

Figure 31-7A

Figure 31-7B

✪✪✪ Question 24

What is the most common type of strain used in the assessment of two-dimensional (2D) speckle tracking?
- **A.** Acoustic strain
- **B.** Eulerian strain
- **C.** Lagrangian strain
- **D.** Natural strain

✪✪ Question 25

A 41-year-old woman with a diagnosis of recurrent triple marker negative breast cancer who has received a cumulative dose of anthracyclines of 450 mg/m² undergoes an echocardiogram including strain imaging. The left ventricular ejection fraction is low normal. On the basis of the radial strain imaging (**Figure 31-8**), what would be the most likely course of treatment for this patient?
- **A.** Proceed with the last dose of anthracyclines (50 mg/m²)
- **B.** Discontinue anthracycline
- **C.** Start the patient on beta blockers
- **D.** Discontinue anthracycline and initiate beta blockers

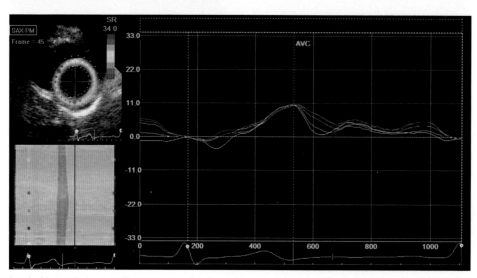

Figure 31-8 (Reprinted with permission from Klein AL, Asher CR. *Clinical Echocardiography Review: A Self-Assessment Tool.* 2nd ed. Philadelphia, PA: Wolters Kluwer; 2017.)

✪✪✪ Question 26

A 52-year-old man is referred for an echocardiogram after receiving 550 mg/m² of doxorubicin (Adriamycin) for the treatment of a tibial sarcoma. His ultrasensitive troponin I was 20 pg/mL. After reviewing **Figure 31-9** global longitudinal strain (GLS) data, what would be most likely recommended to his oncologist?

A. To interrupt therapy due to abnormal GLS, as there is concern for subclinical LV dysfunction

B. To continue therapy as the GLS and the biomarkers are normal

C. To repeat the GLS in 3 weeks and then discuss changes in clinical management

D. To obtain a cardiac magnetic resonance (CMR) study, as the risk of congestive heart failure is too high, and echocardiography may be unreliable to identify small differences in ejection fraction

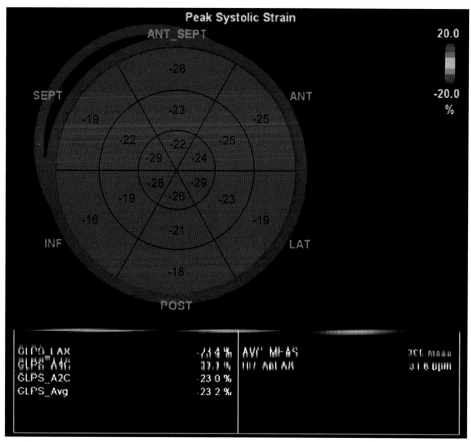

Figure 31-9 (Reprinted with permission from Klein AL, Asher CR. *Clinical Echocardiography Review: A Self-Assessment Tool.* 2nd ed. Philadelphia, PA: Wolters Kluwer; 2017.)

ANSWERS

1. **Answer: B.** The left ventricular apex rotates counterclockwise during systole. Similar to peak myocardial strain, peak apical rotation occurs at or near the end of the T wave on the electrocardiogram (ECG). Rotation is measured in degrees as seen on the y-axis of the display (**Figure 31-10A**). Just the opposite is seen at the base of the left heart with clockwise rotation occurring simultaneously (**Figure 31-10B**). The degrees of rotation at the base and apex are inversely related with normal aging, meaning the apex increases its rotation and the base decreases its rotation, respectively (**Table 31-1**). The apex "untwists" or rotates clockwise during diastole; therefore answer A is incorrect. The apex rotates in one direction during systole; therefore answer C is incorrect. See Takeuchi et al. (2006) and Kaku et al. (2014) for further information on age-related changes in rotational mechanics assessed by two-dimensional and three-dimensional speckle-tracking echocardiography.

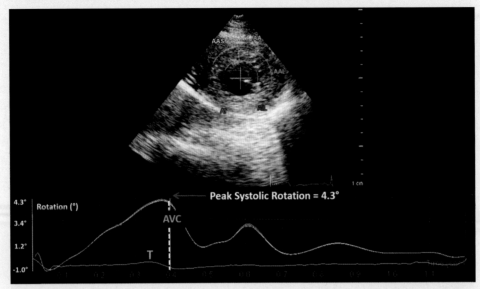

Figure 31-10A Example of left ventricular (LV) apical rotation in a normal 31-year-old woman. In this example, peak apical rotation occurs near the end of the T wave on the ECG. Note the waveforms are positive indicating counterclockwise mechanical movement. Peak systolic rotation in this patient is 4.3°, which is normal for the patient's age.

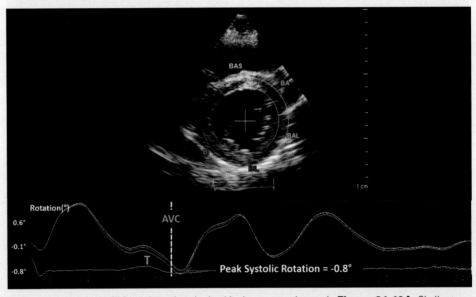

Figure 31-10B Example of left ventricular (LV) basal rotation obtained in the same patient as in **Figure 31-10A**. Similar to peak apical LV rotation, peak basal rotation normally occurs at or near the end of the T wave on the ECG. The peak systolic rotational waveforms are negative, indicating clockwise movement. There is trivial rotation occurring at the base as compared to the apex at end-systole with the base rotating less than one degree (base = −0.8° vs. apex = 4.3°).

2. **Answer: D.** Peak myocardial strains (longitudinal, radial, and circumferential) for both the right and left ventricle occur at or near the end of the T wave on the ECG. The end of the T wave represents aortic valve closure (AVC) or end-systole and is the point of transfer of myocardial energy (potential to kinetic) and peak myocardial deformation. However, peak strains can also normally occur slightly before and after AVC. Peak myocardial strains that occur before AVC can be labeled as "systolic strain (SS)," peak strains that occur at AVC can be labeled "end-systolic strain (ESS)," and

peak strains that occur after AVC can be labeled "post-systolic strain (PSS)" (**Figure 31-11A**).

A recent consensus document published by the European Society of Cardiovascular Imaging and American Society of Echocardiography Industry Taskforce to standardize deformation imaging suggests ESS should be reported as the default parameter for the description of peak myocardial deformation. However, other parameters mentioned above may be reported as well, but need to be labeled in a way that is clear to the end user.

Table 31-1. Age-Related Normal Range of Left Ventricular Rotation and Torsion Using Three-Dimensional Speckle Tracking Echocardiography

	Age Group				
Variable	1-3	20-29	50-59	>60	P
Rotation (°)					
Base	−5.35 ± 2.57	−3.24 ± 2.45[b]	−2.22 ± 2.23[a]	−1.70 ± 2.14[a,b,c]	<.0001
Apex	5.05 ± 3.82	10.35 ± 4.17[a,b]	11.22 ± 5.30[a,b,c]	12.79 ± 4.28[a,b,c]	<.0001
Torsion (°/cm)	1.78 ± 1.10	1.41 ± 0.58	1.46 ± 0.76	1.75 ± 0.66[b]	<.0001

There appears to be less dramatic change in basal rotation compared to apical rotation with aging. As the basal rotation decreases, apical rotation increases. In addition, torsion, which is the base-to-apex gradient in the rotation angle along the long axis (°/cm), appears constant and without significant changes until the sixth decade of life. As the left ventricular ejection fraction does not change significantly with aging, neither does torsion.

Data are expressed as mean ± SD (range).

[a]P <.001 vs. 1 to 3 years.
[b]P <.001 vs. 4 to 9 years (data not shown).
[c]P <.001 vs. 10 to 19 years (data not shown).

Data modified and obtained from Kaku K, Takeuchi M, Tsang W, et al. Age-related normal range of left ventricular strain and torsion using three-dimensional speckle-tracking echocardiography. *J Am Soc Echocardiogr*. 2014;27(1):55-64.

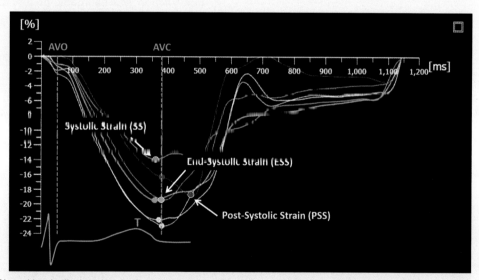

Figure 31-11A Normal longitudinal strain waveforms in a healthy 26-year-old man obtained from the apical 4-chamber view. There are six waveforms that correspond to the base, mid, and apical segments. The period between aortic valve opening (AVO) and aortic valve closure (AVC) is when the myocardium is mechanically contracting, also known as mechanical systole. As ventricular pressure is at its maximum, peak deformation occurs shortly thereafter (toward the end of the T wave). Note the peak strain waveforms occurring before, during, and after AVC.

Measurement of AVC can be determined by several methods such as manually measuring the timing from spectral Doppler or by the ultrasound system's algorithm that identifies minimal systolic volume (that is, end-systole) or valve closure. Via the manual method, a Doppler cursor is placed across the aortic valve from either the apical 5-chamber or long-axis view. Continuous-wave Doppler is then activated, and the signal is optimized by increasing to a sweep speed of 100 mm/s and decreasing the Doppler scale to properly observe the valve closure or "click" artifact. Measurements from the R wave of the ECG to AVC are performed (**Figure 31-11B**).

Normative two-dimensional (2D) strain values are reported in **Table 31-2**.

Recommended ultrasound settings and acquisition for 2D speckle tracking strain imaging:

- Adequate frame rate (FR) (recommended 40-80 fps; higher FR for higher heart rate)
- On-axis imaging (requires tilting/rocking the image [left-to-right] to include both epicardium and endocardium in 2D sector)
- Avoid/reduce foreshortening (moving down a rib space and having the patient breathe in may improve apical imaging)
- Adequate depth (vendor dependent and may require all chambers in view)
- Apnea (Have the patient breathe in or out; whichever improves image quality)
- Decrease sector size as needed (will increase 2D frame rate)
- Decrease 2D harmonic frequencies (with technically difficult studies)
- Avoid or reduce 2D artifacts (may interfere with speckle tracking)
- Obtain/document blood pressure at, or near the time of acquisition of the 2D images (strain is load dependent; may allow for more accurate assessment of global longitudinal strain)

The accuracy of event timing such as aortic valve closure (AVC) must be correct in order to measure end-systolic strain correctly. In the event AVC time is automatically calculated by the ultrasound system, the sonographer should confirm the timing (vertical position) of the AVC demarcation point, as displayed on the strain graph, to ensure it is correctly positioned. It is possible the calculation of AVC is incorrect, occurring too early, resulting in peak strain (and global strain) measurements that are underestimated (**Figure 31-12**).

3. ▶ **Answer: A.** This patient has abnormal apical rotation due to active ischemic disease. Although there are positive waveforms, the values on the y-axis are labeled as degrees; therefore, answers B, C, and D are incorrect. All strain measurements result in a percent change in deformation. Two-dimensional (2D) parasternal short-axis imaging of the apex demonstrated significant dysfunction in all myocardial segments with worsening function in the anterior and lateral wall segments (**Video 31-1**). Findings were consistent with a large LAD territory infarction. The left ventricular (LV) ejection fraction was estimated at 20% to 25%.

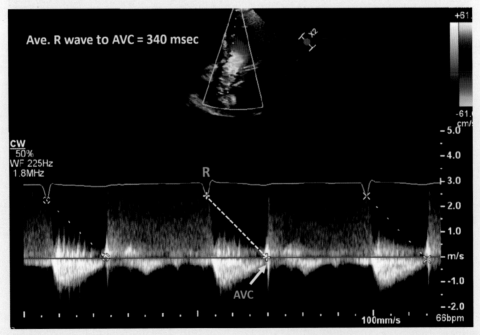

Figure 31-11B Measurement of ECG R wave to aortic valve closure (AVC) by continuous-wave Doppler echocardiography. A time caliper is placed at the center of the R wave and extrapolated to the demarcation point of valve closure or "click" artifact on the aortic valve continuous wave Doppler waveform (arrow). Three measurements of R wave to AVC were made and averaged (Ave). The R wave-to-AVC duration in this patient is 340 msec.

Table 31-2. Normal 2D Values for Global Radial Strain (GRS), Global Circumferential Strain (GCS), and Global Longitudinal Strain (GLS)

Parameter	Mean Value	95% Confidence Intervals	Imaging View
GRS	47.3%	43.6% to 51.0%	Parasternal short-axis papillary muscle level
GCS	−23.3%	−24.6% to −22.1%	Parasternal short-axis papillary muscle level
GLS	−19.7%	−20.4% to −18.9%	Apical long-axis, 4-chamber and 2-chamber views

Mean values are reported as the average from the six segments in each view. Radial strain is reported as a positive value (thickening), and longitudinal and circumferential strains are reported as a negative value (shortening).

Data modified and obtained from Yingchoncharoen T, Agarwal S, Popovic Z, et al. Normal ranges of left ventricular strain: a meta-analysis. *J Am Soc Echocardiogr.* 2013;26(2):185-191.

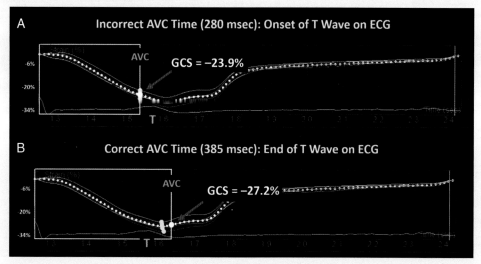

Figure 31-12 Example of incorrect and correct aortic valve closure (AVC) time for measurement of global circumferential strain (GCS) in the same patient. The electrocardiogram (ECG) R wave to AVC measurement (280 ms) was incorrectly calculated in example A, resulting in an underestimation of GCS (−23.9%). In addition, note the peak GCS calculation occurred at the onset of the ECG T wave, which is nonphysiologic. Example B demonstrates a correct R wave to AVC measurement (385 ms), resulting in correct calculation of the peak GCS (−27.2%). Note there was nearly a 14% difference between the two GCS values. Peak GCS should be calculated at the end of the T wave on the ECG.

As described in the answer outline for question 1, rotation can be assessed from the parasternal short-axis views with conventional measurements obtained at the basal left ventricle, LV apex, or both. As expected in this patient, a significant reduction in the apical rotation was demonstrated (**Figure 31-13**). The normal averaged apical rotation for this patient's age is 10.8° ± 4.9°. The averaged rotation from the six segments in this patient was 4.59°, which is significantly reduced due to ischemic disease and myocardial dysfunction.

4. ▶ **Answer: B.** Peak systolic longitudinal strain was applied to the three apical views (**Videos 31-2A** to **31-2C**). Answer A is incorrect because peak strains were measured before end-systole, which occurs at aortic valve closure (AVC). Answer C is incorrect because all peak strains were measured before AVC. Answer D is incorrect because peak strains that occurred after AVC were not mea-

sured. The combined averaged strains from the base, mid, and apical planes create a "global" value, or global longitudinal strain (GLS). Two-dimensional (2D) GLS obtained from the apical 4-chamber (**Figure 31-2A**), 2-chamber (**Figure 31-2B**), and long-axis (**Figure 31-2C**) views in a normal patient with bradycardia (48 BPM). The majority of the peak strains were measured during "mechanical systole," which is the period between aortic valve opening and aortic valve closure (AVC). Otherwise, all peak strains would be measured on the vertical dotted line (AVC) or end-systole (see the answer outline for question 2 for further explanation of measurements of peak strain and event timing). A bull's-eye plot of the peak strains from the three apical imaging planes is displayed (**Figure 31-2D**) including a 17-segment model, which includes the apical cap. The averaged GLS is −19.2%, which is normal.

TEACHING POINT

From the apical views, because the heart is shortening in the long axis, the reported strain values are negative. For example, if the resting, initial length of an object is 10 mm and a change in length occurred and is now 8 mm, the overall change in length is −20%, resulting in shortening of the object:

$$Strain = \left[\left(L_1 - L_0\right) \div L_0\right] \times 100$$
$$= \left[\left(8 - 10\right) \div 10\right] \times 100$$
$$= \left[-2 \div 10\right] \times 100$$
$$= -0.2 \times 100$$
$$= -20\%$$

where L_1 is the length at a given point in time and L_0 is the baseline length.

Just the opposite would occur if the initial length of an object at 10 mm increased by 2 mm to a new length of 12 mm, resulting in a positive change in length of 20%:

$$Strain = \left[\left(L_1 - L_0\right) \div L_0\right] \times 100$$
$$= \left[\left(12 - 10\right) \div 10\right] \times 100$$
$$= \left[2 \div 10\right] \times 100$$
$$= 0.2 \times 100$$
$$= 20\%$$

An important discriminator in determining the type of strain being measured is the magnitude of the values. For example, average GLS values rarely exceed −22% in the normal heart, whereas circumferential strain values are typically much higher (see the answer outline for question 19 for further explanation of normal circumferential strain values).

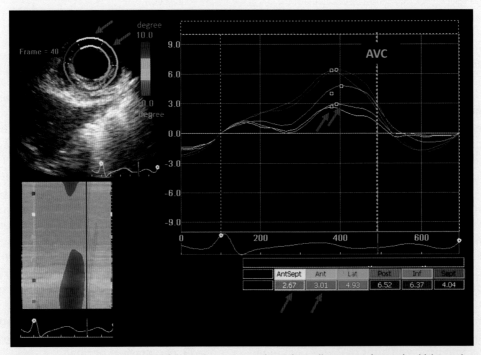

Figure 31-13 Lowest rotational values are reported in the anterior septum and anterior wall segments (arrows), which correlates with the extensive abnormalities in wall thickening seen by 2D imaging. In addition, there is early peak rotation that occurs well before the end of the T wave on the electrocardiogram. The averaged rotation from the six segments was 4.59°, which is significantly reduced due to ischemic disease and myocardial dysfunction. Normative rotational values are reported in **Table 31-1**.

5. **Answer: C.** Several studies have explored the deformation of the ventricle, describing myocyte arrangements as a continuum of two helical fiber geometries. In the subendocardium, the fibers are roughly longitudinally oriented, with an angle of 80° with respect to the circumferential direction of the fibers located in the mid-wall of the thickness of the myocardium. As a result, global longitudinal strain (evaluating the longitudinal fibers) should be the measure of choice when evaluating pathology involving the subendocardium. See **Figure 31-14** demonstrating different methods for assessing myocardial strain.

6. **Answer: A.** The formula for the calculation of myocardial strain includes the change in length divided by the original length (see Technical Tip in the answer outline for Question 4). Answers B-D do not reflect the positive or negative changes that occur within the heart during systole. Depending on the axis of deformation being evaluated, the strain values can either be positive or negative. For example, as the heart contracts or "coils" during systole, the mitral valve annulus displaces toward the apex an estimated 10 to 15 mm normally. This displacement reflects a negative change in the myocardium, creating shortening. Shortening can be measured by longitudinal strain in the apical views, or circumferential strain in the parasternal short-axis views. In addition, as the heart shortens, simultaneous thickening of the heart occurs in the orthogonal axis, which in part, creates thickening of the walls. Thickening of the heart can be measured by radial strain imaging.

7. **Answer: B. Figure 31-3** is an example of normal 2D radial strain imaging in the parasternal short-axis view at the papillary muscle level (left). The homogeneous relatively dark red color coding indicates

the peak thickening from each of the six segments is near 40% or higher. To the right are the peak strain waveforms that occur on or about the end of the T wave and aortic valve closure (AVC). The averaged values from each segment are reported to the far right, with the lowest value in the mid-lateral wall (ML) segment at 38.07% and the highest value in the mid anterior wall (MA) segment at 50.59%. The averaged radial strain is 42.9%, which is normal. Observe how well synchronized the normal heart is with peak radial strains occurring on or about AVC. This is in contrast to the radial strain example in a patient with myocardial disease seen in **Figure 31-15**.

Although circumferential strain may also be obtained from the parasternal short-axis views, answer A is incorrect as the waveforms displayed are positive. Answer C is incorrect as strain rate curves display three peaks, similar to the tissue Doppler imaging trace at the mitral annulus. Answer D is incorrect as longitudinal strain is obtained from the apical views, not the parasternal views.

8. **Answer: D.** Because of low intervendor agreement, two-dimensional (2D) strain data are not interchangeable. The JUSTICE (Japanese ultrasound speckle tracking of left ventricle study) provides reference 2D strain values for the three most commonly used vendors. In their study, they also show statistically significant differences for gender and age. As a result, when reporting longitudinal strain, it is important to take into consideration the vendor used and the gender and age of the patient.

9. **Answer: A.** The apical 4-chamber, apical long-axis, and apical 2-chamber views are required in order to calculate a bull's-eye plot for GLS (**Figure 31-16A**).

Answers B-D are incorrect as parasternal and apical views cannot be combined.

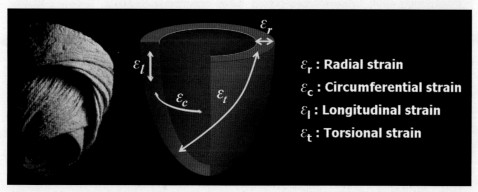

ε_r

ε_r : **Radial strain**

ε_c : **Circumferential strain**

ε_l : **Longitudinal strain**

ε_t : **Torsional strain**

Figure 31-14 Representation of a heart image cast demonstrating the fiber orientation and changes in orientation from the subendocardium to the epicardium (left). Types of strain that can be measured include circumferential, longitudinal, and radial strain (right). In addition, the "torsional" left ventricular strains can theoretically be assessed. (Reprinted with permission from Armstrong WF, Ryan T, eds. *Feigenbaum's Echocardiography.* 7th ed. Philadelphia, PA: Wolters Kluwer Health/Lippincott Williams & Wilkins; 2010.)

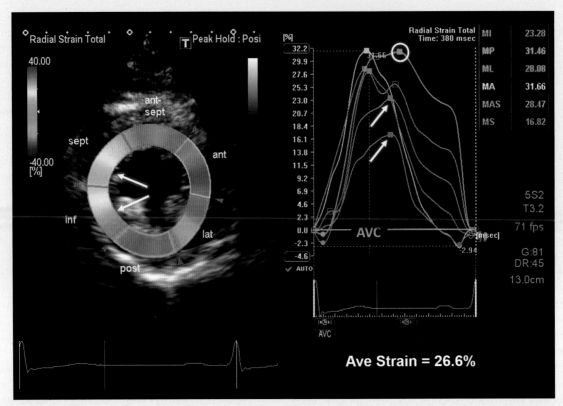

Figure 31-15 Two-dimensional (2D) radial strain imaging obtained at the parasternal short-axis view at papillary muscle level (left), in a patient with right coronary artery territory disease. The heterogeneous color-coding indicates the peak thickenings from the six segments are variably reduced. In addition, the values are much lower as compared to the peak strains in **Figure 31-3**. The orange-to-yellow hue indicates that majority of the strains are near 30%. To the right are the corresponding peak strain waveforms that display significant differences in amplitude and timing. The averaged values from each segment are reported to the far right, with the lowest values in the mid-septal wall (MS) segment (16.82%) and mid-inferior wall (MI) segment (23.28%) (arrows), respectively. Note that the waveforms from these two segments appear different, and peak well after AVC, as compared to the other waveforms. This finding is consistent with postsystolic shortening (PSS) that is pathologic. Note the mid-posterior wall (MP) segment also demonstrates PSS (circle). This may be due to underlying ischemic myocardium that is being tracked at the subendocardial level within the segment. The averaged radial strain is 26.6%. Lastly, observe the increased dispersion (that is, dyssynchrony) of the peak strains that is typically seen in ischemic disease.

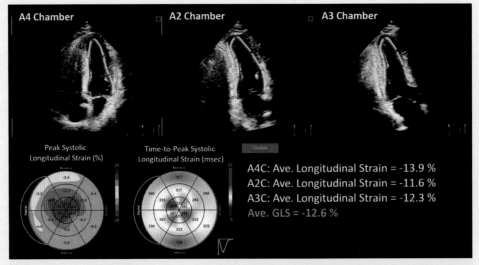

Figure 31-16A The top images show the apical 4-chamber, apical 2-chamber, and apical long-axis views that are obtained in order to calculate GLS. The bottom images are the corresponding bull's-eye plots that include the peak systolic longitudinal strain values (left) and time-to-peak systolic longitudinal strain values (right) obtained from the base, mid, and apical levels. To the far right are the average longitudinal strains from the three apical views. The GLS in this patient is −12.6%, which is abnormal.

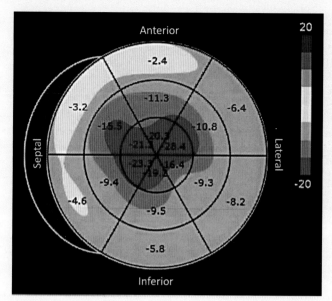

Figure 31-16D Peak systolic longitudinal strain BE plot as seen in **Figure 31-16A**. Note the marked reduction in the basal strains, which then increase at the middle and apical levels. The near normalization (red color) of the apical strains is consistent with "apical sparing" as seen in patients with cardiac amyloidosis.

TEACHING POINT

The bull's-eye (BE) plot shown in **Figures 31-16A** and **31-16B** is consistent with so-called "apical sparing" that can be observed in patients with biopsy-confirmed cardiac amyloidosis (CA). Phelan et al. (2012) studied 24 patients (8 with CA, 8 with hypertrophic cardiomyopathy, and 8 with hypertensive heart disease) with mild to moderate left ventricular hypertrophy (LVH) and adequate image quality to accurately perform longitudinal strain imaging. All patients had an absence of electrocardiographic criteria for low voltages or a pseudo-infarct pattern, which may be seen in patients with CA. The results demonstrated that when the reader was properly trained in identifying this unique strain BE pattern, the classification of CA increased significantly. The overall sensitivity was 86%, specificity was 95%, and overall accuracy was 92% in predicting CA. This BE pattern provides a rapid visual clue to possible CA and further clinical correlation should be considered.

10. **Answer: C.** Reported normal values for GLS vary from −15.9% to −22.1% (mean, −19.7%; 95% CI, −20.4% to −18.9%). Answer B is incorrect as that is the reported normal mean value for global radial strain imaging at the mid-level of the LV from the parasternal short-axis view. Answer A is incorrect because that is the reported normal mean value for circumferential strain at the mid-level of the LV from the parasternal short-axis view. Answer D is also incorrect because the mean value would be too low for any GLS measured in the LV. Note the positive percent values in answers B and D reflect thickening of the LV, whereas answers A and C reflect short-

ening of the heart and are therefore reported as negative values. See Yingchoncharoen et al. (2013) for more information regarding the determination of normal mean strain values and confidence intervals.

11. **Answer: C.** The current expert consensus for multimodality imaging of the adult patient during and after cancer therapy defines subclinical LV dysfunction as a >15% reduction in GLS when compared with baseline. This is based on the findings of Negishi et al. (2013), who showed that a reduction in GLS of 11% (95% confidence interval, 8.3%-14.6%) had the best receiver operator characteristics to predict a subsequent reduction in left ventricular ejection fraction at 1 year of follow-up with a sensitivity of 65% and a specificity of 94%.

12. **Answer: D.** Wall filter or circuit saturation artifact is seen on the spectral Doppler display, and therefore is not a source of 2D imaging artifact. Wall filter or circuit saturation artifact appears as linear signals or spikes above and below the zero-baseline; more commonly, this is referred to as a valve "click" artifact. See **Figure 31-11B** for further explanation of how this artifact may be useful in strain imaging. Answers A-C may all be a source of interference with 2D speckle tracking, resulting in an underestimation of the true myocardial deformation. Note that any artifact that resembles "speckles" can influence or interfere with speckle tracking, and care should be taken to avoid such artifacts.

13. **Answer: A.** The acquisition rate of speckle tracking for the assessment of myocardial deformation is recommended at 40 to 60 fps. Answers B-D are incorrect as the scan line density is increased which may result in an underestimation of peak values. This is particularly important when assessing strain rate imaging, as identifying the true peak values may require higher fps. Conversely, too high fps may result in reduced image quality, due to a reduction in scan line density, resulting in reduced tracking quality.

14. **Answer: D.** Cho et al. (2009) evaluated whether two-dimensional strain offered additional benefit over LVEF to predict clinical events in patients with acute heart failure. Investigators found that global circumferential strain is a powerful predictor of cardiac events and appears to be a better parameter than LVEF in patients with acute heart failure (hazard ratio of 1.15; 95% confidence intervals of 1.04-1.28; P = .006).

15. ▶ **Answer: B.** Longitudinal strain (LS) is currently the most common type of strain imaging modality used for the 2D assessment of RV mechanics (**Figure 31-17**). An apical 4-chamber "RV-focused" view is acquired during apnea (**Video 31-3A**). Longitudinal strain can be applied to the RV free wall (**Video 31-3B**) or may include the septal wall as

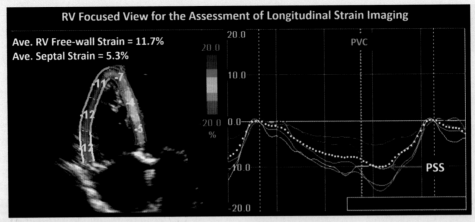

Figure 31-17 RV free wall and septal longitudinal strain imaging in a 52-year-old woman with a history of multivessel disease, including the right coronary artery. 2D imaging demonstrated a significant reduction in longitudinal shortening of both the septum and RV free wall. Note the marked reduction in the RV free wall and septal strain values from base to apex averaging −11.7% and −5.3%, respectively. In addition, the majority of the strain waveforms along with the global peak strain (dotted white curve) occur well after pulmonary valve closure (PVC). These findings are consistent with ischemic disease and postsystolic shortening (PSS), which is considered to be pathologic.

well (**Video 31-3C**). Normal basal RV free wall LS is −25.3 ± 5.9%, mid RV free wall LS is −28.4 ± 4.7%, and distal RV free wall LS is −24.1 ± 4.6%, respectively. See Horton et al. (2009) and Rajagopal et al. (2014) for further information on normative values in RV strain. The algorithms developed for circumferential and radial strain imaging cannot be applied to the right ventricle due to the inability to image the short axis and its noncircular morphology; therefore answers A and C are incorrect. Transverse strain (answer D) could theoretically be applied to the right ventricle to assess "thickening" toward the center of contraction; however, this has not been validated in the assessment of right heart function.

TECHNICAL TIPS

When assessing RV strain, it is important for the sonographer to focus on the septum and RV free wall at the expense of imaging the left ventricle (LV). In addition, the RV free wall tends to include significant artifact that is most likely generated from extracardiac structures that are accentuated during normal respiration. Therefore, as with LV image acquisition, it is imperative for the sonographer to obtain 2D imaging during apnea, free of artifact. See Horton KD et al., **Videos 31-3A** to **31-3C**, and Technical Tips in the answer outline for Question 2 for further information on suggested acquisition for strain imaging. If the measurement of end-systole is being used for the right ventricle, the sonographer must ensure the values established by the system reflect this. This may require the measurement of the electrocardiogram R wave to pulmonary valve closure (PVC) for more accurate estimation of strain. See **Figure 31-12** for an explanation on how to determine accurate event timing and end-systole.

16.  **Answer: D.** The sonographer should instruct the patient to either breathe in or breathe out (until image quality is at its best), then cease breathing during acquisition of the 2D image. **Video 31-4A** demonstrates the effects of normal respiration on the 2D image during acquisition from the apical 4-chamber view. Observe the pronounced lung artifact that is seen in the region of the anterolateral wall during normal respiration; the sonographer instructed the patient to take a small breath in and out and hold it, then acquired the 2D image as seen in **Video 31-4B**. Note the high-quality 2D imaging with no lung interference in **Video 31-4B** as compared to **Video 31-4A**. Longitudinal strain analysis was performed on the two images, demonstrating significant differences in the peak longitudinal strain values in the anterolateral wall from base to apex (**Figure 31-18**). Answers A-C may result in capturing of artifact and are not recommended during 2D myocardial strain image acquisition.

17. **Answer: A.** Myocardial contractility is influenced by conditions such as preload and afterload; therefore strain imaging (a surrogate of contractility) may be influenced as well. Increases in afterload (that is, the resistance the heart must overcome to eject) may result in differences in strain values from study to study. Therefore, blood pressure (BP), particularly systolic BP, may play an important role when interpreting strain values and whether there is an increase/decrease in overall values. It is recommended that the sonographer acquire the BP around the time of acquiring 2D images for strain analysis. Answers B-D are incorrect as these variables have not been shown to influence the overall strain values. The study by Yingchoncharoen et al. (2013) demonstrated in a general linear model

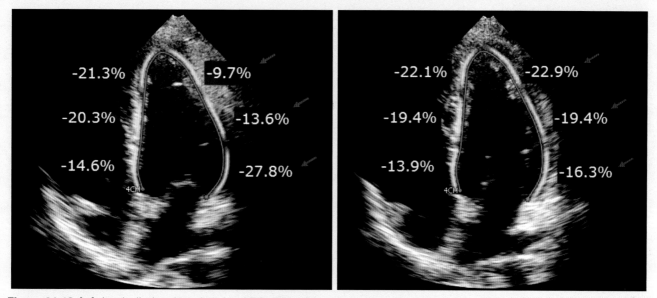

Figure 31 18 Left: Longitudinal strain analysis from **Video 31-4A** in a normal patient during respiration. The anterolateral wall longitudinal strain values are exceptionally high in the basal segment (−27.8%), low in the mid-LV segment (−13.6%), and especially low in the apical segment (−9.7%) (arrows). Just the opposite would be expected in a normal patient, in whom 2D strain values are typically the lowest in the basal segments and highest in the apical segments. **Right:** Longitudinal strain analysis from **Video 31-4B** in the same patient acquired during apnea. The anterolateral wall longitudinal strain values appear to be corrected (arrows) and, as expected, lower values are observed in the basal segments and higher values are seen in the apical segments, respectively. Importantly, no significant differences in the inferoseptal longitudinal strain values are seen between the two data sets.

(meta-regression) that only mean BP was independently associated with higher values of strain throughout twenty-four 2D strain studies in nearly 2600 patients.

18. **Answer: B.** Both longitudinal and circumferential strain measure the overall peak shortening of the myocardium during ventricular systole. Answer A, lengthening in diastole, is the opposite of shortening; answer C, thickening during systole, is the measurement of myocardial deformation by radial strain imaging; and answer D, thinning during diastole, is the opposite of thickening. Note that both lengthening and thinning can be estimated by strain imaging technology but are not currently applied during routine clinical use.

19. **Answer: C.** End-systolic circumferential strain was measured from the base, mid, and apical slice planes in the parasternal short axis view (see **Figure 31-19**). Like longitudinal strain, circumferential strain is a measure of left ventricular shortening; therefore the values are negative. An important differentiator between longitudinal and circumferential strain is the average global strain value, which is typically much higher for circumferential strain. Average normal global longitudinal strain from the apical views rarely exceeds −22%.

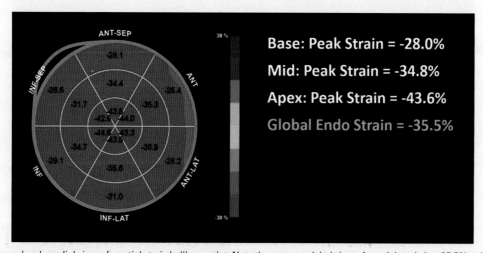

Figure 31-19 Normal endocardial circumferential strain bull's-eye plot. Note the average global circumferential strain is −35.5%, with the lowest strain measured at the base (-28%) and the highest strain measured in the apex (−43.6%).

In addition, normal basal peak longitudinal strain rarely exceeds −20%. The global circumferential strain in this example measures −35.5%. Answers B and D are incorrect as end-diastolic strain is not currently measured and has not been validated as a reliable measure of myocardial performance.

TECHNICAL TIP

When acquiring 2D parasternal short-axis images for the estimation of circumferential strain, the sonographer should pay close attention to image quality. All images should be acquired during shallow breathing or apnea and should be free of significant 2D artifacts. In addition, the images should be acquired as on-axis (circular) as possible (**Videos 31-5A** to **31-5C**). This will ensure that there is no interference from lung artifact and the correct "speckle" vector is being measured. This may improve the reproducibility of the global strain values.

20. **Answer: C.** Normal mean GCS is reported to be -23.3% (see **Table 31-2**). Answer A is incorrect because that is the reported normal mean value for circumferential strain at the mid-level of the LV in the parasternal short-axis view. Answer B is incorrect, as that is the reported normal mean value for global radial strain imaging at the mid-level of the LV from the parasternal short-axis view. Answer D is also incorrect because the mean value would be too high for any GCS measured in the LV. Note the positive values in answers B and D reflect thickening of the LV and are therefore positive values, whereas answers A and C reflect shortening of the heart and are reported as negative values. See Yingchon-

charoen et al. (2013) for more information regarding the determination of normal mean strain values and confidence intervals.

21. **Answer: A.** Radial strain imaging displaying multiple waveforms from a 3D model. Note the strain waveforms are positive, which reflects thickening of the left ventricle during systole. The average strain in this patient is 35%, which is normal.

The clue that this is a 3D model is the VPS (voxels per second) of 26. Unlike a pixel, which represents graphic information in 2D space with its x- and y-axis coordinates, a voxel represents a unit of graphic information in 3D space requiring the z-axis coordinates. Currently, an inherent limitation of 3D myocardial deformation imaging is the relatively low temporal resolution (26 VPS), whereas 2D myocardial deformation is typically acquired at double that rate.

22. **Answer: C.** Circumferential strain rate imaging was obtained at the basal level of the parasternal short-axis view (**Video 31-6**). Unlike strain imaging, which typically includes just one peak (systolic) value reported during the cardiac cycle, strain rate imaging permits three reported measurements, including the systolic (S′) strain rate, early diastolic (E′) strain rate, and late diastolic (A′) strain rate (**Figure 31-20**). Answer A is incorrect because the strain rate is obtained in the parasternal short-axis view, not in an apical (longitudinal) view. Answers B and D are incorrect because like longitudinal strain imaging, radial strain imaging includes one peak that is reported.

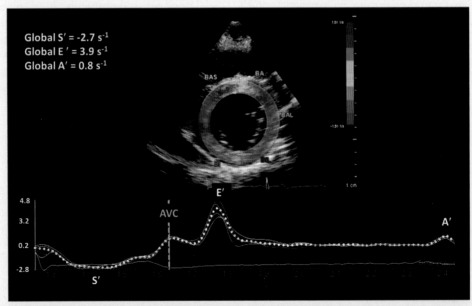

Figure 31-20 Circumferential strain rate (CSR) imaging obtained at the parasternal short-axis mitral valve level in a normal patient with bradycardia. Observe that the three waveforms that can be measured include S′, E′, and A′. As with tissue Doppler imaging, the peaks of the three waveforms are similar in timing. The white dotted line represents the global values that are averaged from the six segments around the left ventricle. The CSR E′ is typically the highest value observed in the normal myocardium; in this example, CSR E′ is 3.9 s⁻¹. Both systolic and diastolic SR can be measured.

23. **Answer: C.** The World Alliance Societies of Echocardiography (WASE) results for lower limits of normal GLS were −17% to −19% in 15 countries studied, except for Korea in whom it was −16% (males), −17% (females), respectively. Lower limits of normal GLS for India was −17% (males), −18% (females); Australia was −17% (both male and female); and United States of America was −17% (male), −18% (female). Therefore, answers A, B, and D are incorrect. Another important observation demonstrated that in the global WASE population, females had higher GLS than males, with the upper limits of normal of −24% in males and −26% in females.

24. **Answer: C.** Lagrangian strain is calculated as the change in length divided by the original length and is the most common type of strain applied to the algorithm for 2D speckle tracking. Answer A, Eulerian strain, and answer B, natural strain, are the same type of strain. The calculation for natural or Eulerian strain is the change in length divided by the instantaneous length. Answer A is not a type of strain applied to ultrasound imaging. Note that the abovementioned strains are named after the two mathematicians Joseph-Louis Lagrange and Leonhard Euler.

25. **Answer: D. Figure 31-8** shows a calculation of radial strain using a short-axis image at the level of the papillary muscles. The calculated radial strain is abnormal at 11% (normal is 40%-60%). As the patient has already received a dose of 450 mg/m², and the radial strain is abnormal, which is suggestive of subclinical left ventricular dysfunction, the most likely course of treatment would be to discontinue anthracycline, switch her to a non-anthracycline–containing regimen, and initiate heart failure therapy.

26. **Answer: B. Figure 31-9** shows the bull's-eye plot reporting normal GLS in this patient. The ultrasensitive troponin I is also normal (<30 pg/mL). Using the data from Sawaya et al. (2012), a GLS < −19% or troponin I >30 pg/mL predicted subsequent cardiotoxicity (that is, a reduction in left ventricular ejection fraction >10% from baseline). As such, it would be appropriate to reassure the referring oncologist and to have him or her continue with the prescribed treatment.

Acknowledgments: We would like to thank Bonita Anderson and Margaret (Koko) Park for including us in this interactive and contemporary textbook. It is an honor to be included in such a publication that we believe is one of the most educational echocardiography textbooks to date. In addition, we would like to recognize the contributions of Juan Carlos Plana Gomez, MD, for his outstanding original work (Chapter 9, Tissue Doppler and strain. In: *Clinical Echocardiography Review: A Self-Assessment Tool*, 2nd ed., edited by Allan L. Klein, Craig R. Asher; 2017) that provided the foundation in writing this chapter. Lastly, we would like to thank the ultrasound industry for their tireless efforts in advancing speckle technology allowing sonographers and clinicians to unlock the "Rosetta Stone" of myocardial deformation.

SUGGESTED READINGS

Amundsen BH, Helle-Valle T, Edvardsen T, et al. Noninvasive myocardial strain measurement by speckle tracking echocardiography: validation against sonomicrometry and tagged magnetic resonance imaging. *J Am Coll Cardiol*. 2006;47(4):789-793.

Asch FM, Miyoshi T, Addetia K, et al. Similarities and differences in left ventricular size and function among races and nationalities: Results of the World Alliance Societies of Echocardiography Normal Values Study. *J Am Soc Echocardiogr*. 2019;32:1396-1406.

Cho GY, Marwick TH, Kim HS, et al. Global 2-dimensional strain as a new prognosticator in patients with heart failure. *J Am Coll Cardiol*. 2009;54(7):618-624.

D'hooge J, Heimdal A, Jamal F, et al. Regional strain and strain rate measurements by cardiac ultrasound: principles, implementation and limitations. *Eur J Echocardiogr*. 2000;1(3):154-170.

Horton KD, Meece RW, Hill JC. Assessment of the right ventricle by echocardiography: a primer for cardiac sonographers. *J Am Soc Echocardiogr*. 2009;22(7):776-792.

Hurlburt HM, Aurigemma GP, Hill JC, et al. Direct ultrasound measurement of longitudinal, circumferential and radial strain using 2-dimensional strain imaging in normal adults. *Echocardiography*. 2007;24(7):723-731.

Kaku K, Takeuchi M, Tsang W, et al. Age-related normal range of left ventricular strain and torsion using three-dimensional speckle-tracking echocardiography. *J Am Soc Echocardiogr*. 2014;27(1):55-64.

Kusunose K, Goodman A, Parikh R, et al. Incremental prognostic value of left ventricular global longitudinal strain in patients with aortic stenosis and preserved ejection fraction. *Circ Cardiovasc Imaging*. 2014;7(6):938-945.

Negishi K, Negishi T, Hare JL, et al. Independent and incremental value of deformation indices for the prediction of trastuzumab-induced cardiotoxicity. *J Am Soc Echocardiogr*. 2013;26(5):493-498.

Negishi K, Negishi T, Kurosawa K, et al. Practical guidance in echocardiographic assessment of global longitudinal strain. *JACC Cardiovasc Imaging*. 2015;8(4):489-492.

Phelan D, Collier P, Thavendiranathan P, et al. Relative apical sparing of longitudinal strain using two-dimensional speckle-tracking echocardiography is both sensitive and specific for the diagnosis of cardiac amyloidosis. *Heart*. 2012;98(19):1442-1448.

Plana JC, Galderisi M, Barac A, et al. Expert consensus for multimodality imaging evaluation of adult patients during and after cancer therapy: a report from the American Society of Echocardiography and the European Association of Cardiovascular Imaging. *J Am Soc Echocardiogr*. 2014;27:911-939.

Plana Gomez JC. Tissue Doppler and strain. In: Klein AL, Asher CR, eds. *Clinical Echocardiography Review: A Self-Assessment Tool*. 2nd ed. Philadelphia, PA: Wolters Kluwer; 2017:chap 9.

Rajagopal S, Forsha DE, Risum N, et al. Comprehensive assessment of right ventricular function in patients with pulmonary hypertension with global longitudinal peak systolic strain derived from multiple right ventricular views. *J Am Soc Echocardiogr*. 2014;27(6):657-665.

Sawaya H, Sebag IA, Plana JC, et al. Assessment of echocardiographic and biomarkers for the extended prediction of cardiotoxicity in patients with anthracyclines, taxanes and trastuzumab. *Circ Cardiovasc Imaging.* 2012;5(5):596-603.

Takeuchi M, Nakai H, Kokumai M, et al. Age-related changes in left ventricular twist assessed by two-dimensional speckle-tracking Imaging. *J Am Soc Echocardiogr.* 2006;19(9):1077-1084.

Takigiku K, Takeuchi M, Izumi C, et al. Normal range of left ventricular 2-dimensional strain: Japanese Ultrasound Speckle Tracking of the Left Ventricle (JUSTICE) study. *Circ J.* 2012;76(11):2623-2632.

Voigt JU, Pedrizzetti G, Lysyansky P, et al. Definitions for a common standard for 2D speckle tracking echocardiography. Consensus document of the EACVI/ASE/Industry Task Force to standardize deformation imaging. *Eur Heart J Cardiovasc Imaging.* 2015;16(1):1-11.

Voigt JU. Incidence and characteristics of segmental postsystolic longitudinal shortening in normal, acutely ischemic, and scarred myocardium. *J Am Soc Echocardiogr.* 2003;16(5):415-423.

Yingchoncharoen T, Agarwal S, Popovic Z, et al. Normal ranges of left ventricular strain: a meta-analysis. *J Am Soc Echocardiogr.* 2013;26(2):185-191.

CHAPTER 32

Ultrasound Enhancing Agents

Contributors: Joan J. Olson, BS, RDCS, RVT and Paul F. Braum, BS, RDCS, RCS, RVT, RVS, ACS

☆ Question 1

The United States of America (USA) Food and Drug Administration (FDA) has approved three microbubble contrast agents for left ventricular opacification and endocardial border detection. The FDA-approved commercial agents are:
- A. Echogen, Lumason, and Definity.
- B. Optison, Definity, and Sonazoid.
- C. Optison, Lumason, and Definity.
- D. SonoVue, Optison, and Definity.

☆ Question 2

Agitated saline, used as an ultrasound enhancing agent (UEA), is effective in all of the following conditions except for:
- A. Detecting a patent foramen ovale.
- B. Detecting a persistent left superior vena cava.
- C. Detecting a pulmonary arteriovenous malformation.
- D. Enhancing the spectral Doppler signal of mitral regurgitation (MR).

☆☆ Question 3

Which of the following lists the proper supplies needed to perform an agitated saline contrast study?
- A. 2 × 10 cc syringes, intravenous (IV) extension with two ports, and a mixture of 10% air and 90% saline
- B. 2 × 10 cc syringes, IV extension with two ports, and a mixture of 10% air, 10% blood, and 80% saline

- C. Three-way stopcock, 2 × 10 cc syringes, 20-gauge IV cannula, and a mixture of 10% air, 10% blood, and 80% saline
- D. Three-way stopcock, 2 × 10 cc syringes, 20-gauge IV cannula, and a mixture of 10% air, and 90% saline

☆ Question 4

Based on expert consensus, what is the definition of inadequate left ventricular (LV) endocardial border resolution?
- A. Failure to detect wall motion in five or greater LV segments in the 17-segment model
- B. Failure to detect two or more contiguous LV segments
- C. Failure to detect three or more contiguous LV segments
- D. Failure to delineate all LV segments in all apical views

☆ Question 5

Based on the most recent Food and Drug Administration (FDA) labeling, what is still considered a contraindication to the use of all ultrasound enhancing agents (UEAs)?
- A. Allergy to blood products
- B. History of hypersensitivity to the agent
- C. Right-to-left intracardiac shunting
- D. Severe pulmonary hypertension
- E. All of the above

585

✪ Question 6

As per the 2014 American Society of Echocardiography (ASE) contrast guidelines for the cardiac sonographer, very low mechanical index (VLMI) represents multi-pulse cancellation sequences that are most effective at mechanical index (MI) values of:

A. <0.2.
B. <0.3.
C. 0.3 to 0.5.
D. None of the above.

✪✪ Question 7

The variables that determine the mechanical index (MI) include:

A. Attenuation and peak negative pressure.
B. Gain setting and peak negative pressure.
C. Peak negative pressure and transmit frequency.
D. Spatial peak temporal average (in Watts/cm²) and transmit frequency.

✪✪ Question 8

During the administration of an ultrasound enhancing agent to delineate endocardial borders, which image adjustment is most likely to enhance the image for improved resolution?

A. Decreasing the imaging frequency
B. Decreasing the mechanical index
C. Decreasing the sector size
D. Narrowing the sector angle
E. All of the above

✪✪ Question 9

When performing contrast imaging and there is shadowing at the level of the basal/mid segments of the left ventricle, which correction method would be appropriate in this instance?

A. Slow down infusion or reduce bolus size and flush rate.
B. Increase the infusion rate.
C. Increase the overall gain.
D. None of the above.

✪✪ Question 10

For which of the following clinical indications has ultrasound transpulmonary contrast not been shown to be beneficial?

A. Detection of endovascular leaks following aortic endograft placement
B. Detection of intracarotid artery plaque and plaque vascularity
C. Detection of left atrial appendage thrombi during transesophageal echocardiography
D. Detection of patent ductus arteriosus in children and adults

✪✪ Question 11

Which statement accurately reflects the current standard on the use of any commercially available transpulmonary ultrasound enhancing agent (UEA) for echocardiography in both pregnancy and pediatrics?

A. Each agent has its own information regarding its use; however, in general, it is acceptable to use them when the benefit outweighs the risk.
B. The use of any of these agents is acceptable and should be used without hesitation.
C. The use of any of these agents is strictly prohibited.
D. There is only one agent approved for use in both pregnancy and pediatrics.

✪✪ Question 12

While administering an ultrasound enhancing agent (Definity) to a patient, the patient experienced back pain. Which of the following statements is false?

A. The back pain usually resolves with discontinuation of the ultrasound enhancing agent.
B. This is considered a precursor to a severe anaphylactic reaction.
C. This is most likely related to the lipid shell of the microbubble.
D. Switching to Optison is an option if additional contrast is needed.

✪✪ Question 13

▶ A 50-year-old man has an echocardiogram for the follow-up assessment of left ventricular (LV) systolic function. Past cardiac history includes an anterior ST segment elevation myocardial infarction (STEMI) with cardiac arrest, percutaneous coronary intervention in the left anterior descending (LAD) coronary artery, hyperlipidemia, and obesity. The previous echocardiogram performed 6 months earlier indicated moderate to severely reduced left ventricular systolic function with a reported ejection fraction of

30% to 35%. Regional wall motion was reported as anterior and anteroseptal wall akinesis with apical dyskinesis. Based on the images provided (**Videos 32-1A** to **32-1D**), which statement is correct?

A. There is apical akinesis with an acute thrombus in the LV apex.

B. There is apical akinesis with an ectopic chordae in the LV apex.

C. There is apical hypokinesis with a vascularized mass in the LV apex.

D. There is lateral wall hypokinesis with an ectopic chordae in the LV apex.

✪✪✪ Question 14

A 50-year-old man presents with shortness of breath. An echocardiogram was ordered and an ultrasound enhancing agent (UEA) was administered. Based on the image provided in **Video 32-2**, which of the following would be the correct diagnosis?

A. Apical hypertrophic cardiomyopathy

B. Left ventricular apical thrombus

C. Noncompaction cardiomyopathy

D. None of the above

✪✪✪ Question 15

A 65-year-old man had an echocardiogram ordered due to increasing shortness of breath and fatigue. Past medical history includes a late presenting inferior myocardial infarction with moderate papillary muscle involvement and subsequent severe mitral regurgitation leading to coronary artery bypass surgery and a mitral valve replacement (MVR). The previous echocardiogram performed 3 months earlier showed severely depressed left ventricular function with an

ejection fraction of 25% to 30%, inferior wall akinesis with a small aneurysm at the base, and a well-seated MVR. Based on **Video 32-3** acquired from an apical 2-chamber view, which of the following statements reflects the correct diagnosis?

A. There is a large inferior wall pseudoaneurysm without rupture.

B. There is an inferior wall aneurysm rupture and containment by the pericardium.

C. There is a pericardial effusion present consistent with Dressler syndrome.

D. There is mechanical MVR dysfunction.

✪✪✪ Question 16

The use of myocardial perfusion (MP) imaging with ultrasound enhancing agents (UEAs) has increased in which of the following settings?

A. Stress echocardiography

B. Chest pain evaluation in the emergency room

C. The evaluation of intracardiac masses

D. All of the above

✪✪✪ Question 17

Ultrasound enhancing agents (UEAs) are recommended to characterize cardiac masses and to integrate all of the information to establish the etiologies of these masses and to potentially avoid diagnostic errors. Based on the apical 4-chamber view images provided in **Figure 32-1**, what is the correct diagnosis for this patient?

A. Metastatic tumor

B. Myxoma

C. Papillary fibroelastoma

D. Thrombus in the right ventricle

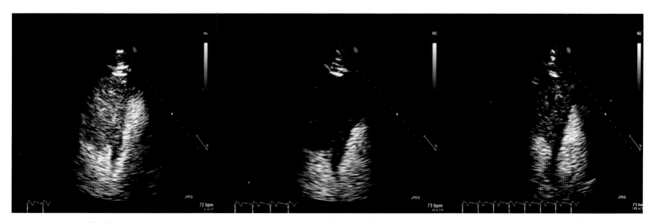

Preflash   Immediate postflash   5 beats postflash

Figure 32-1 Apical 4-chamber view.

✪✪ Question 18

Which of the following is not an advantage of a continuous infusion of an ultrasound enhancing agent (UEA) compared to a bolus injection?

    A. Reduced left ventricular (LV) cavity acoustic shadowing

    B. Reduced far-field attenuation

    C. Quantification of myocardial perfusion

    D. Ease of infusion

✪✪✪ Question 19

Which of the following is an emerging application for the use of ultrasound enhancing agents (UEAs)?

    A. Thrombolysis

    B. Molecular imaging

    C. Targeted drug/gene delivery

    D. Diagnostic ultrasound–induced inertial cavitation

    E. All of the above

✪✪ Question 20

Studies examining the risk versus benefit of ultrasound enhancing agents (UEAs) in acute critical care settings have demonstrated:

    A. The use of intravenous UEAs to be associated with a slight increase in all-cause early mortality.

    B. An increased risk for anaphylactic reactions when compared to an outpatient setting.

    C. A significant reduction in all-cause mortality when contrast is utilized.

    D. Less beneficial effects but no difference in risk when compared to an outpatient setting.

✪✪ Question 21

What specific change in ultrasound enhancing agent composition led to improved transpulmonary passage and left ventricular opacification for the current Food and Drug Administration (FDA)–approved agents?

    A. Change in microbubble shell composition

    B. Change in gas molecular weight

    C. Utilization of nitrogen gas–filled microbubbles

    D. Continuous infusion of contrast instead of a bolus injection

✪ Question 22

The current Food and Drug Administration (FDA) indication for the use of ultrasound enhancing agents (UEAs) is:

    A. Myocardial perfusion.

    B. Doppler enhancement.

    C. Stress echocardiography.

    D. Improvement in left ventricular opacification.

✪ Question 23

The very low mechanical index (VLMI) imaging techniques available on most systems have been shown to permit which of the following off- and on-label clinical applications?

    A. Myocardial perfusion imaging

    B. Improved endocardial border resolution

    C. Detection and evaluation of intracardiac masses

    D. All of the above

✪✪ Question 24

Figure 32-2 is an apical 4-chamber view acquired during an agitated saline injection into an upper extremity vein. The center image was recorded immediately after the first appearance of contrast was seen entering the right atrium (RA); smaller inset image (upper left corner) was recorded several cardiac cycles later. Which answer below supports the likely diagnosis?

    A. Patent foramen ovale (PFO)

    B. Sinus venosus defect (ASD)

    C. Pulmonary arteriovenous malformation

    D. Persistent left superior vena cava

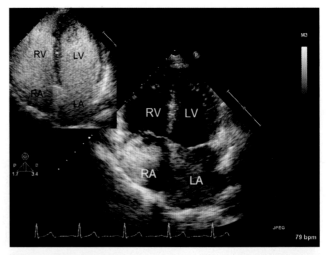

Figure 32-2 (Reprinted with permission from Armstrong WF, Ryan T, eds. *Feigenbaum's Echocardiography.* 7th ed. Philadelphia, PA: Wolters Kluwer Health/Lippincott Williams & Wilkins; 2010.)

CASE 1

A 65-year-old woman post recent abdominal surgery developed a postoperative gastric wound infection and shortness of breath. This was followed by a pulmonary embolism. Cardiac testing included a venous duplex exam that was positive for deep vein thrombosis in the right calf. Additionally, an echocardiogram was ordered.

✪✪ Question 25

▶ Based on the images provided in **Videos 32-4A** and **4B** (apical 4-chamber unenhanced images) and **Videos 32-5A** and **5B** (apical 4-chamber enhanced images), the patient appears to have:

   A. Right ventricular (RV) thrombus with a mobile attachment and a mobile interatrial septum (IAS).
   B. RV hypertrophy, a thickened moderator band, and an IAS aneurysm.
   C. Right and left ventricular thrombi with a mobile IAS.
   D. An RV mass with a left-to-right shunt and a mobile IAS.

CASE 2

▶ A 55-year-old man presents to the emergency room (ER) with tinnitus and an elevated blood pressure of 226/126 mm Hg. The electrocardiogram shows borderline ST elevation in the anterior leads. A stat echocardiogram with an ultrasound enhancing

agent (UEA) was performed to improve left ventricular border delineation and better assess wall motion and systolic thickening.

Images from the initial echocardiogram performed in the emergency room (ER) are shown in **Video 32-6A** (apical 4-chamber view), **Video 32-6B** (apical 2-chamber view), and **Video 32-6C** (apical long-axis view). The patient was taken to the cardiac catheterization laboratory immediately after the ER echo and a stent was placed due to a significant proximal left anterior descending artery (LAD) occlusion. Another echocardiogram was performed 36 hours post cardiac catheterization that included myocardial perfusion imaging with flash (**Video 32-7A**, apical 4-chamber view; **Video 32-7B**, apical 2-chamber view; and **Video 32-7C**, apical long-axis view).

✪✪✪ Question 26

What conclusions can be drawn from the post–cardiac catherization echocardiographic images?

   A. No improvement in the LAD territory noted; scar and thinning remain
   B. Improved perfusion of the LAD territory with no residual wall motion abnormality
   C. Improved perfusion of the LAD territory with residual wall motion abnormality
   D. Perfusion cannot be analyzed as the exam was not correctly performed

ANSWERS

1. **Answer: C.** Although SonoVue is the name of Bracco's agent in Europe, it was called "Lumason" in the USA when approved in 2014. Both SonoVue and Lumason are the same sulfur hexafluoride–containing microbubble. Optison and Definity contain perfluoropropane gas and have been approved for years in the USA.

2. **Answer: D.** Agitated saline as a UEA is very useful for determining both intracardiac and intrapulmonary shunts. It is also useful for determining connections in the venous system such as persistent left superior vena cava. Agitated saline is classified as a UEA but is not a transpulmonary agent. Therefore, its use in anything in the left heart is not viable as its bubbles are too large to pass through the pulmonary capillary bed. This would make enhancing a spectral Doppler signal in the left heart such as MR impossible.

KEY POINT

The vessels within the pulmonary capillary bed are approximately 2 μm in size, and the average bubble created by agitated saline is 3 to 6 μm. The large bubble size eliminates the use of agitated saline in the left heart. The transpulmonary UEAs create bubbles that are 0.7 to 1.1 μm and are easily capable of passing through the pulmonary capillary bed, thus, illuminating the left side of the heart.

3. **Answer: C.** The use of agitated saline as a UEA has been reported as far back as the 1970s. The establishment of best-case practices has evolved over time to reflect the best supplies and optimal techniques that enhance the likelihood of a successful agitated saline enhancement study. Those supplies include two 10 cc syringes, a three-way stopcock, an IV cannula ≥20 gauge, an IV start kit, and an extension set

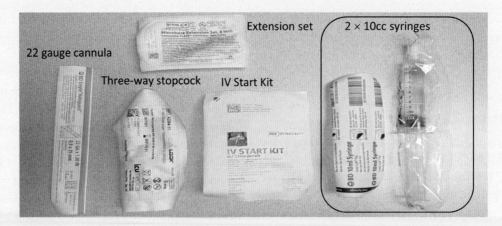

Figure 32-3A

(**Figure 32-3A**). The three-way stopcock enables three-way flow from inlet to outlet, inlet to side port, or side port to outlet; this enables the mixing of the patient's blood with saline and the agitation of the blood and saline mix between both syringes before it is injected into a peripheral vein (**Figure 32-3B**). The optimal preparation of the saline itself is a mixture of 10% air, 10% patient's blood, and 80% saline.

TEACHING POINT

Introducing some of the patient's blood into the saline mixture enhances the agitated saline contrast study by generating smaller microbubbles as well as increasing the concentration of microbubbles injected. Furthermore, there is a greater ultrasound reflection of fragmented red blood cells or scattered cellular content secondary to hemolysis from agitation.

4. **Answer: B.** Although arbitrary, the definition of inadequate border resolution has been defined as inability to delineate two contiguous borders on a noncontrast echocardiogram. Therefore, for the accurate estimation of LV ejection fraction (LVEF) and/or for the accurate analysis of LV regional wall motion, ultrasound enhancing agents should be used when two or more LV segments cannot be visualized adequately.

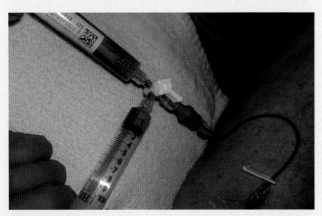

Figure 32-3B

5. **Answer: B.** Since the original Box Warning in 2007, the FDA has removed several contraindications and requirements for monitoring after the administration of contrast. **Table 32-1** lists the three commercially available UEAs approved by the FDA including the contraindications for each. Optison and Definity are also contraindicated in patients with known hypersensitivity to perflutren, while Lumason is contraindicated in patients with histories of hypersensitivity reactions to sulfur hexafluoride lipid microsphere components or to any of the inactive ingredients in Lumason. Therefore, answer B is correct.

Although allergy to blood products (answer A) is a contraindication to giving Optison, it does not pertain to all contrast agents. Since 2016, all three UEAs have announced that the FDA has removed the contraindication for UEAs use in patients with known or suspected right-to-left (answer C), bidirectional, or transient right-to-left intracardiac shunts. Severe pulmonary hypertension (answer D) is no longer a contraindication.

6. **Answer: A.** Tissue cancellation techniques such as multipulse cancellation sequences use very low mechanical index (VLMI) to enhance microbubble contrast and eliminate tissue signals. VLMI contrast imaging is more effective at MI values <0.2. Low MI represents harmonic imaging techniques that are used at MI values <0.3, intermediate MI represents harmonic imaging techniques used at MIs of 0.3 to 0.5, and high MI is any MI that exceeds 0.5. Real-time VLMI techniques are available on nearly all newer commercially available ultrasound imaging systems.

7. **Answer: C.** The MI is a measure of acoustic power. The MI can be defined as peak negative pressure divided by the square root of the transmit frequency (units in megahertz). The adjustment of the MI is especially important in studies using ultrasound enhancing agents, in order to avoid microbubble destruction.

8. **Answer: B.** Decreasing the mechanical index (MI) reduces bubble destruction and allows for sustained

Table 32-1. The Three Commercially Available UEAs Approved by the FDA

Name	Manufacturer/ Vial Contents	Mean Diameter	Shell	Gas	Contraindications
Lumason (sulfur hexafluoride lipid-type A microspheres)	Bracco Diagnostics, 5 mL	1.5-2.5 µm (maximum 20 µm, 99% ≤10 µm)	Phospholipid	Sulfur hexafluoride	Allergy to sulfur hexafluoride
Definity (perflutren lipid microsphere)	Lantheus Medical Imaging, 1.5 mL	1.1-3.3 µm (maximum 20 µm, 98% ≤10 µm)	Phospholipid	Perflutren	Allergy to perflutren
Optison (perflutren protein type A microspheres)	GE Healthcare, 3.0 mL	3.0-4.5 µm (maximum 32 µm, 95% ≤10 µm)	Human albumin	Perflutren	Allergy to perflutren/blood products

Reprinted from Porter TR, Mulvagh SL, Abdelmoneim SS, et al. Clinical applications of ultrasonic enhancing agents in echocardiography: 2018 American Society of Echocardiography Guidelines Update. *J Am Soc Echocardiogr*. 2018;31(3):241-274. Copyright © 2018 by the American Society of Echocardiography. With permission.

imaging times at lower doses. A very low MI (VLMI) has been shown to improve the enhancement of endocardial borders and therefore has a greater sensitivity for detecting wall motion abnormalities with the added benefit of demonstrating bubble uptake in the myocardium itself or myocardial perfusion. Contrast-enhanced myocardial perfusion techniques utilize much lower MIs and have demonstrated greater sensitivity for detecting obstruction in the coronary system when balanced ischemia is present. The remaining adjustments would lead to enhanced bubble destruction and therefore would not lead to image enhancement (**Table 32-2**).

9. **Answer: A.** Bolus injection can result in severe shadowing (an ultrasound enhancing agent artifact called attenuation) of the basal to middle left ventricular cavity; over time the shadowing will resolve as the accumulation of contrast begins to reduce. The best method to correct for shadowing (caused by attenuation from too much contrast) is to slow down the infusion rate or reduce bolus size and flush rate. Increasing the infusion rate (answer B) is incorrect as this would create more shadowing. Increasing or decreasing the overall gain (answer C) will have no effect on eliminating attenuation as overall gain does not cause bubble destruction.

Contrast agent administration should be done with either harmonic low-MI imaging or with VLMI real-time software.

10. **Answer: D.** Intravenous contrast has provided additional information aside from left ventricular opacification by improving both the detection of carotid plaque and plaque neovascularity in carotid ultrasound imaging. It also has been utilized to differentiate spontaneous contrast from thrombus during transesophageal echocardiography and to detect endoleaks following percutaneous vascular stent endografts. It is not utilized for detection of intracardiac shunts, which may require agitated saline but not transpulmonary contrast agents.

11. **Answer: A.** Each agent has its own statement on its use in pregnancy and pediatrics. It is recommended that the package insert for the UEA planned for use is read for specific details. In general, all UEAs come with a statement indicating that their use in echocardiography is not well established and is limited due to lack of data. In this case, the use of these agents is acceptable when the benefit outweighs the risk.

One agent has been approved for use in pediatrics; however, its use has been restricted to general ultrasound for opacifying the liver and urinary tracts and therefore has no relevance to echocardiography. It is important to note that this is the case for many UEAs that are produced in the pharmacy realm and the lack of data does not always preclude its use. The lack of data for the use of these UEAs in pregnancy and pediatrics is common due to the lack of subjects willing to undergo clinical trials while pregnant or to subject their children to the same.

12. **Answer: B.** Back pain is an infrequent complication that has been exclusively seen with intravenous Definity use. It has not been reported with Optison, and thus this ultrasound enhancing agent could be utilized in a patient who experiences back pain with Definity. Although the exact cause for back pain is unknown, it is most likely related to the lipid shell composition since it is not seen with albumin-shelled agents. It should not be considered a precursor to the more severe anaphylactoid reactions, which are rare (reported at less than 1 in 10,000).

13. ▶ **Answer: A.** There is clearly apical dilatation and akinesis in both the enhanced and unenhanced images. The enhanced images (**Videos 32-1B** and **32-1D**) reveal the apical myocardium is thin with no apparent uptake of the ultrasound enhancing agent (UEA), indicating lack of perfusion typical

Table 32-2.

Control	Detail	Effect on Image	Effect on Contrast
Frequency	Adjustable between 2-4 MHz	Increases penetration Decreases resolution	The higher the frequency, the better the image The lower the frequency, the image degrades
Focal zone	Adjustable by size and length	Variable near field, enhances image resolution	Enhances image resolution
Mechanical index (estimate of peak acoustic intensity)	Adjustable (output power)	When high: increases penetration and beam strength When low: decreases beam strength	When high: destroys bubbles and decreases time bubbles are visible When low: destroys less bubbles and increases time bubbles are visible
Depth/field of view	Adjustable depth range for image	Allows imaging at greater depth, requires increased power, and decreases frame rate as depth increases	Increasing image depth reduces the frame rate and therefore reduces the chance of bubble destruction; however, overall image resolution may be compromised
Gain	Adjustable. Has two controls: overall and time-gain compensation	When increased: enhances returning echo image by increasing the echoes that are displayed	Adjusts the amount of amplification of the returning echo signals. Higher gains result in a brighter signal (excessive gain can cause blooming artifact and increased overall image noise level). Lower gains result in a diminished signal (loss of contrast effect)
Dynamic range	Adjustable; controls the range of signals that can be enhanced	Increases or decreases the gray scale that can be displayed	For left ventricular opacification, dynamic range should be set to a lower level For myocardial perfusion imaging, a higher dynamic range will result in lower level signals being seen
Compression	Adjustable related to dynamic range. Compresses or expands the dynamic range	Enhances gray scale setting that can be achieved by dynamic range	Increased dynamic range: Further enhances image Decreased dynamic range: less shades of gray; image appears more contrasty
Sector size	Increases and decreases sector width	When decreased: increases the frame rate while narrowing the image width, thus improves resolution When increased: decreases the frame rate while widening the image width, reduces resolution	When increased: a wider sector width will have a lower frame rate and thus not affect bubble destruction. A narrow sector will have a higher frame rate and potentially enhance bubble destruction
Doppler signals	Spectral signals only (pulsed-wave and continuous-wave)	Quantifies the velocity of flow	Enhances the signal with contrast as a reflector Adjust Doppler gains low to reduce signal to noise ratio (approximately 30% Doppler Gain). Perform once contrast effect is reduced as Doppler enhancement requires very little contrast

Courtesy of Lantheus Medical Imaging; with adaptations.

of infarcted muscle. The nonenhanced images (**Videos 32-1A** and **32-1C**) fail to demonstrate the acute thrombus present in the apex. Fresh thrombus has the same density as blood and is thus sonolucent. This is a great example of the need to use UEAs when there is any wall motion abnormality, especially when the anterior wall or apex is involved. The sonolucent nature of the mass rules out any solid structure such as an ectopic chordae or solid mass (answers B, C, and D). The fact that this is a routine follow-up examination after an anterior apical infarction with no symptoms suggestive of an embolic event is a great reminder of how these agents are a necessity for best clinical outcomes. In this case, the incidental finding led to a new therapy to prevent the possibility of a cerebral vascular accident.

KEY POINT

This case highlights the importance of using a UEA when there is a wall motion abnormality, especially when the apex is involved. The fact that this is a routine follow-up examination of a known anterior infarction with apical akinesis with no symptoms suggestive of an embolic event is a great reminder of the how UEAs are a necessity for best clinical outcomes. In this case, the incidental finding led to a new therapy to prevent the possibility of a cerebral vascular accident.

14. **Answer: C.** Noncompaction cardiomyopathy is uncommon. It is an increasingly recognized abnormality that can lead to heart failure, arrhythmias, cardioembolic events, and death. Due to the alterations of myocardial structure, thickened hypokinetic segments consist of two layers: a thin, compacted subepicardial myocardial layer and a thicker, noncompacted subendocardial layer.

    When left ventricular noncompaction is suspected, UEAs may be helpful in identifying the characteristic deep intertrabecular recesses by showing contrast-enhanced filling of intracavitary blood between the prominent left ventricular (LV) trabeculations (Figure 32-4). The recommendation in suspected noncompaction cases is to use a harmonic contrast setting with a myocardial index at 0.3 to 0.4 to help better delineate the myocardial trabeculations.

15. **Answer: B.** The enhanced apical 2-chamber view clearly demonstrates the appearance of the ultrasound enhancing agent (UEA) within the pericardial

space. This would instantly exclude Dressler syndrome as there should be no UEA within the pericardial space with this condition. The likely reason for the UEA in the pericardial space is a connection between the heart and the pericardium. The inferior wall aneurysm that was present 3 months earlier has grown large enough to rupture and make a connection with the pericardial space. Therefore, this is a contained rupture of an inferior wall aneurysm secondary to myocardial infarction. Without the use of a UEA, it is more than probable that this would have been diagnosed as a loculated pericardial effusion without tamponade physiology or quite possibly even Dressler syndrome.

16. **Answer: D.** The use of MP imaging with UEAs has increased, specifically in the setting of stress echocardiography, chest pain evaluation in the emergency room, and in the evaluation of intracardiac masses. The American Medical Association Current Procedural Terminology (CPT) Panel approved a category III for "myocardial contrast perfusion echocardiography; at rest or with stress, for assessment of myocardial ischemia or viability." The use of real-time very low mechanical index (MI) imaging in patients with chest pain adds additional diagnostic and prognostic information by simultaneously providing perfusion information. If complete replenishment of contrast is observed within 4 seconds in a segment with abnormal regional wall motion (i.e., normal perfusion), this identifies a patient at intermediate risk for cardiac events compared with a high-risk situation in which both a regional perfusion abnormality (delayed replenishment of contrast) and a wall motion abnormality exist. To differentiate a thrombus from an intracardiac tumor, real-time very low MI perfusion imaging with high-MI flash should be used if available. Thrombi are avascular and show no contrast enhancement after a high-MI flash impulse, as opposed to tumors, which may be vascularized

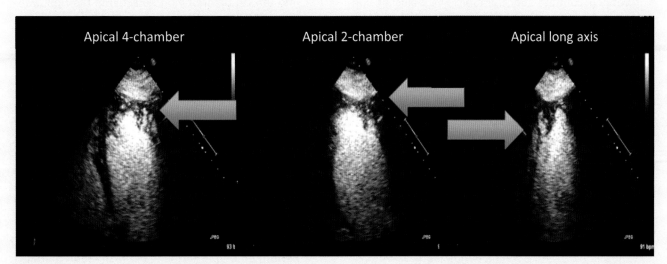

Figure 32-4 Arrows indicate the multiple deep trabeculations of the LV myocardium at the LV apex, which are clearly seen with the use of UEAs.

(when malignant) and will demonstrate proportional degrees of perfusion by flash replenishment real-time very low MI imaging.

17. **Answer: C.** The series of images shown in **Figure 32-1** demonstrate a metastatic tumor in the right ventricle (RV). Suspected intracardiac masses can be a normal variant of cardiac structure such as a false chord, accessory papillary muscle, or heavy trabeculation or can be pathologic such as thrombus, vegetation, or tumor. Echocardiographic perfusion imaging using a very low mechanical index (VLMI) with intermittent-flash (high-MI) technique has been demonstrated to characterize the vascularity of cardiac masses and to assist with the differentiation of malignant, highly vascular tumors from benign tumors or thrombi. Characterization is supported by qualitative and quantitative differences between the levels of perfusion (enhancement) in various types of cardiac masses in comparison to the adjacent myocardium. Malignant tumors show complete enhancement or hyperenhancement of the tumor (compared with the surrounding myocardium), thus, supporting the existence of a highly vascular tumor as in this case. Stromal tumors, such as myxomas, have a poor blood supply and appear partially enhanced. Thrombi or papillary fibroelastomas are generally avascular and show no enhancement. Potential pitfalls exist that may be due to the appearance of partial enhancement of the avascular structures in the far field. It is recommended that perfusion imaging be done in views that allow near-field visualization of microbubble replenishment following the high-MI impulses.

18. **Answer: D.** Continuous infusion of a UEA permits quantification of myocardial perfusion using destruction replenishment curves. Since the concentration of contrast is constant, the 1-exponential function can be utilized to examine contrast replenishment following destructive impulses. This cannot be done following a bolus injection, because of the varying contrast concentration. The bolus of contrast also can produce temporary acoustic shadowing and far-field attenuation that is seen to a lesser degree with continuous infusion.

19. **Answer: E.** All of the applications listed for this question are emerging uses of UEAs. Thrombolysis-specific applications include acute coronary syndromes and ischemic stroke. Molecular imaging is used for ischemic memory imaging, plaque formation, early plaque formation, and myocarditis/transplant rejection. Targeted drug/gene delivery–specific applications include DNA/RNA delivery for atherosclerosis, limb ischemia, myocardial regeneration, and antiangiogenesis in targeted tumor therapy. Diagnostic ultrasound–induced inertial cavitation applications include improved downstream skeletal muscle perfusion ischemic limbs (such as in sickle cell disease) and improved microvascular outcomes in acute coronary syndromes.

20. **Answer: C.** Large propensity-matched clinical outcomes data from the Premier database have demonstrated that patients receiving contrast-enhanced echocardiograms have an actual reduction in mortality when compared to patients receiving noncontrast echocardiograms.

21. **Answer: B.** The change from room air gas to higher molecular weight gases has led to longer persistence of microbubbles (due to reduced diffusivity and solubility) and consistent left ventricular (LV) opacification following venous injection or infusion. Although newer microbubbles contain polymer shells that may produce consistent LV opacification following venous injection, they are not yet approved.

22. **Answer: D.** Although UEAs have been shown to improve reader confidence during stress echocardiography, and to provide myocardial perfusion data that add incremental value, the current FDA approval is only to improve left ventricular opacification. It is not approved for stress echocardiography, Doppler enhancement, or for a myocardial perfusion indication.

23. **Answer: D.** VLMI imaging techniques are available on most commercially available systems (**Table 32-3**). These permit the enhancement of microbubble nonlinear behavior at these very low MIs while simultaneously reducing background tissue signals (which do not exhibit nonlinear behavior at very low MIs). This has been utilized not only to provide improved endocardial border delineation, but also to detect myocardial perfusion and perfusion of intracardiac masses.

24. **Answer: B.** The center image was recorded immediately after appearance of contrast was seen entering the right atrium (**Figure 32-2**). Note that contrast is seen in the RA and left atrium (LA) almost simultaneously. Concurrent early appearance of contrast into the LA before being detected in the right ventricle (RV) is consistent with a sinus venous defect (atrial septal defect) as a result of overriding of the superior vena cava (SVC) with immediate communication to the LA through anomalous right upper pulmonary venous drainage. Equal opacification of all four cardiac chambers is noted in the smaller insert image acquired several cardiac cycles later. Answer A is not correct; with a PFO contrast is usually seen entering RA first and then the right ventricle (RV) before any evidence of bubbles is seen in the left heart. Maneuvers such as Valsalva, cough, or pressing on the abdomen will increase right atrial pressure over left atrial pressure and allow manifestation of the right-to-left shunt. Therefore, agitated saline injection for the detection of a PFO should be performed under normal quiet respiration followed

Table 32-3. Commercially Available Very Low MI Pulse Sequence Schemes and Their Mechanism of Action

Descriptor	Company Manufacturer(s)	Tissue Cancellation Technique	Advantage(s)	Disadvantage(s)
Pulse-inversion Doppler and very low MI[a]	Philips Sonos/iE33 Toshiba Aplio/Xario GE 1.5-, 1.6-, and 1.7-MHz transducers	Alternating polarity	High resolution	Attenuation and dynamic range
Power modulation and very low MI[a]	Philips Sonos/iE33 GE 2.1- and 2.4-MHz transducers	Alternating amplitude	High sensitivity	Resolution, image quality, and dynamic range
Contrast pulse sequencing and very low MI[a]	Siemens Acuson	Both alternating polarity and alternating amplitude	Image quality and high sensitivity	Attenuation and dynamic range
Low MI[b] harmonic (LVO)	All vendors	B-mode; no cancellation	Image quality	Decreasing contrast sensitivity, apical swirling, and no perfusion

LVO, left ventricular opacification.

[a]Very low MI < 0.2.
[b]Low MI < 0.3.

by a second injection including a 10-second held Valsalva maneuver. Answer C is not correct; a right-to-left shunt from a pulmonary arteriovenous malformation (PAVM) would not appear in the left heart immediately after injection, as the shunt from a PAVM will first occur 5 to 15 beats after the bubbles are seen entering the right atrium. This delay represents the time required for the contrast to pass through the arterial bed, the PAVM, and into the pulmonary veins. The bubbles may also be identified originating through the pulmonary vein confluence and not from the interatrial septum. Answer D is incorrect; persistent left superior vena cava (LSVC) can be detected by identification of the contrast entering the coronary sinus before entering the RV. This is best demonstrated in an apical 4-chamber view oriented posteriorly to view the coronary sinus or from a parasternal long-axis view where the dilated coronary sinus and the RV can be seen simultaneously. The injection should be in left arm vein, and when a persistent LSVC is present, contrast can be seen entering the coronary sinus first, followed by the RA and RV.

25. **Answer: A.** The nonenhanced images (**Videos 32-4A** and **32-4B**) suggest possible right and left ventricular thrombi with a very mobile IAS. The RV thrombus has a smaller mobile attachment seen intermittently during the capture. The enhanced images (**Videos 32-5A** and **32-5B**) clearly define a large RV thrombus with a small mobile component and a mobile and aneurysmal IAS. There is no uptake of the contrast agent into the mass itself,

indicating (along with patient history and previous medical information) the mass is likely a thrombus. The left ventricular (LV) cavity appears to be thrombus-free with excellent contractility on the enhanced images. Answer B is incorrect; the RV free wall is not sufficiently delineated in these images to comment on RV hypertrophy and the moderator band is not visible with the large thrombus present. Answer C is incorrect as there is no LV thrombus seen in the enhanced images, although it is suspected in the nonenhanced images. Answer D is not the best choice, as a left-to-right shunt is not clearly identified on the enhanced images.

KEY POINT

Commercial ultrasound enhancing agents (UEAs) can identify as well as rule out suspected thrombus/mass in all four chambers of the heart. This case highlights why lab protocols should include using UEAs regardless of image quality whenever the diagnosis is to rule out a suspected cardiac source of emboli.

26. **Answer: C.** Improved perfusion of the LAD territory is seen with some residual wall motion abnormality remaining. Post–high mechanical index (MI) flash myocardial replenishment of the UEA should occur within 5 seconds during rest and 2 seconds with stress. Note that the areas indicated by the arrows in the post apical 4-chamber (**Figure 32-5A**), apical 2-chamber (**Figure 32-5B**), and apical long-axis (**Figure 32-5C**) views show less reperfusion and some remaining abnormal systolic thickening in

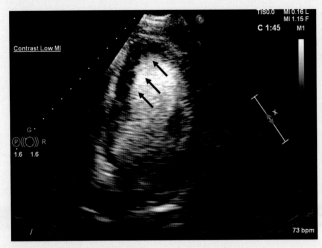

Figure 32-5A Apical 4-chamber view post procedure.

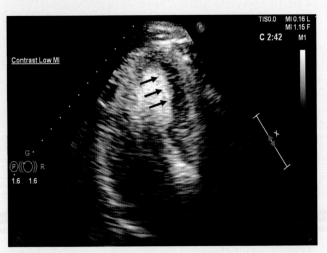

Figure 32-5C Apical long-axis view post procedure.

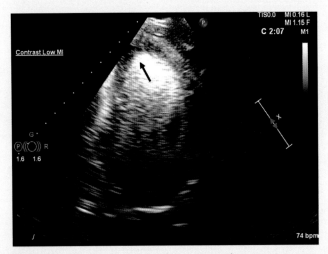

Figure 32-5B Apical 2-chamber view post procedure.

the septal (apicoseptal), inferoapical, and anterior segments, respectively. The true appreciation is best seen in the case study videos (**Videos 32-7A** to **32-7C**). Since the examination was performed only 36 hours post stent deployment, it is a reasonable indicator that the residual wall motion abnormality is likely hibernating myocardium and future improvement is yet to be seen. This postprocedure echocardiogram may also serve as a baseline for future follow-up studies.

Acknowledgments: The authors thank and acknowledge Thomas R. Porter, MD, Joan J. Olson, BS, and Feng Xie, MD (Chapter 11, Contrast-Enhanced Ultrasound Imaging) in *Clinical Echocardiography Review: A Self-Assessment Tool, 2nd ed.*, edited by Allan L. Klein, Craig R. Asher; 2017. The authors also thank Bhavin Patel, Jessica Hypolite, and Ina Butuc for their assistance in providing **Figure 32-3A** and **32-3B**.

SUGGESTED READINGS

Abdelmoneim SS, Bernier M, Scott CG, et al. Safety of contrast agent use during stress echocardiography in patients with elevated right ventricular systolic pressure: a cohort study. *Circ Cardiovasc Imaging.* 2010;3(3):240-248.

Acquatella H. Echocardiography in Chagas heart disease. *Circulation.* 2007;115(9):1124-1131.

Lindner JR, Porter TR, Park MM. *American Society of Echocardiography Guidelines and Recommendations for Contrast Echocardiography: A Summary for Applications Approved by the U.S. Food and Drug Administration.* https://www.asecho.org/wp-content/uploads/2018/07/Contrast-Echo-On-Label-Summary-FINAL-rev.pdf.

Marriott K, Manins V, Forshaw A, Wright J, Pascoe R. Detection of right-to-left atrial communication using agitated saline contrast imaging: experience with 1162 patients and recommendations for echocardiography. *J Am Soc Echocardiogr.* 2013;26(1):96-102.

Mulvagh SL, Rakowski H, Vannan MA, et al. American Society of echocardiography consensus statement on the clinical applications of ultrasonic contrast agents in echocardiography. *J Am Soc Echocardiogr.* 2008;21(11):1179-1201.

Porter TR, Abdelmoneim S, Belcik T, et al. Guidelines for the cardiac sonographer in the performance of contrast echocardiography: a focused update from the American Society of Echocardiography. *J Am Soc Echocardiogr.* 2014;27(8):797-810.

Porter TR, Mulvagh SL, Abdelmoneim S, et al. Clinical applications of ultrasonic enhancing agents in echocardiography: 2018 American Society of Echocardiography Guidelines Update. *J Am Soc Echocardiogr.* 2018;31(3):241-274.

Wei KJ. Utility contrast echocardiography in the emergency Department. *JACC Cardiovasc Imaging.* 2010;3(2):197-203.

CHAPTER 33

Stress Echocardiography: Ischemic and Nonischemic Heart Disease

Contributors: Tony Forshaw, BExSci, M Cardiac Ultrasound and Raymond R. Musarra, ACS, RCS, RDCS

✪ Question 1

A 77-year-old man with multiple cardiovascular risk factors complains of burning chest pain on exertion that is relieved by rest. During exercise echocardiography, which of the following is likely the latest event to be observed?
 A. Chest pain
 B. Regional and myocardial relaxation abnormality
 C. Regional wall motion abnormality
 D. ST-segment depression on electrocardiogram

✪ Question 2

Which row in Table 33-1 demonstrates a normal global and regional response to dobutamine infusion during stress echocardiography?
 A. A
 B. B
 C. C
 D. D

✪✪ Question 3

Which of the following statements regarding the left ventricular (LV) response to exercise is correct?
 A. Athletes have a larger resting LV cavity size with less improvement in contractility post exercise compared with nonathletes.
 B. The LV cavity size should be larger post exercise compared to preexercise to accommodate the increase in stroke volume that occurs with exercise.
 C. There is a reduction in LV cavity size due to the shorter diastolic filling period at higher heart rates.
 D. There is a reduction in LV cavity size post exercise in patients with severe mitral valve regurgitation due to the increased blood volume leaking back into the left atrium.

Table 33-1.

	Endocardial Excursion		LVESV		LVEF		Myocardial Thickening	
	LD	Peak	LD	Peak	LD	Peak	LD	Peak
A	↑	↑	↓	↓	↑	↑	↑	↑
B	↑	↑	↑	↑	↑	↓	↑	↓
C	↑	↑	↑	↑	↑	↑	↑	↑
D	↑	↓	↓	↓	↑	↑	↑	↓

LD, low dose; LVEF, left ventricular ejection fraction; LVESV, left ventricular end-systolic volume.

✪ Question 4

Which of the following would be considered an inappropriate indication for stress echocardiography?

A. Moderate, symptomatic mitral stenosis

B. Severe, asymptomatic aortic stenosis

C. Patient presenting with scleroderma

D. Patient presenting with a coronary calcium score of 480

E. Severe, symptomatic aortic regurgitation

✪ Question 5

Which of the following would be considered an absolute contraindication to treadmill stress echocardiography?

A. Severe mitral regurgitation

B. 3 mm ST-segment elevation in leads V2, V3, and V4 on the electrocardiogram

C. Known obstructive left main coronary artery stenosis

D. Pulmonary artery systolic pressure of 55 mm Hg

E. Resting systolic blood pressure of 210 mm Hg

✪✪ Question 6

Which scenario is indicative of a nondiagnostic treadmill stress echocardiogram for the exclusion of significant coronary artery disease in a 60-year-old female patient with exertional chest pain?

A. The patient completed 7 minutes of the Bruce protocol

B. The heart rate at peak exercise was 112 bpm

C. The patient did not experience her usual chest pain during the test

D. Postexercise image acquisition was completed in 58 seconds

✪ Question 7

A patient develops left-sided chest discomfort during stage 3 of the Bruce protocol. Which of the following additional parameters would necessitate immediate termination of exercise in this patient?

A. New onset left bundle branch block (LBBB) on the electrocardiogram (ECG)

B. Heart rate reaches maximum predicted heart rate

C. 2 mm ST-segment depression in leads II and III on the ECG

D. Systolic blood pressure (SBP) falls >10 mm Hg following an increase in workload

E. SBP reading increases from 180 to 200 mm Hg since last stage

✪ Question 8

Which of the following scenarios would not normally be assessed by stress echocardiography?

A. A patient with known lung sarcoidosis to assess for cardiac involvement

B. A patient whose recent medical examination showed elevated lipids, hypertension, and diabetes

C. A patient complaining of shortness of breath when walking up hills

D. A patient being considered for cardiac revascularization following prior myocardial infarction

E. A patient for the investigation of chest tightness

✪✪ Question 9

A 40-year-old man reports to the echocardiography laboratory for a transthoracic echocardiogram (TTE) due to dyspnea with exertion. The TTE reveals an E/e′ of 10, left atrial volume index of 25 mL/m^2, peak tricuspid valve regurgitant velocity of 2.0 m/s, and a reported ejection fraction of 60%. Based on these results, what additional testing may be helpful in assessing this patient's exertional dyspnea?

A. No additional testing is required as the resting TTE answered the clinical question

B. A diastolic stress echocardiogram

C. Dobutamine stress echocardiogram as patient experiences dyspnea with exertion

D. A perfusion stress echocardiogram with ultrasound enhancing agent

✪✪✪ Question 10

A 44-year-old woman complains of exertional substernal chest discomfort that limits her exercise capacity. She has type 2 diabetes mellitus and hypertension. Her body mass index is 29 kg/m^2. Coronary artery computed tomography angiography shows mild nonobstructive coronary atherosclerosis. Coronary flow reserve assessment is planned using flow velocity measurements in the left anterior descending artery interrogated with pulsed-wave Doppler during the echocardiographic examination. Which of the following is the stress modality of choice in these circumstances?

A. Dipyridamole echocardiography using 0.84 mg/kg

B. Dobutamine echocardiography using 2.5 to 40 µg/kg/min

C. Dobutamine echocardiography using 10 to 40 µg/kg/min

D. Semisupine bicycle exercise electrocardiogram

E. Treadmill exercise echocardiography using Bruce protocol

✪ Question 11

Which of the following statements is correct about the basic concepts of myocardial viability assessment?

    A. Dobutamine stress echocardiography can differentiate viability in the endocardium versus epicardium.

    B. No reflow indicates viable myocardium in the presence of an open epicardial vessel.

    C. Nontransmural infarction of <50% of myocardial thickness does not impair wall thickening.

    D. Q waves on the electrocardiogram indicate an absence of viable myocardium in the corresponding territory.

    E. Stunned myocardium is a state of contraction-perfusion mismatch that can be seen after successful reperfusion therapy.

✪✪✪ Question 12

During myocardial perfusion echocardiography, a microbubble contrast agent is infused at a constant rate. Echocardiographic images are acquired using low-power real-time imaging with intermittent high-energy bursts (flashes) aimed at destroying microbubbles. Which of the curves in **Figure 33-1** best reflects normal replenishment of microbubble contrast after a "flash" in segments not affected by flow-limiting coronary stenosis?

    A. A

    B. B

    C. C

    D. D

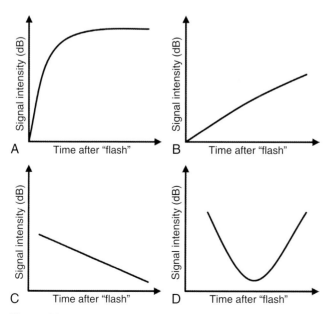

Figure 33-1

✪✪ Question 13

A 71-year-old woman reports for a dobutamine stress echocardiogram as a workup for a transcatheter aortic valve replacement (TAVR). The patient has a history of hypertension, congestive heart failure (New York Heart Association functional class III), a mean aortic valve gradient of 18 mm Hg, an aortic valve area (AVA) <1 cm², a left ventricular ejection fraction (LVEF) of 20% to 25%, and coronary artery disease with percutaneous coronary intervention to the left anterior descending coronary artery. The echocardiographic results are noted in **Table 33-2**. Based on these findings, which of the following statements is most accurate?

    A. Surgery is not indicated as this test demonstrates pseudo-severe aortic stenosis.

    B. Aortic valve replacement is indicated, and perioperative mortality rate is high.

    C. Aortic valve replacement is indicated, and perioperative mortality rate is low.

    D. The results are indeterminate.

Table 33-2.

Measurement	Rest	Low Dose	20 µg/kg/min Dobutamine
LVOT diameter	2.0 cm	–	–
LVOT VTI	11 cm	16 cm	21 cm
SV	44 ml	50 ml	66 ml
AV peak velocity	2.9 m/s	3.2 m/s	4.2 m/s
AV mean gradient	18 mm Hg	27 mm Hg	41 mm Hg
AV VTI	51 cm	70 cm	94 cm
AVA	0.86 cm²	0.72 cm²	0.70 cm²

AV, aortic valve; AVA, aortic valve area; LVOT, left ventricular outflow tract; SV, stroke volume; VTI, velocity-time integral.

✪✪ Question 14

A 72-year-old man reports to the echocardiographic laboratory for follow-up of his stenotic mitral valve. Echocardiographic findings are consistent with moderate mitral stenosis (MS) with a calculated mitral valve area (MVA) of 1.7 cm². The patient reports minimal symptoms and a supine bicycle stress echo is ordered to assess hemodynamics with exercise. Which of the following postexercise findings would be suggestive of hemodynamically significant MS?

A. Increase of MVA

B. Increase in the transmitral gradient of 20 mm Hg

C. Increase in the pulmonary artery systolic pressure (PASP) from 30 mm Hg at rest to 50 mm Hg post exercise

D. Nonlimiting symptoms during stress

Question 15

A 35-year-old man with known mitral valve prolapse, severe mitral regurgitation (MR), and limited symptoms has been referred for stress echocardiography to aid in planning timing of surgical intervention. He had previously walked for 15 minutes on the Bruce protocol despite having severe MR at rest. Which of the following parameters is least useful in this scenario?

A. Left ventricular contractile reserve

B. Patient's symptoms throughout the test

C. Pulmonary artery systolic pressure (PASP) post exercise

D. Severity of MR post exercise

E. Treadmill exercise time

Question 16

An 80-year-old woman with a heavily calcified aortic valve and dyspnea has been referred for further investigation. Based on the data listed in **Table 33-3**, which is the most appropriate test for this patient?

A. Treadmill stress echo using the Bruce protocol to exclude underlying coronary artery disease as a cause of symptoms

B. Dobutamine stress echo with Doppler assessment of the aortic valve function

C. Treadmill stress echo using the Naughton protocol due to previous poor exercise capacity

D. Myocardial perfusion scan with cycle ergometer due to risk of patient on treadmill

E. No further tests are required

Table 33-3.

Parameter	Value
Ejection fraction	20%
Aortic valve area	1.0 cm²
Mean aortic valve gradient	19 mm Hg
Previous stress echo exercise time	4:30 min

Question 17

Which of the following may contribute to a false-positive result during stress echocardiography?

A. Left circumflex disease

B. Suboptimal stress

C. Single-vessel disease

D. Mitral annular calcification

E. Mitral regurgitation

Question 18

A 66-year-old man with normal resting cardiac function walked 7 minutes on the Bruce protocol before stopping with central chest pain and dyspnea. The baseline and post exercise images acquired from the parasternal long-axis (PLAX), parasternal short-axis (PSAX), apical 4-chamber (A4C), and apical 2-chamber (A2C) views were taken by the sonographer at rest (baseline) and within 60 to 90 seconds of test termination and can be seen in **Videos 33-1A** and **33-1B**, respectively. Which coronary artery or arteries is/are most likely diseased?

A. Left main

B. Right

C. Left circumflex

D. Right and left anterior descending

E. Left anterior descending

Question 19

A 64-year-old man presents with intermittent chest pain. He has a strong family history of coronary artery disease. A transthoracic echocardiogram shows left atrial dilatation, normal resting left ventricular wall motion and left ventricular ejection fraction of 55%. Dobutamine echocardiography was ordered and global longitudinal strain values were obtained at baseline, low dose, and peak dobutamine infusion. Which of the following sets of values listed in **Table 33-4** is most consistent with significant coronary artery disease as the cause of this patient's chest pain?

A. Row A

B. Row B

C. Row C

D. Row D

Table 33-4.

	Baseline	5 µg/kg/min (Low Dose)	20 µg/kg/min (Peak)
A	−16%	−16%	−20%
B	−16%	−20%	−15%
C	−19%	−22%	−22%
D	−19%	−20%	−23%

CASE 1

A 65-year-old woman presents for a dobutamine stress echocardiogram for preoperative risk assessment. Resting images demonstrate moderate hypokinesis of the inferior wall with an overall normal ejection fraction of 55%. At low-dose dobutamine imaging (5 mg/kg/min) the inferior wall augments function appropriately; how ever it worsens by peak infusion images (20 mg/kg/min), becoming akinetic with associated ST-segment changes noted in the inferior electrocardiogram leads.

✪✪ Question 20

The response to dobutamine noted in this patient is:
- **A.** Biphasic.
- **B.** Ischemic.
- **C.** Monophasic.
- **D.** Nonphasic.

✪✪ Question 21

Based on the dobutamine stress results above, which statement is true?
- **A.** A flow-limiting stenosis is present with nonviable myocardium.
- **B.** A flow-limiting stenosis is present with viable myocardium.
- **C.** Flow limiting stenosis of a coronary artery is unlikely
- **D.** The myocardium is scarred, which suggests that viability is not present.

✪✪ Question 22

Which of the following responses to dobutamine infusion would be indicative of scarring and lack of left ventricular viability?
- **A.** Biphasic
- **B.** Ischemic
- **C.** Monophasic
- **D.** Nonphasic

CASE 2

▶ A 50-year-old man with known coronary artery disease who received a permanent pacemaker 3 years ago for syncope presents to the emergency department complaining of shortness of breath. He is found to be in pulmonary edema and is admitted to the cardiac care unit. After diuresis he experiences symptomatic improvement. A coronary angiogram reveals severe triple vessel coronary artery disease. A dobutamine stress echocardiogram is performed (**Video 33-2A** to **F**). The study also shows moderate mitral regurgitation.

✪✪ Question 23

Which of the following findings best describes the stress echocardiography results?
- **A.** Biphasic response in the apical segments
- **B.** Inferoseptal wall ischemia
- **C.** Marked viability in the inferior wall
- **D.** Mild viability in the inferolateral wall
- **E.** Right ventricular ischemia

CASE 3

▶ A 58-year-old woman with a history of hypertension presents to the emergency department with atypical left-sided chest discomfort. She is overweight but has no known history of diabetes mellitus or coronary artery disease. The finding from her electrocardiogram (ECG) is unremarkable and the initial set of biomarkers is negative. Her initial blood pressure is 152/90 mm Hg. A stress echocardiogram is performed with the use of an ultrasound-enhancing agent (**Video 33-3A** to **C**). She exercises on the treadmill reaching a workload of 7 metabolic equivalents (METS) and her peak blood pressure is 170/90 mm Hg. Her target heart rate is achieved. The test is ended because of fatigue and mild dyspnea but no chest pain. Her ECG at peak heart rate reveals 2 mm downsloping ST-segment depression in leads II, III, AVF, V5, and V6.

✪ Question 24

Which of the following statements about the stress echocardiogram in this patient is correct?
- **A.** Stress echocardiography has a poor prognostic value in women.
- **B.** Stress electrocardiography is more sensitive to subendocardial ischemia than is stress echocardiography.
- **C.** The electrocardiographic changes represent a false-positive result.
- **D.** There is evidence of ischemia during stress on the electrocardiogram and echocardiogram images.
- **E.** There is global left ventricular hypokinesis post exercise due to a hypertensive response.

CASE 4

▶ A 69-year-old woman presented for preoperative assessment prior to elective cholecystectomy. She exercised for 6 minutes on the Bruce protocol (7.9 METS), achieving 84% of maximum predicted heart rate before stopping with dyspnea and leg fatigue. She did not experience any chest discomfort and there was minor upsloping ST-segment depression. An ultrasound enhancing agent was used to improve endocardial border definition. Apical 4-chamber (A4C), apical 2-chamber (A2C), and apical long-axis (ALAX) images were taken at rest (baseline) and immediately post exercise (**Video 33-4**).

✪✪ Question 25

▶ Which of the following is the best interpretation of the stress echocardiogram images shown in **Video 33-4**?

A. No regional wall motion abnormalities observed
B. Inferior hypokinesis
C. Apical akinesis
D. Lateral and inferior hypokinesis
E. Anterior, apical and lateral hypokinesis

✪✪ Question 26

A subsequent angiogram demonstrated patent coronary arteries without significant stenosis. Which of the following statements is most likely?

A. The stress echocardiogram was indeterminate due to inadequate workload (<85% of maximum predicted heart rate achieved).
B. The stress echocardiogram was actually normal (false-positive stress echocardiogram findings).
C. There is significant left anterior descending artery stenosis that was missed on the angiogram (false-negative angiogram).
D. There is a myopathic response on the stress echocardiogram.

CASE 5

▶ A 34-year-old man with an unremarkable history other than previous exposure to tuberculosis was referred for stress echocardiography following complaints of intermittent sharp chest pain. The patient's resting blood pressure was 120/88 mm Hg and the electrocardiogram (ECG) was normal. During the stress echocardiogram the patient developed burning chest pain described as a level 5 severity on a scale of 10 and requested that the test be terminated after 4 minutes of exercise. The corresponding ECG showed horizontal ST-segment depression in V6, V5, V4, I, II, III, AVF, and AVR, which resolved 3 minutes into recovery. Standard images of the parasternal long-axis (PLAX), parasternal short-axis (PSAX), apical 4-chamber (A4C), and apical 2-chamber (A2C) views were taken by the sonographer at rest (baseline) and within 60 to 90 seconds of test termination (**Video 33-5A** and **B**).

✪✪ Question 27

Which of the following findings best describes the results of the stress echocardiogram?

A. Ischemia involving the apical and lateral segments of the left ventricle (LV)
B. Left ventricular dilatation with regional wall motion abnormalities suggestive of ischemia in the anterior and inferior segments of the LV
C. Left ventricular dilatation with regional wall motion abnormalities suggestive of ischemia in the anterior, apical, and septal segments of the LV
D. No evidence of ischemia in a submaximal stress test

✪✪ Question 28

Which of the following statements best represents the most likely finding of the coronary angiographic study for this patient?

A. There is multivessel disease involving the circumflex and left anterior descending arteries.
B. There is multivessel disease involving the left anterior descending and right coronary arteries.
C. There is nonobstructive coronary artery disease.
D. There is single-vessel disease involving the left anterior descending artery.
E. There is single-vessel disease involving the right coronary artery.

CASE 6

▶ A 72-year-old man presented with anginal symptoms that occurred while mowing the lawn. He has controlled hypertension and an elevated lipid profile, with no other cardiac risk factors. A stress echocardiogram was ordered to rule out ischemia as the cause of his symptoms. Standard images from the parasternal long-axis (PLAX), parasternal short-axis (PSAX), apical 4-chamber (A4C), and apical 2-chamber (A2C) views were taken by the sonographer at rest (baseline) and within 60 to 90 seconds of test termination (**Video 33-6A** and **B**).

✪ Question 29

Which of the following options best describes the echocardiographic findings post exercise?

    A. Anterior hypokinesis

    B. Inferior hypokinesis

    C. Lateral hypokinesis

    D. Septal hypokinesis

✪✪✪ Question 30

Based on these images, where is the most likely site of flow-limiting stenosis that would be identified during coronary angiography?

    A. Proximal right coronary artery

    B. Proximal left anterior descending artery

    C. Obtuse marginal branch

    D. Mid right coronary artery

    E. Distal left circumflex artery

CASE 7

▶ A 70-year-old man with known minor coronary artery disease presented with new onset dyspnea and markedly reduced exercise tolerance. A resting transthoracic echocardiogram was unremarkable, as were the electrocardiogram (ECG) and initial observations. He was a smoker with untreated hypertension, treated hypercholesterolemia, and type II diabetes. A stress echo was ordered, and the patient exercised to a good workload (11.4 METS) before stopping due to dyspnea. He reported no chest pain or anginal symptoms throughout the examination. The ECG developed right bundle branch conduction abnormalities with exercise. There was insufficient tricuspid regurgitation to assess the right ventricular systolic pressure. Standard images from the parasternal long-axis (PLAX), parasternal short-axis (PSAX), apical 4-chamber (A4C), and apical 2-chamber (A2C) views were taken by the sonographer at rest (baseline) and within 60 to 90 seconds of test termination (**Video 33-7A** and **B**).

✪✪ Question 31

Which of the following statements best describes the stress echocardiographic findings post exercise?

    A. There is a dynamic left ventricle and a dilated hypokinetic right ventricle post exercise.

    B. There is excellent cardiac contractile reserve; this is a normal stress echocardiogram.

    C. There is hyperdynamic left ventricular function suggesting dynamic outflow tract obstruction.

    D. There is isolated ischemia of the mid-lateral segments of the left ventricle.

✪✪ Question 32

Which of the following additional findings is most likely, based on the postexercise images?

    A. Restenosis of the left anterior descending artery stent

    B. Severe aortic stenosis

    C. Severe mitral regurgitation

    D. Significant pulmonary hypertension

CASE 8

▶ A 63-year-old woman presents to the stress laboratory for a stress echocardiogram for the investigation of exertional dyspnea. She has a history of hypertension, a family history of coronary artery disease, and general complaints of lower back pain. Her electrocardiogram was normal at rest, and she was mildly hypertensive with a blood pressure of 144/82 mm Hg. She exercised for 2 minutes and 35 seconds on the standard Bruce protocol before stopping due to dyspnea. The peak heart rate was 181 bpm (116% maximal predicted heart rate, and the blood pressure was elevated at 230/104 mm Hg). There were no ST-segment changes during the test or recovery. The patient's E/e′ was 12 at rest, increasing to 16.4 at peak exercise. Standard images from the parasternal long-axis (PLAX), parasternal short-axis (PSAX), apical 4-chamber (A4C), and apical 2-chamber (A2C) views were taken by the sonographer at rest (baseline) and within 60 to 90 seconds of test termination (**Video 33-8A and B**).

✪✪ Question 33

Based on the echocardiographic images provided, which of the following statements best represents the interpretation of this examination?

    A. There is indeterminate diastolic function post exercise due to a marked hypertensive response to exercise.

    B. There are elevated diastolic filling pressures at rest, persisting with exercise, with evidence of ischemia in the left anterior descending coronary artery territory of the left ventricle.

    C. The E/e' is normal at rest, with evidence of exercise-induced elevated filling pressures with exercise, suggestive of a hypertensive response to exercise.

    D. There is echocardiographic evidence of single-vessel disease.

✪✪ Question 34

Which of the following findings best explains the ventricular response to exercise in this patient?

A. Single-vessel flow-limiting stenosis (>50%) causing ischemia
B. Normal diastolic function at rest with exercise-induced diastolic dysfunction
C. Decreased left ventricular (LV) systolic pressure with exercise
D. Compression of subendocardial vessels

CASE 9

▶ A 69-year-old woman with a history of type 2 diabetes mellitus, hypertension, and advanced renal disease presents to the emergency department with an episode of left-sided chest pain lasting 20 minutes. She is admitted and ruled out for acute myocardial infarction. A stress echocardiogram is requested (**Video 33-9A to F**). Her resting blood pressure is 220/100 mm Hg. A dipyridamole stress echocardiogram is performed because of elevated blood pressure. She experiences chest pressure during dipyridamole infusion, but the electrocardiogram does not show ischemic changes.

✪✪ Question 35

Which of the following best describes the stress echocardiography findings?

A. Mild ischemia involving the anterolateral wall
B. Mild ischemia involving the apical septum only
C. Moderate ischemia involving anteroseptal and anterior walls

D. Moderate ischemia involving inferior and inferolateral walls
E. No echocardiographic evidence of ischemia

✪✪✪ Question 36

Which of the following statements is correct about the stress echocardiogram?

A. Dipyridamole stress echocardiography has lower sensitivity than does dobutamine echocardiography.
B. Dipyridamole stress echocardiography has lower specificity than does dobutamine echocardiography.
C. In women, Dipyridamole stress echocardiography is preferred to dobutamine echocardiography as it is less likely to produce a left ventricular outflow tract gradient.
D. The chest pain in this patient is most likely a side effect of dipyridamole.
E. The peak wall motion score index in this patient portends a low risk for cardiac events.

✪✪ Question 37

Based on the stress echocardiogram results, what would be the most likely finding with coronary angiography in this patient?

A. Diffuse disease involving the distal left anterior descending artery
B. Flow-limiting mid left anterior descending artery stenosis
C. Flow-limiting obtuse marginal artery stenosis
D. Flow-limiting right coronary artery stenosis
E. No flow-limiting coronary artery disease

ANSWERS

1. **Answer: A.** The use of stress echocardiography to diagnose flow-limiting coronary artery disease is based on a sequence of events known as the ischemic cascade as shown in **Figure 33-2**. The decrease in blood flow initially produces a perfusion abnormality, diastolic and systolic dysfunction, in that order, and then hemodynamic abnormalities occur. Electrocardiographic changes and symptoms occur late in the ischemic cascade; hence, the sensitivity of these parameters to identify ischemia is lower.

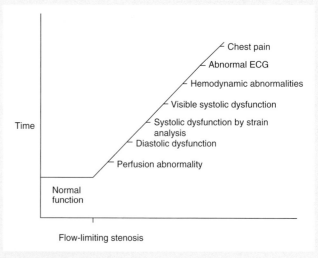

Figure 33-2

2. **Answer: A.** A normal response to dobutamine infusion during stress echocardiography starting with a low dose is a progressive increase in regional endocardial excursion, myocardial thickening, and LVEF as well as a decrease in LVESV. A decrease in regional endocardial excursion and myocardial thickening at peak dose compared with a low dose (as described in row D) indicates myocardial ischemia. Cavity dilation and a decrease in LVEF at peak dose (as described in row B) are uncommon and usually indicate a high ischemic burden.

3. **Answer: C.** With an increasing heart rate, the diastolic filling period becomes shorter, and less volume fills the left ventricle. The cardiac output increases to meet oxygen demands by predominantly increasing the heart rate. The duration of the systolic phase of the cardiac cycle remains relatively unchanged with increasing heart rates. There is a small increase in stroke volume due to an increase in ventricular contractility (inotropic response), but this is not achieved through an increase in LV end-diastolic volume (LVEDV). Typically, the initial increase in stroke volume plateaus at around 50% to 60% of a patient's maximal oxygen uptake and the remaining increase in cardiac output is due to increasing heart rate (chronotropic response). In some elite athletes, there may be a slight increase in LVEDV post exercise due to improved venous return, although this is not typical for most patients. Answer A is incorrect as exercise training adaptations result in an increased resting LV cavity size, but the same physiological changes occur during exercise, resulting in an increase in ejection fraction post exercise. Answer D is incorrect since mitral regurgitation causes an increase in LV end-diastolic volume at rest due to the added volume required to maintain cardiac output as the total LV filling volume is equal to the mitral regurgitant volume + left ventricular outflow tract stroke volume.

4. **Answer: E.** Stress echocardiography as a testing modality may be used for a multitude of indications.

The most common is to rule out ischemia in the patient who may be demonstrating symptoms, such as chest pain or dyspnea, which may be indicative of a flow-limiting coronary artery stenosis (>50%-70% stenotic). In the setting of valvular heart disease, exercise stress testing is not indicated in patients who have severe symptomatic aortic regurgitation as stress testing is only used to assess functional capacity when symptoms are questionable; therefore, answer E is correct. Stress testing may be used to elicit symptoms in patients who may not have symptoms due to self-limiting their daily activities. In the mitral valve disease population, stress echocardiography is indicated in the setting of severe, asymptomatic mitral stenosis, or symptomatic, moderate mitral stenosis (as described in answer A). The end point for stress testing in the setting of mitral stenosis includes stress-induced measurements of a transmitral valve mean pressure gradient >15 mm Hg and a pulmonary artery systolic pressure >60 mm Hg, which would also suggest the valve would benefit from surgical or percutaneous intervention. This may be assessed with either a dobutamine stress test or an exercise bicycle exam, which allows progressive Doppler measurements to be acquired throughout the stress phase of the test. In the setting of pulmonary hypertension (PHTN), stress testing may be helpful for the review of left and right ventricular function, or when there is a suspicion of exercise-induced pulmonary hypertension. A scleroderma patient (as described in answer C) may present for stress testing due to the risk of development of PHTN at rest or with exercise. Patients may also present for stress echocardiography following an elevated coronary calcium score on computed tomography. Regardless of global coronary artery disease risk, a score greater than 400 is an appropriate indication for a stress test (as described in answer D). The more common noncoronary indications for stress echocardiography are noted in **Table 33-5**.

Table 33-5. Common Noncoronary Indications for Stress Echocardiography

Indication	Reason
Microvascular disease (diabetes mellitus, syndrome X, etc.)	Evaluation of coronary flow reserve
Dilated nonischemic cardiomyopathy	Assessment of inotropic contractile reserve
Hypertrophic cardiomyopathy	Gradient provocation and risk stratification
Valvular heart disease	Assessment of exercise tolerance and hemodynamics including pressure gradients and tricuspid regurgitant velocity Differentiation of severe from "pseudo-severe" aortic stenosis in patients with low left ventricular systolic function (dobutamine infusion)
Exertional dyspnea	Assessment of diastolic parameters and tricuspid regurgitant velocity
Post–cardiac transplantation	Detection of transplant vasculopathy

5. **Answer: B.** ST-segment elevation on the electrocardiogram is suggestive of acute myocardial infarction. According to the AHA guidelines for Exercise Standards for Testing and Training (Fletcher et al., 2013), acute myocardial infarction is an absolute contraindication to exercise testing. Stress echocardiography is, however, useful for risk stratification and planning of surgical intervention in patients with severe mitral regurgitation (answer A). The evaluation of the patient with known obstructive left main coronary artery stenosis (answer C) and systemic or pulmonary hypertension (answers D and E, respectively) are relative contraindications only.

6. **Answer: B.** Several criteria must be satisfied to ensure the heart has been adequately assessed during stress echocardiography to rule out obstructive coronary artery disease. These include achieving an adequate exertion level and acquiring postexercise echocardiographic images within an acceptable timeframe. The main parameters for determining level of exertion during stress testing are the percentage of age-predicted maximal heart rate (APMHR) and/or maximal rate pressure product (RPP). The APMHR is simply derived as 220 minus the patient's age with the target threshold being ≥85%. The RPP is derived as the product of the maximal heart rate and maximal systolic blood pressure with the target threshold being ≥25,000. Postexercise echocardiographic imaging should be completed within 1 to 2 minutes (ideally <60 seconds) as inducible wall motion abnormalities can resolve quickly in the recovery phase of the test.

   For this patient, the APMHR is 160 bpm (220 − 60) and target threshold is 136 (85% of 160). However, peak heart rate for this patient was only 112 bpm (70% of the APMHR) which would be considered an inadequate workload and therefore, answer B is correct.

   The completion of 7 minutes on the Bruce protocol (answer A) does not necessarily indicate a nondiagnostic test. While completing 9 minutes (stage 3) on the Bruce protocol has good prognostic value, it is not an indicator of adequate workload with many patients unable to complete 9 minutes of exercise despite exercising at a high intensity for them. The absence of symptoms (answer C) does not indicate a nondiagnostic test, especially when the patient's heart is not placed under enough stress to elicit a response as in this case. Postexercise imaging in <1 minute (answer D) does not indicate a nondiagnostic test.

7. **Answer: D.** A drop in SBP greater than 10 mm Hg from the previous stage, when associated with any other signs of ischemia, is an absolute indication to terminate a test. The onset of asymptomatic LBBB (answer A) or ST-segment changes (answer C) may be a useful diagnostic finding, but do not necessitate termination of the test. An exaggerated hypertensive response (answer E), defined as SBP >250 mm Hg or diastolic blood pressure >115 mm Hg, is a relative indication to cease the test and is at the physician's clinical discretion. The maximum predicted heart rate (answer B) does not necessitate the immediate termination of the test.

8. **Answer: A.** Echocardiographic assessment of cardiac sarcoidosis is performed with a resting echocardiogram examination, not a stress echocardiogram. In these patients, findings suggestive of cardiac sarcoidosis include a reduced ejection fraction (<40%) or nonanatomical distribution of regional wall motion abnormalities. These findings are not transient or provoked by ischemia and therefore stress echocardiography is not indicated in these patients. Appropriate indications for performing a stress echocardiogram may include investigation of angina (answer E), assessment of viability of myocardium prior to revascularization (answer D), investigation of the asymptomatic patient with moderate risk factors (answer B), or the investigation of dyspnea (answer C).

9. **Answer: B.** A diastolic stress test is performed when there is suspicion that a patient may have heart failure with preserved ejection fraction (HFpEF). These patients often present with borderline abnormalities at rest with no echocardiographic findings that would explain dyspnea upon exertion. While a patient may be diagnosed with HFpEF when a resting TTE demonstrates an E/e′ >15 and is not a candidate for a diastolic stress test when E/e′ is <8, a diastolic stress test is useful to differentiate the patients falling between these two groups (that is, indeterminate diastolic function). Patients with normal diastolic function who have preserved annular velocities will increase their cardiac output during exercise without a significant elevation in left ventricular (LV) filling pressures; a patient with abnormal diastology can increase their cardiac output with exercise only by elevating their LV filling pressures. The diastolic stress test protocol may be performed using a bicycle or a treadmill, although the bicycle is preferable as this enables the performance of Doppler measurements throughout the exam. The diastolic stress test protocol includes imaging of the left ventricle, pulsed-wave Doppler interrogation of mitral inflow, tissue Doppler imaging of the mitral annulus, and continuous-wave Doppler assessment of the tricuspid regurgitant signal (TR Vmax) for estimation of the pulmonary artery systolic pressure at rest and during each stage of the test. The test is considered positive for exercise-induced elevated LV filling pressures when the E/e′ increases to >14, the septal E/e′ ratio is >15, and TR V_{max} is >2.8 m/s. If the E/e′ is <10 and TR Vmax <2.8 m/s, the test is considered normal.

10. **Answer: A.** Microvascular dysfunction without flow-limiting epicardial coronary disease can cause angina-like exertional chest pain in different patient

subgroups including patients with diabetes mellitus, hypertension, and syndrome X. During exercise testing, typical symptoms can be provoked along with ischemic ST-segment changes. In contrast to coronary artery disease, wall motion abnormalities may not be an early event in these patients. Pulsed-wave Doppler examination of the mid-to-distal left anterior descending artery has been shown to be highly feasible in the low parasternal long-axis view under the guidance of color Doppler flow mapping and it allows assessment of the coronary flow reserve. Normally, there is at least a twofold increase in the peak diastolic coronary flow velocities with vasodilator infusion (such as dipyridamole or adenosine) compared to rest. Abnormal coronary

flow reserve (≤2) carries diagnostic and prognostic information in certain subgroups of patients. In a large study of patients with negative dipyridamole echocardiography by wall motion criteria, abnormal coronary flow reserve provided independent prognostic information in both diabetic and nondiabetic patients (Cortigiani et al., 2007).

11. **Answer: E.** Stunned myocardium is a state of contraction-perfusion mismatch that can be seen in the setting of acute myocardial infarction after successful reperfusion. If recurrent chronic ischemia occurs, the dysfunctional but viable myocardium is called hibernating myocardium. Hibernating myocardium results from recurrent stunning of the myocardium (**Figure 33-3**, basic concepts of viability).

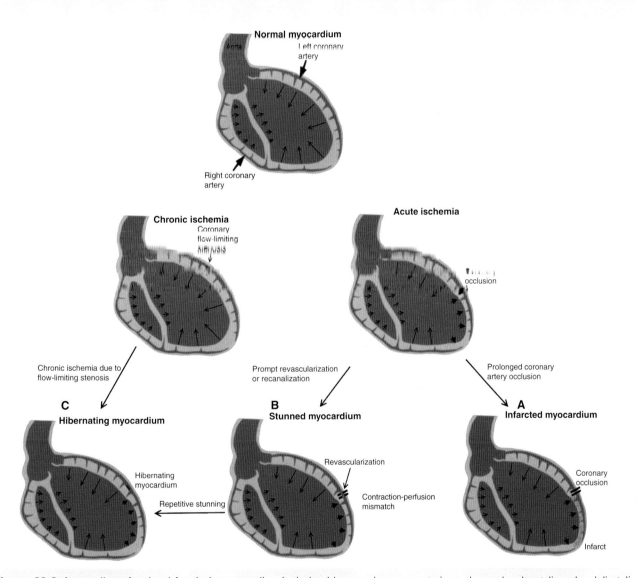

Figure 33-3 A normally perfused and functioning myocardium is depicted by normal coronary arteries and normal end-systolic and end-diastolic volumes. In the middle row on the right, a complete left coronary artery occlusion has occurred in the setting of plaque rupture with acute thrombosis. If the lack of perfusion is prolonged enough, a myocardial infarction ensues, with loss of function, depicted here by a regional increase in end-systolic volume (A). If reperfusion occurs, due to either recanalization or revascularization, the contractility, initially abnormal due to ischemia, may remain impaired in the acute and subacute stages, with subsequent improvement. This phenomenon is called stunning (B). Repetitive stunning leads to a state of chronic myocardial dysfunction called hibernation (C). A chronic flow-limiting coronary artery occlusion leads to downregulation of the regional wall motion abnormality, leading to hibernating myocardium (C).

Dobutamine stress echocardiography cannot differentiate viability in the endocardium versus epicardium (answer A). No reflow commonly results from capillary destruction and it is most consistent with no viability (answer B). A nontransmural infarction of only 20% of the wall thickness can impair wall thickening (answer C). Up to 40% of regions showing Q waves on the electrocardiogram are viable (answer D).

12. **Answer: A.** A quick replenishment is observed in segments not affected by stenosis after a high-energy burst (flash) that destroys the microbubbles within the myocardium. This can be quantified by two parameters: the peak signal intensity and the rate of the signal intensity rise. Graph A is an example of a normal rise of signal intensity to its peak level. Graph B, on the contrary, shows a slower rise and a lower peak intensity, which can be consistent with flow-limiting coronary stenosis.

13. **Answer: C.** This patient meets the criteria for classic low-flow, low-gradient aortic stenosis (AS) with a calculated AVA at rest <1.0 cm², a mean aortic valve gradient <40 mm Hg, and an LVEF <50%. Dobutamine stress echocardiography is indicated in these patients to determine whether true AS exists (depressed LVEF due to severe AS) or whether pseudo-severe AS is present (small AVA due to a poor LVEF). The test begins at a low-dose infusion of 2.5 to 5.0 µg/kg/min, increasing by 5 to 10 µg/kg/min every 3 to 5 minutes; usually to a maximum infusion rate of 20 µg/kg/min. Dobutamine is a positive inotrope and therefore, at low doses this will usually result in increased contractility of the left ventricle; at higher doses, evidence of ischemia may be visualized due to the increased myocardial oxygen demand.

When there is true severe AS, with dobutamine infusion the transaortic velocity will increase to ≥4 m/s, the mean pressure gradient will increase to ≥40 mm Hg, and the calculated AVA will remain severely reduced (<1.0 cm²). In this patient, all these parameters meet the criteria for severe AS and therefore, aortic valve replacement is indicated. Additionally, as contractile reserve has a favorable impact on mortality in this patient population, flow reserve is part of the assessment. An increase of >20% in stroke volume is considered positive for contractile reserve. In this patient, the stroke volume increased from 44 to 66 mL, an increase of 22%. Thus, this patient would be expected to have lower perioperative mortality rate when compared to patients with absent contractile reserve. Therefore, answer C is correct.

Had this been pseudo-severe AS (as described in answer A), the gradients would have increased slightly with the AVA increasing to >1 cm² as the test progressed.

14. **Answer: B.** Stress echocardiography may be helpful in patients with MS who are exhibiting symptoms that are equivocal in nature. While the supine bicycle exercise stress test is the method of choice, treadmill and dobutamine stress tests have been validated as well. Stress echocardiography is appropriate in the asymptomatic patient whose resting echocardiogram is consistent with severe MS. Additionally, patients who are symptomatic may have a stress test when their resting echocardiogram demonstrates mild to moderate MS. Hemodynamically significant MS is observed when the PASP increases to >60 mm Hg or when the transmitral mean gradient is >15 mm Hg. Therefore, an increase in the transmitral gradient to 20 mm Hg (answer B) is the correct answer. An increase in the MVA (as described in answer A) would be indicative of a valve that is more flexible, and therefore less severe. A 50 mm Hg PASP gradient post exercise (as described in answer C) does not meet the cutoff of a 60 mm Hg PASP at peak exercise. Nonlimiting symptoms (as described in answer D) during stress are not an indication for an intervention, although limiting symptoms during stress would be an indication based on current guidelines.

15. **Answer: D.** The severity of the lesion is already documented and is not of incremental value. The functional capacity and patient's exercise tolerance, including the absence of symptoms, is very helpful to formally document the effects of the regurgitation. A significant decrease in exercise capacity with associated symptoms of dyspnea would indicate that the MR is impacting on their activity levels and would suggest intervention is required. The hemodynamic consequence of the mitral lesion can be further quantified by assessing the PASP, which will elevate secondary to the regurgitation applying a back-pressure on the pulmonary circulation. The primary role of stress echo in the assessment of severe MR is the evaluation of cardiac reserve. Normal contractile reserve is defined as an increase in ejection fraction of at least 5% post exercise.

16. **Answer: B.** Dobutamine stress echocardiography with Doppler assessment of the aortic valve would be indicated to further assess the presence of low-flow, low-gradient aortic stenosis (AS). An increase in contractility will result in an increase in gradient and a fixed AVA to indicate true severe aortic stenosis (see answer outline for Question 13). Conversely, a fixed (or even slightly reduced) gradient with an increased AVA would suggest that the low-gradient and the reduced AVA is caused by the poor driving pressure, which is failing to open the calcified valve leaflets; that is, pseudo-severe arctic stenosis. Treadmill echocardiography with either the Bruce protocol (answer A) or the Naughton protocol (answer C) would not be optimal due to the limited

imaging opportunities of the study (typically rest and post), without the progressive data points that are obtained in a dobutamine aortic stenosis study to demonstrate a trend. A myocardial perfusion scan (answer D) will not assess the valve function with increased contractility.

17. **Answer: D.** Stress echocardiography has been shown to demonstrate regional wall motion abnormalities when a luminal obstruction >50% is present. This is due to the increased demand for oxygen by the myocardium during stress echocardiography. The sensitivity of stress echocardiography to detect coronary artery disease is in the range of 75% to 85%, with specificity between 80% and 90%. When the patient reaches a heart rate >85% of their age-predicted maximum, the sensitivity is even higher. Mitral annular calcification (answer D) may result in a false-positive stress echocardiogram as tethering impacts the motion of the mitral annulus, which may reduce the motion of the basal inferior and inferoseptal segments. The remainder of the options are examples of contributors to false-negative exams, which are more common with suboptimal stress tests (as described in answer B) where there is a failure to meet 85% of the age-predicted maximum heart rate. Poor image quality may be avoided through the use of an ultrasound enhancing agent. False-negative findings can also occur with single-vessel disease (as described in answer C), more notably with left circumflex stenosis (as described in answer A) where a smaller amount of myocardium receives inadequate blood supply. Including the apical long-axis views will improve the detection of regional wall motion abnormalities in the left circumflex territory. Mitral regurgitation (as described in answer E) may also contribute to a false-negative finding as patients may have hyperdynamic ventricles, which makes the recognition of regional wall motion abnormalities difficult. Examples of contributors to both false-negative and false-positive exams are noted in **Table 33-6**.

18. **Answer: C.** Wall motion abnormalities occur at and distal to the site of perfusion abnormality/obstruction. A strong understanding of the usual variants of coronary anatomy can aid in the prediction of affected arteries based on the stress echocardiographic findings. **Figure 33-4** demonstrates coronary distribution in relation to segments of the left ventricle.

The postexercise images show normal augmentation of contraction in the anterior and septal segments, which are supplied by the left anterior descending artery. A normal increase in contractility also occurs in the inferior segment, which is supplied by the right coronary artery and possibly the left anterior descending in the apical inferior segment. Hypokinesis is seen in the mid-lateral and posterior basal to mid segments which are supplied by the circumflex artery; therefore, answer C is correct.

19. **Answer: B.** Global longitudinal strain reflects myocardial shortening in the longitudinal direction and therefore is a negative number. Normal values are more negative than −20%. Deformation analysis during dobutamine infusion can provide objective evidence of viability and ischemia. Normally, global longitudinal strain increases with low-dose dobutamine (i.e., becomes more negative) followed by a plateau prepeak dose and possible mild decrease at peak dobutamine dose (row C). Patients with flow-limiting coronary disease also show an increase in global longitudinal strain at low dose, but this is followed by a significant decrease in longitudinal strain at peak dose, sometimes below the baseline value (row D). Also, patients with flow-limiting coronary disease commonly have lower resting global longitudinal strain values compared with controls despite preserved left ventricular ejection fraction.

20. **Answer: A.** A dobutamine stress echocardiogram is the stress test of choice for preoperative risk assessment when the pretest risk assessment is in the intermediate range or higher. A biphasic response (answer A) shows an initial improvement

Table 33-6. Common Causes of False-Positive and False-Negative Results During Stress Echocardiography

False-Positive Results	False-Negative Results
• Hypertensive response to stress • Frequent PVCs, SVT • Microvascular disease (syndrome X) • Nonischemic cardiomyopathy • Aortic regurgitation • Effect of tethering seen with mitral annular calcification or after mitral surgery • Coronary vasospasm • Abnormal septal motion due to pacing, conduction abnormalities, prior surgery, or right ventricular volume overload	• Inadequate level of stress including the use of beta-blockers before stress • Single-vessel disease, especially left circumflex • Concentric left ventricular remodeling • Hyperdynamic state in patients with significant mitral regurgitation or aortic regurgitation • Apical foreshortening • Delays in image acquisition post exercise

PVC, premature ventricular complex; SVT, supraventricular tachycardia.

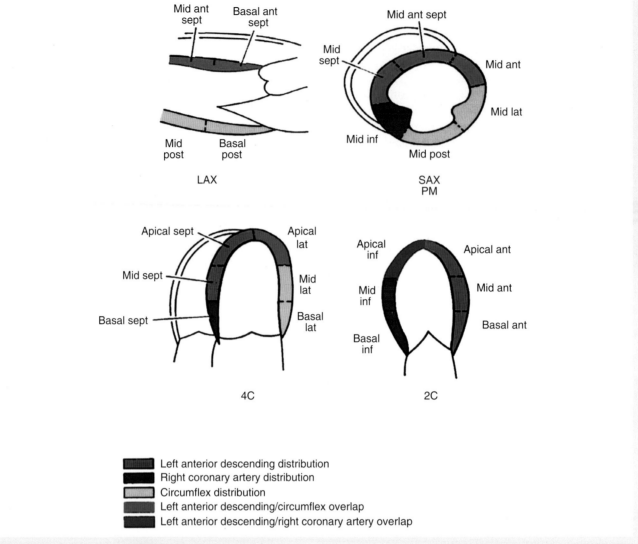

Figure 33-4 This schematic demonstrates the relationship between coronary artery distribution and the corresponding left ventricular segments. With the four standard views, the territories of each of the main coronary arteries can be evaluated, as defined by the color scheme. Areas of overlap are indicated in green. (From Armstrong WF, Ryan T. *Feigenbaum's Echocardiography*. 7th ed. Philadelphia, PA: Lippincott Williams and Wilkins; 2010:485.)

in left ventricular (LV) function following low-dose infusion of dobutamine, which then deteriorates at a higher dose.

An ischemic response (answer B) shows a deterioration in LV function. A monophasic response (answer C) describes a normal response with inotropic contractile reserve where there is an increase in LV contractility and a reduction in LV cavity size resulting in an increase in ejection fraction with each phase of the test. A nonphasic response (answer D) shows no change in LV contractility throughout the test.

21. **Answer: B.** The presence of a biphasic response, which is improved myocardial contractility and systolic thickening with low dose of dobutamine, which then worsens at a high dose of dobutamine, is associated with flow-limiting coronary artery stenosis with viable myocardium.

22. **Answer: D.** As previously stated, there are four characteristic responses to dobutamine infusion. Of these responses, a nonphasic response whereby no change to left ventricular (LV) contractility is seen indicates the presence of scarred myocardium with no viability. Therefore, answer D is correct.

A biphasic response (answer A) whereby function is augmented at low dose and is followed by deterioration at high dose indicates the presence of viable myocardium, but the coronary artery that supplies the myocardium has flow-limiting stenosis. An ischemic response (answer B) whereby function deteriorates indicates the presence of myocardium with stress-induced ischemia due to flow-limiting stenosis. A monophasic response (answer C) whereby improvement is seen at low dose and persists or further improves at high dose indicates viable myocardium with no stenosis of the coronary artery subtending the dysfunctional segment/region.

23. ▶ **Answer: D.** This case illustrates a patient with ischemic cardiomyopathy and severe left ventricular dysfunction with minimal inotropic contractile reserve and without evidence of inducible ischemia. Mild viability in the inferolateral wall is evident with improvement in contractility best seen in the apical long-axis view (**Video 33-2C**), augmenting at low dose and continuing to improve with peak infusion. This finding is also supported in the parasternal views (**Videos 33-2D** and **33-2E**).

The absence of inotropic contractile reserve, consistent with a scarred myocardium, portends a poor prognosis. Patients with significant viability demonstrate improved survival and improvement in left ventricular function after revascularization, beta-blocker therapy, and cardiac resynchronization therapy. This patient is unlikely to benefit from revascularization or beta-blocker therapy. Likewise, it is unlikely that this patient will respond to cardiac resynchronization therapy.

KEY POINTS

▶ Inotropic contractile reserve predicts left ventricular functional recovery after revascularization.

▶ Inotropic contractile reserve predicts response to beta-blocker therapy.

▶ Absence of inotropic contractile reserve portends a poor prognosis.

24. **Answer: C.** The case illustrates a normal stress echocardiogram (as seen on the images) discordant with the stress electrocardiogram results. The specificity of the stress electrocardiogram can be affected by several factors, including left ventricular hypertrophy, preexisting conduction abnormalities, drug therapy, etc. It has been shown that the specificity of ST-segment changes during exercise is lower in women than men. The sensitivity and specificity of stress echocardiography are superior to those of electrocardiography and, given the normal results of the stress echocardiographic images, it can be assumed that the results of the electrocardiogram are falsely positive.

25. **Answer: E.** This case demonstrates a positive finding for exercise-induced left ventricular dysfunction. The left ventricular ejection fraction dropped from 65% at rest to 45% post exercise. There was a clear regional distribution to the wall motion abnormalities, with the apical, anterior, and lateral walls demonstrating hypokinesis (answer E). This is appreciated in the A2C view (anterior hypokinesis), the ALAX view (inferolateral hypokinesis), and the A4C view (anterolateral hypokinesis).

26. **Answer: D.** Based on the stress echocardiogram findings, a stenosis is expected in the left anterior descending (LAD) coronary artery. However, the angiographic findings did not show a corresponding stenosis in the LAD or any of the other coronary arteries. There are several potential causes for a false-positive finding on the stress echocardiogram, most of which relate to a combination of poor image quality and overinterpretation of the findings. Neither seems to be the case in this set of images, with a clear decline in systolic function post exercise; the use of an ultrasound-enhancing agent increases the confidence of the findings as well. Therefore, this most likely represents a myopathic response observed on the stress echocardiogram. It is important to note that in one large study (From et al., 2010), in patients with clear exercise-induced left ventricular dysfunction, almost a third of patients had <50% stenosis by angiography, and most importantly, there was no significant difference in the 4.5-year survival when compared with patients who had >50% coronary artery stenosis. This highlights the importance of stress echocardiography in these patient groups, and to ensure that the findings are not dismissed as merely falsely positive.

27. **Answer: C.** The postexercise images are compared with the resting images to assess changes in left ventricular (LV) cavity size, regional wall motion analysis, and LV ejection fraction. In a normal exam, the LV systolic function improves with a decrease in end-systolic volumes. Although the test was submaximal with the patient exercising 4 minutes, the echocardiographic images demonstrate clear ischemia with an increase in the LV cavity size post exercise and hypokinesis of the apical, mid-anterior, and septal segments (answer C).

28. **Answer: B.** Based on the regional wall motion abnormalities that were seen in the postexercise images, multivessel disease involving the left anterior descending and right coronary arteries is expected (see **Figure 33-4**). Cardiac catheterization demonstrated an 80% proximal left anterior descending stenosis, middle and distal right coronary artery stenoses of 60% and 70%, respectively, 99% ostial stenosis of the posterolateral branch of the right coronary artery, and an 80% stenosis of the posterior descending coronary artery.

29. **Answer: B.** The basal and middle inferior wall segments are hypokinetic, along with the corresponding basal inferoseptal segment. The remaining septal segments were normal.

30. **Answer: D.** Based on the stress-induced regional wall motion abnormalities in the basal and mid inferior wall and basal inferoseptal segments, and as the right ventricle appears unaffected by the ischemia, this suggests that the stenosis is distal to the right ventricular branch of the right coronary artery. This would suggest a mid-level right coronary artery stenosis.

31. **Answer: A.** The postexercise images demonstrate a severely dilated and hypokinetic right ventricle. As a consequence, the left ventricle is underfilled and appears hyperdynamic. Answer B is incorrect since the abnormal right ventricular appearances means that this stress echocardiogram cannot be considered a normal examination. Answer C is incorrect as there is nothing to suggest that the left ventricular outflow tract is obstructing. Answer D is incorrect since the lateral wall is contracting well.

32. **Answer: D.** The postexercise images, particularly evident in the parasternal short-axis view, demonstrate flattening of the interventricular septum consistent with significant pulmonary hypertension. Answer A is incorrect as the left anterior descending artery territory augmented contraction appropriately. Answer B is incorrect since there are no supporting Doppler traces to suggest the presence of severe aortic stenosis. While acute severe mitral regurgitation (answer C) can cause pulmonary hypertension, it would not result in a significantly smaller left ventricular end-diastolic volume when compared to the resting images.

33. **Answer: C.** This patient had a normal E/e' (<15) at rest, which increased to >15 with exercise, demonstrating exercise-induced elevation of left ventricular filling pressures. Additionally, a review of the images shows a hypertensive response to exercise, with left ventricular (LV) cavity dilatation and global systolic dysfunction; this patient also had a reported systolic blood pressure of >200 mm Hg. It is not possible to conclude that diastolic filling pressures are elevated at rest as left atrial volume index and peak tricuspid regurgitation velocity were not measured (answer B). It is unlikely that the response to exercise in this patient is due to single-vessel disease (answer D), as global left ventricular dysfunction, with increases in LV size, is a sign of severe multivessel or left main coronary artery disease. It is important to note that a hypertensive response to exercise may reduce the specificity of the test, resulting in a false-positive reading.

34. **Answer: D.** This patient's left ventricle dilated and became hypodynamic with exercise. This is due to an increase of LV systolic pressure, which compresses the subendocardium, which is the furthest cardiac muscle from the coronary arteries. This has a negative impact on flow and results in subendocardial ischemia. Had this been single-vessel disease with a coronary blockage >50% (as described in answer A), the wall motion abnormality would have been regional in nature instead of the global response as seen in this patient. Had this been caused by decreased LV systolic pressure (as described in answer C), the left ventricle would not have dilated as this echo is indicative of increased LV pressure.

35. **Answer: C.** This case illustrates a patient with moderate ischemia in the mid inferoseptal and anterior walls, as well as the mid anteroseptum and apical segments. Coronary angiography confirmed a severe mid left anterior descending artery stenosis.

36. **Answer: A.** The sensitivity of dipyridamole stress echocardiography for single-vessel disease may be as low as 50%, but its specificity is excellent (88%-100%). The peak wall motion score index is about 1.7, which confers a high cardiovascular risk to this patient (>5% cardiovascular risk events/year). Even though chest pain may represent a nonspecific symptom and a side effect of dipyridamole, the presence of new wall motion abnormalities indicates ischemia.

TEACHING POINT

Wall motion score index is a semiquantitative tool recommended by the American Society of Echocardiography (ASE). Each left ventricular segment should be assessed individually in multiple views based on a 16-segment model for the assessment of left ventricular wall motion. A wall motion score is assigned to each visualized segment and the motion score index is calculated as the average of the scores of all visualized segments. The following scoring system is recommended by ASE: (1) normal or hyperkinetic, (2) hypokinetic (3) akinetic, and (4) dyskinetic. The 17-segment model is recommended to assess myocardial perfusion and is not recommended for the assessment of regional wall motion abnormalities.

37. **Answer: B.** Based on evidence of moderate ischemia in the mid inferoseptal and anterior walls, as well as in the mid anteroseptal and apical segments, flow-limiting mid left anterior descending artery stenosis is expected. Coronary angiography subsequently confirmed a severe mid left anterior descending artery stenosis.

Acknowledgments: The authors would sincerely like to acknowledge Edgar Argulian, MD, MPH, and Farooq A. Chaudhry, MD (Chapter 14, Stress Echocardiography: Ischemic and Nonischemic) in *Clinical Echocardiography Review: A Self-Assessment Tool*, 2nd Edition, edited by Allan L. Klein, Craig R. Asher, 2017.

SUGGESTED READINGS

ACCF/ASE/AHA/ASNC/HFSA/HRS/SCAI/SCCM/SCCT/SCMR 2011 appropriate use criteria for echocardiography. A report of the American College of Cardiology Foundation appropriate use criteria task force, American Society of Echocardiography, American Heart Association, American Society of Nuclear Cardiology, Heart Failure Society of America, Heart Rhythm Society, Society for Cardiovascular Angiography and Interventions, Society of Critical Care Medicine, Society of Cardiovascular

Computed Tomography, Society for Cardiovascular Magnetic Resonance American College of Chest Physicians. *J Am Soc Echocardiogr.* 2011;24(3):229-267.

Cortigiani L, Rigo F, Gherardi S, et al. Additional prognostic value of coronary flow reserve in diabetic and nondiabetic patients with negative dipyridamole stress echocardiography by wall motion criteria. *J Am Coll Cardiol.* 2007;50(14):1354-1361.

Fletcher GF, Ades PA, Kligfield P, et al. Exercise standards for testing and training: a scientific statement from the American Heart Association. *Circulation.* 2013;128(8):873-934.

From AM, Kane G, Bruce C, Pellikka PA, Scott C, McCully RB. Characteristics and outcomes of patients with abnormal stress echocardiograms and angiographically mild coronary artery disease (<50% stenoses) or normal coronary arteries. *J Am Soc Echocardiogr.* 2010;23(2):207-214.

Lancellotti P, Pellikka PA, Budts W, et al. The clinical use of stress echocardiography in non-ischaemic heart disease: recommendations from the European Association of Cardiovascular Imaging and the American Society of Echocardiography. *J Am Soc Echocardiogr.* 2017,30(2).101-138.

Nagueh SF, Smiseth OA, Appleton CP, et al. Recommendations for the evaluation of left ventricular diastolic function by echocardiography: an update from the American Society of Echocardiography and the European Association of Cardiovascular Imaging. *J Am Soc Echocardiogr.* 2016;29(4):277-314.

Ng AC, Sitges M, Pham PN, et al. Incremental value of 2-dimensional speckle tracking strain imaging to wall motion analysis for detection of coronary artery disease in patients undergoing dobutamine stress echocardiography. *Am Heart J.* 2009;158(5):836-844.

Pellikka PA, Nagueh SF, Elhendy AA, Kuehl CA, Sawada SG, American Society of Echocardiography. American Society of Echocardiography recommendations for performance, interpretation, and application of stress echocardiography. *J Am Soc Echocardiogr.* 2007;20(9):1021-1041.

CHAPTER 34

Cardiac Shock and Emergency Echocardiography

Contributors: Anthony Wald, BTech, PDM, GDCT and Kellie D'Orsa, BSc, DMU (Cardiac), GCHELT

✪ Question 1

What is the most common echocardiographic feature of cardiogenic shock?

- **A.** Left ventricular (LV) systolic dysfunction
- **B.** Papillary muscle rupture
- **C.** Right ventricular (RV) systolic dysfunction
- **D.** Significant pericardial effusion causing cardiac tamponade

✪✪ Question 2

A previously healthy 40-year-old woman on oral contraception and in profound shock is brought into the emergency department by the paramedics. She has recently returned home after a long international flight. Four to six hours prior to admission, she had complained of increasing shortness of breath and subsequently collapsed at home. What is the most likely echocardiographic finding?

- **A.** A small exudate pericardial effusion
- **B.** Aortic stenosis with a mean gradient over 45 mm Hg
- **C.** Dilated right heart with leftward septal deviation
- **D.** Wall motion abnormality in the left anterior descending coronary artery territory

✪✪✪ Question 3

A patient with an acute inferior myocardial infarct has now developed fulminant pulmonary edema. What is the most likely complication of the infarct that caused the edema?

- **A.** Aortic dissection
- **B.** Left ventricular apical thrombus

- **C.** Papillary muscle rupture
- **D.** Ventricular septal rupture

✪✪ Question 4

Transmitral pulsed-wave (PW) Doppler is performed on a patient with acute severe mitral regurgitation (MR) who remains in sinus rhythm. Which feature of the PW Doppler waveform is expected?

- **A.** L-wave
- **B.** E/A reversal
- **C.** A-wave greater than 1.2 m/s
- **D.** E-wave velocity greater than 1.2 m/s

✪✪✪ Question 5

While performing a transthoracic echocardiogram (TTE) on a patient with a late presentation circumflex myocardial infarction, the patient develops acute shortness of breath and pulmonary edema and is now in cardiogenic shock. The TTE identifies a ruptured posteromedial papillary muscle. What continuous-wave (CW) Doppler profile is expected across the mitral valve during systole?

- **A.** Dense parabolic shape with a mid-systolic peak
- **B.** Dense triangular shape with an early systolic peak
- **C.** Faint parabolic shape with an early systolic peak
- **D.** Faint truncated shape with a late systolic peak

✪ Question 6

Which is the most common finding in a patient with acute presentation peripartum cardiomyopathy?

A. A normal-sized left ventricle (LV) with normal systolic function and prominent diastolic dysfunction

B. A dilated LV with globally hypokinetic systolic function

C. A dilated LV with normal systolic function

D. A normal-sized LV with regional wall motion abnormalities

✪ Question 7

What is the recommended acoustic window for a transthoracic echocardiogram (TTE) during a cardiac arrest?

A. Apical

B. Parasternal

C. Suprasternal

D. Subcostal

✪✪ Question 8

Transesophageal echocardiography (TEE) is proving to be useful in which of the following emergency scenarios?

A. Acute coronary syndrome

B. Acute pulmonary embolism

C. Cardiac arrest

D. Pericardial effusion with cardiac tamponade

✪✪ Question 9

A patient presents to the emergency department with anterior penetrating trauma to the chest. The patient is hypotensive, tachycardic, and short of breath. Considering the mechanism of injury, which cardiac pathology is most likely to be found on the transthoracic echocardiogram?

A. Aortic dissection

B. Pericardial tamponade

C. Ruptured mitral valve

D. Ventricular septal defect

✪ Question 10

A 74-year-old woman comes to the emergency department after experiencing a significant emotional event. She has significant chest pain, and her electrocardiogram (ECG) shows ischemic-like changes. She is taken to the cardiac catheterization laboratory as an acute coronary syndrome but is found to have normal coronary arteries. Her echocardiogram post procedure is abnormal. What is the most likely echocardiographic finding?

A. Normal left ventricular (LV) systolic function

B. Apical LV hypertrophy with a mid-systolic gradient

C. Preserved basal LV systolic function with apical ballooning

D. Severe septal hypertrophy and hyperdynamic LV systolic function

✪✪ Question 11

What is the most common location for a postdeceleration traumatic aortic injury?

A. Aortic arch

B. Ascending aorta

C. Descending thoracic aorta

D. The region of the aortic isthmus

✪✪ Question 12

▶ A patient presents with a type A aortic dissection. Based on the transthoracic echocardiogram images provided (**Videos 34-1A** to **34-1F**), which coronary artery is most likely to be included in the dissection plane?

A. Left circumflex coronary artery

B. Left anterior descending coronary artery

C. Right coronary artery

✪ Question 13

A patient presents to the emergency department with a stab wound to the anterior chest. Which is the most likely chamber to have been damaged?

A. Right ventricle

B. Right atrium

C. Left ventricle

D. Left atrium

✪✪✪ Question 14

A patient presents with acute shortness of breath and a new early diastolic murmur. He was involved in a high-speed car accident less than 2 hours earlier; he was wearing a seatbelt at the time of the accident. Which valve is the most likely to have been affected?

A. Aortic

B. Mitral

C. Pulmonary

D. Tricuspid

✪✪✪ Question 15

The disappearance of pleural lung sliding on two-dimensional (2D) lung ultrasound imaging associated with a "barcode or stratosphere sign" on the M-mode trace has a high sensitivity and specificity for which lung pathology?

A. Atelectasis
B. Pleural effusion
C. Pneumothorax
D. Pulmonary embolism

✪ Question 16

What is the echocardiographic finding synonymous with electrical alternans?

A. Acute mitral regurgitation
B. Hepatic venous systolic flow reversal due to severe TR
C. Large pericardial effusion
D. Restrictive diastolic filling profile

✪✪ Question 17

Which is not an echocardiographic sign of cardiac tamponade?

A. Plethoric and noncollapsing IVC
B. Exaggerated respiratory variation of 25% across the mitral valve
C. Exaggerated respiratory variation of 35% across the tricuspid valve
D. Right ventricular (RV) systolic collapse

✪✪ Question 18

▶ Based on images shown in **Video 34-2**, the striking abnormality on the parasternal long-axis image is associated with:

A. Aortic dissection.
B. Mitral valve infective endocarditis.
C. Right ventricular infarct.
D. Massive pulmonary embolism.

✪✪✪ Question 19

Which of the following is not a component of the cardiac Rapid Ultrasound for Shock and Hypotension (RUSH) ultrasound examination?

A. Assessment of left ventricular (LV) contractility
B. Evaluation of right ventricular size

C. Exclusion of pericardial effusion and cardiac tamponade
D. Exclusion of significant valvular stenosis/regurgitation

✪✪ Question 20

A 62-year-old male patient who recently underwent orthopedic surgery presents to the emergency department with presyncope and loss of vision in the right eye. The patient is afebrile, in normal sinus rhythm with a heart rate of 85 bpm, heart sounds are normal with no murmurs, and heart size is normal on the chest X-ray. Which is most likely to be found on the transthoracic echocardiogram (TTE)?

A. Left atrial appendage thrombus
B. Left-heart infective endocarditis
C. Paradoxical pulmonary embolism
D. Pedunculated left ventricular (LV) thrombus

✪✪✪ Question 21

Interstitial syndrome is an ultrasound entity caused by pulmonary edema, interstitial pneumonia, acute respiratory distress syndrome, or lung fibrosis. The characteristic ultrasound appearance of this syndrome is the appearance of B-lines. Which of the following is not characteristic of B-lines?

A. B-lines do not move with lung sliding
B. B-lines arise from the pleural line
C. B-lines erase A-lines
D. B-lines look like comet-tail artifacts

CASE STUDY 1

▶ A 54-year-old man presents to the local health center with shortness of breath and chest pain. He states that the pain started 2 months prior and is worse with activity. He has a history of hypertension and lung cancer for which he has been receiving treatment for 1 month. Blood pressure is 140/90 mm Hg, and heart rate is 80 beats/min. Heart examination is without murmurs, rubs, or gallops. Lung examination reveals bilateral rales in the bases. Trace edema is present to the knees. Focused cardiac ultrasound was performed at the bedside (**Videos 34-3A** and **34-3B**).

✪✪ Question 22

▶ Which is the most likely cause of this patient's chest pain?

A. Cor pulmonale
B. Heart failure with preserved ejection fraction
C. Ischemic heart disease
D. Malignant pericardial effusion

CASE STUDY 2

▶ A 34-year-old man with a history of human immunodeficiency virus (HIV) presents to the clinic complaining of fatigue and shortness of breath. He was in his usual state of health 2 months ago, when he began to experience increasing dyspnea with activity, eventually progressing to shortness of breath with rest. Review of systems is positive for decreased appetite, paroxysmal nocturnal dyspnea, night sweats, and lower extremity swelling. He is not receiving antiretroviral therapy. Per his family, he has a long history of alcohol use. Physical examination reveals a thin man in no distress. His respiratory rate is 18/min, heart rate is 110 bpm, and oxygen saturation is 90% on room air. He is without fever; blood pressure is 90/60 mm Hg. Neck veins are distended. Heart sounds are without murmurs, rubs, or gallops. Lower extremities demonstrate 2+ pitting edema to the mid-thigh region. Focused cardiac ultrasound was performed at the bedside on presentation (**Videos 34-4A** to **34-4C**).

✪ Question 23

Which is the patient's most likely diagnosis?

A. Alcoholic cardiomyopathy
B. HIV cardiomyopathy
C. Pericardial effusion causing cardiac tamponade
D. Pneumocystis pneumonia

ANSWERS

1. **Answer: A.** The most common echocardiographic finding in cardiogenic shock is reduced LV systolic function (and a reduced cardiac output).

   Cardiogenic shock occurs most commonly due to acute coronary syndromes and severe multivessel coronary artery disease. However, it should be noted that cardiogenic shock can be caused by many other mechanisms such as papillary muscle rupture (answer B), significant sepsis, and polypharmacological overdose. RV infarction with subsequent RV systolic dysfunction (answer C) and pericardial effusions causing cardiac tamponade (answer D) are also potential causes of cardiogenic shock.

2. ▶ **Answer: C.** Oral contraception and long periods of sitting in the same position such as on a long international flight are risk factors for the development of deep vein thrombosis, which can embolize to the lungs. Classic two-dimensional echocardiographic features of a large acute pulmonary embolism include right ventricular (RV) dilatation with reduced RV systolic function, McConnell sign (akinesis of the RV mid-free wall with preserved contractility or sparing of the RV apex; **Video 34-5A**), and flattening and paradoxical (leftward) motion of the interventricular septum (**Video 34-5B**). Rarely, mobile thrombus in transit may be seen within the right atrium (RA) or RV (**Video 34-5C**). Another Doppler sign associated with acute pulmonary embolism is the "60/60" sign. This sign includes a short RV acceleration time ≤60 ms and a tricuspid regurgitant (TR) pressure gradient ≤60 mm Hg (**Figure 34-1**).

3. ▶ **Answer: C.** Infarction of the left ventricular (LV) inferior wall can lead to posteromedial papillary muscle rupture. The posteromedial papillary muscle has a single supply of blood from the posterior descending artery of the right coronary artery or dominant left circumflex artery. If this blood supply is occluded for any significant period and infarction occurs, a complication can be the rupture of the papillary muscle head (**Video 34-6A**). This can lead to acute severe mitral regurgitation and the development of pulmonary edema (**Video 34-6B**). Papillary muscle rupture of the anterolateral papillary muscle is rarely seen as this papillary muscle has a dual blood supply from the left anterior descending and left circumflex coronary arteries.

4. **Answer: D.** The mitral regurgitant volume and normal stroke volume from the lungs combine to flow across the mitral valve in diastole. Therefore, a peak velocity of 1.2 m/s or higher is a simple supportive sign of severe MR. However, factors such as left ventricular (LV) relaxation, LV filling pressures, atrial fibrillation, and mitral stenosis need to be taken into account.

   An L-wave (answer A) refers to the presence of mid-diastolic flow. This may be seen when there is markedly abnormal LV relaxation. An L-wave may also be seen normally when there is sinus bradycardia; in this instance, the L-wave velocity is less than 20 cm/s. E/A reversal (answer B), which is an impaired relaxation pattern with a low E velocity and A wave prominence, virtually excludes the

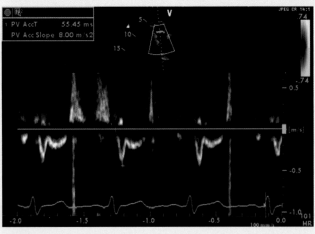 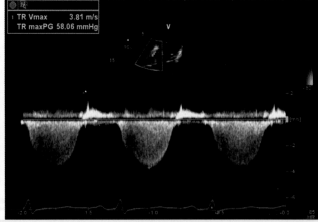

Figure 34-1 The "60/60" sign in a case of acute pulmonary embolism. The RV acceleration time ≤60 ms (left) and the TR pressure gradient ≤60 mm Hg (right).

presence of severe MR. An A-wave velocity greater than 1.2 m/s (answer C) is not indicative of severe MR.

5. **Answer: B.** The CW Doppler profile in this setting is expected to show evidence of acute, severe MR. The density of the CW Doppler signal is proportional to the number of red blood cells within the Doppler beam. Therefore, for a regurgitant Doppler signal, the denser the signal, the more significant the regurgitation volume. Furthermore, the CW Doppler profile of an MR jet reflects the systolic pressure gradient between the left ventricle (LV) and left atrium (LA). When there is acute, severe MR, there is a rise in the left atrial pressure. This results in a decreased LV-LA pressure gradient toward the end of systole. On the CW Doppler signal, this appears as an early peaking, triangular-shaped MR profile (**Figure 34-2**). This appearance is also known as the "V cutoff sign."

6. **Answer: B.** Peripartum cardiomyopathy, previously referred to as postpartum cardiomyopathy, has a poorly understood etiology and is usually diagnosed by process of elimination. Patients typically present during the last month of pregnancy and early puerperium and up to 6 months postdelivery. They can present with typical heart failure symptoms of orthopnea, dyspnea, and fluid retention. Peripartum cardiomyopathy is also associated with atrial and ventricular arrhythmias that can be malignant. Echocardiographic findings include a dilated LV with a global reduction in systolic function (answer B). Transthoracic echocardiography may also detect mural thrombus, mitral or tricuspid regurgitation, right ventricular systolic dysfunction, and pericardial effusion. It is estimated that with conventional heart failure treatment, in over 50% of patients with peripartum cardiomyopathy the LV will return to normal.

7. **Answer: D.** The subcostal window is recommended during a cardiac arrest. Probe positioning for the parasternal window would interfere with effective chest compressions, and the apical window would be challenging due to the amount of chest movement created by vigorous chest compressions. Imaging from the subcostal window provides information that may identify potential reversible causes of cardiac arrest. These reversible causes have been described by a mnemonic known as "H's and T's" (**Table 34-1**). For example, subcostal imaging can assist in the recognition of hypovolemia, pericardial effusion causing tamponade, regional wall motion abnormalities associated with acute coronary syndrome, or an acute pulmonary embolism.

8. **Answer: C.** The positioning of the probe in the esophagus facilitates continuous imaging during external chest compressions. Published case studies have shown that TEE imaging during cardiac arrest has allowed the hand position to be changed on the chest wall to reduce left ventricular outflow tract (LVOT) compression during cardiopulmonary resuscitation (CPR). This ensures an adequate cardiac output. Furthermore, TEE image quality is usually not affected by body habitus or emphysema.

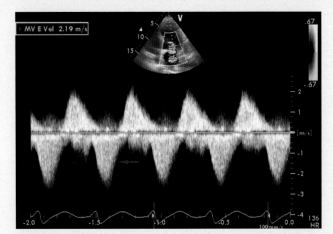

Figure 34-2 An example of a V cutoff sign on the MR CW Doppler signal (arrow). The low MR velocity also suggests a marked elevation in the left atrial pressure.

Table 34-1. H's and T's for Reversible Causes of Cardiac Arrest

H's	T's
Hypovolemia	Tamponade (cardiac)
Hypoxia/hypoxemia	Toxins
Hydrogen ion excess	Tension pneumothorax
Hypokalemia/ hyperkalemia	Thrombosis (pulmonary)
Hypothermia	Thrombosis (coronary)

Cardioversion can also safely take place while the TEE probe is inserted.

9. **Answer: B.** Penetrating chest trauma involving the heart can lead to significant bleeding into the pericardium via perforation of a cardiac chamber, laceration of a coronary artery, or penetrating injury to the myocardium. Cardiac tamponade can quickly evolve due to the rapid accumulation of blood in the pericardial space. Blood in the pericardial space could also clot to form hemopericardium. If the pericardium is largely intact, cardiac tamponade can develop. If the pericardium has a significant disruption, extra-pericardial bleeding could occur resulting in hypovolemic shock.

10. ▶ **Answer: C.** Stress-induced cardiomyopathy or takotsubo cardiomyopathy (TTC) is now well recognized in patients who have experienced a significant emotional or physically stressful event. Typically, symptoms include extreme chest pain and ECG changes are consistent with an acute coronary syndrome. Patients can also experience significant shortness of breath. Cases of stress induced cardiomyopathy have also been reported in patients who have suffered cerebral vascular events, acute asthma attacks, and prolonged surgical events. Classic echocardiographic findings of TTC are normal or hyperdynamic contraction of the basal segments of the left ventricle with varying degrees of hypokinesis of the middle and apical LV segments. In most cases, the apex is significantly dilated and is often dyskinetic (**Video 34-7A**).

Variants of TTC may exist where the apex becomes hyperdynamic, and the basal to middle segments are akinetic; this variant is known as a reversed or inverted TTC. There is also a "ringbark" TTC where only the middle segments of the left ventricle are akinetic (**Video 34-7B**). Left ventricular outflow tract obstruction and right ventricular involvement are other known variants of TTC.

TEACHING POINT

One of the critical characteristics of takotsubo cardiomyopathy is that LV regional wall motion abnormalities extend beyond the distribution of any single coronary artery.

11. **Answer: D.** Traumatic aortic injury is the second most common cause of death (after head injury) in deceleration trauma, with almost 90% of patients who sustain this injury dying at the scene of the incident (Di Marco et al. 2013). The theory behind deceleration traumatic aortic injury is an unequal distribution of forces between the fixed and mobile regions of the aorta. The region of the isthmus is where the ligamentum arteriosum forms after the closure of the ductus arteriosus. This region is a relatively fixed area of the aorta and is thus prone to deceleration injury.

12. **Answer: C.** Based on the images provided, regional wall motion abnormalities are noted in the segments supplied by the right coronary artery (basal inferior septum [**Video 34-1D**], and basal and mid inferior wall segments [**Video 34-1E**]).

TEACHING POINTS

A study of an extensive series of aortic dissections found that the right coronary artery (RCA) was more often involved in the dissection than the left anterior/ circumflex artery (Neri et al. 2001). Coronary artery involvement with aortic dissection has been divided into three classifications. Type A coronary artery involvement is an occlusion of the artery due to the aortic false lumen pressing onto the origin of the artery or pressure from a pericardial effusion inhibiting coronary flow. Type B coronary artery involvement is a retrograde extension of the dissection from the aorta into the coronary artery. Type C coronary artery involvement involves the circumferential detachment of the coronary artery from the aorta due to the dissection. Importantly, the classification of coronary artery dissection should not be confused with the traditional Stanford classification of aortic dissection.

13. **Answer: A.** Due to its anatomical position the most common chamber to be damaged in penetrating anterior chest trauma will be the right ventricle.

TEACHING POINT

In a person who survives a penetrating chest wound, the most common presentation will be cardiac tamponade. The occurrence of tamponade can reduce the bleeding from the laceration. The volume of blood required for tamponade is minimal due to the rapid accumulation of the fluid in the pericardial space. Apart from trying to establish the site of the trauma, sonographers should be aware of regional wall motion defects due to laceration of coronary arteries as well as traumatic injury to the cardiac valves. Due to the mechanism of injury, most victims of direct high-velocity wounds to the anterior chest wall involving the heart (such as gunshot wounds) will not survive.

14. **Answer: A.** Isolated valvular injury is rare. The aortic valve is most often injured, followed by the mitral and tricuspid valves. The mechanism of aortic valve injury is believed to be a sudden increase in intrathoracic pressure due to rapid deceleration, which can lead to a retrograde pressure wave against the aortic valve. This water hammer effect, particularly if suffered in early diastole when the pressure difference across the aortic valve is maximal, causes the valve structure to become disrupted, leading to acute severe aortic regurgitation. The early diastolic murmur found in acute severe aortic regurgitation is due to the rapidly equalization between the aortic and left ventricular diastolic pressures.

15. **Answer: C.** Ultrasound of a normally inflated lung will reveal the visceral and parietal pleura sliding against each other during normal respiration. An M-mode trace of a normal lung will also show the pleura in contact with the aerated lung; this is referred to as the "seashore or sandy beach sign" (**Figure 34-3A**). Clear identification of lung sliding and/or a seashore sign excludes a pneumothorax at that specific point of the lung. The pneumothorax forces a separation between the visceral and parietal pleura due to the accumulating air. This becomes evident on ultrasound by the disappearance of the lung slide on the 2D image and a change in the M-mode signal to a "barcode or stratosphere sign," which appears as a pattern of parallel horizontal lines above and below the pleura highlighting its lack of movement (**Figure 34-3B**). Studies have shown a high sensitivity and specificity for lung ultrasound in the detection of pneumothorax.

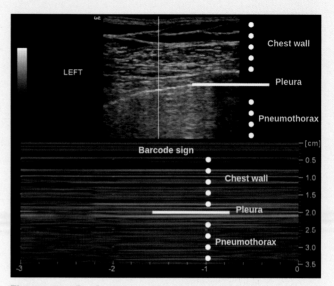

Figure 34-3B "Barcode" or "stratosphere" sign of abnormal lung motion as seen with a pneumothorax. Observe the absence of the "sand" and the presence of a "barcode" below the pleural line. This appearance is characteristic of pneumothorax.

TEACHING POINTS

Lung ultrasound features of a pneumothorax include abolished lung sliding ("barcode" or "stratosphere" sign on the M-mode trace), the absence of B-lines, absence of the lung pulse, and the presence of the lung point. B-lines are essentially ring-down artifacts and therefore appear as long, hyperechoic, vertical lines or streaks throughout the image depth. The lung pulse is a small rhythmic movement of the pleura in synchrony with the heartbeat; this pulse is absent when there is air in the pleural space preventing transmission of movement through the lung to the pleural interface. The lung point is identified as the boundary between normal lung and collapsed lung in the pneumothorax. On M-mode, the lung point is identified by the appearance of alternating lung sliding (seashore sign) and absent sliding (stratosphere sign) during respiration.

16. **Answer: C.** Electrical alternans is the phenomenon where the amplitude of the electrocardiographic QRS complex changes as the heart "swings" within a large pericardial effusion (**Video 34-8**). A large QRS complex is created when the heart is closer to the precordial leads; a smaller QRS complex is generated when the heart swings away from the precordial leads within the effusion. Sinus tachycardia with electrical alternans is highly specific for a large pericardial effusion.

17. **Answer: D.** RV systolic collapse is not considered a sign of cardiac tamponade. The right-sided cardiac chambers collapse as the pericardial pressure increases due to the accumulation of pericardial effusion, which is indeed a diagnostic criterion for

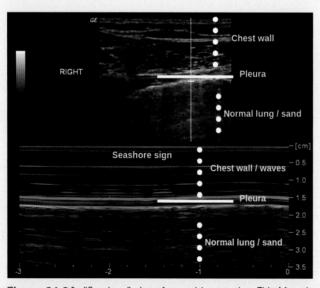

Figure 34-3A "Seashore" sign of normal lung motion. This M-mode trace demonstrates the "sand-on-the-beach" or "seashore" sign that is seen with normal lung sliding.

tamponade, but collapse occurs during the relaxation phase of each of the chambers. The right atrium collapses during ventricular systole and the right ventricle will collapse during ventricular diastole.

TEACHING POINTS

Right atrial (RA) collapse or inversion is seen when the intrapericardial pressure (IPP) exceeds the RA pressure; this usually occurs during atrial relaxation, immediately following atrial contraction, when the RA pressure is at its lowest point. Therefore, RA collapse or inversion is seen during late ventricular diastole or early ventricular systole. RV collapse occurs when the IPP exceeds the RV pressure; this usually occurs during early to mid-diastole when the RV pressure is at its lowest point.

18. ▶ **Answer: A.** The parasternal long-axis view shows an example of a type A aortic dissection. The dissection flap prolapses through the valve in diastole and is associated with severe aortic regurgitation (**Video 34-9**). There also appears to be significant left ventricular hypertrophy, potentially indicating long-standing/untreated hypertension, which is a risk factor for aortic dissection.

    Answer B is incorrect as there are no signs of obvious mitral valve disease. Answers C and D are incorrect since the right ventricle is of normal size and appears to have normal function, thus excluding a right ventricular infarct or a massive pulmonary embolism.

19. **Answer: D.** The RUSH examination is performed in patients presenting to the emergency department with undifferentiated hypotension. The aim of this examination is to rule out or diagnose conditions causing hypotension. The components of the exam include ultrasound imaging of the heart, inferior vena cava (IVC), abdomen (Morison's/FAST abdominal views with thoracic windows), and aorta, as well as scanning for pneumothorax. These components can be recalled with the mnemonic: HI-MAP (H = heart; I = IVC; M = Morison's; A = aorta and P = pneumothorax). This examination may also be considered as a three-part assessment of "the pump," "the tank," and the "pipes." The cardiac or heart portion of the RUSH exam evaluates for pericardial effusion/tamponade, right ventricular failure (as a sign of pulmonary embolism), LV function (whether hypodynamic or hyperdynamic), the IVC (for volume status and an estimation of central venous pressure), and the aorta (to exclude aortic dissection or abdominal aortic aneurysm).

20. **Answer: C.** As the patient has had recent orthopedic surgery, it may be assumed that his mobility has been limited. Therefore, he is susceptible to the development of deep vein thrombosis, which might result in an acute pulmonary embolism. Given the patient's presentation, it appears that he may have suffered some type of systemic embolic event. Therefore, the TTE may reveal a paradoxical pulmonary embolism traversing a patent foramen ovale (answer C).

    Left atrial appendage thrombus (answer A) is unlikely as the patient is in sinus rhythm. Left-heart infective endocarditis (answer B) is also unlikely as the patient is afebrile and heart sounds are normal with no murmurs. Pedunculated LV thrombus (answer D) is unlikely based on the information provided.

21. ▶ **Answer: A.** B-lines are artifacts generated by the juxtaposition of alveolar air and thickening of subpleural interlobular septa in pulmonary interstitial edema; they arise from the pleural line. On 2D imaging, B-lines appear as long, hyperechoic, vertical lines or streaks throughout the image depth as these lines are essentially comet-tail or ring-down artifacts (**Video 34-10**). In the normal, aerated lung, A-lines appear as hyperechoic, horizontal lines arising at regular intervals from the pleural line; these A-lines are erased when B-lines are present. Therefore, answers B, C, and D are all characteristic features of B-lines. Another characteristic feature of B-lines is that they move synchronously with lung sliding; therefore, answer A is not characteristic of B-lines.

TEACHING POINT

The characteristic lung ultrasound features of B-lines are as follows:
• They originate from the pleural line.
• They appear as long, vertical hyperechoic lines throughout the image depth.
• They erase A-lines.
• They move with lung sliding.

The presence of multiple B-lines (≥3) in a region of interrogation is suggestive of the presence of interstitial syndrome.

22. ▶ **Answer: C.** Focused cardiac ultrasound (FCU) images acquired from the parasternal views show that left ventricular systolic function is not preserved (answer B is incorrect). While cor pulmonale (answer A) cannot be excluded with FCU, the normal size of the right ventricle makes it less likely. There is no pericardial effusion (answer D is incorrect). Complete analysis of wall motion is a difficult interpretive skill and belongs in the scope of practice of an echocardiographer. However, a practitioner performing FCU should note obvious wall motion abnormalities such as that present in this example. The parasternal long-axis view shows significant hypokinesis of the posterior wall and the short-axis view shows hypokinesis of the inferior-posterior segments. This FCU study is in no way

definitive, but it helps steer the initial management and next set of diagnostic tests toward ischemic heart disease.

23. **Answer: C.** The patient has cardiac tamponade. Dyspnea in an immunocompromised patient has a broad differential. There are clues from the physical examination that he is in heart failure, leading away from pneumonia, but after physical examination the differential still includes disorders with very different management strategies. The focused cardiac ultrasound (FCU) images obtained by a user with basic FCU training demonstrate within minutes of arriving at the bedside that left ventricular systolic function is preserved and there is a significant pericardial effusion. As the diagnosis of tamponade is clinical, seeing an effusion on FCU should prompt the clinician to check for pulsus paradoxus, which may not have been done initially without suspicion of pericardial effusion. While the ultrasound assessment of tamponade is complex and involves several modalities/views, looking for obvious compression of the right ventricle (seen in the subcostal view) should be noted by an FCU practitioner.

Acknowledgments: The authors thank and acknowledge Marc D. Robinson, MD, and Kirk T. Spencer, MD (Chapter 10, Focused Cardiac Ultrasound) in *Clinical Echocardiography Review: A Self-Assessment Tool*, 2nd ed., edited by Allan L. Klein, Craig R. Asher; 2017. The authors also thank Bonita Anderson for providing the images for question 12.

SUGGESTED READINGS

Anderson BA. *Sonographer's Guide to the Assessment of Heart Disease.* Brisbane, Australia: MGA Graphics; 2014.

Di Marco L, Pacini D, Di Bartolomeo R. Acute traumatic thoracic aortic injury: considerations and reflections on the endovascular aneurysm repair. *Aorta (Stamford).* 2013;1(2):117-122.

Husain LF, Hagopian L, Wayman D, Baker WE, Carmody KA. Sonographic diagnosis of pneumothorax. *J Emerg Trauma Shock.* 2012;5(1):76-81.

Lichtenstein D. Novel approaches to ultrasonography of the lung and pleural space: where are we now? *Breathe.* 2017;13(2):100-111.

Lichtenstein DA, Menu Y. A bedside ultrasound sign ruling out pneumothorax in the critically III: lung sliding. *Chest.* 1995;108(5):1345-1348.

McLean AS. Echocardiography in shock management. *Crit Care.* 2016;20:275.

Miller A. Practical approach to lung ultrasound. *BJA Educ.* 2016;16(2):39-45.

Neri E, Toscano T, Papalia U, et al. Proximal aortic dissection with coronary malperfusion: presentation, management, and outcome. *J Thorac Cardiovasc Surg.* 2001;121(3):552-560.

Spittell PC, Spittell JA Jr, Joyce JW, et al. Clinical features and differential diagnosis of aortic dissection: experience with 236 cases (1980 through 1990). *Mayo Clin Proc.* 1993;68(7):642-651.

Volpicelli G, Elbarbary M, Blaivas M, et al. International evidence-based recommendations for point-of-care lung ultrasound. *Intensive Care Med.* 2012;38(4):577-591.

Volpicelli G. Sonographic diagnosis of pneumothorax. *Intensive Care Med.* 2011;37(2):224-232.

Zhang M, Liu Z-H, Yang J-X, et al. Rapid detection of pneumothorax by ultrasonography in patients with multiple trauma. *Crit Care.* 2006;10(4):R112.

CHAPTER 35

Transesophageal Echocardiography

Contributors: Kenneth Horton, ACS, RCS and Karen G. Zimmerman, BS, ACS, RDCS (AE/PE), RVT

✪✪ Question 1

Which of the following statements regarding probe insertion technique is correct?

 A. Locking control wheels is recommended at the time of probe insertion.

 B. The probe should be inspected for damage before insertion and a live sector image should be on the screen.

 C. The probe should be inserted with the patient flat on his or her back.

 D. Extension of the neck facilitates esophageal intubation.

✪✪ Question 2

Aortic valvular gradients are best obtained using transesophageal echocardiography (TEE) in which view?

 A. Midesophageal view with anteflexion

 B. Midesophageal view with retroflexion

 C. Deep transgastric view at 30° with retroflexion

 D. Deep transgastric view at 0° with anteflexion

✪✪✪ Question 3

Which of the following associations between complication and incidence is correct regarding transesophageal echocardiography (TEE)?

 A. Mortality: 0.1% to 0.2%

 B. Esophageal perforation: 0.4% to 0.9%

 C. Major bleeding: <0.01%

 D. Heart failure: 0.5%

✪✪ Question 4

The pulmonary venous flow pattern demonstrated by transesophageal echocardiography (TEE) in **Figure 35-1** is consistent with:

 A. Large atrial reversal secondary to increased left ventricular end-diastolic pressure.

 B. Mild mitral regurgitation.

 C. Mitral stenosis.

 D. Severe mitral regurgitation.

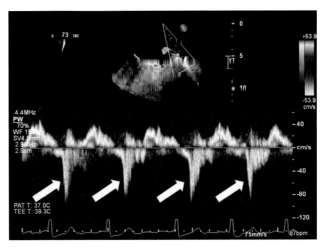

Figure 35-1

✪✪ Question 5

⏵ What is the main pathologic finding in this transesophageal echocardiographic (TEE) midesophageal view (**Figure 35-2A** and **35-2B**, and **Video 35-1**)?

 A. Bileaflet mitral valve prolapse

 B. Flail posterior mitral valve leaflet

 C. Large vegetation

 D. Systolic anterior motion of the mitral valve

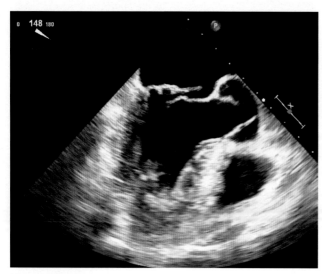

Figure 35-2A

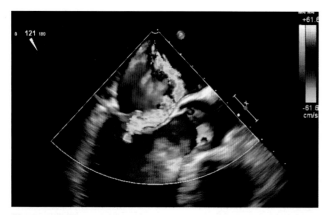

Figure 35-2B

✪✪ Question 6

What normal anatomical structure in the left atrial appendage (LAA), as seen in **Figure 35-3**, could be mistakenly diagnosed as a left atrial appendage thrombus or mass?

    A. Crista terminalis
    B. Eustachian ridge
    C. Foramen ovale
    D. Pectinate muscles

✪ Question 7

What can be used during precardioversion transesophageal echocardiography (TEE) to help distinguish dense spontaneous echo contrast in the left atrial appendage (LAA) from thrombus?

    A. Biplane imaging
    B. Color flow Doppler
    C. Spectral Doppler velocities
    D. Ultrasound enhancement agents (UEA)

✪✪✪ Question 8

What abnormality is noted in this transesophageal echocardiographic (TEE) image acquired from a patient with a bioprosthetic valve and anemia (**Figure 35-4A** and **35-4B** and **Videos 35-2A** and **35-2B**)?

    A. Doppler artifact
    B. Normal "washing jets"
    C. Paravalvular regurgitation
    D. Valvular regurgitation

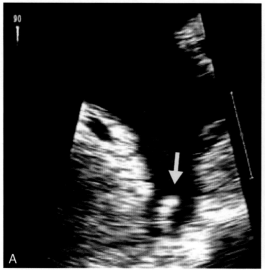
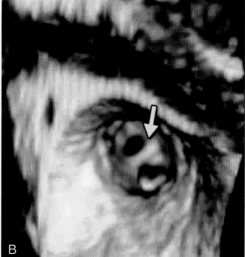

Figure 35-3 A, two-dimensional transesophageal echocardiographic view of the LAA. B, three-dimensional transesophageal echocardiographic view of the LAA. (Reprinted from Beigel R, Wunderlich NC, Ho SY, et al. The left atrial appendage: anatomy, function, and noninvasive evaluation. *JACC Cardiovasc Imaging*. 2014;7(12):1251-1265. Copyright © 2014 American College of Cardiology Foundation. With permission.)

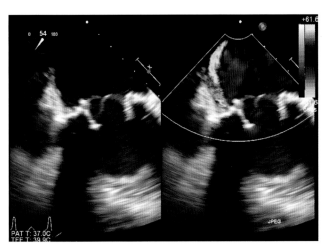

Figure 35-4A

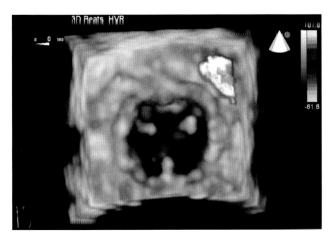

Figure 35-4B

⭐⭐ Question 9

When performing high-level disinfection of a transesophageal transducer, enzymatic cleaning is performed to:

A. Neutralize microscopic accumulation of blood left on the probe.

B. Eliminate any bacteria that came in contact with the probe.

C. Remove inorganic and organic debris that can otherwise remain on the probe's surface and defeat the efficacy of the disinfection.

D. Sterilize the probe.

⭐⭐⭐ Question 10

Which of the following statements regarding the tricuspid valve is correct?

A. The anterior leaflet has the longest radial length.

B. The names of the leaflets are septal, anterior, and inferior.

C. The septal leaflet has the longest radial length.

D. The tricuspid valve is usually visualized only in the midesophageal 4-chamber view.

⭐⭐⭐ Question 11

Which of the following is an absolute contraindication for transesophageal echocardiography (TEE)?

A. Barrett esophagus

B. Esophageal diverticulum

C. History of gastrointestinal surgery

D. History of radiation to the neck and mediastinum

⭐ Question 12

What is the finding in this patient with back pain (Figure 35-5)?

A. Ascending aortic dissection with intramural hematoma

B. Descending aortic dissection with intramural hematoma

C. Descending aortic dissection with mirror image artifact

D. Descending aortic dissection with pericardial effusion

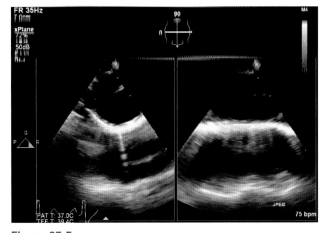

Figure 35-5

⭐ Question 13

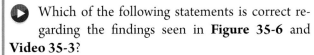 Which of the following statements is correct regarding the findings seen in **Figure 35-6** and **Video 35-3**?

A. It is the most common benign tumor of the heart.

B. It is usually attached to the interatrial septum.

C. Surgery is the treatment of choice.

D. All of the above.

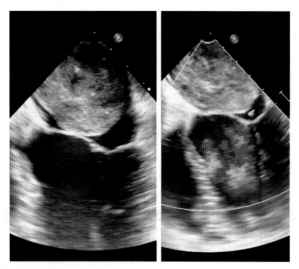

Figure 35-6

✪ Question 14

The midesophageal views of the aortic valve presented in **Figure 35-7A** and **35-7B** demonstrate a:

A. Periaortic abscess.
B. Quadricuspid aortic valve.
C. Noncoronary sinus that has ruptured into the right atrium.
D. Sinus of Valsalva aneurysm of the right coronary sinus.

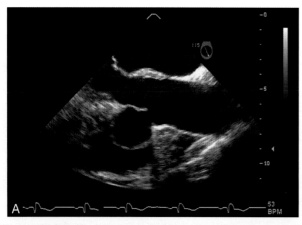

Figure 35-7A (Reprinted with permission from Klein AL, Asher CR. *Clinical Echocardiography Review. A Self-Assessment Tool.* 2nd ed. Philadelphia, PA: Wolters Kluwer; 2017.)

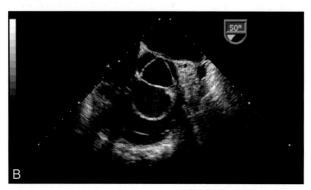

Figure 35-7B (Reprinted with permission from Klein AL, Asher CR. *Clinical Echocardiography Review. A Self-Assessment Tool.* 2nd ed. Philadelphia, PA: Wolters Kluwer; 2017.)

✪✪ Question 15

Which transesophageal echocardiographic (TEE) view is used to obtain the structures noted in **Figure 35-8**?

A. Midesophageal commissural
B. Midesophageal long-axis
C. Transgastric basal short-axis
D. Transgastric two-chamber

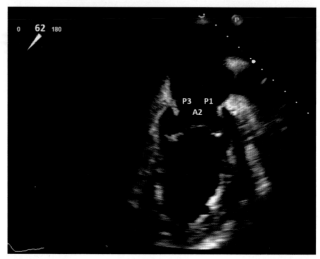

Figure 35-8

✪ Question 16

What is the structure identified by the arrow in **Figure 35-9**?

A. Right upper pulmonary vein
B. Superior vena cava
C. Inferior vena cava
D. Coronary sinus

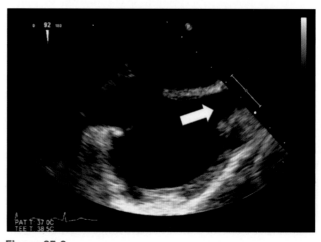

Figure 35-9

✪ Question 17

▶ What is the finding shown in **Figure 35-10** and **Video 35-4**?
   A. Sinus venosus defect
   B. Patent foramen ovale
   C. Ostium secundum defect
   D. Ostium primum defect

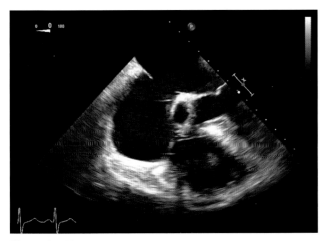

Figure 35-10

✪ Question 18

The pulmonary valve can be best visualized from which of the following standard transesophageal echocardiographic (TEE) views?
   A. Midesophageal short-axis
   B. Midesophageal bicaval
   C. Transgastric right ventricular inflow
   D. Transgastric long-axis

✪ Question 19

At what degree is the transesophageal echocardiographic (TEE) 4-chamber view acquired?
   A. 0°
   B. 30°
   C. 90°
   D. 180°

✪ Question 20

In the midesophageal window, the far field displays more _____ structures due to the probe position within the esophagus.
   A. Superior
   B. Posterior
   C. Lateral
   D. Anterior

✪ Question 21

Which control or manipulation can be used to electronically rotate the imaging plane axially from 0° to 180° on the transesophageal echocardiographic (TEE) probe?
   A. Simply rotating the probe handle
   B. Using the side buttons on the probe handle
   C. Rotating the large wheel on the probe handle
   D. Rotating the small wheel on the probe handle

✪✪ Question 22

▶ Which tricuspid valve (TV) leaflet is identified by the asterisk in this transgastric image (**Figure 35-11** and **Video 35-5**)?
   A. Anterior
   B. Septal
   C. Posterior
   D. B or C

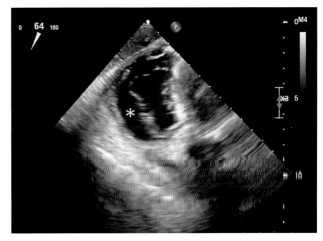

Figure 35-11

✪ Question 23

Which aortic cusp is seen adjacent to the interatrial septum?
   A. Left coronary cusp (LCC)
   B. Noncoronary cusp (NCC)
   C. Right coronary cusp (RCC)
   D. A or B

✪✪ Question 24

▶ The normal variant visualized in this transesophageal echocardiographic (TEE) image (**Figure 35-12**, arrow and **Video 35-6**) is the:
   A. Crista terminalis.
   B. Eustachian valve.
   C. Inferior vena cava (IVC).
   D. Limbus.

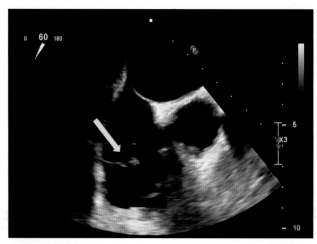

Figure 35-12

✪ Question 25

▶ Based on the images provided (**Figure 35-13** and **Video 35-7**), what is the most likely pathologic finding in this patient?
   A. Ventricular septal defect
   B. Ruptured sinus of Valsalva aneurysm
   C. Patent foramen ovale
   D. Mitral valve prolapse

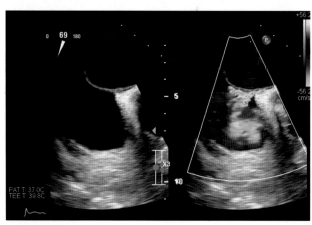

Figure 35-13

✪✪✪ Question 26

The following are appropriate indications for transesophageal echocardiography (TEE) except:
   A. Guidance during percutaneous noncoronary interventions.
   B. Routine assessment of pulmonary veins in patients after pulmonary vein isolation.
   C. Suspected acute aortic pathology.
   D. When transthoracic echocardiography (TTE) is nondiagnostic due to poor-quality images.

✪✪✪ Question 27

Which of the following statements is correct regarding methemoglobinemia after benzocaine topical anesthesia for transesophageal echocardiography (TEE)?
   A. Oxygen saturation is low, arterial partial pressure of oxygen (PO_2) is normal, and there is no cyanosis.
   B. There is no cyanosis, but arterial PO_2 and oxygen saturation are low.
   C. Higher levels (methemoglobinemia level >70%) may result in dysrhythmias, circulatory failure, neurologic depressionand death.
   D. The treatment of choice is 100% oxygen.

✪✪ Question 28

The high-esophageal view of a patient in the operating room in **Figure 35-14** shows a(n):
   A. Left atrial myxoma.
   B. Near field artifact.
   C. Extracardiac tumor invading the left atrium.
   D. Large pulmonary embolism in the main and right pulmonary arteries.

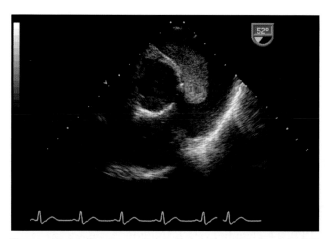

Figure 35-14 (Reprinted with permission from Klein AL, Asher CR. *Clinical Echocardiography Review. A Self-Assessment Tool.* 2nd ed. Philadelphia, PA: Wolters Kluwer; 2017.)

✪✪ Question 29

▶ A transesophageal echocardiogram (TEE) is ordered on a 45-year-old patient with a stroke who had a nondiagnostic transthoracic echocardiogram earlier in the day. What abnormal finding is shown on **Figure 35-15** and **Video 35-8**?
   A. Thrombus in transit
   B. Flail mitral valve leaflet
   C. Aneurysmal atrial septum
   D. Prominent eustachian valve

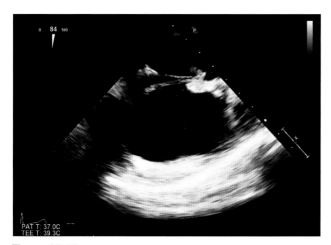

Figure 35-15

✪ Question 30

What is the abnormal pathology seen on **Figure 35-16** and **Video 35-9** in the patient with sudden shortness of breath and elevated white blood cell count?

A. Flail mitral valve
B. Prominent eustachian valve
C. Right atrial appendage thrombus
D. Tricuspid valve endocarditis

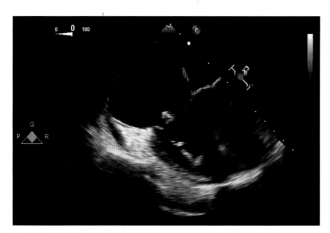

Figure 35-16

✪✪ Question 31

What is the abnormal finding in this patient with a new murmur who is being evaluated for hypotension and hemodynamic instability following a myocardial infarction (**Figure 35-17A** and **35-17B** and **Video 35-10**)?

A. A pericardial effusion with cardiac tamponade
B. A ventricular septal defect
C. Findings consistent with pulmonary embolism
D. Left ventricular lateral wall hypokinesis

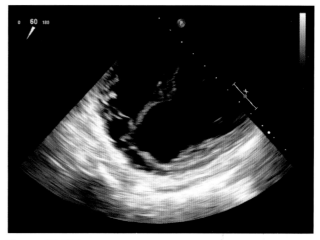

Figure 35-17A

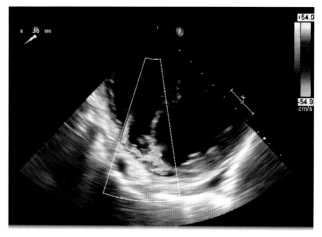

Figure 35-17B

✪✪✪ Question 32

Based on the images provided (**Figure 35-18** and **Video 35-11**), what is the abnormal finding in this patient who underwent aortic valve replacement 2 years ago and now presents with new complete heart block?

A. Infected aortic annulus with abscess
B. Paravalvular regurgitation
C. Prosthetic aortic valve stenosis
D. Sinus of Valsalva-to-right atrium fistula

✪✪ Question 33

How should the atheroma (3 mm thickness) in **Figure 35-19** be graded?

A. Grade 1
B. Grade 2
C. Grade 3
D. Grade 4

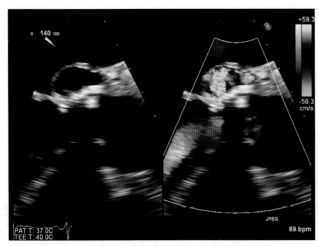

Figure 35-18

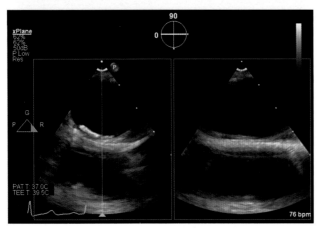

Figure 35-19

✪✪ Question 34

▶ What is the abnormal finding in this patient with elevated left ventricular outflow tract velocities and pressure gradients (**Figure 35-20**, **Video 35-12**)?

    A. Aortic regurgitation

    B. Bicuspid aortic valve

    C. Subaortic membrane

    D. Valvular aortic stenosis

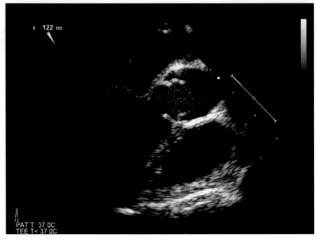

Figure 35-20

✪✪ Question 35

Which of the following medications is not used for conscious sedation and pain relief of a patient undergoing transesophageal echocardiography?

    A. Fentanyl

    B. Midazolam

    C. Narcan

    D. Propofol

ANSWERS

1. **Answer: B.** Some of the most feared complications of transesophageal echocardiography occur during probe insertion. Knobs should never be locked to diminish the possibility of pharyngeal or esophageal injury. In the outpatient setting, the probe should be inserted in moderately sedated patients with the patient in the lateral decubitus position and with anterior flexion of the neck. In the perioperative setting, the probe is usually inserted with the patient supine and under general anesthesia. The probe should always be inspected before insertion, with an image on the screen confirming normal probe function. The American Society of Echocardiography guidelines for performing a Comprehensive Transesophageal Echocardiography Examination have detailed descriptions of the appropriate techniques of probe insertion.

2. **Answer: D.** The evaluation of patients with aortic stenosis using TEE includes visualization of the aortic valve anatomy and planimetry of the aortic valve area. When possible, transvalvular gradients are obtained. However, obtaining accurate transaortic gradients can be technically challenging. It requires a deep transgastric view at 0° with anteflexion of the probe tip (**Figure 35-21**) The objective is alignment of the aortic valve and proximal ascending aorta as parallel as possible with the continuous-wave Doppler cursor. Alternatively, the transducer position can be set at 90° to 100° and the probe slowly pulled back, keeping the anteflexion and the tip adjusted

Deep transgastric five-chamber

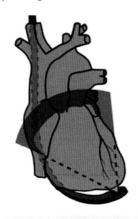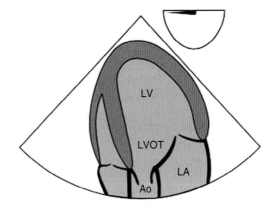

Figure 35-21 Image demonstrating TEE probe location for a deep transgastric view on the left and the corresponding TEE image on the right. (Reproduced with permission of the Oxford University Press through PLSclear, from Sidebotham D, Merry AF, Legget ME, et al. Practical perioperative transesophageal echocardiography. In: *Oxford Clinical Imaging Guidelines.* 3rd ed. Oxford, UK: Oxford University Press; 2018.)

with the lateral knob. These maneuvers are important not only in patients with valvular stenosis but also in patients with hypertrophic obstructive cardiomyopathy.

3. **Answer: C.** TEE is a safe technique in the proper setting and in experienced hands. The overall incidence of complications is very low (0.18% to 2.8%). The highest complication rates (>10%) are hoarseness and lip injury. Mortality occurs in <0.02% and major bleeding in <0.01%.

4. **Answer: D.** Pulmonary venous flow assessment is part of a comprehensive evaluation in patients with mitral regurgitation. **Figure 35-1** shows holo-systolic flow reversal (arrows), which is consistent with severe mitral regurgitation. In patients with mild mitral regurgitation (answer B), usually the pulmonary venous flow is normal with predominant or mildly blunted systolic flow. A large atrial reversal wave is seen in patients with increased end-diastolic pressure (answer A) but this is not seen in this figure as flow reversal occurs during systole. In patients with mitral stenosis (answer C), the typical finding is a slow deceleration slope in the diastolic wave of pulmonary venous flow.

5. **Answer: B.** Degenerative mitral valve disease is the most common cause of severe mitral regurgitation requiring surgery. Echocardiography is the main diagnostic modality to assess mitral valve disease. Although transthoracic echocardiography often offers enough diagnostic information, TEE is the gold standard for anatomical definition. Posterior mitral valve prolapse and/or flail are more common than anterior mitral pathology. A flail leaflet is diagnosed when ruptured chordae are visualized and the tip of the leaflet points superiorly into the left atrium in systole. In cases of posterior leaflet flail, the regurgitant jet is anteriorly directed.

6. **Answer: D.** Pectinate muscles are complex indentations that line the surface of the left atrial appendage (**Figure 35-3A**). Larger pectinate muscles can be mistaken for thrombi. Three-dimensional echocardiography of the appendage may help differentiate the pectinate muscles from small thrombi (**Figure 35-3B**). The crista terminalis (answer A) and Eustachian ridge (answer B) are anatomical structures located in the right atrium. The foramen ovale (answer D) is an opening in the atrial septum that allows for shunting of blood from the right to the left atrium during fetal circulation.

7. **Answer: D.** Using ultrasound enhancement agents (UEAs) during TEE to differentiate spontaneous echo contrast or artifact from thrombus in the left atrial appendage (LAA) is an off-label use of UEAs. Administration of UEAs during TEE can assist in better visualizing the LAA. When administering UEAs for LAA visualization, very small, slow injections of the UEA should be given. Harmonic imaging should be utilized with very low mechanical index (MI) settings (<0.2). Slow injections along with low MI settings should minimize artifacts associated with UEA administration (e.g., attenuation, swirling). When using UEAs to identify LAA thrombus, the thrombus will appear as an area that does not take up the UEA and it will appear black. As shown in **Figure 35-22A** there is an area of possible thrombus in the LAA noted by the arrow. An ultrasound enhancement agent was administered (**Figure 35-22B** and **Video 35-13**) and the presence of thrombus was ruled out. Biplane imaging (answer A), color flow Doppler (answer B), and spectral Doppler velocities (answer C) are all modalities that can be used to better assess the LAA but will not be helpful in differentiating spontaneous echo contrast from thrombus.

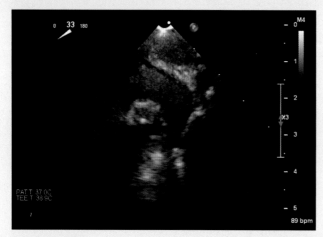

Figure 35-22A

Figure 35-22B

8. **Answer: C.** In patients with bioprosthetic valves, hemolytic anemia may be an indication of a paravalvular leak. The high-velocity flow through the paravalvular leak causes the red blood cells to rupture (hemolysis) leading to anemia. Paravalvular regurgitation can often be visualized on a transthoracic echocardiogram; however, TEE is usually performed to better assess the precise location and severity of the leak. Oftentimes imaging a paravalvular leak requires off-axis planes to localize the leak. Paravalvular regurgitation that results in anemia can often be repaired surgically or with percutaneous techniques.

9. **Answer: C.** Cleaning of a transesophageal probe may vary slightly from facility to facility. However, the basic steps that should be followed should be consistent across all facilities:
   • Point-of-care cleaning is performed immediately after probe removal at the bedside. Point-of-care cleaning should be performed with material that is approved by the equipment manufacturer. After the cleaning is completed, the probe should be placed in a biohazard-labeled container for transport to the cleaning room.

• Enzymatic solutions are protein inhibitor solutions that release enzymes to degrade and loosen biologic material that is on the probe. The enzymatic cleaning should be performed with a solution that is approved for use by the equipment manufacturer. It usually requires that the probe be soaked in the solution for a specified length of time.
• High-level disinfection (HLD) is the process of complete elimination of all microorganisms in or on a device, except for a small number of bacterial spores. Examples of HLD solutions include glutaraldehyde and orthophthalaldehyde (OPA).
• An electrical safety check should be performed on all transesophageal probes prior to their next use on a patient.
• Probes should be stored by hanging in a cabinet free of contact with other objects.

10. **Answer: A.** Although transthoracic echocardiography usually provides diagnostic imaging of the pathology of the tricuspid valve, transesophageal echocardiography (TEE) can offer additional information regarding anatomy and function. This is particularly relevant in patients with suspected endocarditis. It is then necessary to know the anatomy of the valve and the different TEE views used to visualize its different components. The tricuspid valve leaflets are the anterior (with the longest radial length), septal, and posterior leaflets (**Figure 35-23**). The tricuspid valve can be visualized in multiple TEE views beginning with the midesophageal 4-chamber view. Because regurgitant jets are usually not coaxial with the ultrasound beam in this view, it is necessary to explore other angles. The 70° to 100° views are often the best for continuous-wave Doppler interrogation. In patients a with normal-sized aorta, the 150° view is helpful for the visualization of tricuspid valve regurgitation jet size.

11. **Answer: B.** Absolute contraindications to TEE include esophageal or pharyngeal obstruction, esophageal diverticulum, active gastrointestinal bleeding from an unknown source, and perforated

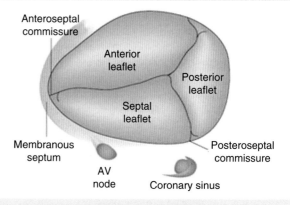

Figure 35-23 (Reprinted by permission from Nature: Shinn SH, Schaff HV. Evidence-based surgical management of acquired tricuspid valve disease. *Nat Rev Cardiol.* 2013;10(4):190-203. Copyright © 2013 Springer Nature.)

Table 35-1. List of Absolute and Relative Contraindications to Transesophageal Echocardiography

Absolute Contraindications	Relative Contraindications
• Perforated viscus • Esophageal stricture • Esophageal tumor • Esophageal perforation, laceration • Esophageal diverticulum • Active upper GI bleed	• History of radiation to neck and mediastinum • History of GI surgery • Recent upper GI bleed • Barrett esophagus • History of dysphagia • Restriction of neck mobility (severe cervical arthritis, atlantoaxial joint disease) • Symptomatic hiatal hernia • Esophageal varices • Coagulopathy, thrombocytopenia • Active esophagitis • Active peptic ulcer disease

GI = Gastrointestinal.

viscus. Relative contraindications include esophageal varices, history of radiation to the neck, Barrett esophagus, and coagulopathy. Absolute and relative contraindications are shown in **Table 35-1.**

12. **Answer: C.** This image demonstrates an aortic dissection in the descending aorta. Note the characteristic dissection flap that separates the true from false lumen. There is also a mirror image artifact noted in the image beyond the aorta. A mirror image artifact appears below a strong reflective surface producing a duplicate image behind the true image.

13. **Answer: D.** The images provided show a left atrial myxoma. Myxomas are the most common benign tumors of the heart. They can be found in any of the heart cavities but most often in the left atrium. Typically, these tumors are attached by a stalk to the interatrial septum. Surgery is usually indicated due to the potential for embolism or obstruction of the mitral valve orifice. In most cases, these are single tumors, although in their familial form, they can be multiple and recurrent. Carney syndrome is an autosomal dominantly transmitted multisystem tumor disorder characterized by myxomas (heart, skin, and breast), spotty skin pigmentation (lentigines and blue nevi), endocrine tumors (adrenal, testicular, thyroid, and pituitary), and peripheral nerve tumors (schwannomas). In Carney syndrome, the cardiac myxomas are also multiple and contribute to the mortality of this disease.

14. **Answer: D.** These images show a sinus of Valsalva aneurysm of the right coronary sinus. This is a rare anomaly, usually congenital although it can be traumatic. Nonruptured aneurysm of the sinus of Valsalva is not associated with symptoms, although it may result in aortic regurgitation. In cases of intracardiac rupture into the right atrium or right ventricle,

acute heart failure and physical findings consistent with severe aortic regurgitation may develop. Once ruptured, the morphology of the aneurysm may change and appears more like a fistulous tract and can be confused with a tricuspid valve vegetation and severe tricuspid regurgitation. The continuous timing of the spectral Doppler waveform helps make the diagnosis of aortic-to-right atrial communication.

15. **Answer: A.** The midesophageal commissural view is obtained with the TEE transducer in the midesophageal window with the imaging plane set to approximately 60°. In this image the P1 and P3 segments of the posterior mitral valve are seen on the medial and lateral aspects of the mitral annulus, respectively. The free-floating A2 segment of the anterior mitral leaflet is seen between the P1 and P3 segments, similar to a trapdoor. Variable amounts of the anterior leaflet are visualized depending on the angulation.

16. **Answer: B.** This is a midesophageal bicaval view. It is usually obtained from the midesophageal window between 90 and 110°. Imaged in this view are the left atrium, right atrium, inferior vena cava, superior vena cava (arrow), right atrial appendage, coronary sinus, and interatrial septum (IAS). This view is commonly used to assess the IAS. In addition, the inferior vena cava and superior vena cava (SVC) inflow are well imaged. Pacemaker leads and indwelling catheters can often be seen entering the right atrium from the SVC. To visualize the right upper pulmonary vein, the probe is rotated clockwise and slightly withdrawn.

17. **Answer: C.** An ostium secundum atrial septal defect (ASD) is located in the central portion of the interatrial septum. The secundum ASD usually

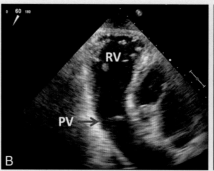

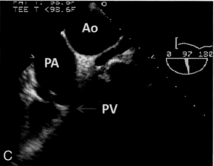

Figure 35-24 Pulmonary valve imaging from the midesophageal right ventricular (RV) inflow-outflow view (A, red arrow), transgastric basal RV view (B, red arrow), and upper esophageal aortic arch short-axis view (C, red arrow). (Reproduced from Hahn RT, Abraham T, Adams MS, et al. Guidelines for performing a comprehensive transesophageal echocardiographic examination: recommendations from the American Society of Echocardiography and the Society of Cardiovascular Anesthesiologists. *J Am Soc Echocardiogr.* 2013;26:921-964. Copyright © 2013 American Society of Echocardiography. With permission.)

arises from an enlarged foramen ovale, inadequate growth of the septum secundum, or excessive absorption of the septum primum. This is the most common type of ASD. Other views that can be used to assess ASDs include the bicaval view (midesophageal window, ~90°-110°) and the midesophageal short-axis view (midesophageal window, ~25°-45°).

18. **Answer: A.** The pulmonary valve is an anterior, and thus, far-field structure for TEE. This can make it more challenging to visualize because of interference from other structures such as the bronchus. The midesophageal short-axis view is one of the most common views for imaging the pulmonary valve. **Figure 35-24** demonstrates the midesophageal short-axis view and other common TEE views that are used to visualize the pulmonary valve. These views are commonly utilized during pulmonary valve transcatheter interventions and to rule out pulmonary valve endocarditis.

19. **Answer: A.** The 4-chamber view (**Figure 35-25**) is obtained with the probe in the midesophageal window at the level of the mitral valve and rotated to

zero degrees. The key structures visualized are the left atrium, right atrium, left ventricle, right ventricle, and mitral and tricuspid valves. The atrial and ventricular septa can also be visualized. The ventricular walls that are displayed in this image are the left ventricular lateral wall and septum and the right ventricular anterior free wall.

This is a very valuable TEE view and most examinations begin with this view. It allows the quick assessment of the size of all four chambers, the function of the left and right ventricles, and gives an initial assessment of the mitral and tricuspid valves. It also allows the assessment of septal and lateral wall motion. Following 2D imaging, color Doppler is used to assess flow through the mitral and tricuspid valves. Slight anterior flexion from this view will bring in the left ventricular outflow tract and aortic valve, resulting in a 5-chamber view similar to that seen on the transthoracic echocardiogram. With retroflexion the coronary sinus will be seen.

20. **Answer: D.** Anatomically, the esophagus is located directly posterior to the left atrium. The midesophageal

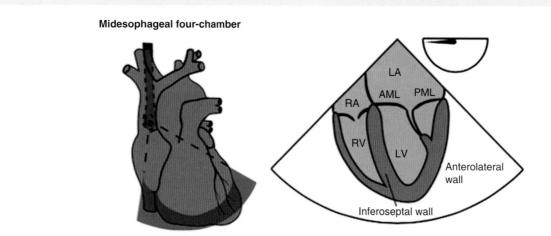

Figure 35-25 Transesophageal echocardiography 4-chamber view. Drawing (left) and echocardiographic image (right) obtained from an upper TEE position with a multiplane probe at 0° rotation. In this view, the apparent apex may actually represent a segment of the anterior wall because of foreshortening of the long axis of the ventricle. (Reproduced with permission of the Oxford University Press through PLSclear, from Sidebotham D, Merry AF, Legget ME, et al. Practical perioperative transesophageal echocardiography. In: *Oxford Clinical Imaging Guidelines.* 3rd ed. Oxford, UK: Oxford University Press; 2018.)

Near field
(close to the transducer)

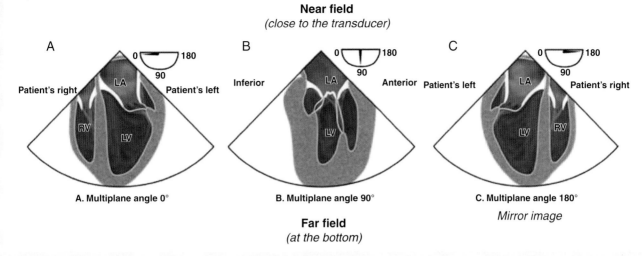

A. Multiplane angle 0°

B. Multiplane angle 90°

C. Multiplane angle 180°

Mirror image

Far field
(at the bottom)

Figure 35-26 Conventions of 2D transesophageal echocardiographic image display. The transducer location and the near field (vertex) of the image sector are at the top of the display screen and far field at the bottom. A, Image orientation at transducer angle 0°. B, Image orientation at transducer angle 90°. C, Image orientation at transducer angle 180°. LA, Left atrium; LV, left ventricle; RV, right ventricle. (Modified with permission from Shanewise J, Cheung A, Aronson S, et al. ASE/SCA guidelines for performing a comprehensive intraoperative multiplane transesophageal echocardiography examination: recommendations of the American Society of Echocardiography Council for Intraoperative Echocardiography and the Society of Cardiovascular Anesthesiologists Task Force for Certification in Perioperative Transesophageal Echocardiography. *Anesth Analg.* 1999;89(4):870-884; and Reprinted from Shanewise JS, Cheung AT, Aronson S, et al. ASE/SCA guidelines for performing a comprehensive intraoperative multiplane transesophageal echocardiography examination: recommendations of the American Society of Echocardiography Council for Intraoperative Echocardiography and the Society of Cardiovascular Anesthesiologists Task Force for Certification in Perioperative Transesophageal Echocardiography. *J Am Soc Echocardiogr.* 1999;12(10):884-900. Copyright © 1999 American Society of Echocardiography and the International Anesthesia Research Society. With permission.)

view is obtained with the transducer at the level of, and behind, the left atrium. Since the probe is posterior to the heart, structures that are visualized in the near field are posterior and structures that are in the far field are anterior (**Figure 35-26**). Multiple long-axis and short-axis views are obtainable from the midesophageal window.

21. **Answer: B.** The TEE probe is a modified gastroesophageal endoscopy probe, typically with a 3- to 7-MHz ultrasound transducer at the tip. The controls on a TEE probe handle usually consists of a large wheel, a small wheel, a wheel locking mechanism, and a series of rotation buttons (**Figure 35-27**). The large

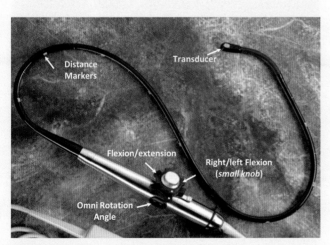

Figure 35-27 Image of a transesophageal transducer showing the controls located on the transducer handle. (Modified from Adams MS. Transesophageal echocardiography: standard views, anatomy and nomenclature. In: *Cardiovascular Sonographer Registry Review.* 2nd ed. American Society of Echocardiography; 2018.)

wheel on the transducer controls the anteflexion (anterior flexion) or retroflexion (posterior flexion) of the transducer tip. The small wheel on the transducer controls the left and right flexion of the transducer tip. There are two buttons that are used to increase and decrease the rotation angle of the imaging plane.

The various views utilized in a transesophageal echocardiogram are obtained by manipulation of the large and small wheels, adjustment of the rotational angle, and physical manipulation of the probe depth and location.

22. **Answer: A.** This transgastric view is obtained with the transducer advanced into the stomach and positioned at the base of the heart. The TV is visualized in short axis at approximately 40° to 60°. The three leaflets of the TV are the anterior, posterior, and septal leaflets. In this view, structures in the far field are anterior in the heart, so the TV leaflet in the far field is the anterior leaflet. This view is instrumental for isolating the origin of tricuspid regurgitation and for planning and performing percutaneous tricuspid valve repair. It is also a good image to determine a pacemaker lead's contribution to tricuspid regurgitation by visualizing if a leaflet is restricted from coapting with the other leaflets during systole.

23. **Answer: B.** The midesophageal short-axis view allows the visualization of all three cusps of the aortic valve (**Figure 35-28**). In a patient with normal anatomy, the noncoronary cusp is always adjacent to the interatrial septum. The right coronary cusp will be adjacent to the right ventricular outflow tract and the left coronary cusp will be closer to the left atrium.

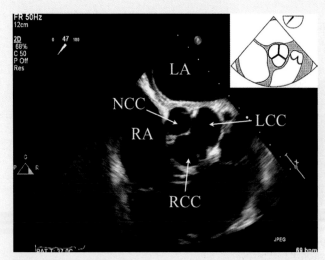

Figure 35-28 Midesophageal aortic valve short-axis view. LA, Left atrium; LCC, left coronary cusp; NCC, noncoronary cusp; RA, right atrium; RCC, right coronary cusp. (Reproduced from Reeves ST, Finley AC, Skubas NJ, et al. Basic perioperative transesophageal echocardiography examination: a consensus statement of the American Society of Echocardiography and the Society of Cardiovascular Anesthesiologists. *J Am Soc Echocardiogr.* 2013;26(5):443-456. Copyright © 2013 Elsevier. With permission.)

24. **Answer: B.** The Eustachian valve is an embryologic remnant of the valve of the IVC. In the embryological circulation, the Eustachian valve directs oxygen-rich blood from the IVC through the fossa ovalis into the left atrium. It is seen as highly mobile filamentous structure in the right atrium (RA). Because of its mobility, it is often misdiagnosed as a right atrial mass or thrombus. The bicaval view is often the best view to see the Eustachian valve and determining its attachment to the IVC/RA junction. At times, the Eustachian valve can be visualized extending from the IVC/RA junction to an attachment point on the interatrial septum. A Chiari network is a similar normal variant and can be distinguished from a Eustachian valve as it has multiple sieve-like fenestrations, has a web-like appearance, and attaches to the upper wall of the RA or interatrial septum.

25. **Answer: C.** The images provided show a patent foramen ovale (PFO). Evaluation of a cardiac source of an embolic event is a common and appropriate indication for performing a transesophageal echocardiogram (TEE). Although a PFO may be discovered and/or confirmed on a transthoracic echocardiogram, a subsequent TEE is often ordered to verify the diagnosis, determine the severity, and rule out an atrial septal defect. The atrial septum is best viewed in the midesophageal bicaval view as the ultrasound beam is most perpendicular to the septum and parallel to any flow across the septum. Color flow Doppler is used to look for flow across the septum and an agitated-saline injection can be performed to determine the direction of the shunt.

26. **Answer: B.** In 2011, the criteria for appropriateness for echocardiography were published (J Am Soc Echocardiogr. 2011;24:229-267). Of the options offered, answer B was considered an inappropriate indication for TEE. After pulmonary vein isolation, routine use of TEE in asymptomatic patients is not indicated. TEE is helpful in the guidance of noncoronary interventions and remains an important tool in the diagnosis of suspected aortic dissection. It is also indicated in patients with suboptimal transthoracic views when visualization of cardiac structures is essential to the clinical decision-making process.

27. **Answer: C.** Methemoglobinemia related to benzocaine topical anesthetic given during TEE is a rare reaction occurring in 0.07% to 0.12% of patients. Methemoglobin levels are elevated due to conversion of iron from a reduced to oxidized form of hemoglobin, which results in a low oxygen-carrying capacity. This results in cyanosis, low oxygen saturation, and normal arterial PO_2. Patients with methemoglobin levels greater than 70% may develop circulatory collapse, neurologic depression, and death. The treatment of choice is intravenous methylene blue 1% solution (10 mg/mL), 1 to 2 mg/kg, administered intravenously slowly for more than 5 minutes, followed by intravenous flush with normal saline.

28. **Answer: D.** This view shows the right ventricular outflow tract (RVOT), the main pulmonary artery (PA), and the right PA branch coursing behind the aorta (**Figure 35-29**). This is a patient with renal cell carcinoma with embolization to the PA. Transesophageal echocardiography (TEE) operators should be familiar with the interrogation of the PAs. The main and right PAs are easier to visualize. Only the very proximal left PA is visualized with TEE.

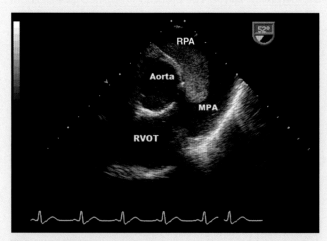

Figure 35-29 RPA, right pulmonary artery; MPA, main pulmonary artery; RVOT, right ventricular outflow tract. (Reprinted with permission from Klein AL, Asher CR. *Clinical Echocardiography Review. A Self-Assessment Tool.* 2nd ed. Philadelphia, PA: Wolters Kluwer; 2017.)

KEY POINTS

▶ The main PA and right PA can be easily visualized by TEE.

▶ The left PA is not well seen with TEE.

29. **Answer: A.** Paradoxical embolus, also known as "thrombus in transit," is an uncommon but life-threatening condition that occurs in patients with a patent foramen ovale (PFO) when a venous thrombus travels into the right heart and crosses the PFO. Patients present with the signs and symptoms of a pulmonary embolism or stroke. The condition has a high morbidity and mortality and urgent treatment is required. Treatment consists of anticoagulation, thrombolysis, and surgical embolectomy.

    Thrombus in transit is best viewed in the imaging planes where the atrial septum is seen (midesophageal [ME] 4-chamber view, ME short-axis view, ME bicaval view). Care must to taken to differentiate the thrombus in transit from other normal variants seen in the right atrium such as Chiari network or Eustachian valve.

30. **Answer: D.** Tricuspid valve vegetations (endocarditis) present as oscillating echo-dense masses attached to the tricuspid valve leaflets. They are most commonly seen in intravenous drug abusers. Other causes of tricuspid valve endocarditis include medical device implantation (pacemakers, defibrillators) as well as venous access (peripherally inserted central catheter [PICC line], dialysis catheters). Tricuspid valve endocarditis can result in leaflet destruction with perforation and flail leaflets. Patients can present with signs and symptoms of right heart failure or pulmonary embolism.

    Multiple views can be used to image the tricuspid valve (midesophageal [ME] 4-chamber, ME short-axis, and transgastric views). In patients with tricuspid valve endocarditis, care should be taken to image all of the other valves for any indication of infection and vegetations.

31. **Answer: B.** Ventricular septal defects (VSDs) are a complication that may develop following a myocardial infarction. They usually develop in the muscular ventricular septum within a few days of transmural infarction. Post myocardial infarction, VSDs have a high mortality if treated conservatively. Often, the VSDs can be visualized on transthoracic echocardiography, but transesophageal echocardiography (TEE) may yield valuable information in planning the surgical or percutaneous repair. TEE can be used to visualize other types of VSDs (e.g., perimembranous). The midesophageal view, transgastric long-axis and short-axis, and deep transgastric views can be utilized to view the ventricular septum. Often off-axis imaging from these views is needed to visualize the ventricular septal defect.

32. **Answer: A.** Aortic annular abscess is a very serious complication of aortic valve endocarditis. It is more commonly associated with prosthetic aortic valves than native aortic valves. It can present in a range of severities from inflammation and swelling of the annular tissue to paravalvular abscess formation encapsulated in the aortic annulus. Severe cases may result in a fistulous communication into the abscess and can result in a left-to-right shunt through the abscess into the right heart structures. As the aortic annulus and proximal ventricular septum become swollen and infected, the atrioventricular node may be affected, resulting in a prolonged PR interval and possibly higher degrees of heart block. Once the diagnosis of aortic abscess is confirmed, urgent surgery is required. Antibiotics alone will fail to control the infection. Surgery involves debridement of the infected tissue and replacement of the aortic valve.

33. **Answer: B.** Grading aortic atheroma by transesophageal echocardiography (TEE) uses a qualitative scale. Areas of the aorta that should be assessed for atheroma include the ascending aorta, aortic arch, and descending aorta. Imaging the aortic arch with TEE is the most challenging part of an aortic assessment because of its location in relation to the esophagus. The ascending and descending aorta are usually better visualized. The ascending aorta is best seen from the mid and upper esophageal windows. The descending aorta can be assessed with the probe deep in the esophagus, rotated so the beam is pointing posteriorly, and slowly withdrawn to view the length of the descending and thoracic aorta. Aortic atheroma is graded according to **Table 35-2**.

34. **Answer: C.** A subaortic membrane is a type of subvalvular obstruction that is caused by a thin, fibrous membrane or ridge that is found in the left ventricular outflow tract just proximal to the aortic valve. They are often crescent shaped, extending from the anterior septum to the anterior mitral valve leaflet. The membrane reduces the area of the outflow tract, resulting in increased outflow velocities and pressure gradients. They are often associated with aortic regurgitation caused by the high-velocity flow damaging the aortic valve leaflets. Careful attention should be taken to visualize the aortic valve leaflets and differentiate the membrane from valvular stenosis. Although a subaortic membrane is often first seen or suspected by transthoracic echocardiography, a transesophageal echocardiogram is performed to determine the extent of the membrane as well as assist in planning for surgical intervention.

35. **Answer: C.** Medications used for conscious sedation will vary depending on local practices and guidelines. Topical anesthesia of the oropharynx is usually achieved with benzocaine, cetacaine, or lidocaine. This is performed to numb the mouth and back of the throat and to decrease the gag reflex during probe insertion. Opioids such as fentanyl (answer A) are used to reduce the discomfort to the patient during probe insertion. Benzodiazepines such as midazolam (answer B) are used to reduce

Table 35-2. Grading System for Severity of Aortic Atheroma

Grade	Severity (Atheroma Thickness)	Description
1	Normal	Intimal thickness <2 mm
2	Mild	Mild intimal thickening (2-3 mm)
3	Moderate	Atheroma >3-5 mm (no mobile/ulcerated components)
4	Severe	Atheroma >5 mm (no mobile/ulcerated components)
5	Complex	Grade 2, 3, 4 plus mobile or ulcerated components

anxiety and relax the patient. Propofol (answer D) is a sedative hypnotic with a rapid onset and recovery time. However, some states prohibit the use of propofol by nonanesthesiologists due to its high risk of apnea.

Narcan (naloxone) has no sedative effects but should always be readily available. It is used to block the effects of opioids in the case of overdose. When administered by intravenous injections it acts within 2 minutes and the effects last 30 to 60 minutes. There must always be adequate staff to monitor the patient's vital signs (blood pressure, pulse, respirations, oxygen saturation) while the patient is undergoing conscious sedation.

Acknowledgments: The authors thank and acknowledge L. Leonardo Rodriquez, MD, for his inspiration based on Chapter 6: Transesophageal Echocardiography in *Clinical Echocardiography Review: A Self-Assessment Tool,* 2nd ed., edited by Allan L. Klein, Craig R. Asher; 2017.

SUGGESTED READINGS

Armstrong WF, Ryan T. The comprehensive echocardiographic examination. In: *Feigenbaum's Echocardiography.* 8th ed. Philadelphia, PA: Lippincott Williams & Wilkins; 2019:chap 4.

Douglas PS, Garcia M, Haines D, et al. ACCF/ASE/ACEP/ASNC/SCAI/SCCT/SCMR 2011 appropriateness criteria for echocardiography: a report of the American College of Cardiology Foundation Appropriate Use Criteria Task Force, American Society of Echocardiography, American Heart Association, American Society of Nuclear Cardiology, Heart Failure Society of America, Heart Rhythm Society, Society for Cardiovascular Angiography and Interventions, Society of Critical Care Medicine, Society of Cardiovascular Computed Tomography, Society for Cardiovascular Magnetic Resonance American College of Chest Physicians. *J Am Soc Echocardiogr.* 2011;24(3):229-267.

Hahn RT, Abraham T, Adams MS, et al. Guidelines for performing a comprehensive transesophageal echocardiographic examination: recommendations from the American Society of Echocardiography and the Society of Cardiovascular Anesthesiologists. *J Am Soc Echocardiogr.* 2013;26(9):921-964.

Hilberath JN, Oakes DA, Shernan SK, Bulwer BE, D'Ambra MN, Eltzschig HK. Safety of transesophageal echocardiography. *J Am Soc Echocardiogr.* 2010;23(11):1115-1127.

Otto CM. Transesophageal echocardiography. In: *Textbook of Clinical Echocardiography.* 6th ed. Philadelphia, PA: Elsevier Saunders; 2018:chap 3.

Rodriquez LL. Transesophageal echocardiography. In: Klein AL, Asher CR, eds. *Clinical Echocardiography Review a Self Assessment Tool.* 2nd ed. Philadelphia: Lippincott Williams & Wilkins; 2017:chap 6.

Sidebotham D, Merry AF, Legget ME, Wright GI, eds. *Practical Perioperative Transesophageal Echocardiography.* 3rd ed. New York, NY: Oxford University Press; 2018.

CHAPTER 36

Interventional and Other Advanced Techniques and Procedures

Contributors: Rick Meece, ACS, RDCS, RCIS and Eric Kruse, BS, ACS, RDCS, RVT

✪✪ Question 1

▶ Which of the following scenarios best describes the findings shown in **Figures 36-1A** and **36-1B** and **Videos 36-1A** and **36-1B**, recently obtained from a patient with an implanted HeartMate II (Abbott) external pump device?

   A. Normal left ventricular assist device (LVAD) function

   B. LVAD power spike

   C. LVAD suction event

   D. Outflow cannula obstruction

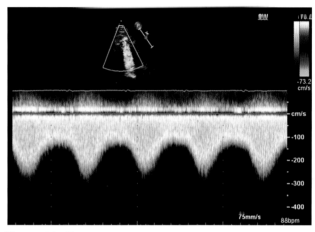

Figuro 36 1B

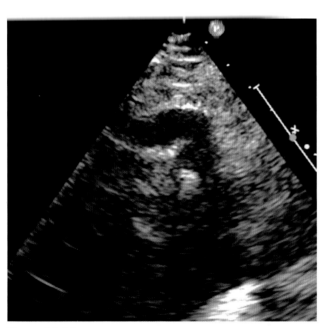

Figure 36-1A

✪✪✪ Question 2

In an echocardiographic assessment of a patient who recently received implantation of a peripheral venoarterial extracorporeal membrane oxygenation (VA-ECMO) device, the 2D imaging and color Doppler demonstrates consistent aortic valve closure. The key observation commonly associated with this abnormal finding is:

   A. An increased right ventricular free wall s′.

   B. A lateral s′ >5 cm/s.

   C. Left ventricular dilatation or enlargement.

   D. A significant decrease in mitral regurgitation.

✪✪✪ Question 3

Which of the following clinical scenarios is associated with a relatively high incidence of right ventricular failure, which may warrant placement of a right ventricular assist device (RVAD)?

A. Post cardiac transplantation
B. Postcardiotomy heart failure
C. Left ventricular assist device (LVAD) insertion
D. Venovenous extracorporeal membrane oxygenation (VV-ECMO) insertion for support
E. Both A and C

✪✪ Question 4

Which of the following intracardiac echocardiography (ICE) catheter locations would be most commonly used as a primary "home view" for proper orientation to surrounding anatomy?

A. Inferior vena cava
B. Right atrium
C. Right ventricle
D. Superior vena cava

✪✪✪ Question 5

An Impella (Abiomed) 2.5 flow assistance device is inserted in a patient admitted with an anterior myocardial infarction and acute cardiogenic shock. During follow-up echocardiographic assessment of the device, which of the following findings would be most concerning?

A. Decrease in left ventricular (LV) function following insertion
B. Increased mitral regurgitation to greater than moderate severity
C. Inlet of cannula >6 cm from aortic annulus
D. LV septal wall dyskinesis with motion toward right ventricle

✪✪ Question 6

Which device is indicated for urgent mechanical circulatory support requiring transseptal cannula placement into the left atrium with a concomitant outflow cannula in the femoral artery?

A. HeartWare assist
B. Impella
C. Intra-aortic balloon pump (IABP)
D. TandemHeart device

✪✪ Question 7

▶ A routine echocardiogram is ordered for a 53-year-old man with a history of increased shortness of breath, significant pulmonary hypertension, and a history of systemic scleroderma. Regarding findings shown in **Figures 36-2A and 36-2B** and **Videos 36-2A to 36-2C**, what potential condition may occur, and what is a good "next step"?

A. Alert the reading physician of possible cardiac tamponade; evaluation for clinical and echo-based evidence for possible urgent pericardiocentesis
B. Possible pulmonary embolism; contact the attending physician as the patient may require an embolectomy
C. Perform an agitated saline study; rule out ventricular septal defect as the cause of RV overload
D. Obtain a 3D full-volume data set for accurate measures of RV volume and function status; possible RV assist device

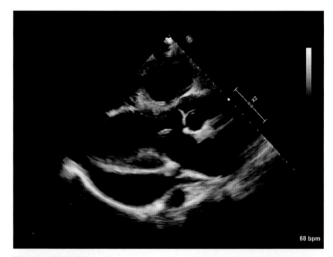

Figure 36-2A

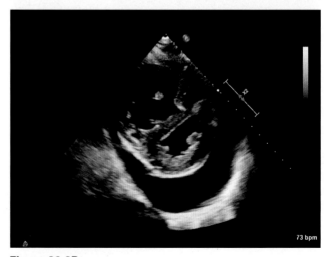

Figure 36-2B

✪✪✪ Question 8

A transthoracic echocardiogram is performed on a patient who recently received a left ventricular assist device (LVAD). Following implantation, the patient continues to experience significant dyspnea with clinical oxygen saturations >94% preceding discharge. Based on the information provided in **Video 36-3**, what is demonstrated as most relevant to the patient's clinical condition?

A. Intermittent aortic valve opening
B. LVAD inlet cannula pump thrombosis
C. Severe aortic regurgitation
D. Severe mitral regurgitation

✪✪✪ Question 9

Echocardiographic assessment of any dynamic aortic valve opening following left ventricular assist device (LVAD) implantation is paramount in evaluating the level of LVAD pump dependence in patients receiving this device. Which of the following complications more commonly develops in the setting of an elevated pump speed?

A. Continuous aortic insufficiency
B. Sinus of Valsalva thrombus
C. Severe mitral regurgitation
D. Aortic valve remains open
E. Both A and B

✪✪✪ Question 10

During the transesophageal echocardiographic (TEE) implantation planning workup for a WATCHMAN (Boston Scientific Corp.) left atrial appendage (LAA) occlusion device, which of the following is the most concerning finding?

A. 21 mm LAA ostial measurement in minor axis
B. 33 mm LAA anterior lobar depth
C. Atrial fibrillation unrelated to mitral valve disease
D. Broccoli-shaped LAA morphology

✪✪✪ Question 11

When deploying a commercially approved WATCHMAN (Boston Scientific Corp.) device in the left atrial appendage (LAA), consideration of the device compression ratio after deployment is important for stable positioning and anchoring of the device. What is the recommended optimal compression ratio?

A. 18% to 30%
B. 8% to 20%
C. Greater than 15%
D. Greater than 20%
E. Both B and D

✪✪✪ Question 12

A patient with a HeartMate II (Abbott) left ventricular assist device (LVAD) and mean arterial blood pressure (MAP) of 90 mm Hg undergoes a ramp speed study to assess for pump thrombosis. Baseline echocardiographic findings demonstrate a left ventricular end-diastolic dimension (LVEDD) of 65 mm, mild mitral regurgitation, no aortic valve regurgitation, and intermittent aortic valve opening. Based on the changes noted at the sequential ramp settings as shown in **Figures 36-3A to 36-3D**, there is:

A. Normal unloading of the left ventricle.
B. Pump thrombosis.
C. Severe aortic insufficiency.
D. Significant systemic hypertension.

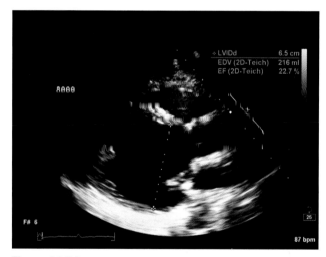

Figure 36-3A

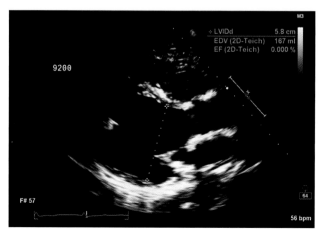

Figure 36-3B

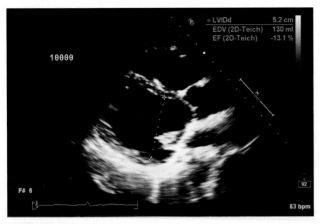

Figure 36-3C

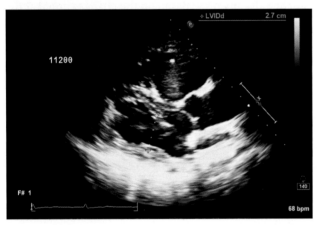

Figure 36-3D

✪✪ Question 13

▶ A 76-year-old woman with a history of lung cancer arrives to the emergency department with a progressive increase in dyspnea. Her initial blood pressure reads 95/64 mm Hg with sinus tachycardia (heart rate of 122 bpm). A previous echocardiogram 4 months ago for labile chest discomfort reported a small pericardial effusion, normal ventricular function, and no significant valve disorder. A repeat bedside echocardiogram is ordered. Based on the images provided in **Videos 36-4A** and **36-4B**, there is a:

A. Moderate pericardial effusion with no validated evidence of cardiac tamponade.

B. Moderate-sized chronic pericardial effusion.

C. Large pericardial effusion with pretamponade findings.

D. Large pericardial effusion with evidence of cardiac tamponade.

✪ Question 14

Which of the following echocardiographic findings is/are important for imaging guidance of a pericardiocentesis procedure?

A. Location of the pericardial effusion

B. Distance from the chest wall to the pericardium

C. Presence or absence of intervening structures

D. Imaging quality of windows available away from the sterile pericardiocentesis site

E. All of the above

✪ Question 15

Following cardiac transplantation, a myocardial tissue biopsy is performed, looking for evidence of rejection. The most appropriate region for bioptome positioning for obtaining a sample of myocardial tissue is the:

A. Septal wall of the right ventricle.

B. Left atrium.

C. Lateral wall of the left ventricle.

D. Free wall of the right atrium.

✪✪ Question 16

▶ A patient presents to the outpatient department for an echocardiogram, cardiac magnetic resonance imaging, and blood work for genetic testing. Test results led to consultation and subsequent scheduling of the patient for a procedure. Based on the images provided (**Figure 36-4** and **Video 36-5**), which procedure might this patient undergo?

A. Left atrial appendage closure

B. Septal ablation for hypertrophic obstruction of the left ventricular outflow tract

C. Transcatheter aortic valve replacement

D. Transcatheter mitral valve replacement

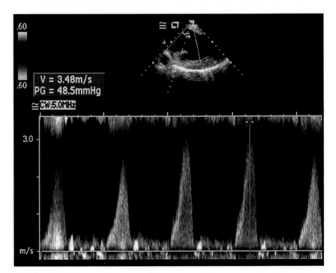

Figure 36-4

✪✪ Question 17

Intracardiac echocardiography (ICE) offers close proximity to structures and high resolution for certain intracardiac procedures. Which frequency range applies to ICE catheter–based transducers?

    A. 1 to 5 MHZ

    B. 5 to 10 MHz

    C. 8 to 12 MHz

    D. 10 to 15 MHz

✪✪✪ Question 18

Use of topographic 3D modeling of the mitral annulus and leaflet morphology has shown value in identifying regions of maximal prolapse in relation to the true annular saddle shape for both surgical and transcatheter mitral interventions. Based on the 3D surgeon's view (**Figure 36-5A**) and 3D topographic navigator model with cut-plane (C-plane) images (**Figure 36-5B**), the primary mitral culprit pathology is:

    A. Flail A2 and A3 segments with P1-scallop prolapse.

    B. A flail A2 segment.

    C. P2-scallop prolapse with a flail A2 segment.

    D. A severe prolapsing A3 segment.

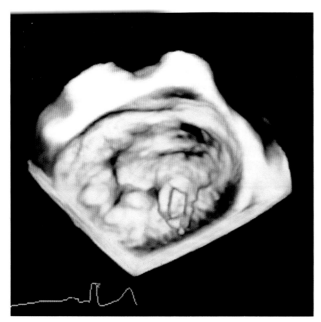

Figure 36-5A

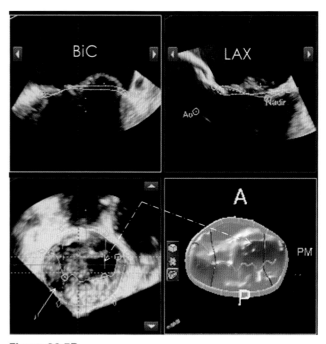

Figure 36-5B

✪✪ Question 19

▶ **Video 36-6** shows a 3D image of a mitral bioprosthetic valve from the left atrial (left) and left ventricular (right) perspectives acquired in an 88-year-old woman. What is the primary pathology and which approach, if any, might address this condition?

    A. Leaflet base perforation; Amplatzer plug occlusion

    B. Leaflet sclerosis and stenosis with no intervention due to age

    C. Endocarditis; requiring high-risk surgical mitral valve replacement

    D. Degenerative calcification with stenosis; transcatheter valve-in-valve replacement

✪✪ Question 20

The gold standard imaging choice for sizing a patient's aortic annulus for transcatheter aortic valve replacement (TAVR) prosthetic valve implantation is computed tomography angiography (CTA) with contrast, due to inherently high-quality spatial resolution and combined use of semiautomated software tools for various diameters, angles, and coronary heights. In some patients, often with renal failure, the CTA contrast agent cannot be used and 3D transesophageal echocardiography (TEE) may be utilized. What is the primary pitfall when considering image acquisition and use of 3D TEE software for annular sizing in TAVR implantation planning?

A. Shadowing artifact across region of interest

B. Tools used to render C-planes are not as robust as CTA

C. Limited operator experience and reproducibility using multiplane reconstruction

D. All of the above

✪✪ Question 21

Which of the following best explains the outflow graft spectral Doppler findings shown in **Figure 36-6** in this patient with a HeartMate 3 (Abbott) ventricular assist device?

A. Normal outflow velocity pattern

B. Interphasic outflow obstruction

C. Diastolic suction event from thrombosis

D. Flow reversal from significant aortic regurgitation

E. High–ramp flow state and mitral regurgitation

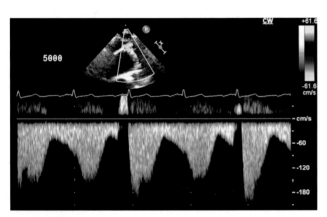

Figure 36-6

✪✪✪ Question 22

▶ A 62-year-old female patient is seen in the emergency room with previous history of multiple left ventricular assist device (LVAD) suction events and increased shortness of breath. The following echocardiographic images (**Videos 36-7A** and **36-7B**) were obtained in the emergency room. Which of the following describes the most likely intervention to address the issue with this patient's LVAD?

A. Increase the LVAD speed

B. Decrease the LVAD speed

C. Leave the LVAD speed and repeat an echo in 6 months

D. Perform bedside echo ramp study to rule out pump thrombosis

✪✪✪ Question 23

▶ A 50-year-old man presents to the emergency room post HeartMate II (Abbott) (external pump) implantation. The patient's left ventricular assist device (LVAD) parameters were: flow +++, power 11.4 watts, and a pulsatility index (PI) of 4.0 with the pump speed of 9800 rpm at the time of admission to the emergency room. The patient's normal baseline LVAD parameters are: flow 5.1 to 6.1 L/min, power 6.0 to 6.5 watts, and PI of 4.5 to 5.0 with pump speed of 9800 rpm. The patient's blood cultures were negative. Given the patient's change in LVAD parameters, negative blood cultures, and the echocardiographic findings shown in **Figures 36-7A to 36-7C** and **Videos 36-8A to 36-8C**, which is the most probable diagnosis?

A. Normal LVAD flows

B. Left ventricular outflow tract fluid-filled thrombus

C. Aortic valve vegetation

D. Mitral valve vegetation

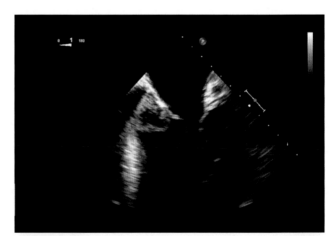

Figure 36-7A

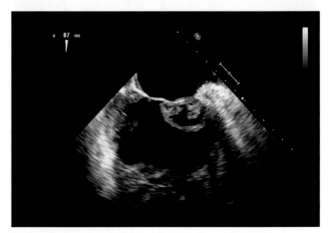

Figure 36-7B

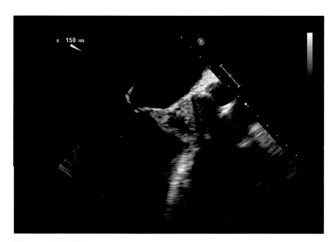

Figure 36-7C

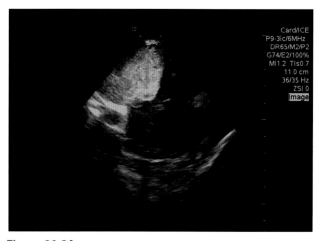

Figure 36-8A

✪✪ Question 24

▶ A 35-year-old woman with a history of a transient ischemic attack and one cerebral vascular accident is undergoing a procedure using intracardiac echocardiographic (ICE) guidance (**Figures 36-8A** to **36-8C** and **Videos 36-9A** to **36-9C**). Which procedure is this patient undergoing?

 A. Left atrial appendage closure
 B. Ventricular septal defect closure
 C. Patent foramen ovale closure
 D. Ventricular tachycardia ablation

✪✪✪ Question 25

▶ A 66-year-old woman with a history of systemic lupus erythematosus, hypertension, and persistent atrial fibrillation arrives for a scheduled procedure. A previous echocardiogram demonstrated moderate left ventricular (LV) hypertrophy, normal LV size and function, severe right ventricular enlargement and poor function, biatrial enlargement, and no significant valvular pathology. Both transesophageal echocardiography and intracardiac echocardiography (ICE) demonstrate no mass or thrombus in the left atrium or left atrial appendage. Which procedure is indicated given the patient history and the images provided (**Figure 36-9** and **Video 36-10**)?

 A. Cardioversion
 B. Patent foramen ovale closure
 C. Left atrial appendage closure
 D. Pulmonary vein isolation

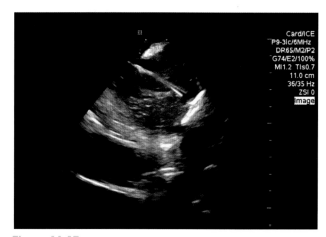

Figure 36-8B

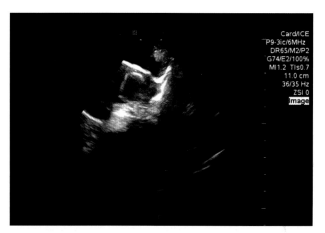

Figure 36-8C

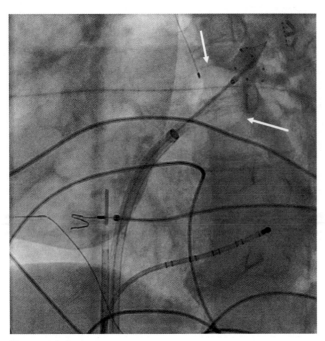

Figure 36-9

✪✪✪ Question 26

▶ 3D and spectral Doppler images provided were acquired immediately following implantation of a MitraClip XTR for severe mitral regurgitation (**Figures 36-10A** and **36-10B** and **Videos 36-11A** and **36-11B**). The potential primary concern to be discussed before permanently releasing the clip is:

A. Adequate posterior leaflet tissue within the MitraClip device.

B. Alignment of clip rotation during grasp.

C. Blunting of right superior pulmonary venous flow velocities.

D. Pressure gradient level across the dual-orifice valve.

✪✪ Question 27

In both MitraClip and left atrial appendage occlusion procedures, the interatrial septal crossing height and angle are critical to ensure that the interventionalist is able to:

A. Place the initial guidewire for catheter placement into the right superior pulmonary vein.

B. Manipulate the procedure catheter for correct device positioning.

C. Avoid transecting a patent foramen ovale.

D. Both B and C.

E. All of the above.

✪✪ Question 28

Most institutions that perform commercial Watchman (Boston Scientific Corp.) left atrial appendage (LAA) occlusion device implantation will have a clinical transesophageal echocardiogram (TEE) for candidacy, evaluation of LAA morphology, screening for any atrial or valve pathologies, and to exclude LAA thrombus. These patients will be NPO (nil per os or nothing by mouth) since midnight, consented for the procedure, cleared by anesthesia for sedation, and may receive 500 mL of intravenous (IV) normal saline within 2 hours before the TEE. What is the primary reason for the IV fluid infusion?

A. Maintenance of adequate left atrial filling and pressure

B. To help prevent patients from experiencing nausea or symptoms of dehydration due to being NPO for many hours

C. To optimize systemic volume loading to reduce occurrence of atrial fibrillation preceding a procedure

D. Enhance IV access point for patency for infusion of anesthetic agents

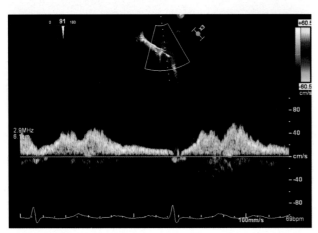

Figure 36-10A

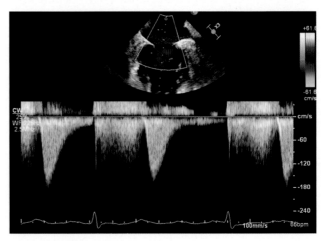

Figure 36-10B

✪✪✪ Question 29

▶ During transcatheter closure of a large-tunnel patent foramen ovale (PFO) with a cribiform Amplatzer device, there is residual transseptal shunting seen with both atrial disks opened and pulled together. Based on the images provided (**Videos 36-12A** and **36-12B**), what suggestions or concerns can the transesophageal echocardiographic (TEE) imaging team articulate to assist in a more complete and effective occlusion?

   A. Use biplane orthogonal 2D imaging to open up the angle of the PFO flow and Amplatzer

   B. View with 3D zoom imaging and color

   C. Note device orientation and shape of disks

   D. Have the interventionalist retract catheter and pull left atrial disk closer to the interatrial septum

   E. All of the above

✪✪✪ Question 30

During routine prescreening imaging for a conscious sedation transcatheter aortic valve replacement (TAVR) procedure with transthoracic echocardiographic assessment, findings included a severely calcified aortic valve, moderate to severe left ventricular (LV) hypertrophy, an LV end-systolic dimension (LVESD) of 2.6 cm, and an LV ejection fraction of 75%. From these findings, which specific risk-based concern should the echocardiographer evaluate immediately following implantation?

   A. Ventricular volume unloading with combined outflow obstruction

   B. Decreased LVESD

   C. Systolic anterior mitral leaflet motion with mitral regurgitation

   D. All of the above

✪✪ Question 31

The use of 3D echocardiography with multiplane reconstruction provides key measurements for transcatheter aortic valve replacement (TAVR) sizing (**Figure 36-11**). Which measurements are the most relevant to TAVR sizing?

   A. Sinus dimensions and area, and left ventricular outflow tract (LVOT) diameter

   B. LVOT diameter, area, and circumference

   C. Sinus dimensions, circumference, and area

   D. Sinotubular junction (STJ), LVOT diameter, and area

   E. Sinus dimensions, circumference, and area, and LVOT diameter

✪ Question 32

▶ In the biplane 2D images of the interatrial septum (**Figure 36-12** and **Video 36-13**), the anatomical nomenclature for regions 1, 2, 3, and 4 is:

   A. 1 = superior, 2 = inferior, 3 = anterior, 4 = posterior.

   B. 1 = inferior, 2 = posterior, 3 = anterior, 4 = superior.

   C. 1 = posterior, 2 = superior, 3 = anterior, 4 = interior.

   D. 1 = posterior, 2 = inferior, 3 = superior, 4 = anterior.

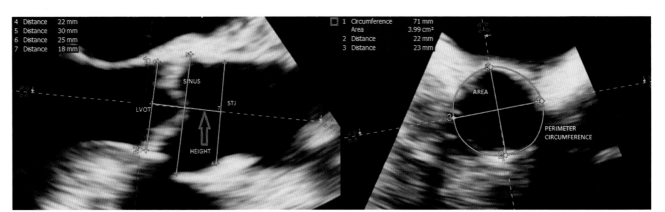

Figure 36-11

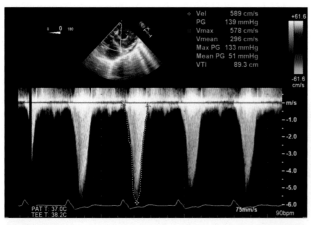

Figure 36-12

✪✪ Question 33

▶ **Figure 36-13** and **Videos 36-14A** to **36-14C** are transesophageal echocardiographic (TEE) images acquired preceding a TEE-guided septal alcohol ablation procedure. What do these images reveal?

A. Nondiagnostic use of intracoronary (IC) contrast

B. Outflow gradients are too high for successful septal ablation

C. The location of the correct septal perforator

D. The location of peak outflow obstruction

✪✪✪ Question 34

In a majority of transseptal interventional procedures performed through femoral venous inferior vena cava access, the cardiologist/surgeon commonly places the initial septal crossing guidewire into the left superior pulmonary vein (LSPV) for nontraumatic anchoring for catheter exchange. This assists in safe insertion of the larger, stiffer catheter for implantation of devices. What is the most common transesophageal echocardiographic (TEE) view and method used to validate correct positioning of the guidewire in the LSPV?

A. Midesophageal (ME) view of mitral valve at 45° and retract TEE probe 1 cm

B. ME bicaval view at 90° and rotate counterclockwise until the vein comes into view

C. High esophageal bicaval view at 110° and rotate clockwise 20°

D. High esophageal view at 0° and manually rotate counterclockwise 40° until the vein comes into view

✪✪ Question 35

▶ In this dual-view 3D data set (**Figure 36-14** and **Video 36-15**), a MitraClip device has been placed at the central mitral valve commissure and has been released from the insertion catheter. Which of the following best identifies concerns in terms of evaluating the success of the procedure?

A. Mitral stenosis

B. Mean pressure gradient

C. Posterior leaflet tissue bridge

D. Pulmonary vein inflow pattern

E. Both A and B

Figure 36-13

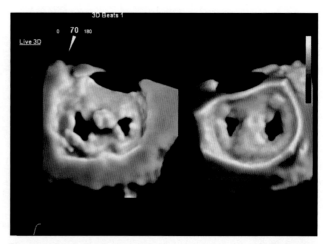

Figure 36-14 Dual view of 3D zoom of mitral valve following central clip placement. The view on the left is from the left ventricular perspective and the view on the right is from the left atrial perspective. A large and relatively wide "tissue" bridge is noted on the posterior leaflet segment, which suggests a good grasping of both leaflets at the A2-P2 region.

✪✪ Question 36

Figures 36-15A and **36-15B** demonstrate use of 3D color Doppler data sets preceding and following placement of a Mitraclip device within the coaptation of the tricuspid anterior and septal leaflets. With a preprocedural regurgitant orifice area (ROA) of 2.17cm^2 and postimplantation ROA of 0.17cm^2, what percent of tricuspid regurgitation (TR) reduction is achieved?

A. 36% reduction
B. 64% reduction
C. 68% reduction
D. 78% reduction

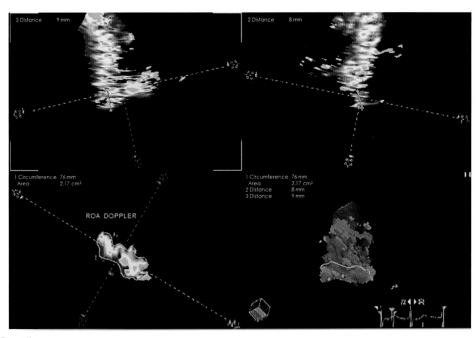

Figure 36-15A Preceding

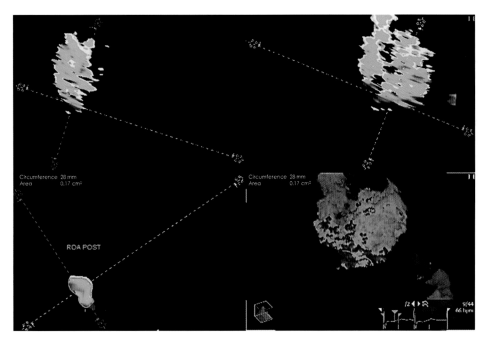

Figure 36-15B Following.

✪✪ Question 37

A 28-year-old female patient is diagnosed at an outlying facility with an atrial septal defect (ASD). Preceding occlusion, the interventionalist requires accurate sizing of the defect in order to achieve good occlusion with low chance of device embolization. Based on the images provided, which method is considered the "gold standard" for sizing of the ASD?

    A. Measurement acquired from **Figure 36-16A**
    B. Measurement acquired from **Figure 36-16B**
    C. Measurement acquired from **Figure 36-16C**
    D. Measurement acquired from **Figure 36-16D**
    E. All of the above

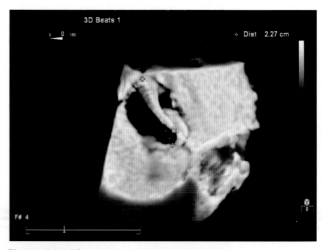

Figure 36-16C

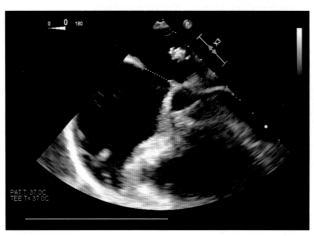

Figure 36-16A

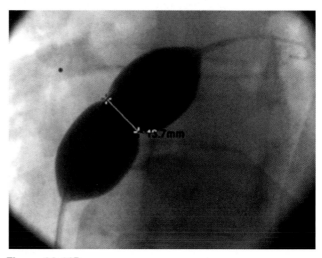

Figure 36-16D

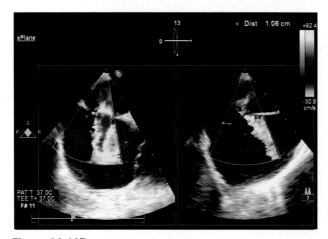

Figure 36-16B

✪✪✪ Question 38

Following MitraClip implantation, residual mitral regurgitation (MR) can be difficult to objectively evaluate. Of the following parameters listed in **Table 36-1**, which three options are most relevant in demonstrating a significant reduction of MR during mitral valve interventions?

    A. 1, 3, 5
    B. 1, 3, 4
    C. 1, 2, 3
    D. 3, 4, 5
    E. 2, 3, 5

Table 36-1.

1. Improved ratio and velocity of pulmonary venous inflow pattern
2. Effective regurgitant orifice area of MR jet using the proximal isovelocity surface area method
3. Direct invasive measurement of left atrial pressure
4. Spontaneous contrast in left atrium
5. Color Doppler jet area

Question 39

A patient readmitted with increased dyspnea at rest recently received a transcatheter aortic valve replacement (TAVR) implantation for aortic stenosis combined with a concomitant mitral "valve-in-valve" (ViV). Images from a follow-up echocardiogram are shown in **Video 36-16.** Which of the following represents the primary finding and the best assessment to establish relevance to her symptoms?

A. Left ventricular volume unloading with hypertrophic obstructive cardiomyopathy; stress echocardiography

B. Prosthetic stenosis; pressure gradients and an aortic valve acceleration time

C. Prosthetic septal wall obstruction; evaluate with spectral Doppler

D. Prosthetic thrombosis; transesophageal echocardiography with color Doppler

Question 40

The transthoracic echocardiographic images shown in **Figures 36-17A** and **36-17B** and **Videos 36-17A** and **36-17B** were obtained immediately following deployment of a 26 mm Sapien 3 transcatheter heart valve (THV) system in the aortic position. Which of the following best describes the result of this implantation?

A. THV deployment is placed too far into the ventricle resulting in severe paravalvular leak

B. Successful deployment of the THV with mild paravalvular leak; nothing further needs to be done

C. Undersizing of the THV for the native annulus resulting in moderate paravalvular leak

D. Incomplete closure of small gaps within the annulus due to protruding calcium in the aortic annulus resulting in severe paravalvular leak

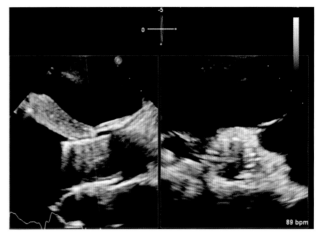

Figure 36-17A

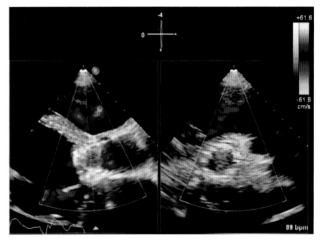

Figure 36-17B

Question 41

Primary components of a vast majority of conventional devices and many surgical implants are often specifically, or a combination of, nitinol (a nickel-titanium alloy), stainless steel, and Gortex material. All have various purposes in the design such as advantages in positioning and deployment and/or are safer and cause less inflammatory responses in patients. Which of the following describes the primary differences in the use of nitinol versus stainless steel for the structural material used?

A. A deployed nitinol device will more effectively reform the target space to the optimal shape for efficacy.

B. When deployed from a compressed state through a catheter, a nitinol device always expands to the manufactured size.

C. Nitinol has the property of "memory" in assuming the original size and design regardless of catheter compression before expansion and release.

D. All of the above.

✪ Question 42

Via transesophageal echocardiography (TEE), what is the primary intracardiac landmark used for orientation and identification of tricuspid valve leaflets regardless of the method or angulation used?

A. Aortic valve
B. Coronary sinus
C. Interatrial septum
D. Ventricular septum

✪✪ Question 43

Which transesophageal echocardiographic approach is most useful in defining the exact location of mitral regurgitant (MR) jets for guiding interventional approaches?

A. 2D biplane imaging
B. 3D zoom color Doppler

C. Multiplane (C-plane) reconstruction from a 3D dataset
D. 2D color compare (color simultaneous or dual) modes

✪✪ Question 44

In performing a 30-day follow-up examination on a patient who received a MitraClip at the central mitral valve commissure, which view(s) is (are) used to measure the pressure gradient across both orifices?

A. Apical 4-chamber and long-axis views
B. Apical 4-chamber and subcostal views
C. Apical 2-chamber view
D. Modified parasternal short-axis view

ANSWERS

1. **Answer: D.** The HeartMate II (Abbott) is a left ventricular assist device (LVAD). The spectral Doppler waveform (**Figure 36-1B**) is markedly echo-dense, showing a peak velocity >2.0 m/s. This indicates potential obstruction along the path of the cursor. The 2D right parasternal image of the outflow graft demonstrates an acute angle with double narrowing and kinking (folding over) of the graft, similar in appearance to a native aortic coarctation (**Figure 36-1A**). Suspicion for obstruction is supported by color Doppler, which denotes a high level of turbulence or aliasing of flow near the region of interest (**Video 36-1A**). The rotational computed tomography imaging shows in high detail the pump apparatus, insertion sites, and abnormal kink in the outflow cannula (**Video 36-1B**).

2. **Answer: C.** There are two primary types of ECMO, one being veno-venous cannulation (VV-ECMO), which is used solely to provide extracorporeal enhanced oxygenation and subsequent respiratory support, decreasing myocardial demand. The second method involves veno-arterial (VA-ECMO) cannulation, which is used to enhance cardiac myocardial efficiency and provide oxygenated respiratory support (**Figure 36-18**). Echocardiography is an essential tool in determining successful emptying and transport efficiency of both ventricles. Identification of ventricular dilatation, decrease in function (no aortic leaflet excursion), increased mitral regurgitation, and visual evidence of decreased flow or stasis (spontaneous contrast or "swirling smoke") of the blood pool within the left ventricle strongly

suggests malfunction of the ECMO device with potential for imminent thrombus formation. This finding may indicate the need for close periodic follow-up of flow dynamics and anticoagulation status.

3. ▶ **Answer: E.** Acute right ventricular failure can develop after a cardiac surgery and especially following cardiac transplantation and LVAD insertion. Due to acute hemodynamic changes in intracardiac end-diastolic pressures and left ventricular volume loading, residual ventricular function is often affected following LVAD insertion. A previously strained right ventricle must adjust to decreased preload and a sudden normalization in cardiac output. This involves geometric changes due to interventricular septum shift and increased pulmonary vascular resistance. Due to chronically stretched myofibrils and associated lengthening, a period of recovery and ventricular remodeling needs to occur. Temporary concomitant RVAD support may be required to allow the right ventricle to gradually acclimate to these changes during the acute recovery phase with a goal of preventing the potential cascade of complications (**Videos 36-18A** and **36-18B**).

4. ▶ **Answer: B.** Intracardiac echocardiography (ICE) is used in interventional cardiology for close proximity real-time visualization of cardiac structures, continuous monitoring of catheter location within the heart, and early recognition of procedural complications, such as pericardial effusion or thrombus formation. ICE catheters are inserted either from below, via a femoral vein, to the inferior vena cava and into the right atrium (RA), or often

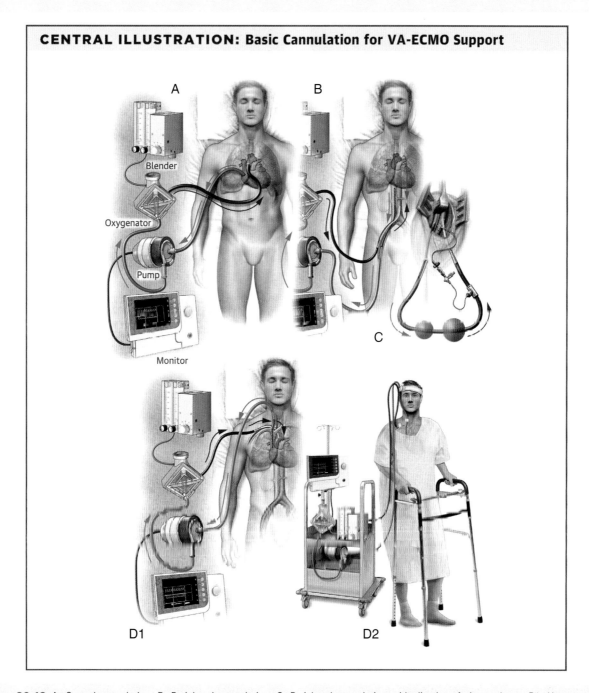

CENTRAL ILLUSTRATION: Basic Cannulation for VA-ECMO Support

Figure 36-18 A, Central cannulation. B, Peripheral cannulation. C, Peripheral cannulation with distal perfusion catheter. D1, Upper extremity cannulation with internal jugular venous cannula and axillary artery arterial cannula. D2, Patients with this configuration may be able to ambulate if clinically appropriate. ECMO, extracorporeal membrane oxygenation; VA, venoarterial. (Reprinted from Keebler ME, Haddad EV, Choi CW, et al. Venoarterial Extracorporeal Membrane Oxygenation in Cardiogenic Shock. *JACC Heart Fail.* 2018;6(6):503-516. Copyright © 2018 by the American College of Cardiology Foundation. With permission.)

from above, via the internal jugular vein, to the superior vena cava and into the RA. Correct positioning is achieved by viewing both fluoroscopy for catheter positioning and ICE imaging for identifying landmarks. In **Video 36-19**, the common "home" with the aortic valve centered in the short-axis view is being obtained (see **Figure 36-19** for labeled structures). Note the RA in the near field and the anterior (Ant) and posterior (Post) orientation of the interatrial septum. ICE maneuvers include advancement,

retraction, anterior/posterior deflection (similar to transesophageal echocardiographic [TEE] flexion), and clockwise/counterclockwise rotation. Three-dimensional ICE matrix transducers are being continually improved in resolution and capabilities competitive with transesophageal imaging for particular transcatheter procedures.

5. **Answer: C.** The Impella (Abiomed) devices are axial-flow pumps inserted retrogradely into the left ventricle from the aorta. The Impella 2.5 system is a

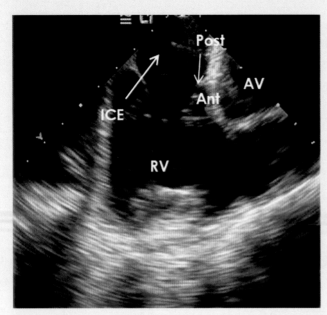

Figure 36-19 Short-axis view with the aortic valve (AV) centered with RV outflow tract (see text for details).

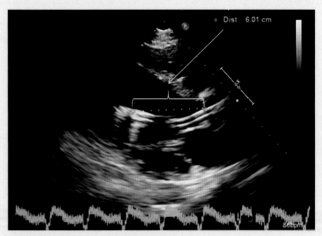

Figure 36-20A

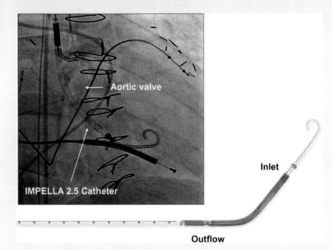

Figure 36-20B Photograph of the Impella 2.5 catheter positioned across the aortic valve. (Reprinted from Dixon SR, Henriques JP, Mauri L, et al. A prospective feasibility trial investigating the use of the Impella 2.5 system in patients undergoing high-risk percutaneous coronary intervention (The PROTECT I Trial): initial U.S. experience. *JACC Cardiovasc Interv.* 2009;2(2):91-96. Copyright © 2009 American College of Cardiology Foundation. With permission.)

temporary ventricular support device indicated for use during high-risk percutaneous coronary interventions or in hemodynamically unstable patients with severe coronary artery disease and depressed left ventricular ejection fraction. The distal LV port of an Impella device should be no more than 4 to 4.5 cm below the aortic annulus and positioned centrally away from papillary muscles (**Figures 36-20A** and **36-20B**). This ensures the inflow ventricular port is well below the outflow tract, limiting interaction with the mitral apparatus and chords to avoid structural trauma and device inefficiency. Impella devices are usually indicated for immediate, short-term (<10 days) management of severe LV dysfunction and are considered a short-term "bridge" device while other options for LV support and management, if any, are evaluated. If the LV inlet is too deep in the ventricle, the aortic outlet may be too proximal to the aortic valve sinuses, creating negative aortic pressure at the valve level. This can induce diastolic flow ischemia or also a condition termed "loop volume overload" within the ventricle, eliminating efficacy of the device. Regarding maintenance of appropriate Impella positioning, patient repositioning (i.e., rolling to the side or elevating the upper torso while an Impella device is inserted) must be carefully monitored to avoid a deleterious change in device position. Point-of-care cardiac ultrasound bedside imaging is an essential tool for reevaluating the Impella position on an as-needed basis.

6. **Answer: D.** The TandemHeart circulatory support device is inserted via inferior vena caval approach into the right atrium, followed by septostomy and subsequent placement of a large left atrial multiorifice port in the center of the left atrium

(**Figure 36-21**). A bypass distal return cannula is placed in the femoral artery, creating a higher rate of return of oxygenated blood to the body. **Table 36-2** lists the advantages of the various conventional hemodynamic support devices and the amount of flow they are capable of, with the TandemHeart device supplying the highest flow rate of the group.

7. **Answer: A.** These images represent signs that can be noted as a result of severe pulmonary hypertension with combined large pericardial effusion with a potential for clinical cardiac tamponade. This particular presentation, which does not show RV diastolic collapse, demonstrates a hypertrophic left ventricle with inhibited filling, left atrial compression, and predictively low cardiac output. Acutely depressed pulmonary pressures relative to the higher end-diastolic pressures from extracardiac compression is often a primary driving force of exacerbated symptoms of extreme orthoptic

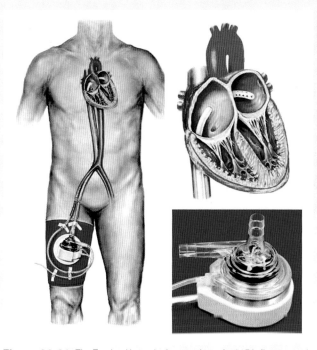

Figure 36-21 The TandemHeart device consists of a 21F inflow cannula in the left atrium after femoral venous access and transseptal puncture and a 15F to 17F arterial cannula in the iliac artery. The externalized centrifugal motor rotates at maximal speed of 7500 rotations per minute, delivering 4 L/min of continuous flow. (From Naidu SS. Novel percutaneous cardiac assist devices: the science of and indications for hemodynamic support. *Circulation.* 2011;123(5):533-543.)

dyspnea. Clinical tamponade would likely result in a need for immediate decompression of the heart via pericardiocentesis.

8. Answer: B. Video 36-3A represents a subcostal view, where improved visualization of the left ventricular apex was achieved. The focal hyperechoic area at the LVAD inlet cannula port detects a small thrombus (**Figure 36-22**, arrows). Additional information in **Video 36-3B** depicts use of an intravenous contrast agent to enhance delineation and differentiate both the inlet and thrombus. This key finding initiated LVAD pump exchange to reestablish effective hemodynamic normalization. **Figure 36-23** describes various confirmatory methods for assessing a state of LVAD thrombosis.

9. ▶ **Answer: E.** (Both A and B). Left ventricular assist devices improve systemic perfusion via creation of a "bypass" of the inefficient native heart "pump" by continuously unloading the left ventricle directly into the ascending aorta. Appropriate pump speed optimization, or a ramp study, is defined according to laboratory results, hemodynamics, and confirmatory echocardiographic findings. M-mode should demonstrate aortic valve leaflets opening at least intermittently, which has been described as inhibiting malcoaptation and long-term leaflet degeneration. Too high pump speed settings can increase intracavity suction enough to keep aortic leaflets from closing, resulting in significant aortic insufficiency (**Figure 36-24A** and **Video 36-20A**), reducing cardiac output and potentially causing myocardial ischemia. An early conventional practice of permanently suturing aortic valve leaflets at the time of implantation ultimately has shown increased risk of thrombosis in the sinuses of Valsalva (**Figure 36-24B** and **Video 36-20B**) and has led to morbidities involving coronary occlusion, cerebral vascular events, or distal embolization. This practice has now been largely abandoned, and more discrete optimization methods are the standard of care.

10. **Answer: D.** The WATCHMAN (Boston Scientific Corp.) device is a percutaneous LAA transcatheter occlusion device used for the prevention of thrombus formation in the LAA that may result in cardioembolic stroke in patients with intermittent or chronic atrial fibrillation. Successful implantation and occlusion generally enable at-risk patients to have cessation of high-grade anticoagulant medical therapy. Suitability for device implantation includes the assessment of the LAA anatomy and morphology, the LAA ostial shape and dimensions, and the "landing zone" diameters at the level of the left coronary circumflex channel. There are described anatomic variants of LAA morphology that tend to divide into true aphid (windsock), biphid (broccoli), and an elongated ostial channel termed "chicken

Table 36-2. Hemodynamic Effects of Mechanical Circulatory Support Devices

Device	Flow	Left Ventricular Preload	Left Ventricular Afterload	Mean Arterial Pressure
Intraaortic balloon pump	0.5 L/min	Slight decrease	Slight decrease	Slight increase
Impella	Up to 5 L/min	Decrease	No change	Increase
TandemHeart	Up to 5 L/min	Decrease	Increase	Increase
Extracorporeal membrane oxygenation	Up to 6 L/min	Decrease	Increase	Increase

From Ergle K, Parto P, Krim SR. Percutaneous ventricular assist devices: a novel approach in the management of patients with acute cardiogenic shock. *Ochsner J.* 2016;16(3):243-249. https://creativecommons.org/licenses/by/4.0/. Copyright © 2016 Authors. Originally published in Ochsner Journal. Available at http://www.ochsnerjournal.org/content/16/3/243.

Figure 36-22

wing" (**Figures 36-25A** and **36-25B**). A patient exhibiting the more complex "broccoli"-shaped LAA morphology suggests multiple lobes and a pectinal network that may be difficult to occlude at the most optimized ostial perpendicular angle. The LAA is best viewed from the midesophageal (ME) views including the ME 0° view, the ME 135° view, the ME 90° orthogonal view, and the bicommissural ME 45°

view. Biplane or 3D multiplane imaging from the 45° acquisition window often yields the most valuable assessment for morphology and dimension measurements. Nonvalvular-disease–related (not related to primary mitral stenosis or regurgitation) atrial fibrillation is a requirement for approved commercial implantation of a Watchman (Boston Scientific Corp.) LAA occluder device at the current time.

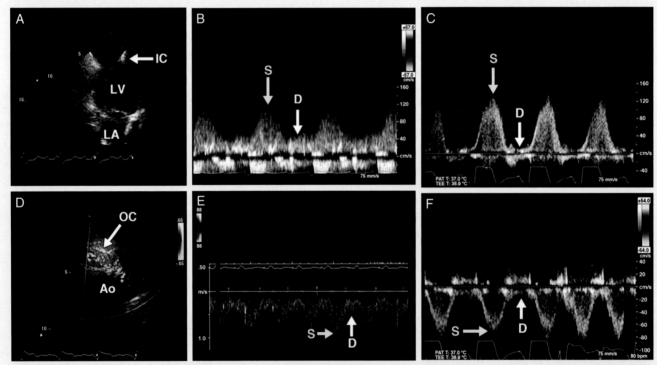

Figure 36-23 LVAD inflow and outflow cannula with Doppler velocity waveforms at baseline and at presentation with intravascular hemolysis (IVH) due to suspected pump thrombosis. Echocardiographic images from a left ventricular assist device (LVAD)-supported patient: A, apical 4-chamber view of the left ventricle (LV) with the inflow cannula (IC) visualized at the apex. B, Doppler velocity waveforms from the IC demonstrating systolic (S) **(yellow arrow)** and diastolic (D) **(white arrow)** flow velocities during normal device function. C, Flow velocities from the same patient at the time of presentation with IVH due to suspected pump thrombosis demonstrating preserved systolic flow velocity with reduced diastolic flow velocity due to impaired device contribution to flow through the pump. D, Right-parasternal view of the outflow cannula (OC) showing flow into the aorta (Ao) from the same patient. E, Systolic and diastolic flow velocities from the OC during normal LVAD function. F, At the time of IVH due to suspected pump thrombosis, again illustrating preserved systolic with reduced diastolic flow velocities. LA, left atrium. (Reprinted from Fine NM, Topilsky Y, Oh JK, et al. Role of echocardiography in patients with intravascular hemolysis due to suspected continuous-flow LVAD thrombosis. *JACC Cardiovasc Imaging*. 2013;6(11):1129-1140. Copyright © 2013 Elsevier. With permission.)

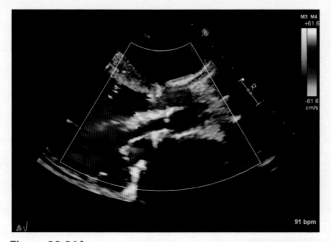

Figure 36-24A

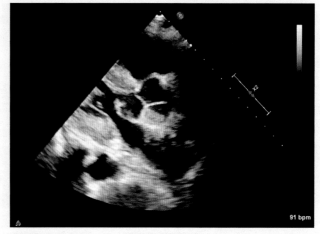

Figure 36-24B

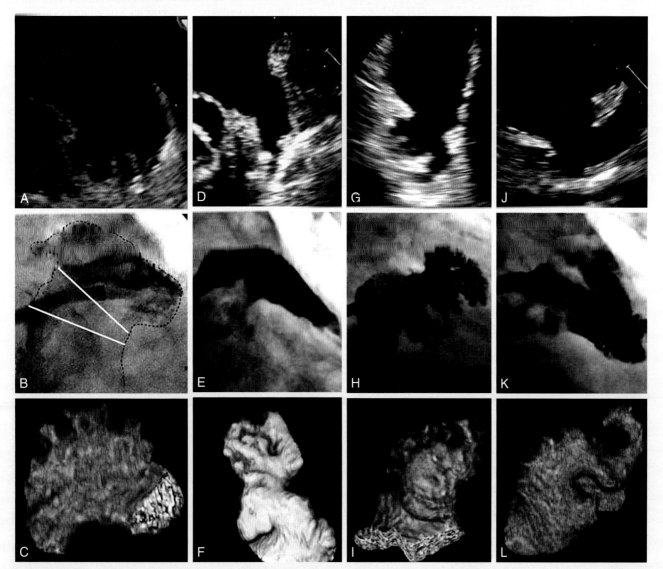

Figure 36-25A Left atrial appendage (LAA) morphologies and modalities. The four different LAA morphologies as shown by transesophageal echocardiography (top), cine angiography (middle), and 3D computed tomography (bottom). Cauliflower (A-C), windsock (D-F), cactus (G-I), and chicken wing (J-L). (Reprinted from Beigel R, Wunderlich NC, Ho SY, et al. The left atrial appendage: anatomy, function, and noninvasive evaluation. *JACC Cardiovasc Imaging.* 2014;7(12):1251-1265. Copyright © 2014 American College of Cardiology Foundation. With permission.)

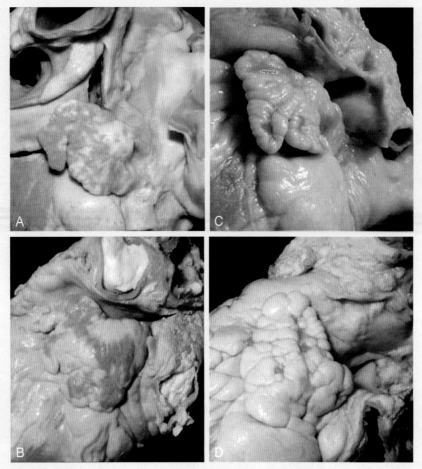

Figure 36-25B Anatomic variants of left atrial appendage morphology. Sample images taken from explanted hearts demonstrating different LAA morphologies (top). A, Chicken wing; B, windsock; C, cauliflower; D, cactus. (Reprinted from Beigel R, Wunderlich NC, Ho SY, et al. The left atrial appendage: anatomy, function, and noninvasive evaluation. *JACC Cardiovasc Imaging.* 2014;7(12):1251-1265. Copyright © 2014 American College of Cardiology Foundation. With permission.)

11. Answer: E The WATCHMAN (Boston Scientific Corp.) device size is chosen to be 8% to 20% larger than the diameter of the LAA body to ensure sufficient compression of the device for stable positioning and anchoring. Hence, the vendor-recommended compression range for this device is a minimum of 8% up to 20%. Based on the angle of implantation, morphology, and depth of the proximal occluder segment compared to the LAA ostium, a larger than nominal sizing may be chosen, resulting in a compression ratio >20% to help ensure no movement or explantation of the device. In the case example shown in **Figures 36-26A** and **36-26B**, there is a maximum landing zone diameter of 19 mm (**Figure 36-26B**) and an average depth of 24 mm; therefore, this patient would likely receive a 24 mm device implantation. This is based on the design of the device, whereby the device-labeled size (mm) dictates the depth that will result in the same proximal width in the noncompressed state. For a 24 mm WATCHMAN (Boston Scientific Corp.) device, the minimum LAA diameter should be > 19.2 mm (20% compression) and the maximum LAA diameter <22.1 mm (8% compression).

12. Answer: A A ramp study is generally performed to ensure optimized hemodynamic exchange and efficiency via speed optimization, to rule out pump thrombosis, and preceding possible explantation (removal) of the LVAD (**Figure 36-27A**). In this study, the "Pre-ramp" baseline LVEDD measure

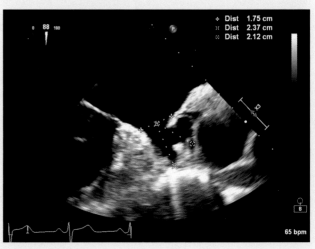

Figure 36-26A

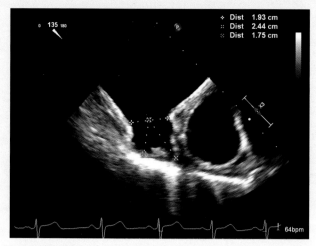

Figure 36-26B

was 65 mm @ 8000 rpm (see **Figure 36-3A**), then sequentially increased to a maximum ramp speed with an LVEDD of 27 mm @ 11,200 rpm (see **Figure 36-3D**). This objectively shows the LVAD pump is unloading the left ventricle too aggressively at the highest rpm with exacerbation of preload suction and underfilling. The ability to rapidly increase such a high slope of change in LVEDD suggests a very unlikely chance of pump thrombosis and a responsive LVAD with normal unloading capability. In the case of pump thrombosis, the resistance of required suction with decreased flow transfer would result in a less sensitive response. Ideally, the LVEDD slope should be >−0.16 when the speeds are adjusted from 8000 to 12,000 rpm in a HeartMate II (Abbott) (**Figure 36-27B**). Other benchmarks include validation

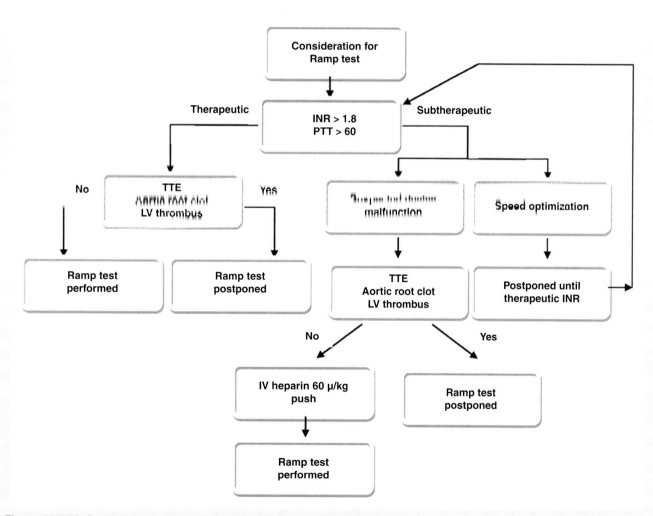

Figure 36-27A Consideration for the ramp test algorithm. Algorithm for consideration of ramp tests based on anticoagulation studies and presence of intracardiac thrombus. Blood pressure should be below 110 mm Hg by Doppler in order to be eligible to start the ramp test. INR, international normalized ratio; IV, intravenous; LV, left ventricular; PTT, partial thromboplastin time; TTE, transthoracic echocardiography. (Reprinted from Uriel N, Morrison KA, Garan AR, et al. Development of a novel echocardiography ramp test for speed optimization and diagnosis of device thrombosis in continuous-flow left ventricular assist devices: the Columbia ramp study. *J Am Coll Cardiol.* 2012;60(18):1764-1775. Copyright © 2012 American College of Cardiology Foundation. With permission.)

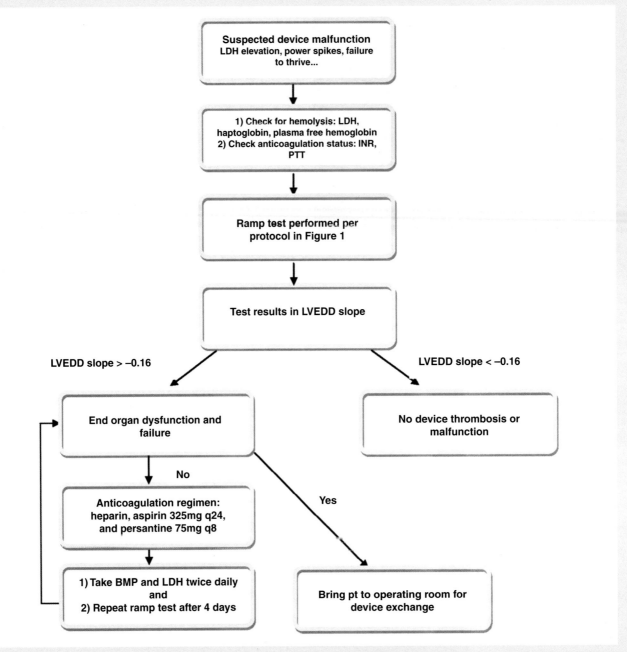

Figure 36-27B Suspected device malfunction algorithm. Suggested management algorithm for patients with suspected device thrombosis. BMP, basic metabolic panel; LVEDD, left ventricular end-diastolic dimension; Pt, patient. (Reprinted from Uriel N, Morrison KA, Garan AR, et al. Development of a novel echocardiography ramp test for speed optimization and diagnosis of device thrombosis in continuous-flow left ventricular assist devices: the Columbia ramp study. *J Am Coll Cardiol.* 2012;60(18):1764-1775. Copyright © 2012 American College of Cardiology Foundation. With permission.)

of aortic valve closure and predicted a decrease in mitral regurgitation. A normally functioning Heart-Mate II (Abbott) LVAD should unload the ventricle via expression of pump demand and achievement of iso-pressure rather than from overly augmenting native left ventricular contractility.

13. **Answer: D.** Cardiac tamponade is primarily a clinical diagnosis. Clinical correlations of tamponade usually include hypotension, a narrow pulse pressure, and severe orthopnea or hypoxia (patient urgency to sit up in order to breathe). This presentation is supportive of true emergent cardiac tamponade. Tamponade may be further confirmed by various echocardiography-based methods, including identification of pericardial effusion and early diastolic collapse of the right ventricular free wall. Early diastolic collapse of the right ventricular free wall may be confirmed from a parasternal long-axis view with M-mode, which offers higher temporal resolution. Modified apical or subcostal views noting the phase of the cardiac cycle based on the electrocardiogram and the duration of collapse may also be obtained. Right-sided inflow resistance may be assessed by evaluating the

inferior vena cava for dilation and lack of inspiratory collapse and paradoxical central hepatic vein flow reversal with respiration.

14. ▶ **Answer: E.** Pinpointing the region and access depth for a loculated pericardial effusion is essential for establishing an appropriate and safe puncture site. The three access points are (anterior) parasternal, (inferior) subcostal, and (lateral) apical. The distance from the chest wall to the pericardium is measured for puncture depth. Any potential for intervening structures or iatrogenic trauma must be clearly defined prior to the procedure. 3D echocardiography with live cut-planes (C-planes) or biplane 2D echocardiography with steerable orthogonal imaging is also helpful. **Video 36-21A** shows the puncture of the needle into the pericardial space, avoiding any intervening structures. **Video 36-21B** demonstrates the needle depth relative to the cardiac chambers to prevent chamber perforation.

Agitated saline may also be injected by the interventionalist to validate needle position within the effusive space before proceeding with fluid extraction (**Figure 36-28**).

15. ▶ **Answer: A.** In general, the safe and consistently accessible region for extracting a myocardial tissue biopsy is from the septal wall of the right ventricle. The apical window allows for the visualization of the bioptome. The bioptome "arrowhead" appearance is somewhat similar to

the opened grip arms of a conventional MitraClip device from an inverted perspective. **Video 36-22A** shows a hyperechoic structure abutting the interventricular septum causing a temporary tenting of the septum; this is the bioptome. **Video 36-22B** demonstrates the benefit of using two orthogonal imaging planes for determining the position of the bioptome. Confirmatory views obtained from different windows and/or scan angles should also be used in order to best localize the bioptome contact point prior to a biopsy sample. Tearing tissue from the free wall of the left ventricle introduces risk of induced arrhythmias or, more rarely, circumflex coronary artery perforation, leading to potential myocardial injury, pericardial effusion, or cardiac tamponade.

16. **Answer: B.** 2D color Doppler images (**Video 36-5**) demonstrate the left ventricle as obtained using intracardiac echocardiography (ICE). ICE is a small catheter ultrasound probe introduced into a cardiac cavity for viewing regions within very close proximity (<4 cm). There is clear evidence of hypertrophy of the basal to middle anterior septum with combined obstructive systolic anterior motion (SAM) of the mitral valve. The peak instantaneous continuous-wave Doppler gradient through this region measured in **Figure 36-4** is 49 mm Hg; however, this gradient is likely underestimated due to suboptimal alignment between the ultrasound beam and the left ventricular outflow tract (LVOT).

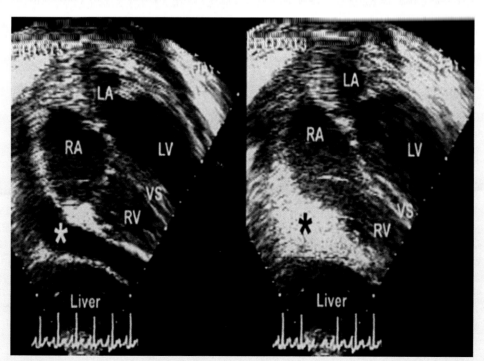

Figure 36-28 Assessment of position of the Teflon-sheathed needle during pericardiocentesis with opacification of the pericardial space (asterisk) after saline contrast injection. LA, Left atrium; LV, left ventricle; RA, right atrium; RV, right ventricle; VS, ventricular septum. (Reprinted from Silvestry FE, Kerber RE, Brook MM, et al. Echocardiography-guided interventions. *J Am Soc Echocardiogr.* 2009;22(3):213-231. Copyright © 2009 American Society of Echocardiography. With permission.)

TEACHING POINT (PRESSURE GRADIENTS IN DYNAMIC LVOT OBSTRUCTION AND AORTIC STENOSIS)

In aortic stenosis, the echocardiographically derived peak instantaneous gradient usually exceeds the peak-to-peak gradient, whereby in hypertrophic obstructive cardiomyopathy, the late rise in velocity from dynamic obstruction yields a more synonymous relationship between peak instantaneous and peak-to-peak gradients (**Figure 36-29**). With the use of continuous-wave Doppler as a surrogate for outflow gradients, the peak instantaneous gradient correlates best for guidance of severity and results regarding a decrease in obstruction following septal ablation.

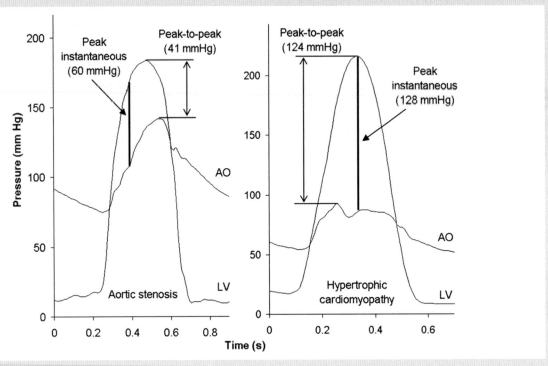

Figure 36-29 Gradient measurement at cardiac catheterization. Continuous high-fidelity left ventricular (LV) and aortic (Ao) hemodynamic tracings were used for evaluation of patients with aortic stenosis (left) and hypertrophic cardiomyopathy (right). Peak instantaneous and peak-to-peak gradient measurements are shown. (Reprinted from Geske JB, Cullen MW, Sorajja P, et al. Assessment of left ventricular outflow tract: hypertrophic cardiomyopathy versus aortic valvular stenosis. *JACC Cardiovasc Interv.* 2012;5(6):675-681. Copyright © 2012 American College of Cardiology Foundation. With permission.)

17. **Answer: B.** The frequency range for commercially available ICE transducer catheters is 5 to 10 MHz, which is an incrementally higher peak frequency capability than that of transesophageal echocardiography (TEE) or transthoracic echocardiography (TTE) (**Figure 36-30**). Use of ICE provides simple access and close-proximity imaging to small, specific intracardiac regions, which is helpful with procedures such as electrophysiology-based ablations requiring guided interatrial septal crossing. Because the ICE transducer is positioned within the chamber of the region of interest (ROI), refraction and attenuation of signals through tissues between the ROI and probe are rarely encountered, in contrast to TTE and TEE. Current ICE catheters must be disposed of following use and may not be cleaned and reused. The decision to use ICE depends on availability, physician training, and preference of the operator. ICE catheters may also be cost-prohibitive depending

on reimbursement guidelines according to payors or institutional policies, only being used on indication-based criteria.

18. **Answer: A.** The images provided show flail A2 and A3 segments with P1-scallop prolapse. The advantages of using 3D mitral modeling as a diagnostic and planning tool include the objective evaluation of accurate morphology and a full assortment of measurements derived from a 3D perspective. Once the accurate "saddle" shape of the annulus is identified, the commissural coaptation line and leaflet segments are traced and seen from the left atrial perspective. Segments that prolapse the most beyond the annular plane (defining true prolapse) are displayed from light pink (mild) to deep crimson red (severe). The 3D zoom live image should have aided in the identification of the central to medial flail regions of the anterior leaflet. The deep red of the modeled P1 lateral scallop demonstrates

Transducer options for optimized imaging by various approaches

Image quality is determined by:

➢ Density and # scan lines (spatial) = amount of returning echoes

➢ Proximity to region of interest

➢ Frequency of returning echoes to and from transducer

➢ Attenuation of signals due to tissues, bone, devices, and distance

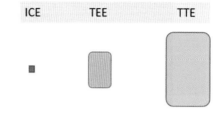

TTE: 2.5 - 5.0 MHz
TEE: 3.5 - 7.0 MHz
ICE: 5.0 - 10 MHz

Figure 36-30

prolapse (see **Figure 36-5B**, lower right panel). Note the "fallout" of the P1-scallop and large A2 segment in the cut-plane leveled at the annulus at lower left, which correlates with the deepest red on the model due to prolapse beyond the level of the C-plane.

19. ▶ **Answer: D.** All surgically implanted bioprosthetic valves, usually between 7 and 15 years, will degenerate regardless of tissue type. Causes of degeneration include endocarditis or systemic factors (e.g., renal failure) shown to accelerate leaflet sclerosis, eventually causing stenosis and/or regurgitation. Many candidate patients now can be offered an option of a transcatheter aortic valve replacement prosthesis within a dysfunctional bioprosthetic valve ring, or "valve-in-valve" procedure. This is approached from transapical access from the left ventricle, or transseptal access from the right atrium, depending on the risk/benefit profile and

optimal appropriateness for access angle and positioning. **Video 36-23** shows an excellent post valve-in-valve result.

20. **Answer: D.** As seen in **Figure 36-31A** (arrows), shadowing and beam attenuation from structures between the TEE transducer and aortic leaflets and annulus make delineating the virtual ring portion just beyond leaflet nadirs or hinge points difficult. **Figure 36-31B** displays minimal shadowing and was properly aligned and traced with a high level of confidence by the echocardiographer.

Techniques such as multiplanar reconstruction (MPR), orthogonal plane shift, and landmark placement (dots) assist in placing four orthogonal points from which a smooth oval may be traced, emulating the predictive shape of a postexpansion TAVR prosthesis stent. 3D MPR techniques take considerable practice in order to assume reliable intraoperator

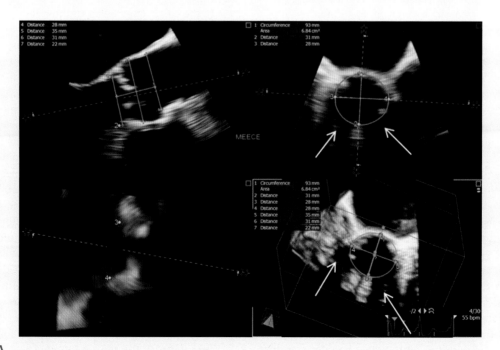

Figure 36-31A

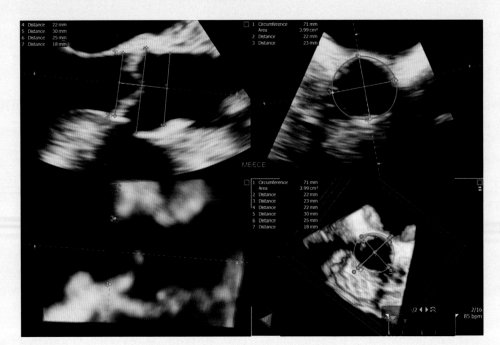

Figure 36-31B

accuracy and minimal variability. The risks for incorrect sizing include dissection in oversizing and regurgitation in undersizing.

21. **Answer: A.** This is the unique and distinct continuous-wave (CW) Doppler pattern of an outflow graft in a patient with internal implantation of the most recently approved HeartMate 3 (Abbott) device. The CW Doppler pattern differs from that of the Heart Mate II and HeartWare devices due to a change using an artificial pulse algorithm. Artificial pulsation is specific to HeartMate 3 (Abbott) to assist a "washout" of the pump with the goal to inhibit thrombus formation as well as facilitate "natural" aortic valve leaflet closure and reduce development of aortic insufficiency.

22. **Answer: B.** The images provided are apical long-axis views focused on the inlet cannula of the LVAD and show a suction effect. Suction events are often the result of left ventricular (LV) unloading from hypovolemia (e.g., gastrointestinal bleed or dehydration), suboptimal inlet cannula positioning, or too high of a pump speed. Therefore, decreasing the LVAD speed will eliminate this suction effect due to the decrease in unloading of the left ventricle. Performing an echo ramp study to rule out a pump thrombosis is also not a correct answer due to the patient's small left ventricular cavity dimension. A small left ventricular cavity dimension is consistent with high LVAD pump speed or a hypovolemic state. If related to an internal bleed or hemorrhage, the source of hemorrhage must be corrected to ensure appropriate LV flow dynamics. Surgical correction is rarely warranted to ensure proper alignment of the inlet cannula with the mitral valve opening, as this

is a known potential issue during implantation and great care is taken to avoid malpositioning of the port.

23. **Answer: B.** The patient's relative numbers suggest an increase in power (see **Table 36-3**). The LVAD power is a measurement of the pump motor voltage and current, and changes with demand on the speed of the pump. The number to look out for in terms of a "power increase" is >10 watts. This patient's LVAD was operating with a power of 11 watts, which generally is considered increased. PI represents the left ventricular pulsatile contribution to the LVAD. The PI was slightly decreased (4.0) compared to the patient's baseline (4.5-5). A decreased PI could indicate a pump thrombosis. The third sign of pump thrombosis is the flow parameter that indicates *+++*on the controller. This is discussed in the question regarding this patient's situation. In any LVAD evaluation, the pump must maintain a fixed number of rpm to ensure proper unloading of the left ventricle. If thrombus is present on the pump rotor, power will increase to maintain the required rpm speed and flow. Given the clinical history and no positive blood cultures, presence of thrombus is the most likely cause for the echo-dense region visualized in the left ventricular outflow tract.

24. ▶ **Answer: C.** This is an ICE guidance procedure for a patent foramen ovale (PFO) closure. **Figure 36-8A** and **Video 36-9A** demonstrate a right and left inter-atrial shunt with aneurysmal septum. **Figure 36-8B** and **Video 36-9B** show the delivery catheter crossing and with partial Amplatzer deployment through the PFO with the first wing of the closure device opened in the left

Table 36-3. Typical LVAD Operating Parameters

	HeartMate II	HeartMate 3	HVAD
Typical speed, rpm[a]	8000-10,000	5000-6000	2400-3200
Speed adjustment increment, rpm/increment	200	100	20
Flow, L/min	4-7	4-6	4-6
Power, W	5-8	4.5-6.5	3-7
Pulsatility index (or HVAD, peak to trough)	5-8	3.5-5.5	2-4 L/min/beat

HVAD, HeartWare ventricular assist device (system); LVAD, left ventricular assist device; rpm, revolutions per minute.

[a]Speeds at the lower range or below the clinical ranges shown above indicate a low level of support is needed and should prompt investigation of native contractility. Speeds above or near the high range described above should prompt investigation for adequate left ventricular unloading, including the possibilities of LVAD dysfunction or native valvular disease that could be affecting unloading.

From DeVore AD, Patel PA, Patel CB. Medical management of patients with a left ventricular assist device for the non-left ventricular assist device specialist. *JACC Heart Fail*. 2017;5(9):621-631.

atrium. **Figure 36-8D** and **Video 36-8C** demonstrate completion of closure of the PFO and dual apposition across the septum. **Figure 36-32** and **Video 36-24** shows 3D rendering of the left atrial disk and apposition against the septum.

25. **Answer: D.** Pulmonary vein isolation via ICE for the treatment of persistent atrial fibrillation is indicated. ICE imaging also guides transseptal access, allowing mapping/ablation catheters to be advanced into the left atrium. Following insertion via right femoral venous access, a pacing/recording catheter is positioned in the coronary sinus with ICE catheter positioned in the right atrium. Pulmonary vein isolation is then performed with radiofrequency ablation or nitrogen gas infusion for cryo-treere. Ablation (as in this case) is performed using 3D electro-anatomic mapping, using ICE for real-time visual monitoring for complications such as a pericardial effusion.

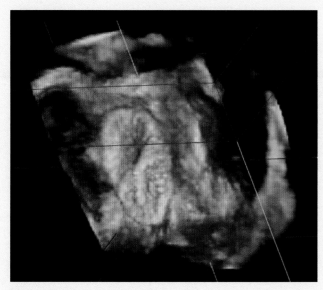

Figure 36-32

26. ▶ **Answer: B.** The MitraClip is a chromium cobalt device with two polyester-covered clip arms designed to grasp both mitral leaflets in a similar fashion as edge-to-edge surgical repair resulting in a double orifice mitral valve if grasping is performed in the central A2-P2 region. These devices are implanted via a transcatheter delivery system that is inserted into the left atrium from the femoral vein via transseptal puncture. Transesophageal echocardiography is used to guide the transseptal puncture and to steer the device to the appropriate mitral valve pathology. A final step preceding leaflet grasping is to view the clip from the left atrial aspect to ensure commissure position (lateral to medial aspect) is as planned, and that clip rotation along the axis aligns the MitraClip arms perpendicular to the leaflet commissural line (**Figure 36-33A**, arrows). If clip rotation is off-axis, or turned too far clockwise or counterclockwise, apposition of leaflets during grasping may flatten and "twist" the shorter posterior leaflet as opposed to the anterior leaflet, opening folds or clefts adjacent to the grasping region, causing malcoaptation that worsens mitral regurgitation. **Video 36-25** shows an opened cleft and malcoaptation lateral to the clip and resultant significant mitral regurgitation seen by color flow Doppler. In this case, the clip was oriented too clockwise, therefore when clamping down, the posterior leaflet pulled medially, opening the clear region of malcoaptation laterally. In addition, the posterior leaflet tissue bridge appears narrow, suggesting a less-than-optimal tissue grasp. The A3 region fallout artifact anteriorly is from shadowing of the device catheter in the sector beam, a common issue in imaging during MitraClip procedures.

27. **Answer: D.** Correcting and validating the exact position for crossing the fossa ovalis during the puncture of the interatrial septum is critical for an optimized angle of the placement catheter, allowing

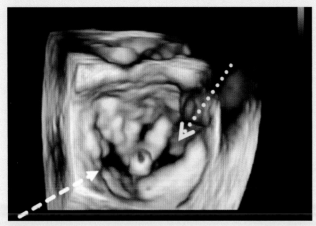

Figure 36-33A Example of an implanted MitraClip at A2-P2 that is malpositioned with too "clockwise" of a rotation angle. This resulted in an opening of a P1-P2 cleft and increased regurgitation. The clip was then turned counterclockwise to a more perpendicular grasp and regurgitation significantly decreased.

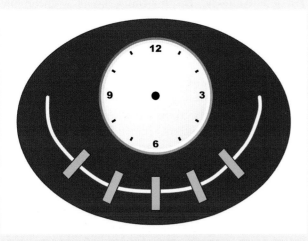

Figure 36-33B This illustration demonstrates the appropriate clip rotational positioning according to anterior "clock" representation along a curved commissural line. This helps to ensure perpendicular leaflet apposition and horizontal alignment of the MitraClip device during implantation. The aortic valve and the mitral valve A2/P2-scallops are located at 12 o'clock when discussing appropriate rotational position of the anterior part of the clip compared to location on the commissural line of coaptation; for example, the lower left of center at 7 o'clock would be 1 o'clock at top.

manipulation of the device catheter, resulting in a successful procedure. For example, crossing too anteriorly and eccentrically through a patent foramen ovale tunnel would likely create an even larger atrial septal defect with extremely difficult manipulation. This could require removal and re-puncture at an optimal placement, leaving two defects and shunts. Both 2D biplane and 3D live imaging are essential tools for determining correct height from the mitral annulus and catheter orientation preceding insertion of the guiding system(s) (**Figure 36-34**). The left upper (superior) pulmonary vein is the primary target for planting the initial guidewire for anchoring and subsequent catheter insertion into the left atrium.

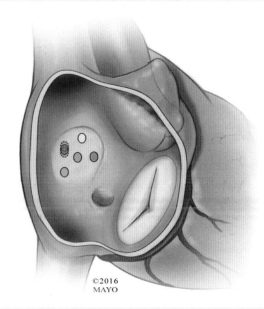

©2016 MAYO

Figure 36-34 Site-specific transseptal puncture for various intracardiac interventions. Red: MitraClip, paravalvular leak closure (a higher crossing site is recommended for medial leaks, and a lower crossing site is recommended for lateral leaks; dashed red circles). Yellow: transseptal patent foramen ovale closure. Blue: percutaneous left ventricular assist device placement, hemodynamic studies. Green: left atrial appendage closure. Orange: pulmonary vein interventions. (From Alkhouli M, Rihal CS, Holmes DR Jr. Transseptal techniques for emerging structural heart interventions. *JACC Cardiovasc Interv.* 2016;9(24):2465-2480. used with permission of Mayo Foundation for Medical Education and Research, all rights reserved.)

28. **Answer: A.** An important aspect of the TEE evaluation for transcatheter LAA occlusion is to accurately assess "real world" morphology and size of the LAA. In an extended NPO state preceding a TEE, patients may not be optimally hydrated, resulting in reduced left atrial volume and pressures. This may underestimate the "native" size of the LAA. Underestimation of accurate LAA dimensions can result in measurement results too small for occluder candidacy. A similar surrogate protocol immediately preceding device implantation is to directly measure left atrial pressure (LAP) following transseptal puncture. A mean LAP of ≥10 mm Hg is a guideline for accurate sizing. **Figures 36-35A** and **36-35B** shows a small appendage with borderline depth for candidacy. **Figure 36-35C** shows the LAA following fluid bolus of 500 cc IV now demonstrating landing zone width and depth of at least 20 mm.

29. ▶ **Answer: C.** The imaging team should always note device shape and orientation, as well as good atrial wall apposition. When both disks are opened and retracted to the septum, there should be close proximity of both disks, appearing relatively flat and parallel to the wall. In this case, there is "doming" of the left atrial disk with very poor apposition and stretching of the central foramen ovale (**Video 36-12B**). In this instance, the interventionalist is likely to adjust and re-deploy to see if this addresses

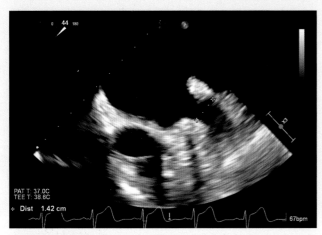

Figure 36-35A

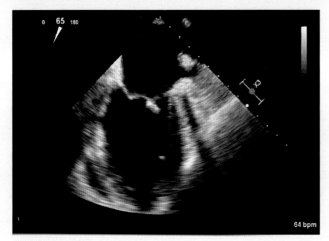

Figure 36-35B

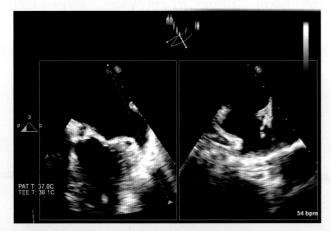

Figure 36-35C

the issue. However, in this case the device system was initially released, resulting in incomplete deployment. A decision was made to retract and remove the defective "domed" Amplatzer and implant another device of the same size and type, which deployed perfectly with excellent occlusion of the PFO. **Video 36-26** shows the device in the correctly released state with tension removed from the septal wall, which now lies flat, straight, and parallel with the occluder.

30. **Answer: D.** Following conversion of a highly stenotic aortic valve to nearly normalized outflow and aortic valve area, there will be an acute decrease in LV end-diastolic pressures synonymous with lowered flow resistance and preload conditions. In an underfilled hypertrophied left ventricle, TAVR implantation can abruptly unload the ventricle, leading to hemodynamic instability with a decreased mean arterial pressure. If the echocardiographer sees signs of ventricular volume unloading with combined outflow obstruction, a decreased LVESD, and/or systolic anterior mitral leaflet motion with mitral regurgitation preprocedure, they should advise the interventionalist and/or anesthesia staff so prophylactic volume loading may be implemented if deemed necessary. **Videos 36-27A** and **36-27B** demonstrate two types of ventricles, a "spade" apical hypertrophy (**Video 36-27A**) and asymmetric septal hypertrophy with systolic anterior motion (**Video 36-27B**), both of which have outflow obstruction at rest with an inherent higher risk of acute ventricular unloading with outflow tract obstruction following TAVR implantation.

31. **Answer: E.** The primary measurement for selecting the appropriate TAVR size is either the area (mm^2) or circumference (mm), depending on which device is being used (i.e., whether stainless steel [balloon-expanded and fixed], or nitinol [self-expanding, no balloon]). The sinus dimensions are also very important. There must be a large enough region of clearance to prevent coronary artery flow obstruction when the calcified native aortic valve leaflets are crushed back into the sinuses by the TAVR device. For example, a sinus to commissure diameter of 27 mm would only allow insertion of a 23 mm Sapien 3 rather than a 26 mm device, as the 26 mm device would prevent calcific leaflets too close to the coronary artery ostia from permitting effective diastolic filling of the coronary arteries, and hinder future catheter access to the coronary arteries.

32. **Answer: B.** The usual view for crossing the interatrial septum (IAS) with a catheter-based baylis wire is from the bicaval view acquired with biplane imaging (90° orthogonal imaging). The transesophageal echocardiographic midesophageal bicaval view delineates the superior and inferior vena caval aspects of the IAS, while the orthogonal short-axis view, often with the aortic valve (AV) in view, delineates the anterior structures (AV and basal IAS) and the posterior IAS. This ensures the interventionalist is aware of optimized positioning and crossing point to the fossa ovalis for a particular procedure (see answer outline for Question 27).

33. **Answer: C.** Location of the correct septal perforator preceding ablation is critical to ensure that regionalized basal septal infarction has the highest chance of removing the obstructive basal septal myocardium. **Video 36-13B** denotes contrast

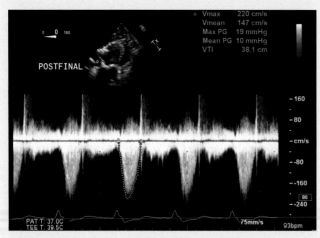

Figure 36-36

enhancement of a larger region that appears to be below the highest sub–left ventricular outflow tract (LVOT) perforator, showing a larger longitudinal perfusion distribution and reduced echogenicity. **Video 36-13C** shows the contrast-enhanced "true" first septal perforator. The region is located more basal and focal to the LVOT and is clearly associated with the primary mitral systolic anterior motion-septal contact point. **Videos 36-28A** and **36-28B** and **Figure 36-36** show a significant reduction in both obstruction and gradients with improved laminar color outflow following ablation.

34. ▶ **Answer: A.** In a "true" ME 45° to 60° bicommissural view of the mitral valve, the left atrial appendage (LAA; on right of sector) and the coronary sinus (on left of sector) should be seen (**Figure 36-37A**). Because the LSPV is slightly superior to the LAA, retracting the probe approximately 1 cm should open up visualization of this vein (**Figure 36-37B** and **Video 36-29**). This can be validated with color Doppler imaging using the color compare (or "color simultaneous" or "dual") modes to differentiate the

vein from the LAA or transverse sinus if the coumadin ridge is not clearly identified. At times, incremental rotation of the plane may be necessary. The actual degree of plane rotation for alignment of a "true" bicommissural view will vary in patients who have cardiac rotation or displacement anatomically.

35. **Answer: E.** Evaluation for mitral stenosis by planimetry and mean pressure gradient are important following a MitraClip. Qualitatively, most operators experienced with MitraClip implantations would likely state this appears to be a good result. There is a wide tissue bridge, suggesting good grasping of both leaflets. Two relatively open orifices are present with good leaflet mobility. Although pulmonary vein inflows are very helpful in being sensitive to changes or reduction in left atrial pressures pre- and post-MitraClip, they are not immediately specific to procedural success. What cannot be derived from the images alone in terms of success are objective measurements related to induced mitral stenosis, which is the most important concern after placing the MitraClip. This can be evaluated by tracing both orifice areas (**Figures 36-38A** and **36-38B**), and as a guideline, ensuring mitral inflow mean pressure gradients are no more than 6 mm Hg, preferably less. In the case where the interventionalist may desire to place a second MitraClip for further reduction of mitral regurgitation, these measures would be essential before proceeding further. Mitral stenosis can be more clinically symptomatic for many patients than regurgitation and is a primary concern for any mitral repair procedure that may cause mitral stenosis.

36. **Answer: D.** There is a 78% reduction of TR severity by 3D vena contracta area. The calculation of percentage reduction is:

$$\text{Percentage reduction}(\%) = (\text{VCA-pre} - \text{VCA-post})$$
$$\div \text{VCA-pre} \times 100 \qquad (1)$$

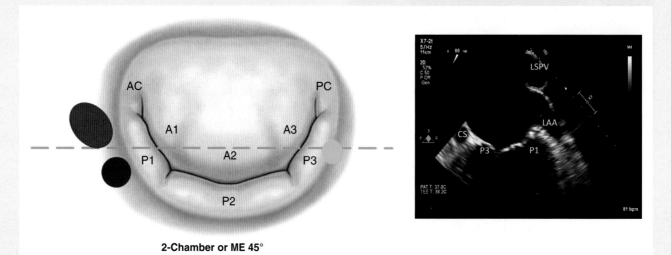

2-Chamber or ME 45°

Figure 36-37A The LAA (green circle) is lateral and the coronary sinus (purple circle) and descending aorta (red circle) are medial.

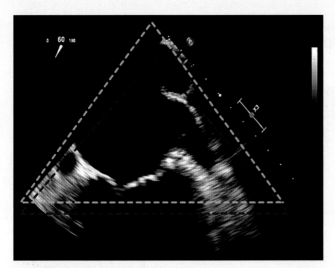

Figure 36-37B The red triangle represents a more inferior positioning of the sector plane, which usually will show the LAA and a slightly cutoff image of the LSPV ostium. To view the fuller depth of the LSPV and insertion of the guidewire, it is necessary to retract to the more superior level of the blue triangle sector position. Color flow Doppler also may aid in validating the echo-free space as being the pulmonary vein.

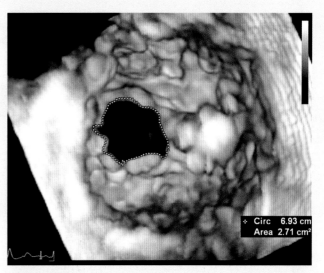

Figure 36-38A Tracing of the direct "en face" view of the medial mitral orifice following clip implantation. Multiplanar reconstruction (MPR) is also used to reduce less-experienced operator subjectivity in alignment of the 3D image on a two-dimensional plane.

where VCA-pre is the original VCA and VCA-post is the VCA post procedure.

The original VCA was 2.17 cm², with a postprocedural VCA of 0.47 cm²; therefore:

$$\text{Percentage reduction}(\%) = (2.17 - 0.47) \div 2.17 \times 100$$
$$= 78\% \qquad (2)$$

VCA area by 3D color flow is just one of the methods for TR severity, but it has gained more interest and relevance for the more complex shape and jet morphology of a trileaflet valve with annular dilatation (**Figure 36-39**).

37. **Answer: E.** All of these methods used in sizing an ASD occluder, with data, have been published in peer-reviewed journals. Many interventionalists prefer balloon sizing for the "waist" diameter (**Figure 36-16D**) because the fully expanded balloon edge may be accurately measured with assumption of a spherical shape that the Amplatzer will impose on the defect itself, and this is combined with very high fluoroscopy spatial resolution. Color Doppler edge to edge (**Figure 36-16B**) also has value in that color will only flow where the true edges of the defect exist (if a nonfenestrated ASD) and should yield effective diameter measurement in agreement to the balloon technique. While the 3D "en face" view has also shown use, the 3D data set acquisition quality, gain settings, dynamic motion, and very thin tissue morphology of the ASD may cause subjective operator error in the measurement. Many like to use 3D multiplanar reconstruction-based C-plane rendering for accurate identification and measurement of the orifice (**Figure 36-16C**). Most would state that the 2D tissue edge-to-edge measurement

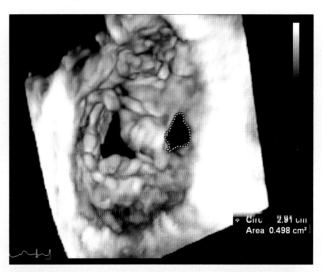

Figure 36-38B Tracing of the "en face" lateral orifice. Both the medial and lateral orifice sizes are combined for a sum equaling total geometric mitral valve area.

(**Figure 36-16A**) is the least reliable technique due to limited appreciation of maximal circumferential or diameter differences on an oval-shaped defect. **Figure 36-40** demonstrates the oval shape of an ASD.

38. **Answer: B.** The 2019 American Society of Echocardiography (ASE) Guidelines for the Evaluation of Valvular Regurgitation After Percutaneous Valve Repair or Replacement elucidate the difficulty and lack of specificity of conventional MR assessment methods for objective measurement of post-clip MR severity. **Table 36-4** and **Figure 36-41** detail the echocardiographic parameters that are assessed during edge-to-edge device deployment to evaluate the severity of residual MR. Of the hemodynamics and TEE parameters useful in determining residual MR severity during mitral valve

CENTRAL ILLUSTRATION: Multimodality Imaging for the Assessment of Tricuspid Regurgitation

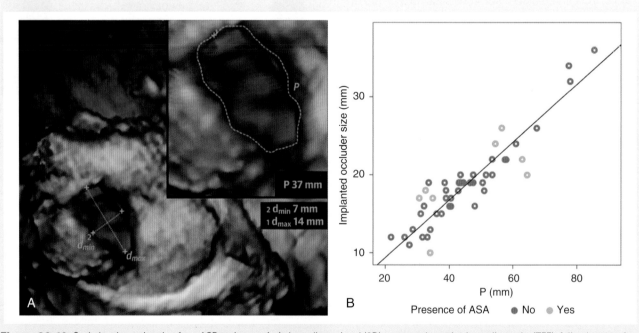

Parameters	Echocardiography (TTE or TEE)		Cardiac Magnetic Resonance	Computed Tomography Angiography
	2D/Doppler	3D/Color		
Structural Parameters				
TV morphology	+++	+++	++	++
RV and RA size	++	+++	+++	+++
SVC and IVC size	+++ (proximal cavae only)	+++	+++	+++
Comprehensive vascular assessment	-	-	+++	+++
Semiquantitative Parameters				
Jet area	+++	+++	++	-
Vena contracta width	+++	+++	++	-
Vena contracta area	-	+++	++	-
Anatomic orifice area	-	+	++	+++
Quantitative Parameters				
Effective regurgitant orifice area	++ (PISA and Doppler SV)	- (see VCA)	-	-
Regurgitant volume	++ (PISA and Doppler SV)	++ (from VCA)	++	-

Figure 36-39 Although echocardiography remains the diagnostic modality of choice for the initial evaluation of the right heart and tricuspid valve, the Venn diagram illustrates the utility and complementary nature of the imaging modalities for certain parameters important in the assessment of tricuspid regurgitation severity. The table shows the relative strengths of each modality for the evaluation of specific parameters. IVC, inferior vena cava; PISA, proximal isovelocity surface area; RA, right atrium; RV, right ventricle; SV, stroke volume; SVC, superior vena cava; TEE, transesophageal echocardiography; TTE, transthoracic echocardiography; TV, tricuspid valve; VCA, vena contracta area. (Reprinted from Hahn RT, Thomas JD, Khalique OK, et al. Imaging assessment of tricuspid regurgitation severity. *JACC Cardiovasc Imaging.* 2019;12(3):469-490. Copyright © 2019 by the American College of Cardiology Foundation. With permission.)

Figure 36-40 Occluder size estimation from ASD perimeter. A, A three-dimensional (3D) transesophageal echocardiography (TEE), full-volume en face view reconstruction. Atrial septal defect (ASD) measurement: maximal diameter (d_max), minimal diameter (d_min), and perimeter (P). B, Linear correlation between the implanted occluder size and atrial septal defect perimeter (P) measured by three-dimensional transesophageal echocardiography; pink dots represent subjects without atrial septal aneurysm (ASA) (*n* = 41), and green dots represent subjects with atrial septal aneurysm (*n* = 8). (Reprinted from Henzel J, Konka M, Wójcik A, et al. Focus on the perimeter and skip the balloon: can atrial septal defect be percutaneously closed without balloon sizing in the era of 3-dimensional echocardiography? *JACC Cardiovasc Imaging.* 2018;11(11):1731-1732. Copyright © 2018 by the American College of Cardiology Foundation. With permission.)

Table 36-4. Hemodynamics and TEE Parameters Useful in Determining Residual MR Severity During Mitral Valve Interventions in the Catheterization Laboratory

Parameter	Parameter Assessing Severity of Residual MR
Invasive hemodynamics	Decrease in regurgitant v wave, LA pressure, and pulmonary pressures are specific signs of reduction in MR severity; consider effects of general anesthesia on MR severity
General echocardiographic findings	
Spontaneous echo contrast in LA	Appearance of spontaneous contrast after MV intervention suggests significant reduction in MR severity
LVEF	Decline in LVEF after MV intervention suggests significant MR reduction in the absence of other causes (ischemia, pacemaker-related, etc.)
Color Doppler	
Color Doppler jet (size, number, location, eccentricity)	• Easy to obtain with a comprehensive, systematic approach • Difficult to assess multiple and eccentric jets • Jet area affected by eccentricity, technical and hemodynamic factors (especially driving velocity)
Flow convergence	• Large flow convergence denotes significant residual MR, whereas a small or no flow convergence suggests mild MR • Difficult to use in presence of multiple jets or very eccentric jets, or may be masked by the device
Vena contracta width	• VCW ≥0.7 cm specific for severe MR • Difficult to use in presence of multiple small jets or very eccentric jets for which orifice shape is not well delineated
Vena contracta area (3D planimetry)	• Allows better delineation of eccentric orifice shape and possibly the addition of VCA of multiple jets • Prone to blooming artifacts
Spectral Doppler	
Pulmonary vein flow pattern	• Systolic flow reversal in >1 vein specific for severe MR • Increase in forward systolic velocity after MV intervention helps confirm MR reduction
MR jet profile by CWD (contour, density, peak velocity)	• Dense, triangular pattern suggests severe MR • May be hard to line up CWD properly in flail leaflet or very eccentric jet after intervention
Mitral inflow pattern	• In sinus rhythm, mitral A-wave–dominant flow excludes severe MR • Decrease in mitral E velocity and VTI suggests reduction in MR severity
Pulsed Doppler of LVOT (deep transgastric view)	• Increase in LVOT velocity and VTI after procedure suggests MR reduction
Quantitative parameters	In general, more difficult to perform; some procedure-specific limitations in quantitation
EROA by PISA	• Not recommended after edge-to-edge repair because assumption of hemispheric proximal flow convergence is violated by the device • PISA often underestimates MR severity in the presence of multiple jets or markedly eccentric jets. • Not feasible in PVR of mechanical prosthetic MV or possibly TMVR (flow masking in LV by TEE)
Regurgitant volume	• Difficult to perform volumetric RVol with pulsed Doppler by TEE

CWD, Continuous-wave Doppler; EROA, effective regurgitant orifice area; LA, left atrium; LVEF, left ventricular ejection fraction; LVOT, left ventricular outflow tract; MV, mitral valve; PISA, proximal isovelocity surface area; PVR, paravalvular regurgitation; TEE, transesophageal echocardiography; TMVR, transcatheter mitral valve replacement; VCA, vena contracta area; VCW, vena contracta width; VTI, velocity–time integral.

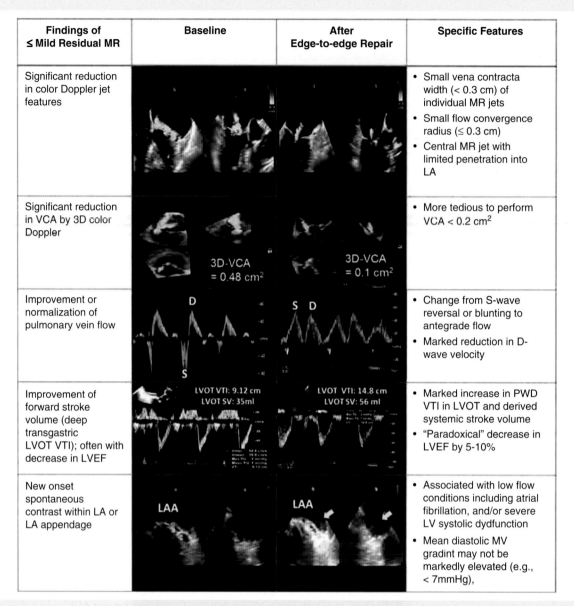

Findings of ≤ Mild Residual MR	Baseline	After Edge-to-edge Repair	Specific Features
Significant reduction in color Doppler jet features			• Small vena contracta width (< 0.3 cm) of individual MR jets • Small flow convergence radius (≤ 0.3 cm) • Central MR jet with limited penetration into LA
Significant reduction in VCA by 3D color Doppler	3D-VCA = 0.48 cm²	3D-VCA = 0.1 cm²	• More tedious to perform VCA < 0.2 cm²
Improvement or normalization of pulmonary vein flow	D S	S D	• Change from S-wave reversal or blunting to antegrade flow • Marked reduction in D-wave velocity
Improvement of forward stroke volume (deep transgastric LVOT VTI); often with decrease in LVEF	LVOT VTI: 9.12 cm LVOT SV: 35ml	LVOT VTI: 14.8 cm LVOT SV: 56 ml	• Marked increase in PWD VTI in LVOT and derived systemic stroke volume • "Paradoxical" decrease in LVEF by 5-10%
New onset spontaneous contrast within LA or LA appendage	LAA	LAA	• Associated with low flow conditions including atrial fibrillation, and/or severe LV systolic dydfunction • Mean diastolic MV gradint may not be markedly elevated (e.g., < 7mmHg),

Figure 36-41 Illustrative echocardiographic parameters of reduction of MR severity to mild after edge-to-edge mitral valve repair. (Reprinted from Zoghbi WA, Asch FM, Bruce C, et al. Guidelines for the evaluation of valvular regurgitation after percutaneous valve repair or replacement: a report from the American Society of Echocardiography developed in collaboration with the Society for Cardiovascular Angiography and Interventions, Japanese Society of Echocardiography, and Society for Cardiovascular Magnetic Resonance. *J Am Soc Echocardiogr.* 2019;32(4):431-475. Copyright © 2019 by the American Society of Echocardiography. With permission.)

interventions, an increased pulmonary venous inflow (velocity–time integral or velocity), a reduction of left atrial pressure (via direct invasive pressure catheter transducer) with a reduction or elimination of the "V" wave, and mild smoke or spontaneous contrast in the left atrium (increase of stasis) coupled with a decreased left ventricular ejection fraction (LVEF) are the best indicators for a significant reduction of MR. Conversely, in presence of spontaneous contrast with preprocedural low LVEF, there also can be induced mitral stenosis, requiring further assessments and potential management.

39. **Answer: C.** This is a small patient with a small ventricle in which the mitral ViV prosthetic stent frame

extends across the left outflow tract in systole. In this case it is important to evaluate the turbulence through the stent; check for true outflow obstruction, TAVR stenosis, or dysfunction; and evaluate both prosthetic valves visually for proper leaflet opening. Continuous-wave (CW) Doppler for pressure gradients and pulsed-wave (PW) Doppler should be sampled below, above, and through the aortic prosthesis (**Figure 36-42A to 36-42C**). The echocardiographer demonstrated no significant increase in flow velocity through the aortic valve (AV) with the PW Doppler sample volume placed at the AV level (**Figure 36-42B**); however, there were increased velocities focally at the septal/stent contact point (**Figure 36-42C**). There is no obstruction of the AV prosthesis

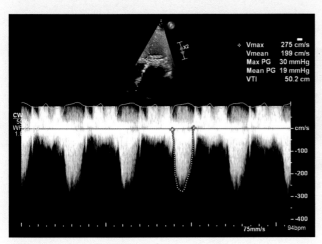

Figure 36-42A CW Doppler.

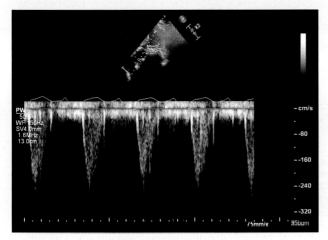

Figure 36-42B PW Doppler with sample volume at the AV.

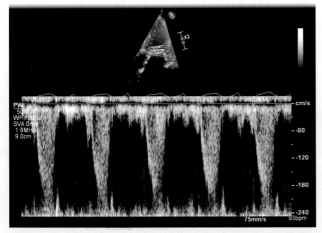

Figure 36-42C PW Doppler with sample volume proximal to the AV.

via CW Doppler (**Figure 36-42A**). While it is possible this patient is mildly unloaded or dehydrated, this speaks to expected turbulent flow from the ViV stent interaction at the septal wall, and possibly evaluating other clinical markers to explain her symptoms, i.e., hemolysis, etc.

40. **Answer: A.** Central intraprosthetic regurgitation is less prevalent than a paravalvular leak following transcatheter aortic valve replacement (TAVR) unless the valve was grossly undersized and subsequently overexpanded. Paravalvular (PV) leaks are most often caused from:
   1. The stent-based open cell geometry allowing for inherent gaps in regions of calcium;
   2. Incomplete closure of gaps due to irregularly calcified leaflets or commissures;
   3. THV vertical positioning remaining too far into the left ventricular outflow tract (LVOT) or above the aortic annulus; and
   4. Undersizing of the THV for the native aortic annulus at maximal expansion.

   In this example, the TAVR prosthesis is deployed too deep, causing malapposition. **Video 36-17A** demonstrates the location of the TAVR leaflets relative to the native aortic valve (AV) leaflets. Poor THV placement can be suggested by noting the depth of metal strut material within the LVOT compared to the aortic and mitral annuli. The color Doppler image is also consistent with severe PV regurgitation, with a maximum circumferential extent of >30% compared to the overall perimeter. The percentage circumferential extent (%Circ) is calculated from a short-axis AV/LVOT plane as:

$$\%Circ(\%) = (JL \div P) \times 100$$

where JL is the length of the jet along the valve curvature and P is the total perimeter (circumference) of the prosthetic valve.

The 2009 American Society of Echocardiography (ASE) Guidelines for the Evaluation of Valvular Regurgitation After Percutaneous Valve Repair or Replacement suggest approximate severity as: mild <10%, moderate 10% to 29%, and severe >30% (**Figure 36-43A**). Other parameters should be used for confirmatory data (**Figure 36-43B**). In this example, there is a suboptimal prosthesis location, a visual circumferential PV leak extent >30%, and a visual vena contracta of greater than 0.6 cm (**Figure 36-17B**). Answer D is incorrect due a complete absence of calcium within the LVOT or aortic annulus.

41. **Answer: C.** One of the most interesting aspects of this nickel-titanium alloy is the springy nature and "memory" that nitinol threads or bands will assume regardless of compression. Due to this property, nitinol devices offer the advantage of not requiring balloon-based expansion and will fit within a particular space and form to the shape of that space, or expand it, based on the radial forces it exerts when deployed. It may not be able to assume its exact original shape when the tissue walls exert higher resistance to expansion than the radial force of the

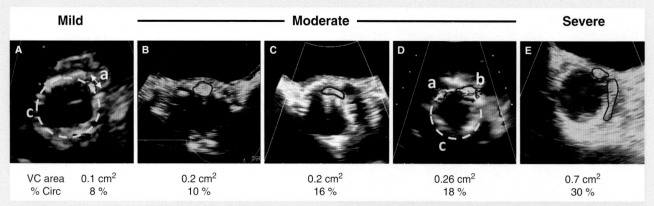

Figure 36-43A Examples of paravalvular regurgitation (PVR) of different degrees of severity using short-axis color Doppler depicting two criteria: vena contracta area (VCA) and % circumferential (Circ) extent of the jet in relation to the total circumference of the prosthetic valve ring. % Circ is calculated as the length of the jet along the valve curvature ("a" in Panel A) divided by the total perimeter ("c" in panel A) as: (a/c)*100. In the case of two jets (D), % Circ would be [(a + b)/c]*100. As the VCA and circumferential extent of the jet increase, AR severity is more significant. However, VCA in TAVR is affected by both circumferential extent and thickness of the PVR, i.e., separation of the valve from the aortic wall. As shown in Panels A and B, the circumferential extent may at times be similar to those of mild regurgitation, but the thickness of the PVR is large, leading to a larger VCA (B). Similarly, Panels B and C depict two lesions of similar moderate severity by VCA but different circumferential extent. These considerations are very important in assessing mild and moderate AR severity and multiple jets (A-D). Once circumferential extent exceeds 30%, PVR is usually severe. (Reprinted from Zoghbi WA, Asch FM, Bruce C, et al. Guidelines for the evaluation of valvular regurgitation after percutaneous valve repair or replacement: a report from the American Society of Echocardiography developed in collaboration with the Society for Cardiovascular Angiography and Interventions, Japanese Society of Echocardiography, and Society for Cardiovascular Magnetic Resonance. *J Am Soc Echocardiogr.* 2019;32(4):431-475. Copyright © 2019 by the American Society of Echocardiography. With permission.)

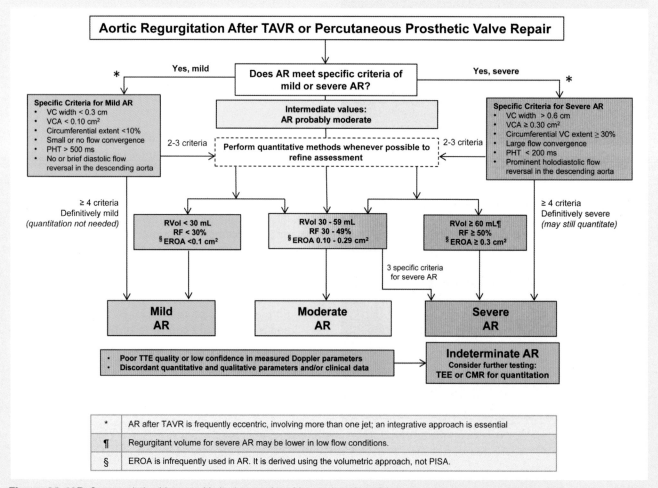

Figure 36-43B Suggested algorithm to guide implementation of integration of multiple parameters of aortic regurgitation (AR) severity after TAVR or prosthetic aortic valve repair. Good-quality echocardiographic imaging and complete data acquisition are assumed. If imaging is technically difficult, consider TEE or CMR. AR severity may be indeterminate due to poor image quality, technical issues with data, internal inconsistency among echo findings, or discordance with clinical findings. (Reprinted from Zoghbi WA, Asch FM, Bruce C, et al. Guidelines for the evaluation of valvular regurgitation after percutaneous valve repair or replacement: a report from the American Society of Echocardiography developed in collaboration with the Society for Cardiovascular Angiography and Interventions, Japanese Society of Echocardiography, and Society for Cardiovascular Magnetic Resonance. *J Am Soc Echocardiogr.* 2019;32(4):431-475. Copyright © 2019 by the American Society of Echocardiography. With permission.)

nitinol bands. This relationship is how the Watchman (Boston Scientific Corp.) device successfully "compresses" the appendage space and occludes it. Nitinol is also used in some designs for transcatheter aortic valve replacement prosthetics, transcatheter mitral valve replacement research-based devices, coronary stents, and Amplatzer occluder devices.

42. ▶ **Answer: A.** In performing clinical and procedural interventional TEE, the use of cardiac landmarks is essential for correctly identifying associated regions and their anatomical location compared to the transducer beam origin and angulation. While the coronary sinus (CS) and interatrial septum (IAS) are clear identifiers of the location of the tricuspid valve septal leaflet, the aortic valve and noncoronary cusp as related to the IAS are more specific for identifying the commissure at the tricuspid annulus base between the anterior and septal tricuspid leaflets (**Figure 36-44** and **Videos 36-30A to 36-30D**).

43. **Answer: B.** All of these imaging methods can successfully delineate the location of MR jets. However, only selections B and D specifically denoted the use of color flow Doppler imaging. Of these two, the 3D zoom color Doppler data set has many advantages over conventional 2D color Doppler imaging. For example, the 3D zoom color Doppler data set may be rotated from both the left atrial (surgeon's view) and left ventricular aspects and multiplane evaluation, where planes may be moved across the commissure to accurately identify the exact location of the largest or primary jet as well as assist in differentiating primary (degenerative valve leaflet)

or secondary (ventricular tethering) components. In **Figures 36-45A** and **36-45B**, there clearly are multiple jets emanating from the central commissure, a suggestion of more secondary components involving leaflet tethering and/or annular dilatation. A known limitation of Live 3D zoom color Doppler is adequate temporal resolution in some patients for truly accurate evaluation of the vena contracta area and proximal isovelocity surface area. This may depend on the conditions (heart rate, size of zoom data set, arrhythmia) at time of acquisition. These issues may be addressed in the future via newer, higher capability transducers and computer processing enabling very high resolution "one beat" acquisition 3D data sets.

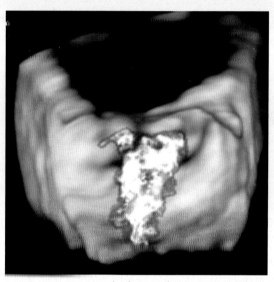

Figure 36-45A 3D zoom color data set of multiple jets of MR from the left atrial or "surgeon's view" perspective.

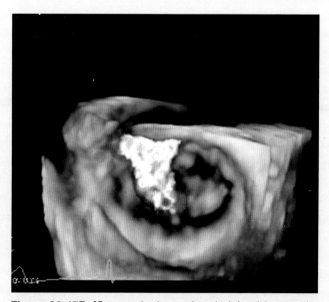

Figure 36-45B 3D zoom color data set from the left atrial perspective showing more focal centrally directed MR jet from A2-P2 region.

Figure 36-44 Use of the biplane subcostal view for the tricuspid valve. Star = aortic valve, left diamond = anterior tricuspid valve leaflet and right diamond = septal tricuspid valve leaflet.

44. ▶ **Answer: C.** Once a MitraClip is permanently placed on the central commissure, the mitral valve will become a "dual-orifice" valve, with one inflow orifice located medially, and the other lateral to the clip. From the apical-4 chamber and long-axis views both orifices can be manually oriented with color Doppler guidance; however, it is very difficult to achieve parallel alignment with flow for accurate continuous-wave (CW) Doppler interrogation with each orifice from these views. While an inferiorly angled parasternal short-axis view would delineate both orifices by color Doppler, again these orifices would be at oblique orientations to the CW Doppler beam and would likely underestimate the velocity and gradient across the orifice. The apical 2-chamber view should enable excellent alignment and demonstration of both orifices and this is the best view for performing CW Doppler, allowing accurate measurements of the pressure gradients across both orifices (**Video 36-31** and **Figures 36-46A** and **36-46B**).

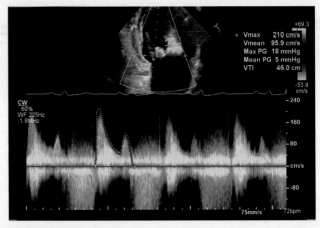

Figure 36-46A Lateral orifice.

Figure 36-46B Medial orifice.

SUGGESTED READINGS

Alkhouli M, Rihal CS, Holmes DR Jr. Transseptal techniques for emerging structural heart interventions. *JACC Cardiovasc Interv.* 2016;9(24):2465-2480.

Beigel R, Wunderlich NC, Ho SY, Arsanjani R, Siegel RJ. The left atrial appendage: anatomy, function, and noninvasive evaluation. *JACC Cardiovasc Imaging.* 2014;7(12):1251-1265.

DeVore AD, Patel PA, Patel CB. Medical management of patients with a left ventricular assist device for the non-left ventricular assist device specialist. *JACC Heart Fail.* 2017;5(9):621-631.

Ergle K, Parto P, Krim SR. Percutaneous ventricular assist devices: a novel approach in the management of patients with acute cardiogenic shock. *Ochsner J.* 2016;16(3):243-249.

Fine NM, Topilsky Y, Oh JK, et al. Role of echocardiography in patients with intravascular hemolysis due to suspected continuous-flow LVAD thrombosis. *JACC Cardiovasc Imaging.* 2013;6(11):1129-1140.

Hahn RT, Thomas JD, Khalique OK, Cavalcante JL, Praz F, Zoghbi WA. Imaging assessment of tricuspid regurgitation severity. *JACC Cardiovasc Imaging.* 2019;12(3):469-490.

Henzel J, Konka M, Wójcik A, et al. Focus on the perimeter and skip the balloon: can atrial septal defect be percutaneously closed without balloon sizing in the era of 3-dimensional echocardiography? *JACC Cardiovasc Imaging.* 2018;11(11):1731-1732.

Keebler ME, Haddad EV, Choi CW, et al. Venoarterial extracorporeal membrane oxygenation in cardiogenic shock. *JACC Heart Fail.* 2018;6(6):503-516.

Kim SS, Hijazi ZM, Lang RM, Knight BP. The use of intracardiac echocardiography and other intracardiac imaging tools to guide noncoronary cardiac interventions. *J Am Coll Cardiol.* 2009;53(23):2117-2128.

Kinno M, Raissi SR, Puthumana JJ, Thomas JD, Davidson CJ. Echocardiography for tricuspid valve intervention. Essentials for understanding echocardiographic imaging in percutaneous tricuspid interventions. *Cardiac Interv Today.* 2018;12(4):62-67.

Naidu SS. Novel percutaneous cardiac assist devices: the science of and indications for hemodynamic support. *Circulation.* 2011;123(5):533-543.

Pislaru SV, Michelena HI, Mankad SV. Interventional echocardiography. *Prog Cardiovasc Dis.* 2014;57(1):32-46.

Silvestry FE, Kerber RE, Brook MM, et al. Echocardiography-guided interventions. *J Am Soc Echocardiogr.* 2009;22(3):213-231.

Stainback RF, Estep JD, Agler DA, et al. Echocardiography in the management of patients with left ventricular assist devices: recommendations from the American Society of Echocardiography. *J Am Soc Echocardiogr.* 2015;28(8):853-909.

Uriel N, Morrison KA, Garan AR, et al. Development of a novel echocardiography ramp test for speed optimization and diagnosis of device thrombosis in continuous-flow left ventricular assist devices: the Columbia ramp study. *J Am Coll Cardiol.* 2012;60(18):1764-1775.

Zoghbi WA, Asch FM, Bruce C, et al. Guidelines for the evaluation of valvular regurgitation after percutaneous valve repair or replacement: a report from the American Society of Echocardiography developed in collaboration with the Society for Cardiovascular Angiography and interventions, Japanese Society of Echocardiography, and Society for Cardiovascular magnetic Resonance. *J Am Soc Echocardiogr.* 2019;32(4):431-475.

CHAPTER 37

Research Methods and Biostatistics

Contributors: Joy Guthrie, PhD, ACS, RDMS, RDCS, RVT and Gillian Whalley, PhD, DMU (Cardiac), BAppSci, MHSc (Hons)

⊛ Question 1

In a recent publication,[1] freshman medical students were screened for cardiovascular risk factors in a study that had the following aim and methods: *"Aim: To screen freshman medical students for rheumatic heart disease and other risk factors that can aggravate the progression of the heart disease. Methods: Freshman (first year) medical students were exposed to full cardiovascular examination. A full cardiac exam was done for 100 students using a portable echocardiography machine."* Which research design was employed for this study?

    A. Longitudinal study

    B. Case control study

    C. Cross-sectional study

    D. Cohort study

⊛ Question 2

Many sonographers suffer from work-related musculoskeletal disorders. To conduct a cross-sectional survey to determine the prevalence of work-related musculoskeletal disorders among sonographers in the United States, what is the correct method for selecting the sample?

    A. Survey all of the sonographers at the hospital/clinic where you work

    B. Survey all of the sonographers who you happen to know

    C. Survey all of the sonographers you have linked to on social media

    D. Survey all of the sonographers registered with the American Registry for Diagnostic Medical Sonography (ARDMS)

⊛ Question 3

Hoffman and Kaplan[2] conducted a study *"designed to determine the reasons for the variability of the incidence of congenital heart disease (CHD), estimate its true value, and provide data about the incidence of specific major forms of CHD."*

What is meant by the "incidence" of a disease?

    A. The proportion of a population with a specific disease

    B. The number of new cases of a disease occurring within a period of time

    C. The ability of a diagnostic test to correctly identify those with a disease

    D. The ability of a diagnostic test to correctly identify those without a disease

⊛ Question 4

Punn et al.[3] published an article entitled "A pilot study assessing ECG versus ECHO ventriculoventricular optimization in pediatric resynchronization patients." They studied nine patients and concluded that *"ECHO optimization of synchrony was not superior to ECG optimization."* What is meant by the term "pilot study"?

    A. A study that includes only a small number of participants

    B. A small preliminary study conducted in order to evaluate the feasibility of the key component(s) of a future, full-scale study

    C. A small study that may provide erroneous results

    D. A small study that does not provide significant results

✪ Question 5

An abstract by Conte et al.[4] reads: "*An 84-year-old man affected by arterial hypertension, diabetes mellitus, chronic renal failure on dialysis, chronic ischemic heart disease, permanent atrial fibrillation, previous AICD implantation about one year before, was admitted to the intensive care unit because of typical chest pain and dyspnea during dialysis treatment with nonspecific ST segment changes at ECG and mild increase of cardiac enzymes. A transthoracic echocardiogram was requested, and it demonstrated a big loculated paracardiac hematoma not easily distinguished from pleural source, with sprays of fibrin localized in correspondence of the free wall of the right ventricle determining a partial compression of the right ventricle with no signs of tamponade.*" What was the research design used by the investigators?

A. Case series
B. Cohort study
C. Qualitative study
D. Single case study

✪ Question 6

The histogram in **Figure 37-1** displays the frequency distribution of echocardiographic measurements of the left ventricular ejection fraction (LVEF) in 221 premature babies (unpublished data collected by Flood & Guthrie). What is the frequency distribution of the LVEF?

A. Normal
B. Positive (right) skewed
C. Negative (left) skewed
D. Bimodal

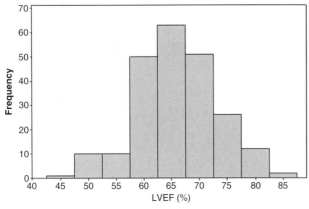

Figure 37-1

✪ Question 7

Conclusions about a sample population can be made using descriptive summary statistics to summarize the data set, such as mean (the average number; calculat-

ed by adding all of the observations and dividing them by the number of observations in the set), median (the middle observation when they are ranked lowest to highest), mode (the most frequently occurring value), and maximum and minimum observed values. When data are normally distributed what assumptions can be made about the data?

A. That the calculated mean, median, and mode are different
B. That the calculated mean, median, and mode are similar
C. That the calculated mean falls exactly in between the observed minimum and maximum values
D. That the calculated median falls exactly in between the observed minimum and maximum values

✪ Question 8

A study by Taniguchi et al.[5] evaluated the link between estimated right atrial pressure (RAP) and liver stiffness (LS). **Figure 37-2** shows the distribution of both parameters. Which is the correct distribution description?

A. Normally distributed with a right skew
B. Normally distributed with a left skew
C. Not normally distributed with a right skew
D. Not normally distributed with a left skew

✪✪ Question 9

The following abstract by Gepner et al.[6] describes a randomized trial of vitamin D: "*Vitamin D (VitD) supplementation has been advocated for cardiovascular risk reduction; however, supporting data are sparse. The objective of this study was to determine whether VitD supplementation reduces cardiovascular risk. Subjects in this prospective, randomized, double-blind, placebo-controlled trial of post-menopausal women with serum 25-hydroxyvitamin D concentrations >10 and <60 ng/mL were randomized to Vitamin D3 2500 IU or placebo, daily for 4 months.*" What do the authors mean by describing their trial as a "randomized, double-blind trial"?

A. Subjects are randomly allocated to receive a treatment or placebo and the researchers know which treatment the participants are receiving, but the participants do not.
B. Subjects are randomly allocated to receive a treatment or placebo and the participants know which treatment they are receiving, but the researchers do not.

C. Subjects are randomly allocated to receive a treatment or placebo and neither the participants nor the researchers know who is receiving a particular treatment.

D. Subjects are randomly allocated to receive a treatment or placebo and both the researchers and subjects know which group they are allocated to.

A. Fat-free mass (the independent variable) and LV mass (dependent variable) are related to each other (positive correlation).

B. Fat-free mass (the independent variable) and LV mass (dependent variable) are related to each other (negative correlation).

C. Increases in fat-free mass (the independent variable) lead to increases in LV mass (dependent variable).

D. Increases in LV mass (the dependent variable) lead to increases in fat-free mass (independent variable).

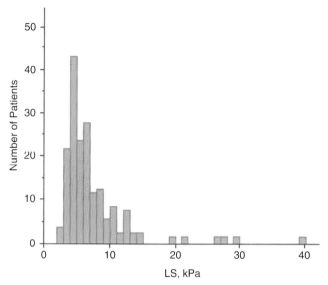

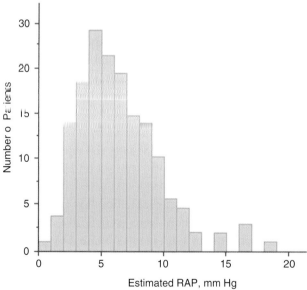

Figure 37-2 (Reprinted from Taniguchi T, Ohtani T, Kioka H, et al. Liver stiffness reflecting right-sided filling pressure can predict adverse outcomes in patients with heart failure. *JACC Cardiovasc Imaging.* 2019;12(6):955-964. Copyright © 2019 by the American College of Cardiology Foundation. With permission.)

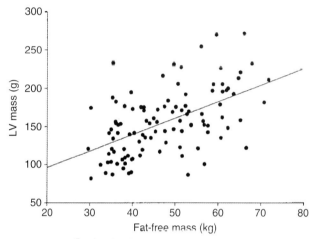

Figure 37-3 (Reprinted with permission from Whalley GA, Gamble GD, Doughty RN, et al. Left ventricular mass correlates with fat-free mass but not fat mass. *J Hypertens.* 1999;17(4):569-574.)

✪✪ **Question 11**

Before starting a research project, researchers will usually conduct a literature review. What is the difference between a narrative literature review and a systematic review?

A. They are the same; a narrative review is simply a written version of a systematic review.

B. They are different; a systematic review always provides an estimate of the effect.

C. They are different; a narrative review contains all relevant literature and a systematic review only includes studies with numeric data.

D. They are different; a narrative review contains some relevant literature and a systematic review includes all relevant literature.

✪ **Question 10**

It is common to plot echocardiography measurements against other measurements to show the relationship between them. In **Figure 37-3**, left ventricular (LV) mass has been graphed against fat-free mass and significant correlation (r = 0.48, *P* < .0001) was observed.[7] What is meant by "LV mass is correlated with fat-free mass"?

✪ Question 12

In clinical research studies, it is often stated that "patients provided informed consent" before taking part in the study. Which of these situations is considered to be a valid description of informed consent?

A. The patient received information to read and signed a consent form agreeing to take part in the research.

B. The patient agreed to a treatment and signed a consent form when they arrived in hospital.

C. The doctor entered the patient's data into a database after the patient left the hospital.

D. The patient was offered a new treatment but only if they consented to be part of a research project.

✪✪ Question 13

It is not always practical for clinical researchers to study an entire target population (e.g., all the patients diagnosed with a specific disease). Therefore, small subsets or groups of individuals are often selected from the target population (known as samples) based on probability. Random sampling is important because it allows for generalization of results. Some commonly used probability-based sampling methods in clinical research are simple random sampling, stratified sampling, systematic sampling, and cluster sampling.[8] What is meant by "cluster sampling"?

A. Every 10th patient is selected from the patients who present with a certain condition.

B. Individuals are selected from the population in such a way that every individual has an equal probability or chance of being selected.

C. The total population is classified into subgroups and a random sample of the subgroups is selected. Participants are then chosen from within each group.

D. The total population is classified into subgroups, perhaps based on location and a random sample is then drawn from each subgroup.

✪✪ Question 14

External validity is an important consideration when undertaking clinical research and this is extremely important in clinical research. For example, in the limitations section of a recent publication by Basile et al.[9] that evaluated the accuracy of lung ultrasonography (LUS) in the diagnosis and management of bronchiolitis in infants, the authors state: "*in this study, experienced physicians in LUS performed the ultrasound evaluations, and the results might not be extrapolated to all pediatricians.*" This raises questions about the external validity of the results. What is meant by "external validity"?

A. Whether conclusions about causes and effects can be drawn from the results

B. Whether the conclusions of the study are generalizable (i.e., applicable to other participants, at other times, and in other places)

C. Whether the results might be correct

D. Whether the results of the study have been tested against known standards

✪✪ Question 15

Reliability or reproducibility of measurements is important in clinical research and in clinical practice. For example, Saul et al.[10] conducted a study concluding that "*Emergency physician sonographers obtained similar Doppler measurements for diastolic function evaluation with very good inter-rater reliability.*" What is meant by "inter-rater reliability"?

A. The measurements obtained in one study were statistically compared with the measurements obtained in a second study conducted in the same fashion.

B. The measurements obtained by a researcher on one occasion were statistically compared against the measurements obtained by the same researcher on two or more other occasions.

C. The measurements were tested against known standards to determine their agreement.

D. The measurements obtained by two or more researchers were statistically compared to determine how much they agreed with each other.

✪✪ Question 16

Panoulas et al.[11] conducted a study to compare the accuracy of making a correct diagnosis of heart disease between two groups of clinicians. The control group used only the findings about the patients' history, physical examination, and electrocardiogram (ECG) to make a diagnosis. The experimental group used the findings of a pocket-size hand-held echocardiographic (PHHE) device to make a diagnosis in addition to the patient's history, physical examination, and ECG. The results of the study are summarized in **Figure 37-4**. What conclusion would be drawn based on the results presented in this figure?

A. The use of PHHE improved the diagnostic accuracy, over and above history, physical examination, and ECG findings.

B. The use of PHHE did not improve the diagnostic accuracy, over and above history, physical examination, and ECG findings.

C. The use of PHHE alone provided the same diagnostic accuracy as the use of history, physical examination, and ECG findings.

D. The use of PHHE alone provided better diagnostic accuracy than the use of history, physical examination, and ECG findings.

✪✪✪ Question 17

Kusunose et al.[12] investigated the role of right ventricular (RV) echocardiographic measurements at rest and during exercise as predictors of progression to mitral valve surgery in patients with asymptomatic mitral regurgitation. They concluded, using a sequential Cox survival model, that RV strain and RV chamber size were important predictors in addition to clinical measurements and left ventricular function based on the data shown in **Figure 37-5**. What conclusion can be drawn from this example?

A. The increasing Chi-square value in each bar (15.9, 28.8, 40.1, 52.2) confirms the significant contribution of each model.

B. The increasing Chi-square value in each bar (15.9, 28.8, 40.1, 52.2) confirms that each of the individual factors contributes more to the predictive model.

C. The increasing Chi-square value in each bar (15.9, 28.8, 40.1, 52.2) confirms that each of the factors contributes more to the predictive model and the P values show that the models are significantly different from each other.

D. The Chi-square tests the significance of each model and the p values on the graph confirm that the models are different from each other.

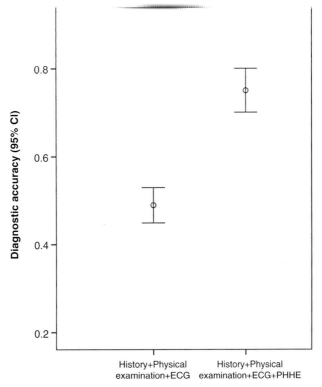

Figure 37-4 (From Panoulas VF, Daigeler A-L, Malaweera ASN, et al. Pocket-size hand-held cardiac ultrasound as an adjunct to clinical examination in the hands of medical students and junior doctors. *Eur Heart J Cardiovasc Imaging.* 2013;14(4):323-330. Copyright © 2012 The Author. Reproduced by permission of Oxford University Press.)

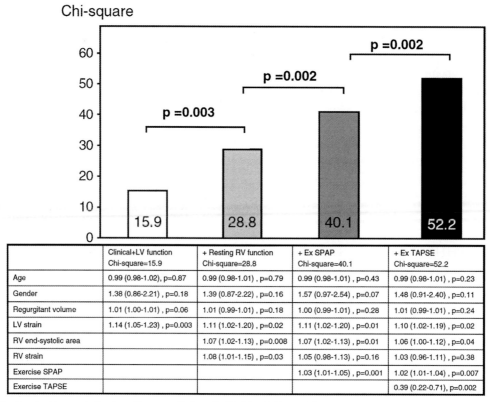

Chi-square

	Clinical+LV function Chi-square=15.9	+ Resting RV function Chi-square=28.8	+ Ex SPAP Chi-square=40.1	+ Ex TAPSE Chi-square=52.2
Age	0.99 (0.98-1.02), p=0.87	0.99 (0.98-1.01), p=0.79	0.99 (0.98-1.01), p=0.43	0.99 (0.98-1.01), p=0.23
Gender	1.38 (0.86-2.21), p=0.18	1.39 (0.87-2.22), p=0.16	1.57 (0.97-2.54), p=0.07	1.48 (0.91-2.40), p=0.11
Regurgitant volume	1.01 (1.00-1.01), p=0.06	1.01 (0.99-1.01), p=0.18	1.00 (0.99-1.01), p=0.28	1.01 (0.99-1.01), p=0.24
LV strain	1.14 (1.05-1.23), p=0.003	1.11 (1.02-1.20), p=0.02	1.11 (1.02-1.20), p=0.01	1.10 (1.02-1.19), p=0.02
RV end-systolic area		1.07 (1.02-1.13), p=0.008	1.07 (1.02-1.13), p=0.01	1.06 (1.00-1.12), p=0.04
RV strain		1.08 (1.01-1.15), p=0.03	1.05 (0.98-1.13), p=0.16	1.03 (0.96-1.11), p=0.38
Exercise SPAP			1.03 (1.01-1.05), p=0.001	1.02 (1.01-1.04), p=0.007
Exercise TAPSE				0.39 (0.22-0.71), p=0.002

Figure 37-5 (Reprinted with permission from Kusunose K, Popović ZB, Motoki H, et al. Prognostic significance of exercise-induced right ventricular dysfunction in asymptomatic degenerative mitral regurgitation. *Circ Cardiovasc Imaging.* 2013;6(2):167-176.)

✪✪ Question 18

Bhatia et al.[13] conducted a randomized control trial in which physicians-in-training were randomized to an educational intervention or a control group in order to determine the effect of the intervention on the use of appropriate transthoracic echocardiography (TTE). Their null hypothesis was that there was no difference between the intervention group and the control group. The results of the statistical analysis to compare the intervention group versus the control group were presented as follows "(13% vs. 34%, P < .001)." What conclusions were inferred from "(13% vs. 34%, P < .001)"?

A. The null hypothesis was rejected. The proportion of physicians using inappropriate TTE was probably lower in the intervention group than in the control group after the education.

B. The null hypothesis was retained. There was probably no difference between the proportions of physicians using inappropriate TTE in the intervention versus the control group after the education.

C. The null hypothesis was rejected. The proportion of physicians using inappropriate TTE was probably lower in the intervention group than in the control group before the education.

D. The null hypothesis was retained. There was probably no difference between the proportions of physicians using inappropriate TTE in the intervention versus the control group before the education.

✪✪ Question 19

A study by Greiner et al.[14] recruited a large cohort (>1200 patients) undergoing right heart catheterization for evaluation of pulmonary hypertension and investigated whether the mean pulmonary artery pressure (mPAP) or the Doppler-derived systolic pulmonary artery pressure (sPAP) predicted survival using a combined end-point of death or heart transplantation. The Kaplan-Meier survival curves (**Figure 37-6A** and **B**) show the impact of pulmonary hypertension on survival. What can be concluded from these graphs?

A. That mPAP <25 mm Hg is associated with better survival

B. That sPAP <36 mm Hg is associated with better survival

C. That both mPAP <25 mm Hg and sPAP <36 mm Hg are associated with better survival

D. That the mPAP must be measured from catheterization to predict survival

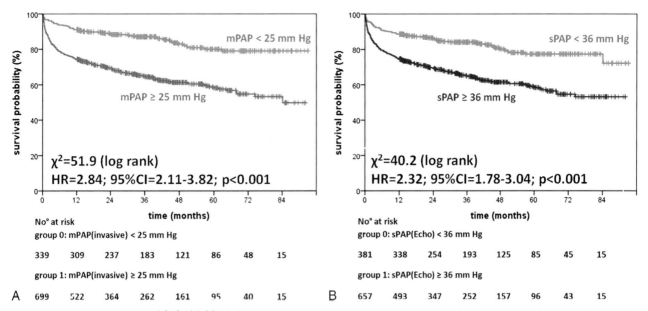

Figure 37-6 (From Greiner S, Jud A, Aurich M, et al. Prognostic relevance of elevated pulmonary arterial pressure assessed non invasively: Analysis in a large patient cohort with invasive measurements in near temporal proximity. *PLoS One.* 2018;13(1):e0191206. https://creativecommons.org/licenses/by/4.0/. Copyright © 2018 Greiner et al.)

STUDY EXAMPLE 1

The following questions relate to a study by Zile and LeWinter[15] when the left ventricular end-diastolic linear diameter (LVIDd) measurements were compared among normal participants, patients with hypertension only (HTN), and hypertensive patients with signs of heart failure with normal ejection fraction (HFNEF). The authors found that LVIDd was normally distributed, but the curve was shifted to the right for the HFNEF group (**Figure 37-7**).

⚛⚛ Question 20

In the graph displayed in **Figure 37-7**, "StDev" refers to "standard deviation." What is the correct description of the standard deviation?

  A. A descriptive statistic referring to the amount of variation in a single set of sample data
  B. A descriptive statistic referring to the central tendency of a single set of sample data (calculated by adding the data values together and dividing them by the number of data values in the set)
  C. A descriptive statistic referring to the middle data value in a single set of sample data
  D. A descriptive statistic referring to the most frequently occurring value found in a single set of sample data

⚛⚛ Question 21

What is represented by the vertical dashed black line on the right of the graph in **Figure 37-7**?

  A. This is the upper 95% confidence interval, meaning 95% of the data for the controls fall below this line.
  B. This is the upper 95% confidence interval, meaning 95% of the data for all participants fall below this line.
  C. This is the upper 95% confidence interval, meaning 95% of the data for all participants fall between this line and the lower confidence interval (not shown).
  D. This is the upper 95% confidence interval, meaning 95% of the data for the controls fall between this line and the lower confidence interval (not shown).

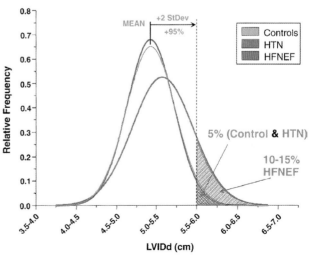

Figure 37-7 (From Zile MR, LeWinter MM. Left ventricular end-diastolic volume is normal in patients with heart failure and a normal ejection fraction. *J Am Coll Cardiol.* 2007;49(9):982-985, with permission from Elsevier.)

✪✪ Question 22

In relation to the graph displayed in **Figure 37-7**, what can be concluded about the impact of hypertension and heart failure with normal ejection fraction (HFNEF) on the left ventricular end-diastolic linear diameter (LVIDd)?

- **A.** That patients with both hypertension and heart failure have larger left ventricular (LV) dimensions compared to controls
- **B.** That patients with hypertension have larger LV dimensions compared to controls
- **C.** That 10% to 15% of patients with both hypertension and heart failure meet the criteria for LV dilatation
- **D.** That 10% to 15% of patients with hypertension meet the criteria for LV dilatation

STUDY EXAMPLE 2

The following questions relate to a meta-analysis that investigated the relationship between restrictive diastolic filling and mortality in patients post–acute myocardial infarction (post-AMI).[16] The authors concluded *"mortality is about four times higher in patients with a restrictive filling pattern than in those with non-restrictive filling patterns after AMI."* The following questions relate to **Figure 37-8**.

✪✪✪ Question 23

Looking at the graph in **Figure 37-8** and the diamond at the bottom, which statement is not correct?

- **A.** The diamond is the estimate of the overall effect.
- **B.** The width of the diamond represents the confidence interval of the overall effect.
- **C.** The height of the diamond represents the confidence interval of the overall effect.
- **D.** The size of the diamond is determined by the sample size.

✪✪✪ Question 24

In the graph in **Figure 37-8**, the columns headed "OR (fixed)" are the odds ratio comparing the two groups of patients with restrictive diastolic filling and with non-restrictive diastolic filling. What does the vertical line signify?

- **A.** The vertical line is equal to an odds ratio of 1 and indicates there are differences between the two conditions.
- **B.** The vertical line is equal to an odds ratio of 1 and indicates there is no difference between the two conditions.
- **C.** The vertical line is equal to an odds ratio of 1 and studies that cross this line should be ignored.
- **D.** The vertical line is equal to an odds ratio of 1 and studies that do not cross this line are the most important.

Study	Restrictive filling deaths/number at risk	Non-restrictive filling deaths/number at risk	OR (fixed) 95% CI	Weight (%)	OR (fixed) 95% CI
Garcia-Rubira	9/26	11/107		3.34	4.62 (1.66 to 12.82)
Nijland	7/12	1/83		0.13	114.80 (11.72 to 1124.08)
Sakata	24/50	9/156		2.70	15.08 (6.30 to 36.07)
Poulsen	3/14	3/44		1.35	3.73 (0.66 to 21.09)
Burgess	2/19	7/83		2.77	1.28 (0.24 to 6.70)
Moller 1	17/26	16/99		2.74	9.80 (3.72 to 25.83)
Cerisano	7/34	2/70		1.23	8.81 (1.72 to 45.15)
Otasevic	8/32	6/74		3.23	3.78 (1.19 to 12.01)
Moller 3	85/167	112/632		27.34	4.81 (3.34 to 6.94)
Moller 2	16/48	30/240		7.93	3.50 (1.72 to 7.13)
Beinart	16/70	47/301		16.27	1.60 (0.85 to 3.03)
Kinova	3/7	9/112		0.72	8.58 (1.66 to 44.46)
Karvounis	3/6	0/27		0.12	55.00 (2.32 to 1302.98)
Moller 4	16/44	7/181		2.07	14.20 (5.36 to 37.61)
Quintana	14/74	43/446		11.80	2.19 (1.13 to 4.24)
Temporelli	17/147	30/424		16.25	1.72 (0.92 to 3.22)
Events/total	247/776	333/3079		100.00	4.10 (3.38 to 4.99)

Test for heterogeneity: χ^2 = 52.42, df = 15 (p < 0.00001), I^2 = 71.4%
Test for overall effect: Z = 14.18 (p < 0.00001)

0.001 0.01 0.1 1 10 100 1000
Favours restrictive filling   Favours non-restrictive filling

Meta-analysis of the restrictive filling pattern after myocardial infarction. Fixed effects model, studies weighted according to sample size. CI, confidence interval; OR, odds ratio.

Figure 37-8 (Reprinted from Whalley GA, Gamble GD, Doughty RN. Restrictive diastolic filling predicts death after acute myocardial infarction: systematic review and meta-analysis of prospective studies. *Heart.* 2006;92(11):1588-1594; with permission from BMJ Publishing Group Ltd.)

✪✪✪ Question 25

In the graph in **Figure 37-8**, the column headed "weight" indicates the contribution to the overall odds ratio. Some studies have been given more weight. Why is this?

A. These are the largest studies with the narrowest confidence intervals.

B. These studies have an odds ratio that is similar to the overall odds ratio of 4.10.

C. These studies are deemed to be of better quality by the reviewers.

D. These studies are the ones that are clearly statistically significant, shown by the fact that the confidence interval does not cross the OR = 1 line.

STUDY EXAMPLE 3

The following questions relate to a study by Malm et al.[17] comparing Simpson's biplane measurements of left ventricular (LV) volumes and LV ejection fraction (LVEF) with and without an ultrasound enhancing agent (or contrast) to LV volumes and LVEF measured by magnetic resonance imaging (MRI). The graph shown in **Figure 37-9**, reproduced from their paper, is described as a Bland and Altman plot after the two statisticians who first published the format. It is one of the better ways to assess agreement between techniques by plotting the difference between two methods against the mean of the two methods. In the LVEF graphs, the open circles are participants with good baseline imaging and the black circles are those with poor baseline endocardial visualization.

✪✪✪ Question 26

Overall, what can be concluded about the use of contrast to measure end-diastolic volume (EDV)?

A. EDV measurements were not improved by the use of contrast.

B. EDV measurements were improved by the use of contrast.

C. EDV measurements by echocardiography (echo) and MRI were similar with and without contrast.

D. EDV measurements by echo and MRI were statistically different with contrast compared to without.

✪✪✪ Question 27

Overall, which of these statements is most supported by the two bottom graphs of left ventricular ejection fraction (LVEF) as seen in **Figure 37-9**?

A. LVEF echocardiographic (echo) measurements are more accurate when contrast is used.

B. LVEF echo measurements are more precise when contrast is used.

C. LVEF echo measurements are more reliable when contrast is used.

D. LVEF echo measurements are more valid when contrast is used.

✪✪✪ Question 28

In the same study, the authors presented the graph shown in **Figure 37-10**, showing the impact of contrast on measurement reliability. What can be concluded from these results?

A. Contrast echocardiography (echo) improved interobserver reliability but not intraobserver reliability.

B. Contrast echo improved intraobserver reliability but not interobserver reliability.

C. Contrast echo did not improve either interobserver reliability or intraobserver reliability.

D. Contrast echo improved both interobserver reliability and intraobserver reliability.

STUDY EXAMPLE 4

The following questions relate to a study by Rigolli et al.[18] investigating the prognostic impact of diastolic dysfunction in patients with chronic heart failure and post-acute myocardial infarction (post-AMI). Survival analysis is commonly used in clinical research to identify factors that are associated with better (or worse) survival. In the graph shown in **Figure 37-11**, the authors divided two groups of patients on the basis of their mitral filling pattern.

✪✪✪ Question 29

Looking at **Figure 37-11**, what does the 1.0 signify on the y axis?

A. This is survival and at the start everyone is alive, so 1.0 is equal to 100%.

B. This is mortality and 1.0 is the starting point in time.

C. This is mortality and 1.0 indicates 100% are alive.

D. This is survival and 1.0 indicates 1% of the patients are alive.

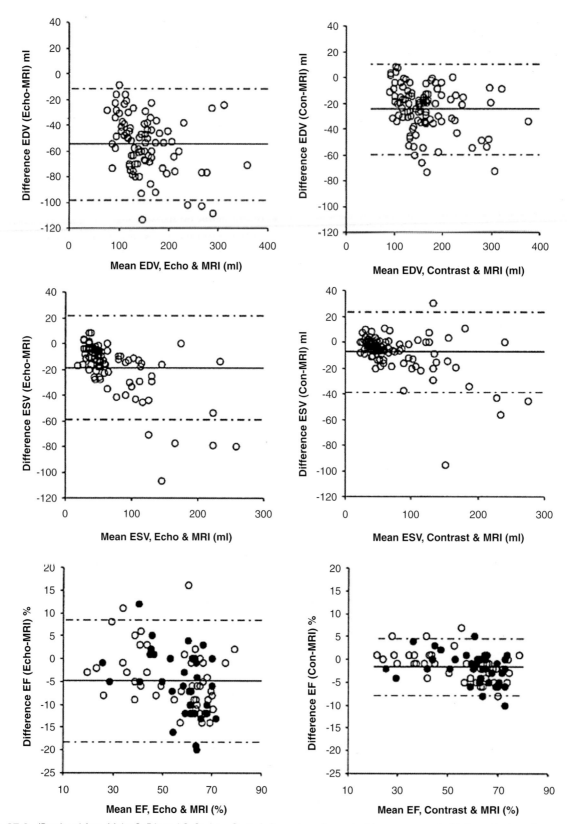

Figure 37-9 (Reprinted from Malm S, Frigstad S, Sagberg S, et al. Accurate and reproducible measurement of left ventricular volume and ejection fraction by contrast echocardiography: A comparison with magnetic resonance imaging. *J Am Coll Cardiol.* 2004;44(5):1030-1035. Copyright © 2004 American College of Cardiology Foundation. With permission.)

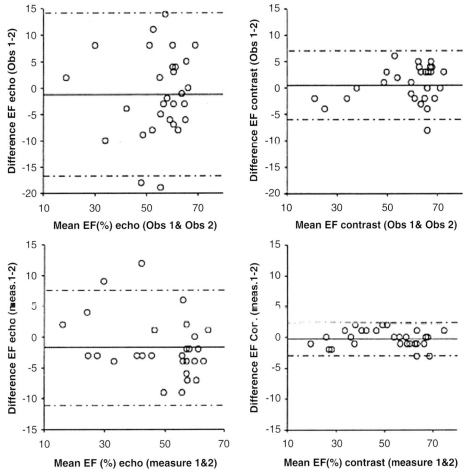

Figure 37-10 (Reprinted from Malm S, Frigstad S, Sagberg S, et al. Accurate and reproducible measurement of left ventricular volume and ejection fraction by contrast echocardiography: a comparison with magnetic resonance imaging. *J Am Coll Cardiol.* 2004;44(5):1030-1035. Copyright © 2004 American College of Cardiology Foundation. With permission.)

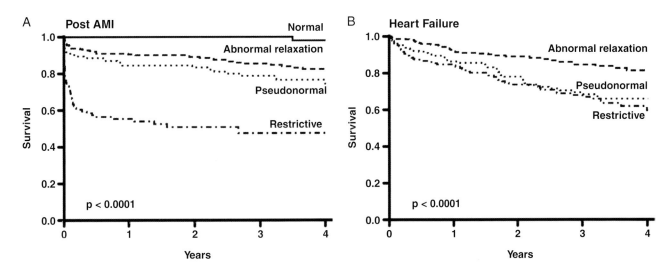

Kaplan-Meier survival diastolic filling pattern E/A in heart failure and post-AMI patients

Figure 37-11 (Reprinted from Rigolli M, Rossi A, Quintanna M, et al. The prognostic impact of diastolic dysfunction in patients with chronic heart failure and post-acute myocardial infarction: can age-stratified E/A ratio alone predict survival? *Int J Cardiol.* 2015;181:362-368. Copyright © 2014 Elsevier. With permission.)

✪✪✪ Question 30

Looking at the data about survival at 30 months in **Figure 37-11**, it can be concluded that mortality in patients with:

A. Restrictive mitral filling is always the highest.
B. Pseudonormal filling is always the highest.
C. Restrictive and pseudonormal filling and heart failure is the same.
D. Restrictive and pseudonormal filling after acute myocardial infarction (AMI) is the same.

✪✪✪ Question 31

Referring to the graph in **Figure 37-11** and looking at the data from the first 6 months, the curves have very distinct shapes. The curves generated from the post–acute myocardial infarction (post-AMI) cohort separate early and the curves from the heart failure group separate gradually. It can be concluded from the first year that:

A. All patients with restrictive mitral filling are at highest risk of death in the first 6 months.
B. Patients with restrictive mitral filling are at low risk of death in the first 6 months if they have had an AMI.
C. Patients with restrictive mitral filling are at high risk of death in the first 6 months if they have heart failure.
D. Patients with restrictive mitral filling are at higher risk of death in the first 6 months if they have had an AMI compared to those with heart failure.

ANSWERS

1. **Answer: C.** A cross-sectional study uses data collected from one sample of subjects drawn from a larger defined population at a specific point in time. In this example, the sample is 100 first year medical students that are drawn from a larger population of university students. A longitudinal study (answer A) is based on data collected from a sample of subjects that are reexamined at another point in time, allowing comparisons to be made on at least two time points. A case-control study (answer B) compares a group of subjects who have a disease (cases) with subjects who do not have the disease (controls). A clinical trial (answer D) tests an intervention (often a treatment, but the intervention can be an imaging test) and includes the capture of baseline data (before the intervention starts) that is compared to postintervention data to determine the impact of the new intervention.

2. **Answer: D.** Prevalence is the percentage (%) proportion of a population who have experienced a specific condition during a given time frame. To conduct a cross-sectional survey to estimate the prevalence of a clinical condition, a representative sample from the entire target population must be drawn upon. In this survey, one wants to obtain information that is representative of all sonographers in the United States, so the sample population should be all sonographers registered with the ARDMS. Answers A, B, and C all represent convenience samples that are not necessarily representative of the entire population of sonographers in the United States. Convenience samples are not recommended because they lead to biased sampling. For example, all the sonographers where you work may have similar exposure to work-related stresses; the sonographers you know may come from a narrow age range; and those that are connected to you on social media may not represent the whole workforce.

3. **Answer: B.** Incidence describes the number of new cases of a disease occurring within a period of time (e.g., per year) and requires knowledge of the number of cases (numerator) and the period of time they were identified (denominator). Answer A is a description of disease prevalence and is usually expressed as the number of cases as a proportion of the population (e.g., per 100,000 population) over a time period. Answer C is the sensitivity of a diagnostic test and is a measure of true positive cases detected. Answer D is the specificity of a diagnostic test and is a measure of the true negatives detected.

KEY POINT

To calculate sensitivity and specificity of a test compared to the gold standard test, use the following table and equations:

Experimental Test	Gold Standard Test Positive Test	Negative Test
Positive test	A (true positive)	B (false positive)
Negative Test	C (false negative)	D (true negative)

$$\text{Sensitivity}(\%) = \left[A \div (A + C) \right] \times 100 \quad (1)$$

$$\text{Specificity}(\%) = \left[D \div (D + B) \right] \times 100 \quad (2)$$

4. **Answer: B.** Pilot studies are conducted to evaluate the feasibility of some crucial component(s) of a full-scale study (in this case the role of electrocardiography [ECG] vs. ECHO ventriculoventricular optimization). Pilot studies should always have their objectives linked with feasibility and should inform researchers about the best way to conduct a future full-scale study. Conducting a pilot study can therefore enhance the likelihood of success of a future full-scale study.[19] Studies that include only a small number of participants (answer A) and/or studies that produce wrong or erroneous results (answer C) or nonsignificant results (answer D) because the number of participants is too small are generally described as "underpowered." Pilot studies can also be underpowered but this is accepted as a likely outcome at the design stage since the primary outcome of the study is not to answer a hypothesis but to inform the future design of a larger project.

5. **Answer: D.** A single case study involves an up-close and in-depth examination of one patient (the case), as well as the related contextual conditions. If several patients with similar presentation or conditions were reported, this would be a case series (answer A). It is not a cohort study (answer B) because cohort studies typically involve the collection of data regarding a specific group of patients (the cohort) over a long period of time and this is only one patient. Although some aspects of this case are described qualitatively, this is not a qualitative research study (answer C). Qualitative research studies involve the collection and analysis of nonnumerical data (for example, by interviewing one or more patients to determine their perceptions, opinions, motivations.

6. **Answer: A.** The frequency distribution of the LVEF is normal, reflected by an approximately symmetrical bell-shaped curve, with the mode (highest frequency value) at the center of the histogram (where LVEF = 65%). Answers B and C are incorrect because they refer to asymmetrical frequency distributions where the mode is not at the center of the distribution and are examples of skewed distributions. Skewed data are not evenly distributed around the central mean, meaning there is an uneven peak (modal value) and the graph has a longer "tail" that may be on either side of the distribution. These graphs are described on the basis of where the tail of the distribution is, for example, a right or positive skewed graph will have a tail on the right-hand side of the graph, and conversely a left or negative skewed graph will have its tail on the left-hand side of the graph. A bimodal distribution (answer D) has two peaks rather than the single peak at the mean seen here. When the distribution of data is skewed or bimodal, the mean, median, and modal values will not be the same as they are for normal distributions and researchers need to use nonparametric analysis techniques that do not make assumptions about an underlying normal distribution.

7. **Answer: B.** The calculated mean, median, and mode are descriptive statistics that are used to summarize a set of data. These numbers will be nearly the same in a large normally distributed data set; however, when a sample is small, small differences may occur. If the mean, median, and mode are widely different (answer A), then the researcher should consider if the data are in fact normally distributed. Normally distributed data have a symmetrical "bell" shape around the central mean, but the observed maximum and minimum values can be different distances from the median. The median is the middle observation when the observations are ranked from minimum to maximum, but there is no underlying assumption that the minimum or maximum values will be equal distances from the median (answers C and D). This is especially true when you have some outlier variables that lie a long distance away from the central numbers.

8. **Answer: C.** Although the data appear to have a cluster of values that form a bell shape around the mode value, both graphs have a long tail to the right. This means that the mean and median values will be different than the modal value. This type of curve is described as having a right or positive skew because a large proportion of the area under the curve will be toward the right. Answers A and B are incorrect because these data are not normally distributed. If they were normally distributed there would be symmetry around the mode. Answer D is nearly correct since the data are not normally distributed, but if the tail of the curve was left skewed, the tail would contain lower values.

9. **Answer: C.** In a *double-blind trial* neither the participants nor the researchers know which participants belong to the treatment group (i.e., exposed to a treatment) and which participants belong to the control group (i.e., not exposed to a treatment). After the study has finished and all data have been collected, the researchers and participants learn which groups the participants were allocated to. This is the optimal trial design as it allows data to be collected without the risk of bias on behalf of the researchers or the participants. Answers A and B are both examples of *single blind trials* where either the researchers or participants, but not both, know if they have received the treatment or the placebo. Single blind trials are not recommended, but they are the only option in some situations, where it is difficult sometimes to keep allocation concealed from researchers. For example, in a surgical trial of tissue versus metal prosthetic valves where the allocation can remain unknown to the participants, it cannot be concealed from either the surgeon or the echocardiographer. And similarly, researchers may remain blind, but participants know what they are receiving, such as

treatment allocation of oral versus self-injection of a medication. Open label trials (answer D) are not ideal as they are subject to bias but are sometimes the only option and occasionally are used in the early stages of researching a new treatment.

10. **Answer: A.** This graph shows that there is a relationship between LV mass and fat-free mass. Fat-free mass is on the x axis and is referred to as the independent variable and LV mass on the y axis is referred to as the dependent variable. This suggests that there is a relationship between the two, that they are correlated with each other in a positive way. A negative correlation would be slanted in the other direction, and higher values in one variable will correlate to lower values in the other (answer B). Correlation should not be confused with causation: correlation only shows the relationship between two variables; correlation cannot confirm that changes in one variable (in this case, fat-free mass) have led to changes in another variable (in this case LV mass) and therefore answers C and D are incorrect as they imply causation. To show causation, a longitudinal study is required, where changes in the independent variable are made and subsequent changes in the dependent variable are observed.

11. **Answer: D.** Both reviews are written and "tell a story," but typically narrative reviews will only contain some relevant research, whereas a systematic review usually contains all relevant research irrespective of the findings. Authors of a narrative review usually choose relevant literature that contributes to the situation they are describing, whereas a systematic review relies on searching multiple databases and identifying all literature on a subject irrespective of the results, publication location, or language, and even includes unpublished results. Answer A is partly correct since both types of reviews tell a story. It is the process by which relevant literature is selected that dictates the type of review. Systematic reviews can and do provide an estimate of effect size (answer B), in which case they are often described as meta-analyses, but some systematic reviews simply report the different studies in an area and because of heterogeneity between the studies (e.g., differences in methods, populations, measurements) they choose not to provide an overall estimate of effect. Systematic reviews can include studies with numeric data (answer C) but they may also include qualitative data (e.g., from interviews). The type of data does not restrict the researcher from undertaking a full systematic review.

12. **Answer: A.** Informed consent for clinical research requires the patient to be given information to read about the study and what is involved for them; the patient should have an opportunity to ask questions before signing a document signaling their agreement to participate in the research project. Simply because a patient consents to receive a type of care

or procedure (answer B) does not imply informed research consent. Similarly, a doctor cannot enter a patient into a study that they have not consented to be part of (answer C) and importantly, patients should not be disadvantaged because they decline to take part in a research project. There should be no impact on clinical care of the patient (answer D).

13. **Answer: C.** This describes cluster sampling, where each randomly selected subgroup of participants is known as a "cluster." Cluster sampling might be based on geographic spread (e.g., randomly selected participants from several towns) or by clinics (e.g., randomly selected participants from several hypertension clinics) or based on a university (e.g., choosing 50 freshman students from a number of universities). Cluster sampling ensures that there is balance for differences that might occur related to where the sample is chosen from. Systematic or interval sampling (answer A) may be useful in situations such as screening a large population where inviting everyone would lead to an unmanageably large group. Instead, potential subjects are ranked such as with an alphabetical electoral roll or employee group. This is preferential to simply recruiting from the start of a list until the sample is achieved, which may lead to selection bias since the end of the list may never be reached. Simple random population sampling (as in answer B) has the best chance of representing the entire population and is ideal. An example might be selecting from an employee database, or from an electoral roll where registration is compulsory. Stratified sampling (answer D) is used when researchers want to achieve an even number of subjects in each group, but the population from which they are drawn have unequal distribution so that simple randomization leads to unbalanced groups. An example of this might be ethnicity, age, or sex, where the researchers may recruit stratified by ethnicity, age, or sex.

14. **Answer: B.** *External validity* means that the conclusions of a single research study can be applied outside the context of that study. Sometimes this is referred to as *generalizability* and describes whether the results can be widely applied, and the same results are likely to be obtained in different settings. In this case, the concern is raised because the study was conducted by only two experienced sonographers leading to the question of whether other sonographers could obtain the same results. Whether cause and effect can be drawn from the results (answer A) is a measure of *internal validity* and depends on the study design. Whether the results look like they might be correct (answer C) is a measure of *face validity* and really is a judgment about whether the study measured what it was intended to. Comparing the results of a study against known standards (answer D) is described as *criterion-related validity* and an example might be to compare the study results with a gold standard test.

15. **Answer: D.** Interrater, or interobserver, reliability is the degree of agreement among two or more observers. Statistically, it measures how much homogeneity, or consensus, there is among the observers' measurements and if there is bias associated with the measurements. Answer A describes test-retest reliability, where measurements are obtained on different occasions and this is an important determinant of how the test will perform in clinical practice. Intrarater or intraobserver reliability (answer B) measures how similar the results are when obtained by the same measurer (observer) when measured on two or more occasions. Answer C describes criterion-related validity and not reliability per se. Tests can produce reliable, yet invalid results. For example, a test can produce the same wrong number consistently and the results would be described as invalid yet reliable.

16. **Answer: A.** Visual examination of the chart indicates that the mean and 95% confidence intervals of the diagnostic accuracy score and 95% confidence intervals for the experimental groups did not overlap and that one group (with the addition of PHHE) had a higher mean accuracy score compared with the control group. If the 95% confidence intervals of two mean scores do not overlap, it can be inferred that there is a significant difference between two mean values at the 0.05 level. Therefore, it can be concluded that the use of PHHE improved the clinical diagnosis of heart disease, over and above history, physical examination, and ECG findings. If there was no difference as suggested by answer B, then the confidence intervals of the two groups would overlap. This study is specifically testing the impact of the addition of PHHE to the current approach that includes history, physical examination, and ECG and therefore the role of PHHE alone (answers C and D) cannot be inferred from this graph.

17. **Answer: C.** The Chi-square statistic in this example is used to show that with each model, the prediction of outcome is improved. A larger Chi-square for the model suggests that the model is better at predicting outcome. The Chi-square is a measure of the whole model, not the individual components and cannot be interpreted fully without the accompanying *P* value, since the significance of the model is unknown and therefore answer A is incorrect. The significance of the contribution of each factor to each model is determined by the table provided in **Figure 37-5.** The p value beside the factor tells you whether it is significantly contributing to each model. Not all the variables in the model are significant, because the factors are sometimes correlated and closely linked to other variables. As described above, the Chi-square is a measure of the model, but not its significance (answer D). The p values do confirm that the models are statistically different to one another.

18. **Answer: A.** The null hypothesis is usually framed as a statement, in this case that there is no difference between the groups after the intervention. The null hypothesis is "rejected" if there is a statistically proven difference (as in this case). When comparing the two groups, there was a difference in the inappropriate use (13% vs. 34%), but this alone is insufficient to reject the null hypothesis. These results need to be considered alongside the p value (*P* < .001), which supports the conclusion that it is highly probable (chance of 1/1000 that this result is occurring from chance alone) that the education program has resulted in lower use of inappropriate TTE in the intervention group (13%) compared to the control group (34%). The researchers would have retained the null hypothesis if the p value had been insignificant (*P* > .05), which is not the case (answer B). Neither C nor D is correct since the null hypothesis was related to the education intervention, not that the groups were different at baseline.

19. **Answer: C.** The authors concluded that either catheterization-based mPAP or Doppler-based sPAP can be used to predict survival to a similar extent, so you can use either measurement to determine survival in patients with pulmonary hypertension. Both measurements are prognostic, with similar hazard ratios and overlapping confidence intervals. It may be tempting to confer more value on the mPAP data (answer A) since the hazard ratio is higher (2.84 vs. 2.32), but both measurements are individually prognostic, with overlapping confidence intervals. These data support using either right heart catheterization or Doppler to assess prognosis, and even though the right heart measurement is more difficult, it can be substituted with the Doppler sPAP, so answer D is incorrect.

20. **Answer: A.** The standard deviation describes the variability (amount of variation or dispersion) among a single sample of data values. A small standard deviation indicates that the sample data are clustered tightly around a small range of values, whereas a large standard deviation indicates that the sample data are spread widely across a large range of values. Answer B describes the calculation of the mean. Answer C describes the median value. Answer D describes the modal value.

21. **Answer: D.** The 95% confidence interval encompasses approximately 2 standard deviations below and 2 standard deviations above the mean. It includes 95% of the data displayed in the curve, meaning that 5% is outside the lower and upper bounds of the confidence interval. This equates to 2.5% within the left tail and 2.5% in the upper tail. Answers A and B are incorrect because the standard deviation applies to both sides of the curve and the 95% is contained between these lines. The 95% confidence interval is between the lower and upper 2 standard deviation lines. Furthermore, this standard deviation is derived from the control data and therefore only applies to that data set. Answer C is partly

correct because it excludes the lower 2.5% that falls outside of the lower 2 standard deviation line but in this case, the 95% confidence interval is calculated from the control data only in order to provide a comparison for the other groups.

22. **Answer: A.** The mean value for LVIDd is in fact similar for the hypertension-only group and control group, but the group with hypertension and HFNEF has a higher LVIDd and more patients: 10% to 15% compared to 5% for the controls and hypertension-only groups, fall outside of the 95% confidence interval. It cannot be concluded that the hypertension-only groups have larger LV dimensions (Answer B) because there is significant overlap between the control and hypertension-only group. The number of 10% to 15% is a measure of the values that fall outside the confidence interval and this cannot be used as a measure of abnormality (answers C and D). The 95% confidence interval shown here applies to this datum only and should not be confused with the reference values that are also often derived using the 95% confidence interval but from highly screened and selective healthy individuals.

23. **Answer: C.** The vertical points of the diamond are the mean of overall effect—if you drew a line through the top and bottom points of the diamond and extrapolated toward the X axis, you could estimate the numeric value of the overall effect. The confidence interval of the effect is indicated by the width of the diamond (answer B). The diamond is an integral part of the graph as it is the measure of overall effect estimate (answer A) and the size of the diamond is an indication of the overall sample size (answer D). The confidence interval is always smaller than the confidence interval of any of the individual studies since it has a much larger sample size (it includes all of the data). The statistical significance of the overall effect is determined by the degree to which the confidence interval of this overall effect overlaps with the line of the odds ratio (OR) of 1.0. In this case, the width of the diamond is far away from the OR = 1.0 line, indicating that the result is significant, and this is confirmed by the numeric values showing that the OR for the difference is 4.1, with a confidence interval from 3.38 to 4.99.

24. **Answer: B.** When comparing two conditions in a meta-analysis, if there are no differences between the two, the odds ratio will be 1.0. A higher odds ratio indicates an increased risk associated with the condition and a lower odds ratio (<1.0) indicates a beneficial reduction in risk. An odds ratio of 1.0 suggests the groups are the same and therefore does not support a difference. When a study's confidence interval crosses the OR = 1.0 line, it means that either the mean OR is close to 1.0 or the confidence interval around that mean extends to include 1.0, but it does not imply anything about the quality of the study. Studies should not be ignored or excluded because their confidence interval crosses the 1.0 line (answer C), but it may mean the study was underpowered. Similarly, the OR and its confidence interval may fall far away from the OR = 1.0 line, but that does not imply the study is better (answer D).

25. **Answer: A.** When calculating an overall effect, the meta-analytical program weights each study on the basis of the sample size and confidence interval of the study effect. The confidence interval is linked to sample size and it can be appreciated that the smallest studies have wide confidence intervals, creating uncertainty about the effect size. In comparison, the larger studies have a tight confidence interval. Answer B is correct that the odds ratios in the four largest studies are similar to the overall odds ratio, but this is not why they carry a higher weight. These studies are the largest and that is why they have been given more weight in the overall calculation. It should be anticipated that their OR is closer to the overall OR, because as the study gets larger, if the selection of participants into that study is unbiased, then the odds ratio will remain similar, but the confidence interval around it will decrease. The reviewers in a meta-analysis should not "judge" a study for quality (answer C) except at the stage of selecting the studies. If the study meets the criteria for inclusion, it should be included. Weighting is performed as described above, not on whether a study is significant or not as suggested in answer D. In this case, two of the four highest weighted studies were not independently statistically significant, as shown by the confidence interval around the estimate overlapping the no difference line (OR = 1).

26. **Answer: B.** Bland and Altman graphs are very useful to compare two techniques. There are three lines that summarize the spread of the data: the solid line, which indicates the mean difference between the techniques, and the two dashed lines that show the 95% confidence interval above and below the mean. In this example above, it can be appreciated that the mean difference between echo and MRI for nonenhanced echo was approximately −50 mL, meaning that echo underestimated EDV by 50 mL on average. With contrast, the solid line crosses the Y axis at approximately −20 mL, which means that the mean echo EDV is closer to that obtained at MRI. This is an improvement but still an underestimation. The other point to note is that the 95% confidence interval around these numbers is between −100 and +10 mL for the noncontrast and reduced to −50 and +10 mL for the contrast EDV measurements and therefore answer A, that EDV volumes were not improved, is not true. The bias indicated by smaller volumes by either echo method compared to MRI means it cannot be concluded that the EDV measurements were similar by echo and MRI (answer C). In order to determine if these differences with contrast were significant (answer D), we would need to perform a

statistical test, but we can see significant overlap in the confidence intervals for the graphs.

27. **Answer: B.** Precision relates to how close two sets of measurement are. In this case, the echo measurements with contrast have a narrower confidence interval, suggesting the contrast-enhanced echo measurements are more precise in comparison to the MRI images. Accuracy (answer A) refers to how close the measurements are. In this example you can see that the mean LVEF is similar by noncontrast echo (−5%) and with contrast (−2%) compared to the MRI LVEF. Reliability, sometimes referred to as reproducibility, is a measure of whether you get the same results under different conditions (e.g., on another day or with another measurer). Reliability is dependent upon the mean value and the standard deviation and is also affected by precision and validity. You could compare echo and contrast echo in this case and say both provide reliable measurements of LVEF and given the mean value is similar and the confidence intervals overlap, you would conclude there was no difference (answer C). Validity is a measure that determines whether the test measures what it is supposed to. In this case the MRI is the gold standard and since the means are the same, both appear equally valid (answer D).

KEY POINT

To understand the difference between accuracy and precision, think of a dart board and the echocardiographic measurements are trying to achieve the center of the board (the true valid measurements). As illustrated in **Figure 37-12**, **A** shows six repeated measurements that all hit the center, with minimal variation. **B** shows six repeated measurements that all hit the same spot, with minimal variation. But the spot is far from the target (and valid measurement). **C** shows six repeated measurements that all hit near the center, but with more variation. The calculated mean may be the similar, but the standard deviation will be wide. **D** shows six repeated measurements that all hit the board without any pattern and far from each other. It is a matter of chance if these measurements are similar.

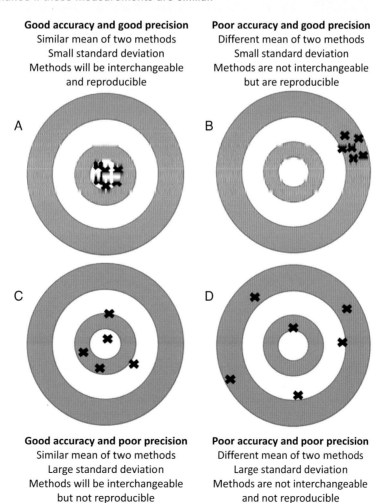

Good accuracy and good precision
Similar mean of two methods
Small standard deviation
Methods will be interchangeable
and reproducible

Poor accuracy and good precision
Different mean of two methods
Small standard deviation
Methods are not interchangeable
but are reproducible

Good accuracy and poor precision
Similar mean of two methods
Large standard deviation
Methods will be interchangeable
but not reproducible

Poor accuracy and poor precision
Different mean of two methods
Large standard deviation
Methods are not interchangeable
and not reproducible

Figure 37-12

28. **Answer: D.** For a test to be useful, in both research and to detect clinical changes, the test needs to be reliable. This means the test gives similar results each time it is performed, allowing for real changes to be detected. There are several factors that contribute to measurement reliability for the echocardiographer; key ones to consider are intra- and interobserver reliability. Intraobserver reliability is the difference a single person gets when they remeasure a set of images (consistency). Interobserver reliability is the difference that arises when two different sonographers measure the same images. In the example above, both are improved with the use of contrast (indicated by narrower confidence intervals compared to the noncontrast echo), but the intraobserver reliability is better than the interobserver reliability.

29. **Answer: A.** This is a Kaplan-Meier survival curve and is used to describe events, in this case death, in different groups over time. Each time a subject in the group experiences an event, the curve dips down. Each curve at 1.0 represents 100% alive. Although this is often described as a mortality curve (answer B), it is in fact a measure of survival as the only subjects left on the curves are the survivors.

30. **Answer: C.** Clear separation of the lines provides an estimate of mortality at any time point (along the x axis). This is broken down into years in this case, and at 30 months (two and a half years), the curves for the post-AMI groups are clearly separated but there is overlap between the pseudonormal and restrictive filling groups. Therefore, it can be concluded that restrictive filling is higher in the post-AMI group but not the heart failure group. The mortality was not similar comparing pseudonormal and restrictive filling and in the post-AMI groups (answers B and D). Although restrictive filling is thought to always be more severe and therefore carries more risk (Answer A), these data do not support that belief in the patients with heart failure.

31. **Answer: D.** The very steep decline in the restrictive filling slope in the AMI group curves suggests that these patients have early events, compared to all of the other groups in which there is a gradual decline in survival. Survival at 6 months is lowest, and therefore mortality is highest in the AMI group with restrictive filling (not the lowest risk as suggested in answer B). While it is true for the AMI groups that the risk of death is highest in the restrictive filling group in this time period, it is not true for the heart failure group, which declines in a linear way (answer A), and in the first 6 months the survival in the AMI group with restrictive filling is higher, not lower (answer C), than the heart failure group.

REFERENCES

Abul Fadi AM, Sobeih AA. Screening university students for rheumatic heart disease. *J Prev Med.* 2018;3(2):13.

Basile V, Di Mauro A, Scalini E, et al. Lung ultrasound: a useful tool in diagnosis and management of bronchiolitis. *BMC Pediatr.* 2015;15:63.

Bhatia RS, Dudzinski DM, Malhotra R, et al. Educational intervention to reduce outpatient inappropriate echocardiograms: a randomized control trial. *JACC Cardiovasc Imaging.* 2014;7(9):857-866.

Conte M, D'Andrea A, Golia B, et al. Iatrogenic delayed cardiac tamponade secondary to intrapericardial hematoma after dialysis catheter placement. *J Emerg Intern Med.* 2018;2(1):18.

Elfil M, Negida A. Sampling methods in clinical research; an educational review. *Emerg (Tehran).* 2017;5(1):e52.

Gepner AD, Ramamurthy R, Krueger DC, Korcarz CE, Binkley N, Stein JH. A prospective randomized controlled trial of the effects of Vitamin D supplementation on cardiovascular disease risk. *PLoS One.* 2012;7(5):e36617.

Greiner S, Jud A, Aurich M, et al. Prognostic relevance of elevated pulmonary arterial pressure assessed non-invasively: analysis in a large patient cohort with invasive measurements in near temporal proximity. *PLoS One.* 2018;13(1):e0191206.

Hoffman J, Kaplan S. The incidence of congenital heart disease. *J Am Coll Cardiol.* 2002;39(12):1890-1900.

Kusunose K, Popović ZB, Motoki H, Marwick TH. Prognostic significance of exercise-induced right ventricular dysfunction in asymptomatic degenerative mitral regurgitation. *Circ Cardiovasc Imaging.* 2013;6(2):167-176.

Malm S, Frigstad S, Sagberg E, Henrik Larsson H, Skjaerpe T. Accurate and reproducible measurement of left ventricular volume and ejection fraction by contrast echocardiography: a comparison with magnetic resonance imaging. *J Am Coll Cardiol.* 2004;44(5):1030-1035.

Panoulas VF, Daigeler A-L, Malaweera ASN, et al. Pocket-size handheld cardiac ultrasound as an adjunct to clinical examination in the hands of medical students and junior doctors. *Eur Heart J Cardiovasc Imaging.* 2013;14(4):323-330.

Punn R, Hanisch D, Motonaga KS, Rosenthal DN, Ceresnak SR, Dubin AM. A pilot study assessing ECG versus ECHO ventriculoventricular optimization in pediatric resynchronization patients. *J Cardiovasc Electrophysiol.* 2016;27(2):210-216.

Rigolli M, Rossi A, Quintana M, et al. The prognostic impact of diastolic dysfunction in patients with chronic heart failure and post-acute myocardial infarction: can age-stratified E/A ratio alone predict survival?. *Int J Cardiol.* 2015;181:362-368.

Saul T, Avitablile NC, Berkowitz N, et al. The inter-rater reliability of echocardiographic diastolic function evaluation among emergency physician sonographers. *J Emerg Med.* 2016;51(4):411-417.

Taniguchi T, Ohtani T, Kioka H, et al. Liver stiffness reflecting right-sided filling pressure can predict Adverse outcomes in patients with heart failure. *JACC Cardiovasc Imaging.* 2019;12(6):955-964.

Thabane L, Ma J, Chu R, et al. A tutorial on pilot studies: the what, why and how. *BMC Med Res Methodol.* 2010;10:1.Whalley GA, Gamble G, Doughty R, et al. Echo left ventricular mass correlates with fat free mass but not fat mass. *J Hypertension.* 1999;17(4):569-574.

Whalley GA, Gamble GD, Doughty RN. Restrictive diastolic filling predicts death after acute myocardial infarction: systematic review and meta-analysis of prospective studies. *Heart.* 2006;92(11):1588-1594.

Zile MR, LeWinter MM. Left ventricular end-diastolic volume is normal in patients with heart failure and a normal ejection fraction. *J Am Coll Cardiol.* 2007;49(9):982-985.

SUGGESTED READINGS

Textbooks

Altman D, Machin D, Bryant T, Gardner M. *Statistics With Confidence: Confidence Intervals and Statistical Guidelines.* 2nd ed. Bristol, UK: BMJ Books; 2000.

Altman D. *Practical Statistics for Medical Research.* 1st ed. Florida, USA: Chapman and Hall/CRC; 1990.

Borenstein M, Hedges LV, Higgins JPT, Rothstein HR. *An Introduction to Meta-Analysis.* West Sussex, England: John Wiley & Sons; 2009.

Bowers D. *Medical Statistics from Scratch. An Introduction for Health Professionals,* 3rd ed. West Sussex, England: Wiley Blackwell; 2014.

Bruce N, Pope D. Stanistreet. *Quantitative Methods for Health Research. A Practical Interactive Guide to Epidemiology and Statistics.* West Sussex, England: Wiley-Interscience; 2012.

Ellis PD. *The Essential Guide to Effect Sizes. Statistical Power, Meta-Analysis, and the Interpretation of Research Results.* Cambridge, UK: Cambridge University Press; 2010.

Gough D, Oliver S, Thomas J. *An Introduction to Systematic Reviews.* 2nd ed. Los Angeles, CA: Sage Publications; 2017.

Greenhalgh T, *How to Read a Paper.* 2nd ed. London, UK: BMJ Books; 2001.

Minichiello V, Sullivan G, Greenwood K, Axford R. *Handbook of Research Methods for Nursing and Health Sciences.* 2nd ed. Melbourne, Australia: Pearson Australia; 2003.

Petrie A, Sabin C. *Medical Statistics at a Glance.* 3rd ed. West Sussex, England: Wiley Blackwell; 2009.

Polgar S. *Introduction to Research in the Health Sciences.* 6th ed. Philadelphia, PA: Churchill Livingstone; 2013.

Rothman K. *Epidemiology: An Introduction* 2nd ed. Oxford; New York, NY: Oxford University Press; 2012.

Journal Papers

Crowther M, Lim W, Crowther MA. Systematic review and meta-analysis methodology. *Blood.* 2010;116(17):3140-3146.

Krousel-Wood MA, Chambers RB, Muntner P. Clinicians' guide to statistics for medical practice and research: part I. *Oschner J.* 2006;6(2):68-83.

Krousel-Wood MA, Chambers RB, Muntner P. Clinicians' guide to statistics for medical practice and research: Part II. *Oschner J.* 2007;7(1):3-7.

Nair T. Medical statistics made easy for the medical practitioner. *Hypertens J.* 2015;1(2):63-67

Thomas E. An introduction to medical statistics for health care professionals: describing and presenting data. *Musculoskelet Care.* 2004;2:218-228.

Thomas E. An introduction to medical statistics for health care professionals: hypothesis tests and estimation. *Musculoskelet Care.* 2005;2:102-108.

Thomas E. An introduction to medical statistics for health care professionals: basic statistical tests. *Musculoskelet Care.* 2005;3:201-212.

Zhou KH, O'Malley J, Mauri L. Receiver-operating characteristic analysis for evaluating diagnsotic tests and predictive models. *Circulation.* 2007;115:654-657.

Websites

The CONSORT Statement: http://www.consort-statement.org/

The STROBE Statement: https://www.strobe-statement.org/index.php?id=strobe-home.

The PRISMA Statement: http://prisma-statement.org/.

COPE (Committee on Publication Ethics): https://publicationethics.org.

NIH Clinical Research Resources: https://www.nih.gov/research-training/clinical-research-resources.

The EQUATOR Network: https://www.equator-network.org/library/research-ethics-publication-ethics-and-good-practice-guidelines/.

The Cochrane Collaboration: https://www.cochrane.org/.

CHAPTER 38

Quality Assurance and Laboratory Management

Contributors: Alicia Armour, MA, BS, RDCS and Karen Helfinstine, MAEd, ACS, RCS, RDCS

✪✪ Question 1

The Intersocietal Accreditation Commission (IAC) for Echocardiography Standards state that appropriate workup for aortic stenosis includes the use of a dedicated nonimaging continuous-wave Doppler transducer from which of the following multiple imaging windows?

    A. Apical, subcostal, suprasternal notch

    B. Apical, suprasternal notch, supraclavicular

    C. Apical, supraclavicular, right parasternal

    D. Apical, suprasternal notch, right parasternal

✪✪ Question 2

As part of the quality improvement process, technical quality review of sonographer performance variability should be evaluated as two studies per modality:

    A. Per month.

    B. Per quarter.

    C. Biannually.

    D. Annually.

✪ Question 3

Participation in a continuing medical education (CME) program:

    A. Improves patient care through acquisition of knowledge and skills.

    B. Assists in the maintenance of clinical competency.

    C. Is essential for the maintenance of professional certification and/or accreditation.

    D. A and B.

    E. All of the above.

✪ Question 4

The following nonimaging information should be included on stress echocardiogram reports:

    A. Target heart rate (HR).

    B. Resting blood pressure and blood pressure response to exercise.

    C. Patient's cardiac symptoms, if any, during examination.

    D. A and B.

    E. All of the above.

✪✪ Question 5

According to the American Society of Echocardiography (ASE) Recommendations for Quality Echocardiography Laboratory Operations guidelines, when performing annual review of 5 to 10 studies for either sonographers or physicians a minimum of _____ of the component images of the appropriate protocol should be performed.

    A. 80%

    B. 90%

    C. 75%

    D. None of the above

✪ Question 6

Which of the following statements regarding the completion of a standardized echocardiographic report is false?

A. Echo laboratories must be careful to avoid too lengthy of a report or one that is too abbreviated.

B. Technically difficult studies should be noted on the report.

C. Amendments to the report do not need to be noted on the original report.

D. The summary should include how the findings correlate to the reason for the study and a statement comparing the current study to previous studies.

✪ Question 7

Regarding the timeliness of the echocardiographic report, which of the following statements is true?

A. Stat reports should be interpreted and communicated by a qualified physician immediately, if possible, and final transcribed reports should be available by the end of the next business day.

B. Stat reports should be interpreted and communicated by a qualified physician within 24 hours and final transcribed reports should be available by the end of the business day.

C. Routine studies should be interpreted by a qualified physician and a report available within 1 business day, while the final transcribed report should be available within 7 working days after interpretation.

D. Routine studies should be interpreted by a qualified physician and a report available by the end of the first business day, while the final transcribed report should be available within 48 hours after interpretation.

✪✪✪ Question 8

Safety is a critical component in all echocardiographic patient studies. Which statement regarding safety is most true?

A. A log of scheduled maintenance for the machine must be kept in the examination room.

B. The transducer face must be examined for tears and possible electrical exposure during the examination and when moving between imaging windows.

C. The ALARA (As Low As Reasonably Achievable) principle should be implemented by adjusting controls and settings for each examination.

D. In addition to cleaning the transducer, the machine should be disinfected and cleaned once a week.

✪ Question 9

Adequate probe preparation and disinfection is mandatory for patient safety. Which of the following statements is true?

A. High-level disinfection procedures should be used for all ultrasound probes.

B. High-level disinfection procedures include soaking the probe in hot water.

C. High-level disinfection can be done while the probe is still connected to the ultrasound machine.

D. High-level disinfection starts with cleaning the probe with a detergent/water solution or a low-level disinfectant.

✪ Question 10

Which of the following would not be included on a standardized transthoracic echocardiographic report?

A. An indication for the study

B. Description of patient behavior during study

C. Sonographer performing the examination

D. Echocardiographic system/machine used

✪ Question 11

When performing a technical quality improvement review for performance variability among sonographers, which of the following should be evaluated?

A. Test appropriateness

B. Report completeness and timeliness

C. Safety of imaging if applicable

D. A and B

E. All of the above

✪ Question 12

Which of the following statements regarding the inclusion of nonimaging data in the stress echocardiographic report is false?

A. The report text must include the blood pressure of the patient at rest and in the recovery phase of the test prior to ending the examination.

B. The report text must include the exercise time and the reason for terminating the test.

C. The report text must include the target heart rate (HR) and the maximum heart rate achieved during the test.

D. The report text must include whether or not the target heart rate was achieved and/or if the level of stress was adequate.

E. None of the above (that is, all statements are true).

✪✪ Question 13

When using ultrasound enhancing (contrast) agents, poor endocardial border delineation is defined as:

A. The inability to adequately visualize any two or more segments in parasternal or apical views.

B. The inability to adequately visualize any two segments in any view.

C. The inability to adequately visualize two or more segments in the parasternal long-axis view.

D. The inability to adequately visualize two or more contiguous segments in any of the three apical views.

✪✪ Question 14

Patient and employee safety is ensured by having in place written policies and procedures. This includes all of the following except:

A. A policy to address technical staff safety, comfort, and avoidance of work-related musculoskeletal disorders.

B. An emergency procedure plan and life-support equipment to cover potential risks to patient safety during special echocardiographic procedures.

C. A policy to address radiation safety for sonographers performing lengthy ultrasound examinations.

D. A written procedure in place for handling acute medical emergencies.

E. None of the above (that is, all policies and plans above are required).

✪✪✪ Question 15

There are numerous processes that can be employed in the development of quality assurance programs for cardiovascular imaging. In the model described by Douglas et al. (*J Am Coll Cardiol.* 2006), there are four distinct domains of process that affect clinical outcome. These domains include:

A. Appropriateness criteria, image acquisition, image interpretation, and results communication.

B. Operator credentialing, appropriateness criteria, image interpretation, and results communication.

C. Operator credentialing, image interpretation, results communication, and customer satisfaction.

D. Patient selection, image acquisition, image interpretation, and results communication.

✪ Question 16

What is quality assurance (QA)?

A. QA is the measurement of degree to which a test satisfies the need.

B. QA is a systematic process used to ensure patient satisfaction and outcomes.

C. QA is a method used to identify deficiencies and errors.

D. QA is a corrective tool used to discipline the team of providers.

✪✪ Question 17

Appropriate use criteria (AUC) for echocardiography specify when it is appropriate to perform a selected echocardiographic examination. Which of the following is considered a rarely appropriate indication for a transthoracic echocardiogram?

A. Clinical symptoms or signs consistent with a cardiac diagnosis known to cause light-headedness

B. Routine surveillance of ventricular function with known coronary artery disease (CAD) and no change in clinical status or cardiac exam

C. Evaluation of suspected pulmonary hypertension including evaluation of right ventricular function and estimated pulmonary artery pressure

D. Routine surveillance (≥1 year) of moderate or severe valvular stenosis without a change in clinical status or cardiac exam.

✪✪ Question 18

Which of the following is considered an appropriate indication for a stress echocardiogram?

    A. Detection of coronary artery disease (CAD) in a symptomatic patient with a low pretest probability of CAD and an uninterpretable electrocardiogram (ECG) or an inability to exercise

    B. Detection of CAD in a patient with acute chest pain and definite acute coronary syndrome

    C. Detection of CAD in an asymptomatic patient with intermediate global CAD risk and an interpretable ECG

    D. All of the above

✪✪ Question 19

The maximal heart rate percentage required to be obtained during a pharmacologic (dobutamine) stress echocardiogram to qualify as a "maximal stress test" is:

    A. 75%.

    B. 85%.

    C. 90%.

    D. 100%.

ANSWERS

1. **Answer: D.** The IAC Standards and Guidelines for Adult Echocardiography Accreditation state that in patients with aortic stenosis the systolic velocity must be evaluated by a dedicated continuous-wave Doppler transducer from multiple imaging windows; specifically, the apical, suprasternal notch, and right parasternal. While the subcostal and right supraclavicular views can be good transducer positions to obtain peak velocities for aortic stenosis, they are not part of the specified windows required as part of the accreditation.

2. **Answer: B.** The Intersocietal Accreditation Commission Standards and Guidelines for Adult Echocardiography Accreditation state under quality improvement measures standards, that a minimum of two cases per modality accredited (transthoracic, transesophageal, and/or stress echocardiography) must be evaluated quarterly (Section 2.1C of the IAC standards and guidelines for Adult echocardiography accreditation).

3. **Answer: E.** It is generally accepted that participation in a continuing medical education program improves patient care through acquisition of knowledge and skills and assists in the maintenance of clinical competency. In many countries, CME participation is considered mandatory for the maintenance of professional certification and/or accreditation. For example, in the United States, Intersocietal Accreditation Commission Echocardiography Standards require technical staff to obtain 15 CMEs over 3 years (Section 1.6A, Continuing Medical Education Requirements of the IAC standards and guidelines for Adult echocardiography accreditation). Other US credentialing bodies require different levels of CMEs depending on when staff was credentialed (American Registry for Diagnostic Medical Sonography requires 30 CMEs every 3 years while Cardiovascular Credentialing International requires 36 CMEs upon second renewal/first triennial renewal).

4. **Answer: E.** The target heart rate, resting blood pressure, and blood pressure response to exercise, as well as a patient's cardiac symptoms (if any) during the exam, should be included on the report. Other required report information includes exercise time, or maximum dose of pharmacologic agent (if used); maximum heart rate achieved; whether or not target HR was achieved and/or if stress was adequate; reason for termination; and summary of stress electrocardiogram findings.

5. **Answer: D.** Under the section "Quality Assessment and Implementation of Quality Improvement Programs —Image Acquisition, the ACE guideline recommends that a minimum of 90% of the component images of the appropriate protocol should be performed. In cases with valvular stenosis, the echo image sets should include all components necessary for quantification of peak Doppler information (e.g., peak gradient, mean gradient, and valve area) in 90% of the cases reviewed.

6. **Answer: C.** This statement is false. As per the ASE Guidelines and Standards document for Recommendations for Quality Echocardiography Laboratory Operations, "If the report is electronically signed, the laboratory must have policies for security and limited system access, use of operational and authority checks, compliance, and privacy enforcement with system administrators. This must include a log of the name, date, and time of all individuals who access, re-access or modify the electronic report."

7. **Answer: A.** According to the American Society of Echocardiography Recommendations for Quality Echocardiography Laboratory Operations guidelines, studies should be categorized as stat or

routine. Stat reports should be interpreted and communicated by a qualified physician immediately, if possible, and final transcribed reports should be available by the end of the next business day. Routine studies should be interpreted by a qualified physician and a report available within 1 business day, while the final transcribed report should be available within 48 hours after interpretation.

8. **Answer: C.** According to the American Institute of Ultrasound in Medicine (AIUM), sonographers should not depend only on the default machine settings for ALARA. Attempts should be made to look at the instrumentation settings to ensure that ALARA is achieved according to body habitus and area being imaged.

9. **Answer: D.** Probes that require high-level disinfection (HLD) should be cleaned first with either soap/running water or a low-level disinfectant. Per the American Institute of Ultrasound in Medicine, "The probes must be disconnected from the ultrasound scanner for anything more than wiping or spray cleaning. Rinse the probe thoroughly with running water, and then dry the probe with a soft cloth or paper towel. Cleaning the probe in this way before HLD is important as the first step in proper disinfection."

10. **Answer: B.** Description of patient behavior during study is not necessary on a standardized report.

11. **Answer: E.** When performing a technical quality review for performance variability among sonographers, quality improvement measures should include (but may not be limited to) the evaluation and review of test appropriateness; technical quality and, if applicable, safety of the imaging; interpretive quality review; report completeness and timeliness; and correlation.

12. **Answer: A.** It is generally accepted (and is a requirement of the Intersocietal Accreditation Commission, Section 3.6.1.1A of the IAC standards and guidelines for Adult echocardiography accreditation) that the stress echocardiographic report text must include the following nonimaging data: (1) exercise time, or maximum dose of pharmacologic agent (if used); (2) target heart rate; (3) maximum heart rate achieved; (4) whether or not target HR was achieved and/or stress adequate; (5) resting blood pressure and blood pressure response to exercise stress; (6) reason for termination; (7) patient's cardiac symptoms, if any, during the examination; and (8) summary of stress electrocardiogram findings.

13. **Answer: D.** Suboptimal endocardial border delineation is defined as the inability to adequately visualize two or more contiguous segments in any of the three apical views. In these instances, ultrasound enhancing agents should be used for the quantification of left ventricular chamber volume and ejection fraction and for the assessment of regional wall motion.

14. **Answer: C.** There is no radiation risk to sonographers performing ultrasound examinations as ultrasound does not use radiation. However, sonographers may be exposed to significant levels of radiation from patients who have both a nuclear test and an echocardiogram on the same day, and also from spending time in catheterization/hybrid laboratories. Therefore, it is recommended that facilities have a formal policy to address radiation safety for sonographers who may be working in this type of environment.

15. **Answer: D.** A quality assurance model for evaluating cardiovascular imaging consists of four distinct domains of process that affect clinical outcome: patient selection, image acquisition, image interpretation, and results communication (**Figure 38-1**). For phase 1 (patient selection), this ensures appropriate patient selection for a study based on evidence or consensus that it is reasonable, will affect medical decision-making, and will lead to quantifiable patient benefits; for phase 2 (image acquisition), this ensures that the study is performed using well-functioning equipment, proficient laboratory staff, and protocols that obtain diagnostic quality images to answer the clinical question; for phase 3 (image interpretation), this ensures that the interpretation is accurate and correct; and for phase 4 (results communication), this ensures that the results are communicated to the referring physician in a complete, clear, clinically relevant, and timely manner to optimize patient management and/or treatment, and ultimately improve health outcomes.

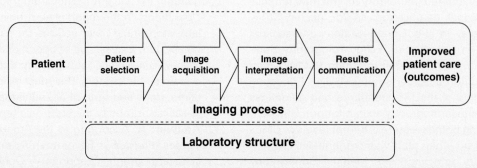

Figure 38-1 Dimensions of care framework for evaluating quality of cardiovascular imaging. (Reprinted from Douglas P, Iskandrian AE, Krumholz HM, et al. Achieving quality in cardiovascular imaging: proceedings from the American College of Cardiology–Duke University Medical Center Think Tank on Quality in Cardiovascular Imaging. *J Am Coll Cardiol*. 2006;48(10):2141-2151. Copyright © 2006 American College of Cardiology Foundation. With permission.)

16. **Answer: B.** QA is a systematic process that ensures patient satisfaction and outcomes. Therefore, the results of the test should be both reliable and diagnostically accurate.

17. **Answer: B.** According to the 2011 AUC for Echocardiography writing group, a request for a transthoracic echocardiogram for the routine surveillance of ventricular function with known CAD and no change in clinical status or cardiac exam is considered rarely appropriate. That is, the test is not generally acceptable and is not a reasonable approach for this indication. For all other options, the test is considered appropriate; that is, the test is generally acceptable and is a reasonable approach for the indication.

18. **Answer: A.** According to the 2011 Appropriate Use Criteria for Echocardiography writing group, a request for a stress echocardiogram for risk assessment in a symptomatic patient with a low pretest probability of CAD and an uninterpretable ECG or who is unable to exercise is considered appropriate. That is, the test is generally acceptable and is a reasonable approach for the indication. For answers B and C, the test is considered rarely appropriate; that is, the test is not generally acceptable and is not a reasonable approach for this indication.

19. **Answer: B.** A heart rate of 85% of the age-predicted maximum heart rate is considered a complete full diagnostic pharmacological stress echocardiogram.

SUGGESTED READINGS

AIUM official statement. Medical Ultrasound Safety. © American Institute of ultrasound in Medicine. Approved 3/16/2008; Reapproved 4/2/2014.

AIUM official statement: Guidelines for cleaning and preparing external- and Internal-Use ultrasound probes between patients, sate handling, and use of ultrasound coupling gel. Approved 5/16/2017. Revised 3/25/2018.

Douglas PS, Garcia MJ, Haines DE, et al. ACCF/ASE/AHA/ASNC/HFSA/HRS/SCAI/SCCM/SCCT/SCMR 2011 appropriate use criteria for echocardiography. A report of the American College of Cardiology Foundation appropriate use criteria task force, American Society of Echocardiography, American Heart Association, American Society of Nuclear Cardiology, Heart Failure Society of America, Heart Rhythm Society, Society for Cardiovascular Angiography and Interventions, Society of Critical Care Medicine, Society of Cardiovascular Computed Tomography, Society for Cardiovascular Magnetic Resonance American College of Chest Physicians. *J Am Soc Echocardiogr* 2011;24(3):229-267.

Lindecker P, et al. Achieving quality in cardiovascular imaging: proceedings from the American College of Cardiology-Duke University Medical Center Think Tank on Quality in Cardiovascular Imaging. *J Am Coll Cardiol.* 2006;48(10):2141-2151.

Gardin JM, Adams DB, Douglas PS, et al. Recommendations for a standardized report for adult transthoracic echocardiography: a report from the American Society of Echocardiography's Nomenclature and Standards Committee and task force for a standardized echocardiography report. *J Am Soc Echocardiogr.* 2001;14(3):275-290.

IAC standards and guidelines for Adult echocardiography accreditation (Published 6/1/2017, Revised 4/27/2018) 9 ©2018 Intersocietal accreditation Commission. All rights Reserved.

Picard MH, Adams D, Bierig SM, et al. Recommendations for quality echocardiography laboratory operations. *J Am Soc Echocardiogr.* 2011;24(1):1-10.

Porter TR, Mulvagh SL, Abdelmoneim SS, et al. Clinical applications of ultrasonic enhancing agents in echocardiography: 2018 American Society of Echocardiography guidelines Update. *J Am Soc Echocardiogr.* 2018;31(3):241-274.

Note: Page numbers followed by "f" indicate figures and "t" indicates tables.